KU-446-832

BASIC SURGERY

vertical gastroplasty

biliopancreatic

steve

Tweariy

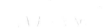

4TH EDITION

BASIC SURGERY

EDITED BY

Hiram C. Polk, Jr., M.D.

Ben A. Reid, Sr. Professor and Chairman, Department of Surgery
University of Louisville
Louisville, Kentucky

Bernard Gardner, M.D.

Professor of Surgery and Director, Division of Surgical Education
University of Medicine and Dentistry of New Jersey
Newark, New Jersey

H. Harlan Stone, M.D.

Program Director, Phoenix Integrated Surgical Residency
Good Samaritan Regional Medical Center
Phoenix, Arizona

with 648 illustrations and 12 color plates

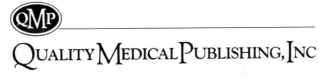

QUALITY MEDICAL PUBLISHING, INC

ST. LOUIS, MISSOURI   1993

ABOUT THE COVER: *Chief of Surgery,* acrylic on canvas, 1990,
61 x 42" by noted surgeon, author, and artist Joe Wilder, M.D.
Dr. Wilder, Professor of Surgery Emeritus at Mount Sinai School
of Medicine in New York, has received international acclaim
for his artistic renderings of surgeons at work, athletes,
and delicate still lifes and landscapes.

Chief of Surgery depicts Arthur H. Aufses, M.D., Chief of Surgery
at Mount Sinai Hospital, and is one of 18 paintings from Dr. Wilder's
"Surgeons at Work" series. Additional information about the artistry
of Joe Wilder may be obtained by contacting the publisher
(see address below).

Cover art copyright © Joseph R. Wilder.

Copyright © 1993 by Quality Medical Publishing, Inc.
All rights reserved. Reproduction of the material herein
in any form requires the written permission of the publisher.

Previously published 1978, 1983, 1987 by Appleton-Century-Crofts.

Printed in the United States of America.

Publisher   Karen Berger

Project Editor   Suzanne Seeley Wakefield

Production   Judy Bamert

Editing Assistant   Kathleen J. Jenkins

Designer   Diane M. Beasley

Quality Medical Publishing, Inc.
2086 Craigshire Drive
St. Louis, Missouri 63146

Library of Congress Cataloging-in-Publication Data

Basic surgery / edited by Hiram C. Polk, Jr., Bernard Gardner, H.
    Harlan Stone. — 4th ed.
        p.   cm.
    Includes bibliographical references and index.
    ISBN 0-942219-29-5
    1. Surgery. I. Polk, Hiram C., 1936-   . II. Gardner, Bernard,
1931-   . III. Stone, H. Harlan, 1930-
    [DNLM: 1. Diagnosis, Surgical. 2. Surgery, Operative.   WO 500
B311]
    RD31.B365   1993
    617—dc20
    DNLM/DLC
    for Library of Congress   92-49686
                                                          CIP

VT/PC/PC
5   4   3   2   1

Contributors

Jannice O. Aaron, M.D.
Associate Clinical Professor, Diagnostic Radiology, University of Louisville; Medical Director, St. Anthony Imaging Center, Louisville, Kentucky

Robert W. Bailey, M.D.
Chief of General Surgery, Greater Baltimore Medical Center, Baltimore, Maryland

Charles M. Balch, M.D.
Professor and Chairman, Department of Surgery, M.D. Anderson Cancer Center and University of Texas at Houston, Houston, Texas

Mitchell H. Bamberger, M.D.
Assistant Professor of Surgery (Urology), Department of Surgery, East Orange Veterans Affairs Medical Center, University of Medicine and Dentistry of New Jersey, Newark, New Jersey

Richard M. Bell, M.D.
Professor of Surgery, University of South Carolina, Columbia, South Carolina

Folkert O. Belzer, M.D.
Professor and Chairman, Department of Surgery, University of Wisconsin Hospital and Clinics, Madison, Wisconsin

Michael L. Bentz, M.D.
Assistant Professor of Surgery, Division of Plastic and Maxillofacial Surgery, University of Pittsburgh, Pittsburgh, Pennsylvania

David G. Bjoraker, M.D.
Associate Professor, Department of Anesthesiology, University of Florida College of Medicine, Gainesville, Florida

F. William Blaisdell, M.D.
Professor and Chairman, Department of Surgery, University of California–Davis Medical Center, Sacramento, California

Kirby I. Bland, M.D.
Professor and Associate Chairman, Department of Surgery, University of Florida College of Medicine, Gainesville, Florida

Anthony P. Borzotta, M.D.
Medical Director, West Wing Intensive Care Unit, Emanuel Hospital and Health Center; Assistant Professor of Surgery, Oregon Health Science University, Portland, Oregon

Jason H. Calhoun, M.D., M. Eng.
Associate Professor of Surgery, Division of Orthopaedic Surgery, University of Texas Medical Branch at Galveston, Galveston, Texas

Frank B. Cerra, M.D.
Professor of Surgery, University of Minnesota, Minneapolis, Minnesota

Lawrence H. Cohn, M.D.
Professor of Surgery, Harvard Medical School; Chief, Division of Cardiac Surgery, Brigham and Women's Hospital, Boston, Massachusetts

John A. Collins, M.D.
Chidester Professor of Surgery, Stanford University Medical Center, Stanford, California

Anthony M. D'Alessandro, M.D.
Assistant Professor of Surgery, University of Wisconsin School of Medicine, Madison, Wisconsin

Mark Deakin, Ch.M., F.R.C.S.
Senior Lecturer in Surgery, Keele University Postgraduate Medical School, North Staffordshire Medical Center, North Staffordshire, England

Richard H. Dean, M.D.
Director, Division of Surgical Sciences and Professor of Surgery, Bowman Gray School of Medicine of Wake Forest University, Winston-Salem, North Carolina

Daniel T. Dempsey, M.D.
Associate Professor of Surgery; Chief, Gastrointestinal Surgery and Research, Temple University, Philadelphia, Pennsylvania

Timothy C. Fabian, M.D.
Professor and Deputy Chairman; Director of Trauma, Department of Surgery, University of Tennessee College of Medicine, Memphis, Tennessee

Lewis M. Flint, Jr., M.D.
Regents Professor and Chairman, Department of Surgery, Tulane University School of Medicine, New Orleans, Louisiana

Donald E. Fry, M.D.
Professor and Chairman, Department of Surgery, University of New Mexico School of Medicine, Albuquerque, New Mexico

J. William Futrell, M.D.
Professor of Surgery, Department of Surgery, Division of Plastic and Maxillofacial Surgery, University of Pittsburgh, Pittsburgh, Pennsylvania

Brian L. Ganzel, M.D.
Assistant Professor, Division of Thoracic and Cardiovascular Surgery, University of Louisville, Louisville, Kentucky

Bernard Gardner, M.D.
Professor of Surgery; Director, Division of Surgical Education, University of Medicine and Dentistry of New Jersey, Newark, New Jersey

Laman A. Gray, Jr., M.D.
Professor of Surgery and Director, Division of Thoracic and Cardiovascular Surgery, University of Louisville, Louisville, Kentucky

James I. Harty, F.R.C.S.I.
Professor of Surgery, Department of Surgery, Division of Urology, University of Louisville, Louisville, Kentucky

Terry C. Hicks, M.D.
Associate Chairman, Department of Colon and Rectal Surgery, Ochsner Clinic, New Orleans, Louisiana

Robert J. Irwin, Jr., M.D.
Associate Professor of Clinical Surgery; Chief, Section of Urology, University of Medicine and Dentistry of New Jersey, Newark, New Jersey

Edwin C. James, M.D.
Professor of Surgery and Dean, Department of Surgery, University of North Dakota School of Medicine, Grand Forks, North Dakota

Peter J. Jannetta, M.D.
Professor and Chairman, Department of Neurologic Surgery, University of Pittsburgh, Pittsburgh, Pennsylvania

John R. Johnson, M.D.
Professor and Chairman, Department of Orthopaedic Surgery, University of Louisville, Louisville, Kentucky

Edwin L. Kaplan, M.D.
Professor of Surgery, The University of Chicago, Pritzker School of Medicine, Chicago, Illinois

Gerald M. Larson, M.D.
Professor of Surgery, University of Louisville, Louisville, Kentucky

Curt E. Liebman, M.D.
Angiography and Interventional Radiology, St. Anthony Imaging Center, Louisville, Kentucky

George W. Machiedo, M.D.
Professor and Vice Chairman, Department of Surgery, University of Medicine and Dentistry of New Jersey, Newark, New Jersey

Donald W. Marion, M.D.
Assistant Professor of Neurologic Surgery, Chief, Head Injury Service, University of Pittsburgh, Pittsburgh, Pennsylvania

Stephen J. Mathes, M.D.
Professor of Surgery, Head of Division of Plastic and Reconstructive Surgery, University of California, San Francisco, California

Martin H. Max, M.D.
Department of Surgery, Conemaugh Valley Memorial Hospital, Johnstown, Pennsylvania

Frank B. Miller, M.D.
Associate Professor of Surgery and Director of Division of General Surgery, University of Louisville, Louisville, Kentucky

William J. Millikan, Jr., M.D.
Professor of Surgery, Texas Tech University School of Medicine, Lubbock, Texas

Anne E. Missavage, M.D.
Assistant Professor, Department of Surgery; Director, Burn Unit, University of California–Davis Medical Center, Sacramento, California

Jerome H. Modell, M.D.
Professor and Chairman, Department of Anesthesiology, University of Florida College of Medicine, Gainesville, Florida

A.R. Moossa, M.D., F.R.C.S.
Professor and Chairman, Department of Surgery, University of California–San Diego Medical Center, San Diego, California

John L. Myers, M.D.
Associate Professor of Surgery and Pediatrics, Division of Cardiothoracic Surgery, The Pennsylvania State University College of Medicine, The Milton S. Hershey Medical Center, Hershey, Pennsylvania

Howard S. Nearman, M.D.
Associate Professor, Departments of Anesthesiology, Surgery, and Reproductive Biology, Case Western Reserve University School of Medicine; Clinical Director of Operative Services, University Hospitals of Cleveland, Cleveland, Ohio

Frank G. Opelka, M.D.
Staff Surgeon, Department of Colon and Rectal Surgery, Ochsner Clinic, New Orleans, Louisiana

Michael D. Pasquale, M.D.
Surgical Critical Care Fellow, Department of Surgery, University of Minnesota, Minneapolis, Minnesota

Paul C. Peters, M.D.
Professor and Chairman, Department of Surgery, Division of Urology, University of Texas Southwestern Medical School, Dallas, Texas

Hiram C. Polk, Jr., M.D.
Ben A. Reid, Sr. Professor and Chairman, Department of Surgery, University of Louisville, Louisville, Kentucky

George Raque, M.D.
Assistant Professor of Surgery, Division of Neurologic Surgery, University of Louisville, Louisville, Kentucky

Linda M. Reilly, M.D.
Associate Professor of Surgery, Department of Surgery, University of California, San Francisco, California

J. David Richardson, M.D.
Professor of Surgery, Department of Surgery, University of Louisville, Louisville, Kentucky

Wallace P. Ritchie, Jr., M.D., Ph.D.
Professor and Chairman, Department of Surgery, Temple University Health Sciences Center, Philadelphia, Pennsylvania

Benjamin F. Rush, Jr., M.D.
Distinguished Professor and Chair, Department of Surgery, University of Medicine and Dentistry of New Jersey, Newark, New Jersey

Christopher B. Shields, M.D., F.R.C.S.(C)
Professor of Surgery, Division of Neurological Surgery, University of Louisville School of Medicine, Louisville, Kentucky

G. Tom Shires, M.D.
Professor and Chairman, Department of Surgery, Texas Tech University School of Medicine, Lubbock, Texas

Jerry M. Shuck, M.D., D.Sc.
Oliver H. Payne Professor and Chairman, Department of Surgery, Case Western Reserve University School of Medicine; Director of Surgery, University Hospitals of Cleveland, Cleveland, Ohio

Hans W. Sollinger, M.D., Ph.D.
Professor of Surgery and Pathology, University of Wisconsin School of Medicine; Director, Pancreas Transplant Program, University of Wisconsin Hospital and Clinics, Madison, Wisconsin

H. Harlan Stone, M.D.
Program Director, Phoenix Integrated Surgical Residency, Good Samaritan Regional Medical Center, Phoenix, Arizona

Ronald J. Stoney, M.D.
Professor of Surgery, Department of Surgery, Division of Vascular Surgery, University of California, San Francisco, California

Stanley E. Thawley, M.D.
Associate Professor, Department of Otolaryngology, Washington University School of Medicine, St. Louis, Missouri

Michael D. Traynor, M.D.
Instructor of Surgery, Department of Surgery, University of North Dakota School of Medicine, Grand Forks, North Dakota

John A. Waldhausen, M.D.
John W. Oswald Professor of Surgery, Chairman, Department of Surgery, The Pennsylvania State University College of Medicine, The Milton S. Hershey Medical Center, Hershey, Pennsylvania

G. Rainey Williams, M.D.
Professor and Chairman, Department of Surgery, University of Oklahoma College of Medicine, Oklahoma City, Oklahoma

Roger W. Yurt, M.D.
Professor and Chairman (Acting), Department of Surgery, Cornell University Medical College; Attending Surgeon and Surgeon-in-Chief (Acting), The New York Hospital, New York, New York

Karl A. Zucker, M.D.
Professor of Surgery, University of New Mexico School of Medicine, Albuquerque, New Mexico

Preface

The traditional approach to undergraduate surgical education has been altered in recent years as a result of various technical and sociopolitical considerations. The blocks of time and effort previously allocated to the surgical sciences in two or more years of the undergraduate medical curriculum have been eroded in many schools. More and more surgical educators and students are required to deal with the cognitive areas of basic surgery in very short periods, often punctuated by major time commitments at the bedside and in the operating room in the care of surgical patients. The stress placed by these curricular changes has been dealt with in various innovative and more or less effective ways. The upshot of these efforts is that it is increasingly difficult to use the standard major texts as first-line educational material for the student. Such books retain great value by virtue of their breadth and depth, since they deal effectively with the spectrum of surgery from its history to its prospects and include all of the specialty areas. Most of the shorter texts have been mere abridgments of the standard works.

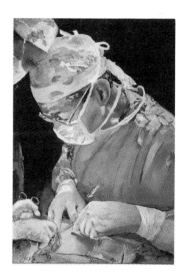

Our Purpose

The purpose of *Basic Surgery* is to present to the student a selected series of common complaints that warrant surgical evaluation or treatment, or both, and to use the *symptom-oriented approach* to direct the student to a clear and concise discussion of the pathophysiology of disease, treatment, repair, and recovery. Because the patient's chief complaint represents his or her first clinical contact with a physician, most of the material is organized around patient presentations. A step-by-step analysis is usually included to illustrate the evolution of diagnosis and treatment. Introduction of the problem-solving method to teaching in medicine has facilitated organization of daily activities toward more accurate diagnosis, more rapid treatment, and more consistently reliable evaluation of results. For these reasons, chapters such as those on abdominal masses and jaundice have been organized accordingly. Nevertheless, some basic surgical considerations have been simplified or omitted, usually because of the relative rarity of an ailment or its overwhelming scope for the undergraduate student. The maintenance of brevity and clarity, as aided by tables and illustrations, has priority in this fourth edition.

What's New in the Fourth Edition?

The organization of chapters reflects our symptom-based approach. Part I discusses some characteristics of surgery, surgeons, and specific broad concepts as applied to clinical practice. The heart of the book, Part II, focuses on a series of patient symptoms that lead directly to surgical assessment of the numerous parameters involved in diagnosis, treatment, and aftercare. Part III covers specific management problems, including postoperative considerations, and presents an overview of several surgical subspecialties.

New chapters have been added, and all chapters substantially updated and rewritten, to reflect the technologic tools and data available to today's surgeons:

- *Diagnostic Imaging of Common Surgical Problems*—emphasizes the partnership between the surgeon and the radiologic consultant in the use of such innovative diagnostic procedures as MRI and CT scanning, radionuclide scanning agents, and ultrasonography.
- *Diagnostic and Therapeutic Laparoscopy*—covers contemporary instrumentation, technology, and an ever-growing range of applications.
- *Critical Care*—discusses life support management, monitoring, and problem-solving for the critically ill patient.
- *Basic Surgical Techniques*—details and illustrates procedures such as administering local anesthetic, placing central venous catheters, intubation, and more.
- *Stroke*—describes the causes, clinical manifestations, and successful management of cerebrovascular disease.
- *Nutritional Support*—includes its theoretic background and current clinical applications.
- *Shock*—all new content emphasizes recognition, monitoring, and treatment of shock as well as adjunctive therapy and management of postshock syndromes.

Other new features make the text more readily accessible to the student and aid comprehension:

- *Key Features*—opens each chapter with a concise summary of content to be covered.
- *Pitfalls and Common Myths*—this new boxed element underscores some of the most frequently encountered mistaken assumptions in surgical patient care.
- *Surgical Pharmacopeia*—provides a brief summary of therapeutic agents, appropriate dosage, indications, and potential complications.
- *New perforated insert section*—offers a pocket-size pull-out of two extremely important areas of surgical pharmacopeia: anesthetic agents and treatment of infection.
- *Algorithms*—used throughout the text to orient students to the problem-solving approach to diagnosis, treatment, and follow-up evaluation of outcome.
- All chapters have been significantly revised and updated or completely rewritten, many by new contributors who bring a broad range of expertise to their topics.

- *Chapter Review*—each chapter ends with a brief self-test to enable students to evaluate their retention of essential information.
- *Question headings*—where possible, section headings have been converted to a question format to sharply focus the reader's attention on the relevance of the content.
- *Use of color*—full-color illustrations have been added to provide real-world examples of what the surgeon will encounter in practice, such as endoscopic evaluation.

Basic Surgery is intended to stand alone or supplement existing major reference works in surgery. In every chapter the bibliography offers carefully selected journal articles, monographs, or chapters within major reference books that we believe provide valuable resource material and in-depth introductions.

Acknowledgments

We wish to express our appreciation and to acknowledge the very specific contributions made by the many individuals who have helped with this book. Clearly, the readers of each prior edition of **Basic Surgery** have contributed much over the years by both formal and informal critiques of the book as well as through their constructive suggestions on how it could be improved. We are likewise indebted to our faculty colleagues (who do not always appear as co-authors) for creating an environment in which this kind of thinking is the norm, for providing countless hours of helpful criticism, and for refocusing our thoughts on the entire spectrum of the surgical sciences.

We are especially grateful to the surgical residents at the University of Louisville who undertook a very detailed review of the Surgical Pharmacopeia sections that appear at the end of most chapters and in the pull-out booklet in the back of the text. They include Drs. Richard W. Bock, Douglas A. Brewer, K. Kent Chevli, Anthony V. Deiorio, Michael J. Doyle, James R. Garrison, Jr., John R. Gosche, Baron L. Hamman, Todd Heniford, Dalton S. Prickett, Christopher J. Theuer, Anne R. Thompson, and Timothy A. Wierson. A special thanks to Wahid Naziri, the Price Fellow of Surgical Research at the University of Louisville, for his thorough and well-organized look at antibiotic therapy, and to Dr. Michael Heine, Associate Professor of Anesthesiology at the University of Louisville, for his excellent compilation of anesthetic and pain-related agents.

We also owe a great deal to individuals in our own offices who have made this book possible and who have worked closely with the contributors and the publishers. They are Margaret Abby and Nancy Dobrovolsky. Both bore a major burden in completing this effort; its consistency and clarity are largely due to their untiring efforts. Finally, we acknowledge the crucial role that Suzanne Wakefield has taken as Project Editor on behalf of Quality Medical Publishing in facilitating and enhancing every idea within the book and the continuing leadership of the President of Quality Medical Publishing, Karen Berger.

Hiram C. Polk, Jr.
Bernard Gardner
H. Harlan Stone

Contents

Introduction: Strategies for Effective Learning and Retention During a
Surgical Clerkship xvii
Richard M. Bell, Hiram C. Polk, Jr.

PART I PREOPERATIVE CONSIDERATIONS

Section One GENERAL APPROACH TO SURGERY

1 Surgical Attitudes, History, and Ethics 3
G. Tom Shires, Hiram C. Polk, Jr.

2 The Mathematics of Clinical Judgment: Including an Evaluation of
Operative Risk 8
Edwin C. James, Hiram C. Polk, Jr.

3 Planning and Managing Anesthesia 28
David G. Bjoraker, Jerome H. Modell

Section Two SPECIALIZED TECHNOLOGIC CONSIDERATIONS

4 Diagnostic Imaging of Common Surgical Problems 61
Jannice O. Aaron, Curt E. Liebman

5 Endoscopy in Surgical Practice 86
Gerald M. Larson, Martin H. Max

6 Diagnostic and Therapeutic Laparoscopy for the General Surgeon 95
Karl A. Zucker, Robert W. Bailey

Section Three PHYSIOLOGIC ASPECTS OF SURGICAL DISEASE

7 Parenteral Fluid and Electrolyte Therapy 122
G. Tom Shires, William J. Millikan, Jr.

8 Nutritional Support 138
Anthony P. Borzotta

9 Respiratory Function and Support 148
Lewis M. Flint, Jr.

10 Surgical Endocrinology 162
Edwin L. Kaplan

11 Gastroduodenal Physiology and Peptic Ulcer Disease 196
Daniel T. Dempsey, Wallace P. Ritchie, Jr.

12 Principles of Surgical Oncology and Tumor Biology 220
Bernard Gardner

13   Transplantation Science and Immunology 237
     Hans W. Sollinger, Anthony M. D'Alessandro, Folkert O. Belzer

PART II   **PATIENT PRESENTATIONS: A SYMPTOM-BASED APPROACH**

14   Intraoral Lesions 257
     Benjamin F. Rush, Jr.

15   Neck Masses 272
     Kirby I. Bland

16   Difficulties in Swallowing 289
     Hiram C. Polk, Jr.

17   Hemoptysis, Cough, and Other Symptoms of Pulmonary Lesions 302
     J. David Richardson

18   Heart Murmurs: Acquired Valvular Heart Disease 315
     Lawrence H. Cohn

19   Heart Murmurs: Congenital Heart Disease 329
     John A. Waldhausen, John L. Myers

20   Acute and Chronic Chest Pain of Cardiovascular Origin 349
     Brian L. Ganzel, Laman A. Gray, Jr.

21   Hypertension 370
     G. Rainey Williams

22   Stroke 379
     Ronald J. Stoney, Linda M. Reilly

23   Lump in the Breast 384
     Bernard Gardner

24   Gastrointestinal Bleeding 403
     J. David Richardson, Bernard Gardner

25   Acute Abdominal Pain 422
     Bernard Gardner, H. Harlan Stone

26   Jaundice 460
     A.R. Moossa, Mark Deakin

27   Abnormal Bowel Movements 481
     Michael D. Traynor, Edwin C. James, Bernard Gardner

28   Abdominal Masses 504
     Frank B. Miller, James I. Harty

29   Hernia 532
     H. Harlan Stone

30   Rectal and Perianal Complaints 547
     Terry C. Hicks, Frank G. Opelka

31   Surgical Masqueraders: Abdominal Pain Rarely Requiring Operation 561
     Bernard Gardner

32   The Ischemic Lower Extremity 571
     Richard H. Dean

33   The Swollen Leg 584
     Anne E. Missavage, F. William Blaisdell

34   Skin and Soft Tissue Lesions 595
     Charles M. Balch, Hiram C. Polk, Jr.

35   Trauma 606
     H. Harlan Stone, Timothy C. Fabian

36   Burns 620
     Roger W. Yurt

37   Pediatric Surgical Emergencies 631
     H. Harlan Stone

38   Head Injuries 653
     Donald W. Marion, Peter J. Jannetta

39   Musculoskeletal Injuries 669
     Jason H. Calhoun

40   Hematuria 684
     Paul C. Peters

41   Obstructive Uropathy and Urinary Tract Infection 694
     Mitchell H. Bamberger, Robert J. Irwin, Jr.

42   The Scrotum 713
     H. Harlan Stone

43   Low Back Pain 719
     Christopher B. Shields, George Raque, John R. Johnson

PART III   POSTOPERATIVE CONSIDERATIONS

Section One   SPECIAL MANAGEMENT PROBLEMS IN THE SURGICAL PATIENT

44   The Approach to the Postoperative Patient 735
     Hiram C. Polk, Jr.

45   Postoperative Fever 745
     Donald E. Fry

46   Shock 757
     George W. Machiedo

47   Surgical Bleeding and Hemostasis 773
     John A. Collins

48   Critical Care 786
     Michael D. Pasquale, Frank B. Cerra

49   Infection 807
     H. Harlan Stone

Section Two   SPECIALIZED PROCEDURES AND BASIC TECHNIQUES

50   Basic Principles of Hand Surgery 830
Michael L. Bentz, J. William Futrell

51   Basic Plastic Surgery 845
Stephen J. Mathes

52   Basic Otolaryngologic Surgery 856
Stanley E. Thawley

53   Basic Surgical Techniques 870
Howard S. Nearman, Jerry M. Shuck

Index 885

COLOR PLATES: Chapter 5 plates follow p. 92; Chapter 22 plates follow p. 380; Chapter 24 plates follow p. 412.

Introduction
Strategies for Effective Learning and Retention During a Surgical Clerkship

RICHARD M. BELL
HIRAM C. POLK, Jr.

KEY FEATURES

This section of the book:
- Offers keys for successful learning during the surgery clerkship.
- Provides tips for balancing demands on your time.
- Reaffirms the principles and precepts of adult education.

This text has been developed with the principles of adult education as the foundation. Unlike the pedagogic model—which is teacher-centered, rigid, and dependent—student physicians are adult learners and therefore must assume the responsibility for their own education. The medical school faculty and others who may serve as mentors function more as "facilitators" rather than as "teachers." Adults' motivation to learn derives from a need to know, usually the need for information or experience necessary to solve some problem. In this environment it is the situation, not the subject matter, that dictates the process.

WHAT MAKES A SURGERY STUDENT SUCCESSFUL?

With such basic educational concepts in mind, the following suggestions may enhance the learning experience during the surgical clerkship.

Accept the Responsibility for Your Own Education! Many of the educational objectives that you have been given were developed by the faculty of your school and represent a consensus of what every physician should know about a disease process. The student, however, should add desired "personal" goals or specific individual areas of interest to those objectives. Decide what *you* wish to accomplish during the surgical rotation.

Plan for the Experience! Learning occurs best in situations in which preparation meets opportunity. Always prepare for scrubbing on or watching an operative procedure by evaluating the patient, reading about the disease process, and reviewing the basic anatomy and physiology of the organ systems involved. It is not necessary to try to learn the technical nuances of surgical procedure, because the objectives of the basic surgical clerkship do not emphasize these. Prepare for the lectures or tutorials in the same fashion. It is prudent to use the time between scheduled activities to get a head start on the next planned session. Make the most of necessary gaps in the day's work schedule.

Take the Time to Critically Evaluate the Learning Experience! Students who are well prepared are usually able to evaluate what they have seen or heard in greater depth than those who are not. In adult learning, the analysis of the learning experience is the core. Ask probing questions, such as: What impressed me the most about what happened in the clinic, lecture, or the operating room today? Does what I saw or heard coincide with my own experience or what I already know? Are there alternatives to the course of action taken? Was my assessment of the situation correct? If so, was my approach the best it could have been? If not, where did I go astray? Considering my own career goals, what information do I need to retain from this clerkship?

When You Don't Understand, Ask! There are no stupid questions. What is unclear to you was also unclear to many of the great masters in medicine at some point in history. Those who ask questions generally find solutions eventually. The level of questioning, however, may indicate the extent of your efforts to find an answer. Equally important is to recognize that there are times and places when asking questions is *not* appropriate.

Periodically Reevaluate Your Needs, Goals, and Objectives for Their Appropriateness! As students increase their clinical acumen and knowledge base, the personal experience that any individual student brings to the learning situation changes. All adult learning is experience centered; therefore, as an individual matures, the depth of understanding changes. Learning goals and objectives must necessarily change as well.

The curricular structure may vary greatly from school to school, yet the goals are similar, if not identical. Graduates are expected to attain a sufficient knowledge base in order to pursue additional training. Further, graduates are expected to develop the necessary skills to continue a lifetime of independent adult learning. As the information explosion continues its exponential growth, physicians who are unable to keep pace in their field may find it impossible to practice in only a few short years after completing their training. If not already developed, this process of continual learning should begin in your clinical years of undergraduate medical education.

Michael Hobsley, Professor of Surgery at the Middlesex Hospital Medical School in London, has enumerated three distinct facets of medical education:

1. The development of the skills involved in gathering information about a particular patient—basically history taking, physical examination, and special investigations
2. The acquisition of knowledge, which is the established facts about diseases and their management
3. Learning to select the correct diagnostic label from one's store of knowledge

Hobsley sums up these three facets in the following excerpts from his book*:

In most medical schools, the emphasis is on items 1 and 2. With regard to item 3, the usual advice given is to construct the differential diagnosis and then narrow down the possibilities. Yet when the medical student becomes a doctor he finds that there are problems with the approach via differential diagnosis.

Firstly, a complete list of all possible diagnoses would usually be very long, and rarely does even the most deliberate and conscientious of doctors draw up such a list. Secondly, no matter how many possibilities the doctor enumerates, it usually transpires that he has forgotten some, of which one may be the correct diagnosis. Thirdly, the concept of the differential diagnosis is only useful if the doctor, having constructed his list, can then afford to sit back and wait for the results of any investigations that he has ordered for their discriminatory value. In other words, if none of the possible diagnoses require urgent treatment. The immediate and pressing problem posed by the patient is: What must the doctor do, or advise, at that instant?

In place of the *differential diagnosis,* the student should develop the concept of the *working diagnosis.* There is a clear-cut distinction between these concepts. Instead of a list of all the possible diagnostic labels in terms of disease, the working diagnosis presents the key to the management of a clinical situation in terms of the action that the doctor should take. Not often is this diagnosis expressed in the form of exact aetiology or pathology. Instead, it is the most accurate description of the patient's problem available to the doctor at that moment, and as such it decides the doctor's immediate management.

■ ■ ■

The guiding principle of this book is our attempt to delve into the mind of the reader (whether medical student, physician house officer, or nurse) and to direct the thought processes that, based on knowledge of the basic sciences and the patient's signs and symptoms, can be used to sketch an outline characteristic of a specific disease. Treatment is then designed to reverse the responsible or associated pathophysiologic derangements rather than to satisfy some memorized or ill-conceived regimen. Always with the patient's benefit in mind, such factual material automatically becomes relevant to the sick and injured and will usually lead to the desired intellectual stimulation that so classically has characterized the surgical sciences.

---

*Reprinted with permission from Hobsley M. Problem-solving in medical education. In Hobsley M (ed). Pathways in Surgical Management, 2nd ed. Baltimore, Edward Arnold Publishers, 1986, pp 3-5.

PITFALLS AND COMMON MYTHS

- Failure to read in a systematic fashion and on a regular schedule.
- Failure to prepare for the next day's scheduled operations, lectures, or seminars.
- Delaying reading until the student is at home and "off for the night."
- You should use odd daytime hours for serious study instead of unproductive bull sessions and aimless discussion of famous cases you have seen or read about.
- Remember that your performance (grades) is evaluated by bedside and operating room conduct as well as by examination scores.

Bibliography

Hobsley M (ed). Pathways in Surgical Management, 2nd ed. Baltimore, Edward Arnold Publishers, 1986, pp 3-5.

PREOPERATIVE CONSIDERATIONS

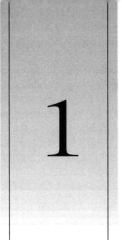

SECTION ONE General Approach to Surgery

1

Surgical Attitudes, History, and Ethics

G. TOM SHIRES
HIRAM C. POLK, Jr.

Surgical historian R.H. Meade has stated, "It is hardly surprising that surgery of a number of parts of the human body had its origin in the treatment of wounds, for in many respects man's environment is a hostile one, threatening him on all sides with insults to the body that is ill adapted to resist force. Aside from the mute testimony of the remains of our forebears, however, the first actual account of the treatment of wounds is to be found in the Edwin Smith Papyrus. According to Breasted, it was written about 1700 B.C., but composed of texts dating back as far as 3000 B.C."

The earliest scientific document ever brought to light is a treatise on surgery. The fascinating Smith Papyrus, now translated and in print, includes the records of 48 cases with discussions of diagnosis, treatment, and prognosis. In his *Great Ideas in the History of Surgery,* Zimmerman stated, "This remarkable book was compiled by an unknown author at a time when medicine was magical-religious, when the vocabulary of science had not yet been created, and when the first groping steps in inductive reasoning were being taken. This volume is as logical as a modern textbook in surgery."

The first real surgical renaissance occurred near the fifth century B.C., when the School of Hippocrates (460 to 377 B.C.) brought the state of the healing art to a position of scientific medicine. This renaissance was so profound that the history of medicine and surgery for the ensuing 2000 years was largely a struggle to regain those peaks of excellence attained during this Golden Age of Greece, 400 years before the Christian era. Insofar as the written word is concerned, in the time between the Smith Papyrus and the monumental works of the *Corpus Hippocraticum* the recorded descriptions are largely ones of treatment of wounds and are generally rather superficial.

The second surgical renaissance coincided with what is generally known throughout the world as *the* Renaissance in fifteenth century Europe following the Dark Ages, although significant contributions were made with the dawning of the Christian Era; certainly, the work of Celsus, *De Re Medica,* is a milestone of description. Celsus provided much of our knowledge of Alexandrian surgery and left the most lucid account of the status of medicine and surgery in the Roman period. However, the Renaissance in Europe did lay the foundation for the monumental works of Harvey, Malpighi, and Paré. Others, aided by the discovery of the microscope, produced a true rebirth of medical and surgical knowledge.

The last half of the nineteenth century was clearly the third surgical renaissance. This period began with the discovery and use of ether in 1842 and chloroform in 1847. Subsequently the work of Pasteur and Lister with antisepsis and asepsis paved the way for modern surgery. The pace of progress in surgery since this third renaissance has been staggering. Many reasons exist for the rapidity and extent of this progress, not the least of which are the coincident advances in science, chemistry, and physiology.

HOW DO WE MEASURE THE SUCCESS OF AMERICAN SURGERY?

If we look at the treatment of wounds as described in the Smith Papyrus, it is clear the only available treatment was the body's natural defenses, even though the ancient physician's powers of observation were outstanding and included a description of the brain and of ligaments. Physiologic observations included pulse patterns and the function of the nervous system. Nevertheless, no technical procedures existed for surgical correction of defects produced by wounds; there was, of course, no anesthesia or asepsis.

If a patient today sustains the same injuries described in the Papyrus, the medical services available for the treatment of those injuries are truly remarkable. The patient can be transported quickly, resuscitated early, given physiologic support in the form of blood, fluid, and electrolytes, and treated with a detailed surgical approach to correct any deficits while he or she is under painless anesthesia and with strictest aseptic technique. In addition, we see complete biologic monitoring and organ support in a variety of forms, whether the deficiency is cardiac, pulmonary, renal, or nutritional. If we look at the contributions to modern surgical practice, it is soon apparent that most of the biologic support systems result from advances in surgery made largely by Americans—although it should be quickly added that such advances were not made by surgeons alone or by Americans alone.

WHAT HAVE BEEN MAJOR RECENT SURGICAL ADVANCES?

As technologic and biologic advances occur in many fields, success becomes more difficult to measure. In a milestone study Comroe and Dripps reported the scientific basis of the support of biomedical research. As that study pointed out, general anesthesia was not used until the 1840s, and it was not until 100 years later that John Gibbon performed the first successful operation on an open heart with complete cardiopulmonary bypass. To establish 10 scientific advances, Comroe and Dripps identified 137 essential bodies of knowledge. They arrived at their conclusions by examining 4000 published articles; 2500 specific scientific reports were particularly important to the development of one or more of the 137 essential bodies of knowledge. From this group of articles, 529 key ones were

selected as prerequisite background to the one major clinical advance in general anesthesia.

Another approach was taken by the Research Committee of the Study of Surgical Services in the United States (SOSSUS), completed in 1975, but was the only work of its kind. As pointed out by Comroe and Dripps, the SOSSUS committee also realized that such discoveries as penicillin, in fields far removed from surgery, have profoundly influenced the care of surgical patients. Similarly, some research performed by surgeons had substantial impact on fields unrelated to surgery, but for most purposes the appropriate definition of surgical research is "research performed by surgeons."

After an extensive survey, the SOSSUS committee identified contributions of important surgical research by general category. For example, the effect on the mortality rate of some important contributions to biomedical-surgical research for a single year is impressive. Fifteen surgical research contributions played a major role in the salvage of a total of 78,538 lives in that year alone. If the number of lives saved were calculated for every year following introduction of a research advance, the total would be even more significant. Furthermore, one must recall that these data were collected in the pretransplant era and that coronary artery surgery was in its infancy.

One major reason for success in research by surgical biologists relates to the funding of biomedical research. Before World War II, research played a relatively minor role in the nation at large and certainly in academic institutions. The total national expenditure for medical research in 1940 was $45 million, of which more than half was expended by private industry. The federal government's investment in biomedical research amounted to only $3 million; today that figure is over $7 billion. Although a number of important advances resulted from medical research during the pre–World War II era, particularly immunization to control infectious diseases, the rate of discovery was very slow by current standards. The 25 years between 1945 and 1970 were a golden era in biomedical research, during which there were steadily increasing financial support of and enormous advances in the prevention and treatment of disease.

The question might legitimately be asked today whether opportunities in surgical research are still available after this explosion of advances in science, technology, and patient care. Meade, in his remarkable book, said, "As medicine has advanced, the role of surgery has decreased. The day will certainly come when surgery will be done only to correct the effects of trauma and congenital abnormalities and advances have been made which may make congenital defects common only in backward areas." Certainly most who have thought about the future of surgery have come to the same conclusions. However, these eventualities probably will not occur in any of our lifetimes. Indeed, there apparently is a new frontier in surgical research that is, in and of itself, renewing and reinvigorating for its parent discipline.

One approach to identifying the frontiers of surgery involves an examination of the major causes of disability and death, the economic costs involved, and the potential capabilities of surgical research to reduce these liabilities.

WHAT IS THE SCIENTIFIC FUTURE OF SURGERY?

We propose that we are now experiencing the fourth great surgical renaissance. If we look at the development of modern surgery in America since the middle of the nineteenth century, we can see the potential for growth in the educational, practical, and technical aspects of surgery almost beyond belief for the next 100 years. In fact, the most spectacular surgical advances and the development of the surgical biologist have occurred only since 1945.

Most of the great advances by surgeons have been built in concert with many other scientists and practitioners from other fields. In addition, the scientific and technologic explosion occurring in this country has evolved in the years since World War II. Perhaps it seems strange to say that the third renaissance lasted only 100 years, but we believe the development of surgical biology that began in 1945 is, in fact, a fourth renaissance and parallels the change in civilization that has been so striking during this period—for example, poliomyelitis has been conquered; man has been to the moon; atomic energy has been developed and harnessed.

The surgical biologist teaches surgery based on all of the old anatomic pathology and on the physiologic and biochemical knowledge that has developed in this technologic age. The practicing surgeon of today is truly a surgical biologist. The remarkable development of technical skills during the past 100 years is ever present. Nevertheless, when we look at the diagnostic acumen, operative support, and postoperative care and supportive systems, including use of blood and blood products, fluids, and electrolytes, nutri-

tional support, and pulmonary-cardiovascular-renal monitoring and support to patients, we recognize that a staggering number of patients are helped to have a better life today than would have been possible even 45 years ago.

Consequently the emergence of surgeons as surgical biologists in the past three decades is and should be recognized truly as the fourth surgical renaissance. Perhaps the key to the future in surgery is the preservation and further development of the role of the surgical biologist.

AN ATTITUDE FOR ACTION

Among medical people, the personality traits of surgeons are considered characteristic and are defined by some as essential for participation in the specialty. As a matter of fact, the traits, however well defined, do not reflect personality nearly so much as an attitude toward illness. That attitude is best characterized as a prompt consideration of alternatives, the formulation of a working hypothesis, and the culmination of that effort in a therapeutic intervention that is both identifiable and often profoundly effective. That effectiveness is more often for good than for bad, but there is also the enormous possibility of producing direct adverse results that more than counterbalance any beneficial effects. The overwhelming characteristic of the early era of surgery, reaching on to present times, has been a concern with life-threatening illnesses. Only within recent decades have we gained the capability to alter the effect of chronic diseases.

Surgery developed as a method of intervention to alleviate illnesses that were not aided by nonoperative means. Although nonoperative therapy was once primitive and largely ineffectual, the need for surgical intervention must have been great; the magnitude of this need is witnessed by the need to balance the benefits of surgical intervention against the remarkable pain that was endured by the patient in the preanesthetic era. Indeed, the implementation of general anesthesia was a major step that enabled the surgical trades to progress to the status of profession and subsequently to become a science. The hazards of surgery persist, but rather than counterbalancing the severe pain associated with such treatment, the possible adverse effects of the procedure, either in the short term as manifested by hospital mortality and morbidity or by an ultimate adverse effect on the disease in question or on some other organ system must be considered. In the following chapter about clinical judgment, this characteristic contrasting of anticipated good and bad is discussed in detail. The activist role assumed in medical practice by surgical disciples requires constant temperance. Unnecessary surgery, however defined, is anathema, and every procedure as promulgated in practice must be approximate to the illness of the patient: never timid when the patient is strong or the illness dangerous but at the same time, not dangerously bold when the patient is weak and the illness mild or chronic.

The leadership provided by surgical thought and testing has provided a seemingly sound foundation for cost-conscious medicine, and numerous adaptations in every surgical specialty have become standard practice. Protecting the continuing and traditional quality of surgical care is a greater responsibility than ever before.

The responsibility for giving meaning to many basic physiologic and anatomic observations has derived from the surgical disciplines. Examples abound, but none is more topical than the evolution of cardiopulmonary support. Indeed, the significance of cardiac catheterization was fully realized only when surgical and supportive techniques advanced to the point of being able initially to palliate and subsequently cure illnesses that could be so defined by the diagnostic intervention. Furthermore, temporary cardiopulmonary support by extracorporeal oxygenation has spawned a secondary series of medical advances that have significance far beyond the cardiac patient. The concept of organ support during treatment is now applied to a variety of illnesses, inevitably exerting a beneficial effect far beyond that anticipated when initially introduced as a palliative measure to deal with complications in cardiac surgical patients. The intensive care unit and all that it has meant to trauma victims and to patients undergoing major treatment for chronic diseases such as cancer are a tribute to the early open-heart surgeons and their recognition of the essentials of moment-to-moment patient care. Respiratory support, which is a keystone of such care, transposed the significance of arterial blood gas studies from the physiology laboratory to the bedside, with a measurable effect on the care of patients with life-threatening illnesses. Indeed, the spinoff derived from the use of extracorporeal circulation with cardiopulmonary bypass and cardiac surgery is ever widening, with its extent still undefined.

The technical capability of organ transplantation has led to a further definition of immunologic processes in man and has stimulated wide basic research in this area that has application far beyond simple organ preservation and transplantation. Clearly, the activist surgeon who was faced with desperate situations developed methods of intervention that evolved from desperate to innovative, acceptable, and ultimately routine. These advances are not very different from the leadership role of surgical thought in defining and literally remodeling current treatment of carcinoma of the female breast. Placing unrealistic and deceiving promises of lesser therapies in the cold light of reality has been the surgeon's duty, but the surgeon has tempered that reality with a marvelous variety of therapeutic options to achieve the ultimate end—a physically and mentally well patient.

WHAT IS THE FUTURE OF THE SURGEON AND THE SURGICAL ATTITUDE?

One may be tempted to suggest that the discipline has reached its peak and there are no further worlds to conquer. Such a belief is consistently wrong, for as fast as the problem of one illness thought to require surgical intervention is solved, technologic and conceptual advances allow the application of surgical endeavors to illness and areas hitherto thought beyond surgical endeavor.

Consider the surgical treatment of thyroid disease and of tuberculous pulmonary tissue, which over the last several decades has been in large measure supplanted by nonoperative means. As these sample areas have allowed surgical interests to move toward the periphery of their present clinical domain, surgery has accepted the enervating challenge of ischemic heart disease and chronic renal disease, areas long thought far beyond the capability or concept of the technical discipline. Consider also the whirlwind changes in treatment of gallstones of the last few years. Lithotripsy promised no surgical incision but at the expense of a high failure rate and lifelong, expensive oral biliary solvent therapy. Laparoscopic cholecystectomy provided what may become a safe and less expensive definitive extirpation of the diseased organ with multiple tiny incisions. Such is the nature of flexible and adaptable science and surgery's capacity to respond to new technology and the public well-being. This ability to grapple with uncertainty and to reach reasoned decisions characterizes the fine clinician and insightful investigator. Indeed, certainty is the enemy of inquiry, and surgical advances depend on an uneasy truce with uncertainty.

The surgical attitude has been and will be critical to continued surgical progress. A surgical procedure that is undertaken today as a desperate and challenging endeavor will become routine in the next decade and obsolete in an era beyond that. In every circumstance a concern for the immediacy of human illnesses allows the continuing application of the concept and the attitude in an ever-broadening and deepening discipline.

AREN'T THERE TOO MANY SURGEONS TODAY?

There has been a longstanding idea that there are too many surgeons, especially general surgeons, in the United States. If there was an element of truth to that belief a decade ago, it has been changed by (1) the attractiveness of surgical superspecialties such as pediatric, vascular, and oncologic surgery, (2) effective control of the number of surgical trainees leaving accredited residencies, (3) the realization that the large "baby boomers" segment of the population is approaching an age that has typically required more general surgical services than ever, and (4) increasing patient demand for less-invasive methods of surgical care. According to some sources, surgeons may well be in *short supply* at the dawn of the twenty-first century. The intermediate-term need for general surgeons is great, and they are increasingly being identified by governmental and provider medical in-services as *the most cost-effective medical practitioners!*

PITFALLS AND COMMON MYTHS

- We fail to think the unthinkable.
- Tomorrow's needs are never fully answered or met by today's technology.
- We fail to think far enough ahead.

BIBLIOGRAPHY

Comroe JH Jr, Dripps RD. Scientific basis for the support of biomedical science. Science 192:105, 1976.

Meade RH. An Introduction to the History of General Surgery. Philadelphia, WB Saunders, 1968.

Polk HC Jr. Presidential address: Surgery of the public good. Ann Surg 209:505, 1989.

Reiss E. In quest of certainty. Am J Med 77:969, 1984.

Shires GT. The fourth surgical renaissance. Presidential address. Ann Surg 192:269, 1980.

Zimmerman LM, Veith I. Great ideas in the history of surgery. Baltimore, Williams & Wilkins Co, 1961.

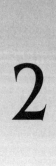

2

The Mathematics of Clinical Judgment

Including an Evaluation of Operative Risk

EDWIN C. JAMES
HIRAM C. POLK, Jr.

KEY FEATURES

After reading this chapter you will understand:
- How to evaluate the applicability of topics in the current literature to your patients.
- The elements of a risk/benefit analysis.
- How we can refine our understanding of operative risk.
- Methods of improving preoperative risk.

Sound clinical judgment has long been the most respected attribute of the capable physician. It is the ability to weigh the many clinical factors bearing on any illness or potential surgical condition to reach the appropriate diagnosis and decide on the optimal course of treatment for the patient. Unfortunately, such a definition provides few clues for the novice—the medical student or surgical resident—on how to develop or otherwise acquire this valuable asset. This chapter reviews the usual components of the clinical decision-making process as exemplified in the surgical setting. A more detailed and exhaustive discussion of many aspects of clinical judgment may be found in Feinstein's classic monograph.

WHAT ARE THE BASIC CONCEPTS?

The most accurate predictor of outcome for a given patient is that of a similar patient population managed in the same way, a tenet totally contrary to the all-or-none concept of risk for any particular patient. The mortality rate of an operation for a given patient is either 0 or 100%. However, the aggregate mortality rate of the next 99 patients, after the same operation, will approach that of the group serving as the clinician's standard. It is the experienced physician's responsibility to treat the patient in the manner that has produced the best overall result in a group of similar patients.

An inexperienced physician must depend on the published reports of others, while endeavoring to develop and maintain the objectivity required for the meaningful interpretation of a personal record of experience. Accurate evaluation of published or reported material is a lengthy and painstaking undertaking. Misinformation may be provided or facts omitted deliberately to show a method (and often the author) off to advantage; however, more often, errors are perpetrated by oversight. The prospective, blind, and/or controlled trial is easy to recognize, and its data are usually carefully substantiated. Other types of studies are prone to error and must be carefully scrutinized.

The following questions are useful in evaluating the work of others, whether it is published or verbal:

- Is the patient population really similar to your own?
- Is the illness staged in clinical terms so that the staging process will be helpful to you before treatment is begun?

- Are the diagnostic and treatment resources similar to your own?
- Are the results too good to believe? The surest sign of invalidity is the report of a large series of operations in which mortality and/or morbidity did not occur.
- Is the follow-up evaluation objective and was it done over a sufficiently long period of time?

DATA BASE

The data base must be applicable to the patient in question and must include appropriate demographic data as well as accurate clinical staging of the illness. Erroneous assessment of the clinical stage, particularly in relation to the patient's chief complaint, has been thoroughly discussed by Feinstein. However, seldom can one identify an appropriately described and documented experience with a significant number of patients exactly like the patient in question. Thus interpolation is a potential error, given an accurate diagnosis, clinical stage, and acceptable data base.

The difficulty of identifying "time zero" in one's patient and in the data cohort is the second most common source of error. Is the starting point the time of the theoretic inception of disease, the first symptom, the initial contact with the physician, or the moment of definitive diagnosis? Obviously, there is no way to compare the conditions of two lung cancer patients (Table 2-1) who initially consult a physician for hemoptysis only (patient A) or for intercostal neuralgia and hepatomegaly (patient B), even though the first five clinical characteristics are identical in both patients.

Although the patients are similar in five specific ways, the patient with hemoptysis is obviously in a much more favorable clinical stage of illness. This is just one example of the stumbling blocks facing the student who fails to thoughtfully analyze the data.

HOW IS OUTCOME BEST MEASURED?

Another variable, the assessment of end results, is subject to fewer errors of interpretation than those just discussed. Although percent survival time, such as 5 years, is a crude criterion of outcome, it can still be useful when treatment options yield greatly differing results.

Measurement of *person-years of life* is a more valid index (Table 2-2). It may be further refined to *well person–years.* As a logical extension of this concept, Spratt suggested that the net value of any clinical process can and should be measured in economic terms—by contrasting, for a given patient, the expense of medical care plus the diminished requirements for further care with his or her enhanced earning capacity as a result of prompt diagnosis and definitive treatment. This concept is not an attempt to measure the worth of human life in dollars and cents, but rather to develop an objective scale by which the beneficial and harmful effects of treatment can be balanced against a constant awareness of the quality as well as quantity of survival.

THE FUNDAMENTAL COMPARISON

An intelligent appraisal of the risks and rewards of a given treatment option, such as an operation, and consideration of the natural history of the illness in question, constitute the fundamental components of clinical judgment. With a very favorable natural history, treatment may not be necessary.

TABLE 2-1 The Effect of Clinical Stage on Survival

	Patient A	Patient B
Symptoms	Hemoptysis	Intercostal neuralgia and hepatomegaly
Sex	Male	Male
Age	55 years	55 years
Tobacco use	40 years	40 years
Site of tumor	Right lower lobe	Right lower lobe
Histology	Squamous cell carcinoma	Squamous cell carcinoma
Percent curable	25	0
Median survival time of those dying (months)	18	4

TABLE 2-2 Influence of Various Treatments on Years of Survival

Condition	Number of Patients	Average Number Years of Life Remaining	Resulting Person-Years	Net Years
A. Normal population aged 75	100	9	800	800
B. Untreated illness	100	2	200	200
C. 1. Medical treatment—good result	50	5	250	
2. Medical treatment—unimproved	25	2	50	
3. Medical treatment—improve initially, then require operation	25	3	75	
a. Decline operation	5	3	15	540
b. Accept operation	20			
(1) Die in hospital post-operatively*	5	3	15	
(2) Survive operation and cured by it	15	9	135	
D. Operation when diagnosis is made				
1. Die in hospital postoperatively*	5	0	0	
2. Improve but succumb to disease	40	2	80	520
3. Well after operation	55	8	440	

*Note that death after operation is more frequent (5/20 = 25%) when operation follows failure of medical treatment as in C.3.b.(1) than when operation is undertaken initially (5/100 = 5%) as in D.1.

The **natural history** of an illness, or its untreated course, is an integral part of every clinical decision. Prior knowledge of the natural history of a particular disease allows one to:

- Identify a clear pattern leading to a definite diagnosis
- Determine the type and urgency of treatment
- Monitor effects of treatment (thereby recognizing ineffective methods)
- Recognize deviations indicating incipient complications

Several illnesses lend themselves to the erroneous assumption that **some treatment** yields better overall survival than does **no treatment.** A case in point would be a lung cancer patient with supraclavicular/scalene lymph nodes that have tested positive (clinical stage IIIb or IV, depending on the presence or absence of distant metastases). Such a case is not amenable to cure, and neither palliative radiotherapy nor pulmonary resection significantly prolongs the patient's life. In fact, either form of treatment may adversely affect the quality of his remaining life. At the opposite end of the spectrum is a patient with a small (≤1 cm in diameter) polypoid lesion in the colon not accessible to the colonoscopist, discov-

ered when a barium enema is done. The probability that the lesion is a benign adenomatous polyp is quite high, while the possibility that it is a cancer is so small that treatment by laparotomy and resection is a far greater risk to the patient than no treatment at all.

Although the great majority of patients for whom operations are proposed are genuinely benefited by them, even the experienced surgeon must guard against false optimism. An objective expression of the natural history of an illness is reflected by the **total person-years** of life remaining at a given point in the illness. Usually this is determined either at the onset of symptoms or time of definitive diagnosis.

Assume the onset of an illness at 75 years of age and that without treatment the mean time until death is 2 years after diagnosis. One may then compute 200 person-years of life among 100 individuals so afflicted but not treated. This is to be compared with 800 person-years to be expected in a normal 100-patient population aged 75 years (Table 2-2).

The results of nonoperative medical management must be considered and compared with no therapy of any sort at one extreme, and immediate, uniform surgical intervention at the other.

Proper analysis of the results of nonoperative medical therapy is complicated by the fact that failures of medical therapy are often still amenable to surgical intervention with significant positive results.

Assume the onset of an illness at 75 years of age (as before). Half of all patients treated nonoperatively live for an average of 5 years, which yields 250 person-years (Table 2-2, group C.1). One-fourth of the patients treated medically are no better off than if no treatment was employed and succumb in 2 years, yielding 50 person-years (Table 2-2, group C.2). The other fourth of patients require operation at a mean time of 3 years after diagnosis and at that point will have contributed 75 person-years to the results of initial medical therapy (Table 2-2, group C.3). Of the 20 patients undergoing surgical procedures, 5 die in the hospital (Table 2-2, group C.3.b[1]), but the 15 survivors live to a normal life expectancy, yielding another 135 person-years of life (15 patients × 9 years). The net results of initial nonoperative care with operation delayed until absolutely necessary is 540 person-years.

The 540 years of life obtained is clearly superior to the 200 additional years that result from no treatment. On the other hand, *sequential medical and surgical therapy* apparently is better than withholding all surgical intervention, with a resultant 390 years (250 plus 50, plus 75, plus 15) of life. The last 15 years are derived from a presumed average 3-year survival after declining surgery for these 5 patients (Table 2-2, group C.3.a). For the sake of clarity, we have excluded the few patients (1% to 2%) who might be harmed by medical therapy, even though this is a necessary and proper component for the precise comparison of therapeutic methods. The harmful effects of surgery, performed on the basis of expected gain in years of living by treatment, is manifested by the loss of additional years of survival in the 5 patients dying after operation (Table 2-2, group C.3.b[1]).

To determine the value of early operative treatment one must take into consideration the common alternatives—that is, no therapy, or nonoperative (medical) management—before a proper decision can be reached. Using the same hypothetical population, one might recommend routine operation following diagnosis for every patient. We have indicated a hypothetical operative (hospital) mortality of 25% (5 of 20 patients) when operation is undertaken after 3 years of unsuccessful medical management. Should surgery be undertaken at an earlier phase in the patient's illness (at a younger age), it may be reasonable to hypothesize an operative risk of 5%. Since these patients die immediately, they live fewer years than those who receive no treatment at all. This regimen leads to a net of 520 years of life for this cohort of patients.

In summary, the example chosen shows that treatment is indicated, that there is relatively little difference in choosing between (1) sequential medical/surgical therapy and (2) immediate operative treatment on a uniform basis, and that both alternatives are better than (3) nonoperative medical management alone.

In the comparative analyses often quoted by surgeons, the results of operations are frequently compared with those of purely medical regimens. This fails to consider that most thoughtful internists realize that operative intervention can contribute greatly to the health of patients who have not been helped by medical management. They ultimately will recommend surgery for a significant number of these patients. The forgoing example clearly shows how staged medical/surgical management provides an added overall benefit to initial nonoperative therapy.

Even the individual who has little skill with figures will perceive the value of this type of analysis, which yields a significant change in end results. *The thoughtful student should focus on a selection of patients who might benefit the most from the optimal utilization of all treatment options.* Ideally, this protocol should include:

- Nonoperative care for those patients who could be expected to do well with medical therapy only
- Withholding surgery from those likely to die as a result

With such clairvoyance, the overall results of treatment would be as shown in Table 2-3. By perfect selection of existing medical and operative therapies, this patient population could approach 78% (626/800) of normal life expectancy in person-years. Unfortunately, in many cases the methodology for prospectively identifying patients most likely to manifest positive end results does not yet exist. However, much of the following data on operative risk are intended to increase the surgeon's accuracy in excluding from operation those patients at high risk of being harmed by the procedure. Although insight on the evaluation of operative risk has increased, there has been little progress in the selection of patients likely to do well with nonoperative therapy.

TABLE 2-3   Computation of Person-Years of Survival Given Perfect Patient Selection

Condition	Number of Patients	Average Number Years of Life Remaining	Resulting Person-Years
Medical treatment—good result	50	5	250
Likely to die after operation	5	0	0
Medical treatment—good result	2	5	10
Medical treatment—unimproved	3	2	6
Well after operation	45	8	360
TOTAL			626

Further consideration of end-results assessment is needed. Obviously a patient may be getting progressively well, remain ill, or die. Analyses of survival or probability of death after treatment may be deceptive, particularly for non-neoplastic diseases.

The changing attitude in recent years toward gastric ulceration is a good example. In the early 1950s, distinguishing gastric ulcer from gastric cancer was a major concern for most physicians. As radiologic technology improved the accuracy of such differentiation was enhanced, and attempts to cure clinically recognized gastric cancer surgically met with limited success. Accordingly, operative treatment of gastric ulcers was relegated to a lower priority. However, while life-and-death issues were clarified, little attention was paid to the natural history of this illness, that is, the overall morbidity of chronic gastric ulceration. Today the pendulum has swung back to early operation, because careful studies have generally showed that:

- Only one third of patients with gastric ulcer remained well after nonoperative medical management.
- One third of patients were chronically ill because of their ulcer disease.
- One third of patients ultimately required operation for control of symptoms.

Although such analyses and comparisons frequently clarify obscure indications for treatment and aid the neophyte in making basic comparisons, results are never better than the quality of the available data that become components of the equation. In the absence of a clearly defined illness, well-controlled prospective clinical trials provide the most efficient and valid comparisons of different methods of therapy for a given situation.

WHAT DETERMINES OPERATIVE RISK?

Although each component of the fundamental comparison may greatly influence the ultimate results of therapy, determination of operative risk is the most important factor in the equation when an operation is proposed.

Mortality

The most important component of operative risk is death after treatment—although not necessarily as a direct result of the surgery. When a patient fails to recover after a diligently performed operation, it is always tempting to attribute the death to the patient's failure to respond instead of searching for a thorough clarification of conceivable errors in judgment or management. The surgeon may be fortunate that by the very decisive outcome of a specific operation, awareness is heightened of the mortality and morbidity attending the procedure. Mortality is absolute, but some physicians attempt to escape direct responsibility for it, whether in descriptions of personal experience or in scientific reports. The proper assumption is that all deaths after operation and before hospital discharge are operative deaths—that they would not have occurred had the surgery not been performed.

A patient who dies of a pulmonary embolus on the seventh postoperative day becomes the surgeon's responsibility because the relative im-

TABLE 2-4 Hospital Mortality for a Given Operation: 65 Years of Surgical Progress

Operation	Hospital Deaths (%)	
	1920-1940	1975-1985
Radical mastectomy	1	0.2
Exploration of common bile duct	16	2
Colon resection	28	5
Laparotomy for intestinal obstruction	37	8

TABLE 2-5 Effect of Urgency of Procedure on Operative Risk

Operation	Hospital Deaths (%)	
	Elective	Emergency
Cholecystectomy	1	4
Cholecystectomy and common duct exploration	2	10
Total abdominal hysterectomy	1	4
Vagotomy and pyloroplasty	1	10
Distal gastric resection	3	20
Colon resection and colon anastomosis	5	18
Resection and graft replacement of abdominal aortic aneurysm	4	30
Femoropopliteal vein bypass graft	2	10
Portacaval shunt	10	50

mobilization, leading to the thromboembolus, most likely would not have occurred without the operation. A death caused by a myocardial infarction on the fourth postoperative day should be considered an operative death because of associated abdominal distention, atelectasis, and respiratory compromise, possibly leading to hypoxia and infarction superimposed on an existing coronary artery stenosis.

The ability to perform an honest assessment of operative risk is as important to the well-qualified surgeon as is the ability to suture wounds securely. It is the ultimate product of multiple factors. Data regarding numerous conditions that affect operative risk are presented in Tables 2-4 through 2-10. For perspective, one should compare the progress made in reducing operative mortality for certain standard procedures within this century (Table 2-4), which reflects not only improved operative skill but also relates to improved overall perioperative care, including

the delivery of anesthesia and enhancements in blood bank technology.

The likelihood of dying after an emergency operation is greater than after the same operation performed electively (Table 2-5). Although mortality and morbidity are primarily a function of the seriousness of the disease or complication requiring operation, hurried preparation and other compromises in technique contribute to the increased risk.

Age (although not necessarily age per se) is also a significant determinant of operative risk. Operative mortality is increased significantly for most procedures at the extremes of life (i.e., the newborn infant and the very elderly patient). To some extent, this increased risk is a function of the types of illnesses that compel the surgeon to operate on a newborn child or a nonagenarian.

Increased operative risk at the extremes of life is particularly apparent for extensive procedures and those conducted on an emergency basis, but

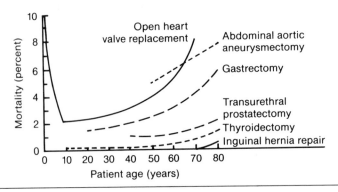

FIGURE 2-1   Mortality in elective operations.

these factors also apply to a lesser degree in elective surgery (see Fig. 2-1). A common error is withholding operation based on *chronologic age* alone in lieu of evaluation of *physiologic age.* Old age per se does not increase operative risk unless there are other associated risk factors, such as a prolonged operative time, or prolonged surgery of the upper abdomen or thorax. If advanced age is to be considered a factor in withholding an operation, it should also be considered an adverse determinant of patient survival without operation.

Another common misunderstanding relates to the *life expectancy of an aged patient.* Table 2-6 provides representative life expectancies for Americans of specific ages. For example, because of abnormal physiologic age, a 55-year-old man with hypercholesterolemia and a previous myocardial infarction is a poorer operative risk for virtually any operation than a well and active 80-year-old man. Furthermore, procedures that incur minimal physiologic dysfunction, in terms of either extent or duration, are nearly as well tolerated by the elderly as by the young. Mastectomy is an example of an operation producing minimal physiologic dysfunction; the operative mortality at 60 years of age and below approximates 1/500 and is 1/300 for patients 60 to 80 years of age.

However, surgeons are undoubtedly cautious, and properly so, in the selection of patients for operation in the older age range. Given a standard operation, the disease for which it is performed becomes a significant determinant of operative risk, probably as much for associated systemic and metabolic aberrations as for technical factors related to the operation itself (Table 2-7).

TABLE 2-6   Average Life Expectancy at a Stated Age

Age (Years)	Remaining Life (Years)
55	22
60	18
65	15
70	11
75	9
80	6
85	4
90	3

In addition, for a given disease, operations of greater magnitude generally bear a greater operative risk (Table 2-8) but can be performed successfully regardless of patient age, with careful perioperative management and lack of technical misadventure. This was demonstrated by O'Donnell et al., who reported an overall 4.7% mortality in 63 octogenarians undergoing resection of unruptured abdominal aortic aneurysms.

Two other important variables contribute significantly to the operative risk attending emergency operations. While the safe or golden interval varies with each disease process, the duration of illness before operation is a significant determinant of survival (Table 2-9). The degree of suppuration or gangrene also exerts a striking effect on survival and, if at all feasible, operation should be recommended before these complications occur. The physician can well imagine the sharply increased operative risk attending emer-

TABLE 2-7   Influence of Disease Requiring Operation on Hospital Mortality for a Given Procedure

Operation	Indication	Hospital Deaths (%)
Partial gastrectomy	Carcinoma	10
	Gastric ulcer	4
	Duodenal ulcer	4
Segmental esophagectomy and primary anastomosis	Carcinoma	20
	Esophagitis	2
	Chemical stricture	4

TABLE 2-8   Influence of Magnitude of Procedure on Hospital Mortality for a Given Operation and a Specific Indication*

Organ	Indication	Operation	Hospital Deaths (%)
Stomach	Carcinoma	Subtotal gastrectomy	8
		Total gastrectomy	15
Biliary tract	Stones	Cholecystectomy	0.6
		Choledochostomy	1.8
Arteries	Atherosclerotic occlusion	Femoropopliteal revascularization	1
		Aortoiliac revascularization	5

*Based on collected series.

TABLE 2-9   Influence of Duration of Illness Requiring Emergency Operation on Hospital Mortality

Duration (hr)	Hospital Deaths (%)		
	Closure of Perforated Duodenal Ulcer	Reduction/ Resection of Intussusception	Appendectomy
0-6	4	1.5	0
7-12			1
13-24	18		1.5
25-48		9	5
48+		26	8

TABLE 2-10 Influence of Degree of Suppuration and/or Gangrene on Hospital Mortality for a Given Operation

Operation	Hospital Deaths (%)
Appendectomy	
Acute inflammation	0
Inflammation and abscess	0.2
Free perforation and peritonitis	4
Cholecystectomy	
Acute inflammation	2
Inflammation and abscess	10
Free perforation and peritonitis	20
Segmental enterectomy	
Nongangrenous	6
Gangrenous without perforation	20
Gangrenous with perforation	40

gency procedures for inflammatory disease of considerable duration (Table 2-10).

Finally, it is logical to assume that the surgeon, the anesthesiologist or anesthetist, the anesthetic technique, and the institution in which the operation is performed all significantly affect operative risk. Although these assumptions may be true, none is easily proved. For example, no statistically significant difference in operative mortality after colon resections for carcinoma could be identified among the several surgeons working in a large midwestern university hospital. However, if the five surgeons performing the fewest colon resections are grouped together for comparison with the three surgeons who performed the greatest number of resections, a significant difference appears favoring the group with the greater amount of experience.

Obviously, the positive relationship between low mortality and frequency of colonic resection for cancer performed by a given surgeon cannot be ascertained. One cannot say that mortality is low because of a larger experience or that the experience is greater because referring physicians are aware of the lower mortality. It is our opinion that the latter factors, experience and referral patterns of surgeons and referring physicians, probably play a significant role.

A lengthy discussion of anesthetics is beyond the scope of this chapter. The experienced surgeon will be concerned about potential deleterious effects in patients with drug sensitivities or allergies and in those with cardiac, liver, or renal disease. Anesthetic drugs may be metabolized or eliminated by the liver or kidney. Alterations or effects of anesthetics on the major serum electrolyte concentrations, particularly potassium, are important. Consultation with the anesthesiology staff is wise when evaluating certain patients suspected to be at risk. For those patients who may become hypotensive (i.e., shock secondary to upper gastrointestinal hemorrhage, third-spacing of fluid in intestinal obstruction), anesthetic management plays a critical role in avoiding hypovolemic shock.

Institutional differences are much more difficult to interpret. In Table 2-11, for example, hospitals A and C have excellent overall mortality figures for three standard procedures, adjusted for operative risk according to a commonly used scale. Hospital D has very poor figures for the two general surgical operations but an excellent one for the gynecologic operation. Hospital B is more difficult to evaluate, with good results after gastric and uterine resections but a poor outcome for cholecystectomy. Patient populations largely influence these results, particularly with reference to the proportion of emergency operations. However, even when one adjusts for these differences according to a preoperative fitness scale, significant differences persist.

Emotional connotations arise when one considers the relative operative risk figures for a given operation performed in a university or a community hospital by an experienced surgeon or by an intern or surgical resident. Few differences exist with respect to the experience of the operating surgeon (surgeon, intern, or resident), which is as it should be because the trainee (intern, resident) is supervised closely, in most university training programs, by an experienced surgeon. In university and community hospitals, there are obvious differences in the patient populations served. However, at a time when operative risk for the treatment of colorectal cancer rarely exceeded 5% on an annual basis in two large midwestern teaching centers, a smaller community hospital reported a mortality of 16% for right colectomy—a difference that is hard to reconcile by differences in patient populations.

An additional factor, which probably has an adverse influence on operative risk, is *preexisting anemia.* Although careful study indicates increased hospitalization, complications, and postoperative mortality for anemic men and in-

TABLE 2-11   Variable Mortality Rates for Three Standard Operations in Six Different Hospitals

	Hospital Deaths (%)		
	Cholecystectomy	Partial Gastrectomy	Hysterectomy
Hospital A	0	1.8	0.3
Hospital B	1.4	1.3	0.3
Hospital C	0.5	1.0	0
Hospital D	4.1	9.8	0.4
Hospital E	6.7	14.3	0
Hospital F	5.5	14.5	0.4

Modified from Moses LE, Mosteller F. Institutional differences in postoperative death rates. Commentary on some of the findings of the National Society. JAMA 203:492, 1968.

creased operative mortality for anemic women, further analysis suggests that it is the severity of the condition requiring the operation that actually affects operative results adversely.

In anemic patients, there are two factors the surgeon should consider:

- The preoperative status of the patient
- The potential for a perioperative hemorrhage

It is hazardous to rely on any routine preoperative hemoglobin (Hgb) level as being safe, since need varies from patient to patient. The patient's overall clinical status, health, and planned operation are important variables in the equation. A hemoglobin level higher than 10 g/dl (and lower than 17 g/dl, because of risk of thrombosis) are desired for all patients undergoing major operations. In the anemic patient, blood volume is a more important consideration than the hemoglobin level. Normal values for both are desired. Several conditions or clinical situations require a more nearly normal hemoglobin level before surgery (higher than 10 g/dl):

- Arteriosclerotic heart disease
- Reduced arterial oxygen saturation
- Age over 50
- Anticipated high blood loss
- Recent myocardial infarction
- Cerebral ischemia
- Reduced exercise tolerance

Patients with chronic anemia, lack of cerebral ischemia, an operation expected to have low blood loss, normal exercise tolerance, and age under 30 may survive an operation with a hemoglobin level below 10 g/dl. A common mistake would be to allow hemoglobin concentrations to drift downward during the course of a long illness and then to use the magic number of 10 g/dl as a transfusion trigger. This would be overtly wrong!

Tissue oxygen delivery is a function of cardiac output, tissue oxygen extraction, and hemoglobin concentration. Since oxygen extraction is often maximal, unnecessarily low hemoglobin concentrations serve only to place an unwelcome burden on a heart that may be less than perfect. Keeping the hemoglobin concentration nearer normal (14 g/dl) than to the magic 10 g/dl is a sign of a physiologically informed physician.

What Is the Risk of Blood Transfusion? The transfusion of blood and blood components is relatively safe with today's blood bank technology and complete screening procedures, but the risk is still not zero. According to Menitove, blood usage in the United States increased steadily through the 1970s and early 1980s, until costs associated with hospital reimbursement and concern regarding transfusion-transmitted diseases, particularly the acquired immunodeficiency syndrome (AIDS), slowed this practice. Adverse reactions to blood and blood component transfusion therapy occur in as many as 10% to 15% of recipients (Table 2-12).

Acute complications (e.g., febrile and allergic reactions) approach a frequency of about 1% per unit of blood transfused. Other acute reactions (e.g., hemolytic, anaphylactic) are much less common. The most serious complication relates to transmission of hepatitis, which occurs with far greater frequency than the much more dreaded complication of AIDS. Eighty percent of transfused hepatitis complications are non-A,

TABLE 2-12 Adverse Effects Associated With Blood and Blood Component Transfusion

	Approximate Frequency*	
	Ratio	**Percentage**
Acute		
Acute hemolytic transfusion reaction	1/25,000	0.004
Febrile, nonhemolytic transfusion reaction	1/200	0.500
Allergic reactions	1/100 to 1/300	0.200 or less
Hypervolemia	Variable	
Noncardiogenic pulmonary edema	1/5000	0.020
Bacterial sepsis	Rare	
Anaphylactic hypotensive reactions	1/150,000	0.0007
Complications of massive transfusions (hemostatic defect, hypothermia, and metabolic abnormalities)	Unknown	
Delayed		
Delayed hemolytic transfusion reaction	1/1500 to 1/9000	0.020 or less
Red blood cell alloimmunization	1/100	1.000
Leukocyte/platelet alloimmunization	1/10	10.000
Hemosiderosis	Unknown	
Graft-v-host disease	Rare	
Posttransfusion purpura	Rare	
Viral hepatitis	1/1500	0.006
Transfusion-associated AIDS	1/36,000 to 1/300,000	0.0007 or less
Transfusion-associated malaria	Rare	

Reprinted with permission from Menitove JE. How safe is blood transfusion? In Smith DM, Dodd RY (eds). Transfusion Transmitted Infections. Chicago, American Society of Clinical Pathology Press, 1991, p 1.
*Frequency is presented as risk per unit transfused.

non-B hepatitis or so-called hepatitis C. Hepatitis B is still reported to occur in about 1% of patients receiving multiple transfusions. A 1991 publication by the American Association of Blood Banks, however, indicates the actual occurrence to be well under 0.1% because of more complete screening techniques.

The use of autologous blood, donated by the patient for his later use, is becoming more common. It is likely that this practice will become even more popular in the future for elective surgery. Autologous blood donation is enhanced by the treatment of the donor (the eventual recipient) with recombinant human erythropoietin. This increases the amount of autologous blood that a patient can donate in preparation for his operation. The use of recombinant human erythropoietin, still in the evaluation stage, is probably too expensive for general use at this time.

Morbidity

Perioperative morbidity must be considered as the second component of operative risk in any therapeutic equation. Morbidity lacks the absoluteness of mortality (0 or 100%) in a given patient and may be ignored or minimized by some surgeons. Psychologic factors, which mitigate against proper categorization of postoperative deaths, are even more significant when dealing with surgical complications. No conscientious surgeon can fail to relate fecal peritonitis arising from a disrupted colonic anastomosis to the operation itself. Less obvious complications are no less important, as the following examples illustrate:

- Phlebitis, leading to pulmonary embolism, following prolonged bed rest in a lumbar laminectomy patient
- Bacteremia arising from a contaminated urinary tract, related to urinary retention and instrumentation, after rectal or hernia operations
- Prolonged ileus requiring nasogastric suction and intravenous fluid and electrolyte therapy, resulting from hypokalemia secondary to the vigorous diuretic therapy of congestive heart failure

CARDIAC RISK FACTORS

Known Risk Factors

Age, previous myocardial infarct, angina, congestive heart failure, hypertension, cardiac dysrhythmia, peripheral vascular disease, cigarette smoking, previous specific cardiac interventions and treatments

Intraoperative Predictors of Cardiac Risk

Surgical factors (site, system, duration, urgency)
Anesthesia (oxygen delivery monitoring)
Cardiac changes (hypertension, hypotension, dysrhythmia)

Postoperative Predictors of Cardiac Risk

Pain and lack of pain control
Fluid shifts, especially hypotension

THE AMERICAN SOCIETY OF ANESTHESIOLOGY (ASA) PHYSICAL STATUS SCALE

Class I	Normal healthy patient
Class II	Patient with mild systemic disease, including smokers
Class III	Patient with severe, but not incapacitating disease
Class IV	Patient with incapacitating disease, constantly threatening to life
Class V	Moribund patient, not expected to live more than 24 hours, with or without surgery
Class E	Emergency; any patient in the above classes who is considered an emergency. The letter E is placed next to the numerical classification because the patient is in a compromised physical state

Modified from James EC, Rhodes BJ, Keller RT, Siegel MB. Evaluation of the preoperative patient. In James EC, Corry RJ, Perry JF Jr (eds). Principles of Basic Surgical Practice. St Louis, CV Mosby, 1987, p 22.

In some instances, the relationship between effect and proximate cause is tenuous. However, one cannot deny that a particular complication would not have occurred had the operation not taken place. How nonfatal complications are related to postoperative death is largely subjective, but they are amenable to reasonably accurate estimation. If the relative weight of an early serious complication with respect to mortality is difficult to assess, the proper evaluation of a late complication is even more difficult to ascertain. In this regard, late anatomic, functional, and psychologic abnormalities owing to treatment, time away from work and other productive endeavors, and length and cost of hospitalization and care are all important considerations.

What Are Cardiopulmonary Risk Factors? Ischemic coronary heart disease is present in many patients of middle and advanced age who require surgery for various illnesses. The direct impact of such illnesses on operative risk is of obvious importance. Conditions of major concern (see the box at left) include congestive heart failure, myocardial ischemia or infarction, hypertension, hypotension, dysrhythmia, and neurovascular problems. Additional risk factors include cigarette smoking and previous specific cardiac interventions and treatments. Cardiac disease severe enough to require digitalis therapy has been shown to significantly increase the morbidity and mortality of operations for carcinomas of the large bowel and lung. Certain changes in the preoperative electrocardiogram are highly indicative of great susceptibility to postoperative myocardial infarction, which suggests that one use specific measures to maintain blood volume intraoperatively and postoperatively and adequate oxygenation and monitoring to avoid this dreaded complication. Intraoperative predictors of cardiac risk include surgical factors such as site, system involved, duration of procedure, urgency, and the method of administering the anesthetic.

The American Society of Anesthesiologists (ASA) classification (see the box at left) is very helpful in the selection of patients with a higher perioperative mortality risk. This well-known risk scale is in general "rougher but broader in scope" than the cardiac risk data of Goldman et al., and all surgeons should be familiar with its implications.

Multifactorial assessment of cardiac risk has become a reliable and objective scheme for predicting such risk. Table 2-13 contains certain cardiac factors weighted for their clinical importance.

TABLE 2-13 Multifactorial Assessment of Perioperative Cardiac Risk

Preoperative Factor	Points	Class/Points	Cardiac Death (%)	Other Comments
S_3 gallop or jugular venous distension	11	Class I 0-5 points	0.2	99% of patients with no or minor cardiac complications
Transmural or subendocardial myocardial infarction within last 6 months	10			0.7% life-threatening complications such as myocardial infarction, pulmonary edema, ventricular tachycardia
Premature ventricular beats > 5/min	7			
Rhythms other than sinus, or presence of premature atrial contractions, on last electrocardiogram	7			
Age > 70 years	5	Class II 6-12 points	2	5% probability of life-threatening but nonfatal cardiac complication
Emergency operation	4			
Intrathoracic, intraperitoneal, or aortic surgery	3			
Evidence of important valvular aortic stenosis		Class III 13-25 points	2	11% probability of life-threatening but nonfatal complications
Poor general medical condition, e.g., electrolyte abnormalities, renal insufficiency, abnormal liver status, or any condition for which the patient is chronically bedridden	3	Class IV ≥26 points	56	22% risk of life-threatening but nonfatal cardiac complication

James et al. suggest these risk indicators:

Evidence for specific pulmonary problems should be identified (Table 2-14). Differential chest examination findings in the normal individual and in patients with abnormal pulmonary conditions are highlighted. Pulmonary function tests help clarify risks suggested by the history and physical examination. For example, a P_{CO_2} greater than 45 mm Hg suggests a likely need for postoperative ventilation. Spirometric readings may suggest the likelihood of postoperative pulmonary complications, that is a maximal voluntary ventilation (MVV) less than 50%, a one-second forced expiratory volume (FEV_1) less than 2 L, an FEV_1 less than 50% of the forced vital capacity (FVC), and an FVC less than 50% of predicted.

These tests, as well as a chest x-ray evaluation and arterial blood gas analysis, should be per-formed on any patient with a significant clinical history of pulmonary symptoms, when perioperative pneumonia risk factors are present, or when a thoracic surgical site is planned. Preoperative risk factors for pneumonia are:

- Low serum albumin (<3.0 g/dl)
- High ASA physical status class
- Smoking history (2x normal risk)
- Chronic pulmonary disease
- Surgical site in the thorax or upper abdomen

If a lung resection is planned, the desired values on pulmonary function tests listed in Table 2-15 should be considered.

James et al. stated that perioperative risk can be minimized by:

TABLE 2-14 Pulmonary Clinical Problems

Problem	Symptoms	Signs	Comment
Hypoxia	Dyspnea and restlessness	Cyanosis, tachypnea	Many causes
Hypocapnia	Dizziness, numbness, paresthesias	Psychomotor impairment, tetany and carpopedal spasm	Usually due to hyperventilation
Hypercapnia	Transient throbbing headache, nausea, palpitations, insomnia	Flushed face, diaphoresis, tachycardia, somnolence	Usually due to hypoventilation
Atelectasis	Fever, dyspnea, chest pain	Normal or decreased breath sounds	Chest x-ray shows streaky densities or collapse of segment, lobe, or lung
Pulmonary infection	Malaise, headache, chills (bacterial, viral), myalgia	Fever, other signs depend on upper or lower respiratory tract etiology	Many causes
Bronchiectasis	Chronic foul-smelling sputum, halitosis	Rales, clubbing	Chest x-ray normal, fibrotic, or cystic
Emphysema (COPD)	Dyspnea, cough, sputum production	Air trapping; decreased breath sounds; increased expiratory phase; occasional rhonchi or rales; percussion hyper-resonance	Chest x-ray normal or hyperinflated bullae; depressed diaphragms
Restrictive lung disease	Dyspnea or exertion	Normal or dry inspiratory crackles	Chest x-ray normal or linear, fibronodular or fibroreticular infiltrates
Asthma	Intermittent dyspnea	Wheezing or absent breath sounds	Chest x-ray usually normal; can simulate COPD
Pleural effusion	Asymptomatic or dyspnea	Decreased fremitus and breath sounds; flat percussion; absence of voice transmission; presence of friction rub	Chest x-ray pleural effusion
Carcinoma	Asymptomatic or cough, dyspnea, hemoptysis, weight loss	None or atelectasis, pneumonia, lymphadenopathy, clubbing	Chest x-ray solitary lesion, hilar mass, mediastinal ade-nopathy

Modified from James EC, Rhodes BJ, Keller RT, Siegel MB. Evaluation of the preoperative patient. In James EC, Corry RJ, Perry JF Jr (eds). Principles of Basic Surgical Practice. St Louis, CV Mosby, 1987, p 23.

TABLE 2-15   Use of Preoperative Forced Expiratory Volume, Maximal Voluntary Ventilation, and Postoperative (Predicted) Forced Expiratory Volume to Determine Extent of Lung Resection

| | Adequate for Designated Resection | | |
| | Preoperative | | Postoperative |
	FEV_1*	MVV†	Predicted FEV_1*
Lobectomy	>1500 ml	>35%	≥1000 ml
Pneumonectomy	>2000 ml	>55%	≥1000 ml

Adapted from Ellison LT. Preoperative evaluation. In Shields TW (ed). General Thoracic Surgery, 2nd ed. Philadelphia, Lea & Febiger, 1983, pp 233-239.
*Forced expiratory volume of 1 second.
†Maximal voluntary ventilation.

- Cessation of smoking even if as late as 1 week before surgery
- Weight reduction
- Improved nutrition
- Incentive spirometry
- Decreased preoperative stay
- Decreased operative time

Perioperative risk is also reduced, according to James et al., by stabilization of the patient's overall medical status and specific treatment for pulmonary problems such as purulent sputum or bronchospasm.

However, undesired consequences of surgery of many diseases should not diminish the physician's appreciation of the effectiveness of operative treatment. Indeed, the contributions of the surgical sciences to patient survival have allowed quantum leaps in the treatment of many illnesses. Reduction of operative risk has been a major factor in this improvement and is as much a result of better selection and preparation of patients for operation as it is of improved technique. Increased operability reflects similar advances with respect to patient selection and operative technique and has similarly contributed to improved survival and quality of life.

HOW CAN ONE ASSESS OPERATIVE RISK MORE OBJECTIVELY?

This is a good question. With the proper interpretation of any single determinant of operative risk, the physician would still be only slightly more helpful to his or her patients than were the leading exponents of shrewd clinical judgment several generations ago. The multiple factors determining operative risk require individual assessment and summation to approach a valid overall risk estimate. Efforts to quantitate such factors, in conjunction with accurate assessment of clinical stage, should provide much-needed objectivity for determining the effects of (1) no treatment versus (2) nonoperative medical treatment versus (3) operative treatment and (4) the role of sequential medical/surgical treatment. Fig. 2-2 presents a cumulative illness rating scale that may be helpful in quantifying degrees of illness. Even such a simple scale as this is a vast improvement over the entirely subjective approach most clinicians have used.

DelGuerico and Cohn described physiologic assessment of cardiovascular reserve as a useful estimate of operative risk by relating the inability to increase cardiac output when challenged by operative or postoperative complications to a much-increased likelihood of death. Not only did that assessment scheme identify patients at high or low risk, it also allowed some patients to move from an unacceptable risk category to an acceptable one by the therapeutic alteration of some determinants of cardiac function (e.g., K^+ dosage, digitalis dosage, correction of anemia).

HOW CAN ONE ASSESS NUTRITIONAL STATUS AND RISK FOR POSTOPERATIVE COMPLICATIONS?

Malnourishment exists to some degree in patients suffering from a number of diseases and acquired conditions, such as cancer, trauma, burns, liver, renal and pulmonary failure, and a

CUMULATIVE ILLNESS RATING SCALE

Instructions: Indicate for each item the term that best describes the degree of impairment. For illnesses that cause impairment on more than one of the items, more than one item must be rated. When more than one illness occurs for a given item, it is the total impairment from these illnesses that is rated. Each system should be rated as follows:

0 = None
1 = Mild
2 = Moderate
3 = Severe
4 = Extremely severe

Cardiovascular-Respiratory System
  1. Cardiac (heart only)
  2. Vascular (blood, blood vessels and cells, marrow, spleen, lymphatics)
  3. Respiratory (lungs, bronchi, trachea below the larynx)
  4. EENT (eye, ear, nose, throat, larynx)
Gastrointestinal System
  5. Upper GI (esophagus, stomach, duodenum, biliary and pancreatic trees)
  6. Lower GI (intestines, hernias)
  7. Hepatic (liver only)
Genitourinary System
  8. Renal (kidneys only)
  9. Other GU (ureters, bladder, urethra, prostate, genitals)
Musculoskeletal-Integumentary System
  10. MSI (muscles, bone, skin)
Neuropsychiatric System
  11. Neurologic (brain, spinal cord, nerves)
  12. Psychiatric (mental)
General System
  13. Endocrine-metabolic (includes diffuse infections, poisonings)

For example: A CVA may impair neurologic, vascular, and MSI. A tumor with metastasis requires a rating on the item describing the primary site of the cancer and a rating on vascular describing the extent of the lymph node involvement.

FIGURE 2-2 Cumulative illness rating scale for assessing degree of illness. (From Linn BS, Linn MW, Gure L. Physical resistance and longevity. Gerontol Clin 11:362, 1969.)

whole spectrum of gastrointestinal disorders (e.g., fistulas, pancreatitis, Crohn's disease, ulcerative colitis). In many of these patients parenteral or enteral nutrition given over an adequate time period is both efficacious and desirable before any form of aggressive operative treatment is carried out (Table 2-16). Enteral nutrition is the method of choice, whenever possible. The physician must exercise good clinical judgment in identifying those patients most likely to experience postoperative complications and who would benefit from perioperative nutritional support.

Questions that should be asked about any patient undergoing a major operation include:

- Has there been deficient nutrition in the past on a chronic basis?
- Is there a debilitating/catabolic disease or condition present?
- What is the patient's current physical status regarding weight loss, muscle wasting, functional edema, skin rash, or neuropathy?

Good clinical skills in performing a thorough history and physical examination are critical in identifying patients suspected of having a deficient nutritional status.

Loss of 10% of body weight or greater, especially if acute, and ***anthropometric indices*** (triceps skinfold thickness, somatic protein status) are useful (but not always reliable) indicators of deficient nutritional status. Some reports have suggested that ***total lymphocyte counts*** of less than $3000/mm^3$ indicate a deficient or compromised immune status, and counts of less than $1500/mm^3$ contribute to postoperative complications and mortality. Other reports have suggested that preoperative ***serum albumin levels*** of less than 3.5 g/dl increase perioperative complications and mortality fourfold. ***Serum transferrin levels*** below 170 mg/dl have been associated with increased risk of sepsis and death in some patients.

The question of accountability has been raised in several recent studies regarding the use or possible misuse of plasma proteins as indicators of malnutrition. Serum proteins, total lymphocyte counts, and skin anergy may definitely point to immune deficiency and malnutrition in some patients. Since these factors are possibly adversely affected by sepsis and other diseases or conditions, such information must be carefully evaluated in assessing a patient's clinical nutrition status.

TABLE 2-16 Results of Parenteral or Enteral Nutrition in Surgical Patients

Indications	Types	Results/Comments
Preoperative	PN	7-10 days effective in reducing postoperative complications and mortality, particularly in malnourished patients undergoing major operations.
Postoperative	PN or EN	Effective in shorter hospital stay and greater wound healing in malnourished patients. PN and EN equally effective.
Cancer	PN	Start 7-10 days preoperatively; effective in reducing major complications, infections, and mortality.
Trauma	PN or EN	EN versus oral—less sepsis and greater nutritional parameters. PN versus EN—equally effective. BCAA*-enriched versus conventional PN: BCAA influences nutrition parameters, but not postoperative morbidity and mortality. Fat plus glucose better for calories than glucose alone.
Burns	PN or EN	PN supplementation of EN, no better than EN alone. High protein intake of benefit in children—greater protein: greater immunoresistance, nutrition parameters, and mortality.
Pancreatitis	PN	Probably not effective (retrospective reports) in reducing complications, may be effective as supportive treatment.
Inflammatory bowel disease	PN or EN	PN effective in inducing remission and avoiding surgery in Crohn's disease. Preoperative PN for 5 days or more reduces postoperative complications. EN effective in Crohn's disease, not evaluated in ulcerative colitis.
Gastrointestinal fistulas	PN or EN	Retrospective reports show greater spontaneous closure and reduced mortality.

Modified from Meguid MM, Campos AC, Hammond WG. Nutritional support in surgical practice: Part II. Am J Surg 159:439, 1990.
PN = parenteral nutrition; EN = enteral nutrition.
*Branched-chain amino acids.

WHAT IS THE ROLE OF PREOPERATIVE LABORATORY TESTING?

Several seemingly legitimate reports are now available that confirm that there can be a sharp reduction in routine laboratory and other tests without adversely affecting patient survival. It appears that virtually billions of dollars are wasted annually on unnecessary testing—testing that bears no relevance to eventual patient outcome after surgery. The most critical predictor for selecting patients requiring laboratory testing, including electrocardiography and chest x-ray evaluation, is a complete history and physical examination. Only those tests that are required for diagnostic purposes or to clarify associated operative risks for given operations should be obtained.

One study recommended, based on calculated costs that would accrue to uncover an asymptomatic, unsuspected medical problem, that only hematocrit, urinalysis, and pregnancy tests (when applicable) be performed routinely.

Narr et al. analyzed the preoperative screening laboratory tests in asymptomatic healthy patients at their institution and found abnormal test results in 160 of 3782 patients. These abnormal test results did not delay the surgical procedures and were not associated with any adverse anesthetic or surgical outcome. Their institution no longer requires routine preoperative laboratory testing for asymptomatic, healthy patients. Obviously, any laboratory test (ECG, BUN, serum creatinine, SGOT, blood glucose, platelet count, pulmonary function test, and so on) that is indicated by the preoperative evaluation, age of patient, or type of operation should be obtained.

The options available at each point of the decision-making process, from diagnosis to deciding treatment options to carrying out these treatment options in an appropriate fashion, are all amenable to computer analysis and further study. A data base containing the results of past therapeutic encounters, both good and bad, helps to define for new patients the most appropriate treatment modality. Such a step-by-step analysis allows evaluation of the elements of clinical judgment implicit in the fundamental comparison of those patients likely to be helped and those who are likely to be harmed by a proposed operation.

The clinician, particularly the surgeon, has an inescapable obligation to improve all of the components of his or her clinical judgment. Each must strive for accuracy of observation and precise and specific medical recording, whether in the patient's chart or in a formal journal report. Most importantly, the surgeon must carefully and thoughtfully interpret existing data with respect to the individual patient.

PITFALLS AND COMMON MYTHS

- Underestimating cumulative effects of age and *occult* multisystem organ impairment.
- Overestimating the value of a selected treatment modality.
- Inadequate assessment of operative risk.
- Underestimating the value of a thorough history and physical examination in clinical decision-making.
- Equating physiologic age with chronologic age in older patients being considered for operation.

- Misuse or lack of use of clinical parameters and plasma proteins as indicators of malnutrition.
- Decision-making that is skewed or slanted because of inaccurate interpretation of clinical data.
- Inadequate recognition and acceptance of one's postoperative complications.
- Too much routine preoperative laboratory testing in a normal, healthy patient.
- "The operative risk for a patient operated on by my chief resident is the same as the world's best reported outcomes."

BIBLIOGRAPHY

Blery C, Charpak Y, Szatan M, et al. Evaluation of a protocol for selective ordering of preoperative tests. Lancet 1:139, 1986.

Borzotta A, Imbembo A. Nutrition. In Lawrence PF (ed). Essentials of General Surgery. Baltimore, Williams & Wilkins, 1988, p 69.

DelGuerico LR, Cohn JD. Monitoring operative risk in the elderly. JAMA 243:1350, 1980.

Dodd RY. Will blood products be free of infectious agents? In Transfusion Medicine in the 1990's. Arlington, Va., American Association of Blood Banks, 1990.

Ellison LT. Preoperative evaluation. In Shields TW (ed). General Thoracic Surgery, 2nd ed. Philadelphia, Lea & Febiger, 1983, pp 233-239.

Feinstein AR. Clinical judgment. Baltimore, Williams & Wilkins, 1967.

Gagner M, Chiasson A. Preoperative chest x-ray films in elective surgery: A valid screening tool. Can J Surg 33:4, 1990.

Goldman L, Caldera DL, Southwick FS, et al. Cardiac risk factors and complications in non-cardiac surgery. Medicine 57:4, 1987.

Greenburg AG, Saik RP, Farris JM, Peskin GW. Operative mortality in general surgery. Am J Surg 144:22, 1982.

Hjortrup A, Sorensen C, Dyremose E. Influence of diabetes mellitus on operative risk. Br J Surg 72: 783, 1985.

James EC, Iwen GW, Demeester TR. Malignant and benign pulmonary neoplasms. In James EC, Corry RJ, Perry JF (eds). Basic Surgical Practice. St Louis, CV Mosby, 1987, p 188.

James EC, Rhodes BJ, Keller RT, Siegel MB. Evaluation of the preoperative patient. In James EC, Corry RJ, Perry JF (eds). Principles of Basic Surgical Practice. St Louis, CV Mosby, 1987, p 23.

Kaplan EB, Sheiner LB, Boeckmann AJ, et al. The usefulness of preoperative laboratory screening. JAMA 253:24, 1985.

Linn BS, Linn MW, Wallen N. Evaluation of results of the surgical procedures in the elderly. Ann Surg 195:90, 1982.

Macpherson DS, Snow R, Lofgren RP. Preoperative screening: Value of previous tests. Ann Intern Med 113:12, 1990.

Meguid MM, Campos AC, Hammond WG. Nutritional support in surgical practice: Parts I and II. Am J Surg 159:345, 427, 1990.

Moore EE, Eiseman B, van Way CW III. Critical Decisions in Trauma. St Louis, CV Mosby, 1984.

Moses LE, Mosteller F. Institutional differences in post-operative death rates. Commentary on some of the findings of the National Halothane Society. JAMA 203:492, 1968.

Moyer CA. The assessment of operative risk. In Rhoads JE, Allen JG, et al. (eds). Surgery: Principles and Practice, 4th ed. Philadelphia, JB Lippincott, 1970, p 232.

Narr BJ, Hansen TR, Warner MA. Preoperative laboratory screening in healthy Mayo Clinic patients: Cost-effective elimination of tests and unchanged outcomes. Mayo Clinic Proc 66:155, 1991.

O'Connor ME, Drasner K. Preoperative laboratory testing of children undergoing elective surgery. Anesth Analg 70:176, 1990.

O'Donnell TF, Darling RC, Linton RR. Is 80 years too old for aneurysmectomy? Arch Surg 111:1250, 1976.

Polk HC Jr. Principles of preoperative preparation of the surgical patient. In Sabiston DC Jr (ed). Textbook of Surgery, 14th ed. Philadelphia, WB Saunders, 1991, p 77.

Rucker L, Frye EB, Staten MA. Usefulness of screening chest roentgenograms in preoperative patients. JAMA 250:23, 1983.

Spratt JS Jr. The measurement of the value of the clinical process to individuals by age and income. J Trauma 11:966, 1971.

CHAPTER REVIEW
Questions

1. List four of the five factors most often responsible for errors in interpretation and application of reports in the literature.
2. What are the true components of operative risk?
3. List seven factors known to influence operative mortality.
4. What is the life expectancy for a 70-year-old?
   a. 2 years
   b. 7 years
   c. 11 years
   d. 15 years
5. The leading cause of postoperative death in the elderly after noncardiac operations is:
   a. Diabetes
   b. Coronary artery disease
   c. Perioperative MI
   d. Congestive heart failure
6. Rank the following events/observations in order of *decreasing* significance in estimation of cardiac risk:
   a. Aortic valvular stenosis
   b. Transmural myocardial infarction 4 months ago
   c. Age >70 years
   d. 8 premature ventricular contractions per minute
7. What is the current risk of transmitting hepatitis B in a patient receiving multiple blood transfusions?
   a. 10%
   b. 2% to 4%
   c. >25%
   d. <0.1%
8. Known preoperative risk factors for pneumonia include:
   a. Surgical site in upper abdomen
   b. High ASA physical status class
   c. Serum albumin <3.0 g/dl
   d. All of the above
9. Pulmonary function test results (PFTs) that predict adequate pulmonary reserve for a pneumonectomy include:
   a. Preoperative FEV_1 of 2000 ml
   b. Maximal voluntary ventilation (MVV) >55%
   c. Predicted postoperative FEV_1 of 1000 ml
   d. All of the above
10. Clinical features suggesting deficient nutritional status in a patient with Crohn's disease include:
    a. Total lymphocyte count <3000/mm^3
    b. Serum transferrin level <170 mg/dl
    c. >10% acute body weight loss
    d. All of the above
11. An otherwise healthy 35-year-old woman scheduled for an elective laparoscopic cholecystectomy should have which of the following preoperative laboratory tests?
    a. Hemoglobin, urinalysis, pregnancy test
    b. Chest x-ray evaluation
    c. Electrocardiogram
    d. None of the above
12. A 22-year-old healthy woman is admitted with an incarcerated femoral hernia. Her ASA physical status class for surgery is:
    a. Class IE
    b. Class III
    c. Class IIE
    d. Class I

13. Common pulmonary clinical features in patients with emphysema (COPD) include all but:
    a. Foul-smelling sputum
    b. Dyspnea, cough, sputum production
    c. Percussion hyperresonance
    d. Increased expiratory phase
14. To be effective in reducing postoperative complications in malnourished patients undergoing major surgery, preoperative parenteral nutrition (PN) should be given for:
    a. 1 to 3 days
    b. 7 to 10 days
    c. 3 to 4 weeks
    d. 12 to 24 hours

Answers

1. a. Population of patients similar to yours
   b. Accurate clinical staging
   c. Similar medical and surgical resources
   d. Objective long-term follow-up
   e. "Too good to be true!"
2. a. Hospital mortality
   b. Early and late morbidity
3. Seven of the following:
   a. Urgency of operation
   b. Age of patient
   c. Degree of suppuration
   d. Nature of illness
   e. Duration of illness
   f. Patient characteristics
   g. Choice of anesthesia
   h. Quality of hospital
   i. Competence of surgeon
4. c. 11 years
5. c. Perioperative MI
6. b. Transmural myocardial infarct 4 months ago
   d. 8 premature ventricular contractions/minute
   c. Age >70 years
   a. Aortic valvular stenosis
7. d. <0.1%
8. d. All of the above
9. d. All of the above
10. d. All of the above
11. d. None of the above
12. c. Class IIE
13. a. Foul-smelling sputum
14. b. 7 to 10 days

3 Planning and Managing Anesthesia

DAVID G. BJORAKER
JEROME H. MODELL

KEY FEATURES

After reading this chapter you will understand:
- Preoperative preparation of the patient and risk reduction.
- Intraoperative management and the physiologic parameters to be monitored.
- The criteria used in monitoring and evaluating abnormalities.
- What constitutes adequate anesthesia and how it is achieved.
- Evaluation of anesthetic methods and agents.
- The requirements to ensure a smooth recovery.

The field of anesthesiology is relatively young, having existed in the United States as a separate discipline for less than 60 years. It began with an almost exclusive concern with rendering patients insensitive to pain during operative procedures. It now also encompasses preoperative preparation, intraoperative physiologic life support, immediate and long-term postoperative care, respiratory therapy, care of the critically ill patient, and the diagnosis and treatment of pain. Subspecialties in ambulatory, pediatric, obstetric, neurosurgical, and cardiothoracic anesthesia and in pain management and critical care medicine have emerged.

PREOPERATIVE PREPARATION
Preanesthetic Evaluation

Obtaining a comprehensive history and performing a physical examination are essential to proper anesthetic care. Although this process commonly occurs immediately before the administration of an anesthetic for emergency surgery, for elective procedures evaluation before the day of surgery in an outpatient clinic setting or in the patient's hospital room allows additional planning, discussion with the surgical team, preoperative testing, and medical consultations to occur without delaying the proposed time of surgery.

In addition to taking the patient's medical history, the anesthesiologist should ask whether the patient or members of his or her family have received anesthesia previously and, if so, whether any untoward events occurred. Of particular concern are delay in awakening, inadequate ventilation postoperatively, muscular weakness, hyperpyrexia, jaundice, hypersensitivity or anaphylactic reactions, and neurologic deficit. The histories of family members may be as important as the history of the patient because conditions such as malignant hyperpyrexia and pseudocholinesterase (required for the rapid metabolism of the succinylcholine, a neuromuscular blocking agent) deficiency are hereditary.

The anesthesiologist should attempt to document all medications taken by the patient, since many medications interact with drugs used during the anesthetic period and may alter the patient's response. Of particular concern are many of the compounds used to treat depression (e.g., monamine oxidase inhibitors and tricyclic antidepressants) and to control cardiovascular response (e.g., beta-adrenergic blocking agents and calcium channel blockers).

Items of special importance in the physical examination include limitation of range of motion, particularly of the neck and jaw, and other features that may complicate airway maintenance and endotracheal intubation. Congenital or acquired abnormalities of the oropharynx, larynx, chest, and cervical spine may dictate using awake endotracheal intubation to ensure a patent airway throughout the operative procedure. Preexisting cardiopulmonary disease must be diagnosed and optimally is treated before using elective anesthesia since the nature of the disease and the physiologic abnormalities it presents frequently influence the anesthetic management of the patient.

The appropriate anesthetic options should be presented, and the patient should provide informed consent. The preoperative discussion also allows the anesthesiologist to allay the patient's fears of the unknown. Patients often express a desire concerning their level of awareness before surgery; some prefer to be fully alert before the induction of general anesthesia, whereas others prefer to be totally unaware the day of surgery. Their choices often may be accommodated by the choice of premedication when it does not superimpose additional risk. An explanation of what the patient will experience during procedures, both while he or she is under local or regional anesthesia and before general anesthesia (e.g., placement of catheters), can greatly reassure the patient. The onset of postoperative pain and what will be done to lessen or control it should also be discussed.

What Laboratory Tests Are Required for Anesthesia?

Although the American Society of Anesthesiologists (ASA) has gone on record that no *routine* laboratory or diagnostic screening test is necessary before induction of anesthesia, the same guidelines recognize that preanesthetic laboratory and diagnostic testing is often essential. Preanesthetic laboratory testing is most efficacious when ordered for appropriate clinical indications based on the patient's preexisting or suspected disease conditions or on specific risk factors such as age or extent of the surgical procedure. For example, the patient who has chronic pulmonary disease in whom postoperative mechanical ventilation might be necessary should have arterial blood analyzed for pH, oxygen tension (Po_2), and partial pressure of carbon dioxide (Pco_2) preoperatively.

Anesthesiology departments and health care institutional committees should develop local guidelines for routine preanesthesia testing in selected patient populations for which the contribution of the tests improves patient outcome. Often the minimal requirement of obtaining a hematocrit or hemoglobin value is required for all patients, with age-related indications for an electrocardiogram (ECG) (e.g., >40 years) and a chest roentgenogram (>60 years) added as necessary. Within these guidelines, the duration of time (e.g., 30 days) that each screening test will be considered current, that is, when a repeat assessment is not required, must also be considered.

ASA Physical Status Classification

Once the history, physical examination, and laboratory results have been reviewed, the anesthesiologist classifies the patient according to the overall severity of systemic disease, including that caused by the current surgical illness. These classes comprise the ASA physical status classification:

- ASA Class I: A normal, *healthy* patient
- ASA Class II: A patient with *mild systemic disease* resulting in no functional limitations
- ASA Class III: A patient with *severe systemic disease* that limits activity but is *not incapacitating*
- ASA Class IV: A patient with *severe systemic disease* that is *incapacitating* and a constant threat to life
- ASA Class V: A *moribund* patient not expected to survive over 24 hours with or without surgery

Recently ASA Class VI has been added for patients who have been declared brain dead and who will undergo surgery for organ donation. An *E* is appended to the classification number if emergency surgery is required.

This physical status classification should not be interpreted as synonymous with risk. Although the higher the number of classification, the more likely an adverse result will occur, there is no direct correlation with risk on a patient-to-patient basis. The often quoted risk ratio of a death directly attributable to the anesthetic of 1 in 10,000 healthy patients may be improving as a result of new monitoring techniques.

Preoperative Medication

The generally recognized goals of using preoperative medications (Table 3-1) are to allay anxiety, to provide analgesia when preoperative pain is present, and in selected patients to provide amnesia. Although marked sedation may be desirable in occasional patients (e.g., children with tetralogy of Fallot, adults with labile hypertension), some prefer no sedation, some cannot tolerate it medically (e.g., patients with respiratory insufficiency or intracranial pathology), or some may shorten their stay in ambulatory care units if they are not premedicated.

The use of intramuscular (IM) barbiturates (e.g., pentobarbital and secobarbital) has given way to use of oral benzodiazepines (e.g., diazepam and lorazepam) because of their potent anxiolytic and antegrade amnesic properties in the absence of significant cardiovascular and respiratory depression. Because of the shorter duration of parenteral midazolam, it has become widely used, even though the effects of a specific dose may vary from patient to patient. Although amnesia may be desirable during and before a procedure, residual obvious amnesia may alarm relatives, whereas more subtle residual amnesia may cause patients' inability to recall discussions of surgical findings and postoperative verbal instructions.

Because of the pain of IM injection of many parenteral preparations, oral administration is often preferred. Although the patient can have nothing by mouth (NPO), taking sips of water (<30 ml) with a tablet 60 to 90 minutes before induction has not been shown to increase the risk of aspiration. For both by mouth (PO) and IM routes, sufficient time, 60 to 90 minutes, must

TABLE 3-1   Common Anesthetic Premedications

Therapeutic Contribution	Specific Drugs	Typical Adult Dose* (mg)	Notes
Anxiety control	Diazepam	5-10 PO	Painful IM; thrombophlebitis IV
	Midazolam	0.5-1 IV increments 2.5-5 IM	Pediatrics: also PO and intranasal routes
	Lorazepam	2-4 PO	Postoperative disorientation and delirium with pain
	Hydroxyzine	75-150 PO	Antiemetic; painful IM
	Pentobarbital	50-150 PO	Delirium with pain
	Secobarbital	50-150 PO	Delirium with pain
Analgesia	Meperidine	50-100 IM	Use if preoperative pain present
	Morphine	5-12 IM	Use if preoperative pain present
Amnesia	Midazolam	0.5-1 IV increments	Antegrade amnesia
	Lorazepam	2-4 PO	Disorientation frequent
Antisialagogue	Glycopyrrolate	0.2-0.3 IV, IM	Reserve for drying before airway procedures
Reduction of gastric acidity	Cimetidine	300 PO at bedtime and in the morning	Side effects possible
	Ranitidine	150 PO at bedtime and in the morning	Side effects unlikely
	Famotidine	40 PO at bedtime and in the morning	Single bedtime dose inadequate for morning procedures
	Sodium citrate	30 ml PO	Used if insufficient time for H_2-blocker effect
Reduction of gastric volume	Metoclopramide	10-20 PO, IV	Also antiemetic
Antibiotics	(Many)		Subacute bacterial endocarditis and surgical wound infection prophylaxis

*Combinations of anxiolytics, analgesics, and amnesics require dosage reduction.

be allowed to achieve a good premedication effect.

The use of anticholinergics (e.g., atropine and glycopyrrolate) preoperatively was common but now usually is reserved for their antisialagogue effects before oropharyngeal or airway surgical procedures and before using endoscopic or special management approaches to difficult airways. Although the preinduction vagolytic effects of anticholinergics are desirable in children, IV or IM administration at the time of induction is preferred.

In patients who are not NPO or who may have gastroesophageal reflux, the risk of regurgitation and aspiration of gastric contents is reduced by decreasing gastric volume to less than 25 ml and increasing gastric pH to greater than 2.5. For scheduled procedures, H_2-blockers are able both to reduce gastric volume and to increase gastric pH. If preoperative time is limited to a few hours, parenteral H_2-blockers may be effective. For immediate surgery, oral nonparticulate antacids will successfully increase gastric pH and slightly increase gastric volume but do nothing about food particles. Since aspiration of particulate antacids containing magnesium and aluminum hydroxides can cause serious pneumonitis, clear antacids such as 0.3 M of sodium citrate (Bicitra or Alka-Seltzer) should be used. Metoclopramide increases gastric motility and relaxes the gastroduodenal sphincter, thereby decreasing gastric volume. Its effect begins in minutes after IV administration and within 30 to 60 minutes when taken orally. Although the routine use of these agents in healthy patients is controversial, serious side effects from short-term use are negligible.

The patient's necessary chronic medications (e.g., antihypertensives, antianginals, bronchodilators, and other cardiovascular medications) generally should be administered preoperatively. Although anesthesiologists frequently order antibiotics for subacute bacterial endocarditis (SBE) prophylaxis, surgeons should choose the appropriate antibiotic prophylaxis for the surgical procedure itself. Steroid coverage must be also provided for the patient possibly unable to respond to stress with appropriate adrenal secretion. An adult dose of 100 mg hydrocortisone IV administered during surgery and 100 mg IV or IM administered postoperatively the day of surgery is typical, with preoperative dosages and the postoperative taper depending on the degree of suppression and nature of the patient's condition.

Why and How Long Should Patients Fast Before Surgery?

The risk of regurgitation and aspiration of gastric contents remains a real threat in the operating room. The usual order for fasting, "NPO after midnight," does achieve the 6 to 8 hours required to empty the stomach in most patients. However, there may be an unpredictable delay in gastric emptying in patients who are obese, pregnant, diabetic, or extremely anxious or who have gastric outlet obstruction, have preoperative pain, are taking narcotics, or have a documented hiatal hernia. Some foods may require 12 hours to leave the stomach, whereas water and crystalloids may require less than an hour. However, a small amount of a caffeine-containing beverage may add significantly more volume and acidity by promoting gastric secretion.

It cannot be assumed the patient for emergency surgery is NPO. If the procedure is urgent (i.e., versus emergent), before administering the anesthetic, 6 to 8 hours should be allowed to elapse after the injury or last food and fluid intake, whichever is more recent, and an H_2-blocker and metoclopramide should be administered. Despite these measures, residual gastric contents may be present, particularly in the presence of pain, fear, or narcotics; thus these patients should still be treated as though they have a "full stomach." If the procedure is truly emergent, metoclopramide IV and a clear oral antacid should be administered. If the procedure is either urgent or emergent, the use of local and regional anesthesia is advantageous because the protective reflexes of the airway will be left intact. If general anesthesia is necessary, performing an awake intubation or rapid-sequence induction should be considered.

Whereas a prolonged NPO period is only bothersome for adults, significant dehydration can result in children. The following regimen permits intake of clear fluids (water, apple juice, clear Jell-O, non-caffeine-containing clear liquids) nearer to surgery:

- Newborn to 6 months: No milk or solids within 4 hours and clear liquids until 2 hours preoperatively
- 6 months to 36 months: No milk or solids within 6 hours and clear liquids until 3 hours preoperatively
- More than 36 months: No solids within 8 hours and clear liquids until 3 hours before surgery

Proper adherence to scheduled surgical times is required if clear liquids will be permitted near the time of surgery. Many centers have not liberalized their regimens to permit adults to ingest clear liquids within 3 hours of surgery because of frequent confusion as to what constitutes a "clear liquid" and the false implication that NPO status is not important.

INTRAOPERATIVE PHYSIOLOGIC SUPPORT
Basic Intraoperative Monitoring

The ASA standards for basic intraoperative monitoring are abstracted below:

- *Oxygenation*
  Inspired gas: oxygen concentration within the breathing system
  Blood oxygenation: pulse oximetry
- *Ventilation*
  Ventilatory adequacy during general anesthesia
    Qualitative: chest excursions, breathing bag observation, auscultation
    Quantitative: carbon dioxide content, expired gas volume
  Endotracheal tube positioning verification: Clinical assessment and end-tidal carbon dioxide
  Continuous ventilator disconnect detection
  Ventilatory adequacy during regional anesthesia and monitored anesthesia care
- *Circulation*
  ECG continuously displayed
  Blood pressure and heart rate at least every 5 minutes
  Continual pulse palpation, heart sound auscultation, intra-arterial pressure monitoring, ultrasound pulse monitoring, *or* pulse plethysmography
- *Body temperature* monitoring capability

In terms of equipment, the efficacy of quantitative carbon dioxide measurement of expiratory gases to document gas exchange and of continuous pulse oximetry to detect hypoxemia rapidly and quantitatively is widely accepted. Established monitoring techniques are also being improved (e.g., continuous ST-T wave analysis of the ECG and trend displays of the parameters included as basic intraoperative monitoring).

Additional monitoring depends on the patient's preexisting disease and on the nature of the surgical procedure. If precise monitoring of muscular relaxants is desired, a device to stimulate a peripheral nerve and to estimate the mus-

cular response to this stimulus should be applied. A Doppler monitor should be placed over the precordium of a patient at risk from air embolus. In such patients use of (1) a multi-orifice central venous catheter with the tip at the superior vena cava–right atrial junction for removing air and (2) a carbon dioxide gas analyzer in the expiratory limb of the anesthesia-breathing circuit to monitor breath-by-breath changes in gas composition also is suggested. An alternative to using the carbon dioxide analyzer is to monitor all exhaled gases with a mass spectrometer. The latter also permits the anesthesiologist to monitor the concentration of all gases within the breathing circuit to ensure that what is being delivered to the patient is appropriate and that equipment is not malfunctioning.

Pulse Oximetry

The pulse oximeter combines the measurement of oxygen saturation by transillumination with photoplethysmography to separate tissue and venous and capillary blood contributions to absorbance from that of arterial blood. Light absorption is measured at 660 nm (at which point reduced hemoglobin exceeds oxyhemoglobin absorption) and at 940 nm (at which point oxyhemoglobin exceeds reduced hemoglobin absorption), with neither source illuminated to assess background light. Brief repeated measurements are made throughout the cardiac cycle so that the peak absorbance, *a*, and the trough absorbance, *b*, of a pulse wave are defined. The absorption that is present at both times is attributable to the absorption of nonarterialized blood and may be cancelled out. Arterial blood saturation is then empirically related to the ratio, *R*, where

$$R = [(a_{660} - b_{660})/b_{660}]/[(a_{940} - b_{940})/b_{940}]$$

Although there are many clinical applications for the continuous measurement of oxygen saturation, it is an insensitive monitor of ventilation. If the inspired oxygen concentration is supplemented, saturations may remain normal during significant hypoventilation and carbon dioxide accumulation. Only late in the course of progressive hypoventilation or airway obstruction will the oxygen saturation decrease.

During anesthesia only 42% of hypoxemic events (oxygen saturation [SaO_2] <73%) in the patient that were detected by pulse oximetry were clinically recognized by personnel blinded to the oximeter data. Intraoperative hypoxemic episodes during intubation, extubation, deliberate one-lung ventilation, and unsuspected endobronchial intubation are easily detected with pulse oximetry. Its use has also been validated in studies of patients predisposed to hypoxemia such as the elderly and obese, patients in the late stages of pregnancy, and in postoperative patients with atelectasis. During transport to the recovery room 19% to 65% of patients have episodes of desaturation below 90%, depending on the duration of time they breathed room air, age, obesity, and the attentiveness of personnel to airway management. Pulse oximetry should also be used during gastrointestinal endoscopies, cardiac catheterizations, many invasive radiologic procedures, and other procedures performed with conscious sedation.

Limitations of Pulse Oximetry Accuracy. Data from commercially available pulse oximeters are limited by physiologic considerations, sources of intrinsic and extrinsic interference, and calibration inaccuracies.

Physiologic Limitations. High oxygen saturation percentages (e.g., 97% to 100%) can be maintained during a substantial deterioration in pulmonary function that would greatly decrease the arterial oxygen tension (PaO_2) (e.g., from 400 to 150). Hypothermia, hypovolemia, or cardiogenic shock may attenuate peripheral perfusion so that the pulse and absorption due to oxyhemoglobin are not detectable in the distal extremity.

Intrinsic Limitations. With the usual dual wavelength devices, only two hemoglobin values can be evaluated: reduced hemoglobin and oxyhemoglobin. Carboxyhemoglobin is interpreted as oxyhemoglobin; so if carbon monoxide is bound to 7% of hemoglobin, a monitor reading of 97% is actually 90% oxygen saturation. Methemoglobinemia, which can occur in patients receiving nitroglycerin or amyl nitrite, will cause readings to converge on 85% for technical reasons. The effect of the injection of dyes such as methylene blue and indocyanine green, which lower readings, is dependent on their concentration in the blood at the detection site and on the absorption spectrum of the dye.

Extrinsic Limitations. Movement interferes with the detection of the pulse and generally will lower the value but is easily appreciated if the monitor displays both the photoplethysmogram and a digital value of saturation. Bright ambient light may increase the background signal enough that the arterial component of absorption becomes too small for processing. The interference from some infrared warming lights, xenon surgical lights, and fluorescent lights may require shielding of the sensor site. Electrocautery does interfere with some early devices be-

cause the current from the photodiode sensor is extremely low and requires preamplification.

Accuracy. The relationship of the R value (defined previously) to saturation is empirically defined using co-oximeter data obtained from desaturating volunteers. Because low saturation observations (e.g., 30% to 70%) are not readily available, most calibrations below 70% are based on few data points or are extrapolated. If low saturations must be measured accurately (e.g., in patients with congenital heart disease), the oxygen saturation in arterial blood should be measured with a co-oximeter.

When Is an Intra-arterial Catheter Indicated Intraoperatively?

The primary intraoperative indications for arterial catheterization are repeated arterial blood sampling and beat-to-beat blood pressure monitoring. With verification of ulnar artery patency by the Allen's test or by Doppler examination, radial artery catheterization with small catheters for short periods of time is performed easily and is safe. With the wide intraoperative use of continuous pulse oximetry and end-tidal carbon dioxide analysis, concerns about ventilation and oxygenation often may be addressed adequately without arterial blood gas measurement, or it may be required less frequently. The invasive measuring system consists of low-compliance tubing connecting the arterial catheter hub to a pressure-sensing transducer, a continuous low-flow heparinized flush system, and an electronic unit that displays a continuous waveform and the digital systolic, diastolic, and mean arterial pressures. Commercial devices that provide beat-to-beat arterial blood pressure noninvasively using radial artery tonometry or a finger plethysmography method are now available.

When Is a Central Venous Catheter Indicated Intraoperatively?

Patients in whom large shifts in fluid volume are anticipated in a brief time or who have sepsis, cardiovascular disease, or respiratory failure and are undergoing major procedures may benefit from insertion of a catheter into the superior vena cava to measure central venous pressure (CVP). CVP is an index of preload to the right ventricle (and the left ventricle in healthy hearts) and of circulating blood volume but requires judgment for correct interpretation, since it is neither specific nor sensitive. A low CVP may indicate either a low blood volume or a normal blood volume if the cardiac output is unusually high.

An elevated CVP may indicate either a high effective blood volume, increased right ventricular afterload (e.g., pulmonary emboli, high pulmonary vascular resistance), right ventricular filling impairment (e.g., pericardial tamponade), tricuspid incompetence, or with concurrent hypotension, probable cardiac dysfunction. Although CVP is a mean pressure measured at end expiration, it increases with controlled ventilation and positive end-expiratory pressure (PEEP).

Cannulation of the central venous circulation can provide the additional benefits of large-bore access for rapid intravenous infusion, a safe site for infusion of vasoactive substances, a sampling site for venous blood, and access to central circulation for placement of other devices (e.g., transvenous pacing catheters or pulmonary artery catheters).

When Is a Pulmonary Artery Catheter Indicated for Intraoperative Use?

For patients in whom CVP monitoring is desirable, but right and left ventricular performance probably will be dissimilar because of pulmonary disease, myocardial ischemia, or other cardiac dysfunction, a pulmonary artery catheter to measure pulmonary artery diastolic pressure (PADP) and pulmonary artery occlusion pressure (PAOP) in addition to CVP may be necessary. If the pulmonary vascular bed, mitral valve, and left ventricular function are normal, PADP, PAOP, mean left atrial pressure, and left ventricular end-diastolic pressure (LVEDP) are approximately equal and reflect left ventricular end-diastolic volume (LVEDV), the optimal measurement of preload for the intact left side of the heart. LVEDP, however, will be elevated in the presence of a normal LVEDV if the ventricle is hypertrophied and noncompliant. PADP and PAOP measured at end expiration require that the alveolar pressure (airway pressure) is less than the pulmonary venous pressure and that the mitral valve functions normally. PADP requires these conditions and normal pulmonary vascular resistance. Usually PADP and PAOP change before CVP, but in the same direction, in patients with hypovolemia and heart failure. Pulmonary artery pressure increases are also often used as a monitor of acute myocardial dysfunction, but they are not specific and are less sensitive than electrocardiography and transesophageal echocardiography.

A pulmonary artery catheter also provides data other than PADP and PAOP. *Cardiac output can be determined by thermal dilution, systemic vascular resistance, and pulmonary vascular resistance, and ventricular function curves can be calculated.* Mixed venous blood may be sampled to determine physiologic intrapulmonary shunting, oxygen consumption, and lactate levels. Continuous mixed venous oxygen content can now be monitored using fiberoptics incorporated into a pulmonary artery catheter to estimate in vivo hemoglobin saturation from reflected light.

Mixed Venous Oxygen Saturation

Mixed venous oxygen saturation ($S\bar{v}o_2$) reflects the *balance between oxygen supply and tissue oxygen consumption.* If the hemoglobin concentration in g/dl (Hb) and arterial oxygen saturation (Sao_2) in percent are measured, mixed venous content ($C\bar{v}o_2$) in capillary oxygen content (Cco_2)/dl and arterial oxygen content (Cao_2) in Cco_2/dl may be estimated by the following:

$$C\bar{v}o_2 = S\bar{v}o_2 \times Hb \times 0.0136$$

and

$$Cao_2 = Sao_2 \times Hb \times 0.0136$$

By substituting into the Fick equation:

$$Cao_2 - C\bar{v}o_2 = \dot{V}o_2/\dot{Q}$$

where $\dot{V}o_2$ is the oxygen consumption in milliliters per minute and $\dot{Q}$ is the cardiac output in liters per minute, mixed venous oxygen saturation in percent may be defined as follows:

$$S\bar{v}o_2 = Sao_2 - [\dot{V}o_2/(Hb \times 0.0136 \times \dot{Q})]$$

According to this equation, a declining $S\bar{v}o_2$ can result from progressive anemia, decreasing cardiac output, arterial oxygen desaturation, or increased oxygen consumption. Even though $S\bar{v}o_2$ is dependent on four parameters, clinicians find it useful because it can be displayed continuously and because the parameter responsible for the change is usually apparent within the context of a specific clinical scenario. Similarly, by measuring $S\bar{v}o_2$, Sao_2, and Hb, either $\dot{V}o_2$ or $\dot{Q}$ can be calculated if the other is known.

How Low May the $S\bar{v}o_2$ Go Without Irreversible Organ Damage? The normal range of $S\bar{v}o_2$ is 68% to 77%. Healthy patients may tolerate transient $S\bar{v}o_2$ measurements below 60%. At less than 50%, oxygen transport to tissue beds is precarious. If $S\bar{v}o_2$ is less than 40%, the limits of compensation are being reached.

Endotracheal Intubation

Equipment Preparation. As a minimum, a suitable laryngoscope and endotracheal tube are required for endotracheal intubation. An oxygen source and a bag-and-mask device for delivering positive pressure ventilation, various sizes of oropharyngeal or nasal airways, a large-bore reliable suction, a syringe for cuff inflation, tape, and benzoin solution to secure the tube are also extremely useful. For the physician who does not intubate frequently, using a laryngoscope with a curved MacIntosh blade (size 3 or 4 for an adult) with a functioning bright light will permit a more panoramic visualization of the distal pharynx and periglottic structures than will use of some straight blades. An ***endotracheal tube*** (7 mm outside diameter [OD] for an adult woman, 8 mm for an adult man) should be fitted with an ***intubation stylet*** that reaches to, but not beyond, its tip and is formed into a hockey-stick shape. A cuffed tube with the integrity of the cuff, pilot balloon, and valve verified is used to seal the adult airway, but a cuff is not used and a small leak is permitted in children less than 8 years of age so that airway edema and injury in the already small-caliber airway may be minimized. If ventilation is adequate before intubation, all the above items, with alternate sizes, extra personnel, a reliable intravenous route, adjunctive drugs, and complete monitoring, should be procured.

Patient Preparation. If the airway is occluded by vomitus or debris, it must be rapidly cleared by suction or gravity drainage. Once cleared, if the patient is hypoxemic or hypoventilating, initial efforts should be made to deliver oxygen and reduce hypercarbia by the method that will do so most rapidly. For the patient with a potentially difficult airway (e.g., the neck is immobilized because of a possible cervical fracture) or for the physician who rarely intubates the airway, endotracheal intubation is rarely the first choice of action. Providing bag-and-mask ventilation with supplemental oxygen until a more skilled intubationist arrives will achieve more for the patient than permitting unsuccessful attempts that can impede remaining ventilatory efforts, cause bleeding or damage to the airway, and cause the patient to struggle and increase catecholamines and oxygen consumption.

Patient Positioning. The major barrier to successful endotracheal intubation is the inability to visualize the vocal cords. The airway may be thought of as having three axes (oral, pharyngeal, and laryngeal) that must be aligned to

visualize the glottic opening and to pass the endotracheal tube into the trachea with confidence (Figs. 3-1 to 3-3). The pharyngeal and laryngeal axes are made parallel by slight neck flexion. For example, the head may be placed on a firm cushion that is approximately 2 to 3 inches thick for an adult (Fig. 3-2) (for infants this step may be omitted because of the large size of an infant's head relative to the thorax). The oral axis is then aligned with the pharyngeal and laryngeal axes by elevating the chin and extending the head

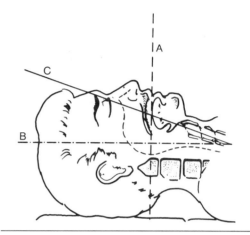

FIGURE 3-1 When the head is in neutral position, the oral (***A***), pharyngeal (***B***), and laryngeal (***C***) axes are not aligned, and visualization of the vocal cords is not possible.

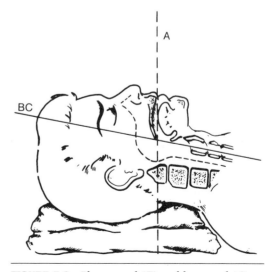

FIGURE 3-2 Pharyngeal (***B***) and laryngeal (***C***) axes can be aligned by placing a cushion under the head to flex the lower cervical spine.

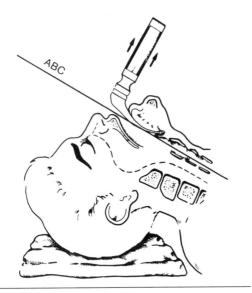

FIGURE 3-3 Extension at the atlanto-occipital joint aligns the oral *(A)*, pharyngeal *(B)*, and laryngeal *(C)* axes. When the tongue and mandible are retracted perpendicular to the airway axes, the larynx can be visualized.

while maintaining the neck flexion (Fig. 3-3). The resulting position of cervical flexion and extension at the atlanto-occipital joint is often called the "sniffing" position. This position is assumed unconsciously just before sneezing to facilitate a large flow of air. Although this position establishes an almost straight line between the mouth opening and the glottic opening, the laryngoscope is used for final alignment of the three axes, maximizing the diameter of the airway and providing proper illumination.

Vocal Cord Visualization. Once the patient is properly positioned, the mouth is opened widely, using a cross-finger technique with the right hand; however, in an anesthetized, fully relaxed patient in the operating room the mouth generally opens involuntarily. *The blade of the laryngoscope is passed gently into the right side of the mouth.* As the blade travels along the tongue, it is swept into a midline position, retracting the tongue to the left. Blade advancement is stopped when its tip is positioned in the vallecula, the junction of the base of the tongue and the anterosuperior surface of the epiglottis. At this time the first significant force is applied with the blade in a direction *perpendicular to the three aligned anatomic axes* described previously. If visualization is not adequate, the larynx may be pushed posteriorly by having an assistant apply pressure to the thyroid cartilage. The blade

must not be used as a lever to pry the base of the tongue out of the line of vision since the teeth will serve as the fulcrum and they will be damaged. The final position (see Fig. 3-3) has been described as "hanging" the patient by the floor of the mouth. The endotracheal tube is then passed through the oropharynx to the right of the blade and is not permitted to enter the path of visualization until its tip reaches the glottic opening. The endotracheal tube is passed until the proximal margin of the cuff is just beyond the vocal cords. As the blade is removed, the length markings on the tube are read at the level of the incisors for future reference and use while securing the tube. The method of positioning described above may not be optimal when other laryngoscope blades are used. With a straight Miller blade, the blade tip is not placed in the vallecula but actually is used to lift the epiglottis.

Other techniques such as blind oral or nasal intubation, fiberoptic intubation, tracheostomy, and retrograde intubation are useful electively in experienced hands but are not beneficial emergently because of the time and skill required. Cricothyrotomy can facilitate rapid emergency entrance into the airway in patients whose anatomy allows identification of the cricoid and thyroid cartilages. Although several excellent commercial cricothyrotomy devices are available, whatever product is available should be examined and its instructions carefully read in advance of its use. In the absence of a commercial device, the cricoid membrane can be punctured emergently by a large-bore intravenous catheter (10, 12, or 14 gauge) that is then connected to a 3-ml Luer-Lok syringe with plunger removed and fitted with an endotracheal tube connector (7.5 or 8 mm OD). Usually oxygen can be forced into the trachea through this device using available ventilation bags, provided that exhalation can occur through the patient's natural airway.

Verification. Although verification that the endotracheal tube is in the trachea usually is easily done, unrecognized potentially lethal esophageal intubation is more likely in neonates and small infants, in patients with low pulmonary compliance, and in trauma patients. Although no method of verification is absolute, a pattern of continuing carbon dioxide elimination displayed on a capnograph is probably the most reliable method. However, during cardiac arrest carbon dioxide delivery to the lung may be so low that exhaled carbon dioxide levels are minimal. Commercially available inexpensive portable devices to detect carbon dioxide have been placed on some resuscitation carts and have been used by emergency medical technicians in the field. Other methods of verification include the following:

- *Observation.* Even during oral intubation, the placement of the tube between the vocal cords cannot always be verified visually. The right and left hemithorax should be observed to rise and fall with ventilation. Although this method is not useful emergently, a benefit of fiberoptic intubation is direct visualization of the trachea and positioning of the tube tip relative to the carina.
- *Auscultation.* Bilateral breath sounds should be auscultated in the anterior to mid-axillary line, and sounds of gas entering the stomach should not be heard.
- *Palpation.* The endotracheal cuff can be identified in the sternal notch by rhythmic compression of the pilot balloon.
- *Instrumentation.* Pulse oximetry is not an acceptable method of verification because desaturation may occur so late that it is not appreciated that esophageal intubation is the cause.

When Should Patients Be Intubated for Anesthesia? Mask anesthesia without endotracheal intubation is an appropriate option for superficial or extremity procedures when the patient is not at risk for regurgitation, upper airway patency is easily maintained, and other indications for intubation do not exist. Indications are based on the patient's condition, the surgical requirements, and anesthetic concerns.

Patient Condition. Medical problems such as respiratory insufficiency, intracranial pathology, or a significant probability of gastric regurgitation justify endotracheal intubation. An upper airway that easily obstructs may require a tube to maintain patency.

Surgical Requirements. Some surgical procedures mandate intubation (e.g., procedures around the head and neck, intrathoracic surgery, and intra-abdominal procedures that could limit diaphragmatic excursion or cause gastric regurgitation and aspiration). If the position of the patient during surgery is other than supine, the airway is usually intubated. Intubation is also usually performed if the surgical procedure is of long duration.

Anesthetic Requirements. Anesthetic techniques that require continuous controlled ventilation or complete muscle relaxation can be carried out more easily, precisely, and safely if intubation, a sealed airway, and a mechanical ventilator are used.

How Is the Patient at Risk for Aspiration Intubated? Some anesthesiologists divide patients at risk for aspiration of gastric contents into two groups. The group at higher risk has conditions that result in the stomach contents' being under pressure, has a stomach containing a large quantity of material, or has active bleeding into the upper airway (e.g., high gastric outlet obstruction, rebleeding tonsils, upper gastrointestinal bleeding). If general anesthesia is imperative, intubating the patient's trachea with a cuffed endotracheal tube while the patient is *awake or very slightly sedated* is recommended for airway protection. The patient's oropharynx can be topically anesthetized, but anesthetizing the larynx and tracheal mucosa to preserve the cough reflex should be avoided.

The other group of patients, those at an intermediate level of risk, have delayed gastric emptying, have not been NPO a sufficient duration of time for gastric emptying to occur, or have a history of gastroesophageal reflux. They can be managed with awake intubation just as the higher risk group or can undergo a *rapid-sequence induction and intubation with cricoid pressure.* During this technique the patient is permitted to breathe oxygen for 2 to 3 minutes to accomplish nitrogen washout. The patient is then given a bolus of thiopental, followed immediately by a 2 mg/kg bolus of succinylcholine. An assistant applies cricoid pressure as soon as the thiopental is administered, and when the patient becomes apneic, the trachea is intubated and the cuff inflated immediately. Ventilation is not performed until after the endotracheal tube is placed because gas may enter the stomach and distend it, increasing the risk of regurgitation and aspiration. If the trachea cannot be intubated on the first attempt, controlled ventilation must be administered to prevent severe hypoxia, but this should be given while cricoid pressure is maintained. The function of cricoid pressure (Sellick maneuver) is to obstruct the esophagus by compressing it between the posterior aspect of the cricoid cartilage and the body of the sixth cervical vertebra. Although highly effective, a Sellick maneuver is not a guarantee that tracheal aspiration can be prevented.

When Should Nasotracheal Intubation Be Used and When Should It Be Avoided?

Indications. Oral placement of an endotracheal tube may be difficult if there are severe restrictions to movement of the temporomandibular joint, the cervical spine, or the atlanto-occipital joint. When prolonged intubation is required in awake patients, the patient is more comfortable and nursing care is facilitated with nasal intubation. Patients requiring awake intubation who cannot tolerate oral laryngoscopy may be intubated nasally.

Complications. Possible complications of nasotracheal intubation include epistaxis, tearing of the pharyngeal mucosa and retropharyngeal dissection, and failure to accomplish intubation. *Contraindications are coagulopathy, obstruction of the nasal passages, and basilar skull fracture.*

Complications of Endotracheal Intubation

During Intubation. Vomiting or regurgitation may lead to aspiration. Trauma may occur in the form of lacerations, edema, hematomas, bleeding, broken teeth, or dislocation of the arytenoids. The endotracheal tube can be placed in the esophagus or mainstem bronchus, or intubation may not be possible. Hypertension, arrhythmias, and myocardial ischemia may occur even in anesthetized, oxygenated, easily intubated patients.

While Intubated. Tube position may change, resulting in extubation or endobronchial intubation. The irritation of the tube may cause persistent coughing, patient agitation, and bronchospasm. Hypertension and coronary ischemia may also occur. Ventilation through an endotracheal tube may fail for mechanical reasons such as tube occlusion by kinking, from defects, or with secretions, because of a cuff leak that prevents the delivery of adequate ventilatory volumes, or because of disconnection of the ventilator circuit.

After Intubation. Initially laryngospasm may lead to hypoxemia. Later a sore throat, hoarseness, and laryngeal edema may be present. Still later vocal cord paralysis may become apparent, and laryngeal granulomas may develop. Long-term intubation is required for tracheal necrosis or stenosis to occur. Hoarseness or dysphonia persisting more than 3 days after extubation is an indication for indirect laryngoscopy.

Goals of Intraoperative Ventilatory Support

In some cases it is appropriate for the patient to breathe spontaneously; however, in most situations, because of drug-induced respiratory depression or muscle relaxant administration, ventilation must be assisted or controlled. When controlling ventilation, usually a tidal volume of 10 to 12 ml/kg at a rate of eight breaths per minute will *remove carbon dioxide adequately* and prevent absorption atelectasis. By monitoring the concentrations of respiratory gases, ventilation can be adjusted to achieve the desired end-tidal carbon dioxide level. If there is a question about the adequacy of ventilation or the magnitude of the arterial to end-tidal carbon dioxide gradient, arterial blood should be analyzed.

For patients in whom an increase in pulmonary venous admixture occurs (e.g., a patient with a pulmonary contusion or with pulmonary edema), application of PEEP is indicated. The exact amount of PEEP to apply is that which minimizes the intrapulmonary shunt without adversely affecting cardiac output. Whenever airway pressures are manipulated to produce adequate ventilation and ventilation-perfusion ratios, these pressures are transmitted to the vascular structures and can thereby decrease venous return.

What Can an Intraoperative Change in Pulmonary Compliance Indicate?

Most emergent pulmonary complications that alter ventilation and gas exchange can be detected by changes in pulmonary compliance.

Compliance Increases. A sudden increase in compliance should alert the anesthesiologist to a significant leak in the breathing circuit. At best, this would produce a loss of ventilating gases and hypoventilation. At worst, an unanticipated extubation or a complete disconnection of the anesthesia apparatus from the endotracheal tube could occur in a paralyzed patient, and the patient would be apneic. Using ventilator alarms, monitoring the carbon dioxide level in the respiratory gas, and monitoring arterial oxygen saturation with a pulse oximeter will alert the anesthesiologist to these potentially disastrous situations.

Compliance Decreases

Airway Causes. Several things can occur with the endotracheal tube per se to cause a decrease in compliance. The tube may kink anywhere along its path but usually does so at the exit from the mouth or nose and in the oropharynx. During the operative procedure the cuff may become overinflated because the gas within the cuff expands when it increases from room temperature to body temperature or because nitrous oxide may diffuse into the cuff and increase its volume. The resulting excessive cuff inflation may cause it to herniate over the end of the tube or encroach on the tube's lumen. The bevel of the endotracheal tube may impinge on the wall of the trachea, or the tube may not be positioned properly within the trachea but is in the right or left main-stem bronchus instead. Obstructions such as thick tenacious secretions or blood within the endotracheal tube can decrease compliance.

Other possible obstructing matter includes endobronchial polyps, tissue from the nose after a nasal intubation, or any foreign body.

Obstructive and Restrictive Processes. Bronchoconstriction causing a decrease in the caliber of the small airways can be secondary to mechanical stimulation such as an endotracheal tube resting on the carina or to a medical event such as bronchial asthma or a pulmonary embolus. A **tension pneumothorax** is the most likely event occurring during anesthesia that could decrease compliance by a restrictive mechanism. Spontaneous tension pneumothorax does occur rarely, but it is more likely after chest trauma, in patients with large pulmonary bullae, or in any patient who has had an internal jugular or a subclavian vein catheter placed. Patients having surgery of the neck, the chest wall, or the kidney also should be considered at risk of pneumothorax. In addition to air externally compressing the lung, **hydrothorax and hemothorax** should also be considered, especially when central venous catheters are used.

Lung Water Accumulation. Interstitial or intra-alveolar pulmonary edema may also decrease pulmonary compliance. Some causes of intraoperative pulmonary edema are an absolute or a relative **fluid overload** as a result of the infusion of excess fluid or the inability of the circulation to handle a normal fluid load, sepsis, or a change in the permeability of the pulmonary capillaries. **Pulmonary contusion** from preoperative trauma or from the trauma of surgery itself also results in a fluid leak. **Aspiration of gastric contents** during anesthesia and **showers of air emboli** can increase pulmonary artery pressure and cause pulmonary edema. Decreasing arterial oxygen tension and increasing intrapulmonary shunt should suggest that lung water accumulation is occurring. Regardless of the cause, ventilation-perfusion ratios and oxygenation frequently can be improved by the manipulation of ventilating pressures, particularly with PEEP.

Goals of Intraoperative Hemodynamic Management

The general goals of hemodynamic management are to establish and maintain adequate perfusion of all organs with blood containing sufficient oxygen and other metabolic substrates (e.g., glucose). Hemodynamic management must provide resuscitation from preoperative deficits, respond to hemodynamic changes induced by the pharmacologic properties of the anesthetic agents, and respond to fluid shifts and losses that may develop during surgery. Intraoperative fluid shifts can be detected by direct observation, measurement of arterial, central venous, and pulmonary artery pressures, and close monitoring of the quantity and specific gravity of the urine.

Intraoperative surgical events can greatly alter hemodynamics. The inferior vena cava or portal vein may be partially or totally occluded secondary to packing or to a retractor placed during difficult surgical exposure. Administration of drugs into the surgical field (e.g., epinephrine-containing local anesthetics, phenylephrine [Neo-Synephrine], or antibiotic-containing irrigation solutions) may cause severe systemic hemodynamic effects. Manipulation of the brainstem during neurosurgical procedures, traction on the optic nerve during eye procedures, or traction or inflation of the alimentary tract also can alter hemodynamics through central nervous system (CNS) reflexes.

Components of Intraoperative Fluid Therapy

Volume (Excluding Blood Loss). Fluid loading just before and during induction appears large on a milliliter-per-minute basis, but it is necessary to maintain adequate blood pressure during the administration of drugs that can decrease preload, contractility, and afterload. The volume infused is dependent not just on the drugs and dosages selected, but also on the patient's preoperative volume status. A patient with no findings of a volume deficit who receives a maintenance intravenous infusion overnight may require only 2 ml/kg of crystalloid to treat the drug-induced hemodynamic changes; however, a patient without a preoperative intravenous infusion but with the findings of severe hypovolemia may require 15 to 25 ml/kg during induction.

Volume administration related to procedures must meet maintenance requirements and third-space losses. Maintenance requirements composed of sensible losses in the urine and feces, insensible losses in the lungs and skin, and a gain for water from oxidation may be substantially increased or decreased intraoperatively. The third space is a nonfunctional, obligatory extracellular fluid compartment derived from functional extracellular fluid (plasma and interstitial fluid) resulting from tissue trauma. Third-space losses cannot be avoided if the patient is kept normovolemic. Procedure-related needs may range from 1 to 2 ml/kg/hour in eye or ear procedures to 10 to 12 ml/kg/hour during major vascular or major bowel procedures, exclusive of blood loss. Important modifiers of procedure-related volume estimates include renal and cardiac failure, continuing deficit causes noted during the preoperative evaluation, and the site of third-space sequestration (e.g., lung or brain).

Electrolyte Maintenance. The electrolyte composition of intraoperative fluids is selected to maintain or restore normal electrolyte concentrations. For this reason third-space volume is administered as a sodium-containing, balanced salt solution. The lactate and acetate anions in balanced salt solutions that are equivalent to bicarbonate on a one-to-one molar basis are designed to offset the metabolic acid production of normal metabolism. Although potassium historically has been used sparingly intraoperatively and often has been omitted from postoperative fluid orders, depletion of intracellular potassium because of chronic diuretic use would suggest that potassium requirements be individualized. Hypomagnesemia is generally not treated intraoperatively unless accompanied by arrhythmias. Calcium chloride is infused only if citrated blood products are extremely rapidly infused (>100 ml/70 kg/minute) or if large quantities of citrate are administered to patients with severe hepatic dysfunction.

Oxygen-Carrying Capacity. Although deviations from normovolemia during anesthesia are poorly tolerated, bleeding patients do not generally require the replacement of the lost red cells until substantial anemia has occurred, but they do require replacement of the volume lost. The volume of blood lost is replaced with crystalloid solutions in a 3:1 ratio initially (increasing with degree of anemia) or with colloid solutions in a 1.25:1 ratio. During this progressive hemodilution, oxygen delivery is maintained by increases in cardiac output and oxygen extraction. In a healthy, normovolemic person with a normal heart the theoretic maximal dilution occurs when oxygen consumption begins to drop because of insufficient delivery. The corresponding hematocrit level is definitely below 25%, perhaps as low as 10%. However, the practical limit of hemodilution is more often determined by the adequacy of myocardial oxygen delivery, particularly by distal to partial coronary blockage. The heart is the one organ that predictably increases oxygen consumption during acute normovolemic hemodilution because it must increase cardiac output. With coronary artery disease, left ventricular hypertrophy, or severe aortic stenosis, hematocrit levels of approximately 30% can be associated with myocardial ischemia. So the maximal limit of acute anemia is not determined by selecting an arbitrary minimal hematocrit or hemoglobin concentration, but by understanding the patient's preexisting cardiac condition and by vigilant monitoring for signs of coronary ischemia.

Adjuncts. Glucose included in intraoperative fluid therapy will prevent the mobilization of fatty acids and starvation ketoacidosis and will prevent depletion of glycogen stores and the risk of transient hypoglycemia. Claims that 100 to 150 g/day of glucose will decrease protein catabolism by 50% are now disputed. Excessive administration of glucose intraoperatively may result in glucose levels of more than 600 mg/dl, leading to intracellular dehydration of the brain and a diminished level of consciousness, delayed awakening from anesthesia, or hyperosmolar hyperglycemia nonketotic coma. New concerns about enhanced cerebral damage if cerebral ischemia occurs while blood glucose levels are high have resulted in less frequent administration of glucose during surgery and its elimination entirely from the fluid therapy of patients undergoing carotid and intracranial procedures.

Intraoperative colloid administration as a supplement to crystalloid administration is limited because of its much greater cost and the infrequency of situations in which it offers a clear advantage. Albumin, purified protein fraction, and hetastarch may justifiably be used for perioperative volume expansion in recently burned patients, in patients with hypovolemia or septic shock and less than 3 g/dl albumin level, in hemodialysis patients, in patients undergoing pulmonary and neurosurgical procedures, and during cardiopulmonary bypass surgery.

Problems That May Occur With Improper Positioning

The unconscious patient cannot complain about an uncomfortable position, which can lend itself to skeletal, muscular, skin, or even nerve damage. Improper positioning can also complicate both the surgical and anesthetic management of the patient. The patient should be positioned in a comfortable position, pressure points should be padded, and traction or abnormal stress on body parts should be avoided.

Surgical Compromise. The surgeon should be available immediately after the induction of anesthesia either to position the patient for the procedure or to verify that the positioning done by others is appropriate for the specific case. *Late discovery of improper positioning may make the procedure technically more difficult and prolong its duration.*

Airway Compromise. The position of the endotracheal tube may change within the trachea when the patient is turned in to the lateral position or is turned prone. The anesthesiologist must recheck the position of the endotracheal tube whenever the position of the patient changes by carefully listening to the peripheral lung fields bilaterally and also listening over the epigastrium.

Hemodynamic Changes. Changes in position also can interfere with venous return. For example, elevation of the kidney rest may compress the inferior vena cava and lead to a decrease in venous return secondary to pooling of blood in the lower extremities. Similarly, use of a steep reverse Trendelenburg position for upper abdominal procedures and the lowering of the legs from the lithotomy position may decrease venous return. The lumen of major vessels within the chest may be compromised by adjacent masses, and even the heart can be rotated and major vessels twisted secondary to position changes. Thus the anesthesiologist must be constantly vigilant for changes in cardiovascular performance whenever the body position is changed.

Muscle, Skeletal, and Skin Damage. The unconscious patient cannot complain about a position that may be associated with musculoskeletal damage or skin breakdown. Skin over bony prominences such as the heels, medial malleoli, sacrum, thoracic spinous processes, and supraorbital ridges is particularly vulnerable to ischemia and ulceration. Fingers may be crushed when the foot of the surgical table is returned to the horizontal position after lithotomy position, and the feet may be injured from pressure when the operating table is raised and the instrument table is not. In addition to damage from positioning, improperly grounded electrical equipment may burn skin or even cause electrocution.

Nerve Damage. Nerves may be injured by the compression of surgical retractors, compression against the operating table or other unpadded surface, and stretching around bony prominences. Ulnar and brachial plexus injuries commonly are associated with general anesthesia and lumbosacral injuries with regional anesthesia. Nerve damage is the second most common complication related to anesthesia that results in a malpractice suit.

Who Is Responsible for Proper Patient Positioning?

Positioning the anesthetized patient requires considerable attention. In general, patients are positioned to facilitate surgical exposure; however, it is incumbent on the anesthesiologist to inspect all pressure points once the patient is positioned to assure proper padding and to prevent unnecessary hyperextension. *This responsibility is shared with the surgeon and the circulating nurse,* but the anesthesiologist should be the one most attuned to this potential for damage and therefore be the one who insists on appropriate changes.

ANESTHETIC TECHNIQUES
Four Basic Types of Anesthetic Techniques

The four most frequently used anesthetic techniques, in the broadest sense, are *local anesthesia, monitored anesthesia care (MAC), regional anesthesia, and general anesthesia.* Within each of the four categories are several different methods and pharmaceutical agents that may be used alone or in combination. The specific methods and agents used should be tailored to the patient rather than apportioned into routines for specific types of surgical procedures. In many cases when elective surgery is contemplated for a healthy patient, the exact technique and agents used will not be of any particular consequence in determining the risk of intraoperative or postoperative complications. On the other hand, certain medical conditions do contraindicate use of certain drugs and procedures.

Basis for Selection of Anesthetic Technique

The selection of the anesthetic technique (i.e., local anesthesia, monitored anesthesia care, regional anesthesia, or general anesthesia) attempts to satisfy several factors concurrently.

Required Surgical Conditions. The anesthetic technique must satisfy the requirements of the proposed procedure; however, complete scheduling and often additional communication between the surgeon and the anesthetist may be required to meet these needs fully. For example, coincident bone, fascia, or skin harvest from a remote site may preclude using regional anesthesia of a single extremity.

Patient History. An understanding of the current illness, preexisting medical conditions, and prior perioperative difficulties may eliminate some techniques and agents from consideration. For example, a patient with unstable angina may not tolerate incomplete local anesthesia but require the full obliteration of pain that can be achieved with regional or general anesthesia.

Hereditary abnormalities (e.g., malignant hyperpyrexia) dictate avoidance of certain anesthetic agents.

Patient Physical Status. Aspects of the patient's physical condition both related and unrelated to the proposed surgical treatment must be considered. For example, a patient with severe cardiomyopathy and a low ejection fraction may warrant local or regional anesthesia rather than general anesthesia. However, patients who are hypovolemic usually will not tolerate regional anesthetics that produce sympathectomy until the blood volume is restored. In general, the more numerous and severe the patient's medical problems (greater numerical ASA physical status), the more reasonable it is to avoid systemic anesthetic effects by using regional rather than general anesthesia.

Laboratory Results. Some laboratory data may contraindicate an anesthetic technique. For example, a documented coagulopathy is generally a contraindication to regional anesthesia. Electrolyte imbalances suggest that regional anesthesia be used for cases that cannot be delayed; however, excessive sedation used to supplement regional or local anesthesia can lead to respiratory acidosis, which may complicate the underlying abnormalities.

Patient Preference. If a patient has a prejudice for or against a specific technique, this preference is honored if there is no medical consequence and safety is not compromised. If the preference does constitute an unwise choice on medical grounds, a physician is obligated to explain the basis of that concern and present the possible alternatives with their associated risks to the patient. For example, some patients, fearing neurologic damage, have a strong prejudice against spinal anesthesia. Other patients may not be able to tolerate local or regional anesthesia for head or neck procedures because of claustrophobia caused by the sterile drapes.

Physician Preferences. Both the anesthesiologist and surgeon should possess sufficient technical abilities that the safest and most effective techniques that satisfy the factors already listed can be used. Only when the risk and efficacy of the anesthetic techniques do not differ should physicians impose their personal preferences. For example, in teaching environments surgical faculty often prefer freedom to discuss a procedure with trainees without alarming the patient; thus using either general anesthesia or sedation with amnesia-producing drugs is necessary.

Difference Between Local Anesthesia and Monitored Anesthesia Care

With *monitored anesthesia care* the anesthesiologist provides full physiologic monitoring services, provides whatever medical care is necessary to maintain patient homeostasis (e.g., ventilation, treatment of abnormal blood pressures, treatment of cardiac rhythm disturbances), and may provide conscious sedation of the patient while the surgeon performs the procedure with the patient under local anesthesia that the surgeon administers or with no anesthesia at all. Generally, *local anesthesia* means that the surgeon administers the local anesthetic agent, an anesthesiologist does not participate, vital signs are monitored by nursing personnel, and significant treatment to maintain patient homeostasis is not required.

During local anesthesia the surgeon may order administration of sedating drugs either intramuscularly preoperatively or intravenously during the procedure by nursing personnel. The surgeon must carefully consider in advance whether or not he or she can safely manage the patient's sedation and its complications should complications related to the surgical procedure develop. Difficulties with this dual role have led some institutions to develop policies for intravenous conscious sedation when an anesthesiologist is not participating in the care of the patient.

How Is Intravenous Conscious Sedation Administered Properly?

Intravenous conscious sedation is defined as the intravenous administration of sedating drugs with or without narcotics while maintaining the patient's ability to be aroused by verbal commands, to respond appropriately, and to retain protective reflexes. Conscious sedation may be required outside the operating room in locations such as treatment rooms and/or the medical office setting.

Patient Selection. Criteria for including patients whose medical status is suitable for conscious sedation and excluding patients who are not suitable should be followed.

Personnel Qualifications. The minimal qualifications of the person monitoring the patient should also be defined. *For example, the person monitoring conscious sedation should not be the same person who performs the procedure.* He or she should be familiar with the desired and adverse effects of the drugs used, know how to recognize airway obstruction, and be able to correct it. An anesthetist or person certified in ACLS should be available in the immediate area.

Monitoring. Personnel should know how to monitor blood pressure, pulse, and oxygenation, how to recognize abnormalities in these parameters, and how to intervene should abnormalities occur.

Equipment. Requirements include not only a blood pressure monitor, an ECG display, and a pulse oximeter, but also a suction, a positive pressure oxygen delivery system, and an emergency cart with resuscitation drugs and additional airway management equipment.

Procedures. A secure intravenous access should be maintained during the procedure. Drug administration and vital signs must be documented. The patient should go to a monitored recovery area after the procedure and leave the area only when specific discharge criteria are met. Conscious sedation should be included in a quality assurance program.

What Is the Systemic Toxicity of Local Anesthetics?

If local anesthetics will be administered, it must be remembered that high blood levels of the local anesthetics can result from rapid absorption, intravascular injection, or simply excessive dosing. Treating the patient who is to receive substantial amounts of local anesthetics in the same manner as one receiving intravenous conscious sedation usually will provide safe conditions. The safety of infiltration also is enhanced by slow injection (i.e., more than 5 seconds for each 1 ml), frequent aspiration for blood, and asking the patient to report the early symptoms of systemic toxicity (e.g., lightheadedness, tinnitus, circumoral numbness). The maximal single dosages listed in Table 3-2 must be reduced for highly vascular tissues such as oral and intercostal sites of injection. The use of 5 μg/ml epinephrine (1:200,000) increases the single dosage limits by approximately one third and roughly doubles the duration of the local anesthetic effect (Table 3-2).

With high blood levels of local anesthetics, the

TABLE 3-2 Local Anesthetics

Classification and Generic Name	Trade Name	Infiltration Concentration (%)	Maximal Single Dose Plain (EPI) (mg/kg)	Duration After Infiltration* (min)	Uses
Esters					
Procaine	Novocain	1	7 (10)	30-120	I, PN, SA
Chloroprocaine	Nesacaine	1-2	11 (14)	15-90	E, I, PN
Benzocaine	Hurricaine	—	3	—	T
Cocaine	—	—	2	—	T
Tetracaine	Pontocaine; Cetacaine	—	0.3	—	SA, T
Amides					
Lidocaine	Xylocaine	0.5-1	4 (7)	30-360	E, I, PN, SA, T
Prilocaine	Citanest	0.5-1	7 (8.5)	30-360	E, I, PN
Mepivacaine	Carbocaine; Polocaine	0.5-1	4 (7)	45-360	E, I, PN
Bupivacaine	Marcaine; Sensorcaine	0.25-0.5	2.5 (3.2)	120-480	E, I, PN, SA
Etidocaine	Duranest	0.5-1	6 (8)	120-480	E, I, PN

*Minimal duration with plain local anesthetic; maximal duration with epinephrine-containing local anesthetic.
EPI = containing 1:200,000 epinephrine; E = epidural block; I = infiltration; PN = peripheral nerve block; SA = subarachnoid block; T = topical anesthesia.

initial CNS symptoms of lightheadedness, tinnitus, confusion, disorientation, circumoral numbness, and visual and auditory disturbances are followed by muscle twitching, tremors, and generalized tonic-clonic seizures. These signs of CNS excitation may be followed by CNS depression in the form of loss of consciousness, respiratory depression, and apnea.

The cardiovascular system is the other site of major local anesthetic toxicity. During the CNS excitatory phase, hypertension and tachycardia occur. Subsequently, mild to moderate hypotension develops as a result of decreased systemic vascular resistance and decreased cardiac output by direct myocardial depression. Bradycardia, conduction delays, ventricular arrhythmias, and finally circulatory collapse may follow. Resuscitation after bupivacaine overdose may be particularly difficult because of the tenacious binding of bupivacaine to the myocardium.

Other Complications of Local Anesthetic Administration

Allergic reactions to local anesthetics have also been reported but are rare compared with the systemic toxicity of excessive blood levels. Ester local anesthetics much more likely will be allergenic than amide anesthetics (see Table 3-2). Anaphylactic reactions attributed to either ester or amide agent administration actually may be due to methylparaben, an antimicrobial used in multidose vial preparations. Reactions may also be due to the predictable pharmacologic responses to the intravascular injection of epinephrine or to a nonspecific vasovagal response to injection.

Failure to achieve adequate anesthesia may be the result of inadequate placement of sufficient quantities of anesthetic or of attempts to infiltrate ischemic or infected tissue. To avoid reaching toxic levels of a local anesthetic before adequate anesthesia is achieved, a lower concentration of the injected drug or a preparation with 5 μg/ml epinephrine may be used. Only a portion of the surgical field should be infiltrated initially; then additional areas can be infiltrated later when redistribution and elimination have lowered the blood level of local anesthetic. The acidosis of ischemic or infected tissue reduces the levels of the lipid-soluble unprotonated amine form of the local anesthetic, which is necessary to penetrate cell membranes and nerve fibers. The hydrochloride salt solutions of these weak bases are acidic but are rapidly buffered by the tissue to its pH. At normal tissue pH, 7.4, only 5% to 20% of the local anesthetic is in the unprotonated amine form, depending on the agent selected. When tissue pH is reduced, more of the protonated ionic form persists, and less drug is available for nerve penetration.

Consequences of Administering Epinephrine With Local Anesthetics

Vasoconstrictors such as epinephrine are included in many local anesthetic preparations to delay absorption, reduce peak blood levels of the injected local anesthetic, and decrease the potential for systemic toxicity, thereby permitting the use of more local anesthetic. The effect of vasoconstrictors on absorption depends on the local anesthetic selected and the site of drug administration (epidural space versus infiltration). Epinephrine substantially reduces the absorption of the agents listed in Table 3-2 when used in infiltration and peripheral nerve block applications. Absorption of lidocaine is reduced by approximately 30% with 1:200,000 epinephrine, regardless of the site of injection.

Systemic epinephrine effects may lead to hypertension and cardiac dysrhythmias, particularly in those patients who have exhibited these conditions in the absence of exogenous epinephrine. Alpha- and beta-adrenergic blockade may be used to treat serious episodes of hypertension and ventricular dysrhythmias without significant effect on the local vasoconstriction induced by the infiltrated epinephrine. Arrhythmias are less of a problem with pure alpha-adrenergic vasoconstrictors such as 1:100,000 or 1:50,000 norepinephrine (Levophed, 10 to 20 μg/ml) or, more commonly, 1:20,000 phenylephrine (Neo-Synephrine, 50 μg/ml). Epinephrine-induced arrhythmias are enhanced by the concurrent use of halothane inhalation anesthesia. During halothane anesthesia the maximal dosage of epinephrine should be limited to 0.3 ml/kg of a 1:200,000 epinephrine solution in a 10-minute period, not to exceed 0.9 ml/kg of 1:200,000 solution per hour.

Decreased wound bleeding is also an important benefit of vasoconstrictor infiltration. However, if regional or general anesthesia is being used, hemostasis can be achieved with a much more dilute concentration of 1:500,000 epinephrine (2 μg/ml or 1 mg/5 dl) in normal saline solution. Vasoconstriction not only reduces blood flow from the surgical incision but also to adjacent tissue that participates in wound healing. If collateral flow is absent (e.g., to digits, hands, and feet), local tissue hypoxia from sympathetic nervous system–induced increases in oxygen consumption, combined with decreased oxygen delivery, may result in necrosis and gangrene. Therefore if the injection site will not permit collateral flow to distal tissue, the use of vasoconstrictors is contraindicated. If epinephrine-containing solutions will be injected by the surgeon, the anesthetist must be notified before the induction of general anesthesia so that use of halothane is avoided.

Regional Anesthesia

Regional anesthesia is the selective blocking by local anesthetics of nerves that innervate a particular area of the body, thus providing anesthesia in that area independent of the level of consciousness. Single peripheral nerve blocks are particularly useful for superficial procedures in a small area. Groups of peripheral nerves can be blocked individually to provide satisfactory anesthesia for larger areas (e.g., ankle block). Essentially all peripheral nerves can be blocked; however, for larger surgical fields and for some procedures (e.g., a radical mastectomy), the total number of injections, the cumulative quantity of anesthetic needed, and the time required to complete all the blocks would be prohibitive. Fortunately, complete abdominal and lower-extremity anesthesia can be achieved by a single subarachnoid (spinal) or epidural injection. Caudal anesthesia for pelvic, perineal, and anal surgery is achieved by using an epidural anesthetic administered through the caudal canal. Similarly, for the upper extremity, the brachial plexus can be anesthetized by administering single injections at different sites with an interscalene brachial plexus block, a subclavian perivascular or supraclavicular block, or an axillary block.

Advantages of Subarachnoid and Epidural Anesthesia. The major advantages of subarachnoid and epidural anesthesia are relative safety and effective anesthesia without any required alteration in consciousness. When managing patients with a myocardiopathy or low ejection fraction, the myocardial depressant effects of inhalation general anesthetics are avoided. Skeletal muscles can be relaxed by achieving motor nerve blockade. However, with epidural anesthesia the selective persistence of motor function is often possible. The intestines are contracted, and sphincters are relaxed due to sympathetic blockade and unopposed parasympathetic effects (when the block exceeds the T5 level). Blood loss

is often reduced, probably as a result of lower venous pressures. There is a decreased incidence of lower-extremity thrombosis because of the increase in extremity blood flow after the drug-induced reversible sympathectomy. The combined use of epidural anesthesia and postoperative analgesia in high-risk surgical patients may lead to lower morbidity because of an inhibitory effect on the neuroendocrine response to the stress of an operation.

Disadvantages. Spinal and epidural anesthesia are relatively contraindicated in some patients with conditions such as agitation or intoxication, coagulopathy, hypovolemia, neurologic disease, chronic back pain, respiratory failure, and infection or extensive back surgery at the site of proposed block.

Neurologic damage from direct drug toxicity is virtually unheard of because of the purity of modern local anesthetic preparations and the sterility and cleanliness of single-use injection equipment. However, nerve damage related to improper patient positioning, retractor placement, errant needle placement, injection of the wrong material, or progression of coexisting neurologic disease can still occur. Also meningitis, epidural abscess formation, and epidural hematoma remain rare but possible complications. Backache occurs as frequently with general anesthesia as it does after lumbar epidural or spinal anesthesia. Contributing factors are the lack of movement during long procedures and ligament stretching after the paraspinal muscles are relaxed. Postdural puncture headache (PDPH) after subarachnoid puncture or if accidental puncture occurs during epidural anesthesia is unlikely in patients over 45 years of age. In young, particularly postpartum patients, PDPH can be prevented by using small needles (25 gauge or smaller) or special noncutting needle tips and by treating them with either caffeine infusions or a blood patch (10 to 20 ml of autologous whole blood in the epidural space at the level of the puncture).

During spinal or epidural anesthesia the sympathetic nervous system outflow of the spinal cord is blocked at a level several dermatomes higher than the sensory blockade. Hypotension and bradycardia usually remain a problem only if unanticipated hypovolemia or excessive anesthesia occurs and the anesthetist's response is delayed. During abdominal procedures parasympathetic afferent nerve fibers that do not travel in the subarachnoid space may be unopposed, resulting in nausea and vomiting; however, this can be controlled by anticholinergic medication. Unopposed parasympathetic innervation to the urinary tract can contribute to urinary retention.

On occasion neural blockade may be incomplete and insufficient for the procedure, usually as a result of inaccurate placement of the local anesthetic or the procedure's outlasting the duration of the block. Single-dose spinal anesthesia may provide from 20 minutes of anesthesia with procaine to over 3 hours for tetracaine with epinephrine. However, continuous spinal anesthesia, achieved by administering repeated doses of local anesthesia through a subarachnoid catheter, is regaining popularity because of the commercial introduction of 28- to 32-gauge catheters. Continuous rather than single-dose epidural anesthesia is preferred since the anesthesia can be prolonged by injecting more anesthetic agent through the catheter and opioids can be administered via the catheter postoperatively for pain management.

Total spinal anesthesia or an excessively high epidural blockade may require respiratory support once the cervical nerve input to the diaphragm is blocked and, often, circulatory support if a complete sympathetic block is sudden and unexpected. If the dosage or baricity of the anesthetic solution injected into the subarachnoid space is incorrect or excessive mixing with the cerebrospinal fluid (CSF) occurs due to coughing or retching, higher-than-planned levels of spinal anesthesia may result. Overdosage by administering excessive quantities of epidural drug or failure to recognize epidural catheter penetration into the subarachnoid space may result in a high or total block of spinal function. The quantities of local anesthesia injected into the subarachnoid space are extremely small, but epidural drug dosages are near limits for systemic toxicity and will be toxic if accidental intravenous injection occurs due to the penetration of an epidural catheter into an epidural vein.

Advantages of Brachial Plexus Anesthesia. The major advantages of brachial plexus anesthesia are its relative safety and its effectiveness without any required alteration in consciousness. Circulatory and respiratory effects are generally absent. Motor and sympathetic innervation to the upper extremity is also blocked, thereby providing muscle relaxation and increased blood flow that may be desirable after some vascular procedures.

Disadvantages. Brachial plexus anesthesia is relatively contraindicated in some patients with conditions such as intoxication, inability to cooperate, coagulopathy, and peripheral neurologic disease. Axillary lymphadenopathy may require blockage of the brachial plexus by the supraclavicular or interscalene route.

Neurologic damage from drug toxicity is not a concern; however, infection from poor technique, injection of the wrong material, transient neuropraxia from direct needle injury, or progression of coexisting peripheral neuropathies can occur. On occasion brachial blockade may be incomplete and insufficient for the procedure, usually as a result of inaccurate placement of the local anesthetic or failure to block all portions of the brachial plexus (e.g., the musculocutaneous nerve with axillary blocks or intercostobrachial nerve with interscalene blocks). Supplemental injections of poorly blocked areas are usually easily accomplished.

Since the quantities of local anesthetic agent injected are often near the limits for systemic toxicity and near vascular structures, these blocks must be performed in fully monitored patients by physicians able to treat systemic overdoses safely. Unusual complications of interscalene blocks include injection into the subarachnoid or epidural space, yielding a total spinal anesthetic, hoarseness from paralysis of the recurrent laryngeal nerve, Horner's syndrome from stellate ganglion blockade, and ipsilateral phrenic nerve blockade. Use of subclavian perivascular blocks may result in tension pneumothorax or hemothorax with errant needle positioning. Axillary block complications include hematoma formation, causing vascular compression.

General Anesthesia

The major advantage of general anesthesia is that it reliably prevents the patient's experiencing pain and it can be continuously increased or decreased as conditions warrant. The major disadvantage is that all organ systems are "anesthetized," often significantly altering their response. Hemodynamic alterations must be aggressively treated. Often ventilation must be augmented and the airway protected.

Common Intravenous Anesthetic Agents and Their Roles in General Anesthesia. Frequently, the anesthesiologist will not select a single agent but a combination of inhalation and intravenous agents (Table 3-3) to produce the desired level of anesthesia without producing the undesirable side effects that might occur if each agent were used independently. Complete intravenous anesthetic administration is often used in cardiac anesthesia (e.g., fentanyl and a benzodiazepine) and outpatient anesthesia (e.g., propofol with or without alfentanil).

Barbiturates. Thiobarbiturates are commonly used to induce anesthesia since they have a pleasant and rapid onset and their effects dissipate rapidly by redistribution throughout the body (not elimination). Hypotension due to venous pooling and cardiac depression may occur but is partially compensated for by increases in heart rate. Respiratory depression or apnea requiring ventilatory support and maintenance of a patent airway is common.

Opioids. Morphine and meperidine are still used to supplement inhalation anesthesia. The potent synthetic agents listed in Table 3-3 cause less histamine release and less increase in venous capacitance, making them more suitable as a primary anesthetic agent. Cardiac depression is minimal, respiratory depression is severe, and intracranial pressure is reduced.

Benzodiazepines. Each of the agents listed in Table 3-3 is a potent anxiolytic used for premedication and for supplementing general anesthesia. Midazolam may be used for induction of anesthesia. Cardiovascular and ventilatory changes are minimal at low doses. Predictable potent antegrade amnesia is possible with midazolam and lorazepam.

Ketamine. Ketamine is a dissociative anesthetic that provides potent analgesia and amnesia, with muscle tone, ventilation, and the airway patency usually maintained. It can be used as an induction agent or as a complete anesthetic. Central cardiovascular stimulation causes hypertension and tachycardia, which increase intracranial pressure. Unpleasant visual and auditory hallucinations during emergence limit ketamine's use.

Etomidate. Etomidate is a rapid, short-acting induction agent that provides anesthesia with a stable cardiovascular response and only transient apnea. Negative attributes include pain on injection, involuntary skeletal muscle movement, postoperative nausea and vomiting, and adrenal suppression.

Propofol. To maintain its solubility, propofol is packaged in a milky white lipid emulsion used in parenteral nutrition (Intralipid). Propofol is a complete anesthetic, with rapid onset and rapid emergence free from nausea and vomiting or residual sedation. Reduction in systemic vascular resistance with resulting hypotension often oc-

TABLE 3-3 Intravenous Anesthetics

Drug Family and Generic Names	Trade Name	Elimination Half-life (hr)	Notes
Barbiturates			
Thiopental	Pentothal	12	Induction agent
Thiamylal	Surital	12	Induction agent equivalent to thiopental
Methohexital	Brevital	4	Induction agent
Opioids			
Fentanyl	Sublimaze	3.5	IV or epidural administration
Alfentanil	Alfenta	1.5	Bolus or continuous IV infusion
Sufentanil	Sufenta	2.5	Significant heart rate reduction
Benzodiazepines			
Midazolam	Versed	2.5	Induction agent
Diazepam	Valium	30	Thrombophlebitis common
Lorazepam	Ativan	15	Prolonged disorientation
Other Agents			
Ketamine	Ketalar	2	Induction agent; complete IV anesthetic in children, burn patients
Etomidate	Amidate	3.5	Induction agent or complete anesthetic if continuous infusion used
Propofol	Diprivan	2	Induction agent; complete IV anesthetic

curs during induction. Ventilation and airway patency must be supported.

Inhalation Anesthetic Agents. The chemical properties of the inhalation anesthetic agents do differ (Table 3-4). The potency of the agents is quantitated at equilibrium by measuring the minimum alveolar concentration (MAC), the concentration at which the drug prevents movement with superficial surgical stimulation in 50% of patients. The blood-gas solubility coefficients of the inhalation agents determine the rapidity with which the patient becomes anesthetized and recovers from anesthesia. A large inspired concentration of oxygen could be administered with the MAC concentration of the anesthetics listed in Table 3-4, with the exception of nitrous oxide. Only under hyperbaric conditions could nitrous oxide alone achieve complete anesthesia. The lower the blood-gas solubility coefficient, the less soluble the agent is in blood, and the faster the induction and recovery occurs. Nitrous oxide is a compressed gas at ambient conditions; halothane, enflurane, and isoflurane are liquids that must be vaporized. Desflurane, a new rapid-acting potent agent, requires special vaporizers since in a warm operating room or at a high altitude it will boil.

The pharmacologic properties of the inhalation anesthetic agents also differ. Halothane, enflurane, isoflurane, and desflurane all cause a reduction in ventilatory response to carbon dioxide and an increase in respiratory rate, a decrease in tidal volume, and a decrease in minute ventilation. They also reduce blood pressure, depress myocardial contractility, and increase systemic vascular resistance. Enflurane, isoflurane, and desflurane can increase heart rate substantially. Nitrous oxide causes few hemodynamic alterations or respiratory depression at the concentrations usually used. The halogenated ethers, en-flurane, isoflurane, and desflurane, provide some muscle relaxation and excellent cardiac rhythm stability. A modest transient reduction in hepatic cellular function and hepatic metabolic activity occurs with inhalation anesthetics but is not problematic as are the rarely occurring halothane hepatitis and acute hepatic necrosis, which probably are caused by an immune mechanism.

Neuromuscular Blockade in Anesthesia

Profound muscle relaxation can facilitate endotracheal intubation, facilitate some surgical procedures (e.g., intraabdominal ones), and reduce the level of anesthesia necessary to prevent movement. Several intravenous drugs (Table 3-5) are available to block the neuromuscular junction. The historical side effects of histamine release, which causes hypotension and cardiac muscarinic receptor blockade that causes tachycardia, have been reduced or eliminated in new agents.

For many years the degree of muscle relaxation and the need for additional relaxant were based on a subjective evaluation by the anesthesiologist and the surgeon; now, however, the degree of muscle paralysis can be quantified with the use of electric nerve stimulation. This practice improves operating conditions and decreases the likelihood of postoperative hypoventilation or apnea from an overdose of muscle relaxants. Even if a patient's abdominal musculature is completely paralyzed by muscle relaxants, the operating conditions may still not seem optimal to the surgeon. For example, a very obese patient with a low-lying rib cage, a patient with intestinal obstruction and distension, or a patient with an inadequate abdominal incision all might appear "tight," yet the problem with exposure is

TABLE 3-4   Inhalation Anesthetics

Generic Name	Trade Name	Minimum Alveolar Concentration (%)	Blood/ Gas Solubility	Boiling Point* (° C)
Nitrous oxide	—	105	0.47	−89
Enflurane	Ethrane	1.6	1.8	56.5
Isoflurane	Forane	1.2	1.4	48.5
Halothane	Fluothane	0.76	2.3	50.2
Desflurane	—	6-7	0.42	23.5

*At 1 atmosphere.

mechanical and cannot be improved by the administration of additional muscle relaxants.

The disappearance of succinylcholine's effect occurs in 5 to 10 minutes because of its metabolism by pseudocholinesterase, a circulating hydrolytic enzyme that may be congenitally abnormal and ineffective in 1 of 3200 patients. When excessive amounts of succinylcholine are administered, a phase II block may produce prolonged muscle weakness or paralysis for which there is no pharmacologic antidote. Ventilation should be supported mechanically in these patients until the effects of the muscle relaxant are dissipated. Nondepolarizing neuromuscular blockade such as that caused by curare, pancuronium, atracurium, and others may be antagonized by the buildup of acetylcholine at the neuromuscular junction with the administration of an anticholinesterase, neostigmine, or edrophonium. An anticholinergic, glycopyrrolate or atropine, that has no direct effect on the neuromuscular junction is administered concurrently to prevent complications from excessive stimulation of cholinergic muscarinic receptors (e.g., bradycardia, bronchospasm).

POSTANESTHETIC CARE
Hemodynamic Changes

Frequently, as the anesthetic agent is eliminated at the end of the procedure, a significant increase in arterial blood pressure occurs, which may be accompanied by coinciding increases in CVP and pulmonary artery pressures. These changes are due to elimination of the arteriolar relaxation, venodilation, and reduction in catecholamine levels that accompany most general anesthetic regimens. Patients whose hypertension is not adequately controlled preoperatively are more likely to experience hemodynamic lability during induction and emergence from anesthesia. Postoperatively, the patient rarely returns to a basal level of stimulation because of pain from the surgical site and the discomfort of other noxious stimuli such as a full bladder, the endotracheal tube, and the presence of other indwelling catheters. Continued meticulous monitoring, aggressive treatment of unsuitable hemodynamics, and avoidance of a precipitous emergence from anesthesia (e.g., by providing adequate analgesia and avoiding narcotic antagonists) can prevent a stormy wake-up period.

When Should a Patient Be Extubated?

If there is no need for continued mechanical ventilation, generally the endotracheal tube is removed at the end of the procedure when the patient becomes responsive to verbal commands or otherwise indicates cortical brain function. Clinical judgment that adequate spontaneous ventilation has returned and that muscular function is normal (i.e., successful antagonism of

TABLE 3-5 Muscle Relaxants

Generic Name	Trade Name	Histamine Release	Heart Rate
Depolarizing Neuromuscular Blockers			
Succinylcholine	Anectine	+	−
Nondepolarizing Neuromuscular Blockers			
Intermediate-Acting			
Atracurium	Tracrium	+	0
Vecuronium	Norcuron	0	0
Long-Acting			
d-Tubocurarine	Tubocurarine	+ +	0
Metocurine	Metubine	+	0
Pancuronium	Pavulon	0	+
Pipecuronium	Arduan	0	0
Doxacurium	Neuromax	0	0

+ = slight response or increase; + + = moderate response; 0 = no change; − = a slight reduction.

neuromuscular blockers) is used rather than specific laboratory assessment of ventilation (e.g., acceptable arterial blood gas values, vital capacity >15 ml/kg, inspiratory force > − 20 cm H$_2$O). If there were preexisting pulmonary insufficiency or an altered level of consciousness or if pulmonary or neurologic impairment could have resulted from the procedure, the endotracheal tube is not removed until the anesthetic agents are gone and the patient's underlying condition can be evaluated.

In most cases having the patient awake before removing the endotracheal tube is desirable because the risk of aspiration is reduced. However, special conditions such as an open ophthalmologic or tympanic grafting procedure may benefit from extubation while the patient is deeply anesthetized to avoid the possibility of coughing and thus increasing intraocular pressure and venous oozing, respectively. In any case, the patient must be capable of spontaneously supporting a patent airway and adequate ventilation before extubation. Patients in whom there is airway compromise secondary to tissue edema frequently are left intubated until the edema recedes.

Indications for Postoperative Ventilatory Support

Based on the patient's pulmonary condition, the physiologic consequences of the procedure performed, and other anesthetic factors, the anesthesiologist decides whether the patient should be permitted to breathe spontaneously at the conclusion of the procedure or whether mechanical ventilatory support is required during the postoperative period.

Pulmonary Considerations. A patient with underlying respiratory insufficiency who undergoes an anesthetic of long duration or a procedure within the upper abdomen or thorax will often require continued ventilatory support. Postoperatively lung volumes and pulmonary compliance are often decreased, and airway resistance and the work of breathing are increased. In addition, the site of the surgical incision may alter the mechanics of ventilation, secretions may accumulate, and atelectasis often develops. Surgery on the lung itself may mandate postoperative mechanical ventilation unless only a small portion of the lung is involved and the remaining parenchyma functions normally.

Procedural Requirements. Circulatory instability continuing into the postoperative period may demand continued ventilatory support so

that poor ventilation does not contribute to that instability. Similarly, patients with increased intracranial pressure or progressive cerebral edema require controlled hyperventilation to produce hypocarbia, which, in turn, lowers cerebral blood flow and intracranial pressure.

Other Patient Requirements. If adequate muscular strength cannot be restored after the use of neuromuscular blocking drugs, ventilatory support is continued. Ventilation is also supplemented when severe intraoperative hypothermia requires rewarming, which increases oxygen consumption that some patients will not be able to match with adequate oxygen delivery. Intraoperative fluid overload that results in compromised pulmonary gas exchange may also indicate a need for postoperative ventilation, usually with the application of PEEP.

Postanesthesia Recovery Room

For the patient who will not need continued intensive nursing care, the recovery room provides an environment in which trained personnel and adequate monitoring are available to deal with problems occurring during the resolution of anesthesia or resulting from the surgical procedure. Problems often requiring treatment in the recovery room include the following: airway compromise, hypoventilation and hypoxemia, excessive sedation or agitation, hypertension or hypotension, cardiac dysrhythmias, bleeding, oliguria, hypothermia or fever, and nausea and vomiting. During the recovery room stay not only should pain be treated, but an appropriate pain management regimen also should be established that will continue to provide control once the patient is discharged. Some recovery rooms have an anesthesiologist in attendance, whereas others depend on the anesthesiologist and surgeon who treated the patient in the operating room to provide direction.

When Should a Patient Be Discharged From the Recovery Room? Patients should not be discharged from the recovery room to routine hospital care until they have recovered from anesthesia and remained free of any acute complications of the surgical procedure for a reasonable period of time. Both the recovery room admission and discharge status should be agreed on by a physician and the nurse and recorded on the patient's hospital chart. Some hospitals evaluate their patients by a recovery room score (Table 3-6) on admission to the recovery room and permit the nurses to transfer the patients to floor care when a score of at least nine of a possible 10

TABLE 3-6 Postanesthetic Recovery Room Score*

Characteristic	Score	Criterion
Activity	2	Moves all four extremities
	1	Moves two extremities
	0	Unable to move any extremities
Respiration	2	Able to breathe deeply and cough freely
	1	Dyspnea; limited respiratory effort
	0	No spontaneous respiratory effort
Circulation	2	SBP within 20% of preoperative pressure; no ECG change
	1	SBP changed 20%-50% from preoperative pressure; minor ECG changes
	0	SBP more than 50% changed; major ECG changes
Consciousness	2	Full awareness; answering questions
	1	Aroused by hearing name called
	0	No response to auditory stimuli
Color	2	Pink
	1	Pale, dusky, or blotchy
	0	Cyanotic nails, lips, or skin

Modified from Aldrete JA, Kroulik D. A postanesthetic recovery score. Anesth Analg 49:924-933, 1970.
SBP = systolic blood pressure.
*The points scored in each section are added for a maximal possible score of 10.

is achieved. The patient who is not able to return to routine hospital care requires transfer to the critical care unit, where cooperative management between the critical care physicians and the anesthesiologist and surgeon is imperative. For outpatients who will not be admitted to the hospital when criteria for recovery room discharge are met, a transition area is often provided where a patient can wear his or her own clothing, ambulate, eat, drink, visit relatives, and, in general, continue to recuperate until ready to leave.

Postoperative Pain Management

Oral Analgesics. Oral nonnarcotic analgesics have limited potency and require a functioning alimentary tract. Oral opioids have variable efficacy because of their unpredictable absorption. Regrettably, at this time outpatient surgery patients must rely on these modalities. Predictable transcutaneous opioid delivery may be a practical approach for the future.

Intramuscular Analgesics. The traditional intermittent intramuscular administration of opioids markedly undertreats some patients and excessively sedates others, sometimes causing severe hypoventilation. The introduction of a nonnarcotic, potent parenteral analgesic, ketorolac, has provided a new approach to satisfactory

postoperative analgesia in patients with respiratory insufficiency.

Patient-Controlled Analgesia (PCA). The self-administration of opioids intravenously, with the incremental dosage and frequency limitations set by the physician, addresses the wide range of dosage requirements for opioid analgesics from one patient to another. The risk of severe hypoventilation or airway obstruction is low because of a hierarchical response to opioids; that is, either sedation that causes the patient to stop triggering the delivery device or adequate analgesia will occur before airway or ventilatory compromise. However, for this to be true, an individual aliquot must not be excessive, and there must be sufficient time for the effects of an aliquot to occur before another is delivered. A typical dosing regimen for a 70-kg patient is 1.5 to 2 mg of morphine per incremental dose, followed by a 10-minute lockout period (another dose cannot be delivered), or 15 mg of meperidine with a 6-minute lockout period. Necessarily, intravenous access must be maintained. In some patients a basal infusion rate of narcotic is administered (e.g., 0.5 to 2 mg morphine per 70 kg per hour), and the patient adds to this dosage by triggering the delivery device. For patients who have great fear of postoperative pain, patient-controlled analgesia is extremely well received because it allows them to remain in control of their pain.

Peripheral Nerve Blocks With Local Anesthetics. After procedures on the extremities or in thoracic dermatome distributions local anesthetic blocks may be performed for postoperative pain control. The analgesia is profound but of limited duration. The coincident sympathetic nervous system block may promote blood flow to marginally perfused tissues at the surgical site (e.g., skin flaps). However, the motor and sensory deficits in the distribution of the block prevent neurologic evaluation. The blocked extremity must be protected by an informed and capable patient. The degree of analgesia provided is not compatible with adequate monitoring of an extremity that must be enclosed within a cast. Blocks of the brachial plexus, femoral nerve, intercostal nerves, and directly into the margins of the incision often are used. Local anesthetic injection into the interpleural space gives the same effect as intercostal blocks at multiple levels.

Intrathecal and Epidural Opioids. The application of opioids in small amounts (compared with parenteral dosages) to the dorsal horn of the spinal cord produces analgesia in that dermatomal distribution. In practice, narcotics, usually morphine or fentanyl, can be administered by bolus or continuous infusion into the epidural space where they diffuse into the CSF and bind to the spinal cord receptors or can be injected into the CSF directly. Because of migration of the drug within the CSF, lumbar epidural administration may be used to treat thoracotomy pain or, in general, pain from any site in the thoracic, lumbar, or sacral distributions. However, the more closely the site of administration and the dermatomal distribution of the pain are matched, the less opioid that is required, and the side effects are reduced. The lack of sedation and continuous course of analgesia are the main attributes of epidural opioids. Because motor blockade does not occur, early mobility is possible. Since sympathetic fibers also continue to function, postural hypotension is not a problem. Although combinations of very dilute local anesthetic solutions with opioids can increase analgesia, motor weakness and partial sympathetic block can become problems.

Complications of Intrathecal and Epidural Narcotic Administration. As greater quantities of drug are infused (e.g., to achieve pain relief after thoracotomy by injection into the lumbar epidural space), central opioid symptoms increase. Central effects include nausea, pruritus, sedation, and respiratory depression. Interest-ingly, simultaneous naloxone infusion often decreases CNS symptoms but does not eliminate analgesia. Patients receiving spinal opioids must always be monitored for respiratory depression, which fortunately is slow enough in onset that conscientiously counting the respiratory rate hourly will detect impending difficulty. Urinary retention is a potential problem with spinal opioids just as with local anesthetics. Providing postoperative anticoagulation after vascular procedures or for other medical indications is not compatible with the presence of an indwelling epidural catheter. Maintaining the epidural catheter in situ for several days postoperatively is not associated with an increased risk of epidural abscess or tract infection provided that aseptic technique is carefully observed during catheter insertion. Surgeons must also be aware that analgesia may be so effective that postoperative surgical complications that would otherwise be indicated by severe pain may be masked.

Anesthesiologist's Postoperative Visit

All patients, except perhaps those outpatients who leave the hospital soon after their procedures, should be visited postoperatively by the anesthesiologist. During this visit the anesthesiologist evaluates the patient for complications attributable to anesthesia and institutes appropriate therapy. This visit allows the anesthesiologist to observe the consequences of his or her evaluation and management of preoperative findings and provides the patient with the opportunity to inform the anesthesiologist of his or her perceptions of the anesthetic experience. Should the patient have displayed any adverse reaction to the procedure, the anesthesiologist must discuss it with the patient and provide information that the patient should then give to a future anesthesiologist should anesthesia again be necessary.

MEDICOLEGAL CONSIDERATIONS
Informed Consent

The patient deserves to have all anesthetic options presented (e.g., regional versus general anesthesia) when more than one approach is appropriate. Ancillary procedures (e.g., epidural catheter or pulmonary artery catheter insertion) should also be explained. Depending on psychologic makeup, one patient may want every step of the procedure explained in detail, whereas another will request only a superficial explanation because the details create excessive anxiety. From a medicolegal standpoint, it is difficult to know exactly what constitutes *informed consent,* an approval to proceed with the proposed plan that is made with knowledge of its possible consequences. It is unlikely that any patient is unaware that severe complications can occur during anesthesia, the worst of which is death. On the other hand, many do not wish to have the details of the potential complications verbalized, and in some cases an attempt to inform patients completely has frightened them to the point that they have refused necessary surgery. In any event, the anesthesiologist should tell the patient both the likely complications (e.g., nausea and vomiting and postoperative pain) and, if the patient wishes such information, the severe but rare hazards of anesthesia (e.g., myocardial infarction and stroke).

Is the Surgeon Liable for the Conduct of Anesthesia Delivered by an Anesthesiologist?

Liability is determined by the court in each specific case; however, the presence or absence of an anesthesiologist influences the judgment. *If an anesthesiologist personally administers the anesthetic, the surgeon should not be held liable for its improper administration.* If the surgeon wishes additional monitors or other safeguards to be used, he or she should request them. However, the surgeon and anesthesiologist both have a duty to protect the patient against the obvious negligence of the other. At the conclusion of anesthesia, there should be a clear understanding between the surgeon and the anesthesiologist as to who will provide subsequent care. Frequently this is a shared responsibility.

Is the Surgeon Liable for the Conduct of Anesthesia Delivered by a Certified Registered Nurse Anesthetist?

If a certified registered nurse anesthetist (CRNA) is involved and if the CRNA is employed and supervised or medically directed by an anesthesiologist, the surgeon's responsibility should be no different from when an anesthesiologist personally performs the anesthesia. If the CRNA is hospital employed but medically directed on site by an anesthesiologist, the same lines of responsibility apply.

The surgeon clearly is the supervisor or medical-directing physician and therefore is liable when a hospital-employed or self-employed CRNA is administering anesthesia and the surgeon is the only physician in attendance. The CRNA may also be held directly liable for negligence in the administration of an anesthetic. However, since the laws regarding nursing practice in most states specify that a nurse anesthetist must administer anesthesia under the supervision of a licensed medical, osteopathic, or dental practitioner, there is no question that in such cases the surgeon is responsible. Unfortunately, many surgeons do not realize this until they are embroiled in a legal suit for alleged malpractice. Denial of such responsibility by the surgeon based on ignorance of the law or limited knowledge in the practice of anesthesia has not been a successful defense.

PITFALLS AND COMMON MYTHS

- Anesthetic techniques and agents must be matched to an individual patient's requirements.
- Safe conscious sedation requires appropriate patient selection; an assistant familiar with the drugs used who is able to recognize and correct airway obstruction; monitoring of blood pressure, pulse, and oxygenation; equipment, including suction, an oxygen delivery system, and an emergency cart; intravenous access; written documentation of vital signs and medications; and a suitable recovery area.

- A pulse oximeter is a useful device to detect hypoxemia, but airway obstruction or hypoventilation can be detected well in advance of hypoxemia by observing the patient and auscultating breath sounds.
- When endotracheal intubation is difficult, remember that oxygenation and ventilation of the patient are the primary goals and they cannot be achieved during extended and unproductive attempts at intubation.
- Who is responsible during anesthesia? Everyone!

SURGICAL PHARMACOPEIA

Drug	Indications	Complications/Comments	Dosage
Anticholinergics			
Atropine	Bradycardia, anti-sialagog	Tachycardia, confusion	0.2-0.4 mg IM, IV bolus, then prn
Glycopyrrolate	Bradycardia, anti-sialagog	Cannot cross blood-brain barrier—hence no CNS adverse effects (sedation or confusion)	0.1-0.4 mg IM, IV bolus, then prn
Scopolamine	Anti-sialagog, amnesia, sedation	Confusion, delirium	0.2-0.6 mg IM, IV bolus, then prn
Anticholinesterases			
Edrophonium chloride	Reversal of neuro-muscular blockade; supraventricular tachycardia	Causes bradycardia (should be given with anticholinergics)	0.5-1 mg/kg IV
Neostigmine	Reversal of neuro-muscular blockade	Causes bradycardia (should be given with anticholinergics)	0.06 mg/kg IV
Antihypertensives			
Esmolol hydrochloride	Short-acting β_1 antagonist (for intraoperative tachycardia, hypertension)	Contraindicated in congestive heart failure	0.5 mg/kg bolus IV, then titrate
Hydralazine	Vasodilator	Can cause reflex tachycardia	5-20 mg q4-6h IV or prn 20-40 mg q6h PO
Labetalol hydrochloride	Selective α_1 and nonselective β_1 and β_2 antagonist	Can precipitate conges-tive heart failure, bronchospasm, A-V block; α/β ratio is $1:3$ for oral and $1:7$ for IV administration	5-20 mg q15min, up to 1 mg/kg IV 200-400 mg q12h PO
Nifedipine	Hypertension, angina, coronary vasospasm		10-20 mg q6-12h PO or SL
Nitroglycerine	Vasodilator: venous at low dose, arterial at higher dose		IV: begin at 10 μg/min, then titrate
Nitroprusside	Arterial and veno-dilator used for hypertension	Can cause cyanide toxicity	1-10 μg/kg/min IV
Barbiturates			
Methohexital (Brevital)	Induction of anesthesia	Mild cardiovascular depression, respiratory depression	1-2 mg/kg IV bolus
Pentobarbital (Nembutal)	Sedation; brain protection	Some respiratory depression	For sedation: 100-200 mg PO, or 50-100 mg IV

Drug	Indications	Complications/ Comments	Dosage
Pentobarbital (Nembutal)—cont'd			For increased intracranial pressure: Load with 15 mg/kg IV, then 1.5 mg/kg/h
Secobarbital (Seconal)	Sedation	Some respiratory depression	100-200 mg PO, or 50-100 mg IV bolus
Thiopental (Pentothal)	Induction of anesthesia	Some cardiovascular depression, respiratory depression	3-5 mg/kg IV bolus
Benzodiazepines			
Diazepam (Valium)	Anxiety, seizures, ethyl alcohol withdrawal	Can cause CNS depression, hypotension; painful with IM or IV injection	2.5-5.0 mg IV q6-8h 5-10 mg PO q6-8h
Lorazepam (Ativan)	Anxiety	CNS depression; may cause hypotension; amnesia	1-2 mg IV q8-12h 1-4 mg PO q8-12h
Midazolam (Versed)	Anxiety	CNS depression, hypotension, amnesia; respiratory depression with subsequent death can occur if given too quickly	0.5-1 mg IV, increasing slowly in $\frac{1}{2}$ to 1 mg increments, up to 5 mg over a 10 min period; 2-5 mg IM
Induction Agents			
Etomidate (Amidate)	Induction of anesthesia	Minimal cardiovascular effects; may provide more hemodynamic stability than other induction agents	0.2-0.3 mg/kg IV bolus
Ketamine (Ketalar)	Induction of general anesthesia; dressing changes	Causes tachycardia and hypertension; can cause cardiac depression in critically ill, catecholamine-depleted patients	For induction of general anesthesia: 1-3 mg/kg IV bolus; 5-10 mg/kg IM bolus For dressing changes: 1-2 mg/kg initially, then 0.25-0.5 mg/kg q10-20min
Propofol	Induction of anesthesia; maintenance of anesthesia	Mild hemodynamic depression	1-3 mg/kg IV bolus
Thiopental, methohexital sodium (see barbiturates)			
Inhaled Anesthetics			
Desflurane	Inhaled anesthetic	Can cause cardiac depression	Titrate

Continued.

Drug	Indications	Complications/ Comments	Dosage
Enflurane	Inhaled anesthetic	Can cause cardiac depression	Titrate
Halothane	Inhaled anesthetic	Can cause cardiac depression	Titrate
Isoflurane	Inhaled anesthetic	Can cause cardiac depression; also causes vasodilation and ↓ systemic vascular resistance; hence overall effect on CO is less than other inhaled agents	Titrate
Nitrous oxide	Inhaled anesthetic of low potency	Can cause ↑ size of air filled spaces (i.e., pneumothorax, bowel obstruction); normally used with another inhaled or IV agent	

Inotropes, Catecholamines, and Sympathomimetics

Drug	Indications	Complications/ Comments	Dosage
Dobutamine hydrochloride	Hemodynamic support β_1 agonist	Tachycardia, dysrhythmias, hypertension	2.5-15 μg/kg/min IV
Dopamine hydrochloride	Hemodynamic support α, β, and dopaminergic agonist; oliguria	Dysrhythmias, hypertension	*Renal effect:* Low doses 2-5 μg/kg/min IV β_1 *effect:* 5-10 μg/kg/min IV α_1 *effect:* ≥15 μg/kg/min IV
Ephedrine sulfate	Hemodynamic support α and β	Dysrhythmias, hypertension	5-20 mg prn IV
Epinephrine	Hemodynamic support, CPR, bronchospasm, anaphylaxis	Dysrhythmias, hypertension	IV: 0.5 μg/min, then titrate 1-2 μg/min—β_2; 4 μg/min—β_1; 10-20 μg/min $\alpha_1 > \beta_1$ or β_2; for anaphylaxis 1:1000 solution: 0.1-0.5 ml q10-15min × 3
Amrinone lactate (Inocor)	Hemodynamic support		1-2 mg/kg load IV, then 2-10 μg/kg/min IV
Norepinephrine bitartrate (Levophed bitartrate)	Hemodynamic support Primarily α_1, some β_1	Often mixed with α_1-blocker for renal protection; hypertension can occur	IV: begin at 1-2 μg/min and titrate
Phenylephrine hydrochloride	Hemodynamic support Primarily α_1	Hypertension can occur	50-200 μg prn IV

Drug	Indications	Complications/ Comments	Dosage
Local Anesthetics *Amides*			
Bupivacaine (Marcaine hydrochloride)	Long-acting regional anesthetic	Seizures; cardiac depression; dosage and route of administration vary with use	Max: 2.5 mg/kg without epinephrine; 3.2 mg/kg with epinephrine
Etidocaine hydrochloride (Duranest)	Long-acting regional anesthetic	Seizures, cardiac depression; dosage and route of administration vary with use	Max: 6 mg/kg without epinephrine; 8 mg/kg with epinephrine
Lidocaine hydrochloride (Xylocaine)	Intermediate-acting regional anesthetic	Seizures, cardiac depression; dosage and route of administration vary with use	Max: 4 mg/kg without epinephrine; 7 mg/kg with epinephrine
Mepivicaine hydrochloride (Carbocaine hydrochloride)	Intermediate-acting regional anesthetic	Seizures, cardiac depression; dosage and route of administration vary with use	4 mg/kg without epinephrine; 7 mg/kg with epinephrine
Esters			
Benzocaine (Hurricaine)	Short-acting topical local anesthetic	Seizures, cardiac depression	Max: 3 mg/kg
Chloroprocaine (Nesacaine hydrochloride)	Short-acting local anesthetic	Seizures, cardiac depression; dosage and route of administration vary with use	Max: 10 mg/kg without epinephrine; 14 mg/kg with epinephrine
Cocaine	Topical local anesthetic	Seizures, dysrhythmias, cardiac depression	Max: 2 mg/kg
Procaine hydrochloride	Short-acting local anesthetic	Seizures, cardiac depression; dosage and route of administration vary with use	Max: 7 mg/kg without epinephrine; 10 mg/kg with epinephrine
Tetracaine hydrochloride (Pontocaine, Cetacaine)	Long-acting local anesthetic	Seizures, cardiac depression; dosage and route of administration vary with use	Max: 0.3 mg/kg for all forms of this drug

Vasoconstrictors

Used in conjunction with some forms of regional anesthesia to:
1. Decrease uptake of local anesthetics and thus its blood level
2. Prolong regional block

Drug	Indications	Complications/ Comments	Dosage
Epinephrine 1:200,000- 1:400,000	Prolongs regional block with local anesthetics	Systemic effects can occur	Add 2.5-5 μg epinephrine per ml of local anesthetic

Miscellaneous Pain Medications

Drug	Indications	Complications/ Comments	Dosage
Butorphanol tartrate (Stadol)	Agonist-antagonist used for pain relief	CNS depression, respiratory depression	1-2 mg q3-6h IV 1-4 mg q3-6h IM

Continued.

Drug	Indications	Complications/ Comments	Dosage
Ketorolac (Toradol)	Potent nonsteroidal anti-inflammatory drug; no CNS or respiratory depression	Can cause renal insufficiency by decreasing synthesis of renal prostaglandins	60 mg loading dose IM or IV, then 30 mg q4-6h IV or IM
Nalbuphine hydrochloride (Nubain)	Agonist-antagonist used for pain relief, sedation	CNS and respiratory depression	5-10 mg q3-6h IV, IM

Neuromuscular Blockers

Drug	Indications	Complications/ Comments	Dosage
Atracurium (Tracrium)	Muscle relaxation	Intermediate-acting (20-45 min); no significant hemo-dynamic effects; may cause some histamine release with larger doses	0.4-0.5 mg/kg IV; may be given as a continuous infusion at 5-10 μg/kg/min
Curare	Muscle relaxation	Intermediate-acting (30-90 min); may cause histamine release, resulting in hypotension	0.6 mg/kg IV q60-90min prn
Pancuronium	Muscle relaxation	Long-acting (60-90 min); may cause 10-15% increase in heart rate and blood pressure	0.1 mg/kg
Pipecuronium (Arduan)	Muscle relaxation	Long-acting (60-90 min)	0.15 mg/kg IV q60-90min prn
Succinylcholine chloride (Anectine)	Muscle relaxation, usually for intubation	Short-acting (5-10 min); may cause life-threat-ening hyperkalemia in patient with burns, paralysis (upper and lower motor neuron lesions), muscular dystrophy, Guillain-Barré syndrome, massive tissue trauma; can cause ↑ ICP	1-2 mg/kg IV bolus
Vecuronium (Norcuron)	Muscle relaxation	Intermediate-acting (20-45 min); no significant hemo-dynamic effects	0.1 mg/kg IV q30-60min prn; may be given as continuous infusion

Opiates

Drug	Indications	Complications/ Comments	Dosage
Alfentanil hydrochloride	Pain relief	Supplement to general anesthesia; respiratory depression; hypoten-sion	8-50 μg/kg prn IV

Drug	Indications	Complications/ Comments	Dosage
Fentanyl citrate (Sublimaze)	Pain relief (analgesia); induction of anesthesia	Respiratory depression, hypotension, nausea/ vomiting; can be given epidurally	1-3 μg/kg prn IV For cardiac anesthesia: 50-120 μg/kg total dose IV
Meperidine hydrochloride (Demerol)	Pain relief	Mild cardiovascular depression, respiratory depression, tachy-cardia	25-100 mg q4-6h IV; 25-100 mg q4-6h IM; 50-100 mg q4-6h PO
Morphine sulfate	Pain, sedation	Respiratory depression, hypotension, nausea-vomiting; can be given epidurally	1-10 mg total dose q4-6h IV, in fractionated doses over a 15 min period 5-10 mg q4-6h IM
Sufentanil citrate	Pain relief, induction of anesthesia	Respiratory depression, hypotension; can be given epidurally	0.2-0.8 μg/kg IV prn For cardiac anesthesia: 20-40 μg/kg total dose IV
Naloxone hydrochloride (Narcan)	Reversal of narcotic respiratory depres-sion or sedation	Can cause sympathetic discharge, reversal of analgesia	0.4 mg or higher IV prn
Miscellaneous			
Droperidol	Nausea/vomiting	Dysphoria or sedation with higher dose	0.625-1.25 mg or higher q6-8h IV, prn
Hydroxyzine hydrochloride (Vistaril)	Sedation, nausea/ vomiting	Minimal respiratory depression; IV injection may cause thrombosis	25-100 mg q4-6h IM; 25-100 mg q6-8h PO
Metoclopramide hydrochloride (Reglan)	Nausea/vomiting	Can cause ↑ gastric emptying and ↑ small bowel peristalsis; contraindicated in small bowel obstruction or gastric outlet obstruction	10-20 mg q4-6h IV, PO
Promethazine hydrochloride (Phenergan)	Nausea/vomiting	Sedation	12.5-25 mg q4-6h IV, IM, PO

BIBLIOGRAPHY

Birmingham PK, Cheney FW, Ward RJ. Esophageal intubation: A review of detection techniques. Anesth Analg 65:886-891, 1986.

Brown DL. Atlas of Regional Anesthesia. Philadelphia, WB Saunders, 1991.

Cousins MJ, Mather LE. Intrathecal and epidural administration of opiates. Anesthesiology 61:276-310, 1984.

Danjani AS, Bisno AL, Chung KJ, et al. Prevention of bacterial endocarditis: Recommendations by the American Heart Association. JAMA 264:2919-2922, 1990.

Ferrante FM, Ostheimer GW, Covino BG. Patient-controlled analgesia. Boston, Blackwell Scientific Publications, 1990.

Grabb WC. A concentration of 1:500,000 epinephrine in a local anesthetic solution is sufficient to provide excellent hemostasis. Plast Reconstr Surg 63:834, 1979.

Kaplan EB, Sheiner LB, Boeckmann AJ, et al. The usefulness of preoperative laboratory screening. JAMA 253:3576-3581, 1985.

Kelleher JF. Pulse oximetry. J Clin Monit 5:37-62, 1989.

Longnecker DE, Murphy FL. Dripps, Eckenhoff, Vandam, Introduction to Anesthesia, 8th ed. Philadelphia, WB Saunders, 1992.

Miller RD. Anesthesia, 3rd ed. New York, Churchill Livingstone, 1990.

Minami H, McCallum RW. The physiology and pathophysiology of gastric emptying in humans. Gastroenterology 86:1592-1610, 1984.

Norfleet EA, Watson CB. Continuous mixed venous oxygen saturation measurement: A significant advance in hemodynamic monitoring? J Clin Monit 1:245-285, 1985,

Sieber FE, Smith DS, Traystman RJ, et al. Glucose: A reevaluation of its intraoperative use. Anesthesiology 67:72-81, 1987.

Stoelting RK, Miller RD. Basics of Anesthesia, 2nd ed. New York, Churchill Livingstone, 1989.

Yeager MP, Glass DD, Neff RK, et al. Epidural anesthesia and analgesia in high-risk surgical patients. Anesthesiology 66:729-736, 1987.

CHAPTER REVIEW
Questions

1. Premedications ordered for a 30-year-old undergoing an open reduction and internal fixation of a recent tibial fracture with general anesthesia would probably *not* include which of the following?
   a. Oral diazepam
   b. Cimetidine
   c. Atropine
   d. Metoclopramide
   e. Meperidine

2. Immediately after extubation the oxygen saturation displayed on the pulse oximeter indicates 80%. This measurement *cannot* be explained by which of the following?
   a. Hypoxemia due to postextubation laryngospasm
   b. Movement artifact
   c. Hypothermia
   d. Interference from warming lights
   e. Inaccurate machine calibration

3. The continuously displayed mixed venous oxygen saturation decreases from 70% to 55% over 15 minutes. This *cannot* be explained by which of the following?
   a. Rapid blood loss
   b. Inhalation anesthesia overdose
   c. A grand mal seizure
   d. Administration of dobutamine
   e. Tension pneumothorax

4. Which of the following is the best immediate indicator of successful endotracheal intubation of the trachea?
   a. Easy movement of gas to and fro
   b. Persistent detection of exhaled carbon dioxide
   c. An endotracheal tube cuff palpated in the suprasternal notch
   d. Vapor in the endotracheal tube on exhalation
   e. Pulse oximetry saturation greater than 90%

5. Which of the following is *not* a beneficial effect of glucose infusion intraoperatively?
   a. Cerebral protection during ischemia
   b. Prevention of the mobilization of fatty acids
   c. Prevention of starvation ketoacidosis
   d. Prevention of hypoglycemia
   e. Enhancement of glycogen stores

6. Which statement is false? Allergic reactions to local anesthetic injections:
   a. Are more common with ester than amide agents.
   b. May be due to methylparaben.
   c. Are often confused with epinephrine effects.
   d. Can cause anaphylaxis.
   e. Include circumoral numbness and tinnitus.

7. Which statement is false? Propofol:
   a. Can provide complete anesthesia.
   b. Is associated with nausea and vomiting.
   c. Is dissolved in a milklike solution.
   d. Permits rapid awakening.
   e. Often causes hypotension.

Answers

1. c	5. a
2. e	6. e
3. d	7. b
4. b	

4

Diagnostic Imaging of Common Surgical Problems

JANNICE O. AARON
CURT E. LIEBMAN

KEY FEATURES

After reading this chapter you will understand:
- The relative values of computed tomography and magnetic resonance imaging.
- The uses and pitfalls of mammography.
- Needle localization of breast lesions.
- How the radiologist can help a surgeon manage the septic patient.
- Radiologic imaging of the endocrine system.
- Ultrasound and interventional techniques.
- How you would utilize diagnostic imaging to evaluate a patient with gastrointestinal bleeding.
- The radiologist's role in the management of vascular occlusions.
- How the radiologist helps in the diagnosis and management of pulmonary embolus.

The partnership between the surgeon and the radiologic consultant has become increasingly important as diagnostic technology and procedures have become more sophisticated and refined. In addition to providing invaluable information for planning surgical procedures, the radiologist can also confirm a diagnosis, provide legal documentation, and may suggest therapeutic alternatives.

The following sections are designed to assist the surgeon in solving surgical problems in the most expeditious and economic fashion. The more recent diagnostic modalities are emphasized, including a comparison of the indications for magnetic resonance imaging (MRI) and computed tomography (CT). The newest radionuclide scanning agents are also discussed. A section on mammography and needle localizations is included because of the potential for problems and misconceptions by both the surgeon and the radiologist with these procedures. The more common or more recent interventional procedures are also included, as are recent innovations in ultrasonography.

The guidelines presented for the work-up of common surgical problems are intended as a convenient reference, not as a comprehensive or inflexible protocol. Other factors such as availability of services, experience of the radiologist, cost, or contraindications to certain diagnostic procedures may significantly alter the ideal diagnostic work-up. Potential pitfalls associated with the procedures are listed at the end of the chapter.

WHAT ARE THE INDICATIONS FOR USING MRI INSTEAD OF CT IN SURGICAL PATIENTS?

Much confusion still exists about whether to use CT or MRI for evaluation of surgical patients; however, some basic principles may assist in the decision-making process.

MRI images are produced by bombarding the body's protons or hydrogen atoms, which have been aligned in a magnetic field, with radio frequency (RF) waves. The RF waves cause the protons to spin as they pick up energy. As they relax when the RF waves are removed, they give off energy or a signal, which is picked up by detectors and is transmitted to a computer, which converts the information into a gray-scale image.

Each tissue produces a characteristic signal and image, depending on how tightly its protons are bound and the influence of certain elements in its surrounding environment. For example, compact bone, which is bound very tightly, gives off little or no signal, producing a signal void. Water protons are loosely bound and produce a very intense signal. Therefore MRI produces poor images of bone structures requiring fine detail, whereas CT scanning produces an excellent image. Conversely, the x-rays used in CT scanning may be diverted or scattered by the dense bone, producing artifacts that distort the images of the adjacent soft tissues. Thus in this circumstance MRI would be the imaging modality of choice. For example, the posterior fossa and temporal tips may have relatively large lesions detected by MRI that are obscured by bony artifacts on the CT scan (Fig. 4-1). Other advantages of MRI over CT include the absence of ionizing radiation and the ability of MRI to scan in multiple planes, without repositioning the patient, an asset in surgical planning (Fig. 4-2).

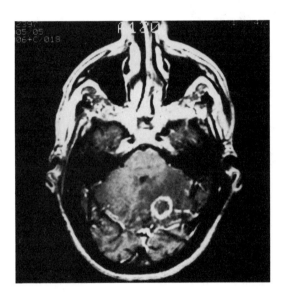

FIGURE 4-1 The best image of the posterior fossa is obtained with MRI because of the absence of bone artifacts, which can obscure pathology on CT scans. This toxoplasmosis lesion is readily apparent on this contrast MRI of a patient with AIDS.

FIGURE 4-2 A sagittal section can be obtained without repositioning the patient using MRI. In this symptomatic patient Arnold-Chiari type I deformity (**arrow**) is readily apparent on the sagittal MRI but is often obscured on CT.

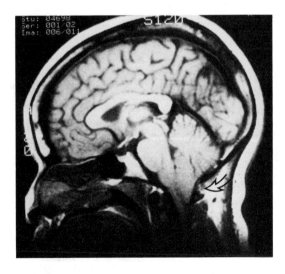

Another disadvantage of MRI is its inability to detect acute hemorrhage, whereas CT is very sensitive in detecting extravascular blood.

The following patients may not be candidates for MRI imaging because of the configuration of the magnet or the adverse effects of the magnetic field: patients whose vital signs are unstable, who have severe claustrophobia, who wear pacemakers, who have metallic foreign bodies, especially in the eye, or who are very obese. Additional problems associated with MRI include lack of training or experience of the radiologist or refusal of payment for certain examinations by third-party insurers. Table 4-1 presents some guidelines that have remained fairly consistent for selecting imaging modalities.

The specificity of MRI continues to improve as more data about the signal characteristics of neoplastic and inflammatory processes become available. The advent of contrast enhancement with gadolinium has significantly increased both the sensitivity and the specificity of the examinations, and its use is probably indicated on a routine basis for MRI of the brain (Figs. 4-9 and 4-10). In some instances using CT and MRI in conjunction greatly increases the specificity of

TABLE 4-1 Guidelines for CT and MRI

MRI More Sensitive and Indicated in Lieu of CT	MRI Equivalent to CT	CT More Sensitive and Indicated in Lieu of MRI
Head and Neck		
Posterior fossa and brain stem pathology	Neck tumor staging	Acute onset of severe headaches
	Salivary glands	Acute stroke
Pituitary and parasellar pathology	Sinuses	Acute trauma
Multiple sclerosis and white matter disease	Laryngeal tumors	Evaluation of bony detail
	Lymphadenopathy	Small calcified lesions
Brain tumor		Temporal bone pathology
Primary and metastases		
Inflammatory disease		
Hydrocephalus		
Dementia		
Chronic headaches		
Seizures		
Visual or hearing loss		
Vertigo/ataxia		
Congenital abnormalities		
AIDS patients		
Parkinson's disease		
Vascular malformations		
Progressive neurologic deficit		
Spine and Spinal Cord		
Congenital abnormalities		Spinal stenosis
Spinal cord and spine tumors		Degenerative arthritic disease of the spine
Spinal cord and spine trauma		Bony abnormalities
Hydromyelia/syringomyelia		
Disk pathology		
Degenerative		
Inflammatory		
Disk herniation (Fig 4-3, *A* and *B*)		
Postoperative		
Diseases of the spinal cord		
Multiple sclerosis		

Continued.

TABLE 4-1 Guidelines for CT and MRI—cont'd

MRI More Sensitive and Indicated in Lieu of CT	MRI Equivalent to CT	CT More Sensitive and Indicated in Lieu of MRI
Spine and Spinal Cord—cont'd		
C1-C2 subluxation and basilar invagination, especially in rheumatoid arthritis		
Thorax		
Congenital heart disease	Pericardial disease	Evaluation of lung parenchyma
Cardiac masses	Aortic dissection	Pleural disease
Mediastinal masses		Rib detail
Hilar masses		
Abdomen		
Liver	Aortic dissection	Liver pathology
Metastases	Aortic aneurysm	Splenic pathology
Hemangiomas	Adrenal mass disease	Pancreatic pathology
Thrombosis of hepatic vein, portal vein		Renal pathology
IVC—thrombosis or tumor		Retroperitoneum for lymphadenopathy abscess (Fig. 4-4)
Status of renal transplant		Gallbladder tumor staging
Renal tumor staging		Clinically suspected abdominal mass (Fig. 4-5)
Diaphragmatic and subdiaphragmatic pathology		Acute intra-abdominal bleeding
Oncology patient for evaluation of residual disease versus fibrosis		
Pelvis		
Cervical carcinoma staging	Bladder carcinoma staging	Pelvic lymphadenopathy
Endometrial carcinoma staging	Rectal carcinoma staging	
Prostate carcinoma staging	Presacral tumor (Fig. 4-6)	
Musculoskeletal System		
Knee		Acute bony injury, especially pelvic and spine fractures
Meniscal, cartilaginous, or ligamentous injuries (Fig. 4-7)		
Baker's cyst or other pathology		
Shoulder		
Rotator cuff tears (Fig. 4-8)		
Joint effusion/other pathology		
Temporomandibular joint—internal derangements		
Soft tissue—tumors/injury		
Bone		
Neoplasm staging		
Metastatic disease		
Osteomyelitis		
Aseptic necrosis of any bone		
Bone marrow disorders		

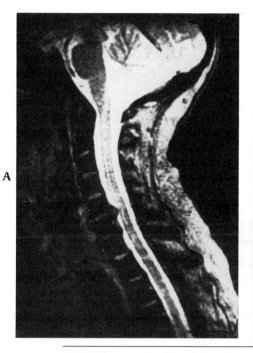

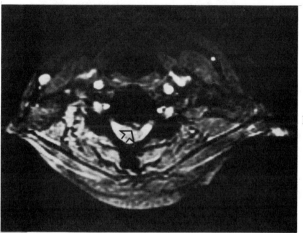

A

B

FIGURE 4-3 MRI of cervical spine showing evidence of degenerative disk disease with a focal central disk herniation seen on both the lateral (**A**) and axial (**B**) sections on this patient.

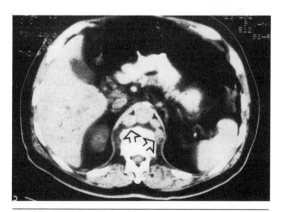

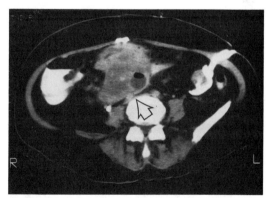

FIGURE 4-4 Both MRI and CT are excellent modalities for tumor staging. This CT of the abdomen shows multiple retrocrural nodes (*arrows*) associated with prostatic metastatic disease.

FIGURE 4-5 Abdominal CT performed on a patient with fever postoperatively demonstrates a large intra-abdominal inhomogeneous mass containing air. This abscess was drained percutaneously with complete resolution.

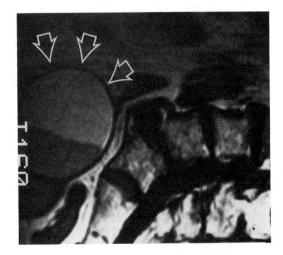

FIGURE 4-6   MRI of the lumbar spine showing a fat-fluid level in a presacral dermoid cyst (*arrows*) incidentally imaged during the lumbar examination.

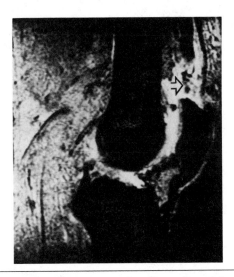

FIGURE 4-7   MRI of the knee showing complete disruption of the quadriceps tendon (*arrow*).

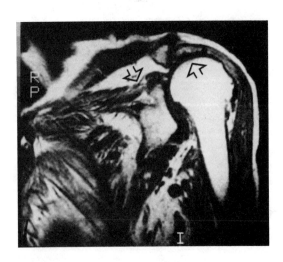

FIGURE 4-8   MRI of the shoulder showing a complete rotator cuff tear (*arrows*).

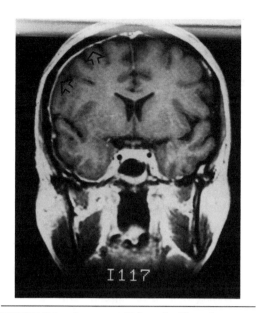

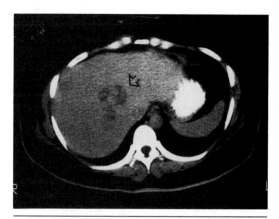

FIGURE 4-11   CT and MRI in conjunction may increase the specificity of an examination. In this young female patient with abnormal liver functions this unusual inhomogeneous lesion (***arrow***) seen on CT was echogenic on ultrasound and had the appearance of normal tissue on MRI and a nuclear medicine liver scan. The findings correlated well with the pathologic diagnosis of focal nodular hyperplasia.

FIGURE 4-9   Contrast MR has significantly increased the sensitivity of MRI scans. This tiny rim subdural hematoma (***arrows***) seen several months after head trauma in a patient with persistent headache was not apparent on non-contrast MRI or a contrast CT of the head.

the examination, with each adding information not available on the other examination (Fig. 4-11).

WHAT IS MAMMOGRAPHY?

Mammography is a radiographic modality for detecting occult breast malignancies in asymptomatic women and is useful in evaluating palpable lesions as well as the remainder of the ipsilateral breast and the contralateral breast.

What Type of Mammographic Equipment Is Best?

Whenever possible, mammograms should be obtained at centers accredited by the American College of Radiology where quality controls are mandatory. Accreditation may be necessary in order to obtain third-party reimbursement. State-of-the-art mammography uses film-screen radiography, which lowers the radiation dosage to the glandular tissue while improving soft tissue contrast.

Availability of real-time ultrasonography using a small parts transducer as a diagnostic adjunct is important, although whole-breast ultrasound is no longer considered a cost-effective diagnostic examination.

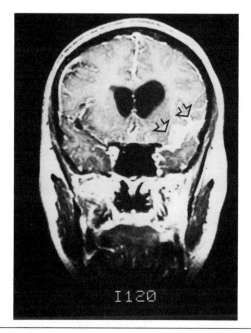

FIGURE 4-10   Contrast MRI shows meningeal enhancement in the sylvian fissure (***arrows***) in this patient with tuberculous meningitis 2 weeks before it was apparent on a contrast CT scan.

What Are the American Cancer Society's Recommendations for Screening Examinations?

The American Cancer Society (ACS) recommendations include the following:

- Age 20 years—begin self-examinations
- Age 20 to 40—medical examination every 3 years
- Age 35 to 40—baseline mammogram
- Age 40 to 49—mammogram every 1 to 2 years; annual medical examination
- Age 50 and older—annual mammogram and medical examination

Bilateral mammography is indicated at any age for a woman with a palpable mass or bloody discharge from the nipple or for whom breast surgery is planned.

What Kind of Cancers and How Many Are Detected on Mammograms?

Eighty-five percent of breast carcinomas are detectable by mammography. Most are adenocarcinomas, 90% of which are ductal and 10% lobular. Conversely, *10% to 15% of breast cancers are not detected on mammography, and a mammogram cannot exclude the presence of breast cancer.*

What Findings on a Mammogram Should Alert the Clinician That the Patient Has a Significant Problem?

- Breast masses. A dense breast mass with a smooth, distinct outline most likely represents a benign lesion such as a cyst or fibroadenoma. However, well-differentiated subtypes of ductal carcinoma such as medullary, mucinous, and papillary carcinomas may have this benign appearance; thus all solid masses greater than 8 mm in diameter are considered suspicious, and performing a biopsy is usually suggested. *Dense breast masses with irregular or stellate shapes or outlines are highly suspicious for malignancies,* and performing a biopsy is recommended.
- Calcifications. Most large calcifications in the breast are associated with benign disease. *Fine, irregular, clustered calcifications are associated with ductal carcinomas, which warrant needle-directed biopsy.*
- Diffusely increased breast density may be associated with diffuse inflammatory carcinoma but more often is seen with mastitis or lymphedema.
- Skin thickening or nipple retraction may be a secondary sign of malignancy.
- A single dilated duct that is associated with a palpable abnormality, bloody discharge, or change from a prior examination may be associated with a ductal malignancy.

What Is the Correct Examination for a Patient With a Bloody Discharge From the Breast?

A mammogram is indicated for a patient with bloody discharge from the breast, but a normal mammogram does not exclude disease. A galactogram in which contrast is instilled into the ducts may outline a lesion in the ducts that cannot be seen on a plain mammogram.

What Procedure Is Followed for a Patient With an Abnormality on Breast Palpation?

See Fig. 4-12.

NEEDLE LOCALIZATION
How Is a Breast Lesion That Cannot Be Felt Removed?

The radiologist can be a tremendous help to the surgeon by placing a needle in or near a nonpalpable suspicious lesion identified on a mammogram (Fig. 4-13, *B*). *Few radiologic procedures have the potential for as much benefit to the patient and the surgeon as a needle localization.* The surgeon, radiologist, pathologist, and patient must all fully understand why and how a needle localization is done, its possible complications, and the limitations of the procedure. Good communication among these individuals is essential to an ongoing successful needle localization program. However, there are many myths about needle localizations.

How Is Needle Localization Performed?

Once a suspicious lesion is identified on a mammogram, the patient is brought to the mammography suite. A scout film using a grid with a hole in it is used to localize the lesion. The breast is prepared with an antiseptic solution, and a local anesthetic agent is injected into the breast. A needle containing a thin, hooked wire is inserted

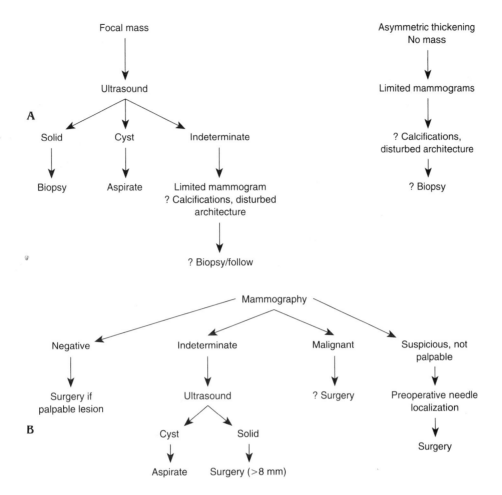

A

Focal mass

↓

Ultrasound

↙ ↓ ↘

Solid | Cyst | Indeterminate

↓ | ↓ | ↓

Biopsy | Aspirate | Limited mammogram
? Calcifications, disturbed
architecture

↓

? Biopsy/follow

Asymmetric thickening
No mass

↓

Limited mammograms

↓

? Calcifications,
disturbed architecture

↓

? Biopsy

B

Mammography

↙ ↓ ↓ ↘

Negative | Indeterminate | Malignant | Suspicious, not palpable

↓ | ↓ | ↓ | ↓

Surgery if palpable lesion | Ultrasound | ? Surgery | Preoperative needle localization

↙ ↘ | | ↓

Cyst | Solid | | Surgery

↓ | ↓

Aspirate | Surgery (>8 mm)

1. A negative mammogram does not obviate the need for a biopsy of a clinically palpable lesion.
2. Ultrasound can differentiate a cyst from a solid mass but cannot differentiate a benign solid mass from a malignant solid mass.

FIGURE 4-12 Algorithm of work-up for examination of a patient with a breast abnormality. **A,** Women who are less than 28 years old or lactating. **B,** Women who are more than 28 years old.

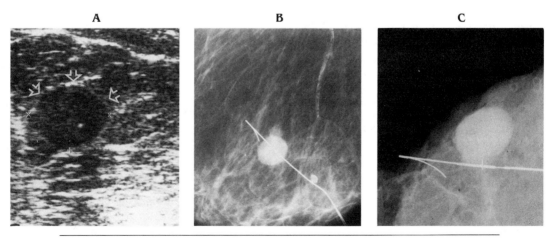

A **B** **C**

FIGURE 4-13 **A,** This breast fibroadenoma (*arrows*), initially believed to represent a cyst, was demonstrated by ultrasound to be a solid lesion. **B,** Needle localization was performed, which assisted the surgeon in removing the lesion. **C,** A specimen radiograph confirmed the presence of the lesion in the specimen.

into the breast through the hole in the grid. The needle may be left in place and secured by the wire, or the needle may be removed, leaving the wire in place, depending on the preference of the surgeon (Fig. 4-13, **B**). Some surgeons believe the flexible wire without the needle is difficult to palpate, making it difficult to dissect along its course.

What Are Some of the Myths About Mammography and Needle Localizations?

Myth: Needle Localizations Are Easy to Perform. In fact, most needle localizations are fairly simple to do; however, lesions in patients with large breasts, very thin breasts, mobile lesions, fibrous changes that divert the needle, or very deep lesions and multiple lesions may be extremely difficult to localize.

Myth: The Lesion Should Always Be at the Tip of the Needle. Ideally, the tip of the needle would be in the lesion; however, the current literature indicates that a lesion that is within 1 cm of the wire or needle is adequately localized. The mammographer may need to relay the location of a lesion to the surgeon as anterior, posterior, medial, lateral, or deep to the wire, and *the surgeon should always review the postlocalization mammogram film before anesthetizing the patient.*

Myth: Radiography of Biopsy Specimens of Noncalcified Lesions Is Not Needed. All biopsy specimens *must* undergo radiography to determine whether the lesion is present in the specimen before closing the incision, unless the surgeon can clearly palpate the lesion in the specimen (Fig. 4-13, **C**). The reported missed lesion rate is 4% nationally. Many surgeons routinely obtain a follow-up limited mammogram of the breast that was biopsied within 4 to 6 months. The radiograph of the biopsy specimen, with the wire in place should accompany the specimen to the pathology laboratory to guide the pathologist when he or she is sectioning the specimen.

Myth: A Special Informed Consent Is Not Necessary for a Needle Localization. There are complications unique to needle localizations. The patient must be informed of the possibility of:

- Fainting secondary to a vasovagal reaction (common)
- Hemorrhage or hematoma (rare occurrence,

usually associated with anticoagulation or bleeding diaphysis)
- Missed lesions (4% rate of failure to excise nationally—very important)
- Transection of the wire (may accidentally occur during localization or during surgery)
- Pneumothorax (extremely rare with experienced mammographers who position needles parallel to the chest wall)
- Reaction to local anesthetic

Myth: A Transected Wire Is No Cause for Concern. Transected wires may migrate and have been reported in distant sites, including the axilla, the back, the popliteal space, and the myocardium. Usually the wire incites a fibrotic response that limits migration. The patient may elect either to obtain a follow-up film in 6 months or to have the fragment removed. Conclusive evidence is not available at this time, but it is generally believed that if migration has not occurred within 6 months, the likelihood of migration is small. Transecting the wire is a technical error and is not malpractice. Not informing patients and not giving them the option of having the wire removed may be malpractice.

Myth: Benign Calcifications Can Be Distinguished From Malignant Ones on the Mammogram. With macrocalcifications or large calcifications, this is true. However, there is increasing evidence that new or changing microcalcifications, regardless of their shape, size, or number, must be considered suspicious for a malignancy, and biopsy is recommended.

Myth: Risk Factors Are Helpful in Mammographic Interpretation. According to Baker in his 5-year Breast Cancer Demonstration Project (California, 1982), *80% of women who have breast cancer have none of the traditional risk factors.*

Myth: A Mammographic Lesion That Has Not Changed After 1 Year Proves the Lesion Is Benign. Although an abnormality that is unchanged over a 1-year period suggests a benign lesion, breast cancer may be stable over a 1-year period, especially in the elderly patient. The recommended follow-up protocol is an initial follow-up examination in 3 to 6 months, then every 6 months to $2\frac{1}{2}$ years, and then an examination annually.

Myth: All Breast Cancers Have Malignant Features on the Mammogram. Unfortunately, 20% of malignant lesions have benign features on the radiograph. Therefore it has become customary to obtain a biopsy or to radiographically follow all solid lesions greater than 8 mm in diameter in spite of their appearance. The universal experience with needle localization of nonpalpable lesions is that for every 10 lesions biopsied, two or three will be malignant.

HOW DO YOU IMAGE A SURGICAL PATIENT WITH FEVER?

When conventional radiography has failed to reveal the cause of fever in a preoperative or postoperative patient, radionuclide scanning may reveal an occult site of infection or neoplasm. *Indium-111 leukocyte* and *gallium-67* scans are the imaging modalities most likely to localize occult infection or neoplasm.

In choosing the appropriate examination, it is helpful to understand the mechanism of localization of each agent. [111]In leukocyte examination requires the tagging of either autologous or homologous white blood cells (WBCs) with [111]In. The labeled cells, when injected into the body, migrate and accumulate at inflammatory foci. [67]Ga has a more complex localization mechanism involving the binding of gallium to transferrin, lactoferrin, ferritin, and siderophores, which are components of both WBCs and bacteria. Infection alters vessel permeability, allowing ^{67}Ga localization even in WBC-depleted patients.

When Is Indium-111 Leukocyte Scanning Used?

[111]In leukocyte scanning is used to localize an acute (<2 weeks old) inflammatory process or confirm a suspected inflammatory site.

When Is Gallium Scanning Indicated?

Indications for ^{67}Ga scanning include localizing or evaluating a chronic inflammatory process such as abscess, osteomyelitis, or diffuse pneumonitis or localizing and staging neoplasms.

Relative sensitivity of ^{67}Ga for tumor localization is as follows:

- Melanoma, >90%
- Hepatoma, >85%
- Lymphoma: Hodgkins, >90%; non-Hodgkins, 60% to 90%
- Lung cancer: squamous cell, >85%; adenocarcinoma, ≈15%
- Testicular carcinoma (seminoma), ≈90%
- Other tumors, 50% or less

What Are the Advantages of [67]Ga Versus ^{111}In in Imaging Inflammation?

[67]Ga is (1) better for detecting chronic inflammatory processes, (2) good at detecting bone and soft tissue infections, and (3) much less expensive.

The use of ^{111}In leukocytes provides the following advantages:

- Minimal to no uptake in healing wounds or incisions; therefore excellent for use in the postoperative patient
- No bowel uptake unless active bleeding is present, making it a good agent for abdominal imaging
- Easier to interpret images, with higher specificity for inflammatory processes
- Possible to tag homologous WBCs in patients with altered functioning of or reduced WBCs

EVALUATING THE PATIENT WITH A SURGICAL ENDOCRINE ABNORMALITY

Information gained by imaging the thyroid, adrenal glands, and testicles can be invaluable to the surgeon in planning the surgical procedure. The pituitary gland and pancreas are discussed in subsequent sections.

What Is the Best Way to Image the Thyroid Gland?

Several recent and significant advances have been made in imaging the thyroid gland. The surgeon should first ask, "Why am I ordering the exam?" The type of examination chosen depends on the information desired. Is there a palpable abnormality? Is it necessary to assess both function and anatomy? Is ectopic thyroid tissue or metastatic disease being sought? The two most commonly used radionuclides are technetium-99m sodium pertechnetate and iodine-123. Use of ^{131}I is currently limited to treatment only or to identification of ectopic thyroidal tissue because of the high radiation dose to the gland. Thallium may be helpful in locating metastatic thyroid lesions.

How [123]I Differs From Technetium Pertechnetate. Tc99m is trapped only by the thyroid and reveals only the configuration of the gland. It is not a quantitative examination (no organification occurs). [123]I, like ^{131}I, can be used to assess both function (uptake) and structure because ^{123}I is both trapped and organified by the thyroid gland.

How Can the Surgeon Specifically Diagnose a Palpable Thyroid Abnormality? (Fig. 4-14, *A* and *B*) Palpable thyroid abnormalities are usually either discrete nodules (Fig. 4-15) or diffusely enlarged glands (Fig. 4-16). By correlating

the size, activity, and configuration of the gland with serum thyroid function tests, one can generate a differential diagnosis. By first assessing thyroid function (T_3 resin uptake, TSH, T_3 and T_4 levels) and deciding whether the patient's thyroid is normal, hypofunctioning, or hyperfunctioning, and then correlating the thyroid activity with the thyroid scan findings as to uptake and

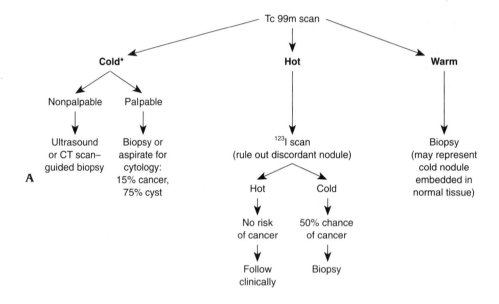

CATCH PALLM (mneumonic for differential diagnosis—for cold nodules): colloid cyst, adenoma, thyroiditis, cancer, hematoma, parathyroid abscess, lymph node, lymphoma, metastases

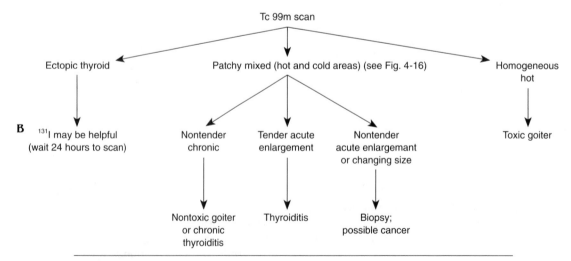

FIGURE 4-14   Chart to guide evaluation of thyroid abnormalities. **A**, Nodule and **B**, enlarged gland.

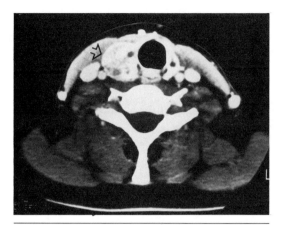

FIGURE 4-15 CT scan of the thyroid demonstrating a well-encapsulated nodule (***arrow***), which was cold on the ^{123}I thyroid scan. The presence of a capsule seen on CT allowed the radiologist to predict correctly that the lesion was benign in a 50-year-old female with a history of thyroid radiation during puberty.

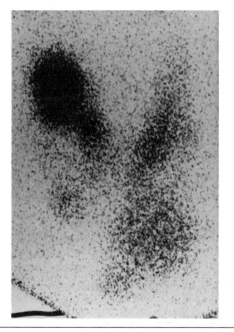

FIGURE 4-16 This ^{123}I thyroid nuclear scan shows a markedly enlarged thyroid and a mixed pattern containing a cold, warm, and hot nodule.

appearance of the gland, the following differential can be generated:

A. Hyperthyroidism with elevated uptake and enlarged thyroid gland
   1. Primary
      a. Diffuse toxic goiter, i.e., Graves' disease (hot gland with homogenous pattern)
      b. Toxic multinodular goiter (mixed pattern) (see Fig. 4-14)
      c. Autonomous thyroid adenoma (discrete area of increased activity; remainder of gland may be suppressed)
   2. Secondary (may be homogeneous or mixed pattern)
      a. Pituitary abnormality
      b. Excess human chorionic gonadotropin (acts like TSH)
      c. Iodine induced
      d. Thyroid carcinoma (rare, <3%)
B. Hypothyroid or euthyroid with increased uptake and enlarged gland
   1. Early Hashimoto's thyroiditis (usually mixed pattern)
   2. Enzymatic defect
   3. Iodine deprivation (mixed pattern)
C. Hypothyroid with decreased uptake and enlarged gland
   1. Thyroiditis (Hashimoto's) (usually mixed pattern)
   2. End-stage Graves' disease (very uncommon)

Nonsurgical Treatment of Thyroid Cancer. Thyroid malignancies can be treated either by surgical resection or ablation of the malignant gland with radioactive iodine. Each thyroid malignancy deserves individualized therapy. The histology of the thyroid malignancy, as determined by biopsy, is a helpful guide to ultimate treatment. Papillary and follicular carcinomas are sensitive to ^{131}I, whereas anaplastic and medullary cell types are resistant.

Ensuring That the Thyroid Gland Has Been Completely Removed. Four to 6 weeks after a "total" thyroidectomy the TSH level should be greater than 50 μU/ml. Contrast CT of the neck or an MRI will usually demonstrate a residual small gland fragment or tumor if the TSH level is not elevated.

How Can the Adrenal Glands Be Evaluated for Neoplasms?

CT and MRI are the most widely used modalities for evaluating the patient for adrenal masses or other neuroendocrine neoplasms. [123]I meta-iodobenzylguanidine (MIBG), used in a nuclear medicine examination, can be a useful adjunct to localize pheochromocytomas and paragangliomas. It has been demonstrated that CT, MRI, and ^{123}I MIBG scintigraphy are similar in their ability to localize pheochromocytomas. Extra-adrenal masses are more difficult to evaluate, and CT with its cross-sectional imaging is of little value. MRI and MIBG are equally effective for evaluating extra-adrenal masses, but MIBG has limited availability because of the lack of approval for clinical uses by the FDA.

A pitfall of MIBG is that many drugs interfere with the uptake of ^{123}I MIBG, and the patient must be prepared with thyroid-blocking drugs before the examination.

How Can the Testes Be Imaged?

The major modalities for imaging the testes and scrotum are ultrasonography and nuclear medicine. CT and MRI are currently reserved for identifying an undescended testicle or staging a testicular malignancy.

The Patient With Acute Testicular or Scrotal Pain. The acute condition of the scrotum is usually defined as acute unilateral swelling with or without pain. A Tc99m nuclear medicine testicular scan, using flow and static phases, is the primary imaging modality for patients presenting with a painful acute scrotum. The technetium scan is the most accurate and expeditious way to differentiate torsion, which requires immediate surgical intervention, from acute epididymitis (Fig. 4-17). In some series Doppler ultrasound plus real-time ultrasound approaches the accuracy of radionuclide scanning for the diagnosis of torsion.

Evaluating a Painless Scrotal Swelling or Mass. Ultrasonography is indicated as the initial radiologic examination of a painless scrotal abnormality. Ultrasound using a small parts transducer can readily differentiate hydroceles (Fig. 4-18) or hematomas from a pathologic condition of the testes such as a neoplasm.

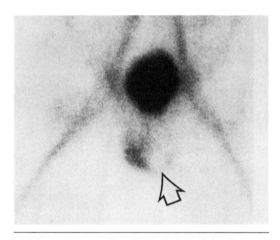

FIGURE 4-17 Nuclear testicular scan shows unequivocally the absence of flow to the left testicle. This was a surgically confirmed torsion of the testes.

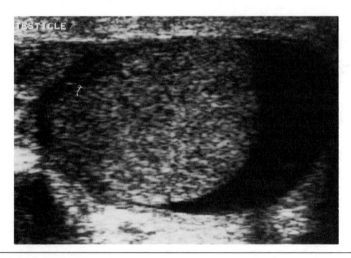

FIGURE 4-18 Ultrasound shows the normal homogeneous tissue characteristics of the testes surrounded by a black rim representing fluid in a hydrocele. Ultrasound is very sensitive for detection of small lesions.

Testicular tumors disrupt the normal homogeneous texture of the testes. Neoplasms are usually seen as heterogeneous echogenic areas of lesser echogenicity than the testes. A pitfall of ultrasound evaluation of the testes is that the sonographic findings are nonspecific and cannot differentiate hemorrhage, infarction, or infection from tumor; however, the false-negative rate for tumor detection is very low. Ultrasound can often locate a tumor in a patient with a normal testis to palpation who has metastatic testicular carcinoma.

Other Testicular Problems Diagnosed by Ultrasound. Scrotal hernias, spermatoceles, and varicoceles all have very specific appearances on ultrasound. Varicoceles may also be seen on a nuclear medicine flow study and may be important in the work-up of infertility in men.

WHAT CHANGES IN ULTRASOUND TECHNOLOGY MAY BE IMPORTANT TO THE SURGEON?

The technology associated with ultrasonography has made many significant advances in the last decade. The overall quality of the images has significantly improved. The new modalities that have become indispensable in contemporary imaging departments include prostatic, endovaginal, and neonatal cranial ultrasound and Doppler imaging of the vessels.

Prostatic ultrasound has become an important tool in guiding the urologist or radiologist in percutaneous biopsies of the prostate. This technique in informed hands is very sensitive for identifying prostatic abnormalities. However, its specificity at times is less than optimal. It can be an important mechanism for monitoring the therapy of prostatic carcinoma.

Endovaginal ultrasound has significantly improved the reliability of ultrasonography for diagnosing ectopic pregnancies (Fig. 4-19), for imaging very obese patients, and for imaging patients in whom the uterus has been removed and the ovaries are difficult to locate.

Neonatal cranial ultrasound has become routine in most neonatology units for evaluating patients for intracranial pathology, including germinal matrix or other intracranial hemorrhages, hydrocephalus, suspected intracranial neoplasms, or suspected central nervous system congenital abnormalities. Use of this method prevents the infant's exposure to repeated relatively high-dose radiation.

Ultrasonic venography of the deep venous system for thrombosis at most institutions has replaced routine venography. This examination is less expensive, and there is no risk of anaphylaxis or other contrast-related complications. The reliability of the examination is quite high in skilled hands. A pitfall in this examination may be obstruction of flow in the pelvis. Superficial thrombophlebitis, although less critical in nature, may at times be difficult to document with ultrasound.

WHAT IS INTERVENTIONAL RADIOLOGY?

With the advent of newer radiographic imaging techniques, the role of diagnostic and therapeutic radiology has been redefined. Interventional radiology is an outgrowth of diagnostic angiography. The radiologist, once only a diagnostician, has recently adapted skills learned while doing angiography to the treatment of some disease entities. Advances in interventional radiology have changed the practice of clinical medicine in many important aspects, intensifying the partnership of the radiologist and the surgeon. This section updates the surgeon on some of the more important and newer diagnostic and therapeutic modalities. Some of the basic indications of diagnostic and therapeutic angiography and interventional radiology are reviewed.

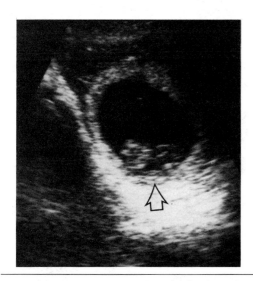

FIGURE 4-19 Arrow points to a fetal pole and gestational sac in the right adnexa. A fetal heartbeat was readily apparent. Endovaginal ultrasound examinations like this one have significantly improved the detection rate of ectopic pregnancies.

What Are the Indications for Percutaneous Drainage and How Is It Performed?

Percutaneous abscess drainage (PAD) is one of the most important interventional procedures performed by the radiologist today. Drainage technique is quite variable but usually involves positioning a needle with imaging guidance and then confirming the needle location. A 0.018-inch diameter guidewire is placed through the fine needle, and a catheter is inserted over the wire. Serial dilation with small catheters is performed to place a soft drainage catheter with multiple side holes into the area being drained. A variety of anchoring devices are available.

Real-time imaging such as ultrasound and/or fluoroscopy is often used in conjunction with CT. Preprocedure imaging provides accurate information to determine a clear access route, the presence or absence of fistulous communications, and the presence of nearby structures that must be avoided. Although ultrasound provides real-time imaging advantages, CT is often superior, particularly in more complex cases.

Indications for PAD have expanded considerably in the past 10 years, and drainage is performed for pancreatic abscesses and pseudocysts, infected and noninfected hematomas, empyemas, lung and mediastinal abscesses, bile collections, necrotic tumors, benign cysts, and even amoebic or echinococcal abscesses. Routine drainage procedures include hepatic abscess, renal abscess, retroperitoneal collections, and collections within the peritoneal compartment, which include subhepatic, subphrenic, and pericolic gutters, common sites for postoperative abscess formation.

Postprocedure bile collections (Fig. 4-20, *A* and *B*) and other benign fluid collections, including renal cysts and urinomas, are among those lesions most easily drained. The presence of an echinococcal cyst or abscess was previously considered a contraindication to PAD but has recently been demonstrated as easily treated in the majority of cases without the development of

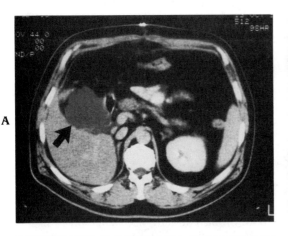

A

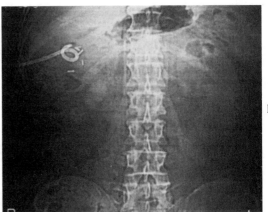

B

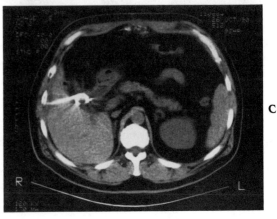

C

FIGURE 4-20 A 56-year-old male, status postcholecystectomy, developed increasing right upper quadrant pain postoperatively. **A,** CT scan of the upper abdomen demonstrates a fluid collection (*arrow*) consistent with a biloma. Using CT guidance, a drainage catheter was placed. **B,** Drainage catheter in the gallbladder fossa. **C,** Resolution of the fluid collection. The tube was removed after 3 days of drainage. The patient's discomfort resolved without development of fever or other difficulty.

anaphylaxis. An obstructed biliary ductal system (Fig. 4-21) and an obstructed ureter are two other common indications for percutaneous drainage and may be coupled with stent insertion and/or stone removal (Fig. 4-22, *C*).

A transgastric approach for pancreatic pseudocyst drainage can be used when the pseudocyst lies directly posterior to the stomach wall and the liver and colon are not interposed between the skin and the anterior stomach wall as demonstrated by a recent CT scan.

Advantages and Disadvantages of Percutaneous Needle Biopsies. CT, ultrasound, or fluoroscopically guided needle biopsies are performed routinely in most hospitals in the United States (Fig. 4-23). The obvious advantages of using an imaging device include:

- Documentation of the presence of the needle in the lesion
- Aid to the surgeon in treatment planning
- Avoidance of injury to adjacent vital structures
- No need for general anesthesia

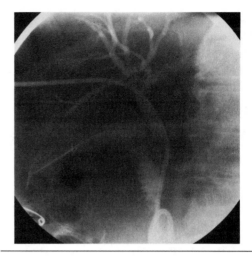

FIGURE 4-21 Percutaneously placed biliary drain with multiple side holes communicating with the common hepatic duct and common bile duct. The drain passes through the ampulla into the duodenum. A retention loop of catheter in the duodenum acts as an anchoring device.

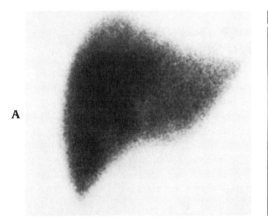

A

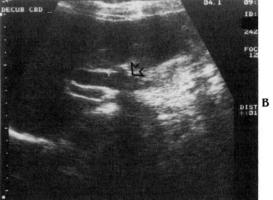

B

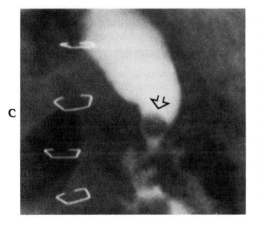

C

FIGURE 4-22 Nuclear hepatobiliary (HIDA) study showing **A,** no activity in the biliary system secondary to high-grade distal common bile duct obstruction in a 19-year-old, 280-pound female after removal of her gallbladder. **B,** Ultrasound in same patient showing markedly enlarged common bile duct (*arrow*) but no clear demonstration of stone. **C,** Retained distal common bile duct stone and partial obstruction of the common bile duct on this image were obtained during follow-up T-tube cholangiography. This stone was subsequently removed percutaneously with fluoroscopic guidance.

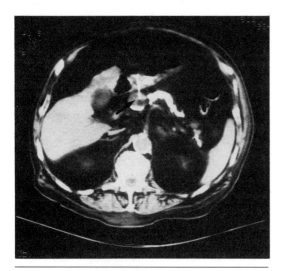

FIGURE 4-23 Percutaneously placed needle within the pancreatic head lesion *(arrow).* Benign-appearing cystic fluid was removed. Note also the dilated pancreatic duct with retained contrast from previous endoscopic retrograde cholangiopancreatography.

Needles used range from a 22-gauge fine needle for aspiration for cytology to a 20-gauge needle for core biopsy, often used in solid organ lesions, to a 13-gauge needle for core biopsy of a bone lesion. Use of real-time imaging such as ultrasound or fluoroscopy is often preferable to fixed imaging such as CT or MRI.

The major disadvantage of the percutaneous biopsy is the small pathologic specimen. *When suspicion for malignancy is high, at least three attempts for percutaneous biopsy are recommended.* If the biopsy specimen shows no malignancy, an open biopsy may be necessary.

How Can Gastrointestinal Bleeding Be Detected With Angiography?

For patients with acute upper gastrointestinal (GI) bleeding, endoscopy is the preferred diagnostic technique if rapid evaluation is necessary. Endoscopy can almost always detect hemorrhage secondary to gastric or duodenal ulceration, gastric malignancy, varices, and gastritis and can usually detect the site of hemorrhage. Arteriography is indicated for the evaluation of acute GI bleeding, often after a positive result from a nuclear medicine bleeding study. Arteriography can detect up to 75% of acute hemorrhage and is ideally suited for both the localiza-

tion and at times the treatment of GI hemorrhage. Embolization material or a vasoconstrictor can be directly injected into the appropriate artery. In a patient with diagnosed gastritis, a vasopressin infusion of 0.1 to 0.4 units per minute is directly injected into the bleeding artery. Patients with hemorrhage secondary to gastric or duodenal ulcer disease appear to benefit most from direct embolization. Angiodysplasia is best treated surgically, although short-term control can be achieved with vasoconstriction or embolization in an attempt to control hemorrhage in patients for whom surgery is relatively contraindicated (Fig. 4-24, *A* and *B*). Embolization is performed as selectively as possible once the site of hemorrhage has been identified. Embolization material, often small pieces of gel foam or small metal coils with attached fibers or even detachable balloons, is placed at the site of hemorrhage. Follow-up arteriography is necessary to confirm hemostasis (Fig. 4-25, *A* to *C*). As in many more specialized radiologic procedures, *a skilled angiographer familiar with interventional techniques and surgical alternatives must perform the diagnostic and therapeutic portion of the study of patients with GI hemorrhage.*

WHEN IS ANGIOPLASTY PERFORMED?

The first article on angioplasty, published by Dotter and Judkins in 1964, predicted a wide range of applications to include coronary, renal, carotid, vertebral, and other sites. Significant medical cost savings have been realized as more and more angioplasty is performed on an outpatient basis. For each anatomic application of angioplasty there exists a separate group of appropriate indications determined by both morphologic and clinical criteria. Patients presenting with lower extremity ischemia require a careful history and physical examination, including noninvasive vascular laboratory studies to determine whether angioplasty is indicated.

Clinical indications for angioplasty include:

- Claudication significantly limiting lifestyle
- Poor wound healing or ischemic ulceration
- Gangrene associated with vascular compromise

Noninvasive studies are routinely used before vascular intervention and provide excellent methods for assessing the success of angioplasty and monitoring vessel patency.

Femoral artery angioplasty and *popliteal artery angioplasty* are often considered together

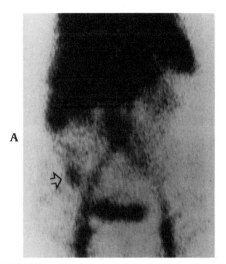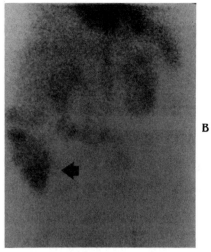

FIGURE 4-24 This 58-year-old male presented with GI bleeding. **A,** Image shows the early angiographic or flow phase of a nuclear-medicine-tagged red blood cell study of GI bleeding. A collection of activity in the right lower quadrant is suspicious for bleeding in the cecum (*arrow*). **B,** Image demonstrates the delayed phase of this bleeding scan at 12 hours, showing increasing activity in the cecum (*arrow*). Surgery revealed angiodysplasia.

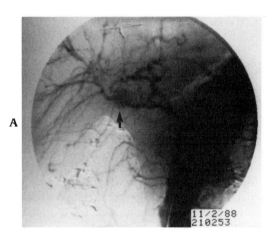

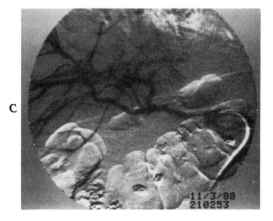

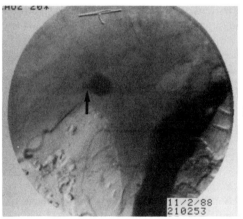

FIGURE 4-25 Embolization can be performed for treatment of bleeding aneurysm. **A,** Right renal arteriogram demonstrates a renal artery aneurysm (*arrow*) in this 65-year-old female with flank pain. Hemorrhage from the aneurysm was demonstrated on CT of kidneys. **B,** Later arterial phase demonstrates more clearly the aneurysm neck (*arrow*) and, **C,** shows no flow into the aneurysm after embolization.

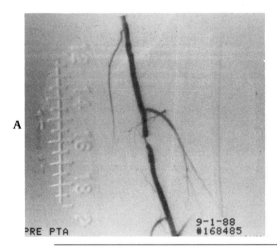
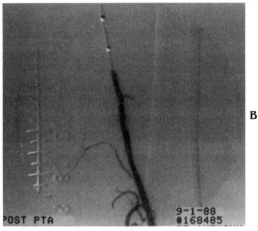

FIGURE 4-26   Patient is a 56-year-old male with claudication of the left leg and an ankle-brachial index of 0.65 on the left by noninvasive testing. **A,** Femoral arteriogram demonstrates tight focal stenosis approximately at 16-cm mark in the distal left superficial femoral artery. **B,** Postangioplasty arteriogram reveals satisfactory dilation of the vessel. Patient had a normal ankle-brachial index and resolution of symptoms after the dilation.

(Fig. 4-26, **A** and **B**). Technically, the antegrade approach is generally used. The vessels are of approximately the same caliber. Postangioplasty patency rates generally compare favorably with those for surgery, especially the 5-year patient survival rate of approximately 48% of all patients undergoing infrainguinal reconstruction. Infrapopliteal artery angioplasty is more commonly limited to patients with ischemic rest pain or disease of greater severity. These procedures are much more demanding technically.

Percutaneous transluminal angioplasty of the renal artery is indicated in patients with renal vascular hypertension either isolated or in conjunction with essential hypertension, in limited cases for improvement of renal function (although this use remains controversial), and in the treatment of posttransplant renal artery stenosis.

WHEN ARE STENTS USED IN THE VASCULAR SYSTEM?

Many clinical trials are currently evaluating the safety, indications, and efficacy of self-expanding and balloon expandable stents in the treatment of atherosclerotic stenosis of the infra-aortic arterial system. The ***Palmaz stent*** has recently been approved for use in the iliac system after a technically less-than-optimal result of balloon angio-

plasty. Although more work is needed, early data are encouraging about the role of this and other stents under investigation.

Nonvascular uses of stents include maintenance of patency of the biliary system secondary to malignant disease; expandable stents for the treatment of inferior vena cava syndrome, superior vena cava syndrome, and other large vein obstructions; and urologic stents in the management of benign prostatic enlargement and associated narrowing of the prostatic urethra. They may also be used in stenting the bronchus secondary to congenital or other brachial stenosis, pancreatic duct stenting secondary to pancreatic duct rupture, or ductal stenosis secondary to pancreatitis.

WHEN ARE LASERS USED INTRAVASCULARLY?

Laser energy is used to create a small channel through which a standard guidewire is placed to facilitate the performance of standard balloon angioplasty. In many trials complication rates have been unacceptably high, and the reocclusion or restenosis rate has been higher than with routine angioplasty. Although several devices may eventually demonstrate acceptable success rates, long-term research is required to show long-term patency rates comparable to currently accepted modalities before laser angioplasty can become the recommended procedure. For the present, laser-assisted angiography is an investigative procedure.

WHAT ARE THE INDICATIONS FOR THROMBOLYTIC THERAPY?

Percutaneously, a thrombolytic agent can be delivered directly into an artery or vein over a period of time to dissolve or promote resorption of a thrombus. The decision to pursue thrombolytic therapy must be made jointly by the referring surgeon and interventional radiologist.

Factors that favor surgical procedure for thrombectomy include:

- Neurologic sensory and/or motor deficit or other signs suggesting that the acutely threatened limb requires emergency intervention
- Limitation of the arteriographic abnormality to a small vessel of the hand or foot (a short trial of thrombolysis may be successful in this instance, but atheroemboli tend not to respond favorably to thrombolytic therapy)
- Recent surgery, hemorrhagic infarction, coagulopathies, GI hemorrhage, or known intracranial aneurysm

Indications for percutaneous thrombolysis include but are not limited to:

- Angiographically documented extensive thrombus or multiple thrombi below the brachial bifurcation or the trifurcation of the calf
- Recurrent thrombosis after surgical thrombectomy
- Treatment in conjunction with angioplasty of documented renal dialysis fistula stenosis or occlusion
- Treatment of extensive pulmonary emboli in patients who demonstrate compromise of cardiac function as the result of increased pulmonary artery pressures
- Thrombotic femoropopliteal occlusions
- Treatment of subclavian and axillary venous thrombosis with or without associated central catheters
- Treatment of thrombosis as a complication of angioplasty or routine diagnostic arteriography
- Treatment of thrombosis of a femoral popliteal graft (almost always successful when using a combination of thrombolysis and corrective angioplasty of the distal stenosis)

INDICATIONS AND PROBLEMS ASSOCIATED WITH PULMONARY ARTERIOGRAPHY

Because of the high morbidity and mortality rates associated with pulmonary emboli and other abnormalities of the pulmonary arterial system, pulmonary arteriography is important for evaluation of a morphologic abnormality of the pulmonary arterial circulation. Although a Swan-Ganz catheter placement, often performed at bedside, can provide important information about the pressures of the right side of the heart as well as pulmonary vascular resistance and cardiac output, pulmonary arteriography remains the gold standard for documenting pulmonary emboli.

Indications for pulmonary arteriography most commonly include strong clinical suspicion of pulmonary emboli. Pulmonary arteriography is often used after a nuclear medicine ventilation and perfusion study. Some controversy exists in the literature about the use of pulmonary ventilation and perfusion studies, but most people agree that pulmonary arteriography is indicated when the probability of embolus on a ventilation-perfusion (V/Q) scan is indeterminate or intermediate. Some advocate that pulmonary arteriography is not necessary in high probability V/Q scans in which there is little debate about the diagnosis or in patients with low probability, since these patients seem not to develop significant sequela secondary to pulmonary emboli. However, the complication rate of intermediate term anticoagulation is so great that most require confirmation.

Pulmonary arteriography is also indicated for patients with vascular malformations and other suspected congenital pulmonary abnormalities. Other rare uses for pulmonary arteriography include evaluation of arteritis, venous occlusion or stenosis, and pulmonary artery aneurysm.

Most limitations of pulmonary arteriography are secondary to technical difficulties. Contrast injection of the main pulmonary artery is contraindicated in patients with elevated pulmonary pressures; for this reason, pressures are often obtained before imaging in patients with suspected pulmonary hypertension. Underlying pulmonary disease may make it impossible for the patient to suspend respiration during filming, thus producing motion artifacts and blurring. Discomfort caused by hyperosmolar contrast injection may even increase patient motion. Newer nonionic contrast agents can help in all of these

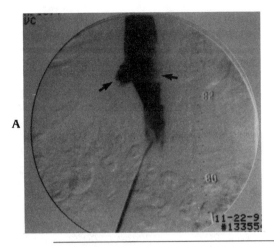
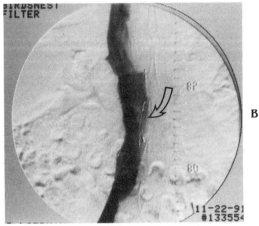

FIGURE 4-27   A, Inferior venacavagram performed before inferior vena cava filter placement shows location of renal veins bilaterally in this 36-year-old male with paraplegia and pulmonary emboli despite adequate anticoagulation therapy. **B,** Cavagram performed after placement of bird's nest filter in the inferior vena cava shows satisfactory position just below the left renal artery *(arrow)*.

technical difficulties while making the study safer.

When Is Inferior Vena Cava Filter Placement Indicated?

The placement of an inferior vena cava filter is indicated in patients with recurrent pulmonary emboli who have a contraindication to anticoagulation therapy or in patients with deep venous thrombosis before major surgery. Increasingly, filters are placed prophylactically in patients with documented prior pulmonary emboli who are undergoing orthopedic surgery or in neurologic patients with lower extremity paralysis. Placement can be performed via venous cut-down, usually through the jugular system or via a percutaneous technique in the femoral or jugular vein. In optimal situations, an inferior vena cavagram is performed to localize the position of the renal veins (Fig. 4-27, **A**). The filter is placed just below the renal veins to trap large clots that would otherwise migrate to the pulmonary arterial system and produce clinically significant emboli (Fig. 4-27, **B**).

The procedure is relatively easy to perform. Once properly trained, the radiologist can place a filter in approximately 15 minutes using only local anesthesia.

Disadvantages of Inferior Vena Cava Filters. Complications of inferior vena cava filters include filter migration in unusual circumstances. This occurrence is rare and usually is associated with placement within an enlarged inferior vena cava. Extremity edema is an uncommon but not rare complication of filter placement associated with thrombosis of the lower extremity venous system. Perforation of the inferior vena cava by a filter has been reported but is rarely significant. Significant recurrent pulmonary emboli, despite proper filter placement, occur in as many as 7% of patients. A slightly increased complication rate has been associated with filter placement through the left femoral vein into the increased angulation at the junction of the inferior vena cava.

PITFALLS AND COMMON MYTHS

Mammography

- Assuming that a palpable lesion is not significant because the mammogram is normal.
- Refusal or reluctance of a patient to get a mammogram because of the discomfort of the procedure may delay diagnosis. Explanation of the need for good compression of the breast tissue and the necessity of some discomfort, but rarely pain, should increase patient compliance.
- Very dense breasts, commonly seen in younger patients, may obscure lesions. Some comment about breast density should be made by the radiologist and should guide the clinician as to the reliability of the mammogram.
- Substandard equipment or positioning may give a false sense of security by producing suboptimal examinations (using American College of Radiology accredited facilities may protect the patient in this instance).

Radionuclide Studies for Fever Work-ups

- A liver-spleen scan for comparison should be performed in conjunction with the infection studies to prevent masking of an infectious process near the liver or spleen by the normal uptake of gallium and indium in these areas.
- Active bleeding may simulate an active inflammatory process with indium-labeled WBCs in the GI tract.
- Bowel activity from swallowed purulent material from the sinuses or respiratory tract may simulate inflammatory process in the intestines.
- Differentiating tumor from inflammation with gallium may be impossible.

Arteriography in Evaluation of GI Bleeding

- Arteriography results may be falsely negative in as many as 25% to 40% of cases with known hemorrhage and positive nuclear medicine GI studies.
- Residual barium from an upper or lower GI examination significantly limits the accuracy of arteriography, because the barium residue obscures the area of hemorrhage.
- In some cases oral contrast from CT examination may also preclude arteriography.

SURGICAL PHARMACOPEIA

Drug	Indications/Complications	Dosage
Vasopressin	Vasoconstrictor used intra-arterially to control bleeding. Must be used cautiously to avoid ischemia.	Varies with indication; 0.1-0.4 units/min IV for hemorrhagic gastritis
Urokinase	Proteolytic enzyme used to lyse thrombi. Systemic anticoagulation results with therapeutic dosages. Cannot be used in patients predisposed to or at risk of hemorrhage.	Varies widely; current doses are up to 4000 U/min IV with frequent follow-up arteriography
Gadolinium (Magnevist)	Intravenous contrast agent for magnetic resonance imaging. Few reported side effects; most common (<5%) is headache.	1 ml/kg of patient's weight to maximum of 20 ml IV
Indium-III	Agent used to tag white blood cells for identifying sites of inflammation.	500 microcuries (μCi)
^{123}I MIBG (metaiodo-benzylguanidine)	Cholesterol derivative that is tagged with radioactive iodine. Used for scanning adrenal glands.	10 microcuries (μCi)

BIBLIOGRAPHY

Adams A, Dondelinger RF. Metallic stents: Vascular and nonvascular uses. Semin Intervent Radiol 8, 1991.

Bassett LW, Gold RH, Seeger LL. MRI Atlas of the Musculoskeletal System. Great Britain, Martin Dunitz, 1989.

Becker GJ, Katzen BT, Dake MD. Noncoronary angioplasty. Radiol RSNA-SCVIR Special Series 170: 921-940, 1989.

Blahd W, et al. Serum thyroglobulin in the management of thyroid cancer. J Nucl Med 31:1771-1773, 1990.

Cragg AH. Update on laser angioplasty. Semin Intervent Radiol 8, 1991.

Davis PS, Wechsler RJ, Feig SA, et al. Migration of breast biopsy localization wire. Am J Roentgenol 150:787-788, 1988.

Hamer MM, Morlock F, Foley HT, et al. Medical malpractice in diagnostic radiology: Claims, comprehension, and patient injury. Radiology 164:263-266, 1987.

Higgins CB, Hricak H, Helms CA. Magnetic Resonance Imaging of the Body. New York, Raven Press, 1992.

Holden R. Fibrinolysis. Semin Intervent Radiol 9, 1992.

Homer MJ, Smith TJ, Marchant DJ. Outpatient needle localization and biopsy for nonpalpable breast lesions. JAMA 252:2452-2454, 1984.

Johnsrude IS, Jackson DC, Dunnick NR. A Practical Approach to Angiography, 2nd ed. Boston, Little, Brown & Co, 1987.

Kadir S. Current Practice of Interventional Radiology. Philadelphia, Brian C Decker, 1991.

Kopans DB. Breast Imaging. Philadelphia, JB Lippincott, 1989.

Kuni CC, Klingensmith WC. Atlas of Radionuclide Hepatobiliary Imaging. Boston, GK Hall Medical Publishers, 1983.

Letourneau JG, Maynar-Moliner M. Duplex sonography and color Doppler: II. Semin Intervent Radiol 7, 1990.

Martin EC. Transcatheter therapies in peripheral and noncoronary vascular disease. Circulation 83(Suppl), 1991.

Meyer JE, Kopans DB. Preoperative roentgenographically guided percutaneous localization of occult breast lesions. Arch Surg 117:65-68, 1982.

Petrillo R, Balzarini L, et al. Esophageal squamous cell carcinoma: MRI evaluation of mediastinum. Gastrointest Radiol 15:275-278, 1990.

Pomeranz SJ. Orthopaedic MRI: A Teaching File. Philadelphia, JB Lippincott, 1991.

Stark DD, Bradley WG. Magnetic Resonance Imaging. St Louis, CV Mosby, 1988.

Taveras JM, Ferrucci JT. Radiology: Diagnosis-Imaging-Intervention. Philadelphia, JB Lippincott, 1991.

VanSonnenberg E, D'Agostino HB, Casola G, et al.

Percutaneous abscess drainage: Current concepts. Radiology 181:617-626, 1991.

Webb WR, Gatsonis C, Zerhouni EA, et al. CT and MR imaging in staging non-small cell bronchogenic carcinoma: Report of the Radiologic Diagnostic Oncology Group. Radiology 178:705-713, 1991.

Weinreb JC, Naidich DP. Thoracic magnetic resonance imaging. Clin Chest Med 12:33-54, 1991.

Zlatkin MB, Reicher MA, Kellerhouse LE, et al. The painful shoulder: MR imaging of the glenohumeral joint. J Comput Assist Tomogr 12:995-1001, 1988.

CHAPTER REVIEW
Questions

1. Mammography is indicated at any age for:
   a. Palpable mass
   b. Bloody discharge
   c. Planned breast surgery
   d. All of the above
2. All of the following are true except:
   a. Mastitis or lymphedema can mimic carcinoma on a mammogram.
   b. A normal mammogram should obviate the need for surgery when the patient has a palpable breast mass.
   c. A mammogram is uncomfortable because of the need to compress the breast tissue.
   d. Very dense breasts may obscure lesions on a mammogram.
3. A mammogram consent form should contain all of the following information except:
   a. Nationally there is a 4% failure to excise nonpalpable lesions localized by a needle.
   b. Fainting secondary to a vasovagal reaction during the needle localization is a common occurrence.
   c. A transected wire does not present a problem and has no implications for future problems.
   d. Reaction to local anesthetic may occur.
4. Choose the best answer with respect to ^{111}In leukocyte examination.
   a. Indicated for localizing melanoma
   b. Indicated for chronic infections
   c. Ideal agent to use postoperatively because it does not have increased uptake or activity at an incision site
   d. Cannot be used in patients with altered or reduced WBCs
5. Hyperthyroidism and an enlarged thyroid gland are associated with all but one of the following:
   a. Diffuse toxic goiter
   b. Toxic multinodular goiter

c. Autonomous thyroid adenoma

d. Iodine deprivation

6. All of the following are true statements except:
   a. Ultrasound is indicated as the initial radiologic examination of a painless scrotal abnormality.
   b. Ultrasound is indicated as the initial radiologic examination in a patient with acute testicular pain.
   c. Ultrasound can differentiate a scrotal hernia from other testicular pathology.

7. All but one of the following are advantages of MRI over CT:
   a. Absence of ionizing radiation
   b. Ability of MRI to scan in multiple planes without repositioning of the patient
   c. Ability of MRI to image acute hemorrhage
   d. Advent of enhancement of contrast with gadolinium has increased both the sensitivity and specificity of MRI examinations

8. Indications for surgical thrombectomy over thrombolytic therapy include all of the following except:
   a. Neurologic deficit associated with vascular compromise
   b. For the treatment of pulmonary emboli in patients who demonstrate compromise of cardiac function secondary to increased pulmonary artery pressures
   c. When arteriographic abnormality is limited to a small vessel of the hand or a foot

9. An angioplasty may be indicated on patients with:
   a. Claudication limiting lifestyle
   b. Poor wound healing or ischemic ulceration
   c. Gangrene associated with vascular compromise
   d. All of the above

10. MRI is superior to CT for imaging all of the following except:
    a. Patients with acute traumatic bony injuries
    b. Posterior fossa lesions
    c. Seizure patients
    d. Acute hearing loss and vertigo

Answers

1. d	6. b
2. b	7. c
3. c	8. b
4. c	9. d
5. d	10. a

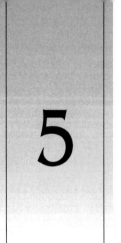

5 Endoscopy in Surgical Practice

GERALD M. LARSON
MARTIN H. MAX

KEY FEATURES

After reading this chapter you will understand:
- The innovations in and applications of diagnostic and therapeutic endoscopy.
- Indications for specialized endoscopic procedures: ERCP, colonoscopy, and PEG.

The introduction of fiberoptic endoscopy to medical practice in the 1970s represents one of the significant developments for the treatment of gastrointestinal (GI) disease in this century. Endoscopic procedures make possible the direct visualization and inspection of the stomach, pancreas, biliary tract, and colon, which were once inaccessible. Endoscopy allows treatment of colon polyps, esophageal varices, bleeding ulcers, common bile duct stones, and many other conditions and spares the patient the major operation formerly required. Videoendoscopy has dramatically improved the quality of the endoscopic picture, and endoscopic ultrasound shows potential for examination beyond the endoscope. In the near future three-dimensional computer imaging may become a routine part of endoscopy.

During the last 15 years endoscopic examination of the GI and biliary tracts has become a valuable diagnostic and therapeutic procedure. The first endoscopes introduced in the 1970s had fiberoptic bundles to illuminate the bowel lumen and then transmit the image through the flexible scope to the eyepiece for viewing. In the past 5 years this technology has changed to video systems, and endoscopes are now designed with a small videochip camera at the tip of the scope

that transmits the image electronically to large-screen monitors and standard videocassette recorders (VCRs). The videoendoscope represents a tremendous advance in endoscopic imaging that provides a large-screen, eye-pleasing picture of the procedure for the physician, assistants, and students. Immediate, high-quality photography and VCR filming of the procedure for documentation of the findings are also possible.

Endoscopic examination enables accurate inspection of the luminal lining of the esophagus, stomach, duodenum, common bile duct, pancreas, duct, rectum, and colon. The scope is introduced through the mouth and is gently advanced into the esophagus. In the esophagus and stomach, endoscopy is often used to evaluate conditions such as esophagitis, gastritis, and ulcer disease. Examples of therapeutic endoscopy include sclerotherapy of esophageal varices and balloon dilation of an esophageal stricture. Colonoscopy often is performed as part of an examination to detect colon cancer, to determine cause of rectal bleeding, and to remove polyps.

INSTRUMENTATION

Endoscopic procedures are performed in specially designed units located in the hospital or in a physician's office. Flexible endoscopes for EGD are slender tubes 9 mm in diameter and 130 cm long that contain a fiberoptic light bundle to illuminate the field and a small videochip camera that electronically transmits the image through the scope to the television monitor and VCR. Standard colonoscopes and flexible sigmoidoscopes are similarly designed except the colonoscope is 180 cm long and the flexible sigmoidoscope is 60 cm.

The scopes contain a working biopsy channel, which is 2.8 mm in diameter, through which biopsy instruments, snares, needle injectors for sclerotherapy, and heater probes or laser catheters can be passed for a variety of diagnostic and therapeutic procedures. The endoscopic retrograde cholangiopancreatography (ERCP) scope is a side-viewing instrument; the light source and the lens are located at right angles to the axis of the scope so that the papilla and the ampulla of Vater can be viewed directly when the scope is positioned in the duodenum. A light source with 300-watt capability is connected to the scope. Scope tips have an irrigation system to keep the lens clean and suction to aspirate luminal contents.

ESOPHAGOGASTRO-DUODENOSCOPY (EGD)
Indications

Upper gastrointestinal (UGI) endoscopy is usually performed to evaluate UGI symptoms and complaints such as heartburn, dysphagia, indigestion, epigastric pain, bleeding, and anemia. The most common conditions that correlate with these complaints include esophagitis, esophageal strictures (benign or malignant), hiatus hernia, gastritis, gastric ulcer, gastric cancer, and duodenal ulcer.

Diagnosis. UGI endoscopy is the most effective individual method of diagnosing UGI tract disease. It is indicated in the same situation as barium studies; however, 20% to 30% of radiologic diagnoses are incorrect or incomplete when compared with endoscopic findings. In our experience, performing endoscopy after obtaining UGI radiographs in nonemergencies changed the clinical diagnosis in 12% of patients and provided the only definitive diagnosis in an additional 12%. Nonetheless, the studies are complementary, and UGI x-ray examination is still used as a preliminary investigation.

The Role of EGD for UGI Bleeding

Esophagogastroduodenoscopy's role is to diagnose the cause of bleeding and to determine whether additional therapy such as endoscopic injection or an operation is likely. UGI bleeding can be a serious medical emergency and is an alarming condition for the patient. The signs of UGI bleeding include (1) vomiting of blood, usually caused by esophageal varices, gastritis, or a gastric ulcer; (2) melena, which is more gradual in onset and generally is caused by ulcers or gastritis in the stomach or duodenum; and (3) rectal bleeding, which also can be a feature of UGI bleeding, especially when the bleeding is considerable. Patients with severe UGI hemorrhage are usually admitted to the intensive care unit for resuscitation and treatment. Endoscopy in such cases can be performed at the bedside in the unit where optimal support is available.

The majority of bleeding episodes are attributable to one of four lesions: duodenal ulcer, gastric ulcer, hemorrhagic gastritis, or esophageal varices. In a national prospective study the sources of UGI bleeding in 2225 patients as determined by endoscopy were duodenal ulcer (24%), gastric erosions (23%), gastric ulcer (21%), and esophageal varices (10%). A review of our own experience and an analysis of the causes of acute UGI bleeding as determined by endoscopy in 115 patients revealed that the same four lesions were responsible for 80% of the bleeding cases (Table 5-1). Endoscopy identified a bleeding source in 92% of patients *(Plate 5-1; color plates follow p. 92).*

Therapeutic Endoscopic Procedures

Sclerotherapy. Sclerotherapy was introduced in 1939, primarily for control of bleeding esophageal varices. It has had a resurgence of popularity in the last two decades, and currently many investigators believe that sclerotherapy is the best initial treatment for esophageal varices because bleeding control is satisfactory and emergency surgery is avoided. In the acute situation the reported success rate ranges from 80% to 95% with a low complication rate. Four trials that compare sclerotherapy with standard medical therapy have been conducted, three of which show that sclerotherapy improves control of variceal bleeding and leads to improved survival overall. In addition, four prospective studies in North America have compared sclerotherapy to elective shunt surgery. Two trials demonstrate comparable survival rates, and one shows improved survival rates with long-term sclerotherapy. Yet sclerotherapy fails in 30% of patients, and surgical rescue with a shunt procedure is necessary.

Ligation. Endoscopic variceal ligation can also be performed for bleeding esophageal varices. The preliminary results appear to show that it is as good as sclerotherapy. The technique is currently under prospective evaluation in randomized trials.

TABLE 5-1 Bleeding Source in 115 Patients

Lesion	No. of Patients (Primary)	%	No. of Patients (Secondary)
Gastritis	48	41	14
Gastric ulcer	19	16	1
Duodenal ulcer	13	13	—
Esophageal varices	11	11	—
Mallory-Weiss tear	6	5	—
Esophagitis	5	4	9
Stomal ulcer	3	2	—
Neoplasm	2	2	—
Duodenitis	0	0	7
Miscellaneous	4	3	—
Undetermined	4	3	—
TOTAL	115	100	31

From Larson GM, Schmidt T, Gott G, et al. Upper gastrointestinal bleeding: Predictors of outcome. Surgery 100:765-772, 1986.

Electrocoagulation. Electrocoagulation relies on electric current to close blood vessels. With monopolar electrode coagulation, current flows from the end of the electrode through the tissue to the patient's grounding plate. With bipolar electrodes, current flows from one microelectrode to another on the surface of the electrode tip. One theoretic advantage for the bipolar device is that it uses much less energy per application than the monopolar method; therefore there is less risk of transmural injury.

Electrocoagulation seems best suited for treating active bleeding from duodenal or gastric ulcers, vascular malformations, and Mallory-Weiss tears. At least five prospective controlled trials of endoscopic electrocoagulation to control UGI hemorrhage have been conducted. Several groups report success rates of 70% or better for stopping active bleeding but with variable impact on patient outcome. The trial reported by Laine is unique in that electrocautery also improved patient outcome and survival rates. Failure of this technique is usually due to difficult exposure of the bleeding ulcer and poor access for the probe. It is important to use a large probe with a 3.2-mm diameter.

Heater Probe. Introduced in 1978, the heater probe simultaneously applies pressure and heat to the bleeding vessel. This probe has been used primarily for patients with bleeding peptic ulcers, and the clinical experience has been encouraging. Johnston et al. retrospectively compared the effectiveness of heater probe and yttrium-aluminum-garnet (YAG) laser in treating patients with active bleeding from peptic ulcer. Hemostatic control was achieved in 19 of 20 patients treated with the heater probe (95%) versus 24 of 35 patients treated with the YAG laser (69%). They comment that the heater probe was considerably faster, more convenient to use, and safer than the laser and that they consider the probe their preferred hemostatic device. Others have compared the bipolar electrodes to the heater probe and found that the results are comparable, with initial control of bleeding achieved in 90% of cases. Repeat treatment is possible with both methods.

Laser. Laser therapy for the GI tract has been available for the past 10 years. The indications for its use are UGI bleeding and neoplasia. The YAG laser is the most powerful coagulator for UGI bleeding of all surgical lasers. The reported experience now exceeds 3600 patients. At least 11 prospective controlled trials of laser photocoagulation for UGI bleeding have been performed. These trials, in general, demonstrate a beneficial effect of laser treatment to stop bleeding and to prevent rebleeding episodes among patients with active bleeding at the time of entry. It has been more difficult to prove that laser therapy alters the requirement for emergency operation, transfusions, or survival. At present, there is no convincing evidence that laser therapy is superior to bipolar electrodes or the heater probe for endoscopic control of bleeding. In addition, the laser system is much more expensive ($50,000 to $100,000 per unit), is not portable, and therefore cannot be taken to the patient's bedside.

Laser treatment of obstructing esophageal cancers is performed endoscopically in patients deemed nonoperable or with recurrent esophageal cancer. Laser fibers are advanced through the biopsy channel of the endoscope to the esophageal tumor. This fiber delivers thermal energy that vaporizes and destroys the superficial layer of the tumor, gradually opening the esophageal lumen so that the patient can swallow better. Multiple treatments are usually required.

Balloon dilation of benign strictures is also a therapeutic application of esophagogastroduodenoscopy. In surgical patients this condition is generally an anastomotic stricture, which may develop after a gastric resection, or an esophageal stricture secondary to gastroesophageal reflux or after a gastric bypass procedure, which is performed for obesity in some cases. The new anastomosis is too snug and is associated with vomiting. Balloon dilation will generally correct these problems. *Placement of feeding tubes* is another application of therapeutic endoscopy and is frequently performed in critically ill ICU patients who are unable to eat and in whom a feeding in the small bowel is preferred. With endoscopic assistance it is possible to put a small feeding tube into the duodenum near the ligament of Treitz to provide nutrition for these patients.

Complications of EGD

Complications include aspiration of gastric content, medication reactions, esophageal perforation (usually at the level of the cricopharyngeus muscle), and cardiopulmonary adverse events. Patient preparation is important, and in most cases these problems can be anticipated and, if not avoided, at least minimized. The incidence of these complications is about 1%. Cardiac and oxygen saturation monitoring during a procedure is often routine.

ENDOSCOPIC RETROGRADE CHOLANGIOPANCREATOGRAPHY

ERCP is performed by passing a side-viewing flexible scope into the duodenum and then placing a small catheter into the ampulla of Vater for injection of dye and radiographic visualization of the common bile duct and the pancreatic duct. The x-ray imaging thus provided will enable diagnosis and treatment of many biliary and pancreatic diseases. Patient preparation and equipment used are similar for standard EGD, but the procedure must be performed in a room equipped with fluoroscopy.

Major Indications for ERCP

Jaundice. Jaundice is caused by either intrahepatic conditions such as hepatitis and cirrhosis or extrahepatic problems such as common bile duct stones or cancer of the pancreas, which causes obstruction to flow of bile in the duodenum. An ultrasound examination of the liver and biliary tree is usually performed before ERCP to determine whether the bile ducts are dilated. Common causes of common bile duct dilation and jaundice are bile duct stones, cancer in the head of the pancreas, pancreatitis with stenosis of the distal common bile duct, and tumors in the ampulla *(Plate 5-2)*.

Pancreatic Disease. ERCP is capable of providing an excellent picture of the pancreatic duct and is very useful for detecting strictures, filling defects, and compression in the pancreatic duct, which can be caused by pancreatitis and in some cases pancreatic cancer. Pancreatitis may be expected based on the patient's clinical history and the presence of elevated pancreatic enzymes.

Epigastric Pain. ERCP is often performed for evaluation of persistent and nondiagnosed epigastric pain. When the more common conditions—esophagitis, peptic ulcer disease, and gallstones—have been excluded, the surgeon-endoscopist is looking for signs of pancreatitis, cancer, or stenosis of the papilla of Vater, which could be causing the symptoms.

Therapeutic Applications of ERCP

Removal of common bile duct (CBD) stones is the most common ERCP procedure. CBD stones generally originate in the gallbladder and migrate through the cystic duct into the CBD (Fig. 5-1). The incidence of CBD stones in patients with gallstones is 10% to 15%. These stones are usually removed at the time of cholecystectomy, but occasionally they are not recognized and become apparent later as "retained" CBD stones. With the recent introduction of laparoscopic cholecystectomy, CBD stones are frequently removed by ERCP before cholecystectomy, since laparoscopic removal of CBD stones is difficult.

ERCP removal of CBD stones begins with the sphincterotomy. With a standard ERCP scope, a catheter with an adjustable cutting wire that is connected to electric cautery is inserted in the ampulla so that the sphincter of Oddi and the ampulla can be carefully cut for a distance of approximately 1 cm. This enlarges the papilla of Vater so that specially designed catheters with balloons or baskets can be advanced into the CBD to retrieve CBD duct stones.

Stent placement is an increasingly common therapeutic procedure for ERCP and is performed to bypass malignant or benign strictures of the CBD. Endoscopic sphincterotomy of the

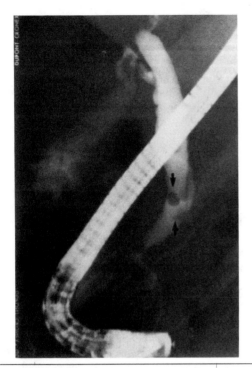

FIGURE 5-1 ERCP study with injection of dye into the common bile duct. The arrows point to a 5-mm stone in the bile duct. This stone was removed by endoscopic sphincterotomy in preparation for laparoscopic cholecystectomy. Note the partially filled gallbladder with gallstones to the left of the scope.

ampulla provides generous access to the CBD, and these stents are placed with fluoroscopic control into the bile duct and passed through the stricture. The stents remain in place until they become clogged, after 4 to 6 months. On an outpatient basis the stent is replaced.

Complications of ERCP

ERCP is associated with the same side effects as EGD, but with the potential complications of pancreatitis, sepsis (cholangitis), and perforation of the duodenal wall. The incidence is 2% to 10%, depending on the series. The pancreatitis is related to the injection of dye into the pancreatic duct plus catheter irritation of the pancreatic duct. Post-ERCP infection and cholangitis correlate with stasis of bile in the CBD. When the duct is obstructed by gallstones or tumor, the static bile is a good medium for infection. Perforation (<1%) may be caused by pushing the catheter through the duodenal wall or by a sphincterotomy that is too long.

COLONOSCOPY

Colonoscopy is the endoscopic examination of the colon and rectum. It is a useful examination to check for abnormalities in the large intestine such as polyps, colon cancer, and colitis. The procedure is performed in the endoscopy suite and is routinely done as an outpatient procedure. The colon must be cleansed well. Bowel preparation consists of laxatives, enemas, and a clear liquid diet over 2 days, or a gut-lavage technique in which the patient drinks a balanced electrolyte solution that contains polyethyleneglycol over 4 hours the evening before colonoscopy. Intravenous medications are given for sedation and analgesia during the procedure.

Indications for Colonoscopy

Colonoscopy frequently begins as a diagnostic procedure to evaluate rectal bleeding or undiagnosed anemia, to clarify abnormalities or filling defects on a barium enema, or to evaluate patients with diarrhea and suspected colitis.

The most common causes of *rectal bleeding* are hemorrhoids, diverticular disease, and angiodysplasia of the colon. Colon polyps and carcinomas often are associated with anemia and the presence of occult blood but generally do not produce acute blood loss. Inflammatory bowel disease is also a cause of rectal bleeding and is usually associated with frequent bowel motions, diarrhea, and other symptomatology of inflammatory bowel disease. Each of these conditions can be seen and identified with colonoscopy.

Constipation and change in bowel habit are also indications for colonoscopy. A prior barium enema examination may demonstrate an abnormality, and colonoscopy is performed to obtain a direct view of the suspected lesion and a tissue biopsy for diagnosis. Patients with diverticulitis may have fever, abdominal distention, left lower quadrant tenderness, and a mass. Medical treatment generally leads to prompt improvement; and colonoscopy can be performed when the diagnosis is in doubt and to rule out cancer.

Flexible sigmoidoscopy and colonoscopy have a role in patients with *inflammatory bowel disease*. Colonoscopy is the examination of choice for diagnosing ulcerative colitis and determining the proximal extension of this disease. Patients with Crohn's disease of the small bowel frequently have anal or rectal abnormalities that require close rectal examination, and an occasional patient will have Crohn's colitis for which colonoscopy is appropriate to make the diagnosis and to determine the extent of the involvement in the colon. In both diseases endoscopy and standard barium enema examination are complimentary. Patients with ulcerative colitis should also have an annual colonoscopy with biopsy because they are at greater risk for developing colon cancer.

For *cancer surveillance* the American Cancer Society recommends that people over the age of 45 years should have a rectal examination, check of the stool for blood, and flexible sigmoidoscopy as part of a cancer screening protocol and a good physical examination. If the stool is positive for blood or a polyp is identified, full colonoscopy is indicated. It is also recommended that patients who have had a colectomy for colon cancer should have follow-up examination of the colon on a regular basis for the first 2 or 3 years because of the likelihood of developing new polyps each year and the 5% to 7% chance of developing a second primary colon cancer within the next 5 or 6 years. There is some controversy about how often the colon should be examined after an operation, but a consensus is that after the first 2 years a check-up every 2 or 3 years can be justified.

Therapeutic Procedures Performed With Colonoscopy

The most frequently performed therapeutic procedure is *polypectomy* performed through the colonoscope *(Plate 5-3)*. It is possible to remove most polyps of up to 3 cm with electrocautery and a snare by this technique. In the past removal of such polyps required an open operation, that is, a laparotomy and then a colotomy or limited resection of the colon segment to remove the polyp, which constitutes a major operation. With colonoscopic removal of polyps, there is virtually no mortality, and the morbidity rate is less than 5% and limited to an occasional episode of bleeding from the polyp stock and a small risk of colonic perforation. Polyps must be removed because they may contain a focus of adenocarcinoma. This risk actually increases as the size of the polyp increases and becomes significant at a diameter of 1 cm, which has a cancer risk of 5%. It is also believed that many polyps are precursors to adenocarcinoma.

Another indication for therapeutic endoscopy includes lower GI bleeding from *angiodysplasia* of the colon. These lesions are vascular malformations in the mucosa of the colon and can cause recurrent episodes of colonic bleeding and

anemia. Some of these lesions can be controlled by *laser coagulation,* which is performed through the colonoscope. Endoscopy of the colon is also used to diagnose and treat *sigmoid volvulus,* a malrotation of a redundant sigmoid that leads to a kinking, obstruction, and eventual perforation.

Limitations of Colonoscopy

Experienced endoscopists are able to pass the colonoscope through the several curves of the colon to reach the cecum in 90% or more of cases. In those instances in which complete colonoscopy is not possible, the limiting factors usually are a very tortuous redundant colon, patient discomfort, or severe diverticular disease.

Relative contraindications to colonoscopy include the presence of peritonitis, a critically ill patient with unstable vital signs, acute diverticulitis, and toxic megacolon. In the elective cases medical conditions such as a recent myocardial infarction, anticoagulation (especially if polypectomy may be performed), and severe chronic obstructive pulmonary disease are also relative contraindications. Active rectal bleeding is no longer considered a rigid contraindication, since blood is a good cathartic and it is often possible to pass the colonoscope, view the colon, and identify the point of active bleeding.

Complications of Colonoscopy

The complications of colonoscopy are *perforation of the colon, colonic bleeding, abdominal distention* and *pulmonary compromise,* and *medication reactions.* Perforation occurs during insertion of the colonoscope when excessive pressure may be used to advance the scope, leading to a tear in the bowel wall at a fixed point. In addition, polypectomy with the snare electrocautery can potentially perforate the bowel wall when the snare is placed too low on the stalk of the polyp and too close to the bowel wall or when excessive current is applied. Fortunately, the incidence of these complications is low (<1%). Explosion during polypectomy with electrocautery has been reported in the past, particularly if the bowel was not well prepared and if hydrogen or methane gas was present. For this reason, a clean, well-prepared bowel is a prerequisite for polypectomy with electrocautery.

FLEXIBLE SIGMOIDOSCOPY

Flexible sigmoidoscopy is similar to colonoscopy except that it is limited to an examination of the anus, rectum, and sigmoid colon for a distance of 60 cm. Sigmoidoscopy is relatively easy to perform, and the preparation is simple, consisting of two Fleet enemas 2 to 3 hours before the procedure. It is the initial screening test for colon cancer surveillance in asymptomatic patients because 40% to 50% of polyps and colon cancers are found in this region. If an abnormality is found within this length of the rectum and sigmoid colon, full colonoscopy is warranted because of the likelihood of an associated lesion higher up in the colon.

PERCUTANEOUS ENDOSCOPIC GASTROSTOMY

Percutaneous endoscopic gastrostomy (PEG), introduced in 1980, has become the procedure of choice for the establishment of a tube gastrostomy in patients not otherwise requiring laparotomy. The most frequent *indication* for the placement of the PEG has been the necessity for feeding patients with severe neurologic impairment because of both congenital and acquired conditions. However, any circumstance requiring tube feedings not adequately provided by the nasoenteral route may be appropriate for a PEG.

Contraindications include patients with total or near-total esophageal obstruction, massive ascites, ongoing sepsis, and extremely short life expectancies. A PEG is not contraindicated in patients with previous abdominal surgery; however, whenever satisfactory transillumination of the abdominal wall by the endoscope cannot be achieved, the procedure should be abandoned.

How Is PEG Performed?

The patient is prepared for PEG as for a routine esophagogastroduodenoscopy; however, the patient is positioned in a supine position, and a dose of preoperative antibiotic is usually given to protect the skin incision against the oral flora carried from the mouth to the abdominal wound. The abdomen is sterilely prepared and draped. After the gastroscope is passed, a brief examination of the esophagus, stomach, and duodenum is carried out to confirm there are no unexpected lesions that would preclude the safe performance of PEG. Then the scope is withdrawn into the body of the stomach, the light is directed in an anterior direction, and the stomach is transilluminated so that the light can be readily visualized through the skin of the anterior abdominal wall. The assistant then pushes on the abdominal wall directly over the light with his or her finger, and the endoscopist should readily see the indentation of the gastric wall during the assistant's palpation.

At this point, local anesthesia is instilled into the skin, and a 1 cm incision is made over this site. A plastic-sheathed needle is pushed into the stomach, with the needle entry observed through the endoscope. A snare passed through the endoscope grasps the plastic sheath. The needle is withdrawn, and a suture or a guidewire, which is provided in the commercially prepared kits, is passed through the cannula into the stomach. The snare is loosened; the suture or guidewire is then grasped with the snare and pulled into the gastroscopic channel; and the gastroscope with the suture is withdrawn, pulling the suture or the guidewire along. The plastic cannula is then withdrawn (Fig. 5-2).

The suture is attached to a gastrostomy tube from the kit. The assistant pulls the suture through the abdominal wall while the surgeon advances the gastrostomy tube through the mouth and into the stomach. The assistant pulls the tube out through the abdominal wall. Next the scope is reinserted so that the placement of the gastrostomy tube in the stomach can be watched *(Plate 5-4).* The G-tube should be close to the gastric mucosa but not excessively tight so that ischemia does not result. The catheter is then secured in place on the anterior abdominal wall. The tube has a valve attached to it so that feedings can begin.

This "pull" technique is the most common method used for PEG. Other techniques include a "push" and an "introducer" technique. These have various advantages and disadvantages that we will not cover here.

The main complication of this procedure is infection of the exit site through the skin. The incidence of such infections has decreased with the use of antibiotics and with the formation of an adequate skin incision so that the tube is not tight at the skin level. A gastrocolic fistula can occur by erosion of the tube into adjacent colon or because of direct inadvertent puncture of the colon by the needle. This usually resolves with withdrawal of the catheter.

Pneumoperitoneum is not infrequent after performance of a PEG but is usually of no consequence. It is secondary to the passage of air around the catheter as it exits the stomach. Overall, the morbidity rate is 5% to 10%, and the mortality rate within 30 days is less than 1%. PEG is a safe and effective means of providing a tube gastrostomy for patients who cannot take adequate nutrition from the nasoenteral route. The candidates must be carefully selected so that this procedure is not overused.

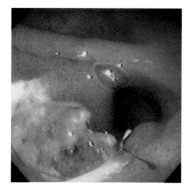

PLATE 5-1

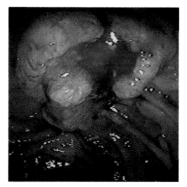

PLATE 5-2

PLATE 5-1 Endoscopic picture of a large ulcer along the greater curvature of the stomach. In the lower left corner of the picture is the white fibrinous exudate, which is also bile stained. This is the ulcer crater and measures approximately 2 × 3 cm. This ulcer is actually located in the anastomosis of a gastroenterostomy, which was performed several years earlier when this patient had a severe injury to the duodenum and head of the pancreas.

PLATE 5-2 ERCP view showing an adenocarcinoma of the ampulla. The patient is a 67-year-old woman who complained of weakness and was known to have occult blood in the stool. Biopsy of this fungating lesion in the duodenum demonstrated well-differentiated adenocarcinoma. The tumor was treated by resection of the duodenum and the head of the pancreas.

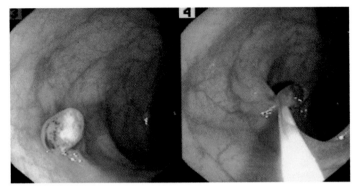

PLATE 5-3

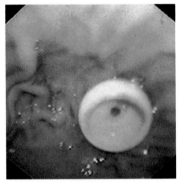

PLATE 5-4

PLATE 5-3   Colonoscopic picture showing a 7-mm adenomatous polyp located in the right side of the colon. The picture on the right shows a snare catheter that has been looped over the polyp and cinched at the base for coagulation.

PLATE 5-4   Endoscopic view of a PEG catheter in the anterior wall of the stomach. The wide tip of the catheter holds it in position while tube feedings are delivered through the central lumina tube, which is also visible.

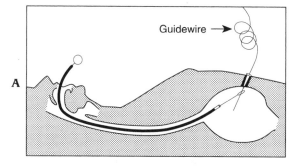
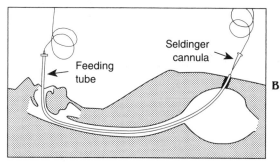

A

B

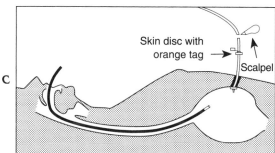

C

FIGURE 5-2   Schematic diagrams of PEG insertion. **A,** The 18-gauge needle has been inserted into the distended stomach. The guidewire is grasped with the colonoscopy snare. **B,** Feeding tube is advanced over the guidewire into the stomach and out through the stomach wall and the anterior abdominal wall. **C,** Proper position of the gastrostomy tube is confirmed by repeat endoscopy. (Courtesy Ross Laboratories, Columbus, OH 43216.)

PITFALLS AND COMMON MYTHS

- Esophagogastroduodenoscopy will not detect the source of bleeding in every patient with UGI bleeding; the accuracy rate is 90% to 95%. In cases of severe bleeding, it is limited by the clinician's inability to clean the stomach of blood and clot for a good look.
- Such therapeutic endoscopic measures as heater probe and sclerotherapy often control the cause of UGI bleeding. Protection is not permanent with one treatment, however, and rebleeding does occur in 10% to 30% of patients. Endoscopic treatment can be used again, but in some instances, such as for a large duodenal ulcer, surgical therapy is more appropriate.
- Total colonoscopy to the cecum is possible in 90% of patients, depending on the skill of the endoscopist. When colonoscopy is incomplete, a barium enema is often obtained to complete the examination.

BIBLIOGRAPHY

Bown SC, Hawes R, Matthewson K, et al. Endoscopic laser palliation for advanced malignant dysphagia. Gut 28:799, 1987.

Cello JP, Grendell JH, Crass RA, et al. Endoscopic sclerotherapy versus portacaval shunt in patients with severe cirrhosis and acute variceal hemorrhage. N Engl J Med 316:11-15, 1987.

Donahue PE, Mobarhan S, Layden TJ, et al. Endoscopic control of upper gastrointestinal hemorrhage with a bipolar coagulation device. Surg Gynecol Obstet 159:113-118, 1984.

Johnston JH, Sones JQ, Long BW, et al. Comparison of heater probe and YAG laser in endoscopic treatment of major bleeding from peptic ulcers. Gastrointest Endosc 31:175-180, 1985.

Juhl GL, Larson GM, Polk HC Jr, et al. Results of colonoscopy in colorectal cancer follow-up program. World J Surg 14:255-261, 1990.

Knutson CO, Max MH. Value of colonoscopy in patients with rectal blood loss unexplained by rigid proctosigmoidoscopy and barium contrast enema examinations. Am J Surg 139:84, 1980.

Kovacs TOG, Jensen DM. Endoscopic control of gastroduodenal hemorrhage. Ann Rev Med 38:267-277, 1987.

Laine L. Multipolar electrocoagulation in the treatment of active upper gastrointestinal tract hemorrhage. N Engl J Med 316:1613-1617, 1987.

Larson GM, Polk HC Jr. Massive upper gastrointestinal hemorrhage. In Scott HW Jr, Sawyers JL (eds). Surgery of the Stomach, Duodenum, and Small Intestine, 2nd ed. Boston, Blackwell Scientific Publications, 1992.

Larson GM, Schmidt T, Gott G, et al. Upper gastrointestinal bleeding: Predictors of outcome. Surgery 100:765-772, 1986.

Max MH, West B, Knutson CO. Evaluation of postoperative gastroduodenal symptoms: Endoscopy or upper gastrointestinal roentgenography? Surgery 86:578, 1979.

Millikan WJ, Henderson JM, Galloway JR, et al. Surgical rescue for failures of cirrhotic sclerotherapy. Am J Surg 160:117-121, 1990.

Ponsky JL, Gauderer MWL, Stellato TA. Percutaneous endoscopic gastrostomy: Review of 150 cases. Arch Surg 118:913, 1983.

Silverstein FE, Gilbert DA, Tedesco FJ, et al. The national ASGE survey on upper gastrointestinal bleeding. II. Clinical prognostic factors. Dig Dis Sci 26(suppl):90-96, 1981.

Stiegmann G, Goff J, Michalezt P, et al. Endoscopic variceal ligation vs sclerotherapy for bleeding esophageal varices: Early results of a prospective randomized trial. Gastrointest Endosc 36:188, 1990.

Sugawa C, Ikeda T, Fujita Y, et al. Endoscopic hemostasis of bleeding of the upper gastrointestinal tract by local injection of 98% dehydrated ethanol. Surg Gynecol Obstet 162:159, 1986.

Westaby D, Williams R. Status of sclerotherapy for variceal bleeding. Am J Surg 160:32-36, 1990.

CHAPTER REVIEW
Questions

1. Name four indications for upper gastrointestinal endoscopy.
2. During a colonoscopy examination it is not always possible for the endoscopist to advance the scope through the entire colon to the cecum. Which of the following answers is *not* a limiting factor or feature?
   a. A tortuous redundant colon
   b. Patient discomfort
   c. A previous cholecystectomy
   d. Severe diverticular disease
3. Which of the following answers is *not* an indication for the placement of a percutaneous endoscopic gastrostomy (PEG)?
   a. A 22-year-old man with a severe head injury has a tracheostomy and is comatose.
   b. A 65-year-old man tripped and fell down the stairs and sustained a subdural hematoma, which was surgically evacuated. He is now slowly regaining consciousness but has developed pneumonia and is receiving tube feedings through a nasogastric tube.
   c. A 47-year-old man was admitted to the hospital with recurrent colon cancer that

has metastasized to the liver. He is jaundiced with ascites, and nutrition has been provided by total parenteral nutrition (TPN).
   d. A 38-year-old woman was severely injured in a motor vehicle accident with femur and rib fractures and a pulmonary contusion and now is gradually recovering from pneumonia and from renal failure caused by acute tubular necrosis. She had DPL during admission but has had no previous abdominal surgery. She is currently receiving 2500 calories per day by TPN.
4. Which one of the following treatments is suitable to perform through an endoscope?
   a. Injection sclerotherapy
   b. Electrocoagulation of bleeding ulcer
   c. Heater probe to a bleeding vessel
   d. Tumor biopsy
   e. All of the above
5. Which finding is *not* a usual indication for ERCP?
   a. Common bile duct stones
   b. Pancreatic cancer
   c. Pancreatitis
   d. Breast cancer
   e. Unexplained epigastric pain
6. What is the incidence of common bile duct stones in patients with symptomatic gallstones?
   a. <5%
   b. 10% to 15%
   c. 50% to 60%
   d. >60%
7. Which conditions *cannot* be diagnosed by endoscopy?
   a. Carcinoma of the cecum
   b. Diverticulosis
   c. Ulcerative colitis
   d. Cholangiocarcinoma
   e. Sigmoid volvulus

Answers

1. Hemorrhage; epigastric pain; clarification or exclusion of questionable radiographic findings; evaluation and biopsy of gastric ulcer; reflux esophagitis
2. c
3. c
4. e
5. d
6. b
7. d

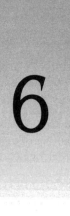

6

Diagnostic and Therapeutic Laparoscopy for the General Surgeon

KARL A. ZUCKER
ROBERT W. BAILEY

KEY FEATURES

After reading this chapter you will understand:
- The technology and instrumentation of laparoscopy.
- How laparoscopy is done.
- The applicability of the procedure to various disease states and its limitations.

The concept of direct, endoscopic visualization of the peritoneal cavity is usually accredited to Georg Kelling of Dresden, Germany. In 1901 he used an existing rigid cystoscope to examine the abdominal cavity of a dog and within a few years began performing this procedure in patients with suspected liver disease. Jacobaeus, a Swedish surgeon of the same era, also reported his clinical experience with this technique and was the first to use the term *laparoscopy*. Over the next several decades laparoscopy became a valuable diagnostic procedure to evaluate patients with chronic abdominal pain, liver disease, ascites of unknown origin, and other intra-abdominal disorders. Although the development of sophisticated noninvasive imaging techniques such as ultrasonography and computed tomographic (CT) scanning has subsequently diminished the diagnostic role of this procedure, it remains a useful modality in patients for whom the diagnosis remains uncertain or visually guided biopsies are required.

The era of therapeutic laparoscopy began in the early 1960s with Raoul Palmer's description of electrocautery destruction of the isthmic and proximal ampulla of the fallopian tubes for elective sterilization. For the past three decades gynecologists have continued to exploit the potential of laparoscopy to treat a number of pelvic abnormalities, and it now represents one of the most commonly performed surgical procedures in North America. General surgeons, however, largely ignored these developments until the description of laparoscopic biliary tract surgery in the late 1980s. The first complete removal of a diseased gallbladder was performed by the French surgeon, Mouret, in 1987, with McKernan and Saye duplicating this achievement in the United States 1 year later. These investigators and others soon realized that laparoscopic management of gallbladder disease could be accomplished with a hospital stay of 1 day or less and with considerably less postoperative discomfort. These patients were able to return to their normal activities within days rather than weeks as is routine after open cholecystectomy. Recognition of the tremendous benefits in overall patient care as compared with open cholecystectomy has now persuaded surgeons to investigate the role of laparoscopic surgery in the management of other commonly encountered intra-abdominal disorders. Currently under development are laparoscopic procedures for acute appendicitis, truncal and selective vagotomy, herniorrhaphy, fundoplication for gastroesophageal reflux, and colon resection for both benign and malignant diseases.

9

WHAT IS REQUIRED TO PERFORM DIAGNOSTIC OR THERAPEUTIC LAPAROSCOPY?

Contemporary surgical laparoscopy has become highly dependent on technology. Modern rigid laparoscopes incorporate both a series of optical lenses for imaging and a system of quartz rods to transmit light into the abdominal cavity. The most popular instruments are 5 and 10 mm in diameter and are designed with either forward-viewing or side-viewing (30 to 50 degrees) lens. Although more difficult to use, angled scopes allow for much greater versatility in visualizing intra-abdominal structures. Some laparoscopes contain a working channel that allows the surgeon to introduce instruments (e.g., operating telescope); however, there is a significant loss of image quality (Fig. 6-1). A light source is connected to the laparoscope via a fiberoptic light cable and is used to illuminate the abdomen (Fig. 6-2). In the past surgeons used the eyepiece of the laparoscope to visualize the peritoneal cavity, but this made it difficult for others in the operating room to monitor the operative procedure and provide useful assistance. In the mid-1980s miniaturized video cameras became available that attached directly to the eyepiece of the laparoscope, allowing observation of the procedure on one or more video monitors (Fig. 6-3). This was a major milestone in the acceptance of endoscopic surgery because it allowed the surgical team to coordinate their efforts to perform more complicated surgical procedures and was proved an extremely valuable teaching tool.

To perform surgery safely within the closed abdomen, it must be distended with gas. Room air, nitrous oxide, and carbon dioxide have all been used to create a pneumoperitoneum. Nitrous oxide is a popular agent for diagnostic procedures because its mild anesthetic properties result in minimal discomfort as the abdomen distends. Room air and nitrous oxide, however, will both support combustion and should not be used in the presence of electrocautery or lasers. Carbon dioxide is inexpensive, readily available, and rapidly absorbed from the blood, which minimizes the risk of gas emboli, although use of this gas does lead to postoperative shoulder pain in 30% to 40% of patients, presumably from irritation of the diaphragmatic peritoneal surface. Most surgeons use carbon dioxide when performing therapeutic laparoscopy. Carbon dioxide is delivered under pressure into the abdomen with the aid of an electronic insufflator (Fig. 6-4). These instruments pump as much as 15 L per minute into the abdomen. They are also designed to allow the surgeon to monitor the pressure within the peritoneal cavity and automatically stop gas flow when a preselected pressure is reached (usually 14 mm Hg or less).

Currently a wide variety of instruments are available for use during laparoscopic surgery, including traumatic and atraumatic grasping forceps, straight and curved dissectors, suction and irrigation cannulas, fanlike retractors, surgical clip appliers, aspiration needles, bowel-grasping forceps, Babcock-like clamps, cotton-tip (e.g., Kittner) dissectors, and needle holders (Fig. 6-5). Many of the dissecting instruments are designed for use with monopolar electrocautery to facilitate the operative dissection and maintain hemostasis. Although widely used, monopolar electric energy can be unpredictable as to the amount of tissue injured. As a result, bipolar cautery instruments, which are less likely to burn distant tis-

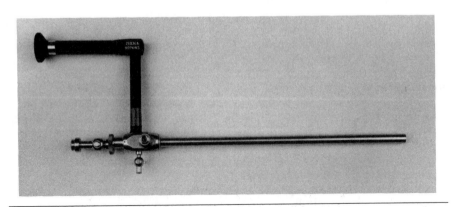

FIGURE 6-1   An operating laparoscope incorporates a small working channel that allows the surgeon to introduce instruments through the same site.

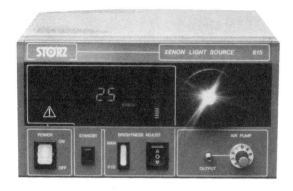

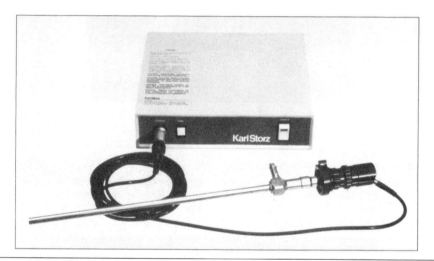

FIGURE 6-2   A light source, fiberoptic cable, and laparoscope are all essential components of the system.

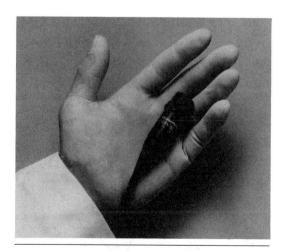

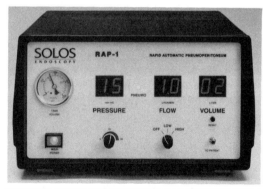

FIGURE 6-4   Contemporary electronic high-flow insufflator device, which can rapidly distend the abdomen with carbon dioxide. Gas flow automatically stops when the preset intra-abdominal pressure is achieved.

FIGURE 6-3   Miniaturized video cameras that can be attached to the eyepiece of the laparoscope.

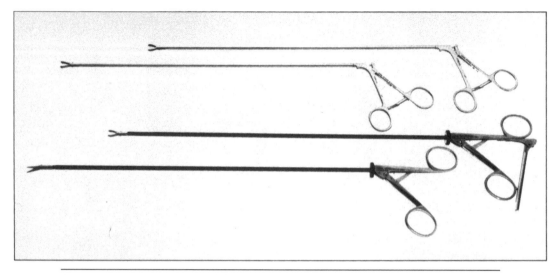

FIGURE 6-5   Representation of the various instruments used during laparoscopic surgery.

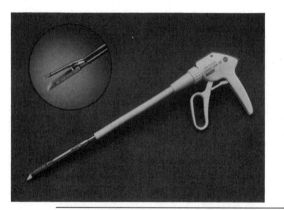 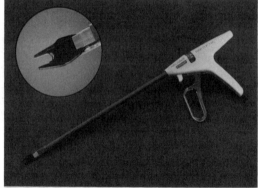

FIGURE 6-6   A variety of automatic stapling devices has been developed that allow surgeons to perform more complicated intra-abdominal laparoscopic procedures.

sues, have recently become popular. Another option for dissection and hemostasis is laser energy. A variety of light frequencies and operating modes (contact versus noncontact) are currently available, all of which have their own unique advantages and disadvantages. Also available are automatic laparoscopic stapling devices, which are similar in many respects to those used in open surgery (Fig. 6-6). These are available in different lengths and staple configurations and can be used for dividing bowel, lung, or vascular structures.

HOW ARE PATIENTS PREPARED FOR LAPAROSCOPIC SURGERY?

Patients are prepared for laparoscopic surgery much as they are for traditional open surgery and therefore must undergo an appropriate preoperative evaluation for possibilities such as cardiopulmonary disease, coagulation abnormalities, and electrolyte disturbances. Operative consent forms must explain the possibility of converting the laparoscopic procedure to an open laparotomy as dictated by the operative findings.

Diagnostic laparoscopy is often performed using a combination of local anesthetics and intravenous sedation. Individuals who are unable to cooperate such as young children or combative adults may require a general anesthetic. Therapeutic laparoscopy generally requires a general anesthetic with complete airway control because this procedure usually lasts longer and requires higher intra-abdominal pressures.

The patient should be placed supine and strapped in position. A foot board is useful since placing the patient in various positions (e.g., Trendelenburg, head up) will allow better visualization of the upper and lower abdomen. Urinary and nasogastric catheters are usually inserted to decompress the stomach and bladder to minimize their risk of injury during insufflation needle or trocar insertion and facilitate examination of the upper abdomen and pelvis. The patient should be prepared in a sterile fashion with the surgical team fully gowned and gloved.

A pneumoperitoneum is established using either a percutaneous approach (i.e., insufflation needle) or an open procedure (i.e., Hassan technique or minilaparotomy). In patients with no complicating conditions or prior abdominal surgery an insufflation needle commonly is used to distend the peritoneal cavity. The umbilical region is the most common location for needle insertion because the abdominal wall is thinnest at this location and all fascial layers are adherent. The needle is placed through a small skin incision and directed toward the lower midline and away from large blood vessels (Fig. 6-7). Placing the patient in a 10- to 15-degree Trendelenburg position allows the small bowel and colon to drop out of the pelvis and lessens the risk of injury. To ensure that the tip of the insufflation needle lies free in the peritoneal cavity, the surgeon generally flushes and aspirates the cavity with saline solution and performs the "Palmer" or "drop" test (fluid is drawn into the abdomen as the abdominal wall is lifted anteriorly). If there is a surgical scar near the umbilicus, a palpable mass, or distended abdominal wall veins (i.e., caput medusae associated with portal hypertension), alternative sites in the middle or upper abdomen (lateral to the epigastric vessels) on either the left or right side may be used. The insufflation needle is then connected to the electronic insufflator and gas introduced at 1 to 1.5 L per minute. If the tip of the needle is in the proper location, the pressure reading should remain less than 8 to 10 mm Hg. If the needle is in a relatively closed space (e.g., intestinal lumen, preperito-

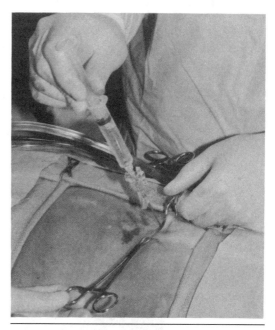

FIGURE 6-7 Insufflation needle with a protective obturator is inserted through a small periumbilical skin incision. From Zucker KA (ed). Surgical Laparoscopy. St Louis, Quality Medical Publishing, 1991, p 150.

neal tissues, omentum), the pressure will increase rapidly to 20 mm Hg or higher. The abdomen is insufflated to a pressure of 14 to 15 mm Hg and the needle removed. A laparoscopic cannula is then inserted with a one-way valve to allow introduction of a variety of instruments into the peritoneal cavity without gas loss.

If extensive adhesions to the anterior abdominal wall may be present, many surgeons prefer using an open technique to establish the pneumoperitoneum. A 2- to 3-cm incision is made in the folds of the umbilicus, and the free peritoneal cavity is entered under direct vision. The larger fascial opening must then be closed around the laparoscopic cannula to maintain an airtight seal. This fascial stitch may be secured to a standard laparoscopic cannula or to modified sheaths with olive-shaped sleeves (to minimize gas leak) and suture wings, which are attached to the fascial stitches (Fig. 6-8). Most diagnostic and therapeutic laparoscopic procedures require additional cannulas to introduce retractors and forceps and are inserted under direct endoscopic guidance to minimize the risk of visceral injury. The location of these entry sites depends on the procedure and the type of instrument used.

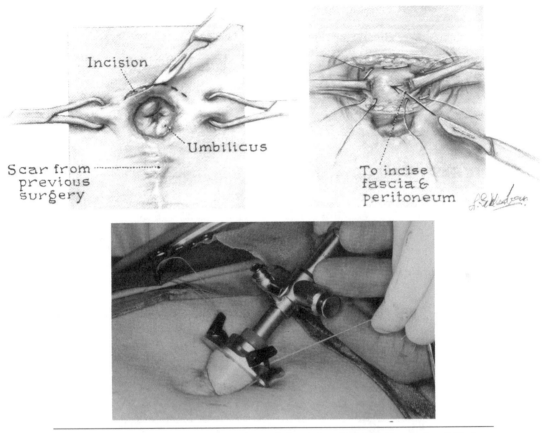

FIGURE 6-8 Open laparoscopy is performed through a slightly larger periumbilical incision. All layers of the abdominal wall are opened under direct vision, and a specially designed cannula is used to prevent gas leak. From Zucker KA (ed). Surgical Laparoscopy. St Louis, Quality Medical Publishing, 1991, pp 89 and 94.

HOW IS DIAGNOSTIC LAPAROSCOPY USED IN GENERAL SURGERY?

Diagnostic laparoscopy has long been used for the assessment of acute and chronic liver disease. More than two thirds of the hepatic surface can be visualized and safely biopsied. Although sonographic- and CT-guided biopsies have essentially replaced "blind" liver biopsy, the use of laparoscopic-directed procedures may still prove advantageous in selected patients, including individuals with small, superficial metastatic nodules that may not be detected with current noninvasive imaging techniques or that are easily interpreted as benign lesions. In addition, radiographic-guided biopsies may miss smaller lesions, or in some patients obtaining larger samples of tissue may be necessary when evaluating disorders affecting hepatic architecture. Com-

plete examination of the liver requires the use of blunt or fanlike retractors to elevate the right and left hepatic lobes. Tissue can be obtained by guiding a percutaneously inserted biopsy needle under laparoscopic guidance or by surgically removing a wedge of tissue that is then extracted through one of the endoscopic cannulas. With either technique hemostasis can be directly assessed. If bleeding occurs, it can be controlled with surgical clips, suture ligation, or electrocautery.

A number of clinicians have advocated the use of laparoscopy for the diagnosis and staging of various intra-abdominal malignancies. This is particularly true if appropriate staging would eliminate the need for laparotomy, for example, in many patients with pancreatic cancer. With this disease only those individuals with a resectable (i.e., curative resection) pancreatic tumor or gastric outlet obstruction should undergo sur-

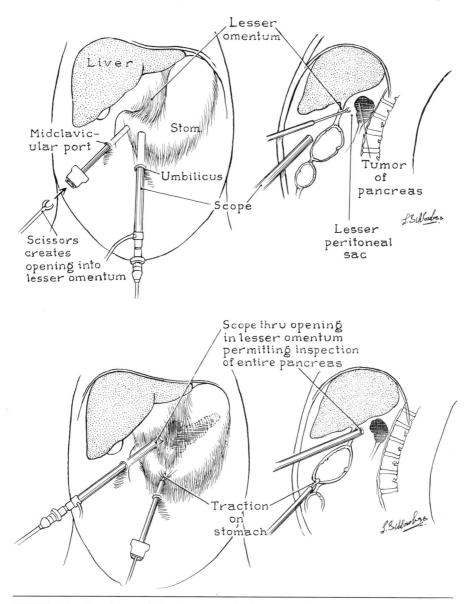

FIGURE 6-9 Opening made in the gastrocolic ligament allows the surgeon to visualize and biopsy the pancreas. From Zucker KA (ed). Surgical Laparoscopy. St Louis, Quality Medical Publishing, 1991, pp 105-106.

gery since adequate biliary palliation can usually be obtained with endoscopic or radiographically placed prosthesis. To select individuals appropriately who might benefit from surgical resection, accurate preoperative staging is necessary. Ultrasonography, CT, magnetic resonance imaging (MRI), and arteriography have been used primarily for this purpose in the past; however, recent data suggest that laparoscopy may contribute significantly to the staging process. This procedure allows for direct visualization of the pancreas, liver, and peritoneal surfaces and apparently is an excellent method of excluding metastatic disease and assessing resectability (Fig. 6-9).

Other malignancies in which laparoscopy has been used for both diagnosis and staging include both Hodgkin's and non-Hodgkin's lymphoma, gallbladder cancer, hepatocellular carcinoma, gastric cancer, esophageal malignancies, carcinoid tumors, cholangiocarcinoma, and leiomyosarcomas. Unfortunately, the role of laparoscopy in the majority of such patients remains unclear because the endoscopic findings usually have not altered the patient's management. Therefore diagnostic laparoscopy should be performed only in selected patients in whom the findings would help dictate subsequent therapy.

A number of clinical investigators have previously advocated the use of laparoscopy in evaluating selected patients after blunt or penetrating trauma. However, until recently very few medical centers were equipped to perform such procedures. With the growing number of trained laparoscopic surgeons, the interest in this application has renewed. The most common indication for laparoscopic intervention is the problematic patient with blunt or limited penetrating trauma for whom it remains unclear where there has been a significant visceral injury. Emergency laparoscopy can be performed in a trauma unit or emergency room setting or in the operating room as a possible prelude to formal laparotomy. The abdomen is prepared and draped using strict sterile technique for the entire procedure. Usually diagnostic laparoscopy for trauma is performed with local anesthesia and minimal intravenous sedation. The basic techniques for establishing a safe pneumoperitoneum are identical to those described earlier. The entire abdominal cavity and pelvis, including the suprahepatic and diaphragmatic spaces, should be examined. The small bowel from the ligament of Treitz to the cecum and most of the colon and proximal rectum can be visualized. The pancreas can be inspected by opening the gastrocolic ligament or through the supragastric route as described earlier. In most patients with evidence of active bleeding or intestinal perforation, a source is easily found. A small laceration of the liver surface or spleen, a torn mesenteric or omental vessel, and other limited injuries often are amenable to laparoscopic control (e.g., electrocautery, laser coagulation, suture ligation). Experience with laparoscopy in patients after blunt or penetrating trauma remains limited. Only a handful of clinical trials have been reported. Although their results have been encouraging, additional studies are necessary to establish its role in such patients.

HOW IS LAPAROSCOPY USED IN PATIENTS WITH SUSPECTED ACUTE APPENDICITIS?

Appendectomy was the first therapeutic gastrointestinal procedure performed under laparoscopic guidance. Since the initial report in 1983 by Kurt Semm of Kiel, Germany, several authors have reported the safety and efficacy of laparo-

scopic surgery in patients with suspected appendicitis. Gotz and his co-workers recently published a series of 625 patients with acute appendicitis, with less than 2% requiring conversion to an open laparotomy (because of operative findings such as dense adhesions). The laparoscopic approach was successful even in situations in which the appendix was retrocecal or deep in the pelvis. Laparoscopic surgery appears to have a number of advantages when compared to traditional open surgery. The entire abdomen can be examined without the need for extending the operative incision. This is particularly useful in those patients with signs of peritoneal irritation but a normal-appearing appendix. In addition, many other intra-abdominal disorders that can mimic acute appendicitis can often be managed with laparoscopic surgery. Infectious wound complications are much less common than in open surgery because contaminated tissues can be removed from the peritoneal cavity without coming in contact with the anterior abdominal wall. A number of authors have claimed that laparoscopic appendectomy is associated with less time in the hospital and a more rapid return to normal activities. In most series patients were able to return home within 24 hours after an uncomplicated appendectomy and return to unrestricted activity within 5 to 7 days. Unfor-

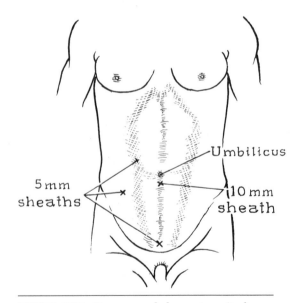

FIGURE 6-10 Recommended puncture site for laparoscopic management of acute appendicitis. The right upper abdominal cannula is used if the ascending colon and cecum require extensive mobilization. From Zucker KA (ed). Surgical Laparoscopy. St Louis, Quality Medical Publishing, 1991, p 229.

tunately, no controlled clinical trials as yet have demonstrated that laparoscopic surgery offers any significant advantage in terms of postoperative recovery.

To perform laparoscopic appendectomy, a pneumoperitoneum is established using either the percutaneous or open technique, and a 10-mm side-viewing laparoscope is introduced through an umbilical cannula. The abdomen is examined to confirm the diagnosis and assess the feasibility of a laparoscopic approach. At least two and often three accessary sheaths are required to mobilize and remove the appendix. The location and size of these cannulas vary, depending on the operative findings and the technique used (Fig. 6-10). A fourth sheath in the right upper abdomen or between the umbilical and suprapubic cannulas is often necessary if the appendix is retrocecal or associated with extensive adhesions. The appendix is identified, freed from the surrounding tissues, and mobilized toward the anterior abdominal wall. Occasionally this step requires division of the lateral attachments of the ascending colon and retraction cephalad of the cecum (Fig. 6-11). The appendix is then held on tension to display the vessels within the

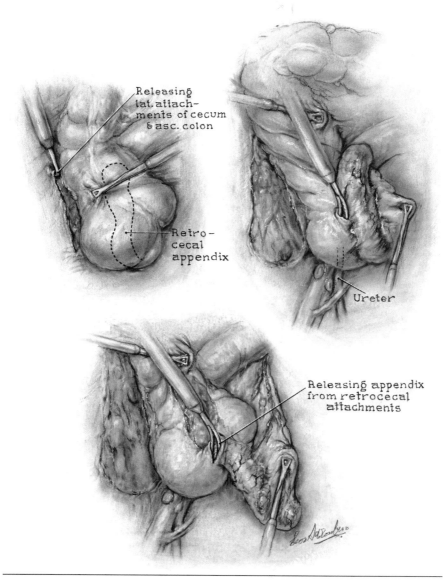

FIGURE 6-11 Medial and anterior mobilization of the ascending colon to expose a retrocecal appendix. From Zucker KA (ed). Surgical Laparoscopy Update. St Louis, Quality Medical Publishing, 1993, p 311.

mesoappendix. Gentle blunt or sharp dissection is used to identify and ligate the vessels, using either surgical clips, suture ligatures, or a laparoscopic stapling instrument (Fig. 6-12, *A* and *B*). The appendix is skeletonized to its juncture with the cecum and ligated with pretied laparoscopic sutures or a stapling instrument (Fig. 6-12, *C-E*). With either technique the base of appendix is not invaginated into the wall of the cecum. Previous clinical studies have shown no advantage with inverting the appendiceal stump; therefore most surgeons performing laparoscopic appendectomy have not performed this maneuver. To date no postoperative complications related to this aspect have been reported.

The appendix generally is removed from the abdomen through the suprapubic or umbilical cannula. All efforts are made to prevent the specimen from coming in contact with the tissues of the abdominal wall. If the appendix cannot be extracted through a standard laparoscopic sheath, it can be placed within a sterile bag and removed through a larger fascial opening. The peritoneal cavity is copiously irrigated and the remaining cannulas removed. The larger fascial defects are closed and the skin incisions approximated with staples or sutures.

An area of controversy concerns whether the surgeon should remove a healthy-appearing appendix when performing laparoscopy for other reasons (e.g., cholecystectomy). Apparently there is little if any benefit in removing the appendix under such circumstances because the risk of subsequent complications from acute appendicitis in such individuals is extremely low. This is in contrast to those patients undergoing laparoscopic surgery for presumed acute appendicitis. Most surgeons have advocated removing a healthy appendix in this situation if there is no obvious source of inflammation elsewhere in the abdomen or pelvis. If a healthy appendix is left in place and the pain recurs, the surgeon may face a diagnostic dilemma and be reluctant to consider appendectomy. Also, there are previous reports that early mucosal appendicitis may on occasion be missed on gross examination alone.

WHEN IS LAPAROSCOPY USED IN PATIENTS WITH GALLBLADDER DISEASE?

In most communities laparoscopic surgery has become the procedure of choice for managing patients with symptomatic gallbladder disease. In those medical centers with extensive laparoscopic experience 90% to 95% of all patients with cholelithiasis are considered candidates for this procedure. Currently the only absolute contraindications to attempting laparoscopic surgery are patients with severe bleeding disorders or generalized abdominal sepsis or peritonitis and women in the latter stages of pregnancy. A list of relative contraindications to attempting laparoscopic surgery is found in the box below. The most commonly encountered relative contraindications are acute cholecystitis and a history of prior upper abdominal surgery. The inflammation and edema that accompany acute cholecystitis often distort the biliary ductal and vascular anatomy, making it difficult to identify important anatomic landmarks. Individuals with a history of previous surgery may have extensive adhesions, which increase the possibility of injury during insufflation needle or trocar insertion and hinder the exposure of the porta hepatis. Although each patient must be evaluated on an individual basis, the most important determinant as to whether such patients can safely undergo laparoscopic surgery is usually the experience of the surgeon.

Patients are evaluated for laparoscopic biliary tract surgery in the same manner as those undergoing open cholecystectomy. A general assessment is made of the patient's health and operative risk, including a careful history and physical examination to exclude other diseases that can mimic biliary colic. An attempt is made to screen individuals for any evidence of choledocholithiasis, including the use of laboratory blood tests (e.g., bilirubin, alkaline phosphatase, aspartate aminotransferase, alanine aminotransferase, amylase) and a high-quality ultrasound to ex-

---

RELATIVE CONTRAINDICATIONS TO ATTEMPTING LAPAROSCOPIC CHOLECYSTECTOMY

Prior upper abdominal surgery
Acute cholecystitis
Morbid obesity
Advanced liver disease
Known abdominal malignancy
Minor bleeding disorders
Inflammatory bowel disease
Inability to tolerate general anesthesia
Early stages of pregnancy
Suspicion of gallbladder cancer

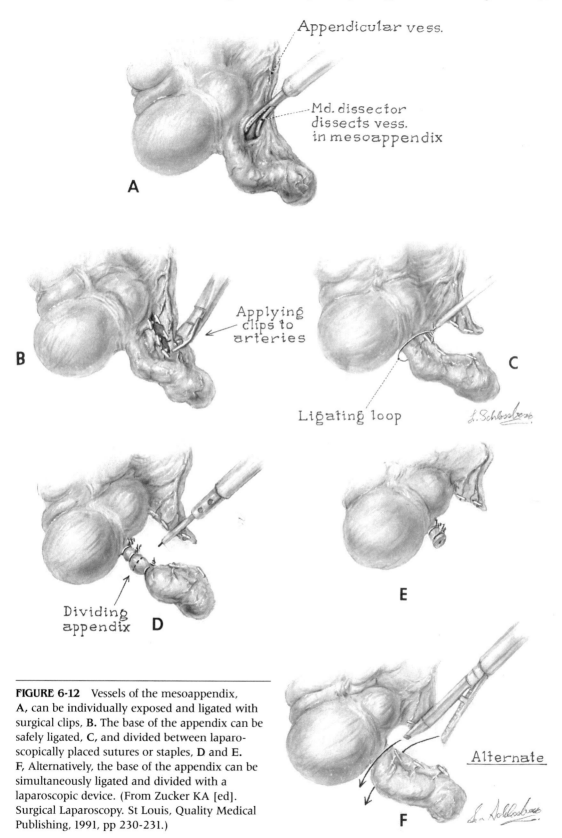

FIGURE 6-12 Vessels of the mesoappendix, A, can be individually exposed and ligated with surgical clips, B. The base of the appendix can be safely ligated, C, and divided between laparo-scopically placed sutures or staples, D and E. F, Alternatively, the base of the appendix can be simultaneously ligated and divided with a laparoscopic device. (From Zucker KA [ed]. Surgical Laparoscopy. St Louis, Quality Medical Publishing, 1991, pp 230-231.)

clude intrahepatic or extrahepatic ductal dilation. If there is strong evidence of persistent choledocholithiasis based on the history, physical examination, laboratory tests, or imaging studies, preoperative endoscopic retrograde cholangiopancreatography (ERCP) is advised. If choledocholithiasis is present, an endoscopic sphincterotomy and stone extraction can be performed at the same setting. Flexible biliary endoscopy has taken on an increasingly important role with the advent of laparoscopic surgery since access to the common bile duct is more difficult with this approach and is not always predictable. Although techniques of exploring the common bile duct have been reported, most surgeons prefer to clear the duct of any known calculi before attempting laparoscopic cholecystectomy.

All patients undergoing laparoscopic surgery should be prepared and draped for the possibility of an open laparotomy. Approximately 5% to 10% of all patients require conversion to open laparotomy, usually because of extensive inflammation and adhesions that prevent accurate identification of the ductal and vascular structures. In patients operated on emergently for acute cholecystitis, this figure may be as high as 20% to 25%.

A pneumoperitoneum is established using either the percutaneous or the open technique. In most patients a total of four laparoscopic cannulas are needed to complete the procedure (Fig. 6-13). In patients with extensive inflammation or adhesions a fifth sheath may be required to provide adequate exposure. After insertion of the 10- or 11-mm umbilical cannula and video laparoscope, the peritoneal cavity is examined for any unsuspected pathology and to determine the feasibility of the laparoscopic approach. When using this four-puncture technique, the surgeon generally stands on the patient's left side with the first assistant positioned directly opposite. In Europe an alternative technique is often used in which the patient is placed in the lithotomy position with the surgeon standing between the patient's legs. The gallbladder and cystic and common bile ducts are exposed by placing atraumatic forceps on the fundus and neck of the gallbladder and retracting the right lobe of the liver cephalad and to the patient's right (Fig. 6-14). The patient is then placed in a 30- to 40-degree reverse Trendelenburg position to allow the small bowel and transverse colon to fall caudad.

The cystic and common bile ducts are identified by dissecting the gallbladder fundus and neck free of any inflammatory adhesions. The entire length of the cystic duct is exposed along with its junction to the common bile duct (Fig. 6-15). Care must be taken to avoid excessive traction on the gallbladder and cystic duct during this dissection because the latter may be easily avulsed from the common bile duct. The cystic artery is usually found posterior and medial to the cystic duct, and care must be taken to identify both the anterior and posterior branches.

Considerable controversy continues about the role of routine versus selective cholangiography during laparoscopic cholecystectomy. Proponents of routine cholangiography state that in addition to excluding the presence of choledocholithiasis, this study also gives the surgeon valuable information about bile duct anatomy. Although several authors advocating selective cholangiography have reported large clinical series with very few problems with bile duct injuries or retained common bile duct stones, most surgeons perform far more intraoperative cholangiography than they did previously with open surgery. Cholangiography is performed by inserting a small catheter into the cystic duct under laparoscopic guidance. Two of the more popular methods either use a specially designed clamp to introduce the catheter and maneuver it into the cystic duct or introduce it percutaneously through the anterior abdominal wall (Fig. 6-16).

After completing the cholangiography, the cystic duct and artery can be ligated with either surgical clips or pretied laparoscopic sutures. Use of suture ligatures is generally recommended if the duct or artery is acutely inflamed and edematous (Fig. 6-17). The gallbladder is dissected from the liver bed using either sharp dissection with a curved scissors, electrocautery, or a laser energy device. The dissection away from the liver bed begins at the neck of the gallbladder and continues upward behind the fundus and dome (i.e., antegrade dissection). This allows the surgeon to maintain adequate exposure by using the gallbladder's attachments to the liver to maintain cephalad retraction of the right lobe of the liver.

Before complete dissection of the gallbladder from the underlying liver bed, the site should be copiously irrigated and inspected for possible bile leakage or bleeding. After the remaining attachments to the liver have been divided, the gallbladder is removed from the abdomen through the umbilical fascial defect. This opening may require enlarging if the stones are very large or the gallbladder wall is very thickened.

The management of patients with choledocholithiasis in this era of laparoscopic surgery has been the focus of intense clinical investigation. As mentioned previously, biliary endoscopy is often performed preoperatively in those pa-

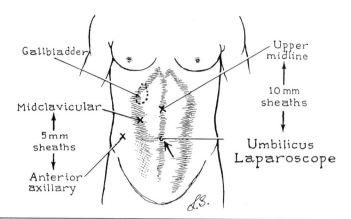

FIGURE 6-13   Recommended puncture sites for laparoscopic cholecystectomy. From Zucker KA (ed). Surgical Laparoscopy. St Louis, Quality Medical Publishing, 1991, p 154.

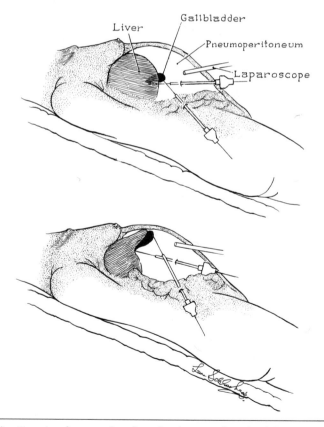

FIGURE 6-14   Grasping forceps placed on the dome and neck of the gallbladder allow cephalad and lateral retraction of the entire right lobe of the liver. From Zucker KA (ed). Surgical Laparoscopy. St Louis, Quality Medical Publishing, 1991, p 156.

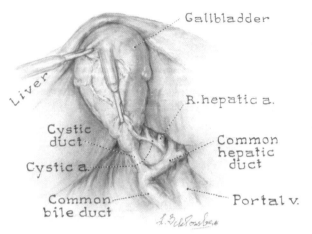

FIGURE 6-15 Entire course of the cystic duct and its juncture with the common bile duct are carefully demonstrated. From Zucker KA (ed). Surgical Laparoscopy. St Louis, Quality Medical Publishing, 1991, p 157.

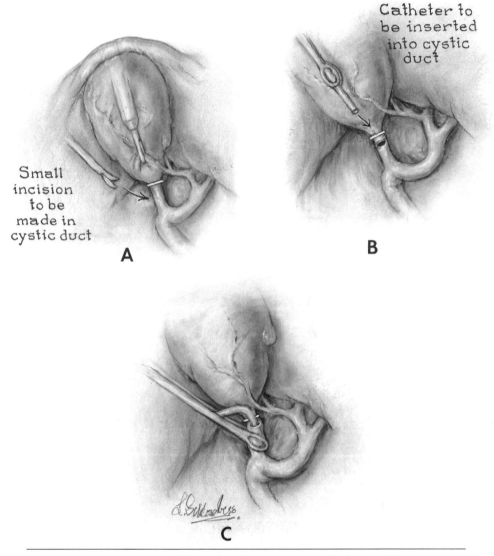

FIGURE 6-16 Laparoscopic cholangiography using a specially designed clamp to introduce and secure the catheter within the cystic duct. From Zucker KA (ed). Surgical Laparoscopy. St Louis, Quality Medical Publishing, 1991, pp 206 and 209.

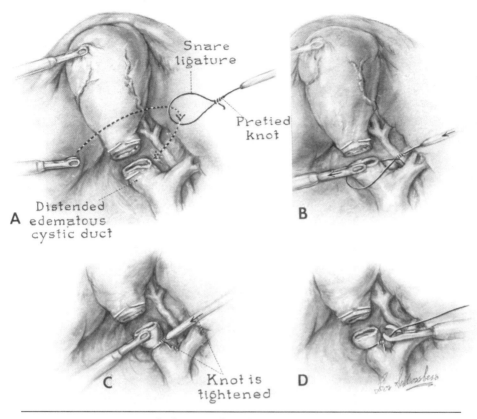

FIGURE 6-17   Sutures applied to an inflamed cystic duct. From Zucker KA (ed). Surgical Laparoscopy Update. St Louis, Quality Medical Publishing, 1993, p 129.

tients suspected of harboring common bile duct stones. An area of controversy has been the management of those patients with filling defects observed on the intraoperative cholangiogram. The two most common options entertained by surgeons in this situation include immediate conversion to open laparotomy and common bile duct exploration or completing laparoscopic cholecystectomy and performing ERCP in the immediate postoperative period. The latter is the most popular approach because biliary endoscopy is extremely successful and avoids the discomfort and prolonged hospitalization associated with open surgery. Some authors have suggested that in selected individuals it may be safe to complete the laparoscopic surgery and not proceed with biliary endoscopy. Patients with no prior history of common bile duct obstruction and who demonstrate only a single small (<3 to 4 mm) defect on cholangiography have been followed successfully, with only a small number requiring subsequent endoscopic intervention.

Efforts to minimize the need for performing an open laparotomy or postoperative ERCP in patients with abnormal cholangiograms have led a number of surgeons to develop methods of extracting common bile duct stones under laparoscopic guidance. The most common technique involves introducing a flexible choledochoscope through the lateral cannula and inserting it into the cystic and common bile ducts (Fig. 6-18). This approach avoids the need for extensive dissection near the common bile duct and thus minimizes the risk of a major ductal or vascular injury. Flexible choledochoscopes are available in diameters as small as 3 mm. They are designed with a deflectable tip that facilitates cannulation of the ductal system and a working channel used to introduce various stone baskets and balloon catheters. A video camera may also be attached to the eyepiece of the choledochoscope to allow the other members of the surgical team to participate. Stones found within the common bile duct are grasped with a stone basket or similar device inserted through the working channel and are removed. The small size of the working channel

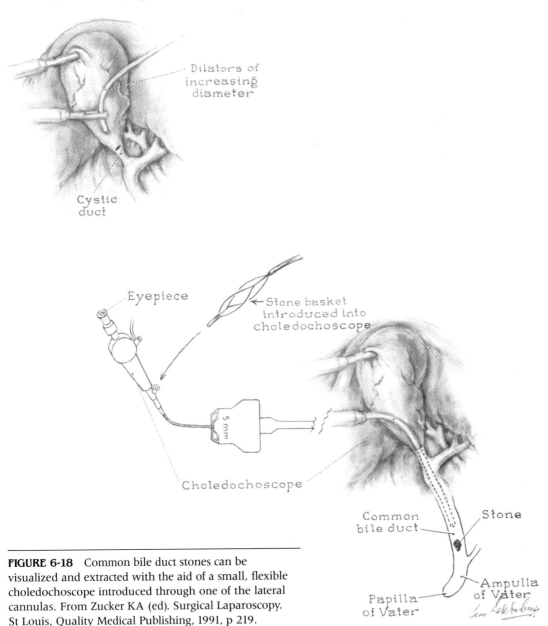

FIGURE 6-18   Common bile duct stones can be visualized and extracted with the aid of a small, flexible choledochoscope introduced through one of the lateral cannulas. From Zucker KA (ed). Surgical Laparoscopy. St Louis, Quality Medical Publishing, 1991, p 219.

does not allow for the extraction of most calculi; therefore the choledochoscope must be removed as each stone is secured. If the stone is too large for removal through the cystic duct lumen, lithotripsy of the stone may be performed, using a mechanical, electric, or laser energy modality.

The main disadvantage of exploring the biliary tract through the cystic duct is that it is not always possible to obtain access to the common hepatic and intrahepatic ducts. The angulation resulting from the cephalad retraction of the gall-

bladder often hinders proximal passage of the choledochoscope. If the stone is not accessible with the scope or proves impossible to remove, the surgeon may elect to leave a guide wire across the common duct and into the duodenum. Postoperatively this will facilitate biliary endoscopy. Another option is to perform a choledochostomy under laparoscopic guidance. This may be done by extending the cystic duct opening down onto the common bile duct juncture or by making a separate anterior choledochostomy

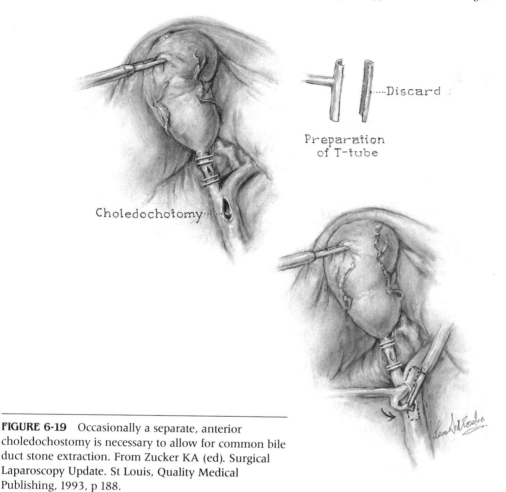

FIGURE 6-19 Occasionally a separate, anterior choledochostomy is necessary to allow for common bile duct stone extraction. From Zucker KA (ed). Surgical Laparoscopy Update. St Louis, Quality Medical Publishing, 1993, p 188.

(Fig. 6-19, *A*). This larger opening into the biliary tract facilitates introduction of the flexible choledochoscope and irrigation and balloon catheters. After ductal exploration a T tube is inserted through the upper abdominal 10- to 11-mm cannula and positioned in the common bile duct under laparoscopic guidance. The T tube is then secured in place with interrupted absorbable sutures and the end brought out through the lateral 5-mm cannula. Reports of successful direct laparoscopic bile duct exploration are limited, but the approach appears safe and effective. Although postoperative ERCP and sphincterotomy remain safe and reliable methods for managing common bile duct stones, most patients prefer not to undergo additional therapeutic procedures after cholecystectomy. Therefore laparoscopic management of choledocholithiasis may soon become the preferred method of managing such patients.

HOW IS LAPAROSCOPY USED IN THE MANAGEMENT OF PEPTIC ULCER DISEASE?

Surgical management of peptic ulcer disease largely has been replaced by medical therapy. Many patients, however, have received either intermittent or continuous drug therapy for their ulcer diathesis since the introduction of H_2-blockers in the mid-1970s. Both physicians and patients have been content to continue indefinite medical therapy when faced with the alternative of major abdominal surgery, even if pharmacologic management provided only partial relief of symptoms. If a laparoscopic procedure were available that allowed the patient to return home within 24 to 48 hours and resume normal activities within a few days and if it effectively controlled acid secretion, surgery would become a more cost-effective and attractive alternative

LAPAROSCOPIC PROCEDURES FOR THE MANAGEMENT OF PEPTIC ULCER DISEASE

Complete Truncal Vagotomy

Thoracoscopic truncal vagotomy with
  endoscopic balloon pyloromyotomy
Transabdominal truncal vagotomy with
  endoscopic balloon pyloromyotomy
Transabdominal truncal vagotomy with
  pyloroplasty

Selective Vagotomy Procedures

Posterior truncal vagotomy and selective
  anterior vagotomy
Posterior truncal vagotomy and anterior
  seromyotomy
Posterior truncal vagotomy and lesser
  curvature excision

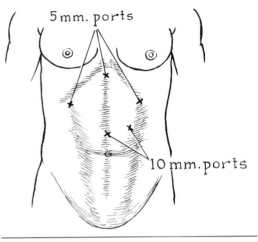

FIGURE 6-20   Recommended positioning of cannulas when performing laparoscopic vagotomy. From Zucker KA (ed). Surgical Laparoscopy. St Louis, Quality Medical Publishing, 1991, p 266.

than lifelong drug therapy. Recently several laparoscopic procedures have been described that reportedly decrease gastric acid production (see the box above). These operations can be categorized as either bilateral truncal vagotomy or selective vagotomy procedures. Unfortunately, there are little published data demonstrating long-term effectiveness for any of these endoscopic procedures in terms of acid reduction and ulcer recurrence.

Bilateral Truncal Vagotomy Procedures

Nonselective vagotomy has been described using both the abdominal and thoracoscopic approaches. Dubois, from the University of Paris, has described a thoracoscopic procedure to identify and divide both vagi. The approach is through the left side of the chest, and endotracheal intubation with a double-lumen tube allows the collapse of the left lung. The patient is placed in the left thoracotomy position and a pneumothorax established by inserting an insufflation needle into the pleural cavity. A 10- to 11-mm cannula is inserted through the fifth intercostal space in the midaxillary line and the video laparoscope introduced. The thoracic cavity is examined and additional sheaths are introduced through the seventh intercostal space (5 mm) along the midclavicular line and in the third intercostal space (10 mm) in the midaxillary line. Dissecting forceps are introduced through the accessary sheaths, and both vagus nerves are identified, with a small segment of each nerve removed for histologic confirmation. The cannulas are withdrawn and the lung fully expanded. At the same time Dubois also performs endoscopic balloon dilation of the pylorus, which partially ruptures the oblique and circular muscles of the pylorus and results in a widely patent channel. This procedure avoids potential problems with gastric stasis after a complete vagotomy has been performed.

A number of surgeons have also performed truncal vagotomy under laparoscopic guidance (i.e., transabdominal approach). The patient lies supine with the surgeon standing on the right or is placed in the lithotomy position with the surgeon positioned between the legs. The head of the bed is elevated 15 to 30 degrees to aid in the exposure of the hiatus. A nasogastric tube decompresses the stomach, and a flexible gastroscope is introduced to distend the esophagus. The endoscope may also be used to transilluminate important anatomic landmarks (e.g., gastroesophageal junction, pylorus). The insufflation needle is inserted through the upper folds of the navel and the pneumoperitoneum established. Four or five laparoscopic trocars and cannulas are required to provide adequate exposure of the stomach and distal esophagus (Fig. 6-20).

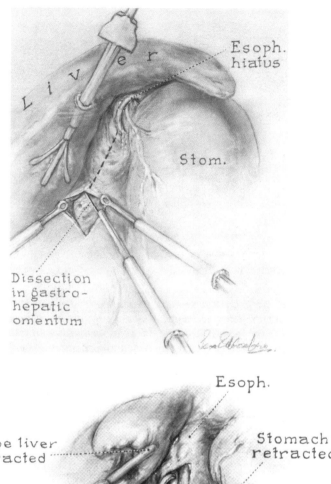

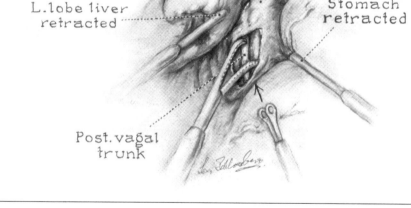

FIGURE 6-21   Exposure of the right (posterior) vagus nerve. From Zucker KA (ed). Surgical Laparoscopy. St Louis, Quality Medical Publishing, 1991, pp 267-268.

The left lobe of the liver is elevated with a fanlike retractor and an opening made in the lesser sac through the gastrohepatic ligament. The right crus of the diaphragm is identified and retracted laterally, with the greater curvature of the stomach pulled to the patient's left (Fig. 6-21). The phrenoesophageal membrane is opened, and further retraction of the gastroesophageal junc-

tion anterior and to the patient's left reveals the posterior mesoesophagus. The posterior vagus nerve is identified along the right posterior aspect of the esophagus and is freed from the surrounding tissues. The nerve is divided between surgical clips and a small fragment removed for histologic examination (Fig. 6-22). The anterior vagus nerve is identified by further incising the phreno-

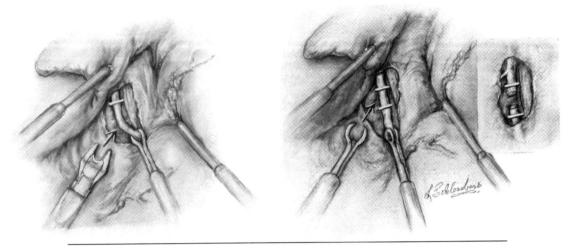

FIGURE 6-22 Ligation and excision of a small segment of the right vagus nerve. From Zucker KA (ed). Surgical Laparoscopy. St Louis, Quality Medical Publishing, 1991, pp 269-270.

esophageal membrane until the left crus of the diaphragm is reached. The nerve is identified and divided between clips, and a small segment is removed.

Pneumatic dilation or laparoscopic-guided pyloroplasty have been recommended to avoid possible gastric stasis. Most surgeons would prefer not to enter the gastrointestinal tract during laparoscopic surgery and therefore have performed endoscopic pyloric dilation.

Selective Vagotomy Procedures

Laparoscopic selective vagotomy offers several distinct advantages over bilateral truncal vagotomy. Antral motility and pyloric function remain intact; thus the need for balloon dilation or pyloroplasty is avoided. Also, the incidence of dumping, diarrhea, and other problems long associated with nonselective acid-reducing procedures should be minimized. Several different laparoscopic procedures featuring selective denervation of the stomach have been reported (see the box on p. 112). Mouiel and his colleagues from the University of Nice, France, were the first group to perform a laparoscopic selective vagotomy procedure in 1989. They modified an open surgical operation described earlier by Taylor that consists of a posterior truncal vagotomy and an anterior seromyotomy. The latter maneuver selectively denervates the fundus of the stomach. Studies by Taylor and others have shown that antral motility and pyloric function are not altered after posterior truncal vagotomy if anterior vagal innervation to this region remains intact. The effectiveness of anterior seromyotomy is based on the observation that the anterior vagal nerve branches course obliquely through the seromuscular layers of the stomach before innervating the fundic parietal cell mass.

The laparoscopic modification of Taylor's procedure is performed with the patient in the lithotomy position with the surgeon positioned between the legs. The gastrohepatic ligament is opened and the posterior vagus nerve divided in the same manner as previously described for truncal vagotomy. The anterior lesser curve seromyotomy is begun at the cardia and extended to within 6 cm of the pylorus (Fig. 6-23). After the seromyotomy is completed, the stomach is distended with methylene blue solution to exclude possible mucosal perforation. The seromuscular defect is then closed with an overlapping (running) absorbable suture to minimize the risks of bleeding and tissue adhesions. Mouiel has reported their results in over 40 patients with intractable ulcer disease with only one failure; however, follow-up remains limited (range, 6 months to 2 years).

A recent modification of this procedure has been developed by Snow and his colleagues in Alabama. The posterior vagus nerve is divided near the hiatus as described by Mouiel; however, a laparoscopic stapling instrument is then used to excise a seromuscular strip of stomach along the lesser curvature (Fig. 6-24). This maneuver, which was previously described by Debass in animals, effectively severs vagal innervation to the anterior stomach. This method appears to take far less time than an extended seromyotomy, and the potential for early or delayed gastric perforation apparently is eliminated.

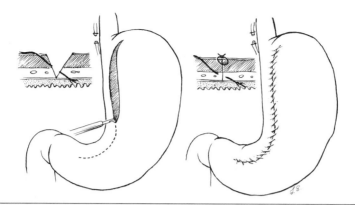

FIGURE 6-23   Selective denervation of the anterior stomach can be accomplished by dividing the branches of the left vagus nerve as they course through the wall of the fundus. From Zucker KA (ed). Surgical Laparoscopy. St Louis, Quality Medical Publishing, 1991, p 273.

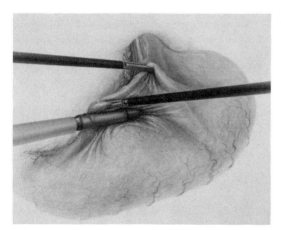
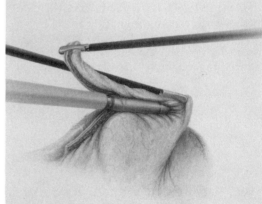
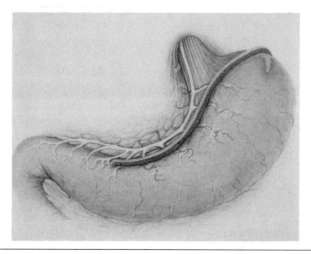

FIGURE 6-24   Alternative method of ligating the vagal nerve branches uses a laparoscopic stapling device to excise a strip of the anterior gastric wall. From Bailey RW. Laparoscopic Management of Peptic Ulcer Disease. Norwalk, Conn, US Surgical Corp, 1992, pp 15-17.

An alternative procedure is posterior truncal vagotomy and selective anterior vagotomy. This procedure is based on a method of selective vagotomy originally described in 1978 by Hill and Barker from the United Kingdom. The patient is positioned supine, and a five-puncture technique is used. The posterior vagal nerve trunk is divided near the diaphragm as previously described. Selective denervation of the anterior stomach is achieved by ligating the fundic branches of the left vagus nerve individually along the lesser curvature (Fig. 6-25). Bailey and his colleagues recently have described their experience in over 30 patients operated on for intractable ulcer disease, and their series also included two treatment failures. As in the previous series follow-up has been limited, with the longest interval less than 2 years.

In the emergency setting laparoscopic surgery may also be indicated for patients presenting within 12 to 24 hours of duodenal ulcer perforation. The abdomen is explored with the laparoscope, which can easily visualize an anterior perforated duodenal ulcer. The peritoneal cavity is irrigated copiously and the perforation closed with interrupted sutures over a vascularized pedicle of omentum. Only a small number of patients have been reported thus far; therefore it is difficult to determine the long-term effectiveness of this approach and to decide which patients are candidates. It is also unclear which of these patients would also be candidates for a simultaneous acid-reduction procedure (i.e., laparoscopic truncal or selective vagotomy).

IS LAPAROSCOPY INDICATED IN THE MANAGEMENT OF ESOPHAGEAL REFLUX?

Symptomatic gastroesophageal reflux represents another common gastrointestinal disorder that is now managed almost exclusively with long-term drug therapy. Previous surgical procedures developed to manage this disease have been shown to control symptoms effectively in 80% to 90% of properly selected patients. Therefore a laparoscopic-guided surgical procedure that could duplicate these results would provide an important therapeutic option for many patients. Various laparoscopic procedures designed to increase lower esophageal sphincter pressure such as placement of a circular prosthesis (i.e., Angle-

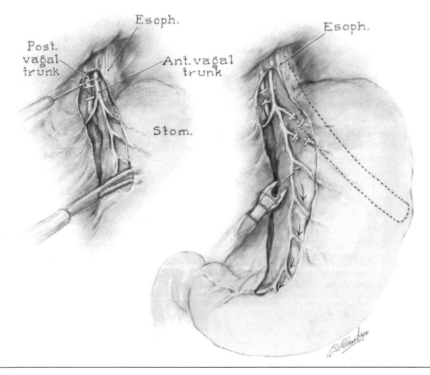

FIGURE 6-25 Selective denervation of the anterior stomach by ligating the vagal branches individually to the lesser curvature. From Zucker KA (ed). Surgical Laparoscopy. St Louis, Quality Medical Publishing, 1991, p 275.

chick), a gastric sling constructed from the falciform ligament, and fundoplication have been proposed. The most successful operative technique, however, is laparoscopic fundoplication, first described in 1991 by Dallemagne et al.

Patients are evaluated in a fashion identical to that for those undergoing open surgery. Evaluation includes upper gastrointestinal endoscopy with multiple biopsies of the distal esophagus and esophageal manometry. The patient is placed in the lithotomy position with the head of the bed elevated 30 degrees. The surgeon is then positioned between the legs of the patient with an assistant standing on each side. A large bougie dilator is inserted to distend the esophagus. A pneumoperitoneum is established and maintained at a maximum of 15 mm Hg. A total of five trocars and cannulas is used. The left lobe of the liver is retracted away from the stomach and the phrenoesophageal membrane opened along the anterior surface of the esophagus. The right crus of the diaphragm is identified and retracted away from the esophagus to allow safe separation of the posterior vagus from the esophagus. The left crus is exposed in a similar fashion and, if present, the hiatal hernia reduced into the peritoneal cavity. If a widened diaphragmatic hiatus is found, separate sutures may be placed across the crural muscles to close this opening (Fig. 6-26, **A**). The short gastric vessels are individually ligated with surgical clips or sutures and divided. After the posterior esophagus and cardia are freed, the greater curvature is pulled from underneath the esophagus and toward the right side of the patient. A second forceps near the right side of the esophagus is used to grasp the gastric wrap and position it anteriorly along the lower esophagus. The two sides of the gastric wrap are then fixed together with interrupted 00 silk sutures (Fig. 6-26, **C**).

Dallemagne's initial report noted that in nine out of 12 patients fundoplication was completed under laparoscopic guidance. Three required conversion to laparotomy for operative compli-

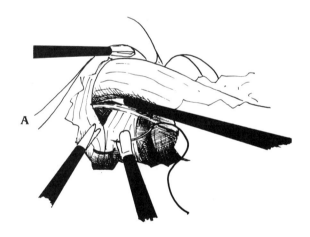

A

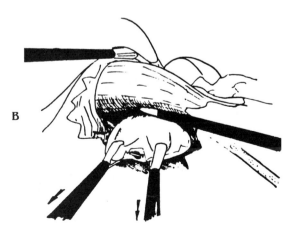

B

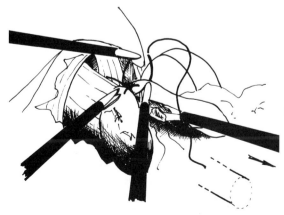

C

FIGURE 6-26 **A**, Widened hiatus can be approximated with sutures placed through the right and left crural muscles. **B**, Greater curvature is mobilized and wrapped around the gastroesophageal junction. **C**, Interrupted silk sutures are passed through both sides of the gastric wrap and the anterior wall of the esophagus. (From Dallemagne B, Weerts JM, Jehaes C, et al. Laparoscopic Nissen fundoplication: Preliminary report. Surg Laparosc Endosc 1:138-143, 1991.)

cations or equipment failure. With additional experience and improved instrumentation, Dallemagne reports that laparotomy now is rarely necessary to complete the procedure. Postoperative follow-up (now in excess of 100 patients) has demonstrated an intact fundoplication in all patients, with dramatic relief of symptoms and healing of previously observed distal esophageal inflammation and ulcers. The follow-up, however, is less than 2 years, and more extensive studies are required to determine the long-term effectiveness of this procedure.

CAN LAPAROSCOPY BE USED FOR BENIGN OR MALIGNANT COLON DISEASE?

Experience gained during laparoscopic management of complicated appendicitis has encouraged a number of surgeons to use these same techniques for resection of diseased segments of the right or left colon. The majority of these procedures require an adjuvant 3- to 5-cm "mini-laparotomy" to perform the anastomosis and/or to remove the specimen. Earlier reports recommended laparoscopic intervention only in those patients with benign disorders of the large bowel such as colonic volvulus or large villous adenomas. Recently, however, laparoscopic procedures for malignant lesions of the colon have been described, but reports of long-term follow-up addressing the effectiveness of this approach as compared to traditional open surgery have not appeared.

Laparoscopic colon resection requires the insertion of at least four or five laparoscopic trocars and cannulas to mobilize the colon and control the mesenteric vessels (Fig. 6-27). Lateral and posterior peritoneal attachments to the colon are sharply divided with scissors, electrocautery, or a surgical laser. The mesenteric vessels can be individually ligated with surgical clips or interrupted sutures or divided with a laparoscopic linear stapling device. For lesions of the right and transverse colon a mini-laparotomy is used to remove the specimen and complete the anastomosis. Generally the umbilical fascial opening is enlarged to allow for evisceration of the ascending colon and terminal ileum. Lesions requiring removal of only a short segment of the descending or sigmoid colon can be managed in a similar fashion. Mobilization of the left colon, however, is more difficult because of the dense and extensive lateral and posterior peritoneal attachments. With more extended resections involving the rectosigmoid colon, the distal bowel is not easily eviscerated for completing the anastomosis. In

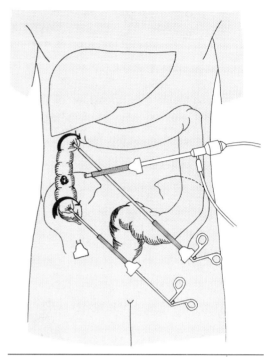

FIGURE 6-27 Cannula placement for laparoscopic-assisted colectomy. A fifth puncture may be placed in the upper abdomen to enhance visualization of the splenic or hepatic flexures. From Zucker KA (ed). Surgical Laparoscopy. St Louis, Quality Medical Publishing, 1991, p 306.

this situation a transanally placed circular stapling device may be used. The rectosigmoid colon is fully mobilized and the mesenteric vessels ligated with staples or sutures. The segment of colon is divided with a linear laparoscopic stapling instrument and extracted through a small left lower quadrant (muscle-splitting) incision (Fig. 6-28). The shaft of the circular stapler is inserted through the anus and maneuvered to the distal staple line. The proximal bowel is brought out through the fascial opening and the anvil of the device inserted and held in place with a purse-string suture. The two ends of the circular stapler are brought together and the anastomosis completed. The shaft of the instrument is removed and the anastomosis examined for its integrity. The mini-laparotomy is then closed and the mesenteric defect approximated with laparoscopically guided interrupted sutures. In a recent publication by Jacobs and his colleagues from Miami, Florida, 20 patients underwent successful laparoscopic colon resection for both benign and malignant disorders. Two thirds of the patients were able to resume an oral

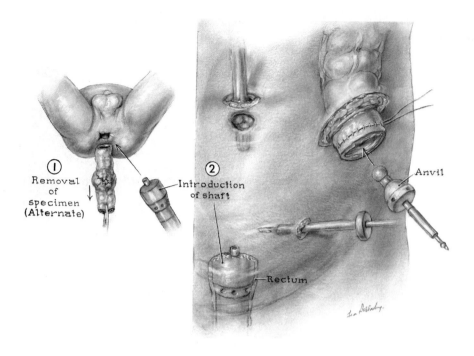

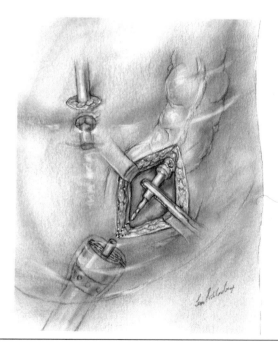

FIGURE 6-28 Low anterior colonic anastomosis is performed with the aid of a circular stapling device introduced through the rectum. From Zucker KA (ed). Surgical Laparoscopy Update. St Louis, Quality Medical Publishing, 1993, p 346.

diet within 24 hours of the operative procedure, and the mean length of the hospital stay was 4 days. Although this report demonstrated the feasibility of laparoscopic-assisted colectomy, it was not randomly compared with patients undergoing traditional open surgery, and the follow-up has been less than 2 years.

IS THERE A ROLE FOR LAPAROSCOPIC HERNIORRHAPHY?

Inguinal hernia repair would seem an unlikely procedure for challenge by laparoscopic enthusiasts. The vast majority of operative procedures for inguinal hernia repair are now conducted in an outpatient setting with the patient under regional or local anesthesia. These procedures are well tolerated, with recurrence rates ranging from as low as 0% to 7% for primary indirect inguinal hernias. Contemporary inguinal hernia repair has been dominated by the extraperitoneal groin approach initially proposed by Bassini in 1884, with various modifications popularized by Halsted, Bull and Cooley, McVay, Lichtenstein, and others. In addition to the recurrence rate, contemporary hernia repairs are associated with a number of inguinal and scrotal complications and require from 2 to 4 weeks for full recovery. Clinical investigators have proposed that laparoscopic transabdominal repair of indirect and direct inguinal hernias may eliminate many of these remaining disadvantages.

In 1982 R. Ger from New York reported the first laparoscopic transabdominal repair in a patient with an indirect inguinal hernia. The defect was repaired by simply closing the internal ring with surgical clips, and after 3 years the patient manifested no evidence of recurrence. A subsequent animal study by Ger showed similar results in 12 dogs. Ger et al. have proposed that the laparoscopic approach has the following advantages: (1) less dissection, (2) decreased incidence of ischemic orchitis, (3) decreased likelihood of bladder injury, (4) elimination of the chance of postoperative ilioinguinal neuralgia, (5) minimal postoperative discomfort, (6) faster recovery time, and (7) identification and treatment during the same procedure of bilateral groin hernias with no additional discomfort.

Several different methods of laparoscopic hernia repair are currently under clinical investigation. Nearly all of these techniques use prosthetic materials to close the neck of the hernia sac. In the technique proposed by Schultz in Minnesota

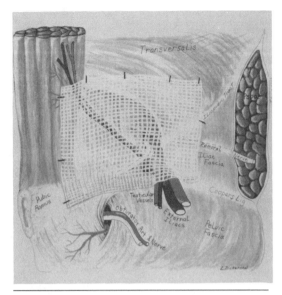

FIGURE 6-29 Laparoscopic herniorrhaphy performed by securing a large prosthetic mesh over the internal inguinal ring. From Zucker KA (ed). Surgical Laparoscopy Update. St Louis, Quality Medical Publishing, 1993.

the peritoneum is incised superior to the defect and a polypropylene plug inserted into the inguinal canal. A similar prosthetic mesh is then placed over the internal ring and the peritoneum closed over both patches with surgical clips or sutures. Corbitt in Florida described a similar technique but included everting the sac into the peritoneal cavity and ligating it close to the internal ring. Unfortunately, a number of early recurrences and complications (e.g., migration of the prosthetic plug) have been reported with this technique.

An alternative approach under investigation by Fitzgibbons and his colleagues in Nebraska is fixation of a large prosthetic graft across the internal ring and pelvic floor without reducing the hernia sac (Fig. 6-29). The mesh is secured in place with a specially designed stapling device. Variations of this technique include placing the mesh beneath the peritoneum to minimize the risk of adhesion to this foreign body. Unfortunately, it is too early to evaluate the results of these approaches, but several multi-institutional studies are currently under way. Until these results are available, laparoscopic management of indirect or direct inguinal hernias should still be considered investigational.

BIBLIOGRAPHY

Berci G, Sackier J. Emergency laparoscopy. Am J Surg 161:332-335, 1991.

Dallemagne B, Weerts JM, Jehaes C, et al. Laparoscopic Nissen fundoplication: Preliminary report. Surg Laparosc Endosc 1:3-9, 1991.

Fitzgibbons RJ, Corbitt JD. Laparoscopic management of inguinal hernia. In Zucker KA (ed). Surgical Laparoscopy—Update. St Louis, Quality Medical Publishing, 1993.

Ger R, Monroe K, Duvivier R, et al. Management of indirect inguinal hernias by laparoscopic closure of the neck of the sac. Am J Surg 159:371-373, 1990.

Jacobs M, Verdeja JC, Goldstein HS. Minimally invasive colon resection (laparoscopic colectomy). Surg Laparosc Endosc 1:11-18, 1991.

Katkhouda N, Mouiel J. A new technique of surgical treatment of chronic duodenal ulcer without laparotomy by videolaparoscopy. Am J Surg 161:361-364, 1991.

Myers WC, Branum GD, Farouk M, et al. A prospective analysis of 1518 laparoscopic cholecystectomies. N Engl J Med 324:1073-1078, 1991.

Petelin JB. Laparoscopic approach to common duct pathology. Surg Laparosc Endosc 1:33-41, 1991.

Pier A, Gotz F, Bacher C. Laparoscopic appendectomy in 625 cases: From innovative to routine. Surg Laparosc Endosc 1:8-13, 1991.

Scott TR, Bailey RW, Flowers JA, et al. Laparoscopic biliary tract surgery: Analysis of 12,337 cases. Surg Laparosc Endosc 2:152-157, 1992.

Warshaw AL. Implications of peritoneal cytology for staging of early pancreatic cancer. Am J Surg 161:8-14, 1991.

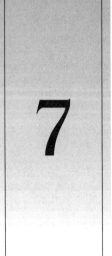

SECTION THREE   Physiologic Aspects of Surgical Disease

7

Parenteral Fluid and Electrolyte Therapy

G. TOM SHIRES
WILLIAM J. MILLIKAN, Jr.

KEY FEATURES

After reading this chapter you will understand:
- The physiology of body fluid and electrolyte spaces.
- Specific electrolyte abnormalities and acid-base balance.
- Fluid and electrolyte management of the postoperative patient.

Proper management of fluids and electrolytes in the surgical patient is an integral and often critical aspect of preoperative and postoperative care. To optimize treatment, the surgeon must appreciate the anatomy of body fluid compartments and understand the normal and altered physiologic responses to disease and surgery. This chapter outlines these principles and incorporates a classification of fluid and electrolyte derangements to guide therapy.

BODY FLUID ANATOMY

As measured by isotopic methods, water constitutes 50% to 70% of total body weight. Body water is divided into three functional compartments: intracellular volume, interstitial fluid, and plasma (Fig. 7-1).

Intracellular Fluid

Intracellular water, which represents 40% of body weight, is largely proportioned to skeletal

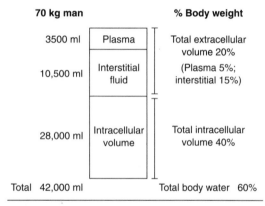

70 kg man		% Body weight
3500 ml	Plasma	Total extracellular volume 20%
10,500 ml	Interstitial fluid	(Plasma 5%; interstitial 15%)
28,000 ml	Intracellular volume	Total intracellular volume 40%
Total 42,000 ml		Total body water 60%

FIGURE 7-1 Functional compartments of body fluids.

muscle. Fig. 7-2 depicts the chemical composition of intracellular fluid, showing that the principal cations are potassium and magnesium, with proteins and phosphates representing the major anions.

Extracellular Fluid

The extracellular fluid compartment, which represents approximately 20% of body weight, is divided into two functional divisions: plasma and interstitial fluid (see Fig. 7-1). Interstitial fluid is further divided into a larger (90%) functional component and several smaller, slowly equilibrating nonfunctional components, which include connective tissue water and transcellular water (e.g., cerebrospinal, joint fluid). The chem-

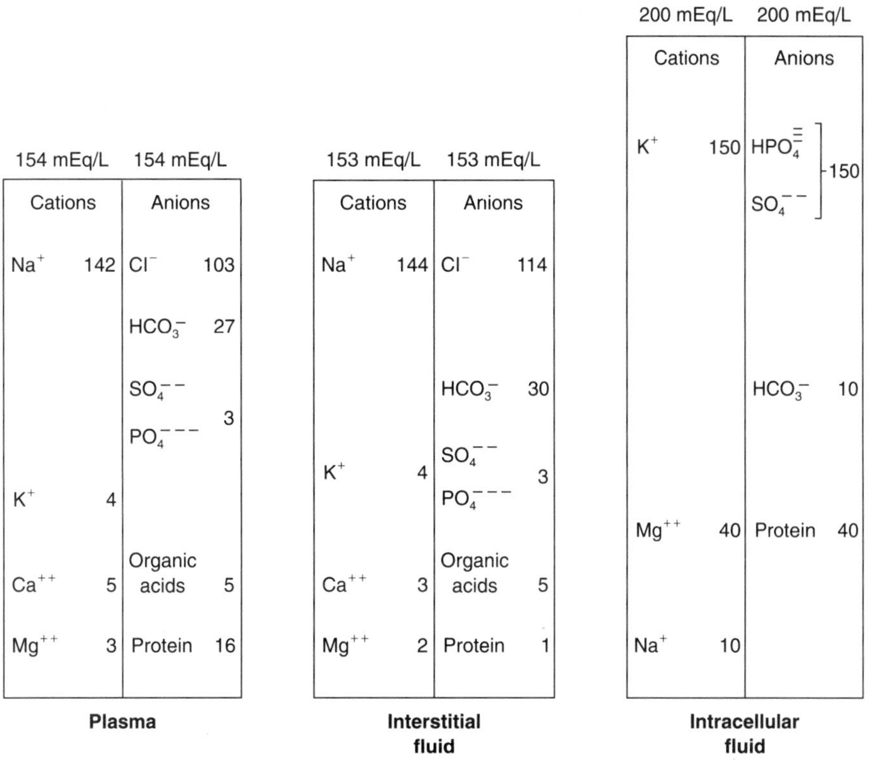

FIGURE 7-2 Chemical composition of body fluid compartments. (From Shires GT, Canizaro PC, Shires GT III, et al. Fluid, electrolyte and nutritional management of the surgical patient. In Schwartz SI [ed]. Principles of Surgery, 5th ed. New York, McGraw-Hill, 1989, p 70. Reproduced with permission.)

ical compositions of plasma and interstitial fluid (see Fig. 7-2) differ slightly but for functional purposes are equivalent. Sodium is the principal cation in the extracellular fluid and the major determinant of plasma osmotic pressure. The principal anions are chloride and bicarbonate.

PHYSIOLOGY OF FLUID AND ELECTROLYTE EXCHANGE

Maintenance of the internal milieu requires coordination of the renal, cardiovascular, pulmonary, gastrointestinal, and integumentary systems. All can be altered by natural disease, trauma, or surgery.

Water Exchange (Table 7-1)

The average 70-kg male consumes approximately 1500 to 2000 ml of free water each day. An additional 500 to 1000 ml are extracted from solid food. Postoperative patients without nutri-

tional support catabolize cells after 5 to 7 days, which releases up to 500 ml/day of intracellular "water of solution." Normal water losses include 800 to 1600 ml in urine, 200 to 300 ml in stool, and 600 ml of insensible water through the skin and respiratory tract. Insensible water loss increases with fever and hyperventilation.

Sodium Exchange (Table 7-2)

The average individual consumes a diet containing 2 to 5 g (88 to 220 mEq) of sodium each day, with any excess readily excreted by the healthy kidney. When extrarenal losses occur or during periods of reduced sodium intake, the healthy kidney can produce urine with less than 1 mEq of sodium per liter. Table 7-3 approximates the average volume and composition of various gastrointestinal secretions. Except for saliva, these secretions are slightly hypotonic or isotonic and can be replaced by isotonic salt solution. However, in postoperative patients who develop con-

TABLE 7-1   Water Exchange (60- to 80-kg Man)

Routes	Average Daily Volume (ml)	Minimal (ml)	Maximal (ml)
Water Gain			
Sensible			
Oral fluids	800-1500	0	1500/hr
Solid foods	500-700	0	1500
Insensible			
Water of oxidation	250	125	800
Water of solution	0	0	500
Water Loss			
Sensible			
Urine	800-1500	300	1400/hr (diabetes insipidus)
Intestinal	0-250	0	2500/hr
Sweat	0	0	4000/hr
Insensible			
Lungs and skin	600	600	1500

From Shires GT, Canizaro PC, Shires GT III, et al. Fluid, electrolyte and nutritional management of the surgical patient. In Schwartz SI (ed). Principles of Surgery, 5th ed. New York, McGraw-Hill, 1989, p 72. Reproduced with permission.

TABLE 7-2   Sodium (Salt) Exchange (60- to 80-kg Man)

Sodium Exchange	Average	Minimal	Maximal
Sodium Gain			
Diet	50-90 mEq/day	0	75-100 mEq/hr (oral)
Sodium Loss			
Skin (sweat)	10-60 mEq/day*	0	300 mEq/hr
Urine	10-80 mEq/day	<1 mEq/day†	110-200 mEq/L‡
Intestines	0-20 mEq/day	0	300 mEq/hr

From Shires GT, Canizaro PC, Shires GT III, et al. Fluid, electrolyte and nutritional management of the surgical patient. In Schwartz SI (ed). Principles of Surgery, 5th ed. New York, McGraw-Hill, 1989, p 72. Reproduced with permission.
*Depending on the degree of acclimatization of the individual.
†With normal renal function.
‡With renal salt wasting.

TABLE 7-3 Composition of Gastrointestinal Secretions

Type of Secretion	Volume (ml/24 hr)	Na (mEq/L)	K (mEq/L)	Cl (mEq/L)	HCO$_3$ (mEq/L)
Saliva	1500 (500-2000)	10 (2-10)	26 (20-30)	10 (8-18)	30
Stomach	1500 (100-4000)	60 (9-116)	10 (0-32)	130 (8-154)	
Duodenum	(100-2000)	140	5	80	
Ileum	3000 (100-9000)	140 (80-150)	5 (2-8)	104 (43-137)	30
Colon		60	30	40	
Pancreas	(100-800)	140 (113-185)	5 (3-7)	75 (54-95)	115
Bile	(50-800)	145 (131-164)	5 (3-12)	100 (89-180)	35

From Shires GT, Canizaro PC, Shires GT III, et al. Fluid, electrolyte and nutritional management of the surgical patient. In Schwartz SI (ed). Principles of Surgery, 5th ed. New York, McGraw-Hill, 1989, p 73. Reproduced with permission.

centration or composition derangements (see later sections in this chapter), measurement of the electrolyte composition of gastrointestinal losses and urine may be required to guide replacement therapy.

CLASSIFICATION OF BODY FLUID CHANGES

Fluid balance disorders can be classified into disturbances of (1) extracellular fluid volume, (2) sodium concentration, and (3) composition (acid-base balance). Although clearly interrelated, therapy is facilitated by analyzing each disturbance individually in the order listed above.

Volume Changes

A deficiency or excess of extracellular fluid volume can usually be diagnosed clinically (Table 7-4) but may require invasive monitoring in patients with preexisting chronic heart disease, renal failure, or cirrhosis.

Routine laboratory studies are usually not helpful in assessing volume changes in the acute phase. For example, serum sodium concentration may be elevated, normal, or depressed in patients with acute volume depletion. Over time, however, laboratory studies can reflect the effects of volume changes as exemplified by a rise in blood urea nitrogen as a result of decreased glomerular filtration rate in volume-depleted patients.

Volume Deficit (see Table 7-4). A deficit in extracellular fluid volume is the most frequently encountered derangement of fluid balance seen in surgical patients and may be due to shed blood, loss of gastrointestinal fluids, diarrhea, or fistulous drainage. More subtle are third-space losses (e.g., in patients with peritonitis) or marked sequestration of extracellular fluid intraluminally and intramurally (e.g., in patients with mechanical bowel obstruction).

Volume Excess. An excess in extracellular fluid volume is usually iatrogenic and can represent failure to recognize preexisting cardiovascular or renal dysfunction. Volume excess is rarely a clinical problem in young patients with healthy hearts and kidneys but is common in older patients with subclinical left ventricular dysfunction. An example is the patient who "spontaneously" develops pulmonary edema 4 days after aortic graft placement because of mobilization of fluid sequestered in the retroperitoneal third space.

TABLE 7-4   Extracellular Fluid Volume

Type of Sign	Deficit		Excess	
	Moderate	Severe	Moderate	Severe
Central nervous system	Sleepiness Apathy Slow responses Anorexia Cessation of usual activity	Decreased tension reflexes Anesthesia distal extremities Stupor Coma	None	None
Gastrointestinal	Progressive decrease in food consumption	Nausea, vomiting Refusal to eat Silent ileus and distention	At operation: Edema of stomach, colon, lesser and greater omenta, and small bowel mesentery	
Cardiovascular	Orthostatic hypotension Tachycardia Collapsed veins Collapsing pulse	Cutaneous lividity Hypotension Distant heart sounds Cold extremities Absent peripheral pulses	Elevated venous pressure Distention of peripheral veins Increased cardiac output Loud heart sounds Functional murmurs Bounding pulse High pulse pressure Increased pulmonary second sound Gallop	Pulmonary edema
Tissue	Soft, small tongue with longitudinal wrinkling Decreased skin turgor	Atonic muscles Sunken eyes	Subcutaneous pitting edema Basilar rales	Anasarca Moist rales Vomiting Diarrhea
Metabolic	Mild decrease in temperature, 97°-99° R	Marked decrease in temperature, 95°-98° R	None	None

From Shires GT, Canizaro PC, Shires GT III, et al. Fluid, electrolyte and nutritional management of the surgical patient. In Schwartz SI (ed). Principles of Surgery, 5th ed. New York, McGraw-Hill, 1989, p 74. Reproduced with permission.

Concentration Changes

The sodium cation is primarily responsible for maintaining the osmotic integrity of extracellular fluid. The signs and symptoms of hyponatremia and hypernatremia can be detected clinically (Table 7-5), especially if changes in serum sodium develop rapidly. More commonly, however, changes in concentration evolve over days in postoperative patients in whom clinical signs may be subtle or masked by medication. Hyponatremia can be especially challenging to manage in patients with heart disease and those with renal or hepatic dysfunction. Assessment of volume status should precede evaluation of concentration derangements.

Hyponatremia. Acute hyponatremia developing over hours is typically seen in patients who sustained a severe closed head injury. In such patients hyponatremia can be lethal because brain intracellular water increases as extracellular osmolarity falls. This edema is additive to the sequestered edema of injury and can rapidly elevate intracranial pressure and cause the patient's death. Hyponatremia is also frequently encountered in postoperative patients who required emergent or urgent operation for trauma or acute surgical illness.

Hypernatremia. Except for burn patients, hypernatremia is rare in adult surgical subjects. As stated previously, significant hypernatremia

TABLE 7-5 Acute Changes in Osmolar Concentration

Type of Signs	Hyponatremia (Water Intoxication)		Hypernatremia (Water Deficit)	
	Moderate:	Severe:	Moderate:	Severe:
Central nervous system	Muscle twitching	Convulsions	Restlessness	Delirium
	Hyperactive tendon reflexes	Loss of reflexes	Weakness	Maniacal behavior
	Increased intra-cranial pressure (compensated phase)	Increased intra-cranial pressure (decompensated phase)		
Cardiovascular	Changes in blood pressure and pulse secondary to increased intracranial pressure		Tachycardia Hypotension (if severe)	
Tissue	Salivation, lacrimation, watery diarrhea "Fingerprinting" of skin (sign of intracellular volume excess)		Decreased saliva and tears Dry and sticky mucous membranes Red, swollen tongue Skin flushed	
Renal	Oliguria progressing to anuria		Oliguria	
Metabolic	None		Fever	

From Shires GT, Canizaro PC, Shires GT III, et al. Fluid, electrolyte and nutritional management of the surgical patient. In Schwartz SI (ed). Principles of Surgery, 5th ed. New York, McGraw-Hill, 1989, p 75. Reproduced with permission.

or hyponatremia frequently accompanies a derangement in extracellular fluid volume.

Mixed Volume and Concentration Abnormalities. Every permutation of mixed volume and concentration abnormalities can occur in surgical patients and reinforces the importance of assessing volume status first. Correction of concentration alterations usually requires different approaches in patients with volume excess compared to those with volume depletion. For example, both of the following patients may have the same degree of hyponatremia: (1) a volume-depleted patient who drinks water while losing large volumes of gastrointestinal fluid and (2) a patient with oliguric renal failure who is receiving hypotonic salt solutions.

A patient with hypernatremia usually presents with a volume deficit, but it can also occur in patients with volume excess as illustrated by those receiving large quantities of isotonic saline solution with restricted water intake. Patients with healthy kidneys usually can self-correct most concentration abnormalities, provided the volume status is adequate to preserve glomerular filtration rate. However, if even moderate volume depletion is allowed to persist over time, oliguric or high-output renal failure can rapidly develop. This is especially true in the geriatric surgical population.

Composition Changes

By definition, composition changes include alterations in acid-base balance plus changes in concentration of potassium calcium, and magnesium.

Acid-Base Balance. The pH of extracellular and intracellular fluids is efficiently maintained within a very narrow range by a series of buffer systems. Protein and phosphate systems control intracellular pH, and the carbonate-carbonic acid buffer system maintains the pH of extracellular fluids. A buffer system is a weak acid or base coupled with its corresponding salt. In the extracellular fluid compartment, endogenously produced strong (completely dissociated) acids such as hydrochloric acid (HCl) combine with base bicarbonate ($NaHCO_3$) to form the sodium salt (NaCl) of the acid plus carbonic acid (H_2CO_3), which is excreted as carbon dioxide (CO_2) by the lungs.

$$HCl + NaHCO_3 \rightarrow NaCl + H_2CO_3 \rightarrow H_2O + CO_2$$

Buffer system capability or function is defined by the Henderson-Hasselbalch equation, which relates pH to the ratio of the salt and its acid:

$$pH = pKa + \log \frac{BHCO_3}{H_2CO_3} = \frac{27 \text{ mEq/L}}{1.33 \text{ mEq/L}} = \frac{20}{1}$$

where pKa is the dissociation constant of carbonic acid and is 6.1. pH will be preserved at 7.4 as long as the 20:1 ratio is maintained. For example, if lactic acid is added to the extracellular fluid, it is buffered by sodium bicarbonate, producing an excess of carbonic acid, which immediately causes an increase in depth and rate of ventilation to clear the excess carbon dioxide and restore the 20:1 ratio. If the process is chronic, compensatory responses by the kidney will increase excretion of acid salts and retention of bicarbonate.

The four types of acid-base abnormalities are presented in Tables 7-6 and 7-7. Unfortunately, complex combinations of acid-base balance are frequently encountered in surgical patients, especially in those in whom the disease process and emergency operation predispose to renal or pulmonary insufficiency and sepsis. Use of arterial pH, partial pressure of carbon dioxide (PCO_2), and plasma bicarbonate allows a more clear-cut definition of the derangement and, coupled with a precise knowledge of the volume status, can actually define therapy.

Respiratory Acidosis. Hypoventilation with retention of carbon dioxide is the cause of respiratory acidosis and frequently occurs in postoperative patients extubated prematurely or who have been aggressively narcotized. Measures to ensure adequate ventilation may require endotracheal intubation with mechanical support. The challenge is greater in patients with preexisting chronic bronchitis in whom elevation in arterial PCO_2 and hypoxia represent the patient's norm. In this subset decreased pulmonary excursion and required doses of narcotics may make early extubation impossible.

Respiratory Alkalosis. Hyperventilation leading to depressed arterial concentration of carbon dioxide is the cause of respiratory alkalosis and commonly occurs before and after surgery. Pain, central nervous system trauma, and hypoxia can produce respiratory alkalosis. The most common cause is partially iatrogenic and is seen in patients receiving mechanically assisted ventilatory support. Usually, in an attempt to reverse hypoxia, the tidal volume and ventilatory rate are increased, producing hypocarbia (<30 mm Hg) and alkalosis. The resultant shift in the oxyhemoglobin-dissociation curve can increase tissue hypoxia. The treatment of hypoxia without hypercarbia is not hyperventilation. Chronic respiratory alkalosis also produces lower serum potassium and calcium levels in patients who frequently are already potassium depleted and can lead to life-threatening cardiac dysrhythmias.

Metabolic Acidosis. Metabolic acidosis results from the overproduction of acid (lactic, ketoacidosis) or failure to excrete the acid load produced by the body (renal failure). It can also occur in surgical patients with excessive losses of sodium bicarbonate from diarrhea or small bowel fistulas. Arterial pH and plasma bicarbonate are depressed as is arterial PCO_2 (compensatory) (see Tables 7-6 and 7-7). The classic model of metabolic acidosis is hypovolemic shock secondary to acute blood loss. Lack of tissue perfusion results in rapid accumulation of lactic acid in a setting of decreased glomerular perfusion, which can temporarily paralyze compensatory mechanisms. The goal of therapy is to restore tissue perfusion by reestablishing extracellular fluid and red blood cell volume. The required vehicles are balanced salt solutions (e.g., Ringer's lactate) and whole blood. Pressors are contraindicated because they exacerbate the basic problem of inadequate tissue perfusion. The overzealous use of sodium bicarbonate to "convert" acidosis is also ill advised. Reestablishing tissue perfusion will clear the lactic acidosis. In addition, short-term acidosis is well tolerated by hypovolemic patients. Induction of alkalosis by sodium bicarbonate shifts the oxyhemoglobin-dissociation curve to the left, thus inhibiting oxygen release at the tissue level. Alkalosis also promotes hypokalemia and promotes ventricular dysrhythmias.

Metabolic Alkalosis. Metabolic alkalosis is caused by loss of fixed acid (e.g., pyloric obstruction with a high nasogastric output) or bicarbonate retention and is almost always accompanied by concomitant deficiency states of potassium and magnesium. Arterial pH and plasma bicarbonate levels are elevated. Compensatory hypercarbia does occur, but the major compensatory mechanism is renal excretion of bicarbonate. The classic model of metabolic alkalosis is the patient with pyloric outlet obstruction from peptic ulcer disease. The loss of large volumes of gastric juice rich in hydrochloric acid produces a hypochloremic, hypokalemic metabolic alkalosis. This condition can be very challenging to treat because extracellular fluid volume losses are usually underestimated and renal mechanisms can worsen alkalosis. In the initial phase of this metabolic alkalosis the kidney will excrete increased amounts of sodium bicarbonate and potassium while retaining hydrogen ion. These added potassium losses compound the preexisting hypokalemia. As extracellular fluid volume depletion worsens, excretion of sodium decreases under the influence of aldosterone, and

TABLE 7-6 Acidosis-Alkalosis

Type of Acid-Base Disorder	Defect	Common Causes	$\dfrac{BHCO_3}{H_2CO_3} = \dfrac{20}{1}$	Compensation
Respiratory acidosis	Retention of CO_2 (decreased alveolar ventilation)	Depression of respiratory center—morphine, CNS injury Pulmonary disease—emphysema, pneumonia	↑ Denominator Ratio less than 20:1	Renal Retention of bicarbonate, excretion of acid salts, increased ammonia formation Chloride shift into red cells
Respiratory alkalosis	Excessive loss of CO_2 (increased alveolar ventilation)	Hyperventilation: Emotional, severe pain, assisted ventilation, encephalitis	↓ Denominator Ratio greater than 20:1	Renal Excretion of bicarbonate, retention of acid salts, decreased ammonia formation
Metabolic acidosis	Retention of fixed acids OR Loss of base bicarbonate	Diabetes, azotemia, lactic acid accumulation, starvation Diarrhea, small bowel fistulas	↓ Numerator Ratio less than 20:1	Pulmonary (rapid) Increase rate and depth of breathing Renal (slow) As in respiratory acidosis
Metabolic alkalosis	Loss of fixed acids Gain of base bicarbonate Potassium depletion	Vomiting or gastric suction with pyloric obstruction Excessive intake of bicarbonate Diuretics	↑ Numerator Ratio greater than 20:1	Pulmonary (rapid) Decrease rate and depth of breathing Renal (slow) As in respiratory alkalosis

From Shires GT, Canizaro PC, Shires GT III, et al. Fluid, electrolyte and nutritional management of the surgical patient. In Schwartz SI (ed). Principles of Surgery, 5th ed. New York, McGraw-Hill, 1989, p 77. Reproduced with permission.

TABLE 7-7 Respiratory and Metabolic Components of Acid-Base Disorders

Type of Acid-Base Disorder	Acute (Uncompensated)			Chronic (Partially Compensated)		
	pH	Pco_2 (Respiratory Component)	Plasma HCO_3^-* (Metabolic Component)	pH	Pco_2 (Respiratory Component)	Plasma HCO_3^-* (Metabolic Component)
Respiratory acidosis	↓↓	↑↑	N	↓	↑↑	↑
Respiratory alkalosis	↑↑	↓↓	N	↑	↓↓	↓
Metabolic acidosis	↓↓	N	↓↓	↓	↓	↓
Metabolic alkalosis	↑↑	N	↑↑	↑	↑?	↑

From Shires GT, Canizaro PC, Shires GT III, et al. Fluid, electrolyte and nutritional management of the surgical patient. In Schwartz SI (ed). Principles of Surgery, 5th ed. New York, McGraw-Hill, 1989, p 77. Reproduced with permission.

*Measured as standard bicarbonate, whole blood buffer base, CO_2 content, or CO_2 combining power. The **base excess value** is positive when the standard bicarbonate is above normal and negative when the standard bicarbonate is below normal.

hydrogen ion losses increase, producing paradoxic aciduria. The goals of therapy are to restore the extracellular fluid volume with an isotonic sodium chloride solution while repleting the potassium deficit. In severe cases infusion of 0.1 N hydrochloric acid may be required to treat a severe metabolic alkalosis. The use of hydrochloric acid solutions requires central venous administration and frequent (every 4 to 6 hours) monitoring of arterial pH, P_{CO_2}, and plasma electrolytes.

Abnormalities in Electrolytes

Potassium Abnormalities (see Fig. 7-2). Over 95% of body potassium is intracellular, and the 50 to 100 mEq ingested daily is largely excreted by the healthy kidney. However, the extracellular concentration of potassium is critical to normal cardiac and neuromuscular function. The catabolic state, injury, acidosis, and hypoperfusion can all cause movement of intracellular potassium to the extracellular fluid compartment and produce hyperkalemia.

Hyperkalemia. Elevated plasma levels of potassium (>6 mEq/L) require immediate intervention or a refractory cardiac dysrhythmia may result. Peaked T waves precede widened QRS complexes, which can evolve to heart block and cardiac arrest unless plasma levels of potassium are decreased. Immediate treatment includes intravenous sodium bicarbonate with glucose and insulin to transport extracellular potassium to the intracellular compartment (1000 ml $D_{10}W$ with 45 mEq sodium bicarbonate plus 20 U regular insulin). Calcium gluconate is also effective emergency treatment because it antagonizes the cell membrane effects of hyperkalemia.

Hypokalemia. Depressed levels of plasma potassium are frequently encountered in surgical patients because the postoperative state predisposes to a loss of gastrointestinal fluids. The evolution of metabolic alkalosis perpetuates potassium depletion. This is particularly true after emergency surgery in which preoperative resuscitation and intraoperative maintenance requires the use of large volumes of isotonic salt solutions to replace losses of extracellular fluid. The kidney is then presented with a filtrate high in sodium that can increase renal losses of potassium in spite of total body deficits. Initially the kidney will increase excretion of potassium until the filtrate concentration of potassium is so low that paradoxic aciduria occurs. Hypokalemia can also be exacerbated by nutritional support because repletion of lean body mass incorporates large supplies of potassium. The treatment of hypokalemia requires anticipation of same and aggressive replacement, which may translate to more than 200 mEq potassium chloride per day. Electrocardiographic (ECG) monitoring is recommended in this setting.

Calcium Abnormalities. The majority of total body calcium is found as calcium carbonate and phosphate in bone. Most ingested calcium (1 to 3 g/day) is lost in stool, with small amounts excreted in the urine (200 mg/day). The normal serum calcium level is 8.6 to 10.4 mg/dl and represents the sum of calcium bound to albumin plus free or ionized calcium. Alkalosis increases the proportion of bound calcium; conversely, acidosis increases the ionized component.

Hypercalcemia. Elevated levels of calcium are rare in surgical patients except for those with bony metastases, hyperparathyroidism, or paraneoplastic syndromes. However, serum calcium levels above 14 mg/dl represent an emergency because death can occur from a refractory cardiac dysrhythmia. The first line of therapy is to restore extracellular fluid deficits with normal saline solution, followed by increasing renal calcium excretion with loop diuretics (furosemide). Steroids, mithramycin, and hemodialysis have all been used to correct hypercalcemia. Urgent surgery represents definitive treatment for patients with parathyroid adenoma.

Hypocalcemia. Serum levels of calcium less than 8 mg/dl define hypocalcemia and are most frequently seen in patients with pancreatitis, high-output fistulas, or necrotizing fasciitis and after removal of a parathyroid adenoma. Symptoms include numbness and tingling of the extremities and the circumoral region. Hyperactive tendon reflexes and a positive Chvostek's sign can be elicited before spontaneous tetany evolves. The QT interval is prolonged on the ECG. Emergency treatment requires intravenous calcium chloride or gluconate. In patients with persistent hypoparathyroidism, oral supplementation with calcium lactate and vitamin D is indicated.

Debate continues about the need for calcium during massive transfusion because few data are available about ionized calcium levels in this setting. However, in patients in whom transfusion requirements exceed 500 ml every 5 to 10 minutes, calcium supplementation is usually suggested. In this rare situation Moore recommends 0.2 g calcium chloride via a separate intravenous access for each 500 ml of whole blood. During massive transfusion, ionized calcium should be monitored along with the QT interval of the ECG.

Magnesium Abnormalities. Total body magnesium approximates 2000 mEq, half of which is in bone. Like potassium, magnesium is an intracellular cation, which during alkalotic states tends to become depleted. Normal dietary intake is approximately 20 mEq/day, most of which is excreted in feces. Normal serum values range from 1.5 to 2.5 mEq/L. A magnesium deficit can exist with normal plasma values, probably because the normal kidney can reabsorb almost all filtered magnesium. Magnesium is required for normal function of many intracellular enzyme systems.

Magnesium Deficiency. Magnesium deficiency is most frequently caused by malabsorptive disorders, diarrheal states, pancreatitis, starvation, high-output intestinal fistulas, primary hyperaldosteronism. chronic alcoholism, and cirrhosis. It also occurs in patients receiving hyperalimentation in whom magnesium input is inadequate and in patients recovering from burn injuries. Symptoms mimic hypocalcemia and include hyperactive deep tendon reflexes and a positive Chvostek's sign. Hypocalcemia and magnesium depletion are frequently coupled. Correction of hypocalcemia requires concomitant correction of hypomagnesemia. Treatment requires anticipation of the deficit. Patients receiving hyperalimentation or prolonged intravenous support should have magnesium supplementation from the onset. When faced by documented depletion, the intravenous route is preferable to intramuscular injection. In symptomatic patients with normal renal function, 80 mEq magnesium sulfate per liter can be given over 4 to 6 hours. In patients without symptoms 80 mEq magnesium sulfate should be given over 24 hours with careful monitoring of plasma levels.

Magnesium depletion can be massive in postsurgical patients, especially those with high-output intestinal fistulas who require intravenous hyperalimentation. Supplemental magnesium (>40 mEq/24 hr) may be required for several weeks. However, as with potassium depletion and treatment of concentration abnormalities, restoration of extracellular fluid volumes deficits must be addressed before adequate repletion of magnesium deficiencies can occur.

Magnesium Excess. Elevated levels of plasma magnesium are usually seen in patients with renal failure and tend to parallel serum potassium and calcium levels. The most common cause is the use of magnesium-containing antacids in patients with depressed renal function. As with plasma potassium, acidosis worsens hypermagnesemia. Symptoms of hypermagnesemia include fatigue, lethargy, nausea, and vomiting. Signs include cutaneous flushing and decreased deep tendon reflexes. Extreme elevations (magnesium level >12 mEq/dl) can cause muscle paralysis, respiratory depression, and cardiac arrest. ECG changes mimic hyperkalemia: elevated T waves, prolongation of the PR interval, and widened QRS segment. Immediate treatment requires discontinuation of magnesium input and correction of acidosis. Intravenous calcium (5 to 10 mEq calcium chloride) may alleviate symptoms, but dialysis usually is required in patients with significant renal dysfunction.

THERAPY
Parenteral Fluid

Table 7-8 lists the commonly available parenteral fluids frequently used to treat surgical patients.

TABLE 7-8 Composition of Parenteral Fluids (Electrolyte Content, mEq/L)

Solutions	Cations				Anions		Osmolality, mOsm
	Na	K	Ca	Mg	Cl	HCO$_3$	
Extracellular fluid	142	4	5	3	103	27	280-310
Lactated Ringer's	130	4	3	—	109	28*	273
0.9% sodium chloride	154	—	—	—	154	—	308
D$_5$ 45% sodium chloride	77	—	—	—	77	—	407
D5W	—	—	—	—	—	—	253
M/6 sodium lactate	167	—	—	—	—	167*	334
3% sodium chloride	513	—	—	—	513	—	1026

From Shires GT, Canizaro PC, Shires GT III, et al. Fluid, electrolyte and nutritional management of the surgical patient. In Schwartz SI (ed). Principles of Surgery, 5th ed. New York, McGraw-Hill, 1989, p 83. Reproduced with permission.
*Present in solution as lactate that is converted to bicarbonate.

The choice of fluid depends on the patient's volume status and the concentration and compositional abnormality to be corrected.

Preoperative Fluid Management

As previously stated, abnormalities in fluid and electrolyte balance can be divided into three components: extracellular fluid volume, concentration, and composition. Every permutation can be found in surgical patients. The safest and most logical approach is to analyze volume abnormalities first, correct same, and then deal with alterations of concentration and composition. Frequently, in patients with healthy kidneys correction of the volume disturbance will concomitantly correct or favorably affect concentration and composition abnormalities.

Correction of Volume Abnormalities. The nature of surgical illness predisposes to volume deficits more frequently than volume excesses except in patients with chronic cardiac or renal disease. In most surgical patients the assessment of volume status can be made on clinical grounds, but in those with comorbid factors such as advanced age, cardiac disease, and renal or hepatic dysfunction, serial measurement of central venous and/or pulmonary artery wedge pressure may be needed. The most common volume disturbance in preoperative patients is an extracellular fluid volume deficit secondary to external losses and sequestration into nonfunctional compartments. Conceptually, this is intuitive, but internal losses are commonly underestimated in preoperative patients. For example, a cirrhotic patient with massive ascites, hypotension, tachycardia, and oliguria may be appreciated to have a massively expended extracellular fluid compartment with a critical deficit in functional plasma volume (decreased effective plasma volume). In contrast, the volume deficit of a preoperative patient with gangrenous bowel obstruction may be grossly underestimated because the volume of fluid sequestered intraluminally, in the bowel wall, and within the "peritoneal burn" is not obvious. Correction of extracellular volume deficits should be aggressive and requires the physician caring for the patient to be a "bedside doctor." Patients with severe volume deficits may require more than 1 L per hour of balanced salt solution (Ringer's lactate) to prepare them optimally for operation. As blood pressure and urinary output increase, infusion rates are decreased. Except in patients with symptomatic concentration abnormalities or severe metabolic alkalosis, hypertonic or iso-

tonic sodium chloride solutions offer no advantage over balanced salt solutions. Similarly, except in patients with symptomatic hypernatremia, D5W is rarely indicated because the glucose load may induce an osmotic diuresis. As previously stated, pressors have essentially no role in the treatment of volume deficits.

Correction of Concentration Abnormalities. Severe hyponatremia (serum sodium <120 mEq/L) or hypernatremia (serum sodium >160 mEq/L) rarely occurs in preoperative patients unless they have significant renal or liver disease (hyponatremia) or have sustained major burns (hypernatremia). Both concentration abnormalities may be symptomatic and require treatment on an urgent basis, especially if the abnormality has developed over a short period of time (hours). Therapy for symptomatic hyponatremia is dictated by the patient's volume and acid-base status. In patients with a volume deficit, hypochloremic metabolic alkalosis, and severe hyponatremia, repletion should be initiated with isotonic (0.9%) sodium chloride solution. Small amounts of hypertonic saline solution (3% or 5%; see Table 7-8) may be required in symptomatic patients whose serum sodium is less than 120 mEq/L. Since the alkalosis and concentration derangement have usually evolved over time, this situation is unusual. If the metabolic alkalosis is profound, extraordinary amounts of potassium chloride and/or hydrochloric acid may be required after extracellular fluid volume has been normalized. In patients requiring hypertonic saline solution, the sodium deficit can be estimated by multiplying the decrease in serum sodium concentration below normal by the estimated liters of total body water.

EXAMPLE: a 21-year-old male with symptomatic hyponatremia who weighs 70 kg and whose serum sodium (Na) level is 119 mEq/L:

Total body water = 70 kg × 0.60 = 42 L

Sodium deficit = (140 − 119 mEq/L) ×
42 L = 882 mEq sodium

Half the deficit can be replaced over 12 hours. Because hypertonic saline solution is hyperosmolar and has the potential of expanding the extracellular fluid compartment, cardiac filling pressures should be monitored during infusion. Hypertonic saline solution is used when there is coexisting metabolic alkalosis. M/6 sodium lactate (see Table 7-8) should be used if metabolic acidosis is the underlying compositional abnormality.

Symptomatic hyponatremia with volume excess almost exclusively occurs in patients with cardiac disease, renal failure, or cirrhosis. In patients with renal failure M/6 sodium lactate may be successful, but peritoneal dialysis or hemodialysis is frequently required. In patients with cirrhosis the problem is somewhat different because the clinical setting usually involves a patient with normal or elevated filling pressures, massive ascites, and renal dysfunction caused by the hepatorenal syndrome. In this subset massive volume paracentesis with concomitant administration of hypertonic saline solution can correct volume status and hyponatremia and reestablish urinary flow.

Clinically significant hypernatremia is rare but can be life threatening. Patients with a volume deficit should be given the combination of half-strength lactated Ringer's and D5W, with care taken not to reduce the serum sodium level too quickly. Rapidly decreasing the serum osmolarity can cause convulsions, coma, and death.

Correction of Alteration in Composition. Correction of abnormalities in volume and concentration usually aids in normalizing alterations in acid-base balance, provided the proper parenteral solution is used (see Table 7-8). In patients undergoing an elective operation, correction of alkalosis is particularly important because anesthesia can worsen the alkalosis by hyperventilation's predisposing to dysrhythmias. Uncorrected alkalosis and volume depletion caused by sequestered extracellular fluid are the two most frequently undetected disorders of fluid and electrolyte balance in preoperative patients.

Intraoperative Fluid Management

Proper intraoperative fluid management begins with adequate restoration of volume deficits and correction of concentration and composition abnormalities before induction of anesthesia. Hypotension elicited by induction defines inadequate preoperative repletion of extracellular fluid volume. Surgeons tend to underestimate operative blood loss. Blood or packed red blood cells should be given for a loss exceeding 500 ml. Intraoperative deficits of extracellular fluid into the wound or to other nonfunctional third spaces (bowel wall, retroperitoneum) are frequently undetected and can produce a postoperative deficit in effective plasma volume.

In patients whose volume status has been adequately restored before the operation, intraoperative fluid requirements during surgery exclusive of blood average 0.5 to 1 L per hour. This volume of extracellular fluid maintenance plus replacement of shed blood is usually adequate in elective operations. In emergency procedures a much greater volume of balanced salt solution may be required to replete deficits in extracellular fluid.

Postoperative Fluid Management

Immediate Postoperative Period. The most common error in the management of postoperative fluids and electrolytes is the assumption that all patients require essentially the same volume and composition of parenteral fluids. Postoperative orders should not be written until the patient is reevaluated in the recovery room, especially with regard to volume deficits.

The general guideline that a systolic blood pressure of 90 mm Hg with a heart rate less than 120 reflects an adequate extracellular fluid volume may apply to an 18-year-old patient with simple appendicitis. The same guideline is usually not adequate to assess a 65-year-old patient with a history of hypertension who has just undergone a 4-hour operation to resect a abdominal aneurysm. Similarly, a urinary output of 30 ml/hr in the recovery room may be adequate provided there is no elevation in blood sugar (>180 mg/dl) inducing an osmotic diuresis. Careful clinical assessment, augmented by monitoring filling pressures in the appropriate patients, is the first step in the management of postoperative fluids and electrolytes. Underestimation of volume deficit is the most common error.

Unexplained tachycardia in the recovery room is more frequently caused by volume deficiency than by pain. Circulatory instability dictates the need for expansion of the extracellular fluid compartment (plasma and interstitial volumes). Unless the patient has severe metabolic alkalosis, replacement of potassium and magnesium is usually not required during the first 24 hours after the operation.

Later Postoperative Period. Management of postoperative fluids is not difficult in the patient with a normal extracellular fluid volume, provided measured losses are replaced and insensible and immeasurable losses are anticipated.

Approximately 1 L of fluid should be administered to provide the volume of urine required to clear the products of intracellular catabolism. This may be given as D5W or hypotonic (0.45%) saline solution. Gastrointestinal losses should be measured and replaced with either isotonic or hypotonic salt solutions (see Table 7-3). Insensible water loss usually averages 600 ml/day but can be more than doubled by postoperative fever or hyperventilation. D5W should be used to replace these losses. Replacement of potassium should begin 24 hours after surgery and include replacement for renal (40 mEq/day) and gastrointestinal drainage losses (see Table 7-3).

Special Postoperative Problems

Volume Excess. Surgical illness and operation are accompanied by an expansion of the extracellular space. Adequate preoperative resuscitation and intraoperative fluid management require additional amounts of balanced salt solutions to maintain effective plasma volume and meet the extra requirements caused by third-space losses. In the late postoperative period young patients with healthy kidneys frequently spontaneously diurese this expanded extracellular fluid volume, provided there is no ongoing catabolic process (e.g., sepsis). Older patients with subclinical cardiac or renal disease frequently cannot mount this diuresis and subsequently develop signs and symptoms of volume excess. The earliest sign is unexpected weight gain after operation. Pulmonary and cardiac signs such as pulmonary edema and congestive heart failure appear late. Proper management of postoperative parenteral fluids and avoiding excessive amounts of isotonic salt solutions will obviate this problem in the majority of patients.

Hyponatremia. Postoperative hyponatremia usually reflects inadequate replacement of extracellular fluid requirements before and during the operation. As in preoperative patients, assessment of postoperative hyponatremia first requires evaluation of extracellular fluid volume status. In older patients volume excess is not unusual and simple free-water restriction will correct the hyponatremia, except in patients with cirrhosis with the hepatorenal syndrome discussed previously. Rarely, hyponatremia occurs in patients in whom water has been used to replace large volume losses of gastrointestinal fluids. Extracellular fluid volume deficit is common in these patients, and correction of volume status with either lactated Ringer's or normal saline solution usually alleviates the hyponatremia.

Hypernatremia. Hypernatremia is a rare postoperative concentration abnormality but is potentially dangerous because extracellular fluid hyperosmolarity can shift intracellular water to the extracellular fluid compartment with adverse affects. Hypernatremia is caused by unexpected losses of water or when free-water losses have been replaced with isotonic salt solutions. The treatment is administration of D5W.

High-Output Renal Failure. High-output renal failure is defined as progressive elevation in creatinine and blood urea nitrogen levels, with concomitant decrease in creatinine clearance in patients producing more than 1000 ml of urine per day. The mechanisms causing high-output renal failure are probably the same as those producing oliguric acute tubular necrosis: hypoperfusion and ischemia. Because the affected kidney continues to produce volumes of urine, providing intravenous therapy is not as difficult as in patients with oliguric renal failure, if care is taken to restrict exogenous potassium and limit sodium input to replace only measured losses. High-output renal failure usually resolves with restoration of urea clearance in 10 days to 2 weeks. Creatinine clearance gradually recovers over weeks to several months.

SURGICAL PHARMACOPEIA

Drug	Indications	Complications	Dosage
3% to 5% saline solution	Hyponatremia; acute, <120 μg/L with volume contraction	Raise serum sodium level only to 125 μg/L; otherwise, leads to brain shrinkage, with confusion, seizure, or coma in volume-expanded hyponatremia	Calculate sodium deficit to serum sodium level of 125 μg/L (3% equals 0.51 μg/L; 5% equals 0.86 μg/L)
Sodium bicarbonate (NaHCO$_3$)	Metabolic acidosis; pH <7.2; hyperkalemia	Watch for hypokalemia and ventricular dysrhythmias	Dependent on level of acidosis or hyperkalemia (one ampule equals 44 μg)

Drug	Indications	Complications	Dosage
Hydrochloric acid (HCl) 0.1 N	Metabolic alkalosis leading to significant hypoventilation	Watch for hyperkalemia with associated ECG changes	1-2 L over 24 hr
Calcium (Ca) gluconate	Cardiotoxic hyperkalemia	Hazardous to patients receiving digitalis therapy if given rapidly	10-20 cc of 10% Ca gluconate over 15-30 min; if ECG is in sine wave or worse, 5-10 cc over 2 min
	Hypomagnesemia, hypocalcemia		1 g Ca gluconate equals 90 mg calcium equals 45 μg calcium
			Give slowly if no cardiotoxicity is present
Insulin with dextrose	Hyperkalemia, >6 μg/L, requiring rapid correction	Watch for hypoglycemia and hypokalemia	20 U regular insulin with 200 cc D50 or 1 L D10W
Sodium polystyrene sulfonate (Kayexalate)	Hyperkalemia requiring slow correction	Takes approximately 24 hours for effect Contraindicated in patients with congestive heart failure, severe HTN, or marked edema; constipation	15 g (4 level tsp) one to four times daily
Furosemide (Lasix) Ethacrynic acid (Edecrin)	Hyperkalemia, hypercalcemia	Watch for hypokalemia and hypocalcemia with resultant cardiac disturbances; ethacrynic acid can produce severe diarrhea, requires concomitant IV hydration	Furosemide: 20-80 mg for hyperkalemia; 80-160 mg for hypercalcemia; can repeat after 6-8 hr Ethacrynic acid: 50 mg IV for hyperkalemia; 100 mg IV for hypercalcemia; can repeat after 6-8 hr
Mithramycin	Hypercalcemia, symptomatic	Give slowly; otherwise increases complications of thrombocytopenia, leukopenia, hemorrhage; 5% increase in liver function test results	25 μg/kg IV daily for 3-4 days
Prednisone	Hypercalcemia resulting from sarcoidosis, vitamin D poisoning, multiple myeloma, or other hematopoietic malignancies	All complications of steroids (infections, ulcers, Cushing's disease, etc.)	50-100 mg/day
Calcitonin	Hypercalcemia, especially with Paget's disease	Short acting; loss of effect as quickly as 2 days; induces nausea and/or vomiting in 10% of patients	100 IU (0.5 cc) subcutaneously or IM daily (up to 8 IU/kg bid)

Continued.

Drug	Indications	Complications	Dosage
Vitamin D	Transient hypoparathyroidism after thyroidectomy or excision of parathyroid adenoma; chronic hypocalcemia, rickets	Watch for vitamin D intoxication in patients with renal failure	0.25-0.5 μg/day
Calcium carbonate ($CaCO_3$) (Tums)	Chronic hypocalcemia	Overdose leads to hypercalcemia (NOTE: also a gastric antacid)	1-2 g Ca/day (1 g $CaCO_3$ equals 400 mg Ca) 500 mg Tums tablet = 200 mg elemental calcium

BIBLIOGRAPHY

Canizaro PC, Prager MD, Shires GT. The infusion of Ringer's lactate solution during shock. Am J Surg 122:494, 1971.

Moore FD, Olesen KH, McMurrey JD, et al. Body cell mass and its supporting environment: Body composition in health and disease. Philadelphia, WB Saunders, 1963.

Roberts JP, Roberts JD, Skinner C, et al. Extracellular fluid deficiency following operation and its correction with Ringer's lactate: A reassessment. Ann Surg 202:1, 1985.

Shires GT, Canizaro PC, Shires GT III, et al. Fluid, electrolyte and nutritional management of the surgical patient. In Schwartz SI (ed). Principles of Surgery, 5th ed. New York, McGraw-Hill, 1989, p 69.

Wong ET, Rude RK, Singer FR, et al. A high prevalence of hypomagnesemia and hypermagnesemia in hospitalized patients. Am J Clin Pathol 79:348, 1983.

CHAPTER REVIEW
Questions

1. The most frequent derangement of fluid and electrolyte balance in the **preoperative** surgical patient is:
   a. Underestimation of deficits in extracellular fluid volume
   b. Metabolic acidosis
   c. Metabolic alkalosis
   d. Respiratory acidosis
   e. Respiratory alkalosis

2. The most frequent derangement of fluid and electrolyte balance in the immediate postoperative period is:
   a. Underestimation of deficits in extracellular fluid volume
   b. Overestimation of intraoperative blood loss
   c. Failure to adequately treat hyperglycemia
   d. Hypomagnesemia
   e. Respiratory alkalosis

3. A patient with an obstructing ulcer of the duodenum has more than 2 L of nasogastric drainage in a 24-hour period. Plasma electrolyte values are sodium, 132 mEq/L; potassium, 2.5 mEq/L; chloride, 85 mEq/L; bicarbonate, 35 mEq/L. Assume normal renal function. Which of the following statements regarding this patient is **not true?**
   a. The patient probably has a deficit of extracellular fluid volume.
   b. Urinary pH could be less than 7.
   c. Initial fluid order should be started with lactated Ringer's solution.
   d. Repletion of potassium deficits may require more than 60 mEq/24 hr.
   e. 0.1 N hydrochloric acid may be needed to correct alkalosis.

4. A 21-year-old previously healthy man is brought to the emergency clinic 20 minutes after sustaining a 45-caliber bullet wound to the femoral artery and vein. His blood pressure is 60 mm Hg systolic, and his heart rate is 156/min. The patient is diaphoretic. Arterial blood gas values obtained in room air show the following: Po_2, 80; Pco_2, 25; pH, 7.30. All of the following are initially required **except:**
   a. Direct pressure to central blood loss site
   b. 2000 ml of lactated Ringer's solution
   c. Type-specific blood
   d. Bladder catheterization
   e. Dopamine at 10 ug/hr

5. Your patient has just been extubated and taken to the recovery room after a 4-hour

emergency operation to correct a bleeding duodenal ulcer. The first arterial blood gas values drawn show the following: Po_2, 60 torr; Pco_2, 85 torr; pH, 7.24. This patient:

a. Should receive 1 L of lactated Ringer's over 30 minutes.

b. Should receive an increase in face-mask Fio_2 from 40% to 60%.

c. Should be encouraged to deep breathe and cough.

d. Should be given one ampule of naloxone (Narcan) intravenously.

e. Should be intubated and placed on mechanical ventilation.

6. Your patient had an emergency placement of a tube graft for a bleeding aortic aneurysm 5 days ago. He complains of severe shortness of breath and has audible rales and a S_3 gallop.

Which of the following results during the initial evaluation after treatment would you not expect?

a. Po_2 of 60 Torr

b. Pco_2 of 60 Torr

c. pH of 7.45

d. Pulmonary artery wedge pressure of 25 mm Hg

e. No change in electrocardiogram

Answers

1. a
2. a
3. c
4. e
5. e
6. b

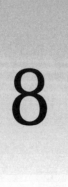

8

Nutritional Support

ANTHONY P. BORZOTTA

KEY FEATURES

After reading this chapter you will understand:
- How to evaluate inadequate nutrition.
- The indications for and routes of administration of nutritional support.
- How to develop a detailed, balanced plan of nutritional support.

Many of the illnesses and injuries subject to surgical treatment, and some operations themselves, alter metabolism, digestion, or appetite. A malnourished patient is at increased risk of complicating infections, wound disruption, and delayed recovery and return to normal activity following operation. Therefore optimal surgical management requires an understanding of nutrition. The objectives of this chapter are to learn how to assess nutritional status, to know the indications for enteral and central parenteral nutritional support, to formulate a sound nutritional support plan, and to select the most suitable route for delivery of nutrients.

WHAT CAN BE DONE TO ASSESS NUTRITIONAL STATUS?
History and Physical Examination

No single test qualifies as a gold standard of nutritional assessment. As always, the history provides many clues. Changes in weight, clothing, or belt size denote weight loss. Recent operations, illnesses, cancer or its therapies, alcohol and drug abuse, prematurity, and the isolation

and loneliness of old age are associated with malnutrition. Prolonged hospitalization requiring multiple diagnostic studies is often associated with a fasting state, the use of hypocaloric intravenous solutions, increased metabolic demands, and reduced oral intake, all factors that are often overlooked in assessing nutritional status.

The physical examination may show malnutrition marked by obvious depletion of fatty contours of the body and wasting of muscle mass (sunken temples, loss of intrinsic hand muscle mass, weakness). A swollen, distended abdomen, high-output fistulas, and dehisced and nonhealing wounds are all markers of a malnourished state. Anthropometric measurements (the height-weight index, creatinine-height index, skinfold thickness measurements, mid-arm circumference and others) have limited value during the acute phase of the patient's hospitalization but are important objective measurements in epidemiologic studies or the long-term follow-up of small populations.

Biochemical Tests

The hepatic secretory proteins, including albumin, prealbumin, transferrin, and retinol-binding protein, reflect the protein synthesis function of the liver, and are markers of visceral protein status. Depressed preoperative protein levels are predictive of postoperative morbidity and mortality. Table 8-1 lists hepatic secretory protein normal values, half-lives, and the degrees of deficiency associated with malnutrition. The shorter half-lives of prealbumin and retinol-binding protein make them ideal markers for short-term,

TABLE 8-1 Hepatic Secretory Proteins Useful in Nutritional Assessment

Protein	Normal Concentration in Serum	Half-Life	Depletion		
			Mild	Moderate	Severe
Albumin	35-55 g/L	20 days	30-35	20-30	≤20
Transferrin	2-4 g/L	9 days	1.5-2	1-1.5	<1
Prealbumin	200-400 mg/L	2-4 days	150-200	100-150	<100
Retinol-binding protein	26-76 mg/L	12 hours			

repeated assessment of nutritional support. They are preferable to transferrin and albumin, which typically require several weeks to demonstrate reliable changes.

Immunologic Tests

Malnutrition is a common cause of secondary immunodeficiency, and infections are the most frequent complication of malnutrition. Cell-mediated, opsonic, polymorphonuclear, and immunoglobulin functions are impaired by undernutrition. Immunologic assessment techniques vary from simply measuring the absolute lymphocyte count (white blood cell count times percent of lymphocytes; normal is $>1.5 \times 10^9$ cells per liter) to flow cytometric analyses of cell function. Delayed hypersensitivity skin tests require the intradermal inoculation of a battery of antigens (mumps, purified protein derivative, Candidan, histoplasmin, streptokinase-streptodornase) to be certain that a patient's anamnestic immune mechanism will be challenged. A normal response is a 5 mm or greater area of induration after 48 hours. Nonresponders are described as **anergic** and are probably at increased risk for postoperative morbidity. Unfortunately, many conditions apart from malnutrition will depress this immune response, including infection, trauma, elective operations, corticosteroids, renal failure, and malignancies.

NUTRITIONAL STATES

Nutritional status is also defined by the metabolic state of the patient. There are four categories:

1. Fed or anabolic
2. Acutely fasted
3. Starvation adapted
4. Stressed or catabolic

A healthy, recently fed individual will be in a net anabolic or protein-building state, with deposition of excess ingested calories into the energy storage forms of fat and glycogen in liver and muscle. Excess amino acid nitrogen is converted to urea and is excreted in the urine. Proteins do not exist in a storage form. All proteins have structural, enzymatic, locomotor, transportation, and other functions. Dr. Francis Moore defined this functional mass of the body as the lean body mass. It can be depleted at varying rates, but losses of 50% or more are lethal.

In the acute fasting state, liver and muscle glycogen is mobilized for energy needs and skeletal muscle proteolysis provides amino acids to the liver for gluconeogenesis. Many body tissues are glucose dependent, and this process provides an essential energy supply. There is a net loss of protein-derived nitrogen into the urine as urea, typically greater than 10 g of nitrogen per day. After days of fasting, metabolism enters a starvation-adapted state marked by enhanced lipolysis or mobilization of adipose energy stores into free fatty acids, which can be converted into ketone bodies. To a large but not complete degree, starvation ketosis supplants glucose oxidation. Urine urea nitrogen excretion falls to less than 5 g per 24 hours, as the body adapts for long-term survival with inadequate nutritional support. Simple starvation of an unstressed individual leads to death in about 230 days, as evidenced by the individuals of the Irish Republican Army who engaged in political fasts in Belfast in the early 1980s.

When an individual is traumatically injured, burned, or suffers a series of septic complications, he enters a catabolic state marked by accelerated protein breakdown. Cytokines and inflammatory mediators released from injured tissues drive this catabolism. Protein losses are most obvious from skeletal muscle, but significant decreases in the protein mass of the heart, lungs, liver, and kidneys also occur. Uncorrected and unsupported, this form of accelerated starvation leads to death in approximately 30 days, as was seen, for example, in burn units before the availability of adequate topical antibiotics and before modern burn wound management methods were developed. In this state of catabolism, nitrogen wasting is greater than 20 g of urea nitrogen per day. Aggressive nutritional support is an essential adjunct in the care of these patients. The acceleration of proteolysis seems to be inevitable once inflammation or infection sets in. However, protein breakdown can be blunted and the anabolic or protein synthesis functions enhanced by provision of adequate protein and energy.

WHAT ARE THE INDICATIONS FOR NUTRITIONAL SUPPORT?

There are four categories of individuals for whom nutritional support should be considered:

1. The *malnourished individual* who needs repletion of energy and protein to restore health or to prepare for operation

2. The *patient unable to eat* at all or whose intake is inadequate for his needs
3. The individual who may be able to eat but for whom *use of the digestive tract is limited,* unsafe, or inadvisable
4. The individual who incurs an *accelerated rate of depletion* that must be supported or reversed

The box below summarizes these indications in some detail. Many more indications for parenteral nutrition existed when enteral support was considered only in terms of oral supplements or nasogastric (NG) tube feeding. Advanced formulations and more aggressive methods of accessing the small intestine have greatly expanded the role of enteral nutritional feeding. Both parenteral and enteral nutritional support can provide a patient with all needed nutritional elements with approximately similar efficacy. Advantages of enteral support are improved intestinal structure and function, adaptation to spontaneous

---

SELECTED INDICATIONS FOR NUTRITIONAL SUPPORT

Enteral

Inadequate oral intake of nutrients for past 5 days
Preexisting malnutrition with inadequate spontaneous oral intake
Major burns (>40% TSA) (duodenal or gastric)
Severe closed head injury (jejunal)
Major trauma (jejunal or gastric)
Adjunctive to radiotherapy or chemotherapy for cancer
Following massive intestinal resection, adjunctive to central parenteral nutrition (gastric)
Prolonged dependence on mechanical ventilation (jejunal)
Low-output enterocutaneous fistulas

Parenteral

Bowel obstruction, including partial obstructions
Prolonged paralytic ileus
Diffuse peritonitis
Short bowel syndrome
Acute hemorrhagic pancreatitis
Multiple abdominal organ traumatic injuries
Extreme prematurity
Necrotizing enterocolitis
Congenital gastrointestinal anomalies: omphalocele, atresias, diaphragmatic hernia
Superior mesenteric artery syndrome
Intractable diarrhea
Malabsorption syndromes
Protein-losing gastroenteropathy (sprue, Ménétrièr's disease)
During treatment of inflammatory bowel disease
Acute hepatitis and reversible liver failure

oral intake, and cost effectiveness. *The gut should always be used when it is intact.*

HOW DOES ONE FORMULATE A NUTRITIONAL SUPPORT PLAN?
Setting Priorities

First, the patient must be adequately resuscitated to ensure that nutrients administered intravenously or enterally will be properly utilized. Second, nitrogen needs should be measured and provided. Third, energy needs should be estimated or measured and provided. Fourth, vitamins and minerals should be provided, because these essential cofactors to intermediary metabolism must be present for optimal utilization of administered nutrients. Fifth, a systematic program for continued monitoring and reassessment of the efficacy of nutritional support must be worked out.

Determining Nitrogen Needs

The simplest and most direct method of measuring nitrogen needs is a 24-hour urine collection to measure urine urea nitrogen (UUN) or total urine nitrogen (TUN). UUN excretion varies with customary nitrogen intake, being greater in a robust football player than in a diminutive elderly woman. The wide variation even among individuals of similar sex and age further underlines the need for actual measurement, rather than relying on estimation.

It is a nutritional law that the body establishes a nitrogen balance and that all nitrogen is excreted in urine, stool, and losses of body substance, and not in the form of gaseous nitrogen. Therefore a urine collection to measure UUN will establish nitrogen loss. Customarily, 3 or 4 g of nitrogen are added to the 24-hour UUN value to account for urinary losses as ammonia and amino acids, in the stool and from the skin. Nitrogen balance is defined as nitrogen intake minus nitrogen excretion and is normally zero. (Nitrogen in grams can be multiplied by 6.25 to give protein in grams.)

Most hospitals are equipped to provide urine urea nitrogen measurements, but in patients with hypercatabolic states the difference between UUN and TUN values increases in an unpredictable fashion. Some authorities now recommend that when possible, TUN measurements be obtained. These measurements should be repeated at least weekly. In patients undergoing rapid metabolic changes it can be done as often as every 3 days. Timed collections as short

as 8 or 12 hours can provide clinically useful measurements. If the patient is receiving no nitrogen or less than the UUN measurement, he will be in negative nitrogen balance.

Calculating Energy Needs

After establishing protein need, the next priority is to calculate energy needs. At any given level of nitrogen intake, supplying an energy source will improve nitrogen balance. In the absence of an energy supply, an unnecessarily large proportion of administered protein is oxidized through the process of *gluconeogenesis*. Energy needs may be estimated on the basis of the Harris-Benedict equations, which determine resting metabolic expenditure (RME). (See the box below.) RME is the energy needed by a person who has fasted overnight, lying supine and breathing quietly. If these values alone are used, inadequate energy needs will be estimated; the results must be multiplied by activity factors to yield estimated total daily caloric requirements. For bed rest, multiply by 1.2; normal activity by 1.3; elective operation by 1.3 to 1.4; for trauma and long bone fractures multiply by 1.4 to 1.5; closed head injury and severe infection by 1.6 to 1.8; and burns of 40% to 100% of total body surface by 2.0. When available, a metabolic cart using the technique of indirect calorimetry will provide a more accurate, individual value. However, an indirect calorimetry measurement over a 10- to 20-minute span of time extrapolated into a 24-hour value must be interpreted in light of the patient's level of activity (agitation or somnolence) and the presence or absence of feeding at the time of measurement, compared with its presence during the rest of the day.

CALCULATING RESTING METABOLIC EXPENDITURE

Resting metabolic expenditure (RME), in kilocalories per day, can be estimated by using the Harris-Benedict equations:

For men
$$66.47 + 13.75 \,(W) + 5 \,(H) - 6.76 \,(A)$$

For women
$$655.1 + 9.56 \,(W) + 1.85 \,(H) - 4.68 \,(A)$$

W = weight in kilograms; H = height in centimeters; A = age in years.

Energy Substrate: Dextrose, Lipids, or Both

In total parenteral nutrition, all energy needs may be supplied in the form of dextrose solutions. The concentration (osmolarity) of solutions determines whether they can be safely administered peripherally (up to 10%) or into a central vein (15% or greater). A minimum of 100 g of glucose per day can prevent starvation ketosis. One way of estimating maximum glucose administration rates is based on the characteristic glucose oxidation rate of 5 mg/kg/min. Glucose administered in excess of the body's ability to oxidize it will lead to lipogenesis and hyperglycemia.

In a patient who develops hyperglycemia with a dextrose energy supply, or whose energy needs are greater than that estimated by the glucose oxidation rate, or who will require parenteral nutrition for more than 4 weeks, lipid emulsions should be used. Up to 40% of total energy needs can be provided as lipid emulsions. The greater caloric density of lipids (9 kCal/g versus 3.6 kCal/g dextrose) makes them an advantageous energy source in patients needing fluid restriction. Lipid emulsions contain the essential long-chain fatty acid, linoleic acid, which if absent can lead to clinical deficiency states after about 6 weeks. Recently, medium chain triglycerides (carbon chains of eight or less) have been introduced into both parenteral and enteral formulations. They are metabolized via pathways different from beta-oxidation of long-chain fatty acids.

Micronutrients

The box below lists vitamins and trace elements necessary for optimal metabolism. Adequate amounts of these micronutrients should be included in all nutritional support prescriptions. Most enteral formulations routinely include them. Deficiency states are unusual in this country but can be induced by inadequate attention to detail and by failing to recognize special needs in specific metabolic states. For example, burn patients should receive an additional 2 mg per day of zinc.

Standard and Specialized Classes of Nutrient Formulations

Categories of enteral and parenteral solutions are listed in the box on p. 143. Each hospital tends to limit the number of commercial brands on formulary, but usually each category is represented. Specialized formulations can be useful in specific disease states. Parenteral and monomeric enteral formulations are composed of individual amino acids whose composition can be tailored. The essential amino acids are tryptophan, threonine, lysine, methionine, phenylalanine, and the three branched-chain amino acids (BCAA), leucine,

---

MICRONUTRIENTS

Vitamins

Essential complex organic compounds, active in minute quantities as coenzymes

Fat-soluble: A (retinol), D (ergocalciferol), E (tocopherol), K (phylloquinone)

Water-soluble: B_1 (thiamin), B_2 (riboflavin), niacin, B_3 (pantothenic acid)
B_6 (pyridoxine), biotin, B_{12} (cyanocobalamin), folic acid
C (ascorbic acid)

Supply: One vitamin pill or one ampule of standard multivitamin preparation for intravenous use will supply the daily vitamin requirements. Vitamin K must be parenterally supplied as a weekly 10 mg intramuscular injection.

Trace elements

Essential, inorganic elements that act as cofactors of enzymatic reactions

Proven essential in man: Iron, zinc, copper, chromium, selenium, iodine, and cobalt

May be essential: Manganese, nickel, molybdenum, fluorine, tin, silicon, vanadium, and arsenic

Supply: A regular diet or a full-strength commercial enteral formula will supply the Recommended Dietary Allowance (RDA). One ampule of commercial trace elements added to parenteral nutrients will supply the RDA.

NUTRITIONAL FORMULATIONS

Enteral

Elemental or Monomeric Formulas

Protein: Hydrolysates (vary from crystalline amino acids to varying percentages of dipeptides and tripeptides)
Carbohydrate: Glucose oligosaccharides, sucrose, maltodextrins
Fat: Small amount of essential fatty acids ± medium-chain triglycerides
Osmolarity: 460 to 800 mOsm/kg (hyperosmolar)
Residue: Minimal (fiber may be added as needed)
Palatability: Poor

Polymeric Formulas—Lactose Free

Protein: Intact, from casein salts or egg whites
Carbohydrate: Starches, glucose oligosaccharides, corn syrup
Fat: 1% to 40% of calories; ± medium-chain triglycerides
Osmolarity: 300 to 750 mOsm/kg (isomolar to hyperosmolar)
Residue: Low to moderate (fiber may be added)
Palatability: Palatable

Polymeric Formulas—Lactose Containing

Protein: Intact, from milk
Carbohydrate: Lactose, corn syrup solids, sucrose
Fat: 10% to 30% as milk fats
Osmolarity: 500 to 1100 mOsm/kg (hyperosmolar)
Residue: Low to moderate
Palatability: Used as oral supplements

Special or Defined Diets

- Blenderized whole foods: intact digestive function needed
- Branched-chain amino acid enhanced (23% to 50% of amino acids), aromatic amino for use in hepatic failure
- High-protein/low-energy ratio for use in stress states
- Essential amino acids ± histidine for use in renal failure

Parenteral

Most hospital pharmacies now provide standardized mixtures of dextrose and amino acids. Concentrations can be varied to suit fluid volume restrictions or particular metabolic states.

Electrolytes are usually standardized, but additional minerals and electrolytes can be adjusted to deal with day-to-day needs.

Lipid emulsions (10% to 20% concentrations)
- 500 ml 10% emulsion over 12 hours twice weekly to prevent essential fatty acid deficiency
- Up to 40% of total caloric requirement can be given in lipid form as a continuous infusion
- Lipids can be safely added to other CPN components to create a 3-in-1 formulation (confirm with pharmacist)

Multivitamins: 1 ampule daily

Trace elements are usually provided as a commercial additive; additional elements may need to be added in specific cases.

isoleucine, and valine. These amino acids cannot be synthesized by the body and must be supplied exogenously for normal protein metabolism to take place. Solutions with increased concentrations of branched-chain amino acids and reduced aromatic amino acids can transiently reverse the encephalopathy of acute liver failure. BCAA-enhanced solutions can significantly improve protein synthesis rates in postoperative or catabolic patients. Mixtures of essential amino acids alone are valuable in patients with acute renal failure, where nitrogen excretion is limited.

Histidine appears to be essential during growth and in renal failure. Glutamine, the amino acid in greatest concentration in muscle and blood, has a vital role in interorgan amide-group transportation, intestinal mucosal cell viability, and gluconeogenesis. Currently it is available only in enteral formulations because of its tendency to precipitate in parenteral mixtures. Dipeptide, tripeptide, and short-chain polypeptide solutions are absorbed more efficiently from the gut compared with free amino acids or intact proteins and may prove to be valuable in catabolic states.

A simple regimen of laboratory surveillance and reassessment is described in the box below.

WHICH ROUTE SHOULD BE USED TO DELIVER NUTRITION?
Central Parenteral Nutrition

Central parenteral nutritional (CPN) support is indicated in a patient who is unable to eat and whose gastrointestinal tract is nonfunctional, nonaccessible, or is involved in disease processes that prohibit enteral feeding. A central venous access site is selected on the basis of ability to obtain and maintain a clean insertion point with minimal movement at the catheter/skin junction and least risk of complications for the patient. This typically means a subclavian route with a single-lumen catheter. Multilumen catheters can safely be used for CPN but are shown to have an increased risk of catheter infection compared with single-lumen catheters. Single-lumen catheters can be maintained for months with careful maintenance. The technique and complications of central venous access are dealt with elsewhere in this text.

STANDARD ORDERS FOR NUTRITIONAL SUPPORT

1. Confirm correct feeding tube or intravenous device placement.
2. Prescribe the formula composition.
3. Prescribe the rate of advancement and target rate of the nutrient.
4. Order a 24-hour urine collection for urine urea nitrogen (UUN) if not already done, and repeat weekly (Sunday 0600–Monday 0600).
5. Intake and output should be recorded each shift.
6. Order laboratory tests to monitor complications and efficacy of nutritional therapy.
   Initial: Chemistry profile, serum magnesium, prealbumin complete blood count (CBC)
   Start up: SMA—6 daily for 3 days
   Maintenance:
       SMA—20 every Monday and Thursday
       prealbumin, magnesium, CBC every Monday
7. Monitor blood glucose every 6 hours during start-up; continue every 12 hours for CPN (or more often as clinically indicated).
8. Enteral-specific orders
   a. Gastric feedings: elevate head of bed 45 degrees
   b. Gastric feedings: check gastric residuals every 4 hours. Hold feedings for 4 hours if the residual is greater than the hourly rate, and notify physician if two consecutive measurements are excessive.
   c. Irrigate feeding tubes with 20 ml of tap water after each intermittent feeding or tid, when tube is disconnected, or before and after medications are administered via tube.
   d. For obstructed tubes not cleared with simple pressure, instill 10 ml of a solution of 1 tablet Viokase, one tablet $NaHCO_3$, and 30 ml of warm tap water; repeat once.
   e. For jejunal feedings, do **not** interrupt for diagnostic tests or NPO status.

Oral and Gastric Feeding

In a patient who is capable of taking foods by mouth, one must determine whether spontaneous oral intake is adequate for measured protein and energy needs. If not, oral supplements should be offered. If intake remains inadequate, tube feeding is needed and a safe route must be chosen (Fig. 8-1). Nasogastric tube feeding is preferred if the duration of nutritional support is to be short term, that is, less than 2 weeks. For longer courses, because of problems in maintaining nasogastric tubes in position, nuisance to the patient, and risks and costs of repeated insertion (particularly in confused or agitated patients), a gastrostomy should be created. This can be done

by an open operation, endoscopy, fluoroscopy, or laparoscopy. The percutaneous endoscopic route is safe, minimally invasive, and quite effective.

The Dysfunctional Upper Digestive Tract

Any *method of intragastric feeding (oral, NG, or gastrostomy) requires the stomach to empty.* If the stomach fails to empty because of atony or obstruction, or if there is evidence of gastroesophageal reflux, aspiration, aspiration pneumonia, or depressed upper airway protective reflexes (e.g., following a stroke, in pseudobulbar palsy, stupor or coma, or even severe, chronic illness), then gastric feeding by any route be-

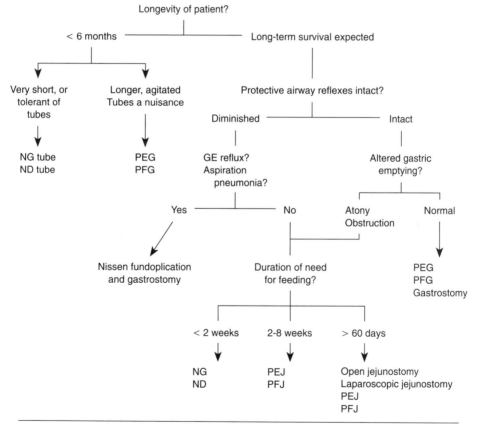

FIGURE 8-1 Selecting an enteral route for a patient who is unable to eat or to eat adequately. *NG:* 8 or 10 Fr. flexible nasogastric tubes; *ND:* 8 or 10 Fr. flexible nasoduodenal tubes, placed with fluoroscopy, pH monitoring, or endoscopic control; *PEG:* percutaneous endoscopic gastrostomy; *PFG:* percutaneous fluoroscopic gastrostomy (requires less sedation than PEG); *PEJ:* percutaneous endoscopic jejunostomy, usually done by passing a fine tube through a gastrostomy tube until its tip ideally lies distal to the ligament of Treitz; *PFJ:* percutaneous fluoroscopic jejunostomy, with or without gastrostomy.

comes a risk to the patient. Rather, access should be made into the small intestine, preferably distal to the ligament of Treitz, which reduces the risk to nil of backwash into the stomach. Nasoduodenal tubes frequently flip back into the stomach and need continuous monitoring and evaluation for proper positioning. Percutaneous endoscopic gastrojejunostomy is a safe and effective way of delivering nutrients with minimal risks. A fine-bore tube is passed through a gastrostomy tube lumen, through the pylorus and duodenum into the jejunum. Placement can also be controlled by fluoroscopy. Laparoscopic techniques are being developed to place jejunal tubes. In patients undergoing major operations on the upper gastrointestinal tract, or following significant multisystem trauma with laparotomy, or in the face of severe head injury, tube jejunostomy should be considered at the time of the original operation or early in the course of treatment. Jejunal feedings can be safely continued even during other operative procedures or diagnostic tests.

PITFALLS AND COMMON MYTHS

- Using estimates instead of measurements of nitrogen and energy needs. Reliance on generic, population-based estimates, especially of nitrogen (protein) requirements, can also lead to seriously deficient nutritional support.
- Failure to reassess protein and energy needs during a course of nutritional support. As a patient improves or incurs complications during a course of therapy, his nutritional needs will change. Failure to measure and modify the nutritional prescription will lead to overfeeding or underfeeding.
- Automatic resort to central parenteral nutrition. Although it often seems easier, CPN is extremely costly compared with enteral feeding. Increasingly, evidence suggests the enteral route improves nutritional and metabolic status with lower morbidity.

BIBLIOGRAPHY

Bursztein S, Elwyn DH, Askanazi J, Kinney JM (eds). Energy Metabolism, Indirect Calorimetry, and Nutrition. Baltimore, Williams & Wilkins, 1989.

Jenkins GM, Baumer T, et al. Enteral feeding during operative procedures. JPEN 15(suppl):225, 1991.

Kinney JM, Jeejeebhoy KN, Hill GL, Owen OE (eds). Nutrition and Metabolism in Patient Care. Philadelphia, WB Saunders, 1988.

McDonald WS, Sharp CW, Deitch EA. Immediate enteral feeding in burn patients is safe and effective. Ann Surg 213:177-183, 1991.

Mullen JL, Gertner MH, Buzby GP, et al. Implications of malnutrition in the surgical patient. Arch Surg 114:121-125, 1979.

Romean JL, Rolandell RH, Wilmore DW. Nutritional support. In American College of Surgeons Care of the Surgical Patient. Vol 1, Critical Care. New York, Scientific American Medicine, 1988.

Scheppach W, Burghardt W, Bartram P, Kasper H. Addition of dietary fiber to liquid formula diets: The pros and cons. JPEN 14:204-209, 1990.

Sitzmann JV. Nutritional support of the dysphagic patient: Methods, risks and complications of therapy. JPEN 14:60-63, 1990.

CHAPTER REVIEW
Questions

1. Name four ways of assessing nutritional status.
2. Compute the energy needs of a 25-year-old male weighing 75 kg, standing 180 cm in height, who has pneumonia following a motor vehicle crash in which two long-bone fractures occurred.
3. Match the patient to the preferred route of nutritional support listed below.
    a. 70-year-old woman recovering from a stroke, who is unable to eat and recently had aspiration pneumonia
    b. 22-year-old man undergoing laparotomy for gunshot wound to stomach, duodenum, and pancreas
    c. 38-year-old woman with exacerbated Crohn's disease and an enterocolocutaneous fistula
    d. 65-year-old man with a large floor-of-the-mouth cancer requiring radiation therapy before resection
    (1) nasogastric feeding tube
    (2) percutaneous endoscopic gastrostomy
    (3) percutaneous endoscopic jejunostomy
    (4) percutaneous fluoroscopic gastrostomy
    (5) operative tube jejunostomy
    (6) central parenteral nutrition

True or false:

4. A 24-hour urine urea nitrogen collection done in the first 24 hours after injury is the only guide needed to determine protein requirements thereafter.
5. A patient with only partial small bowel obstruction, not complete obstruction, is at no risk for malnutrition.
6. Vitamins and trace elements are essential components of a nutritional support prescription.
7. All amino acids have equal nutritional efficacy.
8. Lipid emulsions can be used to supply up to 40% of energy needs.

Answers

1. History-taking, physical examination, measuring serum proteins (albumin, prealbumin, transferrin, retinol-binding protein), anthropometric measurements (height-weight index, arm muscle circumference, triceps skinfold thickness), immune tests (absolute lymphocyte count, delayed hypersensitivity skin tests), timed urine collection for excretion of urea nitrogen
2. $66.47 + 13.5\ (75) + 5\ (180) - 6.76\ (25) = 1828.5$ kCal/day
   $1828.5 \times (1.5\ to\ 1.8) = 2743\ to\ 3291$ kCal/day
   (1.5 to 1.8 is the range of activity factor multipliers applicable to such a patient; selection is based on bedside assessment.)
3. a (3); b (5); c (6); d (2) or (4)
4. F
5. F
6. T
7. F
8. T

9 Respiratory Function and Support

LEWIS M. FLINT, Jr.

KEY FEATURES

After reading this chapter you will understand:
- Some fundamentals of respiratory physiology.
- How to assess abnormalities in pulmonary function.
- Which intraoperative decisions affect postoperative respiratory function.
- Management of postoperative pulmonary complications.

Normal oxygen transport is critically important to the recovery of patients who undergo major operations. After abdominal and thoracic surgical procedures in particular, lung function is frequently distorted, and disorders of oxygenation are ever-present threats to the postoperative patient. The introduction of continuous pulse oximetry monitoring has disclosed significant episodes of hypoxemia during emergence from anesthesia, during transport from the operating room to the postanesthetic recovery area, and in the postoperative recovery period. The frequency of these abnormalities is directly proportional to the seriousness of the patient's illness, and they occur more often after upper abdominal and thoracic surgical procedures.

An understanding of basic respiratory physiology and the most common disorders observed preoperatively and postoperatively allows pre-diction of some complications and rapid, effective treatment of most others.

RELATIONSHIP OF OXYGEN DELIVERY AND CONSUMPTION AND RESPIRATION

Normal function, reaction to stress, and repair depend on cellular metabolic processes that require oxygen and produce carbon dioxide as a by-product. On the average, an individual at rest will use 4 ml of oxygen/kg body weight/min and produce 3.2 ml of carbon dioxide per minute. *The process of acquisition, transport, and utilization of oxygen is called respiration.* The ratio of carbon dioxide production (Vco_2) to oxygen consumption (Vo_2) is the *respiratory quotient,* or RQ. Each cell obtains oxygen by diffusion from the surrounding extracellular fluid, which is replenished by oxygen carried in capillary blood. Carbon dioxide diffuses from the cell and is transported centrally by the venules and veins. The main contribution of the lung to respiration is the exposure of venous blood to atmospheric gases, allowing the uptake of oxygen and the discharge of carbon dioxide. *The gas transfer that occurs in the lung is only one component of the transport mechanism for respiratory gases, which also requires an intact cardiovascular system and normal hemoglobin levels and function.* Cellular use depends on the functional integrity of subcellular biochemical systems. These components and their interrelationship are shown in Fig. 9-1.

Oxygen transport requires integration of several physiologic functions, including the cardiovascular system, the oxygen-carrying capacity of the blood, the lung, and the various cellular subsystems. Both oxygen delivery (DO_2) and VO_2 can be calculated from clinical measurements that can be obtained at the patient's bedside. Arterial catheterization is a routine bedside procedure that permits measurement of arterial oxygen tension (PaO_2) and the hemoglobin level and calculation of arterial oxygen saturation (SaO_2) and content (CaO_2). Mixed venous oxygen tension (PvO_2), saturation (SvO_2), and content (CvO_2) can be determined from individual blood samples drawn from a catheter placed in the pulmonary artery or by using a pulmonary artery catheter with a continuous measuring oxygen

electrode installed. Oxygen delivery and consumption related to body surface area (BSA) can then be calculated according to the following equations:

$$DO_2 = [CaO_2 \text{ (ml/dl)} \times \text{Cardiac output (L/min)}]/BSA$$
$$VO_2 = [DO_2 - (CvO_2 \times \text{Cardiac output})]/BSA$$

The normal relationship between oxygen delivery and consumption and one typical postoperative change in this relationship are depicted in Fig. 9-2. At the breakpoint of the curve to the left of the graph, oxygen consumption becomes dependent on flow (delivery). On the left side of the curve this occurs at an oxygen delivery of approximately 330 cc/min/m². Such a situation arises in the patient who is subject to hypovolemic shock. In critically ill postoperative patients, particularly those with adult respiratory distress syndrome (ARDS; see below), the relationship changes on the right side of the graph, with flow dependency at very high oxygen deliveries. This change occurs because of increased demand at the cellular level in the presence of pathologic redistribution of blood flow away from splanchnic organs and cellular derangements in oxygen use. Accumulation of lactic acid (as lactate) in the blood is evidence of tissue ischemia and increased cellular anaerobic metabolism. It may occur during low oxygen delivery (hypovolemic shock) or high oxygen delivery (ARDS) and is depicted diagrammatically in Fig. 9-3.

In the critically ill patient oxygen delivery is manipulated by first altering flow (cardiac out-

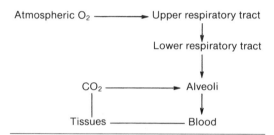

FIGURE 9-1   Graphic depiction of the relationship between oxygen delivery and oxygen consumption. (From Vincent J. Crit Care Med 18:S71, 1990.)

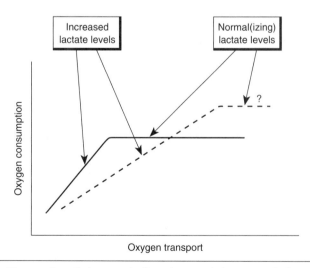

FIGURE 9-2   Changes in cellular metabolism that result in accumulation of lactate in the peripheral blood. (From Carey L. Curr Probl Surg 11, 1971.)

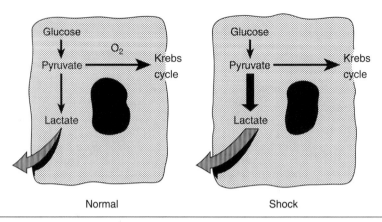

Normal   Shock

FIGURE 9-3   Gas exchange.

TABLE 9-1   Dependence of Oxygen Delivery
on Hemoglobin Concentration

	Oxygen Delivery of 830 ml/min	Oxygen Delivery of 645 ml/min
Hemoglobin	13 g/dl	10 g/dl
Pao_2	100 mm Hg	100 mm Hg
Oxygen saturation	90%	90%
Cardiac output	5 L/min	5 L/min

TABLE 9-2   Effect on Oxygen Delivery of
Simultaneously Altering Cardiac Output and
Hemoglobin Concentration

	Oxygen Delivery of 968 ml/min	Oxygen Delivery of 919 ml/min
Hemoglobin	10 g/dl	12 g/dl
Pao_2	100 mm Hg	100 mm Hg
Oxygen saturation	90%	90%
Cardiac output	7.5 L/min	6 L/min

put) and then oxygen-carrying capacity (hemoglobin and oxygen tension). Tables 9-1 and 9-2 illustrate the effects on Do_2 of altering these factors alone and together. Normal Vo_2 is usually obtained at Do_2 levels of 400 ml/min/m², with additional oxygen made available to tissues by increasing tissue oxygen extraction.

Carriage of oxygen and carbon dioxide occurs by the chemical combination of these gases with hemoglobin and plasma water in addition to physically dissolved gas. These reactions contribute to the buffering capacity of the blood. Knowledge of the means of oxygen and carbon dioxide carriage allows the determination of blood-gas content from easily measured blood-gas partial pressures and hemoglobin levels.

WHAT IS VENTILATION?

Breathing provides for cyclic renewal of respiratory gases within the lung, supplying fresh oxygen to it and carrying carbon dioxide to the exterior; this process is termed ventilation. During ventilation atmospheric gas is introduced into the upper airways (nose, mouth, pharynx, larynx, and trachea) and then into a system of branching conduits (bronchi, segmental bronchi, bronchioles, and terminal bronchioles). During this passage the gas is filtered, warmed, saturated with water vapor, and mixed with gas remaining in the airways from the previous breath. The conducting airways are lined by a mucous blanket, which is constantly swept upward toward the larynx by the cilia of the bronchial cells. Conscious clearing of excessive mucus is accomplished by coughing. No gas transfer occurs within the conducting airways; thus the volume of gas filling this space is called *anatomic dead space.* Because of mixing and the addition of water vapor, the gas arriving at the gas-exchange surfaces (alveoli) has a composition somewhat different from that of atmospheric gas.

Ventilation is under central nervous system control. Changes in ventilation are mediated through changes in the rate of breathing and the depth (volume) of each breath. The volume of a normal breath is called *tidal volume.* The addition of inspiratory reserve volume to the normal tidal volume inflates the lung to total lung capac-

TABLE 9-3   Terms Used in Spirometric Measurements

Term	Symbol	Description
Vital capacity	VC	Maximal volume exhaled after deepest inspiration (includes V_T, IRV, and ERV)
Tidal volume	V_T	Volume inhaled or exhaled during steady-state respiration
Inspiratory reserve volume	IRV	Maximal gas that can be inhaled after a quiet inspiration
Expiratory reserve volume	ERV	Maximal gas that can be exhaled after a quiet exhalation
Residual volume	RV	Volume remaining in lungs after full expiration
Inspiratory vital capacity	IVC	Maximal volume inhaled after full expansion
Forced expiratory volume per time interval in seconds	FEV	Volume exhaled in a given time period during a complete forced expiration (FVC)
Maximal expiratory flow rate	MEFR	Volume exhaled per second, measured between the 200 ml and 1200 ml volumes of the forced expiratory spirogram
Maximal midexpiratory flow	MMF	Volume of air per second exhaled during the middle half of expired volume of forced expiratory spirogram
Maximal voluntary ventilation	MVV	Maximal breathing capacity (in L/min) the individual can breathe with maximal voluntary effort (actual measurement for 12 sec only)

ity. Forcible expulsion of as much of the gas filling the total lung capacity as possible yields a volume called the *vital capacity.* Vital capacity is easily measured at the bedside by use of hand-held respirometers. This volume indirectly reflects pulmonary reserve and may be reduced by as much as 60% after an upper abdominal operation that is done with the patient under general anesthesia. The terminology applied to various lung volumes and capacities appears in Table 9-3.

Inflation of the lung occurs as a result of the work done by the diaphragm and chest wall musculature in producing a subatmospheric pressure at the mouth, causing inward gas flow. This work normally uses very little energy, requiring slightly more than 1% of the resting V_{O_2}. However, disease states can cause marked alteration in the work of breathing. For example, systemic infection and shock can result in markedly increased diaphragmatic blood flow and increased oxygen demand by the diaphragm. For this reason, most patients with severe infections and shock are treated with controlled ventilation using adjuvant ventilators.

The volume of gas inhaled is limited by three components: the impediments to diaphragmatic and chest wall motion, the resistance of airways, and the elastic recoil of the lung. The net effect of

---

FACTORS INFLUENCING EFFECTIVE COMPLIANCE

Intrapulmonary Factors

Edema
Pneumonia
Infiltrative malignancy
Fibrosis

Extrapulmonary Factors

Abdominal distention
Space-occupying process: pneumothorax; hemothorax
Chest-wall restriction

---

these limiting factors can be quantitated as the effective compliance of the lung-thorax system. Effective compliance is expressed as the volume of gas drawn into the lung per unit of subatmospheric pressure generated at the entrance to the airway (ml gas/cm H_2O). Reduction of effective compliance may occur secondary to numerous factors intrinsic or extrinsic to the lung-thorax system. Factors influencing effective compliance are listed in the box above.

Deflation of the lung is a passive phenomenon that normally occurs against a very low resistance. Lung emptying proceeds in a "waterfall" fashion from alveoli to conducting airways along positive pressure gradients generated by the elastic recoil of the lung. Forceful exhaustion during coughing brings into play the diaphragm and abdominal-wall and chest-wall musculature. Alveolar volume decreases rapidly during deflation until the outward forces of the chest wall are equal and opposite in direction to the elastic recoil forces of the lung. Surface-active material (surfactant) lining the bubblelike alveoli prevents alveolar collapse at low alveolar volume and aids in maintaining open airways. Disease states such as neonatal respiratory distress syndrome (hyaline membrane disease) and ARDS can damage surfactant and lead to persistent atelectasis of alveoli. Therefore at the end of deflation a certain volume of gas (functional residual capacity [FRC]) remains in the lung. Forced deflation of the lung by conscious effort expels some, but not all, of this gas (expiratory reserve volume [ERV]). The volume that cannot be expelled is the residual volume (Fig. 9-4).

Disease states that alter deflation of the lung influence pulmonary function by causing early closure of small airways. The inefficiency of lung emptying thus produced manifests as a reduction in the velocity of gases expelled from the airways.

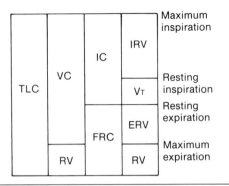

FIGURE 9-4   Lung volumes and capacities. *TLC* = total lung capacity; *IC* = inspiratory capacity.

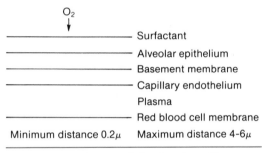

FIGURE 9-5   Diagram of the alveolocapillary membrane.

HOW DOES GAS EXCHANGE OCCUR IN THE LUNG?

Gas exchange takes place in the alveolar ducts and sacs. These chambers are separated by septa containing the capillary latticework. This arrangement vastly increases the surface area available for gas exchange. The components of the membrane separating gas and blood are depicted in Fig. 9-5. Exchange of oxygen and carbon dioxide in the alveoli cannot be quantitated by direct measurement, since pulmonary capillary blood and alveolar gas cannot be accurately sampled. Information gained from sampling of blood entering (venous) and leaving (arterial) the lung and analysis of inhaled and exhaled gas allow inference of the efficiency of gas exchange.

A brief consideration of concepts that describe that behavior of gases and gaseous mixtures in aqueous solution is necessary for an understanding of alveolar function. Dalton's law (gases present in a mixture exert a partial pressure related to their fractional concentrations) is applicable to atmospheric gases; that is, the sum of all partial pressures must equal atmospheric pressure (P_B). Gases outside the airway system are quantitated according to their fractional concentrations. Thus inhaled gas concentrations are expressed as F_I, with a further subscript denoting the type of gas, followed by a decimal for the fractional concentration (F_{IO_2}, F_{IN_2}), e.g., atmospheric gas at sea level has an F_{IO_2} of 0.21 ml/mm Hg and a partial pressure (P_{O_2}) of 159 mm Hg. The partial pressure of any gas is derived by multiplying P_B by the fractional concentrations of the gas.

The sum of gas partial pressures in the alveoli must equal P_B. Alveolar gas differs from inhaled gas in that it is saturated with water vapor and is in equilibrium with pulmonary capillary carbon dioxide. The addition of these two gases reduces the partial pressure of the other gases correspondingly. The composition of "average" alveolar gas is calculated in terms of alveolar partial pressures (P_A), using the alveolar air equation:

$$P_B = P_{AO_2} + P_{ACO_2} + P_{AH_2O} + P_{AN_2}$$

Each term in the equation can be derived or directly measured. It was noted previously that

TABLE 9-4   Partial Pressure of Alveolar Gases (Breathing Air)

Gas	Partial Pressure (mm Hg)
Oxygen	100-110
Nitrogen	600-670
Carbon dioxide	33-43
Water vapor	47

alveolar carbon dioxide is in equilibrium with capillary carbon dioxide. Blood-gas partial pressures can be easily measured because arterial P_{CO_2} (Pa_{CO_2}) represents the carbon dioxide tension after equilibration with alveolar gas, PA_{CO_2}. The known contribution of water vapor at body temperature is 47 mm Hg. The equation then may be rearranged:

$$P_B - PA_{CO_2} - PA_{H_2O_2} + PA_{N_2}$$

Since the partial pressures of oxygen and nitrogen are related to their fractional concentrations, the following alveolar air equation may be written for atmospheric gas at sea level when Pa_{CO_2} of 40 mm Hg has been measured:

$$760 - 40 - 47 = PA_{O_2} + PA_{N_2}$$

OR

$$673 = PA_{N_2} = 673 \times 0.79$$

THEN

$$PA_{N_2} = 673 \times 0.79$$

AND

$$PA_{O_2} = 673 \times 0.21$$

Typical alveolar-gas partial pressures are listed in Table 9-4. Pa_{O_2} is highly variable in normal patients and tends to decrease with age. Sixty-year-old patients, for example, frequently have Pa_{O_2} levels in the 60 mm Hg range. The presently available evidence indicates that gases diffuse from alveoli and the blood along pressure gradients that come rapidly to equilibrium.

WHAT ARE THE BASICS OF PULMONARY PERFUSION?

Examination of the typical PA_{O_2} and Pa_{O_2} values reveals that complete equilibrium between alveolar gas and capillary blood is not reflected by mixed arterial P_{O_2}. This discrepancy, called the *alveolar-arterial gradient for oxygen*

$(A - aD_{O_2})$, usually has a value of 30 to 40 mm Hg. The normally occurring $A - aD_{O_2}$ results from the contribution of blood that has not participated fully in gas exchange because of passage by an alveolus that is underventilated with respect to blood flow or because of passage through minute, normally occurring venoarterial shunts. *The effects of gravity on the upright lung cause relative underventilation and overperfusion of alveoli in the lower portion of the lung. Similarly, analysis of exhaled air reveals a lower P_{CO_2} (PE_{CO_2}) than would be expected if equilibrium were reached between arterial carbon dioxide and all gas residing in the lung and airway system.* The arterial exhaled air gradient for carbon dioxide is normally 12 mm Hg and is primarily caused by the fact that dead-space gas is not exposed to capillary carbon dioxide and dilutes the carbon dioxide contained in alveolar gas. Since arterial gas tensions are easily measured, most postoperative disorders of ventilation and perfusion are initially considered abnormalities of $A - aD_{O_2}$ or $A - aD_{CO_2}$.

WHAT IS THE RELATIONSHIP BETWEEN VENTILATION AND PERFUSION?

The maintenance of normal oxygenation and carbon dioxide elimination depends on the arrival of gas and blood at the exchange interface, that is, the matching of ventilation ($\dot{V}$) and the blood flow ($\dot{Q}$). Abnormalities of ventilation-perfusion matching manifest as abnormally large values for the gradients described previously. The contribution to the $A - aD_{O_2}$ of ventilation-perfusion mismatching is eliminated by raising the F_{IO_2} to 1 mm Hg. This maneuver raises the PA_{O_2} in all ventilated, perfused alveoli to a level sufficient for eradicating the effects of mismatching. Any resulting $A - aD_{O_2}$ is due to the contribution of blood that has not participated in gas exchange (venous admixture effect). Venous admixture can result from passage through an anatomic venoarterial shunt such as those found in patients with congenital cardiac and pulmonary anomalies. In patients with acute lung disease, however, most venous admixture results from continued perfusion of nonventilated (e.g., collapsed or atelectatic) alveoli.

Abnormalities of the arterial–exhaled air carbon dioxide gradient (dead-space effect) are caused by reductions of blood flow with respect to ventilation (e.g., after hemorrhage), which increase the volume of gas not exposed to blood carbon dioxide. This additional dead space is called *alveolar dead space.*

HOW DOES THE LUNG PARTICIPATE IN ACID-BASE BALANCE?

Carbon dioxide elimination plays a primary role in the regulation of the body acid-base status because of its reaction with plasma water:

$$CO_2 + H_2O \leftrightarrow H_2CO_3 \leftrightarrow H^+ + HCO_3^-$$

Total ventilation determines the input of carbon dioxide into this reaction. Depressed ventilation results in increased P_{ACO_2} and P_{aCO_2}, driving the reaction to the right and increasing hydrogen ion concentration. The result is lowered pH, or acidosis. The acidosis resulting from decreased ventilation is called respiratory acidosis. Increased ventilation removes carbon dioxide and decreases the hydrogen ions. The result is an elevated pH. This is respiratory alkalosis.

The important aspects of respiratory function are summarized by noting the interdependency of ventilation, blood flow, and blood function. Direct measurements of blood-gas tensions and inhaled and exhaled gas concentrations are possible and allow derivation of alveolar-gas composition. The difference between measured arterial and derived alveolar oxygen tensions reveals the effect of shunt and ventilation-perfusion mismatching. The arterial–exhaled gas gradient for carbon dioxide indicates the dead-space effect. These gradients are basic to an understanding of respiratory dysfunction in surgical patients. The lung also influences hydrogen ion concentration by altering carbon dioxide in a major buffering system. Respiratory acidosis and alkalosis can be diagnosed by measuring the arterial pH and P_{aCO_2}.

WHAT IS THE CLINICAL APPROACH TO PULMONARY FUNCTION ASSESSMENT?

A complete preoperative respiratory evaluation is required whenever major surgery is contemplated. In general, this evaluation entails a complete history and physical examination augmented by appropriate roentgenographic and laboratory studies.

Certain historical and physical findings occur commonly in patients with pulmonary diseases (e.g., the history of wheezing in asthmatic pa-

tients, the cough and sputum production of chronic bronchitis, and the hemoptysis that often precedes other clinical manifestations of pulmonary neoplasms). Exposure to cigarette smoke and industrial toxins should be quantitated both as to daily dosage and duration (e.g., two packs per day for 20 years). Physical examination may reveal an increased anteroposterior chest diameter, indicating obstructive lung disease. In a patient with acute pneumonia rapid respirations and chest pain are common.

After the initial history and physical examination are obtained, roentgenographic evaluation of the chest is performed. Anteroposterior and lateral views are obtained routinely. Evaluation of these films yields valuable information about the type and extent of lung disease.

Although emergency operations may require curtailment of the complete pulmonary evaluation, as much information as possible should be obtained for an adequate evaluation of the influence of pulmonary function abnormalities on surgical risk.

HOW IS THE PREOPERATIVE PULMONARY EVALUATION CONDUCTED?

Preexisting chronic lung diseases frequently occur in surgical patients. They are called *obstructive* or *restrictive*, according to the predominant physiologic defect (this type of classification does not preclude combinations of defects):

Obstructive lung diseases	Restrictive lung diseases
Asthma	Chest wall injury
Emphysema	Neuromuscular disease
Bronchitis	Tumors, infections, acid aspiration, and cardiac failure

The physiologic abnormalities in obstructive disease result from inefficient lung deflation that occurs because of early closure of diseased small airways. *A history of heavy smoking, allergy, or exposure to irritants is frequently discovered. Chronic cough with sputum production is a prominent feature of chronic bronchitis. Examination of the patient reveals the effects of inefficient lung emptying, an increased anteroposterior chest diameter, decreased chest expansion, and prolonged exhalation. Wheezing during early exhalation indicates airway closure. The chest radiograph classically reveals a large intrathoracic gas volume in relation to body size, flattening of the diaphragm, and abnormally large distances between ribs.*

Patients with obstructive lung disease characteristically show increases in resting lung volume (FRC). The retardation of exhalation is evidenced by a reduction in the velocity of the gas expelled by a forced exhalation. In addition, the response to exercise may be altered in patients with significant loss of functioning tissue. At rest, arterial gas tensions may be normal or may show retention of carbon dioxide (increased Pa_{CO_2}), which results from severe disturbances of ventilation-perfusion matching.

Frequently the functional abnormalities of obstructive disease are delineated by simple bedside tests. Obstruction to gas flow is indicated if forced exhalation is prolonged, especially if early wheezing is noted. The inability to extinguish a match at a 6- to 8-inch distance by forced exhalation without pursed lips is evidence for an important reduction in exhalation velocity. Restrictive lung diseases are diagnosed primarily by the physical examination.

Factors extrinsic to the lung that produce restrictive defects increase the work of breathing with normal or reduced lung volume. Hypoventilation with carbon dioxide retention may occur, with severe restriction of diaphragmatic and chest-wall motion (i.e., abdominal distention and massive obesity).

Pulmonary function studies confirm the diagnosis in patients with restrictive defects. Total lung capacity is usually low because of the unusually large amount of energy required to fully expand the chest. VC is thus reduced.

Intrinsic lung diseases such as pneumonia that are caused by bacterial or viral infection can also lead to restrictive defects. Compliance is reduced, and the work of breathing is increased. A rapid, shallow breathing pattern occurs. Low Pa_{CO_2} and inefficient oxygenation are prominent features. Many important postoperative pulmonary complications fall into this category.

Pulmonary function testing and blood-gas evaluation are indicated if any evidence of preexisting lung disease is discovered. In addition, the evaluation of blood-gas tensions may be of value preoperatively in patients without lung disease in whom an extensive operation is planned. Baseline values thus obtained may be important in the management of postoperative pulmonary complications.

Formal evaluation in the pulmonary function laboratory may be necessary for patients who demonstrate significant chronic lung disease.

Pulmonary function testing may also be valuable in candidates for major thoracic, cardiac, or abdominal surgery. In general, pulmonary function testing requires special equipment and trained technical personnel. Information may be gained that will quantitate the patient's ability to ventilate adequately (VC plus maximal voluntary ventilation), the level of maximal ventilation (maximal voluntary ventilation), lung deflation (maximal midexpiratory flow rate), and the efficiency of gas exchange (measurement of diffusion capacity and shunting).

Additional information is obtained using cardiac chamber pressures and cardiac function data (cardiac output) recorded after bedside catheterization of the right side of the heart. The Swan-Ganz flow-guided balloon catheter allows pressure measurements in each of the right heart chambers. Left ventricular function is assessed by recording changes in pulmonary capillary wedge pressure after various maneuvers such as volume loading (saline solution or blood infusion).

The additional risk factors imposed by pulmonary disease are modified by the type of operation planned. Emergency surgery is accompanied by increased risk because of the frequent inability to evaluate pulmonary function thoroughly and to correct preexisting defects. In addition, the process that makes emergency surgery necessary may be accompanied by acute pulmonary disease (e.g., the pneumonia that complicates splenic rupture).

When elective or emergency operations require direct entry into the thoracic cavity and removal of functioning lung tissue, additional risk is imposed. In many instances preoperative pulmonary function studies and blood-gas examination aid in determining the amount of lung tissue that can be removed safely.

Many postoperative respiratory complications can be prevented by vigorous preoperative therapy. In patients in whom preexisting lung disease is discovered, an aggressive program directed toward improvement of pulmonary function should be pursued. Irritants such as cigarettes are removed and any respiratory infection quantitated and treated. Drug therapy may include use of bronchodilators and antibiotics. Physical therapy such as use of a deep-breathing apparatus may speed convalescence. The intermittent positive-pressure breathing device is a useful means of delivering bronchodilators and mucolytics to the patient with chronic pulmonary disease, particularly if that patient has used the device previously. For the majority of patients, however, the intermittent positive-pressure breathing treatment as it is applied in most hospitals is of little use in preventing postoperative pulmonary complications. Preoperative training in the use of the incentive spirometer provides a superior method for obtaining complete lung expansion in the patient without a prior history of pulmonary disease. This device uses the patient's ability to generate negative intrathoracic pressure to provide for total alveolar inflation. Because the device induces relaxation of the abdominal muscles, incisional pain is minimized. Intraoperatively, the functional status of the pulmonary system is monitored by following hemodynamic variables (blood pressure and heart rate) and arterial blood-gas tensions. Tidal volume measurements may reflect the adequacy of ventilation.

WHAT INTRAOPERATIVE FACTORS INFLUENCE PULMONARY FUNCTION?

The majority of postoperative pulmonary disorders occur in patients with preexisting lung disease. In addition, a number of previously healthy individuals who sustain injury or who undergo complex elective surgery develop pulmonary complications. The choice of anesthetic management, operative approach, and postoperative therapy influences postoperative pulmonary function.

The anesthetic management of a patient with lung disease is directed toward optimal support of functioning lung tissue. General anesthesia entails a period of unconsciousness when protective reflexes are ablated. In patients with severe chronic lung disease its use may predispose them to loss of functioning lung units resulting from alveolar collapse or aspiration of gastric contents. In such patients the use of regional anesthesia such as an epidural or spinal block may be preferred; however, spinal anesthesia includes muscle paralysis below the level of anesthesia. High spinal block may thus decrease ventilation because of associated muscle weakness. In general, the operation performed rather than the anesthetic technique used determines postoperative pulmonary function.

The choice of the operative incision directly affects pulmonary function. Thoracic incisions disrupt the functional integrity of the chest wall. Associated pain leads to lowered tidal volume and alveolar collapse. Thus the sequence of events following chest incision is qualitatively similar to traumatic chest injury.

The atelectasis and pneumonia that may complicate direct chest injury and intra-abdominal inflammation are directly related to the extent of damage to the chest wall and the underlying lung. Alterations in pulmonary function after chest injury result from derangements of the mechanical function of the chest. The introduction of air (pneumothorax) or blood (hemothorax) into the pleural space reduces and maldistributes the gas entering the lung with each breath. Hypoxemia (low Pa_{O_2}) results. If uncontrolled, this process may lead to massive restriction of ventilation and hypercarbia (increased Pa_{CO_2}). Direct damage to the lung produces atelectasis and hemorrhage into the lung tissue, resulting in failure of gas exchange units and ventilation-perfusion mismatching. If a sufficient amount of lung tissue is damaged, hypoxemia results.

The placement of abdominal incisions in proximity to the thoracic cage (e.g., subcostal or upper midline) produces similar functional defects. When wound complications occur (e.g., infection and/or breakdown), pulmonary dysfunction is augmented.

WHAT ARE COMMON POSTOPERATIVE PULMONARY COMPLICATIONS?

Postoperatively, repeated physical examinations and chest radiographs are extremely valuable. However, external evidence of pulmonary function problems may be subtle in postoperative patients. Incisional pain, apprehension, or drug effects predispose to an abnormal breathing pattern. A high index of suspicion and early aggressive efforts to achieve a diagnosis are thus important considerations. Continuous pulse oximetry supplemented by periodic measurements of arterial blood-gas tensions must be used in patients at risk for pulmonary complications. Direct measurement of tidal volume and blood-gas tensions leads to early diagnosis of respiratory difficulty.

Efforts directed toward early diagnosis of pulmonary complications may be therapeutic in themselves. The patient who is subjected to daily chest examinations by his or her physician is forced to move in bed, sit up, take deep breaths, and perform other maneuvers that lead to full expansion of the lungs, coughing, and clearance of retained secretions. The following variables are those usually monitored in seriously ill post-operative patients:

- Vital signs
- Cardiac monitor
- Central venous pressure
- Urinary output
- Daily weight
- Arterial cannula: blood gases and pressure
- Sequential pulmonary functions

In postoperative patients severe respiratory failure results from hypoventilation (muscle paralysis, airway obstruction) or impaired oxygenation as a result of various intrapulmonary factors. Initial signs of respiratory failure include increased respiratory rate, use of accessory muscles of respiration (suprasternal or intercostal retraction, flared nares), and stridor or noisy inspiration caused by laryngeal obstruction. During the immediate postanesthetic recovery period such signs may be masked by anesthetic effects, making direct measurement of arterial gas tensions and tidal volume mandatory during postanesthesia recovery.

When persistent respiratory failure is diagnosed, artificial ventilation, using a volume ventilator, is indicated. This device allows delivery of preset tidal volumes and fine adjustments of the oxygen content of inspired air. Access to the airway in the patient requiring ventilation is obtained by inserting plastic, cuffed endotracheal tubes. They can be passed into the trachea via the nasal or oral route. The gas delivery system is closed by inflating a cuff attached to the tube. The cuff is positioned in the trachea below the larynx and above the carina. Pressures within the cuff should be maintained below 22 mm Hg to ensure that tracheal necrosis, which leads to tracheoesophageal fistula, innominate artery erosion, or tracheal stenosis, is avoided.

Artificial ventilation is required whenever spontaneous ventilation is inadequate. Table 9-5 lists the indications for oxygen therapy and for instituting artificial ventilation in surgical patients.

Mechanical ventilation should be discontinued as soon as feasible. The withdrawal of artificial ventilation, or "weaning," is usually begun in a gradual manner as soon as the criteria for instituting ventilatory support are no longer met. Bedside measurements of VC and negative inspiratory force (NIF) allow identification of patients suitable for weaning. Inspiratory pressure and FIO_2 should be reduced to minimal levels consistent with normal oxygenation. Nutrition and muscular strength are preserved insofar as possible, and when VC exceeds 30 ml/kg and NIF exceeds -20 cm H_2O, a trial cessation of artificial ventilation is warranted.

In selected patients innovations such as positive end-expiratory pressure (PEEP), continuous positive airway pressure (CPAP), pressure support ventilation, and intermittent mandatory ventilation (IMV) may be indicated to optimize therapy or hasten weaning. Table 9-6 details the usual forms of ventilator therapy used in surgical patients.

Atelectasis is the most common pulmonary complication encountered in the early postoperative course. This condition, which results from alveolar collapse in some areas, is usually caused by inefficient ventilation and clearing of secretions during anesthesia. The most graphic example of severe postoperative atelectasis is encountered in the patient who is placed in the lateral position for thoracotomy. The lung, which is dependent during the procedure, may be poorly ventilated. Because of its dependent position, the "down" lung is difficult to suction efficiently; thus pooling of airway secretions may

TABLE 9-5 Indications for Specific Respiratory Support

Area	Measurements	Normal Range	Physiotherapy and Oxygen	Intubation and Ventilator
Mechanics	Respiratory (per min)	12-25	25-35	>35
	Vital capacity (ml/kg)	70-30	20-15	<15
Oxygenation	$A-aDO_2$ (mm Hg)	50-200	200-350	>350
	PCO_2 (mm Hg)	100-75 (air)	200-70 (O_2)	<70 (O_2)
Ventilation	PCO_2 (mm Hg)	35-45	45-60	>60

TABLE 9-6 Forms of Ventilator Therapy

Modality	Abbreviation	Indication
Assisted ventilation	—	Ineffective ventilatory effort
Controlled ventilation	—	Inefficient ventilation, delirium, coma, etc.
Positive end-expiratory pressure	PEEP	Persistent hypoxia; $FIO_2 > 0.5$
Continuous positive airway pressure	CPAP	End-expiratory pressure without artificial ventilation; to improve weaning
Intermittent mandatory ventilation	IMV	When spontaneous ventilation is desired with periodic ventilator breaths; usually during weaning
Pressure support ventilation	—	When support of the patient's spontaneous ventilation effort by clinician-selected levels of airway pressure is desired

occur. Tachypnea and respiratory distress occur soon after thoracotomy, with a radiographic picture of the consolidation of the down lung providing confirmation of the diagnosis. Bronchoscopic aspiration and aggressive efforts to clear secretions are necessary in such patients. Atelectasis is aggravated by the depression of cough and deep breathing secondary to incisional pain.

The main clinical feature of early postoperative atelectasis is fever. Physical examination may reveal areas of poor ventilation in the lung and "crackling" sounds during breathing. The chest radiographs and blood-gas examination results may be normal. Therapy for atelectasis is directed toward improvement of cough, encouragement of deep breathing, and early ambulation. In this setting nasotracheal suction is the therapeutic mainstay for improvement of cough and removal of retained secretions. However, in particularly severe cases bronchoscopy may be required to reexpand the lung totally. Preoperative preparation of the patient for such eventualities is important in preventing severe atelectasis. In such settings preoperative training with the incentive spirometer has its greatest value. *The most important complication of atelectasis is pneumonia, which results from microbial invasion of atelectatic alveoli. Fever, leukocytosis, increased sputum production, and the appearance of infiltrates on chest x-ray film confirm the diagnosis.*

Pulmonary embolization is a rare but important postoperative complication. Changes in coagulation dynamics accompany most major operations, and intravenous clotting can occur, especially in lower extremity veins. Portions of the clot may dislodge and migrate in the venous circulation, becoming entrapped in the pulmonary vascular bed. If these entrapped emboli cause pulmonary infarction, chest pain, dyspnea, shock, and occasionally sudden death may result. Blood-gas analysis reveals low PaO_2. Definitive diagnosis is often difficult, especially if emboli are small and multiple. Radiologic aids to diagnosis such as chest radiography, isotope scanning, and angiography are valuable.

Prevention of stagnation of blood in lower extremity veins by means of early ambulation may aid in preventing thrombosis. Once embolization has occurred, judicious use of drugs that alter clotting is indicated. In some patients blockage of further emboli using intracaval filter devices may be indicated.

WHAT IS ADULT RESPIRATORY DISTRESS SYNDROME?

ARDS is a condition characterized by progressive failure of oxygenation caused by edema of pulmonary tissues and exudation of fluid into the alveolar chambers. This entity has recently received renewed interest. It represents, in all likelihood, the uniform response of the lung to a variety of insults, some of which are listed in the box on p. 159.

The clinical picture of ARDS is characterized by arterial hypoxemia, loss of pulmonary compliance, and a roentgenographic picture of bilateral bronchopneumonia. Patients who have needed massive fluid therapy for resuscitation of hemorrhagic shock may become hypoxemic in

CAUSATIVE FACTORS IN ADULT RESPIRATORY DISTRESS SYNDROME

Microembolization: primary; secondary
Sepsis: extrapulmonary; intrapulmonary
Diffuse intravascular coagulation
Direct pulmonary injury: obvious; occult
Fluid overload
Aspiration of blood, saliva, or gastric
    content

the early postresuscitation period as a result of fluid overload. This form of hypoxemia should not be confused with ARDS, since the process is easily reversed by intermittent positive-pressure breathing and diuresis. No permanent structural damage to the lung occurs.

True ARDS presents as a relentless hypoxemia associated with loss of pulmonary compliance. Ventilator therapy is frequently indicated. The decision to use oxygen therapy or artificial ventilation in patients with ARDS is based on trends of clinical variables associated with the disease process. Mild hypoxemia is treated by oxygen enrichment alone, using humidified oxygen delivery through face masks or nasal prongs. Nasal oxygen catheters should be used with caution, since misplacement of a nasal cannula into the esophagus may result in acute gastric dilation. If hypoxemia progresses, transnasal or transoral intubation of the trachea is necessary, and ventilatory support using a volume ventilator is instituted. A pattern of ventilation is selected to supply the patient with slow, deep inspirations to ensure adequate response to the ventilatory therapy. Improved alveolar inflation and recovery of lost lung compliance lead to correction of the hypoxemia in most cases. However, if initial ventilator therapy fails to evoke an adequate response, alveolar inflation can be improved by raising mean intrapulmonary pressure. An efficient means of doing this is to raise end-expiratory pressure (using PEEP). PEEP is frequently required in the ranges of 5 to 10 cm to clear the progressive atelectasis associated with ARDS. Tracheostomy may be required for long-term ventilatory support.

Although ventilator therapy is the mainstay for support of oxygenation in patients with ARDS, it will usually fail to cure the problem unless an underlying cause for the condition is sought, found, and corrected. The most common obscure cause for ARDS is undetected invasive infection. Such infection may reside in the abdomen after surgery, within the lung itself, or in some other obscure site. Timely excision or drainage of the infection results in correction of the pulmonary problem.

Despite aggressive therapy, the mortality rate from established ARDS is 40% to 60%. Postmortem examinations of lungs in patients who succumb to this process disclose pulmonary edema, congestion, alveolar collapse, and bacterial invasion of lung tissue. The precise mechanism by which remote infection predisposes the lung to this pneumonic process is not clear. There is increasing evidence that remote infection produces aggregation of leukocytes, platelets, and/or other debris that in turn produce microembolic injury to the lung via the pulmonary capillary endothelium. Evidence of adhesion of leukocytes to endothelium with subsequent damage, increased permeability, and edema formation is frequent in patients with ARDS.

Pulmonary infection frequently supervenes in the patient with adult respiratory distress syndrome, requiring postoperative intensive care. Despite this fact, antibiotic therapy should be withheld until culture evidence of infection allows specific antibiotic therapy. When possible, single drugs to which the infecting organisms are sensitive should be used.

PITFALLS AND COMMON MYTHS

- The most common cause of confusion in a postoperative patient is hypoxia.
- Everyone has roughly the same serum sodium level. The Pa_{O_2} is highly variable.

- Individual baseline measurements vary with age.
- Look and listen to the patient before changing the ventilator settings.

Drug	Indications	Complications	Dosage
Aminophylline or theophylline	Bronchodilator for moderate to severe reversible broncho-spasm; increases diaphragmatic con-tractility; may help in weaning a patient from a ventilator	Requires frequent determinations of plasma levels; desired level, 10-20 μg/ml Side effects usually begin at plasma levels >20 μg/ml and include headaches, dizziness, nervousness, nausea, vomiting, epigastric pain, dysrhythmias, and convulsions States that prolong half-life: Drug interactions—macrolide antibiotics, furosemide, cimeti-dine, and beta-adrenergic blocking agents Disease states—alcohol-ism, cigarette use, congestive heart failure, liver dysfunction	Loading dose: 5.8 mg/kg at a rate of 25 mg/min Maintenance dose: 0.4-0.9 mg/kg/hr
Albuterol	Bronchodilator, selective beta-2 agonist; produces minimal dysrhythmias	May produce a slight decrease in blood pressure, with compen-sating tachycardia	1 to 2 inhalations every 4 to 6 hr
Metaproterenol	Bronchodilator with selective beta-2 activity (long-acting, 3-5 hr)	Tachycardia, hypotension; tolerance and refractory to frequent adminis-tration	0.3 ml (10-15 mg) of a 5% solution in 2.5 ml of normal saline solution bid to qid
Atropine	Parasympathetic agent antagonist that causes bronchodilation and a decrease in secretions	Bradycardia, cycloplegia and glaucoma, respira-tory depression, and decreased gastric motility	0.05-0.1 mg/kg of a 1% solution
Acetylcysteine (Mucomyst)	Mucolytic agent useful in treating patients with mucoid plugs and inspissated secretions	Nausea, vomiting, and bronchospasm have been reported	1-10 ml of 20% solution nebulized into a face mask q2h to q6h (should be given with a bronchodilator)
Heparin	Therapy for proven pulmonary embolus	Bleeding, hematoma, anaphylaxis, thrombo-cytopenia	Loading dose: 50-75 units/kg, then 10-20 units/kg qh (adjust based on partial thromboplastin time [PTT])

BIBLIOGRAPHY

Scalea T, Goldstein A, Phillips T, Stillman R. Respiratory problems. In Stillman R (ed). Surgery: Diagnosis and Therapy. Norwalk, Conn, Appleton & Lange, 1989, pp 161-178.

Weissman C. Perioperative respiratory physiology. J Crit Care 6:160-171, 1991.

Vincent J, Van Der Linden P. Septic shock: Particular type of acute circulatory failure. Crit Care Med 18:S70-S74, 1990.

CHAPTER REVIEW
Questions

1. What three clinical bedside tests may be used to diagnose the patient with severe obstructive lung disease?
2. Name four lung function tests that are characteristically abnormal in patients with restrictive pulmonary disease.
3. List four intraoperative factors that may reduce respiratory function postoperatively.
4. How is the diagnosis of postoperative pneumonia made?
5. What are the main pathophysiologic characteristics of ARDS?

Answers

1. a. Limited prolonged forceful expiration, with decreased velocity and possibly a wheeze
   b. Inability to extinguish a match at 6 to 8 inches
   c. Marked reduction in exercise tolerance (inability to climb a flight of stairs because of respiratory failure)
2. a. Total lung capacity
   b. Vital capacity
   c. Compliance
   d. Work of breathing
3. a. Inadequate ventilation (atelectasis)
   b. Aspiration of gastric contents
   c. Choice of incision
   d. Choice of anesthetic agents
4. a. Increased sputum production
   b. Fever
   c. Leukocytosis
   d. New infiltrates on chest x-ray film
5. a. Hypoxemia
   b. Loss of compliance
   c. Fluffy infiltrates on chest x-ray film
   d. Presence of an underlying cause (shock, trauma, infection)

10 Surgical Endocrinology

EDWIN L. KAPLAN

KEY FEATURES

After reading this chapter you will understand:
- The approach to diagnosing thyroid nodules.
- Treatment options for hyperthyroidism.
- Appropriate management of thyroid cancer.
- Diagnosis and treatment of parathyroid, adrenal, and gastrointestinal endocrine abnormalities.
- The important guidelines in treating adrenal masses.
- A basic review of the physiology of the endocrine system, which you should supplement by additional study.

Diseases of the endocrine system are among the most interesting and important seen by both physicians and surgeons. Traditionally the endocrine system has been considered to include the pituitary, thyroid, parathyroid, and adrenal glands and the testes and ovaries. More recently it has been recognized that the gastrointestinal tract also contains large numbers of different amine- and peptide-secreting cells and thus should be considered an endocrine organ as well. This chapter deals with the tumors and diseases of the endocrine system that are commonly treated by surgeons.

THYROID

Diseases of the thyroid present the largest number of problems seen by the endocrine surgeon. They primarily include nodules of the thyroid and the diffuse toxic goiters associated with Graves' disease.

Important Anatomy

The thyroid is composed of two lobes connected by an isthmus that lies on the trachea approximately at the level of the second tracheal ring. The gland is enveloped by the deep cervical fascia.

The arterial supply to each thyroid lobe is twofold (Fig. 10-1). The superior thyroid artery, which is the first branch to arise from the external carotid artery, enters each thyroid lobe at its superior pole. The inferior thyroid artery comes from the thyrocervical trunk, a branch of the subclavian artery. This artery enters the thyroid lobe laterally on each side. Each thyroid lobe is drained by three sets of veins—the superior, middle, and inferior thyroid veins. They drain into the jugular and innominate veins bilaterally.

The two nerves on each side of the lobe should be carefully preserved by the surgeon who is performing a thyroidectomy (Fig. 10-2). Both originate from the vagus nerve. The first and most important is the recurrent laryngeal nerve. On the left side this nerve loops around the aorta and ascends in the tracheoesophageal groove to the larynx. On the right side this nerve loops around the subclavian artery and ascends once more to enter the larynx. Division or excessive trauma to either of these nerves leads to vocal cord paralysis on the affected side since the recurrent nerve innervates most of the intrinsic muscles of the larynx. Bilateral damage leads to bilateral vocal cord paralysis.

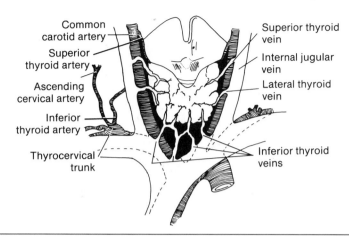

FIGURE 10-1   Surgical anatomy of the thyroid gland. The superior and inferior thyroid arteries and the venous drainage of the thyroid are shown.

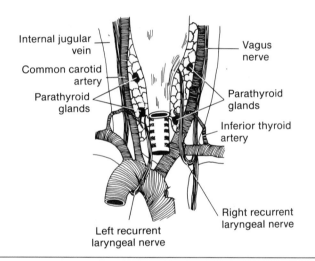

FIGURE 10-2   Anatomy of the thyroid gland, posterior view. Note the relationship of the inferior thyroid arteries, parathyroid glands, and the recurrent laryngeal nerves. The superior laryngeal nerve is not shown in this diagram.

The external branch of the superior laryngeal nerve, another branch of the vagus nerve, runs near the superior pole vessels and can be damaged when they are ligated. Since this branch innervates the cricothyroid muscle, its damage leads to impairment of fine tunings of the voice; thus one's singing voice or voice projection is impaired if these nerves are damaged.

Two parathyroid glands are usually found on the posterior surface of each thyroid lobe. These are small structures, but they are very important in the control of serum calcium homeostasis. It is vital that their integrity and viability be maintained during thyroidectomy or else severe hypocalcemia will result, which can be a life-threatening complication.

Normal Thyroid Physiology

Two types of endocrine cells are present within the thyroid gland: (1) the parafollicular, or C cell, and (2) the follicular cell. C cells are neuroectodermal in origin and secrete calcitonin (thyrocalcitonin) and other substances. As is described later, medullary carcinoma of the thyroid is derived from these C cells. The second cells of the thyroid, the follicular cells, produce the thyroid hormones—thyroxine (T_4) and triiodothyronine

(T_3). The follicular cells have the unique ability to trap and concentrate iodide from the serum (Fig. 10-3). A concentration gradient of iodide of 20 to 1 or more is found in normal individuals, whereas in patients with Graves' disease, a form of thyrotoxicosis, gradients of 500 to 1 have been identified between the cells and the serum. Within the follicular cells, iodide is oxidized to iodine by a peroxidase enzyme and then the iodine is incorporated into the amino acid tyrosine to form either monoiodotyrosine (MIT) or diiodotyrosine (DIT). Coupling then occurs to produce either T_4 or T_3, and these hormones are stored as thyroglobulin within the colloid.

The synthesis and release of thyroid hormone are controlled by a finely tuned hypothalamic-pituitary-thyroid feedback system (Fig. 10-4). When diminished levels of T_4 or T_3 are present in the serum, the hypothalamus secretes thyrotropin-releasing hormone (TRH), which travels to the anterior pituitary by the hypothalamic-pituitary portal circulation. TRH stimulates the release of thyroid-stimulating hormone (TSH) into the systemic circulation, which results in a greater synthesis and release of thyroid hormones. When excessive concentrations of T_3 or T_4 are present in the serum, a negative-feedback system shuts off the secretion of TSH, hence decreasing the rate of synthesis and release of T_3 or T_4 from the thyroid gland. Thus in the healthy individual the secretion of thyroid hormones is controlled within narrow limits. The thyroid hormones affect the body's general metabolic rate and influence a wide variety of enzyme systems.

How Is Thyroid Function Tested?

As demonstrated in Table 10-1 and Fig. 10-4, a number of different tests are available to evaluate

TABLE 10-1 Principal Diagnostic Tests of the Thyroid

	Abbreviation	Normal Range
Direct and Indirect Measures of T_4 and T_3 Supply		
Serum thyroxine	T_4	4.9-12.0 μg/dl
Free thyroxine	FT_4	2.8 $\pm$ 0.5 ng/dl
Resin triiodothyronine uptake	RT_3U	Varies with laboratory 20%-30%
Free thyroxine index	$FTI(T_7)$	Varies with laboratory 6.4-10.5
Serum triiodothyronine	T_3	115-190 ng/dl
Radioactive iodine uptake	RAIU	Varies with laboratory <22%
Serum thyroid-stimulating hormone	TSH	Varies with laboratory 0.4-4 μU/ml
Thyroxine-binding globulin capacity	TBG	12-20 μg T_4/dl $\pm$ 1.8 μg
Measures of Autoimmunity		
Antithyroglobulin antibodies	TGHA	Titer <1/20
Antimicrosomal antibodies	MCHA	Titer <1/20
Long-acting thyroid stimulator	LATS	Negative
Thyroid-stimulating immunoglobulins	TSI	Negative
Measures of Thyroid and Pituitary Responsiveness		
T_3 suppression test		Decrease 50% of control or to normal
Thyrotropin-releasing hormone (TRH) stimulation test		Peak TSH 10-30 μU/ml at 20-30 min
TSH stimulation test		Double RAIU or above 10%
Assessment of Thyroid Anatomy		
Thyroid isotope scan	Scan	Homogeneous distribution; normal size, shape, and position
Computerized tomographic (CT) scan		Homogeneous distribution; normal size, shape, and position
Ultrasonic scan		Uniform tissue density
Fine-needle aspiration with cytologic examination		Non-neoplastic-appearing cells

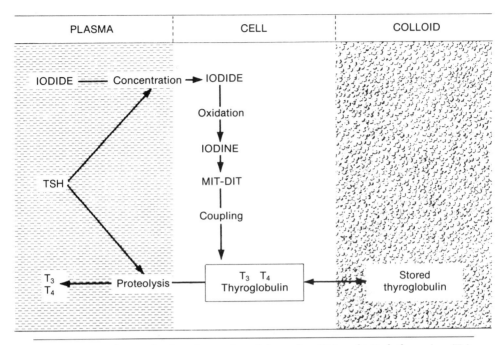

PLASMA	CELL	COLLOID

IODIDE ══ Concentration → IODIDE

Oxidation

IODINE

MIT-DIT

Coupling

TSH

T_3
T_4 ← Proteolysis ← T_3 T_4 Thyroglobulin ← Stored thyroglobulin

FIGURE 10-3   The synthesis and secretion of thyroxine *(T_4)* and triiodothyronine *(T_3)*.

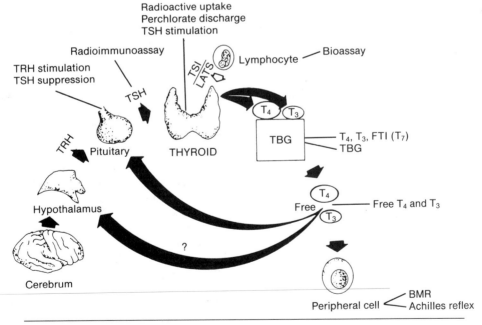

Radioactive uptake
Perchlorate discharge
TSH stimulation

Radioimmunoassay

TRH stimulation
TSH suppression

TSI/LATS   Lymphocyte — Bioassay

TSH

TRH

Pituitary   THYROID

T_4 T_3

TBG — T_4, T_3, FTI (T_7)
— TBG

Hypothalamus

Free T_4
T_3 — Free T_4 and T_3

?

Cerebrum

Peripheral cell — BMR
— Achilles reflex

FIGURE 10-4   The physiologic regulation of thyroid hormone secretion and the thyroid tests that measure these parameters are illustrated.

thyroid function and thyroid topography. Serum levels of TSH, T_4, and T_3 can be measured very accurately. Measurement of the circulating TSH level and free thyroxine index (FTI or T_7) is the easiest and best way to assess thyroid function status in most patients. When patients are thyrotoxic, for example, the FTI value is high, and the circulating TSH level is suppressed. On the other hand, if a person is hypothyroid, the FTI value is low, and the circulating TSH value is high.

Common Benign Nodules of the Thyroid

It is estimated that 4% of the U.S. population have a nodular thyroid gland. Each solitary nodule must be properly evaluated because of the possibility that it may represent a cancer of the thyroid. Benign nodules are classified in the following way.

Colloid Nodules. Colloid nodules can occur because of an iodine deficiency; however, in most instances in the United States no cause is found. The lesions present as single or multiple nodules within the thyroid gland. On gross examination of a cut section, this lesion has a glassy appearance because of the large amount of colloid that is present. On histologic examination macrofollicles with areas of hemorrhage, cystic degeneration, and hyperplasia can be seen.

Adenoma. Adenomas, benign neoplasms, often are classified as microfollicular, follicular, and fetal types, according to their microscopic pattern. Grossly, they appear as solid lesions that are well encapsulated.

Thyroiditis. Lymphocytic (Hashimoto's) thyroiditis is considered an autoimmune disease against the individual's own thyroid tissue. Areas of localized thyroiditis may present as a single nodule; however, more commonly a diffuse, bilateral disease is present. The thyroid has a firm, lobulated feel and may contain single or multiple nodules. A pyramidal lobe is frequently present. On histologic section many lymphocytes may be seen infiltrating within the thyroid parenchyma. Progressive destruction of the follicular cells takes place. Antimicrosomal (MCHA) and antithyroglobulin (TGHA) antibodies usually circulate and can be detected in the serum of most of these patients. Although most individuals have normal thyroid function early in the disease, as more thyroid tissue is destroyed, hypothyroidism generally occurs.

Acute thyroiditis is an uncommon condition. It is caused by a bacterial infection of the thyroid.

A congenital pharyngeal sinus tract is sometimes present.

Granulomatous thyroiditis can be of viral origin. In this rare condition a painful gland with thyrotoxicosis may be present. Giant cells and granulomas are present on histologic examination.

Cysts of the Thyroid. True cysts of the thyroid are very rare. Most cystic lesions represent degenerated colloid nodules. Parathyroid cysts also can occasionally be found within the thyroid parenchyma.

Malignant Lesions of the Thyroid

Cancer of the thyroid comprises an interesting group of diseases, each of which has a different incidence, rate of spread, pathogenesis, treatment, and prognosis. In the United States approximately 1200 deaths occur each year from thyroid cancer. Thus thyroid cancer ranks only thirty-fifth among cancers causing death. However, two high-risk groups have been identified: (1) individuals who received low-dose external irradiation to the head and neck area and (2) those who belong to families in which medullary cancer of the thyroid is present. These groups are discussed in greater detail in the sections that follow.

What Diagnostic Tests Can Differentiate Benign and Malignant Thyroid Nodules?

It is essential to take a careful history and to conduct a physical examination. A history of low-dose irradiation to the neck is, perhaps, the most important fact that can be obtained. On physical examination most cancers are felt as hard and irregular lumps. Enlarged, abnormal lymph nodes in the lateral neck or adjacent to the thyroid strongly suggest malignancy.

Thyroid function tests are not very useful as diagnostic tests since most patients with thyroid cancer are euthyroid. However, in the presence of hyperthyroidism, it is less likely a nodule will be a cancer. Radioactive scans (Fig. 10-5) can be helpful. Today most scanning of the thyroid is done with iodine 123 or technetium 99m since these isotopes result in a low radiation dose to the thyroid. Most cancers of the thyroid appear as "cold" on thyroid scan; however, so do most of the benign lesions listed previously. Thyroid cancers represent only approximately 10% of all cold nodules.

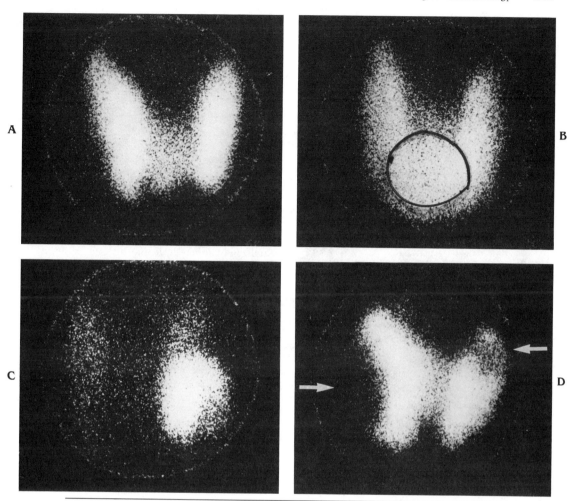

FIGURE 10-5   Radioiodine (isotope) scans of the thyroid gland. **A,** Normal scan. **B,** "Warm" nodule, which has the same isotope uptake as the surrounding tissue. **C,** "Hot" nodule. The isotope concentrates in the palpable nodule, and very little of the remaining normal thyroid gland is seen. Thyroxine is secreted autonomously from the hot nodule and suppresses the secretion of pituitary thyroid-stimulating hormone. Thus the remaining thyroid gland is suppressed. **D,** A "cold" nodule on each side is identified.

Ultrasonography can be used to differentiate solid from cystic lesions (Fig. 10-6). Since most cancers are solid, this differentiation can be somewhat helpful. Core-needle biopsy of the thyroid, using a Vim-Silverman or a Tru-cut needle, yields a core of tissue that can be examined microscopically. This procedure has the disadvantage of causing bleeding and other morbidity in some patients.

More recently cytologic evaluation of the aspirate of a nodule obtained by a small-gauge needle (fine-needle aspiration) has gained greater usage (Fig. 10-7). As shown in Fig. 10-8, four types of results can be obtained. If the result is consistent with colloid nodular disease, no operation is performed unless compression of the trachea or esophagus is present. If the finding is sheets of follicular cells, all patients should be operated on since follicular adenomas and carcinomas cannot be differentiated by this technique. Furthermore, a finding of carcinoma should lead to early operation. If an inadequate

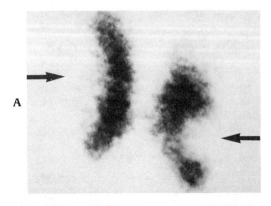

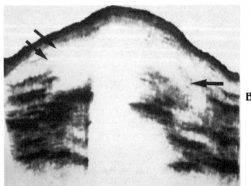

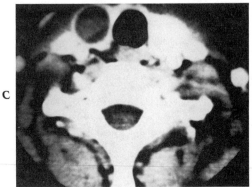

FIGURE 10-6 Multiple thyroid nodules as visualized by different diagnostic tests. **A,** On isotope scanning a "cold" nodule of both the left and right lobe is seen. **B,** On ultrasonography (transverse section) the nodule of the left lobe *(one arrow)* exhibits some echoes and is therefore partially solid, whereas the nodule on the right *(two arrows)* has no echoes and is therefore a cyst. **C,** On computed tomography with contrast infusion the left lobe is seen as solid, whereas the nodule on the right side is clearly cystic.

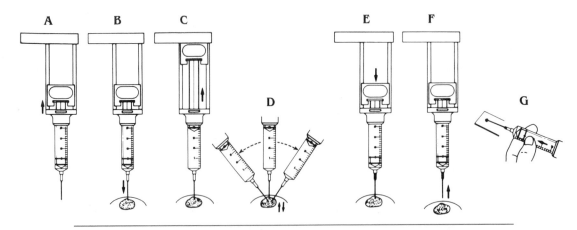

FIGURE 10-7 Top, left to right: Technique for fine-needle aspiration biopsy. **A,** Aspirate 1 to 2 ml of air into syringe to loosen plunger and facilitate expiration of contents after aspiration. **B,** Insert needle into lesion without aspiration. **C,** Retract syringe piston to provide maximal suction. **D,** Make several passes at different angles, withdrawing needle to near the surface before redirecting. Bottom, left to right: **E,** Release suction passively. **F,** Withdraw needle. **G,** Express needle contents onto a glass slide. (From Ahmann AJ, Wartofsky L. The thyroid nodule. In Becker KL [ed]. Principles and Practice of Endocrinology and Metabolism. Philadelphia, JB Lippincott, 1990, p 315.)

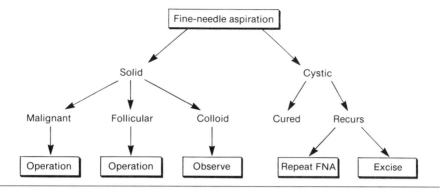

FIGURE 10-8   Current algorithm for diagnosis of a thyroid nodule. This scheme uses needle aspiration with cytologic examination as the primary tool for diagnosis. (Courtesy Dr. Jon van Heerden.)

specimen is obtained, the test should be repeated. Fine-needle aspiration with cytology is the best test for evaluation of a thyroid nodule.

In summary, *of greatest concern are thyroid nodules that are solitary, recent in origin, found in young individuals or men of any age, and cold on scan and solid on ultrasound. A prior history of low-dose irradiation to the head or neck indicates a cancer of the thyroid is more likely. A definitive diagnosis of cancer can best be made preoperatively by fine-needle aspiration of the nodule with cytologic examination.*

What Are the Different Types of Thyroid Cancers?

Papillary Cancer. Approximately two thirds of all thyroid cancers are papillary, and 90% of such lesions occur in young individuals. Papillary cancer is approximately three times more common in females than in males. Its usual course is rather benign in the young, but it is much more aggressive in patients over 50. Seventy-five percent of individuals have no symptoms when the nodule is discovered. On physical examination 20% to 30% have enlarged lymph nodes, which might lead to the diagnosis. Grossly, these tumors often can be seen to infiltrate the surrounding thyroid tissue. Microscopically, papillary projections are present with a fibrovascular stroma. The cells have crowded vesicular nuclei. Small calcium deposits called *psammoma bodies* or calcospherites are commonly found. Multicentricity of papillary cancer is microscopically found in up to 80% of instances. Metastases to the lymph nodes are

found in 50% to 60% of cases. The usual mode of spread is first to the lymph nodes and later to the lungs, bones, or elsewhere.

Follicular Cancer. Follicular cancer occurs with increased frequency in older individuals, especially in the fourth to sixth decade. It occurs more frequently in females than in males. Multicentricity within the gland is less frequent than in papillary cancer. The usual mode of spread is not to the lymph nodes but rather by the hematogenous route. Thus lung and bone metastases are the most common types, and sometimes symptoms of metastatic disease are the first to present.

Grossly, follicular cancer usually is seen as a hard, single nodule. Microscopically, follicles with cells that are crowded and abnormal are seen. Capsular and vascular invasion is common.

Is There a Relationship Between Irradiation to the Neck and Thyroid Cancer? In 1950 Duffy and Fitzgerald first recognized that low-dose external irradiation to the head or neck area would lead to a higher-than-normal incidence of papillary and follicular cancers. Most cancers occur after exposure of 15 Gy or less to the thyroid area, but a dose of as little as 0.065 Gy has been demonstrated to cause an increase in the incidence of thyroid cancer. Irradiation was given for several main reasons: (1) to shrink the thymus (an enlarged thymus was thought to press on the trachea and cause sudden crib death); (2) to shrink the tonsils and adenoids; and (3) to treat acne vulgaris during adolescence. Others were treated for cervical lymphadenitis, hemangiomas, and other miscellaneous reasons. In addition to thyroid cancer, low-dose external irradiation causes an increase of benign and malignant salivary gland tumors, basal and squamous cell cancers of the skin, meningiomas and malignant brain tumors, and even breast cancer. Even parathyroid adenomas result from this irradiation. The usual latency period is 20 to 35 years from irradiation to tumor recognition.

By far, most of the thyroid cancers in irradiated patients are papillary, but some are follicular. At the time of surgery for either a single nodule or for multiple nodules, approximately 35% to 40% of these irradiated patients have been found to have cancer of the thyroid. This compares strikingly with the 15% incidence of cancer in nonirradiated patients who were operated on for a single, cold, and suspicious nodule before the use of needle-aspiration biopsy.

What Is the Proper Treatment of Papillary and Follicular Cancers? When no history of irradiation is present, a lobectomy of the thyroid should be performed during surgery on any suspicious nodule (Fig. 10-9). The tissue is submitted to a pathologist while the patient is still anesthetized, and a frozen section is performed. If it is considered benign, no further operation is performed. If it is shown as a papillary cancer on frozen section, a near-total or a total thyroidectomy should be performed if the primary cancer is 1 cm in diameter or greater or if metastases are present. Any abnormal lymph nodes within the central compartment (i.e., near the thyroid or in the tracheoesophageal groove) are removed. Finally, a modified radical neck dissection is performed only if enlarged, pathologic lymph nodes are present in the lateral triangle, that is, the area lateral to the carotid artery. This operation removes the lymph node–bearing tissue from the lateral triangle of the neck but preserves the motor nerves running through this compartment, including the phrenic nerve, spinal accessory nerve, the brachial plexus, and the sternocleidomastoid muscle. In most instances the jugular vein can be preserved as well. Hence this operation results in a better cosmetic and functional result than a classic radical neck dissection.

Patients with a history of irradiation who have single or multiple nodules are treated similarly except that a near-total thyroidectomy is performed in all patients at the initial operation because of the higher incidence of cancer and because benign and malignant lesions are known to occur in the same gland of such patients.

All patients with papillary or follicular cancer should be treated for life with thyroid hormone to suppress circulating TSH to low or undetectable levels. TSH stimulation appears to accelerate the growth of thyroid cancer. Furthermore, metastatic papillary and follicular thyroid cancers will take up radioiodine in 70% to 80% of instances after the thyroid gland has been removed. A total body radioiodine scan is per-

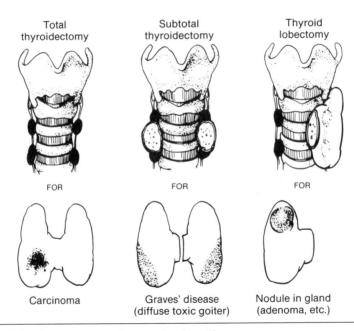

FIGURE 10-9   Common operations on the thyroid.

formed 3 to 4 weeks after thyroid replacement is stopped. If metastases are identified, the patient can be treated with high-dose radioiodine (iodine 131) which concentrates the radiation treatment into the area of metastases. External irradiation to the neck and elsewhere is sometimes helpful. Chemotherapy is used primarily for tumors without iodine uptake and for late-stage disease. The best single drug is doxorubicin (Adriamycin), and multiple agents are often used.

The prognosis for patients with papillary and follicular cancer is quite good when the patient is less than 45 to 50 years of age, the histology is well differentiated, there is no local invasion of tumor into the trachea or esophagus, there are no distal metastases, and the nuclear DNA pattern is diploid. Such patients have approximately a 2% mortality rate. Poor prognosis is predicted when a patient is older than 50 years of age at the time of diagnosis, the tumor is poorly differentiated, the nuclear DNA pattern is aneuploid, local invasion is present in the neck, distant metastases are present, and the primary tumor is quite large. Such individuals have a 50% to 70% mortality rate from the tumor. Of interest is the fact that in patients with papillary cancer, lymph node metastases per se do not confer a poor prognosis.

Anaplastic (Undifferentiated) Cancer of the Thyroid. Anaplastic cancer is one of the most virulent cancers found in man. It commonly occurs in middle or old age. The usual clinical course is rapidly downhill, with rapid growth of a thyroid mass in the neck, lymph node metastases, and peripheral dissemination. Pain, fever, and malaise are common, and dyspnea, dysphagia, and tracheal obstruction are not uncommon. Microscopically, sheets of cells are found that demonstrate many mitoses. A large cell (spindle cell) type is common; a small cell variant often is thought to represent lymphoma.

Usually these lesions are very far advanced when they are diagnosed; in such cases only a needle biopsy for diagnosis may be needed. If surgery can be performed on them early when they are still contained, a total thyroidectomy should be performed. A tracheostomy is sometimes necessary because of tracheal invasion or recurrent laryngeal nerve damage. Radioiodine is not concentrated by these anaplastic tumors, but external irradiation to the neck may temporarily shrink these lesions. Finally, chemotherapy with vincristine, doxorubicin, and chlorambucil is being tried, often in combination with radiation therapy. These regimens may lead to short-term remissions, but the long-term prognosis is extremely poor. Most patients die within 1 to 2 years after the diagnosis is made despite all therapy.

Medullary Cancer of the Thyroid. In 1959 medullary cancer of the thyroid was first classified as a separate type of malignancy. Soon after, it was demonstrated that these tumors arise from thyroid C cells; hence they are calcitonin-secreting tumors. These tumors are hard and gritty and may occur unilaterally in sporadic cases, but they almost always occur bilaterally in familial cases. C-cell hyperplasia, a precursor of medullary cancer, also has been identified, particularly in familial cases. These tumors spread first to the lymph nodes of the neck and mediastinum and then systemically to the lungs, liver, adrenals, and bones. Microscopically, sheets of uniform cells may be present. Sometimes they look like carcinoid tumors; however, in other cases a spindle cell variant is present. These are the only thyroid lesions that contain amyloid. When biopsy results from lymph nodes are negative, the prognosis is better, but with positive results, only a 40% 10-year survival rate has been found.

Associated Endocrine Disturbances

Diarrhea. Diarrhea is present in approximately one third of the advanced cases of medullary cancers. This diarrhea is very similar to that of a carcinoid syndrome. It is believed caused by either serotonin, prostaglandins, calcitonin, or kinins, each of which has been associated with this tumor.

Cushing's Syndrome. Cushing's syndrome, caused by ectopic production of adrenocorticotropic hormone (ACTH) by the tumor, may also occur.

Familial Medullary Carcinoma Syndrome (Sipple's Syndrome; Multiple Endocrine Neoplasia [MEN], Type IIA). In its entirety, MEN, type IIA, consists of bilateral medullary carcinoma, bilateral pheochromocytomas, and parathyroid hyperplasia (see the box on p. 172). C-cell hyperplasia of the thyroid and adrenal medullary hyperplasia are believed precursors of frank cancer and pheochromocytomas. This syndrome is transmitted as an autosomal dominant trait, which means that 50% of the children with a family member with this syndrome probably would be affected. Hence it is important to screen these families very carefully by measuring calcitonin levels and to treat the tumors as soon as they are diagnosed.

MEN, Type IIB. This disease is found in children or young adults. Individuals with medullary cancer of the thyroid or C-cell hyperplasia also have neuromas of the tongue, conjunctiva,

MULTIPLE ENDOCRINE NEOPLASIA, TYPE II

Type IIA (MEN, IIA)	Type IIB (MEN, IIB)
Bilateral medullary carcinoma of the thyroid (MCT) gland	Bilateral medullary carcinoma of the thyroid gland
Pheochromocytoma(s)	Pheochromocytoma(s)
Parathyroid hyperplasia	Parathyroid disease (rare)
No specific phenotype	Specific ganglioneuroma phenotype
Familial inheritance as a mendelian autosomal-dominant trait	Can occur in mendelian autosomal-dominant pattern
Variable rate of MCT progression, generally less aggressive than MEN, IIB	Generally rapid MCT progression

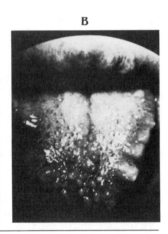

FIGURE 10-10   A, Typical marfan-like appearance of a patient with the MEN, type IIB, syndrome. B, Note the thickened lips and neuromas of the tongue that are diagnostic of this syndrome.

lips, and the buccal mucosa (Fig. 10-10) and ganglioneuromas of the bowel. The diagnosis is often suspected because of the neuromas of the tongue or conjunctivae. They also usually have a marfanlike appearance, with long extremities, high arches of the feet, and kyphoscoliosis. Furthermore, although they often have associated pheochromocytomas or adrenal medullary hyperplasia, they rarely have parathyroid hyperplasia. The medullary cancer is usually much more aggressive in patients with MEN, type IIB, than with MEN, type IIA.

How Is Medullary Thyroid Cancer Diagnosed? The finding of an elevated basal or stimulated serum calcitonin concentration is virtually pathognomonic of a medullary thyroid cancer. Calcium and/or pentagastrin infusions serve as provocative tests in borderline cases. Thus calcitonin is an excellent and a very important tumor marker. Carcinoembryonic antigen (CEA) is also a very good tumor marker. In individuals who have a known medullary cancer or who are at risk, serum calcium and urinary catecholamine concentrations should also be evaluated to rule out the possibility of an associated pheochromocytoma or hyperparathyroidism. The pheochromocytomas should be operated on first, if they are present, since they are a particular hazard during anesthesia. Later, a total thyroidectomy should be performed, and nodes of the central compartment should be removed. A lateral neck dissection should be performed if enlarged nodes are present in that area. Especially aggressive surgery is used with this tumor because thyroxine does not suppress it and radioiodine is not concentrated. External irradiation and chemotherapy are of some usefulness, but surgical excision of the tumor is most important. Postoperatively, serum calcitonin and CEA levels should be obtained at intervals to ascertain the presence, absence, and progression of the tumor.

THYROTOXICOSIS

Thyrotoxicosis refers to a syndrome caused by oversecretion of thyroid hormones. It may occur

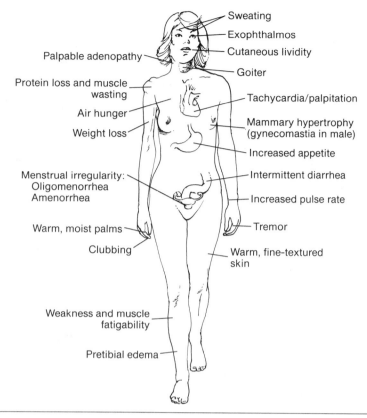

Sweating
Exophthalmos
Cutaneous lividity
Goiter
Palpable adenopathy
Protein loss and muscle wasting
Tachycardia/palpitation
Air hunger
Mammary hypertrophy (gynecomastia in male)
Weight loss
Increased appetite
Intermittent diarrhea
Menstrual irregularity: Oligomenorrhea Amenorrhea
Increased pulse rate
Warm, moist palms
Tremor
Clubbing
Warm, fine-textured skin
Weakness and muscle fatigability
Pretibial edema

FIGURE 10-11   Clinical manifestations of Graves' disease.

as a result of a toxic nodular goiter, a hyperfunctioning adenoma (a "hot" nodule), or very rarely a struma ovarii (i.e., hyperfunctioning thyroid tissue within an ovarian teratoma). However, the most common cause of thyrotoxicosis today in the United States is Graves' disease.

Graves' Disease

Graves is the eponym used in the English-speaking world to describe the syndrome of diffuse toxic goiter with thyrotoxicosis. Graves, an Irish physician, described this syndrome in the early English medical literature.

The signs and symptoms of Graves' disease are illustrated in Fig. 10-11. Note that in addition to having thyrotoxicosis, these patients also may have exophthalmus, a diffuse goiter, and pretibial myxedema, all of which are considered manifestations of a generalized autoimmune disease. This triad is not found in the other forms of thyrotoxicosis. Individuals with Graves' disease also have a relative lymphocytosis, lymphoid infiltration of the thyroid parenchyma, and round-cell infiltration of the retro-ocular muscles and

fat. In addition to elevated levels of serum T_4 and FTI, antithyroid antibodies can be detected frequently in the serum of such patients. Furthermore, long-acting thyroid stimulator (LATS) and thyroid-stimulating immunoglobulins (TSI) are found in many individuals and are considered by many investigators the cause of the thyrotoxicosis since serum TSH levels are uniformly low in these individuals. Most Graves' disease is found in women; the female-to-male ratio is 8:1. Although a traumatic event has been postulated to trigger the onset of this disease, the treatment is medical and not psychiatric therapy.

How Can Graves' Disease Be Treated? Three forms of treatment regimen are available: antithyroid drugs, radioactive iodine, and surgery (Table 10-2). No therapy is without complications, and each has good and bad features. Although subtotal thyroidectomy was used in most patients in the past, the current trend by most endocrinologists in the United States is to treat more patients with radioiodine therapy.

Antithyroid Drugs. Most individuals are treated initially with a thyroid-blocking drug (e.g., propylthiouracil [PTU] or methimazole).

TABLE 10-2   Treatment of Toxic Diffuse Goiter

Method	Dose	Onset of Response	Complications	Remarks
Antithyroid drugs				
Propylthiouracil	300-600 mg/day	2-6 wk	Rash, drug fever— 4%-8% Agranulocytosis— 1½%	Size of gland decreases Monitor results with T_3 and T_4 levels
Methimazole	30-60 mg/day		Recurrence of hyperthyroidism in 75% after discontinuing medication	Prolonged remission in 25% Patient must be closely followed
Iodine	5 drops, bid	Rapid blocking of hormone release	Temporary effect	Rarely used alone
Surgery	Subtotal (90%-95%) excision of gland	Immediate	Mortality <1% Permanent hypo-thyroidism—30% Recurrent hyper-thyroidism <10% Vocal cord paralysis—1% Hypoparathyroidism—1%	Safe for use in younger patients and pregnant women
Radioiodine (^{131}I)	5-10 mCi	Several months	Permanent hypo-thyroidism, 50%-70% with delayed onset; recurrence possible	Close long-term follow-up needed Avoid in children or pregnant females

This therapy is often given as a trial for 6 months to a year and then stopped. Although initial reports were more promising, currently only approximately 25% of my patients have a prolonged remission after stopping this medicine. In the others the disease recurs, necessitating the use of other definitive therapy. From 4% to 8% of individuals develop a side effect such as skin rash, leukopenia, and hepatic dysfunction to these antithyroid drugs. Agranulocytosis is a very serious complication. Finally, to be effective, these medications must be taken every 6 to 8 hours, but many patients are noncompliant.

Radioactive Iodine Therapy. This treatment is very attractive because no operation is necessary and the cost of treatment is less than that of an operation. However, iodine 131 cannot be given to pregnant women since it could destroy the fetal thyroid. Furthermore, there are other theoretic and, in some cases, practical considerations about its use. They concern the possibility of future genetic changes due to the radioactivity when given to young, fertile individuals and the possibility of an increased incidence of thyroid cancer or leukemia after a long latency period (as with external irradiation). These risks have largely been disproved. However, many patients remain afraid of the potential effects of radiation. Furthermore, after radioiodine therapy, hypothyroidism occurs in a large number of patients so that by 10 years after treatment, 70% or more of individuals require thyroid replacement therapy. Often hypothyroidism occurs insidiously after a number of years. When lower-dose regimens of radioiodine are used to prevent this latter difficulty, treatment to a euthyroid state is prolonged in many individuals, and the theoretic risk of thyroid cancer is increased. For these reasons I generally do not use radioactive iodine treatment for children or for young adults.

Surgical Therapy. Subtotal thyroidectomy does not have any of the potential risks of radioiodine therapy. Furthermore, the time to regaining a euthyroid state is the shortest of all therapeutic regimens. However, patients must undergo a general anesthetic and an operative procedure.

The complications of surgery for thyrotoxicosis should be very low, and this is the case when patients are operated on by an experienced neck surgeon. Both permanent hypoparathyroidism and recurrent nerve injury are the major risks of this procedure. Each has occurred in approximately 1% of my patients. No mortality from a thyroid operation has occurred at the University of Chicago Medical Center during the last 20 years. Thyroid storm has been essentially eliminated in these patients by proper preparation for surgery.

What Is the Proper Way to Prepare Patients for Surgery? Since the early 1920s it has been recognized that iodide therapy blocks the output of thyroid hormone. It also decreases the vascularity of the toxic thyroid gland. Thus even today some mildly toxic individuals can be safely prepared for surgery by treatment with a saturated solution of potassium iodide or Lugol's solution alone.

The beta-adrenergic blocker, propranolol, may also be used alone or, better still, in combination with iodide. Propranolol slows the heart rate to normal and eliminates the tremor. Thus many groups have advocated treating with propranolol for 1 week or less and operating while the patient is still grossly toxic, but with the peripheral manifestation of the disease blocked. I too use this regimen on rare occasions for patients who cannot take other medications. However, I believe it is safer to restore individuals to a euthyroid state when possible with antithyroid drugs (e.g., PTU or methimazole) and then add iodide for 8 to 10 days before the operation. Propranolol can be used as well. Although this preoperative regimen of achieving a euthyroid state is longer, it apparently is safer.

Surgical Procedure. At operation, a subtotal thyroidectomy is performed, which usually leaves the posterior portions of each thyroid lobe intact to protect the recurrent laryngeal nerves and the integrity of the parathyroid glands (see Fig. 10-9). My goal is to leave a total of approximately 4 to 5 g of well-vascularized thyroid tissue in each patient at the end of the procedure. After surgery approximately 60% to 70% of patients are euthyroid while off all medications. Recurrent thyrotoxicosis has occurred in less than 10% of patients. These results are considered quite satisfactory.

PRIMARY HYPERPARATHYROIDISM

Hyperparathyroidism is a condition in which there is an oversecretion of parathyroid hormone. In patients with primary hyperparathyroidism the serum calcium level is elevated because of an adenoma in approximately 85% of cases, because of hyperplasia approximately 15% of the time, or, rarely, because of a carcinoma of the parathyroid glands. In patients with secondary hyperparathyroidism oversecretion of parathyroid hormone is compensatory for a low serum calcium concentration. This occurs most commonly today in patients receiving dialysis for chronic renal failure, but it can also occur in patients with rickets (vitamin D insufficiency) and in patients with some malabsorption syndromes.

Recognition of the prevalence of primary hyperparathyroidism has increased markedly in recent years. It is estimated that this condition is diagnosed in one in every 500 patients who enter a hospital. Primary hyperparathyroidism is also the most common cause of hypercalcemia in an outpatient population.

Patients with primary hyperparathyroidism manifest hypercalcemia, hypophosphatemia, and increased calcium and phosphate in their urine. These findings have been referred to as "the classical triad" for diagnosis of primary hyperparathyroidism.

Parathyroid hormone (PTH) has three basic actions, all of which tend to elevate the serum calcium concentration: (1) it causes bone resorption through osteocytic osteolysis and by increasing osteoclastic activity; (2) it acts on the gut to increase the absorption of calcium; and (3) it acts on the kidneys to increase the tubular resorption of the filtered calcium ion and to decrease the proximal renal tubular resorption of phosphate ion. Thus more calcium and less phosphate are conserved.

The cellular action of PTH apparently is mediated through the adenyl cyclase, cyclic-adenosine monophosphate (cAMP) system. In recent years the importance of vitamin D has been recognized. Clearly, the action of PTH on the gut and on bone requires the presence of vitamin D metabolites.

How Is the Serum Calcium Level Regulated?

Serum calcium levels in humans are normally regulated within very narrow limits. The primary control mechanism is through the parathyroid glands. In healthy individuals, when the serum ionized calcium level is diminished, the parathyroid glands secrete more hormone. Increased circulation of PTH then acts on the gut, kidney, and bone to raise the serum calcium concentration to normal. Conversely, when hypercalcemia occurs, PTH secretion is lessened, thus permitting the serum-ionized calcium level to return to normal.

Calcitonin has never been proved an important physiologic regulator of serum calcium levels in humans. Thus in humans the major control of serum calcium homeostasis is affected by the interaction of PTH and vitamin D metabolites.

Clues to the Diagnosis of Primary Hyperparathyroidism

Although most of the original patients with primary hyperparathyroidism had severe bone disease, it was soon realized that more patients had renal stones (Table 10-3). Peptic ulcer, pancreatitis, fatigue, hypertension, arthritis, arthralgias, and mental disorders later were recognized as associated with this condition. Today, because of the common use of multiphasic chemical screening, many patients are diagnosed who are relatively asymptomatic.

What Are the Harmful Effects of Hypercalcemia?

Hypercalcemia, per se, causes a number of clinical manifestations. Among them are nausea, vomiting, constipation; polyuria and polydipsia; fatigue, weakness, stupor, and coma; depression and psychosis; and metastatic calcification. Thus if a patient with breast cancer, for example, rapidly deteriorates, rather than considering the possibility that this deterioration is due to brain metastases, one should first test to determine the serum calcium level. If the serum calcium level is elevated, the restoration of this value to normal can lead to a remarkable recovery in many instances.

TABLE 10-3   Initial Manifestations of Hyperparathyroidism*

Condition	No. of Patients (%)
Hypercalcemia on screening test (routine physical examination)	40 (8)*
Renal stones	28
Symptoms of hypercalcemia (weakness, constipation, lethargy, polyuria, polydipsia)	7
Peptic ulcer disease	5
Hypertension	4
Bone disease	4
Diabetes mellitus	3
MEN I	3
Thyroid disease	3
Pancreatitis	2
Lump in neck	1

From Clark OH, Way LW. The hypercalcemic syndrome: Hyperparathyroidism. In Friesen SR, Bolinger RE (eds). Surgical Endocrinology. Philadelphia, JB Lippincott, 1978.
*Eight percent of the patients were completely asymptomatic.

Differential Diagnosis of Hypercalcemia

The most common cause of hypercalcemia in patients in a hospital setting is malignancy with bone metastases (Table 10-4). A bone scan is much more efficacious than routine bone x-ray examinations in diagnosing early cases of this type. Certain malignancies such as squamous cell cancers of the head and neck and lung, hypernephromas of the kidney, and some cholangiocarcinomas of the liver, secrete PTH-like substances and thus cause hypercalcemia. A new peptide, parathyroid-related polypeptide (PRP), has been found to cause this hypercalcemia and can be measured in the blood of many patients with these tumors. Thiazide diuretics can elevate the serum calcium concentration, and their use should be stopped before a diagnosis of primary hyperparathyroidism is made. Multiple myeloma, sarcoidosis, and other granulomatous diseases can also result in hypercalcemia, as can taking too much vitamin D or vitamin A. Other less common causes of hypercalcemia are leukemia, hyperthyroidism, myxedema, addisonian

TABLE 10-4   Causes of Hypercalcemia

Condition	Approximate Frequency (%)
Malignancy	35
Breast cancer	
Metastatic tumor	
PTH-secreting tumor (lung, kidney, others)	
Multiple myeloma	
Acute and chronic leukemia	
Hyperparathyroidism	28
Artifact (e.g., laboratory error, dirty glassware, cork stopper, tight tourniquet)	10
Vitamin D overdose	8
Thiazide diuretics	4
Hyperthyroidism	3
Milk-alkali syndrome	3
Sarcoidosis	3
Miscellaneous	6
Immobilization	
Paget's disease	
Addison's disease	
Idiopathic hypercalcemia of infancy	
Dysproteinemias	
Vitamin A overdose	
Myxedema	
WDHA syndrome	

From Clark OH, Way LW. The hypercalcemic syndrome: Hyperparathyroidism. In Friesen SR, Bolinger RE (eds). Surgical Endocrinology. Philadelphia, JB Lippincott, 1978.

crisis, immobilization, the milk-alkali syndrome, and acromegaly.

How Is Primary Hyperparathyroidism Diagnosed?

The most important parameter for establishing the diagnosis of primary hyperparathyroidism is a simultaneous elevation of the serum calcium and parathyroid hormone levels. Circulating PTH is measured by radioimmunoassay. In other hypercalcemic states (e.g., sarcoidosis) the serum PTH concentration is low or nondetectable. Ectopic hyperparathyroidism due to tumor can be diagnosed by measuring elevated levels of circulating PRP and demonstrating the tumor, usually in the chest, kidney, or liver. Hypophosphatemia is present in approximately 80% of patients with hyperparathyroidism, but that percentage varies somewhat with dietary factors. A chloride to phosphate ratio greater than 33 is confirmatory. The alkaline phosphatase level is elevated only if significant bone disease is present. Renal tubular resorption of phosphate is decreased; this measurement is made by comparing the creatinine clearance by the kidney with the phosphate clearance. Urinary AMP is also elevated in individuals with this disease.

A number of radiologic findings have also been described but are usually recognized only when severe bone disease is present. They include resorption of the lateral third of the clavicle, cystic changes of osteitis fibrosa, and subperiosteal bone resorption of the phalanges and distal tufts of the fingers. This latter finding is pathognomonic of hyperparathyroidism when it is present. Dental x-ray examination can also be helpful since the lamina dura, a fine rim of bone that surrounds normal teeth, is absent in patients with primary hyperparathyroidism.

Pathology of Primary Hyperparathyroidism

Most pathologists agree that a single adenoma is the cause of 80% to 85% of all cases of primary hyperparathyroidism and that chief cell hyperplasia comprises most of the remaining cases.

Carcinoma of the parathyroid is the cause of less than 1% of all cases of primary hyperparathyroidism. Parathyroid cancer spreads locally to lymph nodes and finally spreads systemically to lungs and bones. If it is recognized at the time of operation, a wide local resection should be performed, removing the lobe of the thyroid and the parathyroid gland. All abnormal lymph nodes should be removed. Care should be taken not to enter the capsule of the carcinoma since local seeding may occur. Patients with carcinoma of the parathyroid have a very poor prognosis if metastatic disease is present. Death occurs not from tumor spread itself but from persistent hypercalcemia with all of its sequelae since this is difficult to control by drugs or chemotherapy.

Where Are Abnormal Parathyroid Glands Found?

Approximately 85% of parathyroid adenomas are found in "normal" locations near the thyroid gland. The upper parathyroid glands are derived from the fourth branchial pouch and are usually found adjacent to the thyroid gland approximately one third of the distance from the upper pole. However, when these glands become enlarged, they frequently are found more inferiorly and posteriorly, even behind the esophagus or in the posterior superior mediastinum. The lower parathyroid glands are derived embryologically from the third branchial pouch, the same branchial organ as the thymus. Normal glands are found adjacent to the lower pole of the thyroid, but roughly 40% of these glands are found within the thymic tongue, inferior to the thyroid gland. Thus it is not uncommon to find adenomas of the lower gland present within the thymus gland, even within the anterior mediastinum. Finally, parathyroid adenomas can be found within the carotid sheath and lateral to it at the carotid bifurcation, and 1% to 3% of all adenomas are located within the thyroid gland.

Can Parathyroid Adenomas Be Localized Preoperatively?

Only 1% to 3% of enlarged parathyroid adenomas can be palpated preoperatively. However, recent advances have permitted the correct preoperative location of approximately 80% of parathyroid glands. Ultrasonography is useful in the neck area (Fig. 10-12); a parathyroid gland appears hypoechoic (i.e., with fewer echoes than the thyroid gland). The thallium-technetium scan can show an enlarged parathyroid gland in the neck but is especially useful in identifying ectopically placed adenomas (Fig. 10-13). Comput-

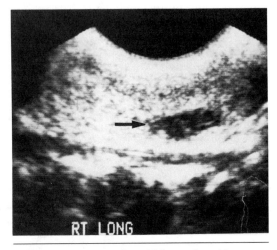

FIGURE 10-12 Intrathyroidal parathyroid adenoma recognized preoperatively by ultrasonography. Note that enlarged parathyroid glands appear almost cystic by this technique.

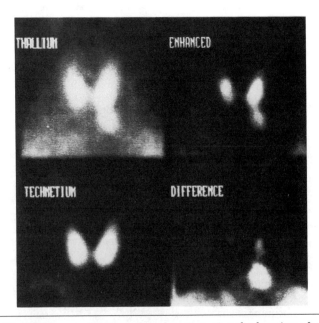

FIGURE 10-13 Thallium-technetium scan demonstrating the location of an intrathymic parathyroid adenoma. *Top left,* thallium 203 goes to the thyroid and to the large parathyroid gland. *Lower left,* Technetium 99m images only the thyroid gland. *Lower right,* The difference, obtained by computer subtraction of the two images, represents the parathyroid adenoma within the thymus.

erized tomography (CT) scans and magnetic resonance imaging (MRI) techniques (Fig. 10-14) can also be useful. Angiography and venous catheterization, with PTH sampling of selective blood samples, also play a role in some very difficult cases. These latter two tests are invasive, however, and complications may be associated with their use.

Because preoperative localization tests are costly and because they are only 80% accurate, most investigators do not recommend their use before an initial parathyroid exploration, for experienced parathyroid surgeons can find and cure 95% to 97% of cases at the time of the first exploration. However, reoperations for primary hyperparathyroidism are much more difficult. All agree that parathyroid localization is imperative before these reexplorations.

What Are the Principles of Exploration?

When operating on a patient for primary hyperparathyroidism, the surgeon must keep the field as bloodless as possible. A transverse "collar" incision is made. Meticulous, careful dissection is necessary. It is important to examine both sides of the neck and try to locate each parathyroid gland. If one parathyroid gland is clearly enlarged and the others are normal, the large gland is considered an adenoma. The adenoma is removed, and a biopsy specimen is obtained from one of the other parathyroids. Frozen sections of

tissue are used to confirm the fact that parathyroid glands were located. If more than one gland is enlarged, this represents hyperplasia. In such instances a subtotal parathyroidectomy is performed, which means the removal of most of the parathyroid mass. A part of one gland, well vascularized, is left in situ. Sometimes a total parathyroidectomy with an autotransplant of parathyroid tissue to the arm is used instead, especially for the hyperplasia associated with familial syndromes. Each normal parathyroid gland weighs 35 to 50 mg. Enlarged parathyroid glands may weigh several times more than normal, up to 10 to 15 g.

If an abnormal parathyroid gland cannot be located initially during neck exploration, a search of all of the ectopic sites should be carried out—high in the neck to the hyoid bone, along the carotid sheath, within the thyroid lobe itself, and into the anterior and posterior mediastinum. In the hands of expert parathyroid surgeons, 95% or more cases of hyperparathyroidism will be cured during the initial neck exploration. A sternotomy should not be done at the first operation unless the patient is in a very serious condition because of the hyperparathyroid state. Rather, a reassessment of the diagnosis and institution of localization procedures should be performed before reexploring the patient and doing a sternotomy. If a patient has had an inadequate neck exploration elsewhere, it is appropriate to reexplore the neck again, for most of these glands can be found and removed through a cervical approach.

What Are the Complications of Thyroid and Parathyroid Surgery?

Hemorrhage. The greatest danger of bleeding is a hematoma in the neck, which can cause tracheal compression and respiratory insufficiency. Once it is diagnosed, the hematoma should be evacuated immediately, even at the bedside if necessary.

Hypoparathyroidism. Removal or devascularization of the parathyroid glands can lead to hypocalcemia in the postoperative period. Hypocalcemia can cause tingling of the fingers, carpopedal spasm, tetany, and convulsions if not treated. Thus the serum calcium level must be followed closely after the operation. Transient postoperative hypocalcemia may require intravenous calcium and oral calcium treatment; for permanent hypoparathyroidism, a lifetime of calcium and vitamin D therapy is necessary.

Recurrent Laryngeal Nerve Injury. If unilateral, this injury results in vocal cord paralysis

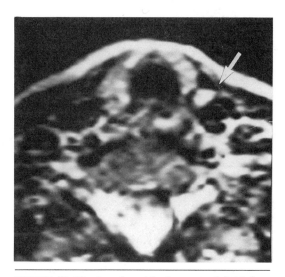

FIGURE 10-14 Parathyroid adenoma of the left side of the neck (***arrow***) located by magnetic resonance imaging (MRI).

on the ipsilateral side. This paralysis generally produces hoarseness and some difficulty in coughing. If a bilateral recurrent nerve injury occurs, bilateral vocal cord paralysis results, often necessitating a tracheostomy because of respiratory embarrassment. Fortunately, damage to a recurrent laryngeal nerve may be transient, and recovery may occur even after 6 to 9 months.

Superior Laryngeal Nerve Injury. Since this nerve innervates the cricothyroid muscle, damage may result in impairment to the singing voice or in the ability to project a loud voice. Often these defects improve after several months.

Thyroid Storm. Thyroid storm may occur soon after an operation on a thyroid gland with thyrotoxicosis if the gland has not been prepared adequately and may be due to a release of excessive amounts of thyroid hormone. Fever, tachycardia, stupor, and possibly death can occur if appropriate treatment is not instituted. The use of propranolol, reserpine, adrenocortical steroids, antithyroid drugs, glucose, and generalized cooling should be instituted. Fortunately, this syndrome rarely occurs today if patients are correctly prepared for operation.

TUMORS OF THE ADRENAL GLANDS

The normal adrenal gland contains two types of tissue, the adrenal cortex and the adrenal me-

dulla. The cortex is divided into three portions: (1) the outermost area, or zona glomerulosa, is the site of mineralocorticoid production; (2) the central area, or zona fasciculata, is the site of production of glucocorticoids; and (3) the innermost layer, or zona reticularis, is the site of sex hormone production. The adrenal medulla is a completely different organ, which is derived from neuroectoderm. This area is a site of epinephrine and norepinephrine production. Thus tumors that arise from different sites of the adrenal gland have different signs and symptoms. The surgical anatomy of the adrenal glands is shown in Fig. 10-15.

What Is Cushing's Syndrome?

Cushing's syndrome is a collection of signs and symptoms that are due primarily to overactivity of glucocorticoid production (Fig. 10-16). The same syndrome can be reproduced by exogenous administration of excessive cortisol. Patients typically have a characteristic appearance—moon faces, buffalo hump, central obesity, and thin extremities. Purple striae and easy bruisability are common. Women with this disease manifest loss of scalp hair, acne, facial plethora, and increased body and facial hair. Hypertension, cardiomegaly, and renal calculi may also occur.

Chemistry changes include normal or ele-

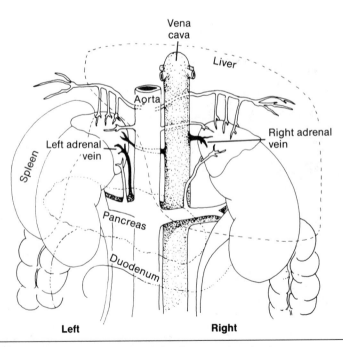

FIGURE 10-15   Anatomy of the adrenal glands (posterior view).

vated serum sodium levels and decreased serum potassium levels caused by the effects of mineralocorticoids on the kidney. There is also a decrease in lymphoid tissue, lymphocytes, and eosinophils and an increase in polymorphonuclear leukocytes in the blood.

Pathophysiology of This Condition. Seventy percent of all cases of Cushing's syndrome are caused by adrenal cortical hyperplasia, which results from an ACTH-producing tumor of the anterior pituitary. Usually it is a small benign tumor, referred to as a *pituitary microadenoma*. This process has been named after Dr. Harvey Cushing, a neurosurgeon who originally described the condition. The tumor of the pituitary secretes excessive amounts of ACTH, which causes hyperplasia of the adrenal cortex and the resulting increase in serum cortisol levels (Fig. 10-17). Another 10% of patients have adrenal cortical hyperplasia caused by ectopic secretion of ACTH. Many tumors (e.g., medullary cancer of the thyroid, carcinoid tumors, lung cancer) secrete ACTH ectopically. Ectopic ACTH production results in hyperplasia of the adrenal cortex

and increased cortisol production. Finally, adenomas of the adrenal cortex comprise 10% to 15% of these cases, whereas carcinoma of this location is the cause of another 5% to 10%. Benign and malignant tumors are autonomous and are not under the control of the pituitary. Thus blood cortisol levels are increased, and ACTH is decreased.

Diagnosis of Cushing's Syndrome. Normally ACTH and cortisol are secreted in a diurnal rhythm. Both levels are highest during the night and in the early morning hours before awakening and are the lowest in the late afternoon. With Cushing's syndrome the diurnal variation of these hormones is lost, and cortisol remains high throughout the day. By measurement of the blood cortisol and ACTH levels at different times during the day, these abnormalities can be diagnosed. Measurement of urinary free cortisol levels are also helpful, for they are also elevated in patients with Cushing's syndrome.

How Are Adrenal Tumors Differentiated From Adrenal Hyperplasia? The differentiation between adrenal hyperplasia and tumor can be made first by blood testing. With a pituitary microadenoma or the ectopic ACTH syndrome, circulating levels of ACTH and cortisol are both elevated (see Fig. 10-17). This is also true in cases

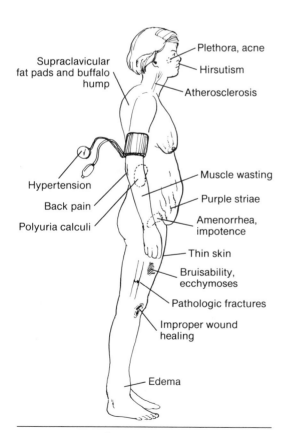

FIGURE 10-16 Characteristic findings of Cushing's syndrome.

Supraclavicular fat pads and buffalo hump
Plethora, acne
Hirsutism
Atherosclerosis
Hypertension
Back pain
Polyuria calculi
Muscle wasting
Purple striae
Amenorrhea, impotence
Thin skin
Bruisability, ecchymoses
Pathologic fractures
Improper wound healing
Edema

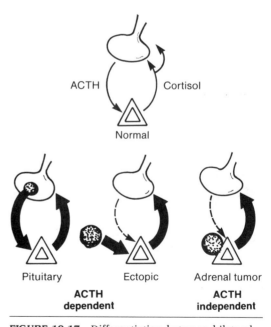

ACTH   Cortisol
Normal

Pituitary   Ectopic   Adrenal tumor
ACTH dependent   **ACTH independent**

FIGURE 10-17 Differentiation between bilateral adrenal cortical hyperplasia (due either to a pituitary ACTH-secreting microadenoma or to ectopic secretion of ACTH) and an adrenal cortisone-producing tumor can be made by measuring circulating ACTH and cortisol levels.

of ectopic ACTH secretion. Adrenal adenomas or carcinomas, on the other hand, secrete cortisol autonomously. Thus in these cases serum cortisol levels are elevated, and ACTH values are low.

Additional differentiation can be made by the use of dexamethasone suppression. If patients with proved Cushing's syndrome are given 8 mg of dexamethasone for 3 days, those with either an adrenal adenoma or carcinoma or others with the ectopic ACTH syndrome will not suppress their levels of blood or urinary cortisol, whereas those with pituitary microadenomas will suppress these concentrations.

Further differentiation can be made by examination of the adrenal gland area by MRI or CT scan (Fig. 10-18). An iodocholesterol scan can also be helpful (Fig. 10-19). Radioiodinated cholesterol is given to the patient and is incorporated into the actively secreting adrenal cortex. If uptake is unilateral, an adenoma or carcinoma is present; if the uptake of the isotope is bilateral, this is diagnostic of adrenal cortical hyperplasia. Finally, an adrenal mass can be imaged by retrograde venography (Fig. 10-20).

MRI examinations can also visualize the pituitary microadenoma in up to 80% of cases in which it is present. Further localization of the pituitary microadenoma can be made by measuring blood levels of ACTH in each sphenoid sinus after passing catheters to these locations.

What Is the Proper Treatment for Cushing's Syndrome? If an adenoma or carcinoma of the adrenal cortex is the cause of the Cushing's syndrome, this tumor should be operated on and removed. Similarly, if the cause of the Cushing's

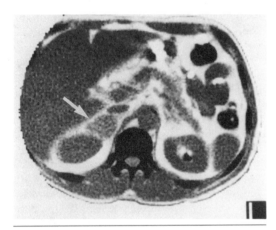

FIGURE 10-18   Computerized tomography demonstrating a right adrenal mass (*arrow*).

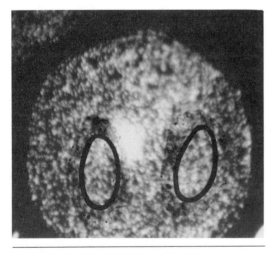

FIGURE 10-19   Iodocholesterol scan demonstrating unilateral uptake of isotope. When the position of the kidneys is superimposed, this uptake localizes a left adrenal mass.

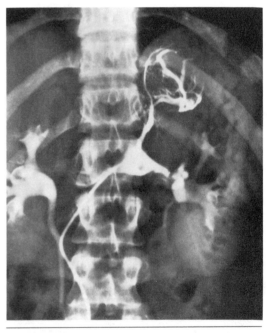

FIGURE 10-20   Retrograde venogram imaging a left adrenal tumor. A catheter was inserted upward through the vena cava, into the left renal vein, and finally into the left adrenal vein. Dye was carefully injected into the catheter and revealed the adrenal cortical tumor on the left side.

syndrome is ectopic production of ACTH, that tumor (e.g., carcinoid of the lung) should be removed if possible; otherwise, the oversecretion of cortisol can be blocked medically.

Some differences of opinion still exist as to what is the proper treatment for adrenal hyperplasia caused by a pituitary microadenoma. The usual treatment in the past was bilateral total adrenalectomy. This therapy necessitates a lifetime of steroid replacement, however. In addition, patients may develop Nelson's syndrome (i.e., hyperpigmentation and enlargement of the pituitary gland) after a bilateral adrenalectomy. This is a serious situation.

Irradiation to the pituitary has also been used as primary treatment for Cushing's disease, especially in children. Such treatment has resulted in some remissions of the disease. However, the technique that has gained greatest favor is the microsurgical resection of the pituitary microadenoma by a transsphenoidal route. In this technique the surgeon approaches the pituitary through the nasal septum. The sphenoid bone overlying the pituitary is removed, and the pituitary gland is seen (Fig. 10-21). The microadenoma is selectively removed, leaving the rest of the pituitary intact. In the best hands, 80% to 90% of patients are cured of Cushing's disease by this technique. Long-term results, including the incidence of recurrence, are not fully known, but some recurrence of disease has occurred. The advantages of this technique are low morbidity and mortality from the operative procedure in these very sick patients and the fact that no replacement therapy of cortisol is required if the microadenoma can be removed and the rest of the anterior pituitary is left intact.

For cancer of the adrenal cortex that cannot be removed, effective treatment sometimes can be obtained by the chemotherapeutic agent O^1P^1DDD, a specific adrenocortical poison. However, adrenocortical cancer has a very poor 5-year survival rate, and ketoconazole, a cortisol inhibitor, can also be used when all of the tumor cannot be removed.

What Is the Correct Preoperative and Postoperative Management? When operating on a patient with either an adrenal cortical adenoma or carcinoma or with bilateral hyperplasia that has resulted in Cushing's syndrome, treatment with adrenal cortical steroids perioperatively and postoperatively is imperative. If a bilateral total adrenalectomy is performed, the patient requires steroid therapy for the rest of his or her life. Similarly, after removal of an adenoma or carcinoma, the adrenal cortex of the opposite adrenal gland is suppressed and will regain its function only after a considerable period of time. Thus such patients also require steroid therapy perioperatively and postoperatively for varying periods of time, even longer than a year. Eventually, in most of them the replacement therapy can be discontinued.

On the day of operation, cortisol or cortisone, 300 mg, is given, one half intramuscularly and one half intravenously. Over the next few days these amounts are rapidly decreased. Oral cortisone acetate can be given as soon as oral feedings are resumed. A maintenance dose is usually 37.5 to 50 mg of cortisone per day, given as 25 mg in the morning and 12.5 mg in the evening. Others prefer to use prednisone therapy instead (Table 10-5). The comparable maintenance doses of prednisone are 5 mg in the morning and 2.5 mg in the evening. In addition, I usually add fludrocortisone acetate (Florinef), approximately 0.1 mg per day. This is a very potent mineralocorticoid and results in the retention of sodium and excretion of potassium from the body. The patient must always be instructed to increase the oral dose of cortisone during times of stress, infections, or trauma. The cortisone should be given intramuscularly if vomiting occurs. Despite their ongoing therapy, these patients can lead long and healthy lives as long as they take their steroids.

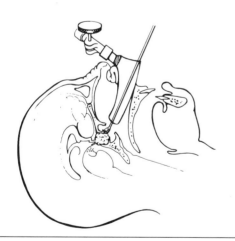

FIGURE 10-21 Transsphenoidal approach to the pituitary. The ACTH-producing microadenoma is selectively removed, leaving the remaining pituitary gland intact. (From Seljeskog EL. Hypophysectomy in Cushing's disease. In Najarian JS, Delaney JP [eds]. Advances in Breast and Endocrine Surgery. Chicago, Year Book Medical Publishers, 1986, pp 477-485.)

TABLE 10-5   Glucocorticoid Equivalencies

Glucocorticoid	Approximate Equivalent Dose (mg)	Relative Anti-inflammatory Potency	Relative Mineralocorticoid Potency	Half-life Plasma (min)	Half-life Biologic (hr)
Short Acting					
Cortisone	25	0.8	2	30	8-12
Hydrocortisone	20	1	2	80-118	
Intermediate Acting					
Prednisone	5	4	1	60	18-36
Prednisolone	5	4	1	115-212	
Triamcinolone	4	5	0	200+	
Methylprednisolone	4	5	0	78-163	
Long Acting					
Dexamethasone	0.75	25-30	0	110-310	36-54
Betamethasone	0.6-0.75	25	0	300+	

ALDOSTERONOMA

Normal aldosterone secretion is controlled by three different mechanisms: (1) ACTH secretion from the anterior pituitary, (2) the serum potassium concentration, and (3) of greatest importance, the renin-angiotensin mechanism (Fig. 10-22). Within the kidney are cells called the *juxtaglomerular apparatus.* A fall in the intravascular volume or pressure within the afferent arteriole leading to these cells results in a release of renin into the circulation. Renin plus angiotensinogen, which is produced by the liver, forms angiotensin I, which is converted to angiotensin II and finally to aldosterone. Aldosterone acts on the distal renal tubule to cause retention of sodium and increased excretion of potassium ions in the urine.

What Is the Clinical Syndrome of Primary Hyperaldosteronism?

In the mid-1950s Conn described the syndrome of primary hyperaldosteronism, which bears his name. Patients with an aldosteronoma demonstrate elevated blood pressure, the absence of edema, and a low serum potassium concentration and frequently manifest polyuria, polydipsia, muscle weakness, and occasionally tetany due to low calcium and magnesium levels from a metabolic alkalosis. They also have a diabetic glucose tolerance curve in many instances. The removal of an aldosteronoma leads to a correction of the hypertension in most instances.

Aldosteronomas are almost always benign. They are much smaller than most of the other adrenocortical tumors and are generally 2 cm in diameter or less. Almost all of the tumors are unilateral.

How Is an Aldosteronoma Diagnosed?

Patients with an aldosterone-secreting tumor have hypertension and hypokalemia, even after thiazide diuretics are discontinued. The diagnosis is confirmed by finding an elevated serum and urinary aldosterone output in the presence of a low serum renin level. Because of an expanded blood volume, the serum renin concentration is low and remains so despite a low sodium diet, the administration of diuretics, or other manipulations that normally raise the serum renin concentration. In addition, a urinary potassium output of greater than 50 mEq per day while the patient is on a high sodium diet is also diagnostic.

The patient's response to spironolactone (Aldactone) therapy is helpful diagnostically and prognostically. A rise in serum potassium concentration of 1 mEq/L or greater with a fall in blood pressure confirms the diagnosis and suggests that removal of the aldosteronoma will lead to a resumption of normal blood pressure postoperatively.

The tumors can sometimes be seen on CT or MRI examinations. If the tumor is too small for

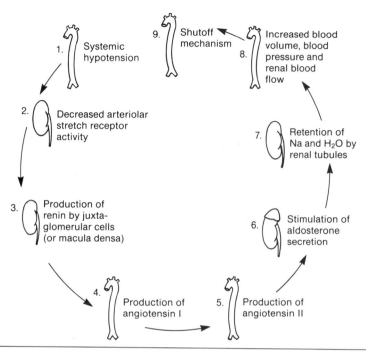

FIGURE 10-22   Renin-angiotensin system and normal aldosterone secretion.

viewing by these methods, its location can often be determined by measuring aldosterone concentration in blood taken from each adrenal vein. Each adrenal vein is catheterized and aldosterone measured from the blood. The aldosterone concentration is highest on the side of the tumor. Retrograde adrenal venography can also be performed (see Fig. 10-20). Finally, the iodocholesterol-131 scan can be used with dexamethasone suppression (see Fig. 10-19). Unilateral adrenal activity suggests strongly that a tumor is present on that side.

An aldosteronoma must always be differentiated from bilateral hyperplasia, for most investigators do not operate for the latter condition. Furthermore, primary hyperaldosteronism must always be differentiated from secondary hyperaldosteronism, which occurs in patients with congestive heart failure, anasarca, and renal artery stenosis. In these situations the aldosterone concentration in the blood and the urine is high; however, circulating renin concentration is also high.

Important Operative Considerations

Since aldosteronomas are usually small, the site of the tumor must be localized preoperatively. Generally at the time of operation the entire adrenal gland containing the adenoma is removed. The blood pressure usually returns to normal within several days to several weeks after the removal of the tumor unless severe renal vascular changes have already occurred because of the hypertension.

PHEOCHROMOCYTOMAS

Pheochromocytomas are tumors derived from the adrenal medulla and from the sympathetic nervous chain from the neck to the pelvis. In the latter location they are generally called paragangliomas. They occasionally occur in the bladder, and a common extra-adrenal position is near the aortic bifurcation at the site called the organ of Zuckerkandl.

What Are the Clinical Signs and Symptoms?

Pheochromocytomas are clinically very dangerous tumors because of the catecholamines—epinephrine and norepinephrine—they secrete. Patients with pheochromocytomas exhibit hypertension, either constant or paroxysmal or both. Attacks of hypertension are often accompanied by excessive perspiration, headaches, palpitations, tachycardia, pallor, nausea, trembling, nervousness, anxiety, chest pain, postural hypotension, or epigastric pain. These symptoms are due to excessive circulating catecholamines. Norepinephrine is an alpha-adrenergic agonist, and its primary manifestations are vasoconstriction and hypertension. Epinephrine acts primarily as a beta-adrenergic stimulator that causes vasodilation, an increase in the heart rate (tachycardia), an increase in ventricular conductivity often resulting in dysrhythmias, dilation of the bronchial musculature, and an increase in blood glucose levels. Thus the symptoms can differ in each patient according to which catecholamine is excessively secreted. In general, the tumors of the sympathetic chain secrete primarily norepinephrine, whereas those of the adrenal beds secrete both epinephrine and norepinephrine. Catecholamines are synthesized from the amino acid L-tyrosine, which is metabolized to L-dopamine, L-norepinephrine, and, finally, to L-epinephrine.

How Is Pheochromocytoma Diagnosed?

One of the safest and most effective ways to diagnose a pheochromocytoma is to study the urinary catecholamines after instituting a special diet (Table 10-6). Elevations of the output of urinary epinephrine or norepinephrine, metanephrine or normetanephrine, or vanillylmandelic acid (VMA) are diagnostic of a pheochromocytoma. Blood catecholamine levels can be measured and may be helpful; however, since anxiety or stress results in an increase in circulating catecholamines, the drug clonidine is used to eliminate elevated levels caused by fear or fright. In addition, the hematocrit level is often elevated, the blood glucose concentration is frequently increased, and the serum potassium level can be decreased.

Pharmacologic studies may also be done to aid in the diagnosis in difficult cases, but only under the strictest of controls. If phentolamine (Regitine), 1 mg, is given intravenously, a rapid decrease of blood pressure and even shock may occur. Stimulation tests using either glucagon or histamine may be used. However, when a tumor is present, a rapid rise in blood pressure may occur. A physician must be present to treat the hypertension or hypotension quickly and effectively or great harm might occur; thus these are very dangerous tests if great care is not taken. During these tests circulating catecholamine levels are measured.

Can Pheochromocytomas Be Localized Preoperatively?

Radiologic studies are very useful for localization of the tumors preoperatively. A chest film should always be obtained to rule out a posterior mediastinal mass. A CT scan (see Fig. 10-18) or MRI examination (Fig. 10-23) can be very helpful.

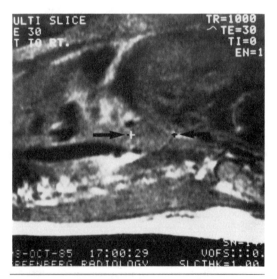

FIGURE 10-23 MRI examination demonstrating an extra-adrenal pheochromocytoma *(arrows)* that was present at the level of the aortic bifurcation in a woman who was 6 months pregnant. Note the fetus within the uterus anterior to the tumor. (From Greenberg M, et al. Extraadrenal pheochromocytoma. Detection during pregnancy using MR Imaging. Radiology 161:475-476, 1986.)

TABLE 10-6 Normal Values for 24-Hour Urinary Excretion of Catecholamines and Metabolites

	Normal Excretion Rate
Norepinephrine	<100 μg
Epinephrine	<50 μg
Vanillylmandelic acid (VMA)	2-10 mg
Normetanephrine and metanephrine	0.3-0.9 mg

The patient must be prepared with an alpha-adrenergic receptor blocking drug before any invasive testing is done since severe hypertension might occur. A new scanning technique using ^{131}I metaiodobenzylguanidine (^{131}I MIBG) is very effective as a localization tool (Fig. 10-24). MRI and ^{131}I MIBG scans are the two best localization tools for pheochromocytomas.

How Should Patients Be Prepared Preoperatively?

One of the most important recent therapeutic advances for a pheochromocytoma is the routine use of alpha-adrenergic receptor blockade for 10 days to 2 weeks before surgery for a pheochromocytoma. Phenoxybenzamine (Dibenzyline) is generally used. It permits the blood pressure to return to normal, hypertensive episodes are eliminated, and the blood volume is increased to normal. Beta-adrenergic receptor blockade with propranolol (Inderal) is also important if tachycardia or dysrhythmias are present. Alpha blockade always should be started before beta blockade.

How Should Patients Be Managed Intraoperatively?

To operate safely, the anesthesiologist or internist manipulating the infusion of drugs during the operation must be excellent in his or her field. Proper monitoring of the patient is essential. An arterial catheter for measurement of blood pressure, a central venous or Swan-Ganz catheter for determining the state of the heart, several other intravenous lines for administration of colloid or crystalloid, a Foley catheter, and an electrocardiogram are used. Transesophageal ultrasonography to monitor the heart is also very helpful.

The surgeon must dissect the tumor gently. Manipulation of the tumor during operation causes catecholamine release and hypertension. As soon as the adrenal vein is ligated, severe hypotension may occur, especially if the patient has not received adequate alpha blockade preoperatively. If hypertension occurs, phentolamine (Regitine) or nitroprusside should be infused intravenously. If hypotension occurs, norepinephrine is infused and the vascular space filled with colloid and crystalloid. It is clear that adequate preparation, careful monitoring, and excellent anesthesia are critical to the success of the surgical removal of a pheochromocytoma.

Although these tumors are usually benign and are found within the adrenal fossae, in the adult approximately 10% are extra-adrenal, 10% are bilateral or multiple, 10% are part of the MEN-II syndromes, and 10% of those in the adrenal bed are malignant. Malignancy is generally determined by the presence of local invasion or distant spread. In extra-adrenal tumors close to half will prove malignant if prolonged follow-up care is given.

In general, an anterior abdominal approach should be used, which permits exploration not only of both adrenal beds but also of the intra-abdominal sympathetic ganglia. The surgeon must treat the tissue very gently since manipulation and rough handling cause the release of catecholamines. Therefore "remove the tissue from the tumor, not the tumor from the surrounding tissue."

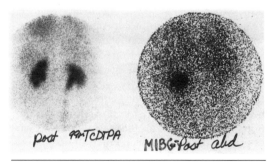

FIGURE 10-24 Localization of a left adrenal pheochromocytoma by MIBG scanning; ^{131}I MIBG scan demonstrates a single focus of activity. *Left,* Technetium 99m was given to demonstrate the position of the kidneys.

What Other Endocrinopathies Are Associated With These Tumors?

It must be remembered that pheochromocytomas may be part of the MEN, type IIA and type IIB, syndromes. As such they may sometimes be associated with medullary carcinoma of the thyroid and parathyroid hyperplasia. Serum calcitonin, calcium, and parathyroid hormone levels should be determined. Pheochromocytomas in such instances are usually bilateral. In children as many as 40% of all pheochromocytomas are bilateral. If so, a bilateral adrenalectomy is usually necessary since the lesions are often multicentric. In the MEN type II syndromes adrenal medullary hyperplasia, a bilateral condition, is the precursor of the pheochromocytomas. If a unilateral adrenalectomy is done to permit the child to grow with normal adrenal cortical function, the other side invariably will develop a pheochromocytoma, necessitating its removal in the future. Thus most investigators favor a bilateral adrenalectomy in patients with the MEN syndrome, even if only one side demonstrates a tumor, for to do so is believed much safer.

What Are the Operative Approaches for Adrenalectomy?

Four general approaches to the adrenal gland are available. The first is the anterior approach. It gives access to both adrenal glands; however, complications include pancreatitis and ileus, since the pancreas must be mobilized to reach the left adrenal gland. Second is the posterior approach, which is performed by removing the eleventh or twelfth rib in the back and entering the retroperitoneal space. The advantage of this technique is that the peritoneal cavity is not entered. Complications of this technique include pneumothorax, since the pleural cavity is often entered, and pancreatitis if this organ is traumatized. The third and fourth approaches, lateral and thoracoabdominal, give good exposure to one side. The latter operation is reserved for large tumors of the adrenal gland such as carcinomas in which a wide resection is mandatory. This incision has the disadvantage of involving both the thorax and the abdominal cavity.

Gastrointestinal and Pancreatic Endocrine Tumors. The pancreas and gastrointestinal tract are now recognized as a very important part of the endocrine system. Tumors from these endocrine cells often elaborate amines and peptides, which result in complex and interesting clinical syndromes.

CARCINOID TUMORS AND THE CARCINOID SYNDROME

Carcinoid tumors were first described in the late 1800s. The name means "resembling carcinoma." However, patients with these tumors have a better prognosis than those with true adenocarcinomas of the bowel. Carcinoid tumors occur from the esophagus to the rectum and also in the thymus, lung (formerly called *bronchial adenomas*), and the ovary (Fig. 10-25). Although each carcinoid tumor should be considered a malignancy, the virulence varies greatly according to the site of origin. For example, appendiceal carcinoid tumors have a very favorable prog-

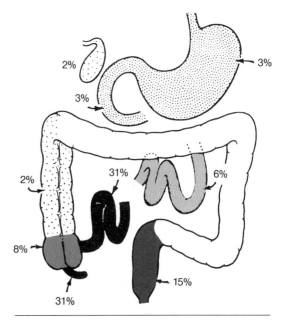

FIGURE 10-25   Incidence of carcinoid tumors in different areas of the body. (From Welsh JP, Malt RA. Management of carcinoids of the gastrointestinal tract. Surg Gynecol Obstet 145:223-227, 1977. By permission.)

nosis, but colonic carcinoids result in a mortality rate not too different from that of adenocarcinomas of that organ.

What Are the Carcinoid Syndromes?

Carcinoid tumors are unique since they can result in what is called a *carcinoid syndrome*. The signs and symptoms of the classic carcinoid syndrome are shown in Table 10-7. In general, flushing with hypotension, diarrhea, asthma, and lesions on the right side of the heart—tricuspid insufficiency—and pulmonic stenosis are present. This syndrome usually is associated with massive liver metastases from a midgut primary tumor, especially from the distal ileum. The endocrine manifestations were originally believed caused exclusively by secretion of serotonin; however, more recently the possible role of motilin, substance P, and other tachykinins as well as prostaglandins has been entertained.

Variant carcinoid syndromes, which are associated with foregut carcinoid tumors (stomach and bronchial), may be due to histamine, 5-hydroxytryptophan, or the tachykinins. Most carcinoid syndromes are diagnosed by the findings of

TABLE 10-7 Symptoms and Signs of the Classic Carcinoid Syndrome

	Mean Incidence (%)
Major Manifestations	
Hepatomegaly	70
Cutaneous flushing	75
Vasomotor changes	
Hypotension	
Diarrhea	70
Endocardial lesions	50
Bronchoconstriction	20
Venous telangiectasis	50
Edema	52
Minor Manifestations	
Pellagra	5
Peptic ulcers	5
Arthralgias	6
Fibrosis	
Retroperitoneal	
Peyronie's disease	
Myopathy	

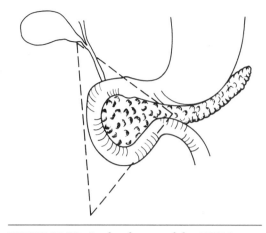

FIGURE 10-26 In the absence of the MEN-I syndrome, most gastrinomas are found in the "gastrinoma triangle." (From Stabile BE, et al. The gastrinoma triangle: Operative implications. Am J Surg 147:25, 1984.)

increased concentrations of 5-hydroxyindole acetic acid (5-HIAA) in the urine. Elevated serotonin levels can also be measured in the blood. Treatment with the somatostatin analog is very helpful in diminishing the flushing, diarrhea, and vasomotor changes of the carcinoid syndromes. Chemotherapy with streptozocin and 5-fluorouracil (5-FU) may offer some remissions.

GASTRINOMAS AND THE ZOLLINGER-ELLISON SYNDROME

In 1955 Zollinger and Ellison described the association of a very virulent peptic ulcer diathesis and a non-beta pancreatic islet cell tumor. It was later shown by Gregory of Liverpool, England, that these tumors secreted the hormone gastrin. Excessive gastrin circulates in the bloodstream and stimulates the growth and hyperfunction of the parietal cells of the stomach. Thus large amounts of gastric acid are made, and peptic ulcers are produced in both normal and abnormal locations of the upper gastrointestinal tract. Bleeding, obstruction, perforation, and diarrhea commonly occur in such patients.

Most gastrinomas are found in the pancreas or in the submucosa of the duodenum (Fig. 10-26). Sixty percent of them are malignant. Tumors can be multiple, especially in patients with the MEN-I syndrome (pancreatic and pituitary tumors with parathyroid hyperplasia causing primary hyperparathyroidism), or diffuse hyperplasia of all of the pancreatic islets may occur. Thus it is difficult to remove all of the tumor in most cases. Before the discovery of histamine (H_2) blockers or omeprazole, a hydrogen ion pump inhibitor, a total gastrectomy was recommended for all patients. Since the advent of cimetidine, ranitidine, and omeprazole, however, the therapy has changed. These antagonists effectively inhibit gastric acid secretion in many individuals with the Zollinger-Ellison syndrome. Currently, greater attempts are being made to remove the gastrinomas, since patients do die of tumor spread and from complications of severe ulcer disease. Complete cures of this syndrome have occurred as a result of removal of the gastrinomas, especially those from the duodenal sweep. Approximately 25% to 30% of patients with the Zollinger-Ellison syndrome have a gastrinoma as part of the MEN syndrome of pancreatic, parathyroid, and pituitary disorders.

A gastrinoma is diagnosed when serum gastrin concentration is elevated in the presence of massive gastric acid secretion. Secretin and calcium infusions result in a rise in serum gastrin levels if a gastrinoma is present.

INSULINOMAS

As the name signifies, insulinomas are insulin-secreting tumors of the pancreas. Approximately 90% are benign. They are usually single; however, multiple tumors are frequently associated with MEN, type I, syndrome.

What Is Whipple's Triad for Diagnosis of an Insulinoma?

Since insulin is secreted autonomously by insulinomas and is not regulated by the serum glucose level, (1) hypoglycemia occurs during times of fasting or exercise (low blood sugar levels usually result in changes of behavior and may cause convulsions, stupor, and even death); (2) at the time of symptoms, the blood glucose concentration is 45 mg/dl or less; and (3) symptoms are relieved by IV infusion of glucose or by oral glucose consumption. Many insulinomas are diagnosed by finding a low blood sugar level in a patient who appears to have had a stroke.

What Is the Current Way to Diagnose an Insulinoma?

The diagnosis of an insulinoma is made by demonstrating an inappropriately elevated serum insulin level at the time of fasting hypoglycemia. Elevated circulating peptide and proinsulin levels are also present. Provocative tests with tolbutamide or calcium infusion may also be helpful; however, prolonged fasting is still the diagnostic test of choice.

Can Insulinomas Be Localized?

Localization of the tumor by CT scan or arteriography (Fig. 10-27) is greatly helpful to the surgeon since these lesions are frequently small. Percutaneous transhepatic catheterization of the veins of the pancreas, with sampling of blood (Fig. 10-28) and hormone analysis, appears useful in localizing some tumors. Intraoperative ultrasonography is often helpful in locating a tumor that is not palpable (Fig. 10-29).

What Is the Operative Approach to an Insulinoma?

Treatment of an insulinoma consists of removal of the tumor either by enucleation or by pancreatic resection as appropriate. After the successful removal of the tumor, the serum glucose homeostasis returns to normal in most cases.

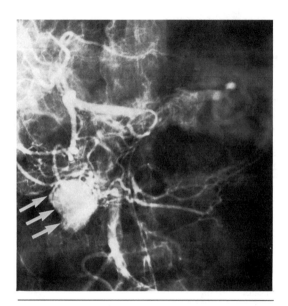

FIGURE 10-27   Celiac artery angiogram in a patient diagnosed with hyperinsulinism demonstrating a tumor "blush" in the area of the head of the pancreas *(arrow)*. An insulinoma was removed from this location at operation.

WATERY DIARRHEA SYNDROME

Profound *w*atery *d*iarrhea, severe *h*ypokalemia, and gastric *a*nacidity or hypoacidity are the symptoms of a person with watery diarrhea syndrome (WDHA), also termed Verner-Morrison syndrome. Diabetes and hypercalcemia may also occur.

Although the diagnosis is often difficult to make, most individuals with WDHA ultimately have been found to have a malignant islet cell tumor of the pancreas. Islet cell hyperplasia has also been described. The same syndrome may result infrequently from a ganglioneuroma or other retroperitoneal neural tumors, from an oat cell carcinoma of the lung, or from extrapancreatic sites.

Most tumors secrete a vasoactive intestinal peptide (VIP); hence the term *vipoma* usually is used to describe the syndrome. However, other peptides have been implicated as well. Treatment consists of removal of the tumor when possible. Medical therapy with corticosteroids or with the somatostatin analog is frequently beneficial in stopping the severe watery diarrhea. Chemotherapy for this and other endocrine gut tumors has been somewhat successful using streptozocin and 5-FU.

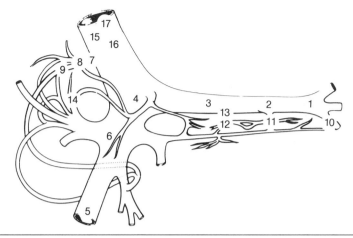

FIGURE 10-28   To perform percutaneous transhepatic catheterization of the pancreatic veins, a catheter is introduced into the liver, and the portal vein is cannulated. A catheter is introduced into the large and small veins draining the pancreas. Blood is sampled at the sites numbered in the diagram, and hormone analysis, in this case for insulin, is performed. An elevated concentration of insulin in this case suggests that the insulinoma is nearby. (From Ingemansson E, et al. Localization of insulinomas and islet cell hyperplasia by pancreatic vein catheterization and insulin assay. Surg Gynecol Obstet 146:725, 1978. By permission.)

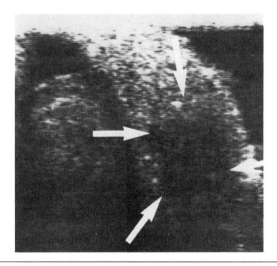

FIGURE 10-29   Location of an insulinoma by intraoperative ultrasonography. The pancreatic endocrine tumor *(arrows)* appears hypoechoic when compared to the surrounding normal pancreas.

GLUCAGONOMA SYNDROME

Glucagon-secreting tumors of the pancreas have been described. A syndrome associated with hyperglucagonemia has been found in many of these individuals. In its entirety it consists of:

- Necrolytic migratory erythema (a specific, superficial skin rash that often is recognized by dermatologists) (Fig. 10-30)
- Diabetes mellitus
- Anemia
- Weight loss

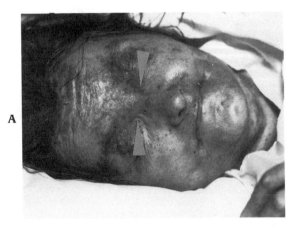

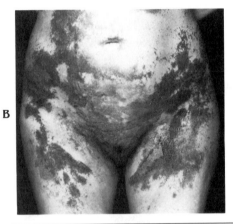

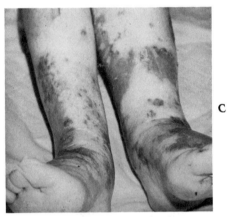

FIGURE 10-30 Appearance of necrolytic migratory erythema in several patients with a glucagon-secreting tumor of the pancreas. When this rash is found in a patient with diabetes mellitus, always think of the possibility of a glucagonoma. **A,** Characteristic rash of face. **B,** Rash of groin area. Note the circular lesions in some areas. **C,** Note the edema and swelling of the left leg associated with hypoproteinemia and venous thrombosis. (From Becker SW, et al. Cutaneous manifestations of internal malignant tumors. Arch Dermatol 45:1069, 1942. © 1942 American Medical Association.)

- Cheilosis and stomatitis
- Hypoaminoacidemia
- Venous thrombosis

This syndrome is diagnosed when a tumor mass of the pancreas is found along with elevated circulating glucagon levels in an individual with diabetes mellitus and the specific skin rash, necrolytic migratory erythema.

Most of these tumors are malignant. However, when these tumors can be completely removed, all of the manifestations of this syndrome disappear and revert to normal. Thus many investigators believe all of the symptoms and signs are due to the severe catabolic effects of increased circulating glucagon levels. Whenever a patient with

diabetes mellitus has a diffuse skin rash, the possibility of a glucagonoma should be considered. Symptomatic improvement, with healing of the rash and improvement of protein metabolism, also follows treatment with the somatostatin analog.

OTHER APUDOMAS

Islet cell tumors that secrete pancreatic polypeptide and somatostatin have also been described in the literature. Undoubtedly other peptides, other tumors, and other syndromes will be recognized in the near future. The endocrine system of the gastrointestinal tract remains a very fruitful area for study.

SURGICAL PHARMACOPEIA

Drug	Action	Indications/Comments	Dosage
Phenoxybenzamine hydrochloride (Dibenzyline)	Alpha-adrenergic blocker	Helps control hypertension of pheochromocytoma—use only preoperatively	Start with 20-40 mg/day PO/IV; increase 10-20 mg/day until hypertension is controlled; used for 7-14 days preoperatively
Propranolol hydrochloride (Inderal)	Beta-blocker	Tachycardia and/or dys-rhythmia associated with pheochromocytoma (administer only *after* alpha blockade); tachycardia and tremors in Graves' disease	30-40 mg/day in 3-4 doses PO/IV
Dexamethasone	Suppresses ACTH	Suppression of pituitary microadenoma (differentiate Cushing's disease from adrenal adenoma)	8 mg PO qid × 3 days
Mitotane o,p'-DDD (Lysodren)	Adrenal cyto-toxic agent	Inoperable adrenocortical carcinoma	2-6 g/day in divided doses tid or qid PO; increase up to 10 g/day for up to 8 months
Cimetidine (Tagamet)	H_2-blocker	↓ Gastric acid secretion in Zollinger-Ellison syndrome	300 mg PO qid; may ↑ up to 2400 mg/day
Ranitidine hydrochloride (Zantac)	H_2-blocker	↓ Gastric acid secretion in Zollinger-Ellison syndrome	150 mg bid PO up to 6 g/day
Omeprazole (Prilosec)	Hydrogen ion pump inhibi-tor	Inhibit gastric acid secretion in Zollinger-Ellison syndrome	60 mg once daily PO up to 120 mg tid PO
Cortisone acetate		Use in perioperative and postoperative manage-ment of adrenal adenoma or hyperplasia	300 mg IM or IV preopera-tively; 100 mg IV tid for 1 day then tapered to final oral maintenance dose of 25 mg at 9 AM/12.5 mg at 9 PM
Somatostatin Analogue (Sandostatin)	Suppresses secretion of serotonin and gastroentero-pancreatic peptides	Hypersecretion in carcinoid, VIPoma, glucagonoma	100-600 μg/day IV in 2-4 divided doses until symptoms are controlled
Spironolactone (Aldactone)	Aldosterone antagonist	Treatment of hyperaldo-steronism resulting from bilateral adrenocortical hyperplasia	100-400 mg/day PO

BIBLIOGRAPHY

DeGroot LF, Larsen PR, Refetoff S, et al. The Thyroid and Its Diseases, 5th ed. New York, John Wiley & Sons, 1984.

Feldman JM. Carcinoid tumors and the carcinoid syndrome. Curr Probl Surg 26:12, 1989.

Kaplan EL. Surgery of the Thyroid and Parathyroid Glands. Edinburgh, Churchill Livingstone, 1983.

Kaplan EL, Michelassi F. Endocrine tumors of the pancreas and their clinical syndromes. In Nyhus LM (ed). Surgery Annual, Vol 18. Norwalk, Conn, Appleton-Century-Crofts, 1986, pp 181-223.

Kaplan EL, Udekwu A. The carcinoid syndromes. In Friesen SR, Thompson NW (eds). Surgical Endocrinology Clinical Syndromes, 2nd ed. Philadelphia, JB Lippincott, 1990, pp 181-209.

Manger WM, Gifford RW, Hoffman BB. Pheochromocytoma: A clinical and experimental overview. In Hickey RC (ed). Current Problems in Cancer. Chicago, Year Book Medical Publishers, 1985, pp 1-89.

Melby JC. Diagnosis and treatment of primary aldosteronism and isolated hypoaldosteronism. In DeGroot LF (ed). Endocrinology, 2nd ed. Philadelphia, WB Saunders, 1989, pp 1705-1713.

Moss NH, Kaplan EL. Insulinoma and nesidioblastosis. In Howard JM, Jordan GL, Reber HA (eds). Surgical Diseases of the Pancreas. Philadelphia, Lea & Febiger, 1987, pp 814-828.

Prinz RA, Sugimoto J, Lorincz AL, et al. Glucagonoma. In Howard JM, Jordan GL, Reber HA (eds). Surgical Diseases of the Pancreas. Philadelphia, Lea & Febiger, 1987, pp 848-859.

Seljeskog EL. Hypophysectomy in Cushing's disease. In Najarian JS, Delaney JP (eds). Advances in Breast and Endocrine Surgery. Chicago, Year Book Medical Publishers, 1986, pp 477-485.

Stabile BE, Morrow DJ, Passaro E Jr. The gastrinoma triangle: Operative implications. Am J Surg 147:25, 1984.

Yashiro T, Salti GI, Kaplan EL. Primary hyperparathyroidism in the 1990's—Choice of surgical procedures for this disease. Ann Surg 215:300-317, 1992.

CHAPTER REVIEW
Questions

1. What is the most reliable tool for the diagnosis of a thyroid nodule preoperatively?
2. What is the best definitive treatment for a patient with Graves' disease?
3. How is the diagnosis of primary hyperparathyroidism made?
4. What is the pathology associated with primary hyperparathyroidism?
5. What is the surgical treatment of bilateral adrenal cortical hyperplasia associated with Cushing's disease?
6. Why is bilateral total adrenalectomy less favored for this condition?
7. Why should a patient with a pheochromocytoma be prepared before the operation?
8. Are all pheochromocytomas within the adrenal glands?
9. What is the MEN-II syndrome?
10. When should an aldosteronoma be suspected?
11. How is the Zollinger-Ellison syndrome diagnosed?
12. How is an insulinoma diagnosed?
13. How is a glucagonoma diagnosed?
14. What is the most common primary site for a carcinoid tumor that is associated with a classic carcinoid syndrome?

Answers

1. Although isotope scanning and ultrasound examinations have been used in the past, by far the single best test for diagnosis of a thyroid nodule is fine-needle aspiration with cytologic evaluation. A good cytologist will diagnose more than 90% of nodules correctly. Furthermore, because it is safe, the test can be repeated if uncertainty remains.
2. Virtually all patients with Graves' disease are first treated with antithyroid pills, often for 6 months to a year. When this medication is stopped, 70% to 75% of patients become thyrotoxic again. Hence most older patients are treated with radioiodine therapy. Most younger individuals are treated with subtotal thyroidectomy.
3. An elevation of serum calcium and parathyroid hormone concentrations is diagnostic of primary hyperparathyroidism. In most assay systems the hypercalcemia found with other tumors is associated with a low or borderline serum parathyroid hormone value. Elevated levels of parathyroid-related peptide (PRP) can be found in many patients with carcinomas of the lung or with hypernephromas who manifest hypercalcemia.
4. Approximately 85% of patients in this group have an adenoma, which is defined as a single gland enlargement. Approximately 15% have multiglandular disease, called *hyperplasia*. All patients with the MEN-I and MEN-II syndromes have hyperplasia. Less than 1% of patients has a parathyroid cancer.
5. Cushing's disease is caused by a microadenoma of the anterior pituitary gland that secretes excessive amounts of ACTH. The favored treatment is transsphenoidal resection

of the pituitary microadenoma if an excellent neurosurgeon trained in this technique is available.

6. After this procedure the patient has to take adrenal cortical steroids for life and runs the risk of developing Nelson's syndrome, which is hyperpigmentation and a rapid growth of the pituitary tumor.

7. Pheochromocytomas secrete norepinephrine and epinephrine and are very dangerous tumors. Severe hypertension and hypotension can occur intraoperatively. These harmful effects can be somewhat minimized by preparing the patient with alpha blockade preoperatively. Beta-adrenergic blockers are added to control tachycardia and dysrhythmias. Still, excellent care is needed intraoperatively.

8. No, at least 10% of all pheochromocytomas are extra-adrenal. They occur from the neck to the pelvis and can develop in any site in which sympathetic ganglia are present.

9. The MEN-II syndrome consists of the genetic association of medullary carcinoma of the thyroid (or C-cell hyperplasia), pheochromocytomas (or adrenal medullary hyperplasia), and primary hyperparathyroidism caused by parathyroid hyperplasia.

10. An aldosteronoma is suspected in patients with hypertension who have severe hypokalemia caused by loss of potassium in the urine. Stop administration of all thiazide diuretics and measure circulating renin and aldosterone levels. A high aldosterone level with a low renin concentration is very suggestive of a state of primary hyperaldosteronism. Studies should be done to differentiate an aldosteronoma from bilateral hyperplasia.

11. The necessary first step is the demonstration of a high serum gastrin concentration with a high output of gastric acid in a patient with severe peptic ulcer disease. It is important to determine that gastric outlet obstruction is not present and that the individual did not have a prior gastrectomy with a Billroth II reconstruction. Finally, an elevation of the serum gastrin concentrations after secretin infusion makes the diagnosis very secure.

12. Although Whipple's triad was important in its day, the most important diagnostic test today is the recognition of an inappropriately elevated serum insulin concentration at the time of profound hypoglycemia. The connecting peptide level should also be elevated on the same sample, proving that the insulin secretion comes from the pancreas and not from injected insulin.

13. Glucagon is a highly catabolic substance. Hyperglucagonemia results in hyperglycemia caused by gluconeogenesis and also by symptoms of severe protein wasting. Necrolytic migratory erythema is a specific skin rash that is diagnostic of this condition. Always think of the possibility of glucagonoma in any diabetic with a skin rash.

14. The most common site of the primary tumor is the ileum. By the time a carcinoid syndrome is present from a gastrointestinal primary site, the liver almost always has massive metastatic disease that overwhelms its capacity to metabolize serotonin or other substances responsible for this syndrome.

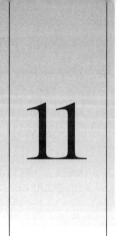

11

Gastroduodenal Physiology and Peptic Ulcer Disease

DANIEL T. DEMPSEY
WALLACE P. RITCHIE, Jr.

KEY FEATURES

After reading this chapter you will understand:
- The anatomy of the stomach and duodenum and the basics of gastric physiology.
- Current information about gastrointestinal hormones and their normal and abnormal production.
- Gastric and duodenal ulcers.
- The factors that influence the operative approach to treatment of duodenal and gastric ulcers.

The stomach, duodenum, and pancreas act together as an elegantly coordinated unit to effect digestion of foodstuffs. Although the overall process is integrated, each organ plays a very specialized role. The stomach elaborates a caustic acid and a powerful proteolytic enzyme that act together to digest protein. It also mixes and grinds ingested foodstuffs and delivers them in an orderly fashion into the duodenum. This organ in turn, in concert with the pancreas, adjusts intraluminal pH and osmolarity, promotes further hydrolysis of protein and carbohydrate, and alters dietary fat into an absorbable form. On occasion this process can go awry, resulting in autodigestion of the gastric or duodenal mucous membrane and leading to the development of a "peptic" ulcer—an interruption of the integrity of the mucosa caused by the action of acid and pepsin.

SURGICAL ANATOMY OF THE STOMACH AND DUODENUM

The normal stomach is bounded superiorly by a physiologically competent esophageal sphincter and inferiorly by a readily demonstrable pyloric sphincter. The wall of the stomach has four layers: the outer serosa, a coat of smooth muscle fibers, the submucosa, and an inner mucous membrane. By convention, the external surface of the organ has been divided into anatomic regions based roughly on the cell types contained in the subjacent mucosa (Fig. 11-1). The body (corpus) contains the vast majority of the stomach's complement of parietal cells, the source of hydrochloric acid and intrinsic factor, and of

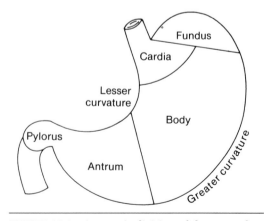

FIGURE 11-1 Anatomic division of the stomach.

chief cells, the source of pepsinogen. Additional cell types include surface epithelial cells, which secrete mucus for lubrication, mucous neck cells, precursors of both surface epithelial cells and parietal cells, and mast cells, which contain histamine as well as other amines. The cardia and fundus differ from the corpus only in that there are fewer parietal and chief cells. The antrum is the principal site of the gastric G cells, the source of the secretory hormone gastrin.

The duodenum curves about the head of the pancreas in a C shape, beginning at the pylorus and ending just proximal to the ligament of Treitz. In its course it receives the common bile duct and both the minor and major pancreatic ducts. Except for the absence of peritoneum on its posterior surface, the wall of the duodenum is analogous to that of the stomach. It is the widest segment of the small intestine. Several mucosal cell types can be identified in the duodenum, including absorptive cells lining intestinal villi, goblet cells secreting mucus, a few G cells, and Brunner's cells, which secrete a mucoid alkaline fluid.

The blood supply to the stomach and duodenum (Fig. 11-2) is remarkable for its rich anastomotic interconnections. The pancreatic duodenal arcades represent the major anastomotic connection between the celiac and superior mesenteric arteries. Parasympathetic (cholinergic) innervation is derived from the vagus nerve, while sympathetic (adrenergic) fibers reach the stomach through the celiac plexus. It is intriguing to recall that the majority of fibers contained

in the vagus nerve are sensory fibers carrying information from the gut to the brain.

PHYSIOLOGY OF GASTRODUODENAL DIGESTION AND ABSORPTION

The principal energy sources for cell work (carbohydrates, fats, and proteins) cannot be absorbed in their dietary forms. Therefore the intermediate process known as digestion must first convert such foodstuffs into their absorbable components. The basic digestive reaction underlying this conversion is hydrolysis, wherein specific enzymes split larger molecules into absorbable basic units, adding water to the reaction. In general, the gastroduodenal region is primarily responsible for initiating digestion, while absorption takes place further down the intestinal tract. Exceptions include alcohol, electrolytes, and ferrous iron, which can be absorbed directly from the stomach.

Carbohydrates

Dietary carbohydrate is primarily starch, lactose, and sucrose. Digestion is initiated when salivary amylase hydrolyzes complex sugars to maltose and isomaltose. Hydrolysis continues in the stomach until thorough agitation of gastric chyme produces sufficient acid mixing to inactivate the enzyme. The greater part of ingested carbohydrate is hydrolyzed under the influence of pancreatic amylase in the duodenum (Fig.

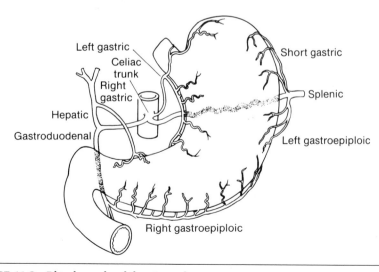

FIGURE 11-2 Blood supply of the stomach.

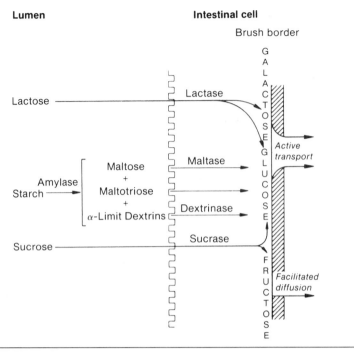

FIGURE 11-3   Digestion of carbohydrates.

11-3), which reduces polysaccharides to disaccharides and to lactose and sucrose. These sugars are further reduced to monosaccharides by the enzymes maltase, isomaltose, lactase, and sucrase, which are present in the brush borders of the intestinal mucosal cells. For the most part only monosaccharides are absorbed, and this occurs principally in the jejunum.

Proteins

Dietary proteins are usually long-chain polypeptides. Reduction to absorbable component amino acids is initiated in the stomach by the release of the preenzyme pepsinogen. Activation to pepsin requires the presence of gastric acid and does not occur at a pH greater than 3.5. Pepsin is an exopeptidase so that the end products of pepsin digestion are proteoses, peptones, and polypeptides, but not amino acids. In the duodenum, further digestion by pancreatic trypsin, chymotrypsin, and carboxypeptidase occurs (Fig. 11-4). Secretion of these enzymes is the result of the presence of partially digested proteins and fat in the duodenum, which causes the release of cholecystokinin-pancreozymin (CCK-PZ). This hormone, along with vagal stimulation, is a potent stimulus to pancreatic enzyme output. Each

enzyme is secreted as an inactive precursor that is subsequently activated by the duodenal hormone enterokinase. As the resultant dipeptides, amino acids, and smaller peptides travel farther down the small intestine, aminopolypeptidases and dipeptidases located in the brush border complete the degradation of protein to amino acids, which are then freely absorbed.

Fats

Dietary fats are principally triglycerides—neutral fats composed of three fatty acids linked to glycerol. Fat digestion occurs primarily in the small intestine (Fig. 11-5). Since enzymes that hydrolyze triglyceride are not soluble in fat, they can work only on the surface of a fat globule. Thus the available surface area is first increased by fragmenting large fat globules into many smaller units. This process, known as emulsification, is primarily caused by the action of bile salts in reducing surface tension of the larger fat globules.

In direct response to vagal stimulation and in indirect response to CCK-PZ released by the presence of protein and fat in the duodenum, pancreatic lipase is secreted into the duodenal lumen. Triglycerides are then hydrolyzed to fatty acids

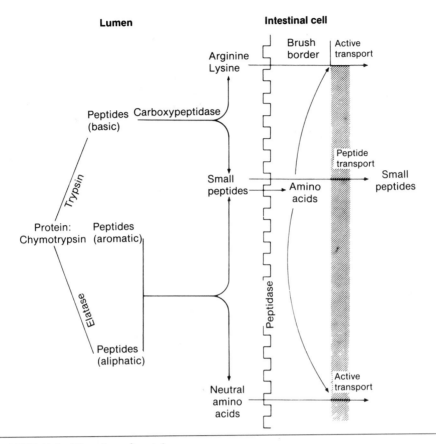

FIGURE 11-4 Digestion of proteins.

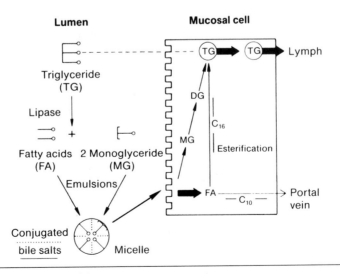

FIGURE 11-5 Digestion of fats.

and a few monoglycerides. However, unlike carbohydrate and protein digestion, hydrolysis alone is not sufficient to ensure absorption, because the free fatty acids and monoglycerides must first be rendered water soluble. Conjugated bile salts are equipped with both a water-soluble and a fat-soluble terminal. A configuration of bile salts with the fat-soluble terminal dissolved in the fat and the water-soluble terminal exposed is known as a micelle. Absorption of fats, which takes place primarily in the jejunum and ileum, is possible only because the external surface of the micelle is water-soluble. The fat-soluble vitamins A, D, E, and K are concomitantly absorbed by clinging to micellar interstices.

PHYSIOLOGY OF GASTRIC MOTOR ACTIVITY

Motor activity in the stomach is the result of autonomic and hormonal modulation of intrinsic gastric electrophysiologic activity. The stomach must simultaneously serve as a commodious reservoir for large volumes of ingested solids and liquids while ensuring that this material is delivered in an orderly fashion to the duodenum. The former function is accomplished primarily by the motor activity of the proximal portion of the stomach, the latter by the distal portion of the stomach. From a resting volume of 100 ml or less, the body of the stomach may increase to a volume of 1500 ml without an appreciable rise in intragastric pressure. This phenomenon, known as receptive relaxation, is dependent on vagal nerve integrity. If receptive relaxation cannot occur, as after vagal denervation of the proximal stomach as a result of parietal cell vagotomy, any sudden increase in gastric volume increases intragastric (IG) pressure and promotes accelerated gastric emptying of liquids.

In contrast to this controlled relaxation in the proximal stomach, vagal stimulation increases the frequency and magnitude of antral contractions. Such contractions propel ingested solid material against a closed pylorus and at the same time repropel that material back into the proximal stomach, thereby producing a mixing and grinding action. Eventually the pylorus opens to an integrated antral peristaltic wave (the antral-pyloric pump), which permits gastric emptying of solids. Therefore, by controlling the rate of relaxation in the proximal stomach and the magnitude and type of contraction in the distal stomach, the vagus nerve plays a dominant role in determining the rate of gastric emptying of both

liquids and solids. Gastric motor activity may be profoundly changed by tumor, ulcer, or operation. In humans, only the hormone motilin has a blood level that correlates with gastric motility. Erythromycin appears to act as a motilin agonist and may dramatically improve gastric emptying in certain patients with gastroparesis.

In the duodenum, wide fluctuations in temperature, pH, or osmotic pressure of gastric chyme initiate a neurohumoral reflex arc that inhibits gastric motility. However, the most profound reduction in gastric motility occurs when fat enters the duodenum. Cholecystokinin (CCK) has been shown to inhibit gastric emptying at physiologic doses.

PHYSIOLOGY OF GASTRIC ACID SECRETION

Total daily gastric secretory volumes approach 1500 ml and are composed principally of water and the ions hydrogen, sodium, potassium, chloride, and bicarbonate. There is a parietal and nonparietal cell component, both of which are nearly isotonic, with major differences in ionic composition (Table 11-1). Copious losses of gastric juices are usually best replaced by normal saline and potassium chloride. Organic constituents of gastric juice include intrinsic factor, several organic acids, mucus, and pepsin. Under basal conditions, a small amount of gastric acid is continually produced, presumably as a result of tonic vagal stimulation. Gastric acid is an important antimicrobial barrier. Achlorhydric patients have unusually high concentrations of gastric bacteria and may be more susceptible to enteritis and pulmonary infections.

There are three discernible yet totally integrated phases of gastric acid production (Table 11-2). The first is properly called the vagal or cephalic phase. The sight, smell, or thought of food elicits increased cortical and hypothalamic neural signals, which are transmitted through the vagus nerves to the stomach. Acid production resulting from vagal excitation is mediated primarily by direct vagal stimulation of parietal cells to release hydrochloride. The vagus also stimulates gastrin release, but this does not contribute significantly to the overall acid response seen during the cephalic phase. In addition, vagal stimulation excites gastric mucus production and releases the preenzyme pepsinogen, which, in turn, is fully activated as the pH falls to 2.0. Although the magnitude of the acid response to the vagal phase surpasses that produced by other phases, its duration is short. Therefore it accounts for only 20% (approximately) of the total volume of acid produced by a meal.

The gastric phase of acid secretion is initiated when food enters the stomach and continues during the several hours required for gastric emptying. The primary mediator of this phase is a polypeptide hormone, gastrin, which is released from antral mucosa by mucosal contact with partially digested proteins. Antral distension may also play some role. Gastrin is absorbed into the bloodstream and subsequently stimulates parietal cells to increase acid production. Pepsinogen release is also facilitated. Gastrin also stimulates mucosal somatostatin cells which inhibit acid secretion. The gastric phase accounts for approximately 70% of the total acid output in response to a meal.

Even after complete gastric emptying, acid production continues as long as gastric chyme remains in the proximal small intestine. The postulated mediator of this intestinal phase (enterooxyntin) has not been isolated. In any case, the intestinal phase accounts for only 5% to 10% of total acid output seen following a meal.

Although it is convenient to regard gastric acid production as occurring in isolated and sequential phases, such an arbitrary separation of factors is artificial. Instead, despite the fact that it contains separate receptors for histamine, gastrin, and acetylcholine, the parietal cell should be regarded as the final common pathway for acid production in response to several stimulatory mechanisms that coexist and overlap (Fig. 11-6). It is clear that all physiologically relevant parietal cell agonists work via the hydrogen potassium ATP-ase as a final common pathway. This is evident from both animal and human experiences with the potent H^+/K^+ ATP-ase inhibitor omeprazol, one dose of which completely blocks acid secretion for up to 24 hours. Another important characteristic of acid secretion is potentiation between agonists, that is, the administration of two agonists (e.g., histamine and gastrin), results in acid secretion that is greater than the sum of acid produced in response to either alone. Furthermore, histamine receptor blockers (H_2-blockers, e.g., cimetidine, ranitidine, and famotidine) inhibit the acid secretory response not only to histamine but also to acetylcholine and gastrin.

Once initiated, gastric acid production does not proceed indefinitely (Fig. 11-7). Passive inhi-

TABLE 11-1 Gastric Electrolytes: Approximate Composition (mEq/L)

	Parietal	Nonparietal
H^+	149	—
Na^+	4	135
K^+	17	8
Cl^-	166	120
HCO_3^-	—	25

Modified from Makhlouf GM, McManus JPA, Card WI. A quantitative statement of the two-component hypothesis of gastric acid secretion. Gastroenterology 51:149-171, 1966.

TABLE 11-2 Phases of Gastric Acid Secretion

Phase	Initiator	Pathway	Mediator at Parietal Cell
Cephalic	Feeding hypoglycemia	Vagal	Acetylcholine gastrin
Gastric	Distention Luminal amino acids and peptides	Vagovagal and local reflexes Direct stimulation G cells	Gastrin*
Intestinal	Small bowel distention Amino acid absorption	Hormonal Direct stimulation G cells	Entero-oxyntin† Gastrin

Modified from Debas HT. Peripheral regulation of gastric acid secretion. In Johnson LR, et al. (eds). Physiology of the Gastric Intestinal Tract, 2nd ed, vol 2. New York, Raven Press, 1987.
*Mediator for antral gastrin release by vagal reflexes unknown.
†A variety of "candidate entero-oxyntins" have been suggested but as yet this hormone has not been identified.

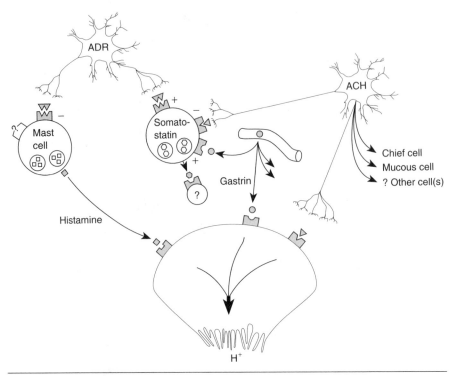

FIGURE 11-6   Model for regulation of acid secretion by canine parietal cell, illustrating the three receptors for the acid secretory agonists histamine, gastrin, and acetylcholine. This model also explains the clinical observation that H_2-blockers also inhibit gastrin-mediated acid secretion by blocking the potentiating and amplifying H_2-receptor on the parietal cell, perhaps unmasking gastrin's inhibitory influence via the somatostatin cell. (From Soll AH, Berglindh T. Physiology of isolated gastric glands and parietal cells: Receptors and effectors regulating function. In Johnson LR, et al. [eds]. Physiology of the Gastrointestinal Tract, 2nd ed, vol 1. New York: Raven Press, 1987, pp 883-909.)

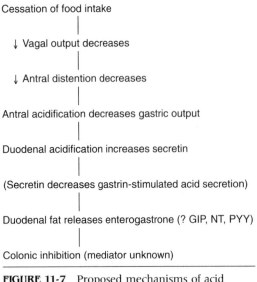

Cessation of food intake

↓ Vagal output decreases

↓ Antral distention decreases

Antral acidification decreases gastric output

Duodenal acidification increases secretin

(Secretin decreases gastrin-stimulated acid secretion)

Duodenal fat releases enterogastrone (? GIP, NT, PYY)

Colonic inhibition (mediator unknown)

FIGURE 11-7   Proposed mechanisms of acid inhibition.

bition of secretion occurs as stimulatory mechanisms spontaneously decrease with time. In addition, active inhibitors exist that function as negative feedback systems. When the pH of material in contact with the gastric antrum falls below 2.5, gastrin release is almost completely inhibited in a normal person. If antral pH rises above 5, gastrin release is again stimulated.

Transfer of acidified gastric content and fat into the duodenum markedly inhibits gastric acid production, as does the presence of hyperosmolar chyme. Both secretin, a hormone released from the duodenal wall in response to a fall in intraluminal pH, and CCK-PZ released by intraluminal fat and protein, inhibit the release of gastrin as well as its effect on the parietal cell. In addition, secretin leads to neutralization of acid chyme by stimulating pancreatic bicarbonate output. That other duodenal hormones may play an important role in inhibition of gastric acid production seems likely.

Gastrointestinal Hormones
(Table 11-3)

Over the past two decades there has been an explosion in our knowledge and understanding of gastrointestinal endocrinology. A meaningful discussion of all important aspects of this increasingly complex and clinically relevant field is beyond the scope of this text. However, the serious student of surgery should be familiar with the names and physiologic actions of gut hormones, especially where they currently affect patient care.

Somatostatin is a 14-amino acid peptide produced by a variety of neural and endocrine cells throughout the CNS and alimentary tract. As its name implies, it inhibits a variety of body functions including endocrine and exocrine secretion, mesenteric blood flow, and GI motility. With the development of the synthetic somatostatin analog octreotide, use of this gut hormone to treat a variety of GI maladies has become common. The current and future potential applications of this subcutaneously administered agent are listed in the box at right. Octreotide is rapidly becoming the drug of choice for malignant carcinoid syndrome and vasoactive intestinal polypeptide (VIP)–secreting tumors. It may also be useful in treating chronic pancreatitis and pancreatic fistulas. Its use may be relatively contraindicated in acute pancreatitis, however, since both human and animal studies suggest no benefit and possible exacerbation of this disease with somatostatin analog.

Motilin is the only hormone whose serum levels have been shown consistently to correlate with GI motor activity. Apparently erythromycin binds reversibly to motilin receptors and increases peristalsis. Recently this agent was shown to be useful in the treatment of diabetic gastroparesis, and there are some anecdotal reports of success with this agent in treatment of postgastrectomy stasis and primary gastroparesis.

Cholecystokinin can be administered to patients unable to eat (e.g., those with short gut or difficult fistulas) to facilitate gallbladder emptying. This may decrease the incidence of pathologic conditions of the gallbladder in this group of high-risk patients. *Glucagon* is commonly used by practicing radiologists, gastroenterologists, and surgeons primarily for its property of inhibiting smooth muscle contraction. Thus it inhibits spasm in the colon, facilitating contrast radiography and colonoscopy; it is also useful in cholangiography for overcoming a spasm of the sphincter of Oddi. Hypersecretion of *gastrin* is a

---

CLINICAL USE OF OCTREOTIDE

Effective (FDA approved)

Carcinoid syndrome
VIPoma

Probably Effective

Dumping syndrome
Pancreatic fistula
Enterocutaneous fistula
Esophageal varices

Experimental

Intestinal obstruction/ileus
Chronic pancreatitis
Antineoplastic
Pain relief
Tumor imaging

Not Effective

Acute pancreatitis
Nonvariceal GI bleeding

Modified from Hurst RD, Modlin IM. The therapeutic role of octreotide in the management of surgical disorders. Am J Surg 162:499-506, 1991.

---

common clinical finding that may lead to the development of gastroduodenal ulcer, but as yet there is no commercially available gastrin antagonist or inhibitor for use in these patients.

DUODENAL ULCER

Although the incidence of duodenal ulcer disease has decreased markedly in the Western world during the past 50 years, it is still a relatively common disorder, afflicting nearly one in ten adults in the United States at some time in their lives. Men in the middle decades of life are more frequently affected than women. The disease is usually a chronic one, characterized by frequent exacerbations and remissions. Nevertheless, in its uncomplicated form, duodenal ulcer is a relatively benign condition. As a consequence, 90% of patients can be adequately managed nonoperatively.

Pathophysiology

Although a unifying hypothesis has yet to be developed, much has been learned about the pathophysiology of duodenal ulcer disease in the past decade. However, the old axiom "no acid, no

TABLE 11-3 Gastrointestinal Hormones

Hormone	Major Source	Major Actions
Gastrin	Antral G cell	↑ Acid secretion ? Important trophic hormone
CCK	Duodenum, jejunum, brain	↑ Pancreatic (enzymes) secretion ↑ GB contraction + ↓ SO tone Other GI smooth muscle effects Enhances release of other GI hormones Candidate enterogastrone ? Appetite control
Secretin	Duodenum, jejunum	↑ Pancreatic HCO_3 secretion ↓ Serum gastrin except with ZE
Somatostatin	CNS; D cells in islets; somatostatin cells	Decrease by paracrine regulation secretion of gastric acid, insulin, glucagon ↓ Pancreatic exocrine secretion ? Decreased mucosal blood flow Inhibits release of most GI hormones Inhibits GI motility
Motilin	Duodenum/jejunum	Modulates GI myoelectric activity
GIP	Duodenum/jejunum	↑ Glucose-stimulated insulin secretion ↓ Stimulated acid secretion
Serotonin	E-C cells throughout gut	Modulates intestinal secretion and motility ? ↓ Gastric acid secretion
Neurotensin	Small bowel, ileum, > jejunum > duodenum	↓ Acid after fat (enterogastrone) ? Mediator of other effects of ingested fat (e.g., ↓ gastric emptying, ↑ pancreatic secretion)
PP	Pancreas	? Modulates pancreatic secretion
Peptide YY	Ileum and colon	? Enterogastrone ?↓ Pancreatic secretion
VIP	Colon, ileum and rest of gut	Vasodilation ↑ Intestinal secretion ↑ Pancreatic secretion ↓ Gastrin release ↓ SS release
Substance P	Gut (neurons) CNS	Smooth muscle contractions ↓ Bile flow ↑ Pancreatic flow Vasodilation
Enteroglucagon	Gut Pancreas	↓ Gastric acid secretion
Bombesin	Stomach Pancreas	Modulates release of other GI hormones ↑ Gastric and pancreatic secretion ? Satiety agent

From Stabile BE, Morrow DJ, Passaro E Jr. The gastrinoma triangle: Operative implications. Am J Surg 147:25-31, 1984.

What Stimulates?	What Inhibits?	Clinical Relevance
Antral distention Luminal peptide, aa, Ca^{++} Bombesin Catecholamines	Low gastric pH Somatostatin Prostaglandins	Acid hypersecretory states
Partially digested fat and protein Bombesin	?	GB emptying
Intraduodenal HCl	↑ Duodenal pH	Secretin stimulation test
Meal with fat and protein	? Cholinergics ? Substance P Serotonin	Carcinoid Islet tumor Fistula
Intraduodenal acid Intraduodenal alkali Intraduodenal fat Bombesin IV fat	Somatostatin, IV glucose, aa	E-mycin
Intestinal nutrients Vagotomy Beta-adrenergic stimulation	Alpha-adrenergic	?
Intraduodenal fat Intraduodenal acid Vagal input	Somatostatin	Carcinoid
Fatty meal	? Intraduodenal bile	?
Protein meal	Atropine	?
Enteric fat and other nutrients	?	?
Vagal stimulation	Alpha-adrenergic	VIPoma WDHA syndrome
Meal		? Dumping
Duodenal food Duodenal pH	?	?
Vagal stimulation	GIP	?

ulcer" is still true, and a gastroduodenal ulcer in an achlorhydric patient is malignant until proven otherwise. Most conventional therapies for duodenal ulcer disease are aimed at reducing the amount of acid produced by the stomach. This is so because as a group (although not necessarily as individuals), patients with duodenal ulcer contain twice the number of parietal cells in their stomachs as do normal persons. For this reason, they elaborate more acid in the basal state, when stimulated with exogenous secretogogs (histamine or pentagastrin), or following a meal. Acid is also delivered more rapidly into the duodenum and persists in that location for a longer period. Although no differences in basal serum gastrin levels are apparent, patients with duodenal ulcer demonstrate a greater gastrin response following ingestion of protein. In general, pepsin responses parallel acid responses in these individuals.

A defect in the acid "brake" on antral gastrin release has also been identified. It requires a lower intragastric pH to inhibit meal-stimulated gastrin release in duodenal ulcer patients compared with healthy persons. Secretin and CCK-PZ responses appear normal. Recently the defensive properties of the gastroduodenal mucosa have been the subject of increased attention among investigators interested in the pathophysiology of peptic ulcer disease (see the box below). While it is relatively easy to demonstrate the significance of the factors in a variety of animal models of mucosal injury, it is difficult to gauge the importance of these findings for human disease. Nevertheless, two agents that stimulate mucosal defense (sucralfate and misoprostol) have proved useful in the treatment of acid peptic ulcer disease in certain subsets of patients. It is clear that many of these defensive

factors are interrelated. Defective mucosal bicarbonate secretion has been demonstrated in patients with duodenal ulcer. The role of *Helicobacter pylori* infection in peptic ulcer disease remains controversial. The majority (85%) of patients with active ulcer disease have evidence of mucosal *Helicobacter* infection. Successful treatment of the infection with antibiotics heals the ulcers as successfully as H_2-blocker therapy and ulcer recurrence is almost always associated with recurrent *H. pylori* infestation. However, the great majority of patients with *H. pylori* infection never develop peptic ulcer disease, and the epidemiology of peptic ulcer differs from that of *H. pylori* infection. Thus the controversy continues.

Diagnosis

The most common presenting symptom in duodenal ulcer is a "gnawing, burning" midepigastric or right upper quadrant pain, aggravated by fasting, often awakening the patient at night and usually relieved by food or antacids. Occasionally the pain radiates straight through to the back, heralding penetration of the ulcer into the pancreas. Vomiting is an unusual feature, unless gastric outlet obstruction coexists. Definitive diagnosis is usually established by an **upper gastrointestinal series** or **endoscopy** showing the actual ulcer crater or markedly deformed duodenal bulb as a result of scarring. Sampling for *H. pylori* should be considered. Endoscopy is particularly useful in evaluating patients with ulcer symptoms following gastric surgery.

OTHER TESTS

Since more than one third of patients with proven duodenal ulcer will demonstrate normal acid responses, routine gastric secretory analysis is probably not indicated. However, **acid secretory tests** are still useful in the evaluation of some patients with duodenal ulcer disease, especially in those with recurrent or complicated ulcer disease. **Basal acid output (BAO)** measured after a 12-hour fast should be less than 4 mEq/hr. Values over 10 mEq/hr suggest gastrinoma. **Maximal acid output (MAO)**, a good index of parietal cell mass, is measured after IV histamine or pentagastrin and averages about 30 mEq/hr or less in normals. If BAO approaches MAO (i.e., BAO/MAO > 0.6), gastrinoma is likely.

Increasingly, fasting **serum gastrin measurements** are being made in patients with documented duodenal ulcer disease. Increasing success in the medical and surgical treatment of gas-

---

GASTRODUODENAL DEFENSIVE FACTORS

Bicarbonate secretion
Mucous secretion
Mucosal blood flow
Epithelial restitution
Intact surface epithelial cell structure and
  function
? Afferent sensory neurons
? Prostaglandin synthesis and availability
? Free radical scavengers
? Growth factors

trinoma by expert gastroenterologists and surgeons probably justifies this approach, provided that the ordering physician is aware of the other causes of hypergastrinemia *and* has access to expert consultation. However, serum gastrin measurement is imperative in patients with high BAO, recurrent ulcer postoperatively, endocrine tumor, or a strong family history of duodenal ulcer. The surgeon should never operate on a patient for duodenal ulcer while ignorant of the fact that the patient has a gastrinoma.

Before elective operation for intractable ulcer symptoms, the surgeon should rule out other potential causes of the upper abdominal symptoms. This will optimize the postoperative result and may stay the surgeon's hand in patients with other concomitant abnormalities that may herald a poor postoperative result. Tests useful in this regard include ultrasonography to rule out gallbladder disease and nuclear scintigraphy to evaluate esophageal, gastroduodenal, and biliary motor dysfunction.

Management

As indicated previously, most patients with duodenal ulcer can be successfully managed without surgical intervention. Although the role of diet in ulcer healing remains controversial, the role of cigarette smoking is clear. Healing rates are higher and recurrence rates lower in patients who stop smoking. Around the world a variety of agents are used in the medical treatment of duodenal ulcer (see the box at right and Surgical Pharmacopeia, p. 217). Because of their convenience, safety, and efficacy the H_2-receptor antagonists have become the mainstay of nonoperative therapy in the United States. These agents markedly inhibit basal and stimulated acid output and effect both symptomatic relief and endoscopic healing of duodenal ulcer in more than 80% of patients. Unfortunately, relapse is common (75%) once medication is discontinued, although the disease does not recur in more virulent form. Thus in some patients H_2-blocker therapy may be required for life. Long-term suppressive medications should be given to patients at increased risk for major morbidity from ulcer recurrence (see the box at right). Use of the most potent antisecretory agent, omeprazole, for treatment of peptic ulcer in nongastrinoma patients is controversial. While it is at least as efficacious in healing as the H_2-blockers, long-term use is expensive, may lead to overgrowth of gastric bacteria as a result of achlorhydria, and has been associated with the development of gas-

tric carcinoid tumors in rats. Generally operation is reserved for those few patients with duodenal ulcer for whom medical therapy fails and/or who develop one of the four cardinal complications (perforation, hemorrhage, obstruction, intractability).

GASTRIC ULCER

Three types of benign gastric ulcer occur in the stomach, according to Johnson. The most common (65%) is the type I ulcer, which can occur anywhere in the stomach at or above the proximal border of the antrum. It is usually situated at or near the angularis incisura on the lesser curvature and is always associated with antral gastritis. Type II gastric ulcer (20%) often occurs in the distal portion of the stomach and is associated with active duodenal ulcer disease or a scarred duodenum (i.e., inactive duodenal ulcer disease). Antral stasis may play a role in the development of type II gastric ulcer. Type III gastric ulcer is a prepyloric ulcer (15%). Type II and III gastric ulcers are etiologically akin to duodenal ulcer and are managed in the same way. Type I gastric ulcer, however, is a pathophysiologically distinct entity, occurring in older patients, many

---

DRUGS FOR DUODENAL ULCER

Antacids
H_2-blockers (cimetidine, ranitidine, famotidine, etc.)
Sucralfate
Colloidal bismuth
Proton pump inhibitors (omeprazole)
Prostaglandins

RISKS FOR MAJOR MORBIDITY FROM ULCER RECURRENCE

>65 years of age
Smoking
NSAID use
Frequent recurrence ($\geq$ 2/yr)
History of complication
Major concomitant illness
? Immunosuppression

of whom are salicylate abusers. It affects women as often as men, is usually associated with normal or reduced secretion of acid, and is characterized by frequent relapse following initially successful nonoperative management (>50%). Current evidence favors the hypothesis that this most common type of gastric ulcer is a result of excessive regurgitation of duodenal contents through an incompetent pylorus that in turn causes an extensive gastritis and an attendant decrease in mucosal resistance to ulceration. *Helicobacter pylori* may be a permissive factor. In South America (and perhaps increasingly so in this country), many gastric ulcers tend to be situated very high on the lesser curvature in the region near the gastroesophageal (GE) junction (Csendes type IV gastric ulcer).

Diagnosis

Symptoms of gastric ulcer are similar to those of duodenal ulcer, except that food may exacerbate rather than relieve the typical pain, which is often experienced in the epigastrium to the left of the midline. Gastric ulcers are readily detected by an upper gastrointestinal series. The key diagnostic consideration is to differentiate type I benign gastric ulcer from ulcerating gastric cancer. Gastric secretory studies are of little value in this regard. A competent radiologist can make this distinction in 80% of instances. However, gastroscopy with multiple biopsies (≥8) and brushings for cytologic studies has become the standard for determining benignity and should be performed in all patients with gastric ulcer. If malignancy is confirmed, operation is mandatory, because if gastric cancer is resected early, before it spreads to lymph nodes, the 5-year survival rate approximates 40%. In contrast, 5-year survival is only 5% when the lymphatic system has become involved.

Management

After malignancy has been ruled out by the appropriate endoscopic studies, patients with noncomplicated gastric ulcers of all types are initially treated similarly to patients with duodenal ulcer (i.e., with H_2-receptor blockers). It must be remembered, however, that gastric ulcers tend to heal more slowly than duodenal ulcers. However, because of the specter of gastric malignancy, healing must be assessed and a low threshold for repeat endoscopy and biopsy maintained. Most benign gastric ulcers should show signs of significant healing (ulcer size decreased by at least 50%) after 8 weeks of effective medical therapy. If a good-quality barium study shows complete healing of the gastric ulcer with no other abnormalities, the patient may be carefully followed. However, the clinician should be aware that benign gastric ulcers may be associated with a gastric malignancy elsewhere in the stomach, and even malignant gastric ulcers can show significant signs of healing.

For these reasons, many practitioners prefer endoscopic follow-up in patients with gastric ulcers. If after 8 weeks of adequate treatment a persistent ulcer cavity is present, repeat biopsies and brushings should be taken. If these yield negative results the patient may be treated for another 8 weeks. If the ulcer has not healed at this time, even if it is benign, the patient should be considered a candidate for surgery.

Although H_2-receptor blockers have become the standard medical treatment of uncomplicated gastric ulcer, it should be remembered that other drugs, such as sucralfate, antacids, and prostaglandin analogs may be useful for treating these patients. Additionally, a very important part of the medical treatment is to insist that the patient cease the use of tobacco and alcohol and if possible also NSAIDs (see the box on p. 207). The recurrence rate of gastric ulcer in patients who have healed one ulcer remains high, especially in elderly persons, those who smoke or regularly consume alcohol, and in those who take nonsteroidal anti-inflammatory drugs or aspirin. Since the morbidity of recurrent gastric ulcer in this population has been shown to be significant, it is not unreasonable to maintain patients on some sort of prophylaxis against recurrent gastric ulcer. This should consist of either H_2-blocker therapy, diligent use of sucralfate, or perhaps in some patients prostaglandin analogs (misoprostol).

NSAIDS AND PEPTIC ULCER

Nonsteroidal anti-inflammatory drugs (NSAIDs) such as aspirin, indomethacin, and ibuprofen are the most commonly consumed drugs in the world. Not surprisingly, they are associated with a significant number of adverse events, including morbidity from peptic ulcer. NSAID therapy is associated with the development of gastric ulcer in about 15% of patients, while duodenal ulcer is less common (in 5%). However, most patients who regularly take these agents have evidence on endoscopic evaluation of injury to the gastroduodenal mucosa. It is sobering to realize that the recent increase in hospitalizations for bleeding gastric ulcers has paralleled the increased consumption of NSAIDs in this country. In one study patients admitted to hospital with bleeding or perforated gastric or duodenal ulcers were more than twice as likely to be taking NSAIDs when compared with age-matched controls. In another study more than 80% of deaths from ulcers occurred in patients taking NSAIDs. NSAID ulcers also tend to be silent until they bleed or perforate.

Prophylaxis against NSAID ulcer is controversial, as is the efficacy of H_2-receptor blockers in this regard. However, with the development of more potent antisecretory drugs (e.g., omeprazol) and physiologically specific agents (e.g., prostaglandin analogs), most experts recommend prophylaxis in high-risk patients taking NSAIDs—the elderly, women, and smokers. Treatment of established peptic ulcers in patients taking NSAIDs is essential and if possible should include cessation of NSAIDs. If this is not possible, a duodenal ulcer can be healed with H_2-receptor blockers, but the more recalcitrant NSAID gastric ulcer should probably be treated with misoprostol or omeprazol.

Indications for Operation in Peptic Ulcer Disease

The indication for operation in patients with duodenal and gastric ulcer disease are quite similar, although malignancy is rarely an issue in the former and obstruction infrequently complicates the latter (see the box below).

Hemorrhage. About 20% of patients with peptic ulcer disease will develop significant UGI bleeding, a complication that accounts for about

40% of all ulcer mortality. Most of these patients will have significant symptoms before bleeding begins, except that patients taking NSAIDs frequently present with bleeding or perforation as the first manifestation of their ulcer disease. Depending on the patient population, patients with bleeding peptic ulcer account for over half of all patients admitted to hospital with UGI bleeding.

Work-up and management of patients with bleeding peptic ulcer depend on the acuity and severity of hemorrhage. Hematemesis or melena require IV fluid resuscitation and urgent endoscopy. The mortality rate for bleeding ulcer is about 10% (stable over the past 40 years); death occurs almost exclusively in the 25% of patients in whom bleeding persists or recurs after initial treatment. Predictors of bad outcome include advanced age, shock, hematemesis, hematochezia, a blood pressure on presentation <90 mm Hg systolic, endoscopic stigmata of recent hemorrhage, and transfusion requirements greater than 8 to 10 units. Patients with any of these criteria require ICU admission, as well as expert endoscopic and surgical care. In selected cases, endoscopic treatment of bleeding ulcer with a technique of thermocoagulation (laser, bicap cautery, heater probe) or injection (sclerosant or vasoconstrictor) may allow a safer elective operation. Occasionally, angiography is of diagnostic and/or therapeutic use.

Operation should be considered in patients at risk for continued bleeding or rebleeding. Acute bleeding requiring 4 or more units of blood should prompt serious consideration for operation, as should prior history of a bleeding ulcer, a visible vessel on endoscopy, giant ulcer, or shock. For a bleeding duodenal ulcer, suture ligation of the bleeding vessel may be combined with vagotomy and drainage or vagotomy and antrectomy. For a bleeding gastric ulcer, resection is preferable (since it excises the ulcer), but a biopsy and oversewing combined with vagotomy and drainage are acceptable in an unstable patient.

Perforation. Perforation usually complicates anterior duodenal or gastric ulcers, although posterior gastric and posterolateral duodenal perforations do occur. This complication of peptic ulcer occurs less commonly than bleeding but is probably more dangerous, with an overall mortality rate of about 15%. Associated hemorrhage is uncommon, but if present suggests another posterior ("kissing") ulcer that should be sought and treated by operation. Antecedent ulcer symptoms may be absent. Early operation is mandatory, and the need for operation is usually obvious because most patients have peritonitis.

INDICATIONS FOR OPERATION IN PEPTIC ULCER DISEASE

Duodenal Ulcer

Bleeding
Perforation
Obstruction
Pain (i.e., "intractability")

Gastric Ulcer

Failure to heal (i.e., suspect cancer)
Bleeding
Perforation
Pain

Pneumoperitoneum evidenced on upright chest and abdominal x-ray films is present in about 85% to 90% of patients. Parenteral antibiotics are given immediately and aggressive fluid resuscitation is begun. For perforated duodenal ulcer, options at operation include closure of the perforation (usually with a "Graham patch" of omentum), with or without a definitive ulcer procedure (usually truncal vagotomy and drainage, although parietal cell vagotomy is a viable alternative). Contraindications to definitive ulcer operation include shock and exudative peritonitis. Indications for definitive operation include prior ulcer history or risk factors such as use of NSAIDs, tobacco, or alcohol.

The high rate of clinical exacerbation (>70%) in patients with previous ulcer symptoms treated by simple closure alone, together with the recognition that most patients can safely have closure and definitive operation, has swung the pendulum of surgical treatment for perforated duodenal ulcer toward definitive operative care.

Perforated gastric ulcer is associated with higher mortality than perforated duodenal ulcer, partly because the patients tend to be older. Furthermore, some perforations occur posteriorly, causing a lesser sac infection that is hard to eradicate. Furthermore, the bacterial load in the stomach and exuded gastric juice may be greater in these patients, since many are relatively achlorhydric. The operation of choice for perforated gastric ulcer is excision, usually by gastric resection. This is usually easier (and perhaps safer) than simple closure for what often are large perforations. Also, it is probably adequate treatment for the 10% or so of patients originally thought to have a perforated benign gastric ulcer who turn out to have a perforated cancer. *Closure without biopsy is condemned.*

Obstruction. As an indication for operation, obstruction is usually a complication of duodenal ulcer; obstruction from gastric ulcer suggests malignancy. Development of gastric outlet obstruction complicating a duodenal ulcer is heralded clinically by distention and frequent episodes of vomiting of undigested food. Obstruction resulting from scarring represents the endpoint of the repeated bouts of exacerbation and healing so characteristic of the disease. It must be differentiated from edema and functional obstruction secondary to a reactivated acute ulcer, because the former requires operation, whereas the latter may not. Once the diagnosis of obstruction is made, this differentiation is best accomplished in the hospital by using prolonged nasogastric decompression and intravenous H_2-blockers. Endoscopy is most useful in ruling out

cancer. After 5 to 7 days of such therapy, gastric emptying is reassessed. Ordinary barium studies are usually adequate to accomplish this task. If obstruction persists, operation is indicated. The most useful procedures in this regard are probably truncal vagotomy and gastrojejunostomy or vagotomy and antrectomy. The several days of gastric decompression have not been wasted, since this maneuver serves to restore tone to the dilated stomach and ameliorates the not uncommon postoperative delay in the return of gastric motor function.

In patients with duodenal ulcer, *intractability* implies persistence of disabling pain despite maximal nonoperative support. In patients with gastric ulcer, intractability usually implies failure to heal and this suggests gastric malignancy. There are probably few benign intractable ulcers, but there are many patients with intractable ulcers (i.e., individuals with peptic ulcer disease) who are either unwilling or unable to follow the rigidly prescribed lifestyle associated with an effective medical regimen. Such a differentiation is probably immaterial, because the end result is always incapacitation or nonhealing.

It is commonly held that individuals operated on for intractable duodenal ulcer are likely to have persisting symptoms or to develop disabling postgastrectomy syndromes. This is a misconception, because the results achieved following operations for pain are indistinguishable from those obtained when the same procedure is employed for one of the other indications, provided the diagnosis is secure. Parietal cell vagotomy and truncal vagotomy and drainage (TV&D) are good surgical options for intractable duodenal ulcer. An intractable or nonhealing gastric ulcer should be treated with partial gastrectomy to include the ulcer.

CHOICE OF OPERATION FOR DUODENAL ULCER

Which of the several available operations to use in a given patient with duodenal ulcer has been the subject of intense debate for decades. Before the advent of controlled clinical trials these discussions were characterized by more heat than light. It is now apparent that differences in the alleged virtues and disadvantages of each are less than previously thought. In general, currently acceptable operative procedures can be classified into two main groups—those that involve primarily a resection of the portion of the stomach and those that involve partial or complete interruption of visceral afferent vagus nerve fibers (Fig. 11-8). In the paragraphs that follow, each is discussed briefly in terms of its rationale, technique, advantages, and disadvantages.

Truncal Vagotomy and Drainage

In the TV&D procedure, currently the most popular operative approach to duodenal ulcer disease in the United States, the stomach is deliberately totally denervated, thereby interrupting the cephalic phase of secretion while maintaining the intactness of the gastric reservoir. As noted previously, however, the motor function of the stomach is also affected: gastric emptying of liquids is hastened, and, more importantly, gastric emptying of solids is delayed. Accordingly, some concomitant procedure to promote gastric drainage is necessary.

The addition of gastroenterostomy to truncal vagotomy allows gastric contents to exit directly into the jejunum. The gastroenterostomy must

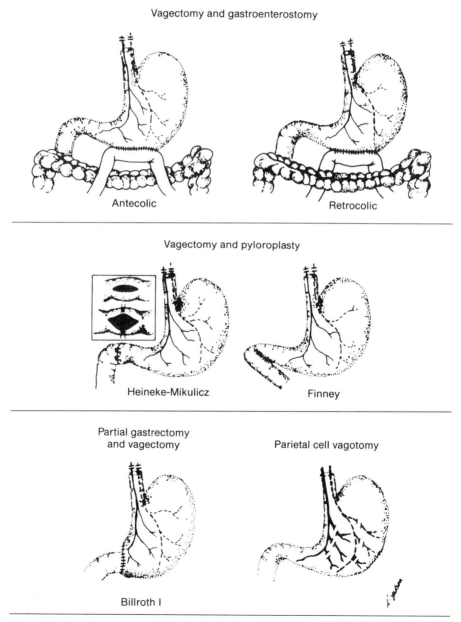

Vagectomy and gastroenterostomy

Antecolic   Retrocolic

Vagectomy and pyloroplasty

Heineke-Mikulicz   Finney

Partial gastrectomy and vagectomy   Parietal cell vagotomy

Billroth I

FIGURE 11-8 Common gastric operations.

be placed in the most dependent region of the stomach to minimize gastric residue. Another type of drainage procedure, the pyloroplasty, is more commonly practiced. The several types available (Heineke-Mikulicz, Finney, Jabouley) essentially enlarge the exit from the stomach. Clear-cut superiority of one drainage procedure over another has not been established.

At present it seems clear that truncal vagotomy and drainage is one of the safest procedures available, is associated with minimal weight loss postoperatively, and carries the same risk of dumping (see below) as does truncal vagotomy combined with resection. Its principal disadvantage is that the threat of recurrent ulcer disease is high: 5% to 8% in 5 years, 10% to 15% in 10 years, and perhaps as high as 30% in 15 years.

Truncal Vagotomy With Hemigastrectomy

This procedure is currently a mainstay in the operative treatment of duodenal ulcer disease. In theory, its virtue is that it abolishes both the cephalic and gastric phases of gastric acid secretion. In fact, its efficacy may relate more to the fact that complete antrectomy seems to provide additional protection if vagus section is incomplete, a common problem when truncal vagotomy is utilized. As illustrated in Fig. 11-8, gastrointestinal continuity can be restored either by gastroduodenostomy (Billroth I) or by closure of the duodenal stump and gastroenterostomy (Billroth II). This procedure is associated with the most admirable "cure" rate of any currently acceptable operation (greater than 99% at 5 years), but unfortunately carries a somewhat higher mortality rate than do the other operations.

Parietal Cell Vagotomy

The objective of this more recently introduced procedure is to denervate only the proximal parietal cell containing portions of the stomach, while maintaining innervation of the antrum and pylorus and remainder of the alimentary tract. In this way, a drainage procedure is unnecessary and normal rates of gastric emptying of solids are achieved. Dumping and diarrhea are minimized. Although simple in concept, parietal cell vagotomy is difficult to execute well, since it requires precise definition of the anterior and posterior antral nerves, which must be preserved, and extensive periesophageal dissection. The operation is inappropriate in a patient with cicatricial pyloric obstruction or with prepyloric ulcer. It may also be a poor choice for a patient

with an ulcer refractory to the blocker therapy. Without question, postoperative dumping is almost totally avoided by the procedure. On the other hand, several studies suggest that a recurrence rate comparable with or higher than that of truncal vagotomy and drainage can be anticipated. Posterior truncal vagotomy with anterior highly selective vagotomy produces ulcer healing and good functional results. This procedure has the advantage that it can be performed laparoscopically.

POSTGASTRECTOMY SYNDROMES

Several late complications may be manifested after an uneventful recovery from gastric surgery. These postgastrectomy syndromes are summarized in Table 11-4. One or more may be seen in 20% of patients. Fortunately, the great majority of such remote complications are readily controlled by nonoperative means. Two of the more vexing are discussed in detail below.

Dumping Syndrome

This syndrome, which occurs in moderate to severe degree in 5% to 10% of patients following gastric operations, consists of a constellation of vasocutaneous (tachycardia, sweating, pallor) and intestinal (bloating, cramping, explosive diarrhea) symptoms shortly following ingestion of a meal. Its pathophysiology relates to the fact that in the absence of either a commodious gastric reservoir or a restraining pylorus (or both), ingested food is inadequately diluted in the stomach and hyperosmotic chyme is delivered rapidly into the small intestine. Here dilution occurs at the expense of the plasma volume, visceral distention ensues, and a variety of humoral agents, including serotonin, bradykinin, and possibly vasoactive intestinal peptide, are released, with the clinical end result indicated. The vast majority of patients with the syndrome can be managed by nonoperative means. Treatment consists of frequent, small, carbohydrate-poor feedings and avoidance of liquids with meals.

Although anticholinergic, antihistaminic, and serotonin antagonists may be tried, the most promising agent for the treatment of severe early dumping is octreotide. This agent is administered subcutaneously before meals and may also be useful in late postprandial dumping thought to be caused by abnormalities in glucose tolerance. If despite such measures the patient is still severely handicapped by the dumping syndrome, a short antiperistaltic segment of jejunum interposed between the residual stomach and proximal intestine to delay gastric emptying has been recommended; it is difficult to be sure of the value of this procedure.

Recurrent (Marginal) Ulcer

Postoperative development of an ulcer in the small bowel in approximation to the gastro-enteric stoma is generally referred to as a marginal ulcer. Such ulcers develop after operation in less than 1% to more than 25% of patients, depending on the initial procedure employed and the length of follow-up, and are heralded by a recurrence of typical ulcer symptoms. Although patients with preoperative hypersecretion of acid are at greater risk, secretory studies are not sufficiently discriminating for diagnosis, which is best made by endoscopy. Recurrence is usually related to incomplete vagotomy. Gastrinoma and MEN type I (see below) must be ruled out, and retained antrum searched for. In the past, reoperative therapy has been clearly superior to nonoperative management. However H_2-receptor blocking agents may alter this view. A recent trial revealed complete healing in all cimetidine-treated patients (versus 13% with placebo). Therefore a trial with H_2-blockers is warranted before undertaking reoperation.

Zollinger-Ellison Syndrome

The *Zollinger-Ellison syndrome (ZE)* consists of massive acid hypersecretion, refractory often virulent peptic ulcer disease, and gastrin producing tumor. Abdominal pain with or without diarrhea is the most common symptom. Multiple ulcers, ulcers in an unusual location (jejunal), or multiple recurrences of peptic ulcer should all suggest the diagnosis. However, because of increased awareness of the importance of this syndrome in acid-peptic disease, most patients diagnosed with ZE today have a typical duodenal ulcer. Reflux esophagitis is an increasingly common presentation.

Although clinical history, radiographic signs (e.g., multiple ulcers, giant rugal folds), or gastric analysis (BAO/MAO >0.6) are suggestive, the diagnosis of ZE is best made by elevated serum gastrin. Other causes of hypergastrinemia (achlorhydria, retained antrum, G cell hyperplasia, vagotomy) can be ruled out by gastric analysis and secretin stimulation test. An increase in serum gastrin of 200 pg/ml or greater after IV secretin is diagnostic of gastrinoma if gastric pH is low.

Gastrinomas occur sporadically (80%) or in association with multiple endocrine neoplasia syndrome type I (20%; see below). Most sporadic gastrinomas occur in the gastrinoma triangle (Fig. 11-9); pancreatic head, duodenum, lymph nodes, and antrum are the common locations. Currently about a third of patients with gastrinoma have metastatic disease at the time of diagnosis. Although the more potent antisecretory drugs have made the management of acid hypersecretion easier, a diligent evaluation to localize a gastrinoma should be made since surgical resection may be curative. Useful preoperative tests include ultrasound, CT scan, arteriography, selective intra-arterial secretin injection with hepatic venous gastrin measurements and MRI scanning. Useful intraoperative tests include ultrasonography and endoscopy.

Patients with ZE syndrome and sporadic gastrinoma should have operation and tumor resection. In experienced hands the tumor will be found in 70% to 100% of patients. Since multiple tumors are not unusual, a thorough exploration is necessary. Lymph node metastases should be removed. Although some patients with liver metastases may benefit from partial hepatectomy for debulking, most patients with diffusely metastatic disease are best managed nonoperatively. If tumor cannot be found, parietal cell vagotomy should be performed, since this may decrease the requirement for antisecretory medication. We add this low-morbidity procedure even in patients undergoing curative resection for gastrinoma. Total gastrectomy, once the mainstay of surgical therapy for ZE syndrome, is now rarely indicated because of the efficacy of antisecretory

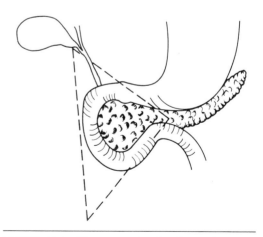

FIGURE 11-9 The anatomic triangle in which gastrinomas are most often found. (From Stabile BE, Morrow DJ, Passaro E Jr. The gastrinoma triangle: Operative implications. Am J Surg 147:25-31, 1984.)

TABLE 11-4 Postgastrectomy Syndromes

Type	Symptoms	Relation to Meals
Early satiety	Upper abdominal fullness, discomfort, eructations	Toward end of meal
Dumping	Upper abdominal bloating, cramping, nausea, vomiting, weakness, palpitations, syncope, flushing, sweating, diarrhea	15 min-1 hour after meals
Late postprandial hypoglycemia	Palpitations, weakness, syncope, sweating	2-3 hours after meals
Malabsorption	Steatorrhea, wasting, avitaminosis	No temporal relation
Diarrhea	Abdominal distension, with occasional cramp, followed by diarrhea	30 min-1 hour after meals
Anemia	Weakness, easy fatigability	No temporal relation
Acute complete afferent loop obstruction	Cramping, abdominal pain, and projectile vomiting, peritonitis	No temporal relation
Chronic partial afferent loop obstruction	Upper abdominal distension and discomfort; relief by bilious vomiting	Between meals, usually 1-2 hours after meals
Alkaline gastritis	Burning epigastric pain unrelieved by antacids; bilious vomiting	No temporal relation
Marginal ulcer	Burning epigastric pain relieved by antacids	Symptoms often relieved by food ingestion

Pathophysiology	Nonoperative Treatment	Operative Treatment
Small gastric pouch fills rapidly and results in gastric distension	Multiple small feedings	Enlargement of gastric pouch with small bowel or colon
Rapid gastric emptying and hyperosmolarity of food, and hypermotility of small intestine result in sequestration of fluid into jejunum, jejunal distension, and abnormal vascular homeostasis	Multiple small feedings of isosmolar diet low in fluid volume and carbohydrates, anticholinergics, postcibal recumbency	Rarely indicated; antiperistaltic jejunal interposition, possibly conversion of gastroenterostomy to Roux-en-Y limb
Rapid absorption of carbohydrate to hyperglycemic levels with correspondingly rapid insulin response, inappropriately high levels of insulin result in subsequent rebound from hyperglycemia to hypoglycemia	Multiple small feedings low in freely hydrolyzed and absorbed carbohydrate, between-meal carbohydrates	Not required
Restricted food intake due to postgastrectomy syndromes and/or fear of same, jejunal bacterial overgrowth, pancreaticocibal asynchrony, reduced allowable absorption time, altered proximal jejunal mucosa	Conduct thorough metabolic studies and give appropriate therapy	Rarely required except to correct a blind loop
Occurs in procedures associated with vagectomy, possibly as a consequence of bile salt deconjugation	Cholestyramine, anticholinergics, low fluid intake, rule out steatorrhea and dumping	Rarely indicated; antiperistaltic jejunal interposition
Achlorhydria and duodenal bypass may result in poor iron absorption, loss of intrinsic factor or bacterial destruction may result in poor B_{12} or folate absorption	Parenteral iron or B_{12} and folic acid as required	Not required
Overly long afferent loop insinuates behind efferent loop producing complete small bowel obstruction; pancreatitis and duodenal gangrene	None	Fixation or shortening of afferent loop; rarely pancreatico-duodenectomy is required
Sudden decompression of partial duodenal obstruction with regurgitation into stomach and bilious vomiting	None	Jejunojejunostomy or conversion of Billroth II to Billroth I
Regurgitation of alkaline intestinal contents back into gastric pouch; damage possibly due to effect of bile salts and back diffusion of hydrochloric acid	Bile salt-binding agents	Conversion of gastroenterostomy to Roux-en-Y limb; vagotomy must be complete!
Continued postoperative excess secretion of acid due to incomplete vagectomy, inadequate resection, retained antrum, Z-E or MEN, type 1 syndrome	Duodenal ulcer treatment regimen	Correct specific cause

therapy and because of the success of gastrinoma resection in centers with physicians experienced in the procedure.

About 20% of patients with ZE syndrome have multiple endocrine neoplasia type I (Wermer's syndrome). These patients have multiple adenomas (of pituitary, parathyroid, and pancreas). In these patients gastrinomas are almost always multiple and frequently microscopic. Thus abdominal operation is rarely curative and, although controversial, is probably best avoided. Treatment of hyperparathyroidism by parathyroidectomy in these patients makes the acid

peptic disease much easier to manage. The definition of malignant gastrinoma is problematic but usually means the tumor has metastasized to the lymph nodes, liver, or, rarely, to bone. Analysis of DNA and hormones produced by gastrinomas may predict clinical behavior more accurately in the future. However, most sporadic tumors left untreated will eventually metastasize. Important prognostic factors include resectability and MEN status. Undoubtedly, better pharmacologic management of acid hypersecretion has decreased the often fatal complications of uncontrolled ulcer diathesis.

PITFALLS AND COMMON MYTHS

- *Gastric cancer management.* We continue to see patients who have been managed as having a benign gastric ulcer who turn out to have gastric cancer. This could be avoided by aggressive endoscopy with biopsies and cytologic brushings together with an upper GI series (which often complements endoscopy) in all patients with signs and symptoms of gastric ulcer. Gastric resection should be *seriously* considered in all patients who fail to heal after a trial of good medical therapy.

- *Delay in surgery for a bleeding ulcer.* While it is clear that most patients with bleeding peptic ulcer will stop bleeding "permanently," it is also increasingly clear that some patients are at very high risk for rebleeding and death. Most such patients can be identified by rather simple clinical and endoscopic criteria and should be operated on earlier, not later. *Experienced surgeons and endoscopists should be involved in the management of these patients from the time they enter the hospital door.*

- *Poor patient selection.* It is tempting for both patient and surgeon to ascribe all sorts of upper abdominal complaints to peptic ulcer. However, the endoscopic or radiologic presence of a gastric or duodenal ulcer does not necessarily mean that the patient's complaints result from this malady. This is particularly relevant for patients being considered for operation to treat intractable or recurrent peptic ulcer and may be one reason why the results of operation in some patients are suboptimal. Preoperative evaluation of the following may be useful and will help to maximize operative results: gastric emptying, gallbladder function and biliary excretion, duo-

denogastric reflux, *Helicobacter* infection, and gastroesophageal reflux.

- *Overuse of the Roux-en-Y gastrojejunostomy.* This operation should probably be reserved for patients with intractable bile vomiting who have intragastric bile acid concentration greater than two standard deviations above the norm. Most of these patients have had previous gastric surgery (Billroth I or II). The Roux-en-Y operation delays gastric emptying dramatically in some patients; it is also inherently ulcerogenic. Thus the operation is best used infrequently for specific indications. Complete vagotomy decreases the risk of marginal ulceration and generous gastrectomy may decrease the incidence of postoperative gastric stasis.

- *More is better.* This is probably not true in surgery for peptic ulcer disease. Considering the safety and effectiveness of H_2-blockers or omeprazole for recurrent ulcer, it is probably more rational to do a safer, lesser ulcer operation with a higher risk of recurrence than to do a larger operation with a lower recurrence rate but more long-term morbidity and higher operative mortality.

- *One operation for all.* Operative treatment for duodenal and gastric ulcer disease must be individualized. Vagotomy and antrectomy may be the right operation for an obese noncompliant man with an intractable duodenal ulcer, but an asthenic young woman who wishes to become pregnant and thus stop her maintenance ulcer medication might be better treated with (laparoscopic?) parietal cell vagotomy.

SURGICAL PHARMACOPEIA

Drug	Indications	Complications	Dosage
Cimetidine (Tagamet)	Peptic ulcer disease	GI symptoms, confusion, rash, headache	300 mg qid or 800 mg hs PO
Ranitidine (Zantac)	Other hypersecretory conditions		150 mg bid or 300 mg hs PO
Famotidine (Pepcid)	Gastroesophageal reflux?		20-40 mg qhs PO
Nizatidine (Axid)			300 mg qhs or 150 mg bid PO
Omeprazole (Prilosec)	Active duodenal ulcer Severe erosive esophagitis Zollinger-Ellison syndrome	GI symptoms, headache, rash	20 mg PO daily for 4-8 weeks
Octreotide acetate (Sandostatin)	Metastatic carcinoid tumor Vipomas Intestinal fistulas	Gallstones, GI symptoms Musculoskeletal pain Headache, dizziness	100-600 μg/d in 2-4 divided doses IV
Misoprostol (Cytotec)	Prevention of NSAID-induced gastric ulcers	Abortifacient property in pregnancy; GI symptoms	200 μg qid PO
Sucralfate (Carafate)	Peptic ulcer disease	Decreased bioavailability of digitalis, phenytoin (Dilantin), tetracycline GI symptoms	1 g qid PO or bid PO
Metoclopramide hydrochloride (Reglan)	Diabetic gastroparesis Antiemetic Gastroesophageal reflux	Restlessness, drowsiness, fatigue, extrapyramidal symptoms, depression, tardive dyskinesia	10 mg PO tid
Glucagon	Diagnostic aid in radiology and facilitation of endoscopy	Nausea, vomiting	0.5 units IV or 2 mg IM

BIBLIOGRAPHY

Adami H-O, et al. Recurrences 1 to 10 years after highly selective vagotomy in prepyloric and duodenal ulcer: Frequency, patterns, and predictors. Ann Surg 199:393-399, 1984.

Amdrup E, Andersen D, Hostrub MD. The Aarhus County vagotomy trial; Parts I and II. World J Surg 2:85, 1978.

Boey J, et al. Risk stratification in perforated duodenal ulcers: A prospective validation of predictive factors. Ann Surg 205:22-26, 1987.

Davis Z, Verhuyden CN, Van Heerden JA, et al. The surgically treated chronic gastric ulcer: An extended follow-up. Ann Surg 185:205, 1977.

Debas HT. Peripheral regulation of gastric acid secretion. In Johnson LR, et al. (eds). Physiology of the Gastric Intestinal Tract, 2nd ed, vol 2. New York, Raven Press, 1987.

Elashoff JD, Grossman MI. Trends in hospital admission and death rates for peptic ulcer in the United States from 1970-1978. Gastroenterology 78:280-285, 1980.

Fromm D. Complications of Gastric Surgery. New York, John Wiley & Sons, 1977.

Herrington JL, Davidson J. Bleeding gastroduodenal ulcers: Choice of operations. World J Surg 11:304, 1987.

Howard TJ, et al. Gastrinoma excision for cure: A prospective analysis. Ann Surg 211:7-14, 1990.

Hunt PS. Surgical management of bleeding chronic peptic ulcer: A 10-year prospective study. Ann Surg 199:44-50, 1984.

Hurst RD, Modlin IM. The therapeutic role of octreotide in the management of surgical disorders. Am J Surg 162:499-505, 1991.

Jensen DM. Economic and health aspects of peptic ulcer disease and H_2 receptor antagonists. Am J Med 81 (Suppl 4B):42-48, 1986.

Jordan PH, Thornby J. Should it be parietal cell vagotomy or selective vagotomy-antrectomy for treatment of duodenal ulcer? Ann Surg 205:572-590, 1987.

Katkhouda N, Mouiel J. A new technique of surgical treatment of chronic duodenal ulcer with laparotomy by videocoelioscopy. Am J Surg 161:361-364, 1991.

Makhlouf GM, McManus JPA, Card WI. A quantitative statement of the two-component hypothesis of gastric acid secretion. Gastroenterology 51:149-171, 1966.

Mulholland MW, Debas HT. Chronic duodenal and gastric ulcer. Surg Clin North Am 67:489-507, 1987.

Rabeneck L, Ransohoff DF. Is *Helicobacter pylori* a cause of duodenal ulcer? A methodologic critique of current evidence. Am J Med 91:566-572, 1991.

Silen W. Gastric mucosal defense and repair. In Johnson LR, et al. (eds). Physiology of the Gastrointestinal Tract, 2nd ed, vol 2. New York, Raven Press, 1987.

Soll AH, Berglingh T. Physiology of isolated gastric glands and parietal cells: Receptors and effectors regulating function. In Johnson LR, et al. (eds). Physiology of the Gastrointestinal Tract, 2nd ed, vol 1. New York, Raven Press, 1987.

Soll AH, Isenberg JI. Duodenal ulcer disease. In Sliesenger MH, Fordtran JS (eds). Gastroduodenal Disease, 3rd ed. Philadelphia, WB Saunders, 1983.

Soper NJ, et al. Long-term clinical results after proximal gastric vagotomy. Surg Gynecol Obstet 169:488-494, 1989.

Stabile BE, Morrow DJ, Passaro E Jr. The gastrinoma triangle: Operative implications. Am J Surg 147:25-31, 1984.

Stabile BE, Passaro E Jr. Recurrent peptic ulcer. Gastroenterology 70:124, 1976.

Thompson JC, et al. Gastrointestinal Endocrinology. New York, McGraw-Hill, 1987.

Vinayek R, et al. Zollinger-Ellison syndrome. Recent advances in the management of gastrinoma. Gastroenterol Clin North Am 19:197-217, 1990.

Welch CE, Rodkey GV, Von-Ryll Gryska P. A thousand operations for ulcer disease. Ann Surg 204:454-467, 1986.

Zollinger RM. Gastrinoma: Factors affecting prognosis. Surgery 97:49-54, 1985.

CHAPTER REVIEW
Questions

1. A 40-year-old man with chronic upper abdominal complaints has hypergastrinemia. He has never been operated on. What is the differential diagnosis and how would you rule out gastrinoma?

2. What would be your treatment of choice for the following patients?
   a. An overweight, otherwise healthy 50-year-old man with prepyloric and duodenal ulcers resistant to ranitidine.
   b. A 35-year-old woman with duodenal ulcer that has been well managed on cimetidine for 4 years. She now wants to become pregnant.
   c. A 40-year-old man with MEN-1, hypergastronemia, and moderate esophagitis.
   d. A 70-year-old woman with a nonhealing type I gastric ulcer.

3. A patient did well for 6 months after vagotomy, antrectomy, and Billroth II gastrojejunostomy for intractable duodenal ulcer. Now she presents with intractable vomiting. What is the differential diagnosis?

4. Your work-up of the patient in question 3 reveals recurrent (marginal) ulcer. What are the possible causes? What should the treatment be?

Answers

1. Differential diagnoses of hypergastrinemia include decreased gastric acid (pernicious anemia, atrophic gastritis, gastric ulcer, H_2-blockers, omeprazole, postvagotomy), increased antral G cell mass (G cell hyperplasia), retained antrum (i.e., on "duodenal stump" after Billroth II gastrectomy) and gastrinoma. In the latter, gastric analysis would reveal low pH, high BAO, BAO/MAO >0.6; the gastrin level would increase significantly in response to an IV secretin bolus.

2. a. Vagotomy and antrectomy has the lowest recurrence rate and any nutritional side effects would probably be well tolerated in

an overnourished patient. Vagotomy and drainage is a reasonable alternative and becomes the procedure of choice if the ulcer disease prevents safe handling of the duodenum.

b. Parietal cell vagotomy

c. H_2-blockers or omeprazole. Pancreatic resection should be avoided, since gastrinomas are multiple, often microscopic, and rarely completely excised.

d. Distal gastrectomy

3. Recurrent ulcer, partial small bowel obstruction, gastric hypomotility and stasis, afferent loop syndrome, bile reflux gastritis

4. Possible causes of recurrent ulcer after ulcer operation include incomplete vagotomy, inadequate gastrectomy, retained antrum, gastrinoma, long afferent limb (e.g., inadvertent gastroileostomy) or missed cancer. This can usually be sorted out by endoscopy and biopsy, barium study, serum gastrin measurement (basal and secretin stimulated), and gastric analysis (before and after sham feeding).

12 Principles of Surgical Oncology and Tumor Biology

BERNARD GARDNER

KEY FEATURES

After reading this chapter you will understand:
- How cancers develop.
- What molecular events are involved in oncogenesis.
- The role of the host.
- The significance of tumor doubling time.
- Some of the factors that determine success in treatment of solid neoplasms.
- Why staging is important.
- The important preoperative and operative steps in determining curability.
- The importance of interaction with other disciplines in the management of the cancer patient.

Surgical oncology has developed because of the need for the surgeon to understand both the fundamental principles of cancer growth and spread and the chemotherapeutic and radiotherapeutic interactions with surgery to provide the cancer patient with a total multidisciplinary treatment plan that will yield the greatest chance of cure.

It is desirable for the surgeon to lead the cancer patient's treatment throughout his or her care, relinquishing that responsibility only when the capability of other specific modalities to manage part of the patient's illness and/or complications becomes apparent. Although it is not possible to establish the precise treatment schedule for all tumors in this chapter, examples are cited to illustrate some of the salient principles of current surgical cancer treatment.

ONCOGENESIS

Classically the development of human cancer was attributed to a two-event process involving the presence of an initiator state (which could be genetic) and contact with a promoter agent (which could be environmental). Experimental work has yielded a plethora of information indicating a complex process that may involve multiple steps.

Transformation of healthy cells to neoplastic ones has been accomplished in the laboratory by a number of agents; see Table 12-1 for a list of common carcinogens seen clinically. The steps involving the development of clinical cancer on a molecular basis involve acceleration of growth kinetics by activation of growth-accelerating oncogenes or loss of suppressor oncogenes, which subsequently lead to growth-factor production. Chromosome losses, duplications, or other anomalies then may result in gene displacement or amplification, leading to unrestrained cellular growth (see below).

In the normal growth cycle, cells leave a resting stage (G0) when appropriately stimulated to enter G1, representing a stage of preparation before DNA synthesis. The S phase (DNA synthesis) is followed by the G2 phase preparatory to mitosis (Fig. 12-1). *Cellular replication is usually controlled;* for example, regrowth of a liver after resection stops when the previous dimensions have been reached, or fibroblast generation ceases when scar formation covers a wound. *Neoplastic cells fail in this control mechanism, and the growth and mitosis continue unabated.* Measurements referable to the growth cycle

TABLE 12-1   Examples of Suspected Carcinogen-Induced Human Cancer

Agent	Geography	Cancer Type
Aflatoxin	Africa	Liver cell
Mycotoxin		
Low-fiber, high-fat diet	United States	Colon
Parasites	Egypt, Rhodesia (***Schistasoma hematobium***)	Bladder
	China, Japan (***Clinorchis sinensis***)	Cholangiocarcinoma
Radiation	Probably universal	Thyroid, breast (?)
Smoking cigarettes	Universal	Lung
Vinyl chloride	United States	Liver
Alkylating chemotherapy	Universal	Leukemia

TABLE 12-2   Examples of S Phase in Various Human Tumors as Determined by Flow Cytometry

Tumor	S Index (%)
Papillary thyroid	1
Melanoma ⎫	
Breast cancer ⎭	5
Colorectal	18
Testicular	40

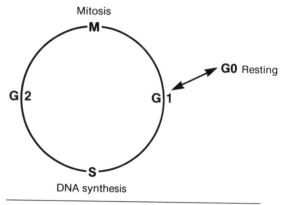

FIGURE 12-1   Cell cycle (representation).

have been made in cancerous tissue by use of *flow cytometry.* This technique involves the analysis of particles flowing single file past a detector to determine certain preset characteristics. For analysis of tumor biology, single-cell suspensions are prepared from fresh or fixed tissue and stained to determine DNA content. The mechanisms may involve fluorescent dyes detected by optical scanners or electronic equipment designed to pick up laser-stimulated excitation converted to an electronic impulse that can be analyzed. The methods involve careful preparation of the cell suspensions. By referring to an internal standard, the G1 DNA content gives an indication of modal chromosome number. Most human cancers are aneuploid, which can be detected rapidly by this technique. Its use, however, as a prognostic indicator has not been borne out in some studies.

The method can also estimate the percentage of cells in S phase. This is correlated with a thymidine-labeling index. A high percentage of S-phase cells may be an adverse prognostic feature (Table 12-2), but further confirmatory studies are required.

Kinetics can be analyzed by using sophisticated techniques of fluorescent labeling of specific antibodies to identify specific oncogenes or thymidine incorporation reflecting intermitotic time and DNA synthesis.

MOLECULAR EVENTS

Stimulation of the cells to unrestrained growth involves a host of molecular events currently being unraveled. *Growth factors* are small peptides that bind to specific cell receptors, leading to either proliferation or inhibition of growth. Many factors have been identified (Table 12-3) that may lead to transformation of cells to neoplastic forms in experimental systems (and presumably clinically). Indication or presence of receptors is vital for the function of growth factors. They represent a membrane component with an extracellular receptor end and intracellular activation end. The latter stimulates the appropriate enzyme systems responsible for increased

TABLE 12-3   Examples of Relationship of Growth Factors to Human Cancer

Growth Factor (GF)	Human Cancer	Action or Relationship
Platelet-derived GF (PDGF)	? Breast	Part of amino acid sequence found in simian viral oncogene affects DNA synthesis in cultured fibroblasts
Epidermal GF (EGF)	Breast, colon, squamous, gastric, bladder, astrocytoma, ovary	Correlated with advanced gastric cancer; correlated with stage and grade of bladder cancer; inverse correlation with estrogen receptor (breast)
Transforming GFα (TGFα)	Breast	50% homologous to EGF; hormone-sensitive breast cancer cells secrete TGFα; blocked by tamoxifen
Transforming GFβ (TGFβ)	Breast	Different structure than TGFα; may be inhibitor of growth; may be related to angiotensin factor; present in extra-cellular matrix
Fibroblastic GF	Breast, esophagus	Related to angiotensin factor; present in extracellular matrix
Insulin growth factors I and II	Breast, sarcoma	Enhanced autocrine growth stimulation
Bombesin	Small cell lung cancer	May lead to increased levels of c-**fos** and c-**myc** proto-oncogenes

growth by stimulating DNA replication or down regulation (depending on the particular growth factor). *Oncogenes* (tumor-forming genes) are transduced from normal host genes (*proto-oncogenes*) and *represent a family of unique DNA sequences whose abnormal expression is associated with development of malignant cell behavior.* Because they originally were identified in a tumor-forming virus, the terminology uses a *V* for oncogenes isolated from viruses and *C* for those isolated from host DNA. Recent experimental technical advances have led to the identification of oncogenes in certain tumors, and some characterization of their activity into three major categories: *growth factor–like oncogenes, signal-transduction oncogenes,* and *nuclear oncogenes.* These new gene identification techniques using chromosome (DNA) probes, monoclonal antibodies, and the more recently developed polymerase chain reaction have led to studies using fixed tissues in which oncogene expression or amplification can be correlated with clinical cancer behavior (Table 12-4). Results of such studies are too recent to report here and require confirmation.

The molecular events described thus far account for *tumor aggressiveness.* Additionally, the production of proteins that stimulate local angiogenesis or proteolytic activity to facilitate tu-

mor spread are also gene induced and add to the inherent properties of the tumor cell in its fight for dominance over the host.

DEFENSE MECHANISMS

Most cancers arise as a single clone, leading to the presumption that a single mutated cell is involved. Recent studies, however, have identified polyclonal families of cells within a cancer that may account for escape from various immunologic and chemotherapeutic attacks. Whether these cells all derived de novo or whether the rapidly dividing tumor cells developed mutations within the colony is not clearly known at present.

A search for a specific tumor antigen that would characterize a particular tumor and lead to a successful immunologic attack against it has not been uniformly successful. At most, clinical cancers are weakly antigenic. *Antibodies to various specific tumor antigens (monoclonal antibodies)* have been used to identify foci of tumor deposits by attaching a radioactive label to the antibody and scanning for emissions. This has been useful for tumors producing certain fetal antigens (carcinoembryonic antigen [CEA] in some colon cancers and alpha-fetoprotein in some hepatomas) but not uniformly so. Treat-

TABLE 12-4   Examples of Relationship of Oncogenes to Human Cancer

Oncogene	Human Cancer	Action or Relationship
c-*myc*	Breast, Burkitt's lymphoma, stomach	No correlation with disease status, although more than 30% of breast cancer patients have amplification; stimulates G1 phase to S phase
n-*myc*	Neuroblastoma, retinoblastoma, breast	Amplification correlates with stage in neuroblastoma
c-*erb* B2 (same as HER-2/*neu*)	Breast, gastric, kidney, ovary	Amplification correlates with breast cancer nodal status and survival (needs confirmation); more common in node-positive breast cancer
ras family	Found in high percent of cancer of colon, thyroid, pancreas	Presence correlates with stage of gastric cancer; enhanced P21 expression in invasive breast cancer compared to in situ; increased P21 in metastases from colon cancer

ment of such cancers by attaching toxins or chemotherapeutic agents to the antibody has also not yielded uniformly good results. A large body of research continues along these lines.

Thus results of treatment using humorally derived antibodies (B-cells) has not been successful, and much attention has been directed at a cellular immune attack. The primary candidate for this defense is the T cytotoxic cell, which has the capacity to lyse foreign cells. These *effector T-cells* lyse virus-infected cells, mainly through the production of T-cell cytokines such as *interleukin-2* (IL-2). Presumably they attack oncogene-induced cancers. The *T-regulator cells* help B-cells produce antibody and also produce IL-2 but are down regulated by *T-suppressor cells*. T-cell activation is stimulated by *interleukin-1* (IL-1) and certain nonspecific mitogens (i.e., phytohemagglutinin). The interest in T-cell stimulation derives from current data on uncontrolled tumor growth in patients with T-cell depletion (e.g., patients with AIDS) and the fact that the molecules encoded by oncogenes may constitute tumor antigens.

Interferons comprise a family of proteins that can induce antiviral responses. Recombinant forms have been produced in sufficient quantities to allow the development of human treatment protocols. Greatest success has been with hairy cell leukemia and chronic myelogenous leukemia.

Nonspecific immunity refers to the ability of peripherally circulating cells (usually lymphocytes) to lyse a variety of cells, including tumor cells without prior sensitization. *Natural killer* (NK) cells may play a role in tumor lysis and resistance to metastatic spread. Killer cells are lymphocytes with distinctive surface markers that may allow them to lyse antibody-coated tumor cells. *Macrophages* may play a role that has not yet been clearly defined in cellular cytotoxicity.

IL-2 produced by stimulated T-cells subsequently stimulates B-cells, NK cells, and lymphokine-activated killer cells and is currently under clinical review as an adjunct in the treatment of cancer patients.

Growth Rate of Cancers

The growth rate of a malignant tumor depends on innumerable factors that presently are either unknown or poorly recognized. In its simplest sense the growth rate is composed of three main elements:

1. Cell division time
2. Growth fraction (percent of cells in active division)
3. Rate of cell loss

Only estimates of these elements are measurable in the clinical situation, so evaluations of tumor growth are fraught with possible errors. Expressed in the usual terms, however, the rate of growth varies with the age of the cancer. Early cancers (small bulk) that tend to have a higher percentage of actively growing cells will approach exponential growth, whereas large-bulk cancers will have a higher rate of cell loss (outgrowth of the vascular supply), leading to a growth plateau. The biphasic growth pattern is similar to a *gompertzian growth curve* and is usually described in this fashion.

Effective systemic therapy initially depends on having cells in an actively dividing state. This reasoning has led to the use of debulking procedures before the use of systemic chemotherapy treatment in some cancers. By the same token, cancers with rapid growth rates (e.g., Ewing's sarcoma) can be shrunk by the use of preoperative chemotherapy, leading to the use of more limiting and less deforming operative procedures as part of a treatment for cure.

The factors that affect growth rate can be divided for convenience into two main categories: (1) inherent properties of the tumor (tumor aggressiveness) and (2) host defense mechanisms. The relationship between tumor aggressiveness and host defenses can be expressed as an equation related to growth rate as follows:

$$\text{Growth rate} = \frac{\text{Tumor aggressiveness}}{\text{Host defenses}} = \frac{1}{\text{Doubling time}}$$

The useful concept of doubling time can be related to the clinical parameters of tumor growth that affect the treatment regimens used for primary and secondary attacks on the cancer. In effect, the longer the doubling time of a particular cancer, the slower its growth rate will be and vice versa.

Growth rates of cancers vary widely and in fact may vary considerably within a particular site. To apply a clinical perspective to this concept, assume that a particular breast cancer arises from a single cell. How long will it take to reach clinically detectable size (i.e., 1 cm)? From measurable data, an average doubling time of approximately 30 days can be predicted for many breast cancers. Using this figure, the length of time such a cancer would have to be present before diagnosis may reach 6 to 8 years. During this long subclinical phase, the factors of tumor aggressiveness and host defense mechanisms have been battling, and the resultant doubling time is a measure of the likelihood of successful treatment. In breast cancer the size of the primary tumor reflects this doubling time fairly accurately. *Of equal significance is the relationship of the doubling time to the free interval after treatment, which is a clue to the length of follow-up necessary before a cure can be assumed.* If a particular breast cancer is completely removed and micrometastases remain, assuming a similar doubling time, the presence of recurrent disease will not be clinically evident for 6 to 8 years.

Therefore 5-year survival data for breast cancer are meaningless in determining the effectiveness of a particular treatment, and longer follow-up must be maintained. Differences between two treatment schemes may therefore be evident only after a 10-year follow-up period.

The reverse of this concept is also useful. For example, if we know that colon cancer rarely recurs after 3 tumor-free years, we can assume that micrometastases in such cases are related to a more rapid doubling time. Therefore colon cancer is probably a more rapidly growing cancer than breast cancer (see the box below).

Propensity to Metastasize

The fact that cure rates are very similar between the two sites is probably related to the fact that, although colon cancer grows faster than breast cancer, it metastasizes late in its natural history, whereas the slower-growing breast cancer metastasizes much earlier in its natural history (see the box on p. 225). This leads to the clinical observation that colon cancer can be attacked aggressively with local treatment (node-positive colon cancer patients have a higher survival rate than node-positive breast cancer patients), even if the tumor is bulky, whereas bulky breast can-

---

SLOW-GROWING AND FAST-GROWING CANCERS

Slow-Growing Cancer

Long incubation period (long doubling time)

Long free period before recurrence

Late recurrence common

Patients continue to die of cancer after 5 years

(Symptoms may persist for years before patient deteriorates)

Fast-Growing Cancer

Short incubation period (rapid doubling time)

Short free period before recurrence

Rare late recurrence

Few deaths after 3 years (after resection), death rate approaches that of normal population

(Classically, patients go into rapid downhill course once symptoms have developed)

cers are not amenable to aggressive local attack. The same factor accounts for the reputed successes of surgical treatment of recurrent colon cancer or single metastases, but such attempts to treat breast cancer have on the whole been unsuccessful (see Tables 12-1 through 12-4).

For many years it has been known that multiple events are necessary for metastases to develop from a primary cancer. Included in these events are the breaking off of single cells or clumps of cells and their circulation to a favorably disposed site, where they attach to an arteriole and produce a fibrin clot. Invasion through the vessel wall and within the tissue and establishment of a vascular supply for nutrients and subsequent growth may depend on numerous additional factors. Current studies are continuing to help us understand the relationship of immune surveillance and other host defenses to prevent successful metastases. Therefore discussion about tumors' having late or early metastases reflects an interplay of multiple events.

EARLY AND LATE METASTASES

Early Metastases

Once tumor reaches certain size, rarely curable
Good correlation between size and survival
Potential for site involvement is widespread
Local recurrence does not influence survival (usually treatment of local recurrence doomed to failure)
Resection of metastatic nodules will not influence survival

Late Metastases

Poor correlation between size of primary and survival (may be better related to local aggressiveness, depth of invasion)
Large massive tumor may still be curable (including direct extension to neighboring organs)
Usually metastasizes to only a few sites
Local recurrence may be resected (or treated) for cure
Success is possible with resection of metastatic lesions

Precancerous Lesions

Selected lesions predictably progress to invasive cancer often enough to justify definitive treatment before development of overt cancer. Examples are listed in Table 12-5.

BIOLOGIC BASIS FOR CANCER SURGERY
Curability of Solid Neoplasms

Recent studies in both clinical and experimental settings have shown that micrometastases may occur very early in the course of some cancers. Indeed, they do occur in the course of many solid malignancies that are locally advanced and are considered the major cause of treatment failure after seemingly adequate curative local surgical procedures have been undertaken.

The significance of the systemic effects of "early" cancers is not well understood. However,

---

TABLE 12-5   Surgery to Prevent Cancer

Underlying Condition	Associated Cancer	Prophylactic Surgery
Cryptorchidism	Testicular	Orchiopexy
Polyposis coli	Colon	Colectomy*
Familial colon cancer	Colon	Colectomy*
Ulcerative colitis (long-standing)	Colon	Colectomy*
Multiple endocrine neoplasia (types II and III)	Medullary cancer of the thyroid	Thyroidectomy
Familial breast cancer	Breast	Mastectomy*
Familial ovarian cancer	Ovary	Oophorectomy

Modified from Mulvihill JJ. Cancer control through genetics. In Avighi FE, Rao PN, Stubblefield L (eds). Genes, Chromosomes, and Neoplasia. New York, Raven Press, 1980.
*Extent of resection and/or reconstruction depends on individual variables.

clinical observations of cancer behavior have led to treatment regimens directed at the local tumor that have produced cure rates unapproached by systemic treatment alone. Little can be gained by a semantic argument about whether any patients with cancer are ever cured. Disease-free intervals of 5 or 10 years after treatment of most solid cancers are associated with so few clinical recurrences that it is safe to assume the patient will never be bothered by that tumor again. For our purposes, *cure is defined in terms of the tumor-free interval for the specific cancer associated with a negligible chance of recurrence.* The actual interval involved depends on several characteristics of a specific cancer.

Knowledge of the stage of disease, the specific biologic behavior, the potential pattern of spread, and the propensity for early microfocal metastatic dissemination of any given cancer should dictate its therapeutic management. In certain malignancies (e.g., oat cell lung cancer, osteogenic sarcoma, anaplastic thyroid cancer, Ewing's sarcoma) dissemination frequently occurs near disease inception. These tumors, characterized by a very high biologic potential for metastases, should be treated with a combination of local and systemic therapy at the outset. At the other extreme, certain tumors (e.g., desmoids, basal cell cancers, chordomas) with an inherent low biologic potential for metastases are curable primarily by using adequate local treatment. When such tumors are locally advanced, extended ablative surgical procedures with or without regional adjuvant radiation therapy may be required.

The majority of solid malignant tumors possess varying degrees of an intermediate inherent potential for metastases, with the *risk of microfocal regional or distant dissemination generally increasing with the advancing clinical and pathologic stage of disease.*

Fig. 12-2 illustrates the concept that most cancers progress clinically from a local to a regional to a disseminated phase in their natural history. Within the framework of this history, the rapidity with which the cancer disseminates beyond regional lymph nodes will define its associated survival rate. For example, esophageal and pulmonary carcinomas with cure rates under 5% disseminate early according to this scheme. At the other end of the spectrum is papillary thyroid cancer and squamous cell carcinoma of the skin, which have prolonged local and regional phases, leading to higher cure rates (>80% at 10 years). *The concept is useful because it indicates the need to attack a cancer during its local and re-*

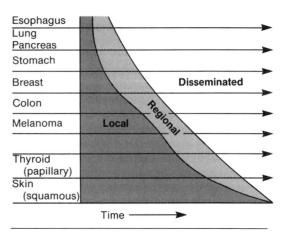

FIGURE 12-2 Clinical behavior of malignancies in terms of progressive development of local, regional, and disseminated stages. The 5-year survival rates correlate with the time in the natural history of the disease when dissemination occurred.

gional phases, since agents that can be used successfully after dissemination in the vast bulk of solid cancers are not available (among the exceptions are choriocarcinoma and some testicular carcinomas). This concept has led to a general approach that involves *wide local excision with resection of the primary lymphatic drainage* (en bloc, if possible) as the treatment of most carcinomas that are diagnosed early and that may be highly curable by adequate local therapeutic modalities alone (surgery or radiation) but, when treated at a later, locally advanced stage, are known to have a high propensity for either regional recurrences (e.g., squamous cancers of the head and neck), distant metastases (e.g., melanoma, breast cancer), or both (gastrointestinal cancer, pancreatic cancer). *Accurate histopathologic diagnosis, precise disease staging, and knowledge of patterns of metastatic tumor spread* provide the necessary insight into the choice and extent of local therapy and the need for either additional regional and/or systemic adjuvant therapy.

Requirements for Wide Resection

With the proven tendency for implantability and transplantation of malignant cells and the propensity for easy seeding of viable tumor cells into an incised wound, *it is essential that an en bloc tumor resection with wide margins be performed whenever feasible.* When a tumor is transected or resected by curettage or in pieces, the treatment field becomes grossly contaminated with viable tumor cells, and miliary recurrences may result. "Conservative" local enucleations of a malignant tumor neglect frequent pseudopodal projections that often penetrate adjacent tissues and may not encompass tumor extensions along perineural, fascial, or muscular planes. The surgeon must adhere to the basic and fundamental principles of a complete en bloc cancer resection of a primary malignant tumor with adequate free margins to avoid the tragic consequence of treatment failure secondary to an otherwise totally preventable local recurrence. It is also essential that the first therapeutic attempt offer the best opportunity for cure. Tumor recurrence after inadequate surgical resections or radiotherapy apparently are associated with a higher incidence of eventual widespread dissemination and ultimate treatment failure. Evidence suggests that the selected population of viable residual tumor cells after unsuccessful surgery or subcurative radiotherapy may be more virulent than the cells of the primary tumor. At least in animals, a significant reduction of a large viable tumor cell population results in an alteration of cell proliferation kinetics, with an increase in the growth fraction and shortening of tumor cell generation time in residual tumor foci.

The ease with which tumor cells separate from the main mass necessitates careful operative techniques to minimize subsequent direct implantation in a wound or suture line. The use of tapes on either side of a colon cancer before

manipulation is a mandatory part of such an operation. To avoid implantation from instruments into a graft donor site, particular care must be taken not to enter the tumor field in any manner. This leads to the principle of wide local excision and particular attention to margins during resection. Inadvertent entry into a malignant "curable" cancer is a sign of poor discipline on the part of the operating surgeon and decreases the chance of cure.

CLINICAL MANAGEMENT
Clinical Staging

The clinical staging of cancers is vital before treatment plans are designed (see the box below). A knowledge of the likely sites of metastases will lead to an appropriate search for metastases that could limit operability. The use of preoperative adjuvants such as chemotherapy or radiotherapy or the avoidance of an operation may be mandated by such a work-up. Sampling of suspicious tissue (e.g., ascites or supraclavicular nodes) is important before the operation is undertaken, since the results may influence the choice of procedure. The surgeon-oncologist must decide preoperatively whether the planned procedure should attempt to cure or to palliate.

The Preoperative Conference

Preoperative evaluation of the patient should be made by a multidisciplinary team. Medical on-

---

TNM SYSTEM OF CLASSIFICATION OF TUMORS

T = Primary Tumors

TX	Tumor cannot be assessed
T0	No evidence of primary tumor
Tis	Carcinoma in situ
T1, T2, T3, T4	Progressive increase in tumor size and involvement

N = Regional Lymph Nodes

NX	Regional lymph nodes cannot be assessed clinically
N0	Regional lymph nodes not demonstrably abnormal
N1, N2, N3, N4	Increased degrees of demonstrable abnormality of regional lymph nodes

M = Distant Metastasis

MX	Not assessed
M0	No (known) distant metastasis
M1	Distant metastasis present
	Specify site of metastasis _____

cologists and radiotherapists are always part of the evaluation team, and whenever possible, general internists, pathologists, and radiologists are included. *Whenever possible, a preoperative diagnosis should be established based on biopsy results.* This is of urgent importance in all soft tissue masses. A preliminary work-up to exclude obvious sites of metastases is completed.

The value of multimodality treatment for some cancers is clear. When that treatment is likely, preoperative consultation with all concerned is warranted, and a single plan that all disciplines accept and adhere to should be selected. In general, each discipline must do its part to perfection; adjuvant chemotherapy and/or radiotherapy cannot convert an inadequate operation to a proper one.

A clinical determination of curability is made and the general condition of the patient evaluated. A treatment plan is outlined that may consist of preoperative chemotherapy for some sarcomas, radiotherapy for large bulky cancers (e.g., of the rectum), or primary surgery followed by adjuvant therapy. Patient risks with each treatment plan are evaluated, although curative treatment is rarely denied. The pathologist is forewarned about the frozen sections he or she likely will be asked to evaluate, and any questions about previous biopsy diagnoses are clarified. If preoperative treatment is suggested, the exact schedule is determined so that operation can be performed at an optimal time, when the patient is free from the complicating systemic effects of chemotherapy and radiotherapy.

The possible operative findings that may modify treatment are discussed (e.g., the discovery of unsuspected metastases, unresectability), and the subsequent intraoperative conduct is planned. In some cases the resection of metastases, the placement of arterial cannulas, or palliative resection must be accomplished. Even modification of the preoperative surgical preparation may be necessary (e.g., treatment of thyroid cancer by total thyroidectomy, followed by radioactive iodine scan postoperatively, may necessitate use of a noniodophore skin preparation). Intraoperative radiotherapy by external beam or seed implantation is now being used in some centers. This therapy may necessitate extensive planning preoperatively, and the long-term merits are not yet known.

A precise preoperative diagnosis in patients with soft tissue sarcoma is imperative, since treatment may consist of amputation, muscle group excision, or wide local excision, depending on the exact histology. Rehabilitation of the patient should be considered before such resections are undertaken. The preoperative conference therefore provides a forum for discussion, coordination, and treatment planning and also provides for a schedule of treatment free from clinical surprises.

Preoperative Preparation of the Patient (Table 12-6)

Since many of the treatments for cancer involve extensive surgery, chemotherapy, or radiotherapy, every effort must be made to ensure that the patient is in the best possible condition to withstand the chosen therapy. A general medical evaluation is conducted by the surgeon and rarely requires specialty assistance (e.g., insertion of a pacemaker). The effects and timing of preoperative chemotherapy and/or radiotherapy are evaluated. A general assessment of fluid balance, anemia, and weight loss (nutritional deficit is almost always present) is made and evaluated with respect to the planned procedure. Specific methods of bowel preparation and hematologic evaluation of the jaundiced patient are standard procedures. However, the preoperative use of hyperalimentation is recommended in the debilitated patient or in one who has lost more than 15 pounds. A 2-week course resulting in 3000 to 3500 calories given daily by central intravenous catheter leads to a weight gain of 6 to 10 pounds in most patients. Postoperative complications such as anastomotic leak or dehiscence of the wound are rare in patients so prepared. Particular attention must be paid to the timing of the operation after radiotherapy (e.g., for head and neck cancer) or to the use of preoperative chemotherapy to avoid postoperative necrosis of flaps, delayed healing, or infection.

Conduct of Operation

Determination of Stage. Every attempt must be made at the time of operation to assess the extent and spread of the cancer. Complete operative exploration is mandatory. *Confirmation by frozen section* of suspicious lymph nodes must be made if the presence of cancer in them will alter the operative approach. A biopsy of metastatic nodules in the liver should be done routinely to avoid confusion later. *If the operation will be abandoned because of the spread of the cancer, histologic proof of the diagnosis is mandatory.* This is not always necessary if resection will be undertaken. Currently intraoperative evaluation of the liver using sonography and

TABLE 12-6 Physiology of the Cancer Patient

Abnormality	Treatment
Tumor acts as a nitrogen trap because of its rapid growth at the metabolic expense of the rest of the body; the patient is in negative nutritional balance and serum albumin may be low Weight loss is prominent because of the tumor growth and possible loss of appetite or partial intestinal obstruction; impairment of wound healing often accompanies operations on cancer patients	Evaluate serum albumin Give IV hyperalimentation preoperatively Supplement the patient preoperatively with vitamin C, 500 mg daily Vitamin B supplementation is warranted if starvation or prolonged IV feedings are present
Although total blood volume is usually normal, anemia due to bleeding is often present; most pronounced in gastrointestinal cancers	Measure blood volume; replace red cell deficit as necessary preoperatively with packed cells; fluid repletion is occasionally necessary
In the elderly patient associated cardiovascular and pulmonary disease may be present, which should be treated preoperatively	Check chest x-ray film, ECG, BUN, and electrolytes if vomiting is present; with associated pulmonary disease preoperative respiratory care, including use of assisted respiration, may be helpful
Rule out obvious possible sites of metastases such as liver, lung, and bones where indicated	Check chest x-ray film and liver chemistries; CT liver scan with contrast is frequently useful
Special associated conditions may be present (e.g., jaundice)	Administer vitamin K as Mephyton, 50 mg IV slowly, for several days in jaundiced patient; check prothrombin time
These patients may have a tendency toward peripheral thrombosis	Check for evidence of thrombophlebitis—wrapping of legs to increase velocity of blood flow in the extremities may be indicated intraoperatively and postoperatively
Debilitated patients have lowered resistance to postoperative infection; anticipate possible contamination of proposed operation (e.g., gastrointestinal resection)	Use antibiotics preoperatively and intraoperatively when indicated

sterile probes has revealed small lesions that alter the prognosis or treatment or both. Similarly use of radioactive monoclonal antibodies has helped diagnose small foci of metastatic colon cancer. These new techniques require fuller evaluation to assess their clinical significance.

Biopsy of a primary tumor is rarely done unless the resulting diagnosis will alter the extent of resection (e.g., lymphoma versus carcinoma) or the cancer is not resectable (e.g., pancreatic carcinoma).

Although the inefficiency of regional lymph nodes as filter traps has been suggested, there are considerable prognostic and therapeutic implications derived from the knowledge of tumor involvement of draining nodes when dealing with specific epithelial and endothelial tumors, which possess a recognized tendency toward lymphatic spread. *The presence of nodal metas-tases is correlated with a decreased survival rate and identifies the patient in need of further adjuvant therapy.* In patients with positive nodes an anatomic node dissection is performed to decrease the tumor cell burden to a minimal number of remaining viable cells that ultimately may be eliminated by a combination of host beneficial factors (immunologic and/or others) and adjuvant regional or systemic therapy.

Adherence to an anatomic en bloc lymph node dissection rather than to "node-plucking" procedures will minimize tumor-cell seeding that may result in local miliary recurrence in those patients with tumor metastases already present in regional lymphatics. If the dissected nodes are found free of metastases, such information can be relied on with greater prognostic significance when the nodal dissection has been performed in an orderly anatomic sequence that provides a more accurate sampling than when lymph nodes were randomly "plucked out."

Curative Operation. When it is determined that resection for cure is feasible, it is undertaken without hesitation. The preoperative decision about the type and extent of operation will have already been made, and they are discussed in the respective sections of this book.

Nonoperative Treatment. The definitive treatment of neoplastic disease by irradiation and drugs is well documented, but a detailed discussion of their indications, effectiveness, and limitations is far beyond the scope of this book. Each alone, as is true for surgery, cures some cancers, whereas other cancers require the most carefully integrated forms of combination therapy (see Fig. 12-3 and the Surgical Pharmacopeia table). Sadly and obviously, some tumors are refractory to all treatment (Table 12-7).

Immunotherapy is based on the concept that the cancer itself is immunogenic and that nonspecific or specific immunotherapy will aid in its control. Although there have been impressive accomplishments in some animal neoplasms, clinical use to date has been very disappointing.

Palliative Operation. The most difficult decisions made at the operating table concern the cancer that cannot be resected because of its invasion into a vital structure or its fixation to the retroperitoneum or spine. Under those circumstances *it is important to determine precisely whether the cancer is truly unresectable by taking appropriate frozen sections.* Even the presence of resectable liver involvement may not necessarily preclude an attempt at cure. This evaluation is difficult and should be made by an experienced surgeon. It is very common to operate on a patient again at a later date and find a resectable lesion associated with profuse adhesions or infection, both of which add formidable risk to the procedure.

Palliation should be undertaken when life can be prolonged or a patient made more comfortable. Exceptions may be made when the surgeon thinks that the patient will live less than 6 months. Obstruction of the gastrointestinal tract is an absolute indication for palliation. Obstruction of the biliary tract is a relative indication, but palliation should be accomplished when feasible.

Palliation also includes the removal of the primary cancer when obstruction is an expected development (e.g., colon or gastric cancer in the presence of liver metastases).

Debulking Procedures. Subtotal resection of cancer in a noncurative setting may be advisable if it facilitates chemotherapy later. Some examples are removing the bulk of ovarian cancer (including omentum) or resecting a segment of infiltrated intestine that might be expected to perforate under intensive chemotherapy. Most of these situations will have been discussed in the preoperative conference. With intensive chemotherapy, such debulking procedures often provide both significant palliation and longevity in highly selected patients.

TABLE 12-7 1980 Estimated Cancer Incidence and Death by Site and Sex*

Site	Incidence (%)		Death (%)	
	Male	Female	Male	Female
Skin	3	2	2	1
Mouth	4	2	3	1
Breast	—	26	—	18
Lung	22	11	35	19
Colon and rectum	14	16	11	14
Pancreas	3	3	5	5
Prostate	19	—	10	—
Ovary	—	4	—	5
Uterus	—	11	—	4
Urinary	9	4	5	3
Leukemia and lymphomas	8	7	9	9
All other	18	14	20	21

Modified from CA 36(1):9, Jan/Feb 1986.
*Excluding nonmelanoma skin cancer and carcinoma in situ.

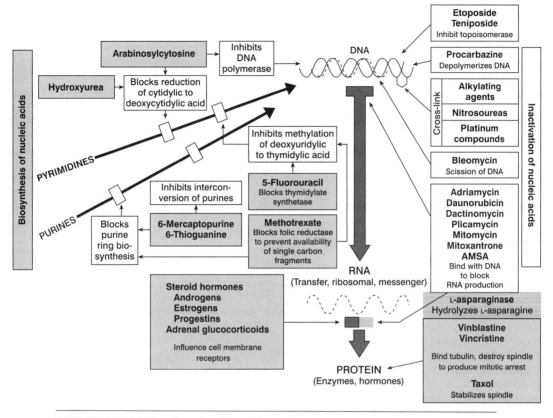

FIGURE 12-3 Mechanism of action of chemotherapeutic agents. (From Krakoff IH. Cancer chemotherapeutic and biologic agents. CA 41:268, 1991.)

Preparation for Adjuvant Treatment. The preoperative conference will have determined the need for adjuvant treatment, depending on the operative findings. The use of steel clips for labeling the dimensions of the field is recommended.

When intra-arterial chemotherapy will be used, the opportunity to place appropriate indwelling catheters should not be lost. Rarely, intraoperative interstitial radiation (implantations) must be planned preoperatively and carried out at operation.

Surgery as an Adjuvant. The primary treatment of a patient may be chemotherapy or radiotherapy, and an operation is needed to provide the adjuvant treatment such as local excision of a primary tumor, removal of endocrine organs, or operative staging for lymphoma. A preoperative plan must be followed, and the surgeon should be familiar with what is needed during the operation such as confirming the stage or delineating

the extent of tumor involvement, obtaining tissue for special studies (e.g., estrogen-binding protein) or diagnosis, protection of structures from future radiation (e.g., ovaries), relief of acute emergent problems (e.g., urinary or gastrointestinal obstruction), or preparation of tissues for radioimplantation. Table 12-8 should be viewed as a generalization regarding the relative advantages and disadvantages of the various cancer therapies.

Maintenance of Records

Frequently only the surgeon can delineate the true extent of a disease and indicate the resection margins and which lymph node groups were removed. The surgeon must orient the specimen for the pathologist and should personally review the pathology report and clarify any discrepancies.

The surgeon's responsibility is to indicate

TABLE 12-8 Comparison of Therapeutic Approaches for the Treatment of Cancer

Type of Treatment	Selectivity	Control		
		Of Primary Tumor	Regional	Systemic
Ideal	++++	++++	++++	++++
Surgery	+	++++	+	0
Radiation	++	+++	++	0
Chemotherapy	++	++	++	++
Immunotherapy	++++	+	++	+

From Wood WC, Cohen AM. Oncology. In Nardi GL, Zuidema GO (eds). Surgery. Essentials of Clinical Practice, 4th ed. Boston, Little, Brown, 1982, p 309.
0 = no effect; + = poor; ++ = fair; +++ = good; ++++ = excellent.

TABLE 12-9 Reported Survival After Resection of Pulmonary Metastases According to Site of Primary in Selected Cases

Site of Primary	No. of Patients	Five-Year Survival Rate (%)
Carcinoma		
Head and neck	83	22-44
Breast	80	13-52
Colon	131	0-30
Rectum	7	52-57
Bladder	36	33-50
Kidney	62	20-62
Testicle	93	31-50
Uterine cervix	73	19-40
Melanoma	73	0-33
Sarcoma		
Soft tissue	149	20-35
Osteogenic	99	27-31

Modified from Ultmann JE, Phillips TL. Treatment of metastatic cancer. In DeVita VT Jr, Hellman S, Rosenberg SA (eds). Cancer: Principles and Practice of Oncology. Philadelphia, JB Lippincott, 1982, pp 1534-1581.

clearly on the chart the clinical and pathologic stage of a disease and whether resection was palliative or curative. Subsequent accurate record keeping by the tumor registrar will depend on a clear surgical notation in the chart and on the dictated operative note. Changes in the pathologic diagnosis or any differences between the frozen and permanent sections should be brought directly to the attention of the responsible surgeon, who must then give the information to other members of the oncology team.

Follow-up Care

The primary physician should be responsible for follow-up care of the patient to ensure good coordination of treatment. In most cases this will be the surgeon, and although the responsibility may be shared with other oncologists, the surgeon is obligated to make sure that follow-up is pursued after other regimens are concluded. Such follow-up should specifically recognize the primary site and stage of the cancer and the propensity, timing, and likely sites of recurrence and/or metastases.

The surgeon must establish rapport with the patient and family and frequently with the referring physician, and this contact should be maintained throughout the patient's subsequent treatment regimen. If cancer should recur, the surgeon may decide to transfer this responsibility to other oncologic specialists, but only after clearly explaining the circumstances to all concerned.

The alert physician must recognize that certain remote metastases, in the absence of overt disseminated disease, are highly amenable to re-resection (Table 12-9). Notable organs, which yield reasonable cure rates in highly selected cases, are the lung and liver.

Ethical Considerations

The physician's role is to eradicate disease, relieve pain, and provide comfort. In the case of the cancer patient, the surgeon's fulfillment of these responsibilities is taxed to the utmost.

Should the patient be told he or she has cancer? Although conditions in each case may modify the surgeon's attitude, the patient and at least one family member ordinarily should be told the diagnosis. The prognosis is always discussed in the most optimistic terms with the patient, indicating the vast number of surgical, radiotherapeutic, and chemotherapeutic treatments available and the positive results that can be obtained. There is no substitute for a patient-doctor relationship built on honesty and trust.

PITFALLS AND COMMON MYTHS

- Failure to plan the treatment with appropriate *preoperative* consultations (multidisciplinary).
- Diagnosing inoperable or unresectable disease without appropriate biopsies (histologic proof).
- Inadequate physiologic preparation of the patient.

- Delay in definitive treatment.
- Failing to be honest and forthright with the patient as to the diagnosis.
- Not using postoperative adjuvant treatment when indicated.
- Invading the tumor field during resection (inadequate resection).

BIBLIOGRAPHY

Alfonso A, Gardner B. Principle of Cancer Surgery. New York, Appleton-Century-Crofts, 1981.

Arbeit JM. Molecules, cancer and the surgeon. Ann Surg 212:3-13, 1990.

Carney D, Sikora K. Genes and cancer. New York, John Wiley & Sons, 1990.

Claman HN. The biology of the immune response. JAMA 258:2834-2840, 1987.

Gardner B. The relationship of delay in treatment to prognosis in human cancer. In Ariel IM (ed). Progress in Clinical Cancer. New York, Grune & Stratton, 1978, pp 123-134.

Goya T, Miyazawa N, Kondo H, et al. Surgical resection of pulmonary metastases from colorectal cancer. Cancer 64:1418-1421, 1989.

Leffal LD Jr. Presidential address. Surgical oncology, expectations for the future. Cancer 42:2925, 1980.

Merkel DE, McGuire WL. Ploidy, proliferative activity and prognosis: DNA flow cytometry of solid tumors. Cancer 65:1194-1205, 1990.

Pardee AB. Principles of cancer biology: Biochemistry and cell biology. In DeVita VT, Hellman S, Rosenberg SA (eds). Cancer Principles and Practice of Oncology, 2nd ed. Philadelphia, JB Lippincott, 1985.

Sugarbaker EV, Ketchum AS. Interdisciplinary cancer therapy: Theory and practice. In Hardy JD (ed). Rhoades Textbook of Surgery. Philadelphia, JB Lippincott, 1977, pp 423-441.

Tubiana M, Pejovic MN, Koscielzy S, et al. Growth rate, kinetics of tumor cell proliferation and long term outcome in human breast cancer. Int J Cancer 44:17-22, 1989.

Wong RS, Passaro E Jr. DNA technology. Am J Surg 159:610-614, 1990.

SURGICAL PHARMACOPEIA

Common Chemotherapeutic Agents

Drug	Classification	Indications	Complications	Dosage
Bleomycin (Blenoxane)	Cytotoxic antibiotic	Testicular cancer, lymphoma, head and neck cancer	Pulmonary fibrosis, leukopenia fever, mucositis	15 mg IV, IM, or subcutaneously twice weekly
Chlorambucil	Alkylating agent	Hodgkin's disease, nonHodgkin's lymphoma, ovarian or breast cancer	GI upset, bone marrow suppression	0.1-0.2 mg/kg/day orally
Cisplatin	Alkylating inorganic salt	Ovarian or testicular cancer, transitional and squamous cell cancer	Bone marrow depression, ototoxicity, nausea, vomiting, nephrotoxicity	80-120 mg/m^2 IV every 3 weeks
Cyclophosphamide (Cytoxan)	Alkylating agent	Burkitt's lymphoma, Hodgkin's and other lymphomas, multiple myeloma, breast, ovarian, or oat cell cancer, neuroblastoma, Ewing's sarcoma	Hemorrhagic cystitis, bone marrow suppression, nausea and vomiting, alopecia	2-4 mg/kg/day orally for 10 days, 1 g/m^2 IV per cycle
Dactinomycin (actinomycin D)	Cytotoxic antibiotic	Wilms' tumor, testicular cancer, choriocarcinoma, soft tissue sarcomas	Nausea, vomiting, GI upset, stomatitis, bone marrow depression, alopecia	0.04 mg/kg/day IV weekly
Doxorubicin	Cytotoxic antibiotic	Lymphoma, transitional cell carcinoma of the bladder, breast or testicular cancer, sarcoma	Stomatitis, alopecia, bone marrow depression, cardiotoxicity	60 mg/m^2 IV every 3 weeks
Fluorouracil (5-FU)	Antimetabolite	Colon, gastric, breast, ovarian, or pancreatic cancer	Stomatitis, GI upset, bone marrow depression, cerebellar atoxia	15-20 mg/kg IV per week, 15 mg/kg orally weekly
Methotrexate	Antimetabolite	Choriocarcinoma, breast cancer, Burkitt's lymphoma, testicular cancer, squamous cell cancer of head, neck, and lung	Stomatitis, hepatic fibrosis, GI upset, bone marrow depression	40-60 mg/m^2 IV per week, 2.5-5 mg/day orally

Drug				Dosage
Phenylalanine mustard (melphalan)	Alkylating agent	Multiple myeloma, breast or ovarian cancer	Bone marrow suppression, GI upset, development of later malignancies	0.25 mg/kg/day orally for 4 days per cycle
Vincristine (Oncovin)	Vinca alkaloid	Wilms' tumor, neuroblastoma, Hodgkin's and other lymphomas, choriocarcinoma, Ewing's sarcoma, testicular or breast cancer	Neuropathy, alopecia, toxic to subcutaneous tissues if extravasated	1.5 mg/m^2 IV per week

Drugs Commonly Used in Cancer Management

Drug	Dosage
Antiemetics	
Diphenhydramine (Benadryl)	25-50 mg orally or IM q6-8h
Prochlorperazine (Compazine)	5-18 mg IM or IV q6-8h
Lorazepam (Ativan)	0.5-2 mg orally or IM bid
Metaclopramide (Reglan)	10-15 mg orally tid before meals
Pain Control	
Oxycodone (Percocet, Percodan)	1 tablet q6h prn
MS Contin (morphine)	Depends on total daily dose of morphine
Morphine SQ	10 mg subcutaneously q4-6h prn
Acetaminophen (Tylenol) with codeine, 30 or 60 mg	1 tablet q4h prn
Duragesic patches	Individualized

Drug	Dosage
Comfort	
Diazepam (Valium)	2-10 mg orally or IM q4h
Diphenoxylate/atropine (Lomotil)	2 tablets q6h × 4, then 1 tablet q12h prn
Alprazolam (Xanax)	0.25-0.5 mg, then 1 mg orally qid
Triazolam (Halcion)	0.125-0.25 mg qhs prn
Temazepam (Restoril)	15-30 mg orally qhs prn

CHAPTER REVIEW
Questions

1. The flattening of the gompertzian growth curve for solid neoplasms is due to:
   a. Decreased DNA metabolism.
   b. Increased thymidine uptake.
   c. Increased cell loss.
   d. Altered cell cycle time.
2. Five-year survival rates are of little value in establishing cure rates for breast cancer because:
   a. Growth rate is slow, necessitating a long interval for metastases to become evident.
   b. Metastases are frequent to all organs.
   c. Growth rate is fast, narrowing the free interval.
3. Under what conditions should isolated metastases be resected?
4. When should a chemotherapist (medical oncologist) be asked to see a patient with resectable cancer? Why?
5. Why may cancers' differing growth rates have similar survival statistics?
6. What are growth factors?
7. Name two methods of determining the presence of liver metastases at operation other than inspection and palpation.
8. What is the primary determinant of an adequate local resection?
9. List three postoperative complications more common in cancer patients.
10. When is histologic proof of the diagnosis of cancer mandatory?
11. What are two reasons for palliative operations?
12. List six circumstances in which the operation becomes an adjuvant to primary treatment for cancer.

Answers

1. c
2. a
3. When dealing with a late metastasizing cancer such as of the colon or if the malignancy is very responsive to chemotherapy and reduction in tumor burden is desirable
4. Preoperatively but after a biopsy has been taken. In an accessible tumor, chemotherapy or a combined approach for debulking of metastatic disease or the placement of catheters for infusional chemotherapy may be contemplated.
5. They may have different metastatic potential.
6. Growth factors are small peptides that bind to specific cell receptors, leading to either proliferation or inhibition of growth.
7. a. Intraoperative sonography
   b. Biopsy with specimen obtained under sonography
   c. Radioactive monoclonal antibody probes
8. Surgical margins free of tumor
9. a. Infection
   b. Wound dehiscence
   c. Phlebitis
10. When the cancer is unresectable
11. a. To prolong life
    b. To increase comfort of patient
12. a. Obtaining biopsy specimen for diagnosis
    b. Endocrine ablation for breast cancer
    c. Obtaining tissue for special studies
    d. Relief of emergent problems
    e. Preparation of tissues for radioimplantation
    f. Debulking before chemotherapy
    g. Staging

13 Transplantation Science and Immunology

HANS W. SOLLINGER
ANTHONY M. D'ALESSANDRO
FOLKERT O. BELZER

KEY FEATURES

After reading this chapter you will understand:
- The history of organ transplantation and preservation.
- The basic immunology of transplantation.
- The mechanism by which the immune response is suppressed.
- Operative considerations in the transplantation of specific organs.

HISTORICAL ASPECTS

Transplantation is the process of taking a graft—cells, tissues, or organs—from one individual, the donor, and placing it into another individual, the recipient or host. If the graft is placed into its normal anatomic location, the procedure is called *orthotopic transplantation* (e.g., heart transplants). If the graft is placed in a different site, the procedure is called *heterotopic transplantation* (e.g., kidney transplants).

Although attempts at transplantation date back to ancient times, the impetus behind modern transplantation was World War II and the Battle of Britain. Royal Air Force pilots often were severely burned when their planes crashed. The mortality rate associated with burns corresponds to the size of the area of skin that has been injured, and the survival rate can be improved if burned skin is replaced. For this reason British doctors turned to skin transplantation from other human donors as the mode of therapy.

However, attempts to replace damaged skin with skin from unrelated donors were uniformly unsuccessful. Over a matter of several days, the transplanted skin would undergo necrosis and fall off. This problem led many investigators, including Nobel Prize winner Peter Medawar, to study skin transplantation in animal models. These experiments established that failure of skin grafting was caused by an immunologic reaction, termed *rejection.* Once it was established that this inflammatory response was immunologic in nature, investigations were carried out to understand further the mechanisms of the immune response to transplantation antigens. In addition, attempts were made to suppress this response after organ transplantation through the use of immunosuppressive drugs. Furthermore, surgeons continued to refine techniques in organ transplantation, and over the past years successful transplantation of the following solid organs has been accomplished: kidney, heart, liver, pancreas, heart and lung, single lung, small bowel, and combined liver, pancreas, and small bowel ("cluster" operation).

The box on p. 238 reviews the milestones in transplantation over the past 50 years.

ORGAN PRESERVATION

Optimal use of organ transplantation for patients with end-stage organ diseases requires using cadaveric organs that must be shared on a national basis. This requires the use of effective, safe, and reliable methods to preserve the organ ex vivo for

MILESTONES IN TRANSPLANTATION

1940-1950

1943 Gibson and Medawar: Description of human skin graft rejection
1945 Owen: Red cell chimerism in nonidentical cattle twins

1950-1960

    Billingham, Brent, Medawar: Description of immunologic tolerance
    Mitchenson, Gowens: Role of small lymphocytes in transplant rejection
1954 First successful kidney transplant in Boston, Massachusetts
    Schwartz and Damashak: Discovery of 6-mercaptopurine

1960-1970

    Woodruff and Anderson: Description of the immunosuppressive efficacy of antilymphocyte
      globulin
1963 First liver transplant by Starzl in Denver, Colorado
    Discovery of immunosuppressive efficacy of prednisone
1966 First pancreas transplant in Minneapolis, Minnesota
1967 First heart transplant in Cape Town, South Africa
    Description of major histocompatibility antigens by Dausset

1970-1980

1972 Discovery of cyclosporin A by Borel
1978 Initiation of first clinical trials with cyclosporin A by Calne

1980-1990

    Introduction of OKT3, the first monoclonal antibody in clinical use
    First successful heart-lung transplant at Stanford University
    Discovery of University of Wisconsin preservation solution
    Introduction of FK 506
    First clinical use of RS-61443 in organ transplantation

---

periods of time up to at least 2 days, although currently most organs are transplanted within approximately 24 hours after procurement.

Preservation of the organ begins at the time a donor is identified, and the donor must be adequately maintained, hemodynamically, so the organ is not injured before procurement and preservation. Injury could occur because of cardiovascular instability and hypotensive episodes. The adequacy of the organ must be assessed by clinical measurements of organ functions before procurement. The nutritional status of the donor may play a role in the quality of the organ, and such factors as fatty infiltrations in the liver or long periods in the intensive care unit can affect the quality of preservation and function of the organ after transplantation. During the operation to remove the organs, warm ischemia must be reduced to a minimal amount of time (<5 minutes), and the organs must be cooled rapidly,

either in situ or by a well-timed back-table flushout (Fig. 13-1).

A high level of care is necessary both in maintenance of the donor and during the donor operation to obtain optimal organs for preservation and transplantation. Sometimes this high level of support is not available, and caution must be used in assessing the quality of the organ before preservation.

Key factors in successful organ preservation are related to hypothermia and the composition of the organ preservation solution. In simple cold storage of organs, they are rapidly cooled to approximately 4° C by flushout of the vascular system with an appropriate organ preservation solution. The flushout should remove blood as completely as possible, be delivered at a pressure that is not damaging to the organ (usually 60 to 100 cm H_2O), and in a volume that is not excessive. The volume for each organ is variable, but

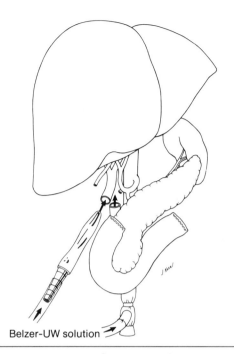

Belzer-UW solution

FIGURE 13-1 In situ flushing of kidneys (not shown), pancreas, and liver during organ retrieval. The liver is flushed through the aorta and the portal vein.

in general, the liver is flushed with approximately 2 to 3 L, the kidney with 200 to 500 ml, and the pancreas with a similar amount. The organ is then placed in a sterile container and kept cold (0° to 4° C).

Hypothermia is beneficial because it slows metabolism. Organs exposed to normothermic 37° C) ischemia remain viable for only relatively short periods of time (for most organs, 1 hour or less). In warm ischemia the absence of oxygen leads to a rapid decline in the energy content (adenosine triphosphate [ATP]) of the organ, a redistribution of electrolytes across the cell membrane, and a decrease in biosynthetic reactions. However, biodegradable reactions continue, including the accumulation of lactic acid, a decrease in intracellular pH, proteolysis, and lipolysis (lipases and phospholipases). These events contribute to changes in the concentrations of intracellular metabolites and structural alterations in cellular membranes that contribute to loss of viability on restoration of blood reperfusion of the organ. With hypothermia the degradative reactions are slowed. A 10° C decrease in temperature, in general, slows down the metabolic rate by a factor of approximately 2 (1.5 to 3). Therefore cooling an organ from 37° C to ap-

proximately 0° C slows metabolism by a factor of 12 to 13.

Hypothermia, however, is not sufficient to give adequate preservation for the time necessary for optimal use of cadaveric organs. In addition, the organ must be flushed with an appropriate preservation solution. Two factors contribute to an ideal preservation solution: (1) the presence of impermeant molecules that suppress hypothermic-induced cell swelling; and (2) an appropriate biochemical environment. Impermeants are agents that remain outside the cells and are sufficiently osmotically active to retard the accumulation of water by the cell. Under conditions of cold storage (cold ischemia), there is a loss of ATP, which is necessary to drive the ion pumps (sodium-potassium-ATPase, sodium) required to maintain normal cell volume. In addition, hypothermia slows the activity of the ion pumps but has little effect on the permeability of the cell membrane electrolytes. Thus there is a relatively rapid accumulation of sodium in exchange for potassium, a loss of the electric potential across the membrane, and the entry of chloride down its chemical gradient. This results in the accumulation of water in the cell, and this cell swelling apparently is a major detriment to successful preservation of organs.

In 1969 Collins et al. developed a preservation solution (Collins solution) that was effective for 30-hour storage of the dog kidney. This solution has been used for kidney preservation for the past 23 years. The composition of this solution is shown in Table 13-1. The solution contains a high concentration of potassium, which was originally thought beneficial in organ preservation because it would retard the loss of potassium from the cell. However, it is now clear that a solution containing a high concentration of sodium is equally effective. In addition, this solution contains a high concentration of glucose, which is an effective impermeant in the kidney and suppresses cell swelling. It is the presence of glucose that makes this solution effective for kidney preservation.

Other cold-storage solutions have been developed, including the hypertonic citrate solution and phosphate buffered sucrose (see Table 13-1). Hypertonic citrate uses a high concentration of citrate, sulphate, and mannitol as impermeants, and phosphate-buffered sucrose depends on sucrose and phosphate as agents to suppress hypothermic-induced cell swelling.

Although these solutions are effective for human kidney preservation for up to 48 hours, they are not as effective for the preservation of other organs. The reasons are not entirely clear but

TABLE 13-1 Composition of Cold Storage Solutions*

Composition	Collins	HOC	PBS	UW
Potassium phosphate, monobasic (KH_2PO_4)	15.1 mM	—	—	25 mM
Potassium phosphate (K_2HPO_4)	42.5 mM	—	—	—
Sodium phosphate (Na_2HPO_4)	—	—	53.6 mM	—
Sodium phosphate, monobasic (NaH_2PO_4)	—	—	15.5 mM	—
Potassium chloride (KCl)	15 mM	—	—	—
Sodium bicarbonate ($NaHCO_3$)	10 mM	—	—	—
Glucose	140 mM	—	—	—
Magnesium sulfate ($MgSO_4$)	30 mM	83.1 mM	—	5.0 mM
Potassium citrate	—	28.1 mM	—	—
Sodium citrate	31.8 mM	—	—	—
Mannitol	—	188 mM	—	—
Sucrose	—	—	140 mM	—
Lactobionate	—	—	—	100 mM
Adenosine	—	—	—	5 mM
Allopurinol	—	—	—	1 mM
Raffinose	—	—	—	30 mM
Glutathione	—	—	—	3 mM
Starch	—	—	—	50 g/L

HOC = hypertonic citrate; PBS = phosphate buffered sucrose; UW = University of Wisconsin.
*These solutions have a final pH of approximately 7 to 7.4 and osmolality of 320 to 350 mOsm/L. Starch is hydroxyethyl starch, and glutathione is the reduced form.

apparently are related to differences in permeability properties of the cell membranes of these other organs. These solutions are suitable for only short-term preservation of the liver, pancreas, and heart: approximately 4 to 8 hours. Saccharides such as glucose, mannitol, or citrate do not appear ideal for suppression of cell swelling in extrarenal organs. In 1987 a new preservation solution was developed (University of Wisconsin solution [UW solution, ViaSpan]) that successfully preserved the pancreas of the dog for up to 72 hours (see Table 13-1). This solution was also effective for preservation of the kidney and the liver; recently this solution has provided relatively good heart preservation.

The UW solution contains lactobionic acid as the primary impermeant. Lactobionic acid has a relatively large molecular mass (358 daltons) and is negatively charged; thus it remains outside most cells and suppresses hypothermic-induced cell swelling. In addition, this solution contains raffinose, a trisaccharide, and hydroxyethyl starch, a colloid. Thus, by effectively suppressing cell swelling, successful pancreas, liver, kidney, and heart preservation has been obtained for periods of up to 24 to 72 hours. The UW solution is effective for preservation of human organs, including the liver, pancreas, and heart.

Although impermeants are important components of cold storage solutions, other components of preservation solutions are also important. The UW solution contains adenosine to stimulate ATP synthesis during reperfusion (transplantation) of the organ. During cold storage there is a degradation of ATP to purines (hypoxanthine, inosine, xanthine), which are rapidly washed out of the cell during reperfusion. Thus the tissue lacks sufficient purine precursors for the regeneration of ATP. Adenosine is an effective precursor; thus, by loading the cell with adenosine during preservation, ATP synthesis is stimulated during reperfusion. ATP is necessary as an energy source for the restoration of normal cell functions and for cellular repair of preservation-induced injury. Allopurinol is added as an inhibitor of xanthine oxidase. During ischemia xanthine dehydrogenase, which uses pyridine nucleotides as electron acceptors, is converted to xanthine oxidase, which uses oxygen as an electron acceptor. Xanthine oxidase catalyzes a reaction (conversion of hypoxanthine to xanthine and to uric acid), which forms a superoxide anion. This oxygen-free radical can be metabolized further to hydrogen peroxide and hydroxyl radicals, which are cytotoxic. The suppression of xanthine oxidase by allopurinol is thought to contribute to the suppression of the formation of oxygen-free radicals during reperfusion and to suppress this form of cellular injury. Glutathione is an essential peptide involved in the scavenging of hydrogen peroxide. During cold storage the cell loses glutathione. The UW solution contains glutathione, which is important in successful long-term liver and heart preservation.

Thus there apparently are three principles of successful organ preservation by simple cold storage: (1) hypothermia; (2) an appropriate physical environment created by impermeants that suppress hypothermic-induced cell swelling; and (3) an appropriate biochemical environment created by metabolites and inhibitors that facilitate restoration of normal metabolism during reperfusion. In the future the development of new information about the mechanisms of hypothermic-induced cell injury will lead to refinements in current organ preservation solutions that will allow even longer-term and better quality organ preservation.

In addition to the method of simple cold storage, organs can be preserved by continuous hypothermic perfusion. This method, developed by Belzer et al. in 1967, uses a machine to pump continuously a perfusion fluid through the organ. In this way oxygen and substrates are continually delivered to the organ, which maintains metabolism, including the synthesis of ATP and other molecules and ion pump activity. In addition, end products of metabolism are removed from the organ. With this method, the liver and kidney can be safely preserved for periods longer than those possible by cold storage. The liver has been preserved successfully for up to 3 days and the kidney for up to 5 days. Machine perfusion currently is used in a few centers in the United States and, in general, gives superior results when compared to simple cold storage. With simple cold storage, approximately 20% to 30% of the transplanted kidneys develop delayed graft function. However, with machine perfusion the rate of delayed graft function in most centers is less than 10%. The perfusate is similar to the UW solution described previously except for the impermeant. For continuous perfusion, gluconate is used in place of lactobionic acid.

MAJOR HISTOCOMPATIBILITY COMPLEX

The major histocompatibility complex (MHC) is a gene complex responsible for virtually every aspect of the immune response, including graft

---

TRANSPLANT TERMINOLOGY

Allogeneic graft: Graft transplanted between two genetically different individuals of the same species
Xenogeneic graft: Graft transplanted between individuals of different species
Orthotopic transplant: Transplantation into same location as original organ (e.g., heart, liver)
Heterotopic transplant: Transplantation into different location (e.g., kidney, pancreas)
LRD: Living related donor

---

rejection. In the human it is referred to as the human leukocyte antigen (HLA) complex. Genes of the MHC are responsible for antigen recognition and the cellular interaction involved in the immune response. These genes have been mapped to chromosome 6 in humans. The MHC genes are divided into three classes: I, II, and III. The class I genes encode cell-surface transplantation antigens serving as the primary targets for cytotoxic T-lymphocytes in graft rejection. The class II genes are the immune response genes. They control the level of the response to some antigens, encode a series of antigens that are expressed on lymphocytes, and serve as primary targets for helper T-lymphocytes. Tissue typing, or histocompatibility testing, is used to determine the exact specificity of a given individual's class I and class II antigens. In general, two class I loci (A and B) and one class II locus (DR) are being typed. At the current time, more than 100 A and B and nearly a dozen DR specificities are known.

IMMUNE RESPONSE TO TRANSPLANTATION ANTIGENS

The major cause for graft loss is immunologic graft rejection, which can be either acute or chronic. Since Medawar's discovery of the immunologic nature of the rejection response, numerous research laboratories around the world have contributed to unravel the mechanisms of rejection. Before these mechanisms are discussed, the box above lists some terms commonly used in transplantation biology.

All surface structures of organ transplants carry membrane glycoproteins that are recognized as foreign by the recipient's immune system. After the surgeon has performed the vascular anastomosis and blood flow to the organ is established, these antigens are released into the peripheral circulation and transported to the central lymphoid organs, which include lymph nodes and spleen. There and in the periphery these antigens are phagocytized by cells of the lymphoid macrophage lineage called *antigen-presenting cells (APCs).* After uptake into APCs, donor glycoproteins are broken into small peptides measuring 10 to 20 amino acids within the acidic compartment of endosomal vesicles (Fig. 13-2). After release from these vesicles, the foreign peptide is placed in a groove between the alpha and beta chain of the so-called class II molecules of the MHC. Some investigators believe that the peptide is necessary for the assembly of MHC class II molecules. This complex is then transported to the cell surface where the complex of peptide and MHC class II antigens can be recognized by the recipient's immune system.

The complex of MHC class II and peptide is recognized by the T-cell receptor of helper T-lymphocytes (CD4$^+$ cells) (Fig. 13-3). The T-cell re-

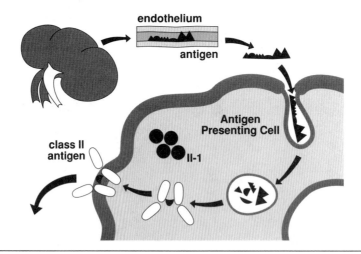

FIGURE 13-2   Uptake of antigen by antigen-presenting cells and presentation by class II MHC.

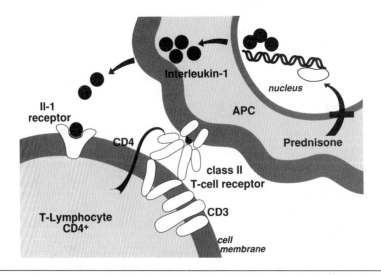

FIGURE 13-3   Recognition of peptide and MHC by T-cell receptor. This interaction is stabilized by CD4 molecule. Interleukin-1 *(IL-1)* is secreted by the antigen-presenting cell *(APC).*

ceptor consists of an alpha and a beta chain with a molecular weight between 40,000 and 90,000, depending on the species. Interaction between T-cell receptor and peptides imbedded in the antigen-binding groove of class II antigens is not enough to result in the activation of CD4$^+$ cells. The interaction between these two complexes is stabilized by the CD4 molecule and several other cell-surface molecules, commonly referred to as "adhesion" molecules. The so-called "CD3 complex," which is in close proximity to the T-cell receptor, apparently also is important in triggering T-cell activation.

Binding of antigen to the T-cell receptor complex stimulates a series of intracellular events that result in the generation of inositol 1,4,5-triphosphate (IP$_3$) (Fig. 13-4). IP$_3$ triggers the intracellular release of calcium ions. Calcium activates the phosphatase calcineurin.

Calcineurin dephosphorylates the cytoplasmatic component of the nuclear factor of activated T-cells (NF-AT$_c$), which facilitates its translocation into the nucleus (Fig. 13-5). NF-AT$_c$ combines with this nuclear cofactor, NF-AT$_n$, to form an activated transcription factor that activates RNA polymerase and regulates the tran-

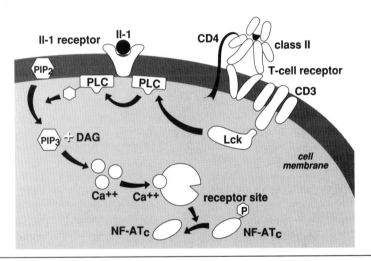

FIGURE 13-4   Binding of peptide and MHC and interaction of interleukin-1 *(IL-1)* with its receptor on CD4$^+$ cells results in a series of intracellular activation events.

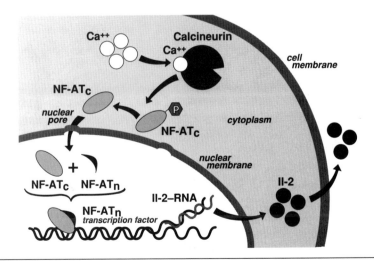

FIGURE 13-5   Activation of NF-AT$_c$ by calcineurin allows entry of this factor into nucleus.

scription of genes and coding of interleukin-2 (IL-2) and other lymphokines and cytokines needed for T-cell activation.

Among the two most important functions of IL-2 is the activation of CD4+ cells, which respond with rapid cell division and clonal proliferation (Fig. 13-6). Furthermore, IL-2 interacts with the IL-2 receptor on killer T-cells (CD8+ cells). These cells become activated and migrate to the transplanted organ where they recognize the original peptide structure to which they were sensitized, attach to the target, and cause cytolytic destruction. The interaction between a CD8+ killer cell and its target organ is mediated through MHC class I antigens. Binding of the MHC complex to the target cell is stabilized through the CD8 molecule.

Once the membranes of killer and target cells are in close proximity, granules located within the cytoplasm of killer T-cells fuse with the cell membrane and empty a pore-forming protein called *perforin* into the small intercellular space. Calcium there changes the conformation of the individual perforin molecules, which then bind to the target cell membrane and insert into it. The monomeric perforin molecules polymerize like staves of a barrel to form pores that admit water and salts and kill the cell.

Although these events describe *acute* or *cellular rejection,* a second type of rejection is of clinical importance. In this process antibodies mediate complement-dependent cytotoxicity (Table 13-2). Humoral rejection again can occur in two forms: hyperacute and chronic. In hyperacute

TABLE 13-2   Types of Rejection

Type	Hyperacute	Acute	Chronic
Time after transplantation	Minutes to hours	7 days to months	Months to years
Mechanism	Antibodies (IgG)	CD4+ and CD8+ T-cells	Antibodies and CD4+ T-cells
Histology	Polymorphonuclear infiltration, interstitial hemorrhage, platelet and fibrin deposition in glomerular capillaries	Lymphocytic infiltration of interstitial tissues, mixed cellular infiltration of small and medium-sized arteries	Fibrosis, vascular absence of small and medium-sized arteries secondary to intense proliferation
Therapy	None	Steroids, ALG, OKT3, FK-506, RS-61443	Steroids(?), RS-61443(?)

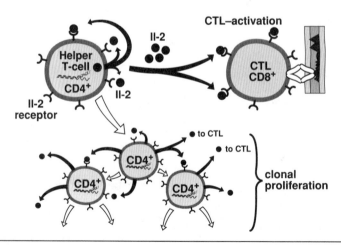

FIGURE 13-6   Activation of CD4+ and CD8+ cells results in clonal expansion.

rejection cytotoxic antibodies are present in the recipient's serum before transplantation. Immediately after the surgeon removes the vascular clamps and restores blood flow to the kidney, these antibodies attack the graft and cause rejection of the transplant within a very short time, usually less than an hour or so. To prevent this type of rejection, recipients are screened before transplantation for the presence or absence of antibodies that can mediate hyperacute rejection. The test system to check for these antibodies is called the *cytotoxic crossmatch.* Recipient serum is mixed with lymphocytes from the donor's lymphocytes or spleen. If after addition of complement the donor's lymphocytes are killed by recipient serum, the crossmatch is called *positive,* and transplantation cannot be performed.

Antibodies, usually of the IgG type, also play an important role in chronic graft rejection. Chronic graft rejection is a slow rejection process, usually occurring several months or years after transplantation. It is also likely that CD4+ cells play a role in this process. Neither hyperacute rejection nor chronic rejection can be treated with immunosuppressive therapy. In contrast, acute rejection mediated by CD4+ and CD8+ cells can be treated very successfully with a wide range of immunosuppressive agents. Even more important is the prevention of the development of an immune response to transplantation antigens through the use of immunosuppressive drugs.

IMMUNOSUPPRESSIVE THERAPY

The mechanism of immunosuppressive drugs has become better understood over the past years. For many years azathioprine and prednisone have comprised the mainstay of immunosuppressive therapy. However, transplant survival rate using these agents in combination therapy rarely exceeded 50% at 1 year. Only since the introduction of cyclosporin A has transplant survival improved significantly, and further improvement is expected with the introduction of new immunosuppressive agents such as FK-506, RS-61443, rapamycin, and deoxyspergualin. These immunosuppressive drugs are described in more detail in the following discussion.

Steroids

The immunosuppressive effect of steroids is incompletely understood but probably relies on interaction at multiple sites in the inflammatory process. Steroids block the production of interleukin-1 (IL-1) by macrophages and inhibit the induction of class I antigens necessary for antigen presentation. Steroids also block gamma-interferon production, neutrophil migration, and lysosomal enzyme release by polymorphonuclear neutrophils. Steroids may also directly inhibit IL-2 synthesis. By blocking the response of leukocytes to chemotactins, inhibitory agents that increase vascular permeability, and by inhibiting vasodilators such as histamine and prostacycline, steroids exert a profound effect to dampen the inflammatory response, and ultimately, to blunt T-cell proliferation. Steroids, however, do not have a significant influence on antibody-mediated rejection.

The adverse effects of steroid therapy are numerous. The acute complications include impairment of glucose tolerance, delayed wound healing, and salt and fluid retention. Patients receiving high-dose steroids may become hypertensive because of salt and fluid retention. Central nervous system effects include insomnia, depression, nervousness, or euphoria. Chronic side effects of corticosteroids include Cushing's syndrome (central obesity, acne, striae, hirsutism, altered facies), cataracts, muscle wasting, and growth retardation in prepubertal children. Further long-term complications include a tendency to develop peptic ulcer disease, osteoporosis, and cataracts. The current trend in transplantation is to minimize the dose of steroids by adding two, three, or four other immunosuppressive agents.

Azathioprine

The antimetabolite azathioprine (Imuran) was synthesized by Nobel Prize winners Hitchens and Ellion from the Burroughs Wellcome Company. Azathioprine is converted in vivo to 6-mercaptopurine, which inhibits purine nucleotide synthesis by altering DNA structure. Azathioprine nonspecifically acts on proliferating lymphocytes and the peripheral nervous system at the level of DNA and RNA synthesis. Its primary toxicity is directed at the bone marrow, and the dose is decreased as the total white blood cells fall or is stopped in a patient with severe leukopenia.

Cyclosporine

Borel, a scientist from the Sandoz Company, demonstrated the potent immunosuppressive properties of cyclosporine, a cyclic undecapeptide isolated from the fungus *Polypocladium infladum gans.* Clinical studies were initiated in 1978 by Calne and Starzl, and in 1983 cyclosporine was approved for use in the United States, resulting in dramatic improvement in the results of all organ transplants, but particularly in liver and heart transplantation. Cyclosporine is metabolized by the hepatic cytochrome P-450 enzymes; therefore blood levels are increased by inhibitors of cytochrome P-450 (ketoconazole, erythromycin, calcium channel blockers) and decreased by inducers of cytochrome P-450 (rifampin, phenobarbital). The mechanism of action of cyclosporine is incompletely understood; cyclosporine reversibly inhibits T-lymphocyte–mediated immune responses. Recent research seems to indicate that cyclosporine, after entering the cells, binds to a protein called *cyclophilin.* The cyclophilline-cyclosporine complex then interacts with the phosphatase calcineurin and blocks the interaction of calcium with calcineurin (Fig. 13-7).

As a result, the cytoplasmatic factor of the cytoplasmatic component of the nuclear factor of activated T-cells cannot enter the nucleus and induce the transcription of messenger RNA for IL-2. Thus the major effect of cyclosporin A lies in its ability to suppress IL-2 synthesis. Cyclosporine seems to inhibit predominantly helper, inducer, and cytotoxic T-cell responses while sparing suppressor T-cells. Cyclosporine causes dose-related nephrotoxicity, probably by a vasoconstrictor effect on the renal microvasculature. Recently it has been postulated that a newly discovered factor, termed *endothelene,* is responsible for this effect. Patients receiving cyclosporine may also develop hyperkalemia, hypertension, and, frequently, neurologic side effects consisting of tremors, paraesthesia, headaches, depression, and, rarely, seizures. Hypertrichosis of the face, arms, and back is seen in approximately 50% of patients.

Antilymphocyte Globulin

The idea of using an antiserum generated by the immunization of an animal with human lymphocytes was first suggested by Metchnikoff in the early 1900s. Antilymphocyte globulin as currently used in clinical practice is a polyclonal serum produced by inoculating horses or goats with human lymphocytes or thymocytes. Two preparations are currently available: ATGAM, produced by the Upjohn Company, and Minnesota antilymphocyte globulin, produced by the University of Minnesota laboratories. Although antilymphocyte sera have been used for many years, their mechanism of action is poorly understood. Most investigators favor the idea that the antibody interacts with this antigen (the recipient T-lymphocyte), causing opsonization and clearance of these cells through the reticular endothelial system. Antilymphocyte sera are usually given through a central line to avoid phlebosclerosis and should be delivered through a filter to prevent administration of insoluble aggregates that may develop with storage. Antilymphocyte globulin may be given in the early posttransplant period as a component of induction therapy or may be administered to treat episodes of acute rejection. In most instances antilymphocyte globulin is used as a part of a multidrug immunosuppressive protocol, usually in conjunction with cyclosporine, azathioprine, and prednisone. Side effects of antilymphocyte sera include chills and fever and the typical skin rash characterized by large, raised, erythematous

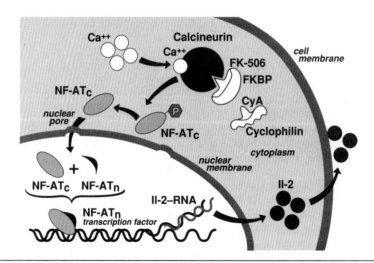

FIGURE 13-7   Mechanism of immunosuppressive action of cyclosporine and FK-506.

wheals on the trunk, neck, and proximal extremities. Thrombocytopenia and leukopenia occur in approximately 10% of patients and require dose adjustment. The use of antilymphocyte globulin has been associated with an increase in the reactivation and development of primary cytomegalovirus infection.

OKT3 Monoclonal Antibody

Whereas ALG is relatively nonspecific, monoclonal antibodies have very specific targets. The technology for the creation of effective amounts of monoclonal antibodies stems from the hybridoma work by Nobel Prize winners Kohler and Millstein. The only commercially available preparation for monoclonal antibodies for use in organ transplantation is the murine monoclonal antibody to the CD3 complex on human lymphocytes, muromonab-CD3 (Orthoclone OKT3). OKT3 is the product of a hybridoma formed from a myeloma cell and a primed murine lymphocyte capable of producing these antibodies. The cell lines are cultured in mouse ascites and the final product purified. There are several ways in which OKT3 is thought to have its effect as an immunosuppressant. The CD3 determinant is a complex of membrane proteins found on the surface of all mature T-lymphocytes that are closely associated with the T-cell receptor. The CD3 complex is thought responsible for transmitting the intracellular message once antigen recognition has occurred. Since OKT3 binds to the CD3 determinant, it prevents activation and, ultimately, the generation of CD8$^+$ killer T-lymphocytes. In addition, after the administration of OKT3 there is a rapid decrease in the amount of circulating lymphocytes. This is most likely a result of opsonization and clearance by the reticular endothelial system of the OKT3 complex. Another possible way in which OKT3 exerts its effect is by modulation of the cell-surface proteins, rendering a T-lymphocyte without a CD3 determinant nonfunctional. In addition to interfering with the generation of cytotoxic T-cells and the modulation of cell-surface proteins, OKT3 blocks the cytotoxic activity of already formed T-killer cells. This is perhaps its most important function. Side effects of OKT3 include pulmonary edema, especially after the first or second dose, fever, and headaches.

FK-506

FK-506 is a macrolide produced by *Streptomyces tseukubakenses,* which was discovered in 1984 in Japan during a search for new immunosuppressive agents. FK-506 is 100 times more potent in blocking IL-2 production than cyclosporine. Its mechanism of action seems similar because FK-506 binds to a protein, FK-binding protein, and this complex again prevents interaction of calcium with the phosphatase calcineurin. Numerous animal studies have demonstrated the superior immunosuppressive potency of FK-506. In patients FK-506 is very effective in heart and liver transplantation for induction and maintenance therapy and in rescue therapy for liver transplants. Major side effects of FK-506 include nephrotoxicity and neurotoxicity.

RS-61443

RS-61443 is an antimetabolite that structurally is a morpholinoethyl ester of mycophenolic acid. This drug inhibits the enzyme inosine monophosphate dehydrogenase and therefore purine de novo synthesis. Because lymphocytes, unlike other cells, do not have a salvage pathway, the action of this drug seems rather selective.

In initial clinical trials at the University of Wisconsin, RS-61443 was administered in conjunction with cyclosporin A and prednisone, replacing azathioprine. In these trials it was shown that with increasing doses of RS-61443, the incidence of rejection episodes in patients receiving kidney transplants was markedly reduced. In addition, RS-61443 was used successfully for rescue therapy in kidney, heart, and liver transplantation. The most remarkable feature of RS-61443 is its low toxicity, in particular, the lack of nephrotoxicity.

Rapamycin

Rapamycin is a macrolide antibiotic derived from *Streptomyces hygroscopicus.* The agent, which initially was described as an antifungal agent, was recently found to have immunosuppressive properties. Rapamycin is structurally very similar to FK-506 but seems to have a slightly different mechanism of action. Rapamycin dramatically prolongs mouse heart and skin allograft survival and rat cardiac allograft survival at very low doses. Clinical trials testing the efficacy of rapamycin will be initiated in several centers in the United States.

Anti-IL-2 Strategies

One very specific approach to achieving immunosuppression is to target activation antigens of lymphocytes involved in allograft rejection. The receptor for IL-2 is important in T-cell activation. There are two approaches to the IL-2 receptor monoclonal antibodies, or so-called *IL-2 toxins.* Clinical experience with monoclonal antibodies directed against the 55-kilo (145-pound) adult and a subunit of the human IL-2 receptor have been tested. The first, called *anti-tac,* is a murine monoclonal antibody, and the second, *33B3.1,* is a rat IgG2A monoclonal antibody. Anti-tac prevents and reduces the frequency of early rejection episodes when used in combination with cyclosporine.

Another approach to the IL-2 receptor is through the diphtheria IL-2 toxin. A combination of protein engineering and recombinant DNA methodologies have produced this IL-2 toxin. The affinity of IL-2 receptor antibodies is inferior to that of IL-2 itself, and these antibodies fix complement poorly; IL-2 toxins are more selectively targeted and more potent agents. When tested in a delayed hypersensitivity model, dramatic specific antigen immunosuppression was observed.

KIDNEY TRANSPLANTATION

In 1992 approximately 140,000 patients in the United States will undergo dialysis treatment for chronic renal failure. Among them, 22,000 will be waiting for a kidney transplant. It is estimated that 9000 to 10,000 kidney transplants will be performed in 1992. In general, the advantages of kidney transplantation versus dialysis include a better quality of life and a longer life expectancy. The surgical technique for kidney transplantation has been standardized for many years now. Usually the kidney is placed into the iliac fossa, with anastomosis of the renal artery to the iliac artery and the renal vein to the iliac vein (Fig. 13-8). Various modifications exist, in particular for kidneys that have several arteries or in recipients with atherosclerotic iliac artery disease. The ureter is implanted into the bladder using an antireflux technique. Most surgeons prefer using the right iliac fossa because of easier access to the iliac vein.

The success of kidney transplantation depends primarily on the relationship between donor and recipient. The best results are obtained in HLA-identical live donor–recipient combinations. Recipients of cadaver kidneys or living-unrelated donor kidneys fare less well. It is estimated that cadaver kidneys have a 50% chance of functioning 10 years after transplantation, whereas the kidneys from HLA-identical live donors have an 80% chance of functioning at the same time interval. The only contraindications

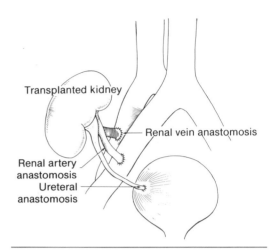

FIGURE 13-8   Kidney transplantation technique.

for kidney transplantation are very advanced age, cancer, and active infection of the recipient. The most common causes of kidney failure in the United States are diabetes, glomerulonephritis, hypertensive nephropathy, and congenital kidney disease. Maintenance immunosuppressive therapy includes cyclosporine, prednisone, and azathioprine. The newer immunosuppressive agents such as RS-61443 and FK-506 remain under investigation.

More than 50% of recipients of cadaveric kidneys will experience acute cellular rejection. This type of rejection is characterized histologically by adherence of lymphocytes to the endothelium of peritubular capillaries and venules, which then progresses to disruption of these vessels, tubular necrosis, and interstitial infiltrates. As rejection proceeds toward irreversibility, there is greater involvement of the vascular elements of the graft. Swelling of the intima and focal fibronecrosis of the media ensue, followed by endothelial cell proliferation and obliteration of the lumina of small arteries by fibrin, platelets, and lymphoid cells. The most reliable diagnosis of acute rejection is made by needle biopsy of the graft, and the most important differential diagnosis is cyclosporine toxicity.

Chronic rejection is a common cause of late graft loss after kidney transplantation. The typical course of chronic rejection is gradual, progressive loss of renal function. It may begin as early as a few months after transplantation but also may occur after years of stable graft function. Patients who have had one or several episodes of acute rejection are more likely to develop chronic rejection. Chronic rejection is manifested histologically by intimal fibroproliferative arterial lesions. These intimal lesions probably stem from repetitive cycles of chronic immune injury to the endothelium, resulting in focal thrombosis and incorporation of thrombus into the arterial wall. Other reasons for graft failure include recurrence of glomerulonephritis and recurrent diabetic nephropathy. Technical complications after renal transplantation include arterial and venous thrombosis, which are usually due to technical error. Renal transplant artery stenosis, manifested by sustained hypertension, is usually a result of a fibrotic process surrounding the transplant artery or the anastomosis. If diagnosed early, this condition can be corrected through either transluminal angioplasty or corrective surgery.

Urinary complications may include ureteral obstruction at the site of the ureteroneocystostomy, sloughing of the ureter, or a leak at the implant site of the ureter. Ureteral stricture usually can be corrected using invasive radiologic techniques, but sloughing of the ureter or leakage must be repaired surgically.

Lymphoceles occur in 5% to 10% of patients after kidney transplantation. Failure to ligate lymphatics crossing the iliac vessels may be the cause of this complication. Unilateral leg swelling on the side of the transplant is usually the first sign. This condition may be associated with a rise in serum creatinine levels if the lymphocele compresses the ureter. Operative correction requires the creation of a window between the lymphocele and the peritoneal cavity.

PANCREAS TRANSPLANTATION

The first pancreas transplant was performed by Kelly and Lillehei on December 17, 1966, in Minneapolis, Minnesota. The indication for pancreas transplantation is type I diabetes, and its purpose is to prevent or stabilize secondary diabetic complications such as retinopathy, neuropathy, and microvascular disease. Pancreas transplantation is performed for three patient groups: pancreas transplantation alone (PA) for patients who do not have significant diabetic nephropathy; simultaneous pancreas-kidney transplantation (SPK) for patients with diabetic nephropathy who receive a kidney transplantation in the same operation (Fig. 13-9); and pancreas transplantation after a successful kidney transplant (PAK). Approximately 600 pancreas transplants were performed in 1991 in the United States, and more than 90% were SPK transplants.

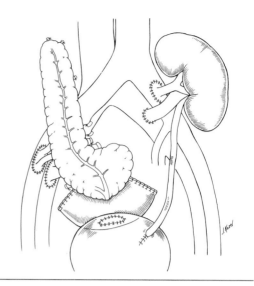

FIGURE 13-9 Combined kidney-pancreas transplantation technique.

The search for the best technique for pancreas transplantation has been a continuing challenge over the past 20 years. In the center of the controversy was the debate on how to manage exocrine pancreatic secretion.

Three surgical procedures are used. The first, pancreas transplantation with enteric drainage, uses anastomosis of the pancreas or pancreatic duct to small bowel. The advantage of this technique is that pancreatic secretions, including bicarbonate, are drained into a physiologic environment. The disadvantage is that the anastomosis between the pancreas and small bowel is prone to leakage, which may result in septic complications. To avoid anastomosis of the pancreas to the draining organ, in 1978 the group from Lyon suggested a second technique, injecting the pancreatic duct with a polymerase substance. This substance hardens after injection into the pancreatic duct, thus obliterating the ductal system. Unfortunately, this may result in posttransplant pancreatitis and pancreatic fistulas. The third—and most popular—technique is drainage of the pancreatic duct into the urinary bladder. Most centers around the world use a whole pancreas transplant with the duodenum anastomosed to the bladder. In this way exocrine pancreatic secretions are excreted in the urine.

This third technique is relatively safe. In addition, urinary amylase can be used as a monitor of pancreas transplant rejection. Currently, the 1-year graft survival rate for SPK transplants is

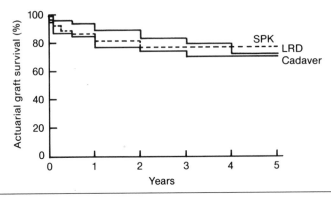

FIGURE 13-10 Simultaneous pancreas-kidney *(SPK)*, primary cadaver, and living related donor *(LRD)* kidney transplants in diabetics; graft survival—University of Wisconsin experience.

75% in the United States (Fig. 13-10). Postoperative complications typical for pancreas transplantation include vascular thrombosis in 3% to 5%, leakage from the pancreaticoduodeno-cystostomy in approximately 10%, bleeding, and peripancreatic infection.

After successful pancreas transplantation, normalization of carbohydrate metabolism occurs. Although freedom from insulin injections undoubtedly improves the patient's quality of life, it is not in itself the purpose of the procedure. The main objective of pancreas transplantation is to reverse or arrest secondary diabetic complications.

The first evidence of the potential beneficial effect from pancreas transplantation on diabetic nephropathy was the observation that patients who receive a combined kidney-pancreas transplant do not develop recurrent diabetic nephropathy in their transplanted kidney. More than 80% of patients undergoing pancreas transplantation suffer from autonomic and peripheral neuropathy. Preliminary data from various centers indicate improvement in motor conduction velocity in the upper and lower extremities and improvement of autonomic neuropathy. With the use of thermography, muscle oxygen tension measurements, and laser Doppler determination, a beneficial effect of pancreas transplantation on microcirculation has been demonstrated. The influence of pancreas transplantation on diabetic retinopathy remains controversial. Quality-of-life assessment after combined kidney-pancreas transplantation has been investigated at several centers in Europe and the United States. There is agreement that patients who have undergone SPK transplantation enjoy a better quality of life than patients receiving a kidney transplant alone. It is estimated that approximately 4000 patients annually in the United States are potential candidates for SPK transplantation. Because of the shortage of organ donors, however, only approximately one fourth will receive a transplant.

ISLET TRANSPLANTATION

Whole-organ pancreas transplantation has emerged as the most effective treatment for type I diabetes; however, it should not be considered the final solution to the problem. A simpler and safer method to restore normoglycemia is transplantation of only insulin-producing beta cells in the form of pancreatic islets or fetal pancreata. In animal experiments with these grafts, reduction of the immunogenicity of the islets has been accomplished. Thus it would be theoretically possible to transplant islets or fetal pancreatic tissue without the need for immunosuppressive therapy. Unfortunately, clinical transplantation of these grafts has met with very limited success. The major problem associated with the transplantation of human islets is related to the difficulty in isolating a sufficient number of islets from one single adult pancreas to restore normoglycemia in the diabetic recipient. The standard islet isolation technique generally includes mechanical separation of the gland, partial digestion using collagenase, and differential density gradient centrifugation to separate the islets from the exocrine tissue. The islets can then be implanted beneath the renal capsule or into the splenic parenchyma or can be injected into the portal vein for engraftment in the liver. Only recently have selected groups been successful in isolating the 300,000 to 500,000 islets sufficient to reverse hyperglycemia. Although more than 100 human islet transplants have been reported from various centers, very few of these grafts ever showed clear evidence of function, and all of them, with the exception of one, have failed. This successful patient is now 18 months past islet transplantation performed in conjunction with a kidney transplant.

LIVER TRANSPLANTATION

Clinical liver transplantation was pioneered by Starzl and Calne, with Starzl performing the first liver transplant in 1963. As of 1980, approximately 200 liver transplants were performed using prednisone and azathioprine as immunosuppressive agents. With the demonstrated benefits of cyclosporin A therapy and a National Institutes of Health conference on liver transplantation in 1983 at which it was decided that liver transplantation was no longer experimental, the number of liver transplants performed in the United States has increased dramatically. Since 1983 when cyclosporin A was introduced into clinical practice, over 10,000 liver transplants have been performed in the United States in approximately 70 centers. Liver transplantation has become accepted as standard therapy for a variety of advanced chronic liver diseases in both children and adults.

The most common indication for liver transplantation in adults is chronic active hepatitis and in children, biliary atresia. Other forms of advanced chronic liver disease such as alcoholic liver disease, sclerosing cholangitis, and primary biliary cirrhosis occur frequently and require transplantation. Our experience and that of others reveal an extremely low level of recidivism among alcoholics after transplantation. In fact, caring for the alcoholic patient with end-stage liver disease who has multiple hospital admissions and variceal bleeds may be more expensive than providing liver transplantation. Fulminant hepatic failure, usually viral in origin, is another common indication for liver transplantation. Since these patients are usually desperately ill, they should be referred to a liver transplant center early in the course of their disease. Patients with hepatic malignancy should also be considered for liver transplantation; however, the long-term prognosis is much less favorable than in patients with benign disease.

If a patient with advanced chronic end-stage liver disease meets any of the following criteria,

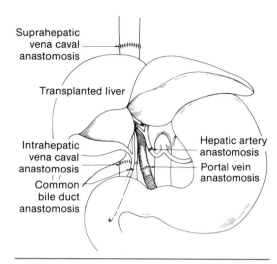

FIGURE 13-11 Most commonly used technique for liver transplantation. The vascular anastomoses are performed in the following sequence: (1) suprahepatic vena caval anastomosis; (2) infrahepatic vena caval anastomosis; (3) portal vein anastomosis; and (4) hepatic artery anastomosis. Common bile duct reconstruction in adults is usually accomplished by end-to-end anastomosis of the donor and recipient common bile ducts. In children a choledochojejunostomy is used.

he or she must be considered a candidate for liver transplantation: (1) total bilirubin level of 15 mg/dl or more; (2) a prothrombin time that is correctable and greater than control by 5 seconds; (3) a serum albumin level of 2.5 g/dl or less; (4) hepatic encephalopathy; (5) variceal bleeding; or (6) intractable ascites.

The most commonly used transplantation technique is shown in Fig. 13-11. Recipient laparotomy is performed with a bilateral subcostal incision extending to the upper midline. The common bile duct, hepatic artery, and portal vein are dissected free. The left triangular ligament is divided, and the vena cava above and below the liver is encircled. Venovenous bypass has been a routine procedure in adults in most liver transplant centers since 1982. Heparin-coated cannulas are placed into the inferior vena cava through the femoral vein and into the portal vein, and venous blood is returned to the axillary vein by using a Biomedicus pump. This procedure gives the operating surgeon the opportunity to complete the hepatic phase and provides support during the anhepatic phase by maintaining the recipient's cardiac output by returning the blood from the subdiaphragmatic portions of the body to the heart.

This advance has markedly reduced the blood product requirements in most patients during the procedure. The usual biliary tract reconstruction involves anastomosing the donor bile duct to the recipient bile duct. Patients with biliary atresia, sclerosing cholangitis, and other diseases in which the recipient common duct is not adequate require biliary reconstruction with a 40-cm Roux-en-Y jejunal loop. Previously, postoperative immunosuppression consisted of various combinations of cyclosporin A, prednisone, azathioprine, and antilymphocyte globulin. Recently, the introduction of FK-506, which has a similar mechanism of action as cyclosporin A, has been shown as nearly 100 times more potent. Currently, a prospective, randomized study comparing FK-506 with cyclosporin A is under way. Liver transplant rejection can be treated with an intravenous bolus of corticosteroids or the monoclonal antibody OKT3. Likewise, FK-506 is available for rescue therapy in patients who have failed conventional antirejection therapy, and it has nearly a 70% rate of rescue.

Both short- and long-term results of liver transplantation in children are better than in adults. Most programs have achieved an 80% to 90% 1-year survival rate for children. In contrast, the overall 1-year survival rate for adults usually is 60% to 80%, depending on the program and the kind of patients receiving surgical treatment at the given institution.

HEART TRANSPLANTATION

The first successful heart transplant was performed in 1967 by Barnard in Cape Town, South Africa. After some years of rather disappointing results, cardiac transplantation gained momentum in the early 1980s after the introduction of cyclosporin A. At the current time, graft survival at 1 year is 85% to 90%. Inclusion criteria for heart transplantation are shown in the box above.

The technique for heart transplantation is now well established (Fig. 13-12). The diseased recipient heart is excised, but the atria are left intact. Implantation of the donor heart includes a running anastomosis of the donor atria to the recipient atria and anastomosis of the ascending aorta and pulmonary artery.

The most common causes of death after heart transplantation include acute rejection, hyperacute rejection, obliterative arteriopathy, and infection. Chronic rejection of the heart is mani-

---

INDICATIONS FOR CARDIAC TRANSPLANTATION

Age: Newborn to 60 years

End-stage cardiac disease, class IV (NYHA)

Normal function or reversible dysfunction of kidneys, liver, lungs, central nervous system

Pulmonary vascular resistance less than 6-8 Wood units or pharmacologically reversible

Absence of active malignancy or infection, recent pulmonary infarction, or severe peripheral or cerebrovascular disease

---

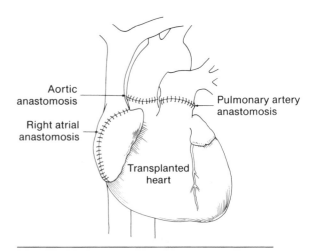

FIGURE 13-12 Orthotopic heart transplantation technique. Aortic, pulmonary, and right atrial anastomoses are shown.

---

fested by recurrent coronary artery disease. A major advance in cardiac transplantation has been made with the introduction of transvenous myocardial biopsy. In most transplant centers transvenous biopsy is performed at routine intervals after transplantation. Immunosuppressive therapy is similar to that for liver and kidney transplantation.

SINGLE-LUNG, DOUBLE-LUNG, AND HEART-LUNG TRANSPLANTATION

Although isolated lung transplantation was first attempted in 1963 at the University of Missis-

**INDICATIONS FOR
SINGLE-LUNG TRANSPLANTATION**

Idiopathic pulmonary fibrosis
Emphysema
Emphysematous alpha-antitrypsin
deficiency
Pulmonary hypertension
Eisenmenger's syndrome

sippi, success eluded thoracic surgeons until 1983 when a patient with idiopathic pulmonary fibrosis survived a single-lung transplant at the University of Toronto. The major indications for single-lung transplantation are listed in the box above.

Single-lung transplantation is usually performed through a posterolateral thoracotomy. The lung with the lowest perfusion ratio is usually selected for transplantation. The actuarial 1-year survival rate for all single-lung recipients reported to the Lung Transplant Registry is 66%. Most of the deaths following single-lung transplantation occur within 60 days and are usually related to poor graft function secondary to infection or the pulmonary sequelae of infection outside the graft (i.e., adult respiratory distress syndrome). Late mortality from isolated lung transplantation is the result of opportunistic infection or bronchiolitis obliterans, a poorly understood process of small airway destruction that is believed a consequence of chronic rejection. Cytomegalovirus disease is a frequent complication of lung transplantation, but successful therapy with antiviral agents has rendered the pathogen less lethal than it was several years ago.

Double-lung transplantation is indicated primarily in the younger patient with bilateral septic pulmonary processes that mandate bilateral pneumonectomy. These processes include bronchiectasis, cystic fibrosis, infected pneumatoceles, and other forms of parenchymal disease associated with recurrent pneumonitis.

The first successful heart-lung transplant was performed in March 1981 by Reitz and his colleagues at Stanford University. The patient lived an active and fulfilling life for more than 5 years. This success launched the revival of clinical heart-lung transplantation. More than 1000 combined heart-lung transplant procedures have been performed in 83 centers. With the introduction of single- and double-lung transplantation, the indications for heart-lung transplantation are changing. Currently in the United States heart-lung transplantation is indicated for patients with cardiopulmonary disease whose heart function is thought irreparable. The Registry of the International Society for Heart and Lung Transplantation reports a 1-year actuarial survival rate of 59% and 5-year actuarial survival of 41%.

The late development of obliterative bronchiolitis limits the overall good results of this procedure. Interestingly, obliterative bronchiolitis is more common after heart-lung transplantation than after isolated lung transplantation. It is hoped that the aggressive use of transbronchial biopsy for the detection of early acute rejection, coupled with the control of an early treatment for cytomegalovirus infection, will result in a significant decrease in this immunologically mediated entity.

BIBLIOGRAPHY

Bach FH, Sachs DH. Transplantation immunology. N Engl J Med 317:489-492, 1987.

Belzer FO, Southard JH. Principles of solid organ preservation by cold storage. Transplantation 45:673, 1988.

Cooper JD, Pearson FG, Patterson GA, et al. Technique of successful lung transplantation in humans. J Thorac Cardiovasc Surg 93:173-181, 1987.

Griffith BP, Kormos RL, Hardesty RL. Heterotopic cardiac transplantation: Current status. J Cardiac Surg 2:283-289, 1987.

Iwatsuki S, Starzl TE, Todo S, et al. Experience in 1,000 liver transplants under cyclosporine-steroid therapy: A survival report. Transplant Proc 20:498-504, 1988.

Krensky AM, Weiss A, Crabtree G, et al. T-lymphocyte–antigen interactions in transplant rejection. N Engl J Med 322:510-517, 1990.

Morris PJ (ed). Kidney Transplantation: Principles and Practice, 3rd ed. Philadelphia, WB Saunders, 1988.

Starzl TE, Hakala TR, Shaw BW Jr, et al. A flexible procedure for multiple cadaveric organ procurement. Surg Gynecol Obstet 158:223-230, 1984.

CHAPTER REVIEW
Questions

1. An allograft is a transplant:
   a. From an individual of a different species
   b. From a genetically identical individual
   c. From a normal anatomic position to an abnormal one
   d. From a member of the same species
   e. That is always rejected hyperacutely

2. The major histocompatibility complex does not include:
   a. HLA A
   b. HLA B
   c. LD
   d. RH
   e. DR

3. Blood transfusions result in:
   a. Decreased kidney transplant survival
   b. A higher incidence of hyperacute rejection
   c. Better tolerance to immunosuppression
   d. Better kidney graft survival
   e. No influence on graft survival

4. A positive crossmatch is:
   a. No contradiction to transplantation
   b. Not as important as matching for HLA antigens
   c. Sure to result in acute rejection
   d. A contraindication for transplantation
   e. Associated with a high stimulation in MLC

5. The best way to induce classical tolerance is:
   a. Injection of enhancing antibodies
   b. Injection of antigens in the neonatal period
   c. Matching donor and recipient for MLC
   d. Generation of suppressor cells
   e. Irradiation combined with ALG

6. One-year graft survival for cadaver kidneys is:
   a. 96%
   b. 45% to 55%
   c. 60% to 90%
   d. 5% to 10%
   e. 25%

7. The preferred arterial anastomosis in adult renal transplantation is:
   a. Aortorenal
   b. External iliac–renal
   c. Internal iliac–renal
   d. Superficial femoral–renal
   e. Common iliac–renal

8. The preferred restoration of urinary continuity in kidney transplantation is:
   a. Ureter–ureterostomy
   b. Ureter–neocystostomy
   c. Ureter–pyelostomy
   d. Crossover ureter–ureterostomy
   e. Pyelo–cystostomy

9. Cyclosporin A:
   a. Suppresses mainly T-lymphocytes
   b. Is a bacterial product
   c. Is a synthetic product
   d. Can only be used in liver transplantation
   e. Cannot be used in combination with other immunosuppressive drugs

10. Pancreas transplantation:
    a. Is more successful than kidney transplantation
    b. Is more successful with islets than with whole organ transplantation
    c. Does not require crossmatching
    d. Has as its major technical problem the management of exocrine drainage
    e. Is associated with a lower mortality than kidney transplantation

Answers

1. d	6. b
2. d	7. b and c
3. d	8. b
4. d	9. a
5. b	10. d

PATIENT PRESENTATIONS: A SYMPTOM-BASED APPROACH

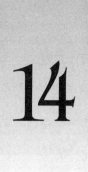

14

Intraoral Lesions

BENJAMIN F. RUSH, Jr.

KEY FEATURES

After reading this chapter you will understand:
- The anatomy of the oral cavity and be familiar with the normal anatomic landmarks and terms.
- Congenital and benign intraoral lesions and a treatment protocol.
- Treatment of traumatic lesions.
- The common sites of oral infection and abscess formation.
- What benign tumors commonly occur.
- How early cancer of the oral cavity is recognized.
- The lymph node drainage sequence for various intraoral locations.
- Single and multimodal treatment of oral cancer.

ANATOMY OF THE ORAL CAVITY

Patients with an intraoral lesion usually come to the surgeon, either directly or by referral, with a specific lesion that requires diagnosis and treatment rather than a complex of symptoms, as occurs in patients who have a pathologic condition of a more internal area. *The anatomic area described as intraoral includes the lips, buccal mucosa, upper and lower gingiva, floor of the mouth, hard palate, and the anterior two thirds of the tongue* (Fig. 14-1). The tongue, by convention, is divided into three anatomic segments.

The *posterior third*, consisting of that portion of the tongue between the circumvallate papillae and the vallecula, is considered to be in the *oropharynx, along with the tonsils, tonsillar pillars, and soft palate.* The anterior third of the tongue is the portion that extends from the tip of the tongue to the point where the tongue is attached to the floor of the mouth. The middle third of the tongue extends from the point where the tongue joins the floor of the mouth backward to the circumvallate papillae.

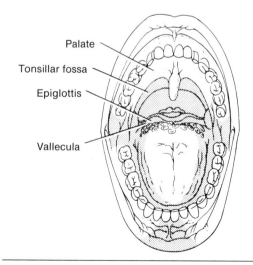

FIGURE 14-1 Anatomy of mouth. Note that shaded areas indicate the common sites of malignancy.

257

How Do You Examine the Oral Cavity?

Although the entire oral cavity is easy to examine visually, it is surprising how often substantial lesions are missed. Physicians should use most of their senses in examining this area. A headlight, a fiberoptic light source, a gooseneck lamp or a dental lamp should be used to bring maximal illumination into the area. A tongue depressor is used to deflect the soft tissues so that each structure can be inspected minutely. The sense of touch should not be neglected, since many oral lesions are submucosal and may only be appreciated by manual palpation; *bimanual palpation is even more effective.* The soft tissues of the cheeks, floor of the mouth, and tongue can be pressed between the gloved finger in the mouth and the other examining hand pressing against the cheek or under the chin so that any intervening mass can be rolled between the examining fingers. The *odor of a necrotic tumor mass* is unmistakable once experienced, and the physician may thus be warned of the presence of a large lesion, even though it is buried somewhere posteriorly in the hypopharynx or nasopharynx.

Although we are discussing primary lesions of the oral cavity, no examination of the area is complete without an inspection of the nasopharynx, hypopharynx, and larynx as well. This requires the use of an oral mirror and headlight or a head mirror reflecting light from a source behind the patient. Even more effective is a fiberoptic nasopharyngoscope passed through the nostril. The ease and accuracy with which fiberoptic devices can be used make them superior tools for examination.

IMPORTANT CONGENITAL LESIONS OF THE ORAL CAVITY
Cleft Lip and Palate

Deformities of the lips and palate are commonly encountered and can be identified by most laymen. They occur in approximately 1 of every 1000 births, and ethnic origin has a substantial influence. Cleft lips and palates are eight times more common in Caucasian babies than in African-American babies. A failure of the central mesodermal tissues of the face to unite between the first and second months of development is represented in the case of cleft lip, and a failure of these tissues to unite between the second and third months results in a cleft palate. Repair of a cleft lip may be done in the newborn, but most surgeons rely on the *rule of 10*—that is, when the baby reaches 10 pounds and the hemoglobin level is 10 g, an event usually occurring at about the tenth postnatal week. At this time the structures are larger and the repair can be performed more accurately. Repair of a cleft palate is usually delayed for 20 to 24 months to permit an easier manipulation of the larger structures. The procedure should not be delayed much later than this, since children who learn to speak with an unrepaired cleft palate will acquire speech defects that may persist throughout their lives. Properly staffed cleft palate clinics include plastic and oral surgeons and speech pathologists, who work as a team.

Retention Cysts

Various retention cysts are found in the lips and oral cavity and usually represent obstructed mucous glands. A special form of retention cysts is the *ranula, which appears as a 2 to 3 cm thin-walled, bluish structure in the floor of the mouth.* Some believe a ranula is a result of congenital or acquired obstruction of Wharton's duct, with rupture of the duct into the submucosal tissues. This lesion can be cured by excision of the dome of the cyst and suture of its margins to marsupialize the floor of the cyst. Cysts of the lips and other intraoral areas are treated by simple excision.

Peutz-Jeghers Syndrome

Peutz-Jeghers syndrome is marked by *multiple melanin spots on the lips and is associated with multiple polyps of the small bowel.* This lesion is inherited, and the only significance of the oral lesion is that it calls attention to the presence of the intestinal polyps that may be associated with bleeding, intussusception, and, very rarely, malignancy.

Lingual Thyroid

In embryonic life, the *thyroid originates at the foramen cecum* and descends into the neck to take up its normal location. Its descent may be halted at any point, and occasionally it fails to descend at all, appearing as a mass in the area of the foramen cecum at the junction of the middle and posterior third of the tongue. *The surgeon must beware of a mass in this location and must not excise it in toto until a biopsy is taken.* Excision of a lingual thyroid will result in an athyroid patient, and the decision to carry out such a procedure should be determined by consideration of the symptoms caused by the mass. If the patient is asymptomatic, the thyroid should be left in situ.

Thyroglossal duct cyst may occur at any point along the route of descent of the thyroid from the level of the tongue down through the hyoid bone to the level of the pyramidal lobe. If such a cyst appears at the level of the foramen cecum, it can be excised—assuming that it has been differentiated from a lingual thyroid by an appropriate biopsy.

Hemangiomas

Hemangiomas may appear in the lips or in any structures of the oral cavity. Simple capillary hemangiomas will often appear in the first few days or weeks of life and seem at first to grow rapidly. By about the ninth month of life the capillaries will begin to sclerose and *the hemangioma will almost always undergo spontaneous resolution* with no other treatment but observation. The eventual product of this evolution is a small, scarred nodule called a *sclerosing hemangioma.* These may sometimes be visualized underneath the translucent mucosa of the oral cavity or palpated beneath the skin but are of no serious clinical importance (Fig. 14-2).

Cavernous hemangiomas, in which the vascular structures form larger lakes, occur in deeper tissues and often involve the tongue. They resolve more slowly but likewise tend to undergo eventual resolution. Related, but much more troublesome, vascular lesions are *vascular malformations* that may be quite extensive. These have completely formed vessels with muscular coats as well as an endothelium and *do not resolve spontaneously.* They can occasionally develop venoarterial shunts, resulting in a rapidly expanding pulsatile destructive lesion called a *cirsoid aneurysm.* Treatment is by excision, which may require multiple operations. Radiation therapy of these mature vessels is of little benefit.

Torus Palatinus

Torus palatinus occurs in the hard palate and is an exostosis occurring along the line of fusion of the hard palate. It may be lobular. The major task of the examiner is to differentiate whether this lesion is benign or malignant. This can be done by simple palpation. The hard feeling of the bone

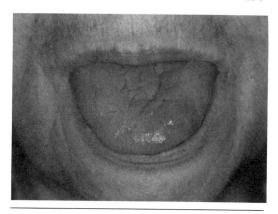

FIGURE 14-2   Hemangioma of tongue in adult. Note lump in left tip of tongue. This was slightly blue and easily compressed.

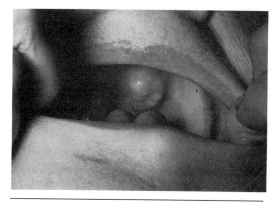

FIGURE 14-3   Torus of the hard palate (torus palatinus).

underlying the thin mucosa is easily recognized. The next task is to convince the patient that this recently found mass has probably been present since birth (Fig. 14-3).

Pierre Robin Syndrome

The Pierre Robin syndrome is a growth defect that produces a small and "undershot" jaw in newborns. A failure of the mandible to grow to its normal size results in poor support for the tongue, which falls back into the pharynx. *Infants with this syndrome may strangle as the tongue occludes the airway.* Treatment consists of suturing the tongue to the anterior lip in such a way that it cannot fall back into the pharynx. As the child grows, the mandible may ultimately achieve normal size or, in some cases, may respond to operative reconstruction.

HOW DO YOU TREAT INJURIES OF THE ORAL CAVITY?
Burns

Patients who have been exposed to fire may demonstrate circumoral or intraoral burns, which usually result from exposure to superheated air. Although these burns may not be serious in themselves, *they should alert the physician to the possibility of respiratory tract burns* that may lead to serious edema in the upper airways and possible subsequent asphyxia. These patients should be admitted to the hospital for observation. *Burned nasal hair* or *soot* in the nasal or oral passages and *elevated carboxyhemoglobin levels* in the presence of hoarseness are all signs that mandate admission.

Chemical burns of the oral cavity may result from attempted suicides or from accidental ingestion of chemicals. The most common offending agent is lye, although acid burns may also be seen. When chemically caused oral burns alert the physician to the possibility of burns in the esophagus and/or stomach, flexible esophagoscopy and gastroscopy should be performed. Patients with such lesions must be observed closely for subsequent esophageal stenosis or gastric perforation.

Electrical burns are often encountered in young children who often explore everything in their environment by putting it into their mouths. Such explorations may lead to biting an electrical cord, with resultant electrical burns of the lips, tongue, and gingiva. These burns may appear superficial initially, but often the damage is greater than is first apparent. These injuries should be treated nonoperatively and observed carefully for 7 to 10 days, at which time the maximal degree of damage should become evident.

Fractures

The subject of fractures of the mandible and maxilla is beyond the scope of this chapter. They can usually be diagnosed by point tenderness, crepitus, and mobility of the fractured part. It is important to note that if permanent adult teeth are lost in the course of trauma, they should be preserved and brought with the patient to the emergency room. Preferably the teeth should be kept moist in an isotonic solution. An easily available household solution is a small glass of milk. If the socket is intact, the oral surgeon can clean and fill the root canal and reinsert the tooth, wiring it into place. If this has been done promptly, the likelihood of saving the tooth exceeds 90%.

Lacerations

The structures of the oral cavities are highly vascular, and lacerations, either as the result of penetrating wounds or of blunt injury, *can lead to profuse, even life-threatening, hemorrhage.* If the patient is unconscious, endotracheal intubation should be done immediately to avoid the morbidity and possible mortality caused by aspirated blood. Initial control of serious hemorrhage can be obtained by placing packing firmly around an endotracheal tube. If hemorrhage does not subside with pressure, the patient's lacerations can be closed with absorbable sutures. Because plain and even chromic catgut tends to lose strength very rapidly in the presence of saliva, the newer synthetic absorbable sutures, which tolerate the oral environment well, are the best materials to use for intraoral suture (Fig. 14-4).

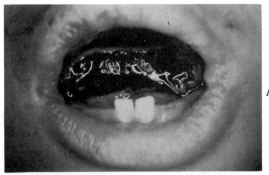

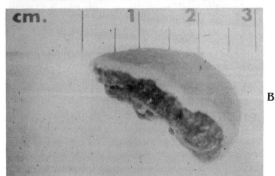

FIGURE 14-4   An example of intraoral injury. **A,** This young child fell while running and actually bit off the tip of her tongue, **B.**

INFECTIONS OF THE ORAL CAVITY

Infections of the oral cavity derive primarily from tonsillitis and from odontogenic sources. With the advent of antibiotics, as well as the use of fluorinated water, both of these sources of infection have decreased markedly over the last several decades. However, swift and rapidly progressive infections are still seen and may be life threatening.

Peritonsillar Abscess

A peritonsillar abscess usually follows one or more attacks of acute tonsillitis. The offending organisms are those normally found in the oral cavity, with the dominant organisms being *Fusobacterium, Bacteroides melaninogenicus,* and multiple species of both aerobic and anaerobic

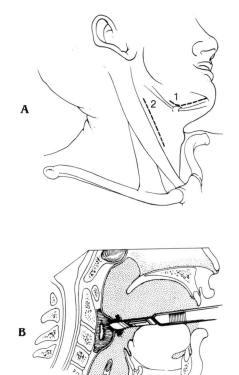

streptococci. *Pus from tonsillar infections tends to accumulate in the peritonsillar space,* lateral and superior to the tonsil itself. The tonsil is forced toward the midline, and the abscess bulges into the oral cavity through the anterior tonsillar pillar and the lateral soft palate. Appearance of this bulge is pathognomonic of peritonsillar abscess (quinsy throat). The abscess should be ***promptly drained*** with a curvilinear incision through the anterior surface of the tonsillar pillar and lateral soft palate. Drainage can be accomplished in adults with the use of local anesthesia. General anesthesia is required for children, who might otherwise struggle, and to avoid frightening the child. In this case, endotracheal anesthesia must be used so that there will be no danger of aspiration of the pus, which could lead to an abscess of the lung. Since the tonsil drains to nodes in the peripharyngeal and retropharyngeal areas, infected nodes may create abscesses in these locations, although these are much rarer sites. Retropharyngeal abscesses are drained through a linear incision in the posterior pharynx and peripharyngeal abscesses are drained by vertical linear incision at the angle of the mandible (Fig. 14-5).

Ludwig's Angina

Ludwig's angina is a rapidly spreading cellulitis in the floor of the mouth that occupies the space above and below the mylohyoid muscle and usually occurs bilaterally. This lesion was very common before antibiotics were developed and often led to suffocation of the patient as a result of swelling in the posterior area of the tongue. In the earlier phases of this infection, treatment with penicillin or first-generation cephalosporin is highly effective. ***Should the cellulitis progress despite the administration of antibiotics, drainage is mandatory to prevent asphyxiation.*** Drainage is usually carried out by a transverse incision at the level of the hyoid, which transects the mylohyoid muscles bilaterally and extends into the submaxillary triangle, to drain the spaces both above and below the muscles and behind the submaxillary glands, which may contain pus. If the collection is unilateral, an incision along the fibers of the digastric muscle will suffice. The pus encountered is often thin and serous. Although predominantly the infection is a cellulitis, this incision will guard against progressive edema in the tongue.

Both tonsillar and odontogenic infections may extend into the fascial planes of the neck and, on rare occasions, may extend down as far

FIGURE 14-5 **A,** Incisions used for drainage of *1,* Ludwig's angina or *2,* parapharyngeal abscess. **B,** Incision for drainage of retropharyngeal abscess.

as the mediastinum. If sepsis continues even with the use of antibiotics and drainage of the usual areas, the cervical fascia medial to the carotids may need to be opened to the level of the clavicle.

Vincent's Angina (Trench Mouth)

Vincent's angina is an ulcerative gingival stomatitis. The bacteria that cause this are usually a mixed oral flora, with a predominance of fusospirochetal organisms. The infection is acute, necrotizing, rapidly spreading, and often associated with a foul odor. Fortunately, the organisms are almost always highly sensitive to penicillin, and such infections are now becoming exceedingly rare.

LESS SERIOUS INFECTIONS OF THE ORAL CAVITY
Herpes Simplex

The lesions of herpes simplex may occur anywhere in the oral cavity but are most commonly found on the lips; they appear as multiple small vesicles and usually rupture to form small ulcers, which are often very tender. The disease is self-limiting, and regression occurs in 5 to 7 days. Unfortunately, some patients are subject to repeated attacks that may be associated with the presence of other viral diseases or periods of reduced immunity. An effective treatment is the use of acyclovir applied as a 5% ointment.

Gingivitis

Gingivitis is an inflammatory lesion of the marginal gingiva, generally chronic in nature. The cause is bacterial plaque at the interface of the gingival epithelium and the teeth. Abscesses form in pockets below this interface and usually contain anaerobic bacteria. Clinical features include gingival discoloration, glossy appearance, hyperplasia or recession, and bleeding. The periodontal bone is eroded and teeth become loose in their sockets. A malodorous breath is noted. This syndrome accounts for the majority of teeth lost in the adult population. If the condition is noted by a physician, the patient should be referred for prompt dental care.

COMMON BENIGN NEOPLASMS

The oral cavity is a fairly common site for various benign tumors. Many of these are congenital, such as hemangiomas, retention cysts, and torus palatinus, as mentioned earlier. Acquired oral lesions include mixed tumors of the minor salivary glands, epulis, polyps, and dermoid cysts.

Mixed Tumors (Pleomorphic Adenoma)

Mixed tumors are of salivary gland origin. The oral mucosa has numerous small salivary glands scattered throughout, sometimes called *ectopic* or minor salivary glands. They are apparently a normal occurrence. These small bits of salivary tissue may give rise to tumors, the most common of which is the so-called mixed tumor. As the name implies, the tumor is made up of several types of tissue. It usually presents as a very *slow-growing submucosal mass covered by intact mucosa.* The benign lesions rarely, if ever, ulcerate and are seen by the physician or dentist because the patient finds and inquires about them. Treatment is by simple excision. Care must be taken, however, that the lesion is completely excised, since local recurrence is common and malignant transformation is a possibility (Fig. 14-6). Mixed tumors occur most commonly in the buccal mucosa and hard palate. Lesions of the hard palate are something of a problem, since the deep margin of the tumor is adjacent to the hard palate itself, and there is a tendency to leave some tumor tissue behind at this margin. It is advisable to remove a small button of hard palate together with the tumor to ensure complete excision.

Epulis (Reparative Granuloma)

Epulis arise at a point of chronic infection in the gingiva, often stimulated by residual tooth root or at the site of drainage of a periapical abscess in

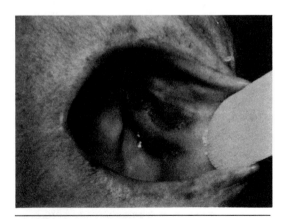

FIGURE 14-6   Malignancy, in this case a mucoepidermoid carcinoma arising from a minor salivary gland in the buccal mucosa.

an unextracted carious tooth. These granulomas may grow to considerable size and will erode the mandible and may involve adjacent teeth. Excision of the granuloma is not curative unless the inciting cause for the persistent chronic infection is eliminated (Fig. 14-7).

Polyps

The polyps most commonly seen in the oral cavity are of traumatic origin. Because of ill-fitting dentures or malocclusion, the buccal mucosa may be traumatized, forming a ridge of scarred tissue or an area of chronic irritation. Patients will sometimes suck on this area repeatedly and, often unconsciously, draw the tissue of the buccal mucosa into a gradually enlarging polyp. Excision of the polyp alone will not cure the problem, since the patient will promptly initiate another lesion through the same behavior. Repair of the dental problem is necessary, as is educating the patient about breaking the habit of sucking on the cheek tissues.

Dermoid Cysts

Dermoid cysts are inclusion cysts similar to those seen in the skin of many areas of the body. They arise through the *implantation* of a small bit of mucosa in the submucosal area. This may be acquired through trauma or can occur congenitally at the site of fusion of embryonic clefts. The implanted mucosa grows to form a small sphere, with what normally would be the external surface of the mucosa lining the sphere. As the mucosa tissues grow and slough off the dead cells on their surface, the cyst accumulates a cheesy,

toothpaste-like secretion and grows slowly. A common site for these lesions is at the midline of the floor of the mouth, and they may gradually grow to substantial size, elevating the tongue and floor of the mouth toward the hard palate. Simple excision is curative, and the cyst can usually be enucleated with ease from the surrounding tissues. One must avoid leaving any small bit of cyst wall that can then generate another cyst.

Odontogenic Cysts

Odontogenic cysts are most commonly seen and treated by dentists and oral surgeons. They lie within the substance of the mandible formed from isolated elements of teeth similar to that described for dermoids, although the contents of these cysts are much thinner and more liquid. Odontogenic cysts are usually diagnosed as a simple unilocular defect on x-ray evaluation of the mandible or, rarely, the maxilla and are easily cured by enucleation of the cyst lining from the substance of the surrounding bone. A space in the bone is left following the removal of the cyst, which ordinarily fills spontaneously with new bone over a fairly short period.

Neuromas

These are very rare lesions in the oral cavity, but if found they have great importance. They often are one of the lesions seen in patients with *Sipple's syndrome, one of the congenital neuroendocrine diseases.* Such patients should be studied for the presence of medullary thyroid, parathyroid hyperplasia, and pheochromocytoma (Fig. 14-8).

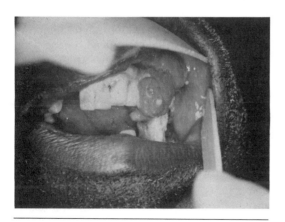

FIGURE 14-7 An epulis of the upper gingiva.

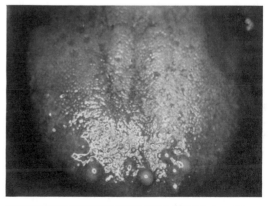

FIGURE 14-8 Neuromas of the tongue in a 20-year-old woman. This is a pathogenic sign of Sipple's syndrome.

WHAT IS THE COMMONEST MALIGNANT LESION?

Ninety-five percent to 98% of all malignant tumors of the oral cavity are epidermoid carcinomas arising from the lining epithelium. The following section is devoted mainly to the recognition and treatment of this lesion.

What Is Its Natural History?

Epidermoid carcinoma of the oral cavity is an excellent example of an environmentally induced tumor, that is, related to lifestyle and behaviors. *Heavy drinking and smoking* appear to be an overwhelming cause for most of the lesions seen today. Such tumors are almost unknown in individuals who neither drink alcohol nor smoke. The interrelationship between drinking and smoking is not fully understood, although it is commonly assumed that tobacco smoke is the inciting carcinogen and that alcohol may act as a stimulatory agent. It is not necessary to be exposed to smoke per se, since the use of nonsmoking forms of tobacco such as chewing tobacco or snuff has been shown to be associated with oral cancer. Nevertheless, smoke appears to contain more rapidly acting carcinogens, since the lesions in smokers appear earlier and more diffusely than in individuals who use nonsmoking forms of tobacco. In individuals using nonsmoking tobacco, the tumors appear directly adjacent to the area where the tobacco is placed, and the lesions tend to appear much later in life, to be more differentiated, and to be more easily treated.

It was once thought that *leukoplakia,* an overproduction of keratin by the epithelial cells of the mucosa that produces a small white patch on the mucosa, represented a premalignant stage of epidermoid tumors. We now know that the *initial evidence of an intraoral cancer is ordinarily a small erythroplastic lesion, which is a small area of reddening in the mucosa.* This change is very subtle and requires close examination under *high-intensity illumination* to demonstrate it. Lesions of this sort are totally asymptomatic and can be detected only by someone with a high index of suspicion and some prior experience with the lesions. Erythroplasia is most commonly found in the floor of the mouth, edge of the tongue, and anterior tonsillar pillars. This reddening may represent an inflammatory response to the "foreign" cells of the neoplasm. Keratosis may also accompany the reaction, and the lesion may be a *mixed red and white color or,* in some cases where keratosis predominates, *may appear as white leukoplakic patch.* This most commonly occurs in the buccal mucosa and lips.

It is important to understand that leukoplakia is a nonspecific reaction to irritation that can be produced by ill-fitting dentures, a rough tooth, biting oral mucosa, or any other chronic irritation. *Leukoplakia is associated with cancer only about 10% of the time.* Erythroplasia is also a nonspecific response to an inflammation of the mucosa which in the short term can be produced by minor trauma or infection. If *erythroplasia persists for 3 or more weeks without evidence of improvement, the underlying cause will be early malignant change in 80% to 90% of adult patients.*

Biopsy of the erythroplastic area will nearly always show some atypia or an in situ carcinoma or, in more advanced cases, microinvasion. The treatment of choice for such lesions is local excision. It is noteworthy that such patients have been exposed to environmental factors (e.g., tobacco smoke) affecting their entire aerodigestive epithelium and that the appearance of the erythroplastic lesion is a marker identifying the individual to be at *high risk for the occurrence of cancer at some other site in the aerodigestive system at a later date.* The risk is as high as 30% for the appearance of an additional lesion over a 5-year period of follow-up.

At some point in the course of the growth of an oral cancer, the lesion begins to spread into adjacent lymph nodes. The time at which this happens appears to be *related to the degree of differentiation* of the tumor; that is, the less differentiated the lesion, the more likely early spread will occur. Tumors of the lower lip and anterior tip of the tongue spread primarily to submental nodes. Lesions of the floor of the mouth, lateral borders of the tongue, gingiva, and buccal mucosa tend to spread primarily to submandibular nodes of the digastric triangle. Lesions in the retromolar triangle and those located at or adjacent to the circumvallate papillae may appear initially in the so-called tonsillar node at the angle of the mandible overlying the jugular vein. Lesions of the hard palate seem to find their way to the lymph nodes much more slowly and, when they do, tend to affect the jugular nodes first (Fig. 14-9). Unlike many common tumors, such as of the breast and lung, spread of oral cancers is usually a very orderly event, with *the nearest adjacent nodes receiving the first metastasis* and growing largest in size and the next lymph node bed becoming involved only after the initial metastasis has grown substantially. As a rule, therefore, the *largest palpable nodes will be high in the neck,* and subsequently involved nodes will be smaller and can easily be palpated along the jugular chain.

Metastasis outside of the area of the head and neck itself is very rare at the time when the patient is first seen. When it does occur, distant metastases usually involve nodes of the mediastinum and the lung. Patients who have had very large tumors and who have had successful local therapy are at risk for distant spread, however. Over a long period of follow-up, a distant metastasis usually will appear in the lung and, more rarely, in the liver or in bone.

Diagnosing Malignant Lesions

The first step in the *diagnosis of intraoral tumors is immediate biopsy.* All areas of the oral cavity are easily accessible for biopsy. Biopsy can be accomplished in an outpatient setting by infiltration of local anesthetic and removal of a piece of the tumor with a small biopsy forceps. Frequently a dermatologist's skin punch is effective

for biopsy of lesions of the tongue. If biopsy is not available to the patient, the ability of the *lesion to take up toluidine blue may be tested.* A mouth rinse of toluidine blue has been developed as an effective screening device with a high sensitivity for early as well as later cancers of the oral cavity. There are a number of false-positive findings since the specificity of the technique is not absolute but the sensitivity is very high. If the lesion does not take up the dye it is a reliable index that it is benign. Any patient who has areas that take up the rinse should be referred immediately for biopsy (Fig. 14-10, *A* and *B*).

Once the lesion has been identified as an epidermoid carcinoma of the oral cavity every effort should be made to evaluate the extent of the primary lesion and its regional metastases. One must remember that *these lesions tend to be multiple,* and *synchronous cancers must be searched for at other aerodigestive sites.* This should include indirect as well as direct endoscopy of the nasopharynx, hypopharynx, and larynx, along with esophagoscopy and bronchoscopy. The search for other primary tumors is more important than a search for distant metastases, which,

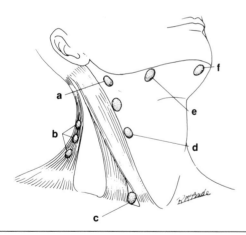

FIGURE 14-9 Cervical nodes initially involved in spread of cancer of the oral cavity and oropharynx. *a,* Superior jugular or "tonsillar node," metastasized from tonsil, posterior third of tongue, and oropharynx; *b,* accessory spinal nodes, metastasized from the nasopharynx; *c,* nodes in lower third of neck, usually from sites below the clavicle (lungs, esophagus, etc.); *d,* mid-third jugular nodes, from larynx, thyroid, and hypopharynx; *e,* submaxillary nodes, from the anterior and internal floor of the mouth and mid-third of the tongue; *f,* submental nodes, from lip and tip of tongue.

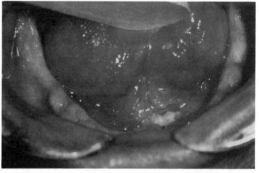

A

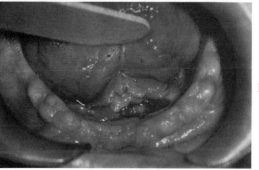

B

FIGURE 14-10 A, Carcinoma of floor of mouth. B, The same lesion showing uptake of toluidine blue.

as we have noted, rarely occur when the patient is first seen. Liver scans, brain scans, bone studies, and bone scans are all futile unless there is some very specific indication, such as alteration in liver chemistry or evidence of bone pain. *CT scan* for all but the smallest lesion is very useful both to demonstrate the extent of the primary lesion and to reveal evidence of nodal involvement not otherwise found on palpation.

The TNM System for Staging Cancer in the Oral Cavity

Over the years, the American Joint Committee for Cancer Staging and End Results Reporting has developed a highly sophisticated, although somewhat complex, system for staging cancers at many sites. Accurate and detailed staging of a tumor permits much more exact prognosis as well as an opportunity to compare the results of treatment of different groups of patients at a single institution and between institutions. This is the TNM system of classification: *T* stands for topography, meaning location of the tumor; *N* stands for the regional nodes; and *M* stands for distant metastases. This is *primarily a clinical system*, so that the presence of nodes and the extent of the primary lesion are determined by physical examination, although the patient may be restaged by pathology as long as the two systems are kept separate. (The current system as it applies to the lips and oral cavity is shown in Fig. 14-14. Not shown in the figure are the subdivisions of N_2, which are: N_2A—metastasis in a single ipsilateral lymph node more than 3 cm but less than 6 cm; N_2B—metastasis in multiple ipsilateral lymph nodes not more than 6 cm; N_2C bilateral or centralateral lymph nodes not more than 6 cm.)

Planning Treatment of Oral Cancer

Although early lesions of the oral cavity can be treated simply by the use of only one modality, more extensive lesions are often treated by two or even three modes of therapy. As a result, precise pretreatment planning by a team consisting of medical, surgical, and radiation oncologists, together with oral surgeons and often speech therapists and prosthodontists, is necessary not only to select the modes of therapy but also to plan reconstruction and functional restoration. In view of the rapid change in size and extent of tumors following each step in multimodal treatment, *restaging and reconsideration of the pa-tient should be done after each course of therapy has been completed.*

Stage I and II tumors of the oral cavity—that is, lesions of 2 cm or less and lesions over 2 cm but not more than 4 cm without apparent nodal disease—can be treated by a single modality and are probably treated equally effectively by either operation or radiation. Considerations of which modality to choose depend on logistics, side effects, and patient preference. At least 15% of such patients will eventually prove to have positive cervical nodes, and there is still some controversy about whether to treat the nodes in the neck, particularly in stage II lesions, or whether to observe and to operate on those patients whose nodal involvement is demonstrated at a later date.

Unfortunately, stage III and IV cancers are much more common than stage I or stage II tumors. Part of the reason for the preponderance of larger lesions is that many patients with these lesions are habitual drinkers and tend to neglect their health or are not aware of the early lesion. It is this group of patients with large and late tumors that requires more than one form of treatment. There seems little argument that *combining radiation and operation* for these lesions produces a better end result. Current fashion is to treat the patient operatively and to follow operation by high-dose radiation therapy both to the primary lesion and to the neck. The type of surgery performed differs with the size and location of the primary lesion. For all of these large lesions, with the exception of those of the lip, *cervical lymph nodes are routinely resected together with the main tumor,* even when the neck shows no malignancy on physical examination, because the incidence of metastatic disease is so high.

Lip. The lip is an exception to the general statements just noted, since external lesions of the lip are easily observed and are usually stage I or II when first discovered. *Metastases to the submental nodes occur uncommonly, with an incidence of about 5%.* Therefore excision or radiation therapy of the primary lesion is the main treatment, and the neck nodes are not resected prophylactically. Even with stage III or IV lesions (Fig. 14-11), lip tumors seem to have a somewhat more favorable prognosis, although lesions at this stage would require multimodal therapy.

Tongue. *Large lesions of the tongue tend to cross the midline and therefore the risk of contralateral metastases exists* (Fig. 14-12). If the mandible is not involved, the tumor, together with a 1 to 2 cm margin of normal tongue, is resected and a radical neck dissection is carried out. The oral specimen is sometimes left connected with the radical neck dissection and the entire specimen is pulled through the floor of the mouth, leaving the mandible intact. The remaining dead space must be filled to permit better function; this is usually done with a myocutaneous flap consisting of muscle and skin that is brought up from the neck or chest wall.

Floor of the Mouth. Stage III and IV cancers of the floor of the mouth are much more likely *to be contiguous with the mandible and require man-*

dibular resection together with neck dissection (see Fig. 14-10, *A*). If they cross the midline anteriorly, there is a risk of contralateral nodal involvement. Similar principles apply to carcinomas of the gingiva, and one can anticipate that the mandible will always be involved whenever there is a gingival cancer.

Upper Gingiva and Hard Palate. Smaller tumors in this area can sometimes be excised with simple local excision, but larger tumors (Fig. 14-13) require removal of the underlying bone, resulting in a defect in the palate or gingival area and communicates with the maxillary sinus. With the largest lesions, an excision of the lower half of the maxillary sinus may be required. Defects in this area allow food and fluids to regurgitate into the nasal cavity and markedly interfere with speech. When an operation in this area is planned, preliminary work with a prosthodontist is essential so that an appropriate prosthesis with an obturator can be constructed; this will close the defect and permit normal speech and mastication. Regional metastases from this area are usually to the jugular chain and for unknown reasons appear to occur much later than lesions in the lower mouth. Therefore, *prophylactic neck dissection is not usually performed;* neck dissection is reserved for patients with palpable cervical nodes.

Chemotherapy

The use of chemotherapy in previously untreated epidermoid tumor of the oral cavity is remark-

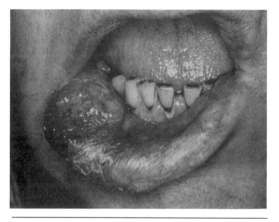

FIGURE 14-11 An advanced epidermoid carcinoma of the lower lip showing adjacent leukoplakia.

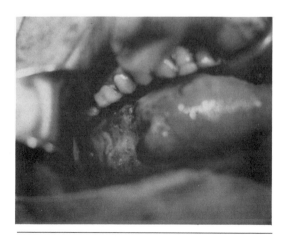

FIGURE 14-12 A deeply invasive epidermoid carcinoma of the middle third of the tongue.

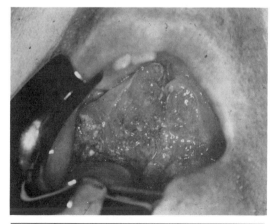

FIGURE 14-13 Epidermoid carcinoma of the hard palate showing "wall-to-wall" spread with involvement of the entire palate.

ably successful in terms of the initial response. Single-drug therapy with **methotrexate** or **cis-platin** produces partial or complete regression in at least 50% of the tumors treated. Even more successful is the use of mixed therapy, with the combination of cisplatin and 5-fluorouracil (5-FU) being the most popular. Partial and complete remission rates are reported as high as 90% with this protocol.

Intra-arterial chemotherapy has also been used for these tumors. The catheter is usually placed in the temporal artery and threaded down to an area just above the carotid bulb. The availability of **implantable pumps** that permit treatment to be continued for many weeks or months without the use of an external apparatus has attracted considerable attention. The implanted pump is recharged with additional drug every 2 weeks. This can be done by injecting the reservoir off the pump with a fine needle inserted through the patient's skin. Unfortunately, the response to these treatments is relatively short lived, and recurrence of the tumor is usually seen from 2 to 8 months after the end of treatment. Because of the dramatic initial response, however, there is considerable interest in the use of these agents in combination with other forms of therapy.

Chemotherapy for cancers recurring after radiation, operation, or a combination of these two modalities is much less promising, and drugs that have been reported to produce regression rates as high as 90% in untreated lesions usually will produce less than 20% to 30% regression rates in recurrent cancers.

Multimodal Therapy

Because of the high response rate of untreated lesions to chemotherapy, there is much interest in the use of initial chemotherapy, followed by radiation or operation or both. If both radiation and operation are used, the sequence is usually chemotherapy, operation, and finally radiation therapy. Such combination therapy takes several months to complete and seems most successful in very large tumors, such as late stage III or stage IV lesions. A number of preliminary studies suggest that these combinations are effective in improving the prognosis in patients with late tumors, but this work is still investigational. Fig. 14-14 reflects an algorithmic approach to treatment of cancer of the oral cavity.

Prognosis

Epidermoid cancers of the oral cavity can be divided into two groups when prognosis is considered. *Lesions of the lips have a substantially better prognosis* for each stage than lesions of the remainder of the oral cavity. Lesions of the remainder of the oral cavity also have a slight variation in prognosis; tumors of the tongue and floor of the mouth have a somewhat poorer prognosis than lesions of the gingiva and buccal mucosa. However, the differences are modest and the entire region can be considered as a group (Table 14-1).

OTHER COMMON CANCERS

Less than 5% of malignant lesions in the oral cavity are of other than epidermoid origin. Of these lesions, the most common are malignant mixed tumor, ameloblastoma, and Kaposi's sarcoma.

Malignant Mixed Tumors

These arise from salivary gland tissue underlying the oral mucosa and occur most commonly in the cheeks and palate, as noted under benign

TABLE 14-1   Five-Year Survival Rates per Stage

	T_1	T_2	T_3	T_4
N_0	Lip: 100% Oral cavity: 76%-83%	Lip: 92% Oral cavity: 63%-67%		
N_1			Lip: 71% Oral cavity: 36%-37%	
N_2 N_3				Lip: 50% Oral cavity: 9%-11%

mixed tumors. The lesions grow slowly and remain localized for long periods. Metastatic lesions are rare, but local recurrence is common and wide excision is mandatory whenever these lesions are removed.

Ameloblastomas

Ameloblastomas are slow-growing lesions occurring in the mandible that are thought to arise from the same cells that form tooth enamel. They appear on x-ray films as multiloculated cysts and grow slowly over a long period, with eventual erosion of the mandibular cortex and invasion into the soft tissue. Metastasis is very rare, but local recurrence is common. Excision of the entire lesion with a margin of normal bone or soft tissue on all sides is important and, if done properly, will cure this lesion.

Kaposi's Sarcoma

A few years ago Kaposi's sarcoma was so rare in the region of the oral cavity that it would not have required comment. However, the epidemic of acquired immunodeficiency disease (AIDS) that has developed in this country has led to the more frequent appearance of a number of rather rare tumors. Kaposi's sarcoma is one of these lesions. In the past, Kaposi's sarcoma was usually heralded by small reddish-brown spots on the feet and lower legs. In AIDS patients, how-

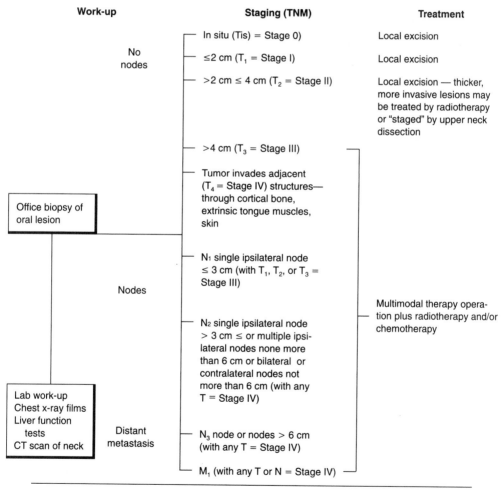

FIGURE 14-14 Algorithm for treatment of oral cancer. The current staging for oral cancer (American Cancer Society, 1988) is shown, with two minor exceptions mentioned in the text under staging.

ever, Kaposi's sarcoma is often found first as a slightly raised purple-red patch involving the hard palate, gingiva, and buccal mucosa or, less commonly, other areas of the oral cavity. The local lesion is very sensitive to radiation therapy or chemotherapy, but the disease is primarily systemic, and, if the patient has AIDS, is universally fatal.

PITFALLS AND COMMON MYTHS

- Failure to biopsy early. Resolution of whether a lesion is benign or malignant should occur as soon as possible, preferably at the first visit. Most oral biopsies can be done as office procedures.
- Overtreatment of early malignant lesions. While this is less common than undertreatment, I have seen very extensive resections proposed for early microinvasive thin lesions that basically involve only the mucosa and in which extensive sacrifices of bone or soft tissue is not necessary.
- Undertreatment of oral cancer. The obverse of the above. Some surgeons shrink from the necessary extensive resections demanded by stage III and IV and even late stage II lesions. They may do too limited a resection or attempt to treat the patient by radiation therapy alone.

- Failure to use multimodal therapy. All stage III and IV patients require treatment by both radiation and operation which yields the best prognosis. Chemotherapy may be added to this regimen, although the degree of added benefit is still unclear. No stage IV cancers should be declared inoperable until reevaluated after a course of combined chemotherapy and radiation, which may "downstage" the lesion.
- Failure to follow the patient adequately for recurrence or the appearance of a second primary lesion. The risk of recurrence is very low after 2 years of follow-up, but second primaries either in the oral cavity or some other portion of the aerodigestive tract occur in up to a third of the patients within 5 years.

BIBLIOGRAPHY

Freund HR. Principles of Head and Neck Surgery, 2nd ed. New York, Appleton-Century-Crofts, 1979.

Lore J. An Atlas of Head and Neck Surgery, 3rd ed. Philadelphia, WB Saunders, 1988.

MacComb WS, Fletcher GH, Healy JE. Intraoral Cavity. In MacComb WS, Fletcher GH (eds). Cancer of the Head and Neck. Baltimore, Williams & Wilkins, 1967.

Myers E, Suen J. Cancer of the Head and Neck. New York, Churchill Livingstone, 1989.

Rush BF Jr. Tumors of the head and neck. In Schwartz S, Shires GT, et al. (eds). Principles of Surgery, 5th ed. New York, McGraw-Hill, 1988, pp 557-602.

CHAPTER REVIEW
Questions

1. Discuss the importance of palpatory examination of the oral cavity.
2. Discuss the significance of clinical staging in oral cavity cancers.
3. A patient presents with metastatic cancer involving a level II cervical node. Where is the most probable site of the primary tumor?
4. A mucosal ulceration of the floor of the mouth is best diagnosed by:
   a. Biopsy
   b. Pain on palpation
   c. Smear and Gram stain evaluation of surface exudate
   d. X-ray examination of the mandible
5. Which of the following abscesses is best drained through a neck incision?
   a. Retropharyngeal
   b. Peritonsillar
   c. Parapharyngeal
6. The most important step in the treatment of all oropharyngeal cancers is:
   a. Pretreatment planning and multidisciplinary consultation
   b. Wide excision with adequate margins
   c. Radium needle implant
   d. Radical neck dissection

Answers

1. Subtle abnormalities in texture and consistency of the oral cavity mucosa in early carcinomas can be detected by careful palpation, often even before their becoming apparent to the naked eye. Proper evaluation of soft tissue swellings, especially in the floor of the mouth and neck, requires careful bimanual palpation.
2. A uniform method of staging cancers in any site is essential for:
   a. Meaningful comparison of end results
   b. Prognostication
   c. Guide to the selection of appropriate treatment
3. The level II group of nodes refers to nodes lying along the upper third of the vein corresponding to the area above the point where the digastric muscle crosses the vein. This nodal group is frequently affected by tumors of the mid-third of the tongue, floor of mouth, lateral gingiva, and buccal mucosa.
4. a
5. c
6. a

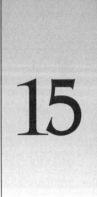

15 Neck Masses

KIRBY I. BLAND

KEY FEATURES

After reading this chapter you will understand:
- The development of and rational treatment for both benign and malignant thyroid nodules.
- The cervical metastatic mass from an unknown primary cancer.
- How to differentiate between the important types of thyroid cancer with respect to individualized treatment schemas.
- An algorithm for a suitable therapeutic approach to neck masses.

Of all illnesses requiring hospitalization in the United States, enlargements in the cervical region of the neck comprise approximately 3%. One half of them are malignant. Even though there is easy access to these neck masses, the differentiation of malignant and benign processes presents a formidable diagnostic challenge to the clinician. Because the patient's age is an important consideration in the evaluation of any neoplastic process, any persistent nontender mass in the neck of an adult should be considered malignant until histologic examination suggests otherwise. The thyroid gland is the most frequent single source of a palpable neck mass; approximately one half of all cervical masses represent a functional pathologic alteration within the thyroid.

Exclusive of benign or neoplastic enlarge-ments of the thyroid, most neck masses are malignant and comprise three functional categories: neoplastic; supraclavicular and congenital cervical; and inflammatory.

Neoplastic Lesions. Malignant tumors represent the majority of lesions; they constitute approximately 85% of the cervical enlargements in this group. Consequently, lesions seen in the lateral cervical area outside the thyroid should be considered neoplastic until histologic review confirms a benign process.

Metastatic Disease. Tumors metastatic from primary foci comprise 80% of all neoplastic neck masses. These lesions most commonly (90%) originate from clinically obvious primary lesions located *above* the clavicle.

Primary Malignancies. Primary tumors that originate within the neck comprise the remaining one fifth of neoplastic masses. Primary lymphoma of the neck comprises 60%; 40% originate in major salivary glands and ducts.

Supraclavicular and Congenital Cervical Masses. Tumors that originate from congenital cervical or supraclavicular lesions constitute another 10% of nonthyroid enlargements.

Inflammatory Masses. Intraoral or cutaneous infections comprise 4% to 5% of cervical masses.

Fig. 15-1 depicts the frequency distribution for benign and malignant cervical masses, and Table 15-1 denotes the frequency and distribution of these masses in 100 theoretic cervical masses in adults. Table 15-2 documents the physical characteristics and anatomic sites of common benign neck masses.

Although inflammatory lesions occur infrequently in adults, they are the most common source of lateral neck masses in children and are usually related to tonsillar infections (Fig. 15-2). Developmental lesions are much more common in children than in adults. In younger age groups the common midline developmental lesions of the neck include dermoid and thyroglossal duct cysts. Lateral developmental masses include cystic hygromas and branchial cleft cysts. In children all persistent, nontender cervical masses larger than 2 cm should be viewed with suspicion. Hodgkin's and nonHodgkin's lymphomas, soft-tissue sarcomas, and thyroid carcinomas are the most frequent malignant neck masses in children. More than 50% of these neoplastic neck masses are malignant lymphomas. Other malignant tumors of the head and neck in children include (in order of occurrence) neuroblastoma, nasopharyngeal squamous cell carcinoma, and malignant melanoma. Tuberculous lymphadenitis (scrofula), once the most common neck mass found in adults, is now rarely seen in the United States.

Inflammatory neck masses are common in teenagers and young adults. Therefore adenopathy from bacterial and viral sources must be considered. Thyroid malignancies are also frequent

TABLE 15-1 Frequency Distribution of All Sources in Theoretic Cervical Masses in Adults

Source	%
Thyroid	50
Metastatic lesion with known primary	31
Primary lymphoma	5
Congenital origin	5
Major salivary gland primary	4
Metastatic lesion with cryptic primary	3
Inflammatory origin	2
TOTAL	100

TABLE 15-2 Common Benign Neck Masses

Location	Physical Characteristics
Lateral, Anterior	
Second brachial cleft cyst	Anterior margin of sternocleidomastoid (SCM) muscle; extends to tonsillar fossa
Torticollis	Newborn: hematoma in SCM; infant: mass with facial asymmetry; child: wryneck with fibrous band of SCM
Thyroid	Follicular adenoma or degenerative cyst of chronic thyroiditis
Carotid artery	Aneurysmal, bulbous mass in elderly
Midline, Anterior	
Aberrant thyroid tissue (supra-, intra-, and infralingual)	Mass at base of tongue
Thyroglossal duct cyst	Infrahyoid inflammatory cystic mass; often in children
Hypertrophied pyramidal lobe	Isolated thyroid enlargement; extends from isthmus toward hyoid
First brachial cleft cyst	Extends along mandible to preauricular area; often inflamed
Teratoma	Irregular mass with airway compression; often in newborn
Submental abscess and cellulitis	Submental space cellulitis and adenitis with progression to abscess
Aneurysm	Aortic arch, innominate artery, or branch at level of sternal notch
Both Midline and Lateral	
Cystic hygroma	Lymphangiocele in infants and children; often occupies entire neck, extends into axilla
Posterior Triangle	
Inflammatory adenopathy	Scalp infection (lice, scabies); viremia (rubella); bacterial inflammation (tonsillitis, pharyngitis)

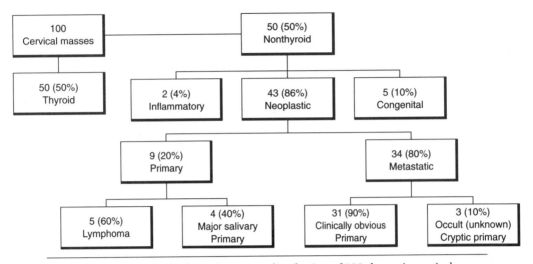

FIGURE 15-1   Cause and relative frequency distribution of 100 theoretic cervical masses.

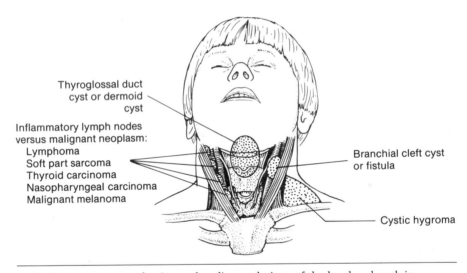

FIGURE 15-2   Common benign and malignant lesions of the head and neck in children.

in this age group and should be part of the differential diagnosis process.

In the over-40 age group any neck mass must be considered a metastatic malignant tumor until proven otherwise (Fig. 15-3). The great majority of all nonthyroid cervical masses represents a metastatic tumor arising from primary neoplasms above the clavicle. The initial management objective should be disclosure of the site of origin of the primary neoplasm to allow for subsequent therapy. In general, an early excisional biopsy of a suspicious cervical lesion through a small incision that can be readily incorporated into subsequent neck dissection wounds is preferable and should be part of the initial assessment of the patient. The scar from the surgical excision of a cervical lymph node harboring squamous cells or glandular tumor cells frequently is the site of tumor implantation and growth. Thus the definitive operative procedure

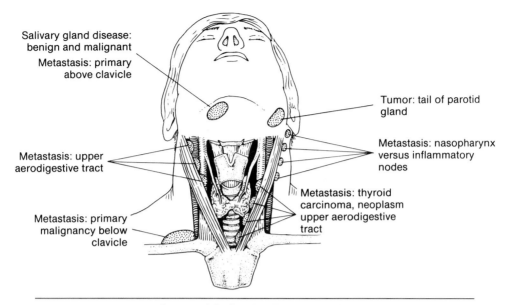

Salivary gland disease: benign and malignant

Metastasis: primary above clavicle

Tumor: tail of parotid gland

Metastasis: nasopharynx versus inflammatory nodes

Metastasis: upper aerodigestive tract

Metastasis: thyroid carcinoma, neoplasm upper aerodigestive tract

Metastasis: primary malignancy below clavicle

FIGURE 15-3 Common lesions of the head and neck in adults.

must include excision of the biopsy scar to reduce (or eliminate) the possibility of recurrence of the local tumor. Although these therapeutic principles have been appreciated for many years, they frequently are ignored, thereby compounding problems for the surgeon who assumes ultimate responsibility for the patient. Deviation from these therapeutic guidelines greatly reduces the possibility of local and regional tumor control and subsequent cure for the patient.

As indicated previously, a thorough history and physical examination of the palpable cervical mass are essential before biopsy. Furthermore, an initial biopsy, either fine-needle aspiration cytology or incisional, performed before a complete physical evaluation is done, is ill-timed and is contraindicated for various reasons:

- Complete evaluation may negate the need for incisional biopsy or fine-needle aspiration.
- Neoplastic cells may be disseminated into an improperly planned incision, the circulatory system, and/or the lymphatic system.
- The primary neoplastic site may remain undisclosed (cryptic), in which case the integrity of an en bloc dissection would not be possible to obtain, possibly altering the therapeutic objectives.
- Thoughtless placement of an incision for biopsy may abrogate the design of an appropriate incision for definitive operation.

The clinician must remember that in the majority of presentations (90%) the primary site for nonthyroid metastatic lesions is obvious. In contrast, a difficult diagnostic challenge may present for the remaining 10% of patients whose lesions are secondary to primary tumors in occult sites. Furthermore, a high index of suspicion for cancer often necessitates obtaining a biopsy specimen from the cervical nodes of those patients in whom the existence of the cryptogenic primary is verified. As with all diagnostic protocols, a meticulous examination for verification and follow-up of the lesion is essential. The occult primary tumor may subsequently become apparent clinically or may become visually detectable at a later examination. In contrast, some occult tumors that give rise to masses seen in the neck may never be identified (clinically or histologically) by the clinician before the patient's demise. Thus the greatest diagnostic challenge presented to the head and neck surgeon is that subset of neck lesions (10% of metastatic lesions) that have a nonthyroid origin (see Fig. 15-1). These metastatic lesions require frequent reevaluation of the patient in an effort to identify the parent neoplasm after evaluation and treatment of the metastatic foci.

A vast network of lymphatic vessels and nodes drains the various organs of the head and neck, skin, and scalp. Before determining the diagnostic approach to an isolated, nonthyroid

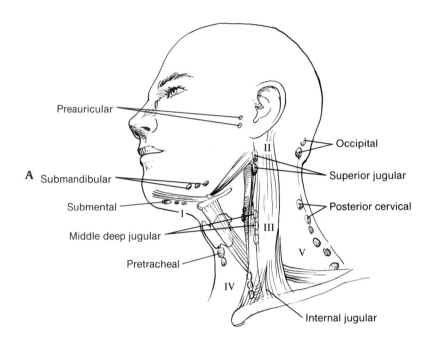

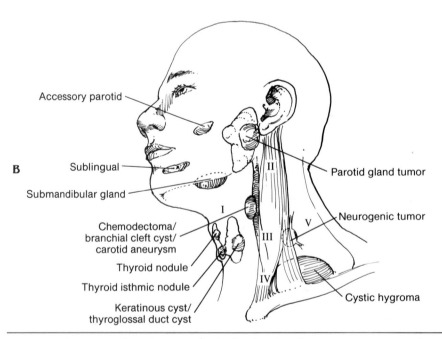

FIGURE 15-4 **A,** Lymph node groups in the head and neck. **B,** Tumors, cysts, and other lesions found in the head and neck.

cervical mass, a basic knowledge of lymphatic drainage of the region and of the frequencies of various head and neck parent neoplasms is required. Fig. 15-4 depicts the common sites of metastases of cancers of the head and neck with regard to specific nodal basins. The lymphatic drainage of all areas of the head and neck is quite specific in terms of anatomic distribution, and the nodal groups' interconnection must be noted. The frequency of metastases from different head and neck regions to specific groups or levels of cervical nodes is quite predictable, although individual variations may exist. Thus, as depicted in Table 15-3, neoplasms of the parotid or minor salivary glands may metastasize to level I or II regional nodal basins. When the parent tumor is of nasopharyngeal origin, palpable nodal disease at levels II and V (e.g., postauricular, posterior cervical, jugulodigastric) is a common clinical presentation. The metastatic potential of the primary neoplasm depends on the lymphatic drainage and its anatomic location and on the histology and stage of the tumor. The propensity for tumors in particular regions within the head and neck to metastasize to specific areas within the anatomic confines of the neck provides clues to the probable site of the occult parent neoplasm. The clinician can often predict the primary site of the metastatic focus after a meticulous head and neck examination, even when the indirect or direct visual examination of mucosal surfaces provides no confirmation of the site(s) of origin.

WHAT IS THE DISTRIBUTION OF PRIMARY NEOPLASMS THAT PRESENT AS A MASS IN THE NECK?

Only 5% of parent tumors go undetected after a meticulous diagnostic search for the primary lesion. Table 15-4 presents the frequency distribution of primary lesions identified after the evaluation of patients with cervical masses of unknown origin. In 329 patients treated for cervical masses originating from unknown nonthyroid primaries, 26% of the lesions eventually were detected; three fourths of the identified lesions were located in the head and neck area, and one fourth originated below the clavicle. Of all primary lesions discovered above the clavicle, 74% originated from the nasopharynx, tonsils, larynx, pharynx, base of the tongue, and related sites. One fifth of primaries detected were infraclavicular sites, mainly the lungs, stomach, and pancreas.

TABLE 15-3   Anatomic Location of Primary Head and Neck Neoplasms Correlated With Common Sites of Metastasis in Cervical Lymph Nodes

Anatomic Location	Level	Nodal Site(s) of Metastatic Tumor
Skin: scalp, face, forehead; parotid, minor salivary glands	I	Occipital, postauricular, facial, submental, parotid
Nasopharynx	II, V	Postauricular, posterior cervical, jugulodigastric, lower posterior cervical
Lateral tongue; posterior tongue; tonsillar fossa, palate	II	Jugulodigastric
Gingiva; lateral floor of mouth	I	Submaxillary
Posterior gingivobuccal sulcus; buccal mucosa; parotid, minor salivary glands	II	Jugulodigastric
Anterior tongue; lower lip; anterior gingivobuccal sulcus; anterior floor of mouth	I	Submental
Larynx, pharynx; posterior tongue; parotid	III	Midjugular
Thyroid, cervical glands	IV	Lower jugular
Any neoplasms arising below clavicle	V	Lower posterior cervical; anterior scalene or supraclavicular

TABLE 15-4 Distribution of Primary Lesions Identified After Initial Treatment of Patients With Cervical Metastases of Unknown Origin*

	Number	Percent
Primary Eventually Detected	85	26
Supraclavicular (head/neck)		(74)
Nasopharynx		
Tonsil		
Base of tongue		
Larynx		
Pharyngeal wall and piriform sinus		
Cervical esophagus		
Nasal cavity		
Retromolar trigone		
Floor of mouth		
Other		
Infraclavicular		(21)
Lung		
Stomach		
Pancreas		
Other		
Miscellaneous		(5)
Melanoma, lymphoma, and lymphosarcoma		
Primary Never Detected	240	73
Lost to Follow-Up	4	1

*Collected and modified from multiple sources for 329 patients.

WHAT ARE THE DIAGNOSTIC APPROACHES NEEDED TO EVALUATE A MASS IN THE NECK?

As discussed previously, obtaining a biopsy specimen from a suspicious neck mass at initial presentation is a common, but potentially serious, error in management. A cervical or supraclavicular mass may be the only clinical manifestation of an occult primary tumor; thus the parent neoplasm must be found and treated to ensure the maximal probability of disease control. The box on p. 279 presents the diagnostic approach to the unknown primary tumor. Using this approach, 90% of patients with cervical masses are diagnosed at the initial physical examination and/or workup. Adherence to the sequence and method of the diagnostic scheme is imperative for successful disease management. Commonly, the position or location of the mass in the neck will indicate specific sites for examination. With the aid of proper instruments and lighting, the goal should be the direct or indirect visualization of all skin and accessible mucosal surfaces of the head and neck.

Sites for Visual Inspection

The sites for visual inspection include the skin, scalp, ears, oropharynx, nasopharynx, and hypopharynx. Digital or bimanual palpation of the areas is emphasized to determine the physical characteristics of the neoplastic growth. The sense of smell is in itself a diagnostic tool because ulcerative or infective lesions may present with the foul odor characteristic of neoplasms.

As emphasized previously, careful planning is essential before performing invasive diagnostic procedures (direct endoscopy and biopsies). The clinician must order appropriate radiographic studies (head and neck plain x-ray films and computed tomograms) before performing surgery or any type of biopsy to avoid the problem of having to interpret images distorted by the hemorrhage and/or edema that can result from the procedure. The physician must also request studies that are ***most commonly diagnostic*** of the primary site and allow evaluation of the anatomic areas most likely to contain metastases. In addition, the clinician may also request special radiographic views that detail contiguous sites to

---

DIAGNOSTIC APPROACH TO A CERVICAL MASS
WITH AN UNKNOWN PRIMARY SITE

History

Inquire about:
Persistent hoarseness, voice change
Dysphasia, pain, sore throat, epistaxis
Prior therapy for skin cancer (e.g., melanoma,
   epidermoid)

Physical Examination

Evaluate:
Face and scalp, skin, ears, neck
External auditory canals
Inspect oropharynx, hypopharynx
Perform comprehensive neck examination,
   indirect laryngoscopy

Radiographic Examination

*To be completed before biopsies or invasive
diagnostic studies are performed:*
Chest x-ray examination (PA and lateral) (all)
Lateral neck views (if suspicious of thyroid
   cancer)
Ultrasonography of neck (select cystic vs. solid
   cervical/thyroid mass)
Facial sinuses/laryngeal—tomograms (all)
Computed tomography of head, neck, larynx
   (select)
Sialogram (select)
Thyroid scan RAI (select)
Esophagogram (select)

Follow-Up Examination and Procedure

Direct laryngoscopy (all)
Esophagogastroscopy (select)
Bronchoscopy (select, with cytology of
   washings)
Fine-needle aspiration of cervical nodes
   (select)
Blind biopsies of base of tongue, nasopharynx
   (select)

Subsequent Evaluations to Consider

Supraclavicular mass:
Upper/lower GI series
Computed tomography/MRI of chest,
   abdomen, pelvis
Endoscopic retrograde
   cholangiopancreatography
Intravenous pyelogram
Cytoscopy, mammography

If primary remains undetected:
Open biopsy—conventional neck incision to
   obtain tissue of cervical mass/nodes for
   frozen section; delay radical neck dissection
   if frozen section results are equivocal

Additional Therapy

Brachytherapy
?? Chemotherapy, external beam radiation

---

identify any ipsilateral mass. To evaluate lesions that originate **below** the clavicle, appropriate studies (e.g., chest radiograms, gastrointestinal barium x-rays, endoscopy, biopsy) are essential.

Following the completion of appropriate and comprehensive radiographic studies, fine-needle aspiration of the cervical mass should be done, for histopathologic identification of a squamous cell or glandular pattern would be invaluable. Furthermore, this procedure will not affect the technical considerations of placement of future incisions. Additionally, the information gained from a fine-needle aspiration often allows the physician to concentrate on procedures that diagnose the common neoplasms that produce squamous or glandular cells. In contrast, this methodology is not applicable for the evaluation of lymphomatous neoplasms. Lymphomas are rarely confirmed by fine-needle aspiration or core-needle biopsies since the volume of tissue required for the flow cytometric analysis usually necessitates an open surgical biopsy.

Once adequate tissue has been obtained at open biopsy, routine stains, immunohistochemical studies, flow cytometric analysis, and perhaps electron microscopy are essential for pathologic interpretation. After procurement of cervical nodal tissue, it may also be necessary to obtain cultures for the identification of bacteria, fungi, and acid-fast organisms.

HOW SHOULD TREATMENT BE INITIATED?

The poor prognosis for metastatic disease may be further complicated in those cases in which the primary tumor remains occult. However, the prognosis differs, depending on the location, number, and size of involved nodes and on the histopathologic cell type. Patients with metastatic lymph nodes in the upper (level II) and middle (level III) cervical regions have a better prognosis than those with metastatic disease in the lower (level IV) cervical and supraclavicular sites. In the absence of a detectable parent neoplasm radical neck dissection is the accepted therapy for an isolated cervical lesion above the supraclavicular space.

This radical procedure has a 2% to 4½% hospital mortality rate as an isolated procedure and is often used in combination with en bloc resections of other organs. The radical neck dissection includes excision of all musculoareolar lymph node–bearing tissue in an area bounded by the midline, the mandible, the clavicle, and the trapezius muscle posteriorly, with resection of the internal jugular vein and the sternocleidomastoid muscle. The carotid artery and the vagus, hypoglossal, spinal accessory, lingual, and phrenic nerves are preserved. The procedure may be modified to conform to various anatomic circumstances. In the absence of antecedent radiotherapy, complications are uncommon, with the preponderance of them confined to the operative site.

The justification for a radical operative procedure demands proof that there is a reasonable chance for control of the disease for a significant number of patients within a defined period of time. Based on previous studies, this radical approach is advised for patients with metastatic epidermoid carcinoma and malignant melanoma. Patients with adenocarcinoma, exclusive of parent salivary gland neoplasms, and lymphomatous lesions are not considered candidates for radical neck operations. Essentially all patients with metastatic adenocarcinoma die of uncontrollable, disseminated cancer and have such limited survival times that the radical procedure is unjustified. Furthermore, patients with nodes of glandular origin in the supraclavicular space are rarely cured by any treatment modality. In these cases an operative approach would be considered only in circumstances in which a reasonable life expectancy is possible after control of the local tumor by irradiation or chemotherapy has failed. In contrast, lymphomatous neck masses are well controlled by radiotherapy and chemotherapy.

A reasonable survival interval for patients with metastatic epidermoid carcinoma treated by radical neck dissection can be expected, even though the primary cancer is not clinically identifiable (Fig. 15-5). Should the primary neoplasm

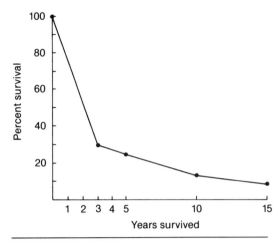

FIGURE 15-5   Survival rate after radical neck dissection for isolated cervical metastatic lesions. NOTE: 15-year survivors have been reported.

be detected subsequently, conventional therapy (surgery or irradiation) can be given. Radiotherapy and operative therapy should not be viewed as competitive modalities for the treatment of patients with cervical metastases associated with an unknown primary. Data suggest that combination modalities may be superior to an operation alone. For instance, partial or radical neck dissection apparently provides adequate therapy for the single node in the submaxillary triangle (level I) and the low subdigastric node(s) (level II). However, radiation therapy provides an equally good result with regard to control of disease and survival. Thus a cooperative attitude between the surgeon and the radiotherapist must prevail to ensure optimal patient management. Large or fixed regional lymph nodes are best treated initially with irradiation, with an optional plan to include some form of partial or radical neck dissection 4 to 6 weeks later should regression of the enlarged nodes not occur after completion of radiotherapy.

The patient with an occult primary should be reexamined at specified intervals in an attempt to identify the parent neoplasm responsible for the neck mass. Random biopsies of the oropharynx and hypopharynx may identify the site of a previously unidentified epidermoid carcinoma. Should such a primary be detected, it should be aggressively treated, for superior long-term and disease-free survival results are best achieved when the parent and secondary lesions have been controlled. Because the nasopharynx may be the original site of high posterior triangle and low posterior cervical metastatic disease (levels II and V), the majority of head and neck surgeons perform routine biopsies of this area. Once squamous cell carcinoma is confirmed, comprehensive irradiation to the nasopharynx should be initiated. This practice serves to eliminate the possibility of the nasopharynx subsequently becoming the site of an occult primary neoplasm. The neck lesion should be exposed, including the biopsy scar within a conventional incision; however, the incision should not compromise the making of a future skin flap if any subsequent radical operation is planned.

SUMMARY

- Cervical enlargements are common physical presentations (2% to 4% of all hospital admissions).
- Approximately one half of all cervical masses are functional alterations of the thyroid gland. Open surgical biopsy is done after the pertinent history and physical and radiographic studies have been obtained.
- Eighty-five percent of cervical enlargements are neoplastic (metastatic lesions, 80%; primary malignancies, 20%).
- Congenital masses comprise 10% of nonthyroid enlargements; inflammatory lesions represent 4% to 5% of cervical masses.
- Patients with adenocarcinoma, exclusive of those of salivary gland origin, and lymphomatous lesions are not candidates for an operation.
- Reasonable survival intervals are expected for metastatic epidermoid carcinoma despite the presence of an occult primary tumor.

CARCINOMA OF THE THYROID GLAND
How Is Carcinoma of the Thyroid Detected and Treated?

Extensive necroscopy studies of previously hospitalized patients indicate that approximately one half of the adult population will harbor one or more nodules in the thyroid. On review, most of these thyroid masses were not palpable. Furthermore, histopathologic evaluation of these occult lesions confirmed that only 2% to 5% of these cryptic lesions were cancer. Thus a minimal risk is connected to these undetectable thyroid nodules.

Palpable nodules of the thyroid are observed in approximately 4% to 5% of the population, and 10% to 20% of these nodules will prove malignant at subsequent thyroid lobectomy (0.6% to 1.0% of total population). Epidemiologic statistics suggest there is an increasing risk of thyroid carcinoma in the United States, but the annual death rate for cancer of this organ in 1991 (1000 cases per year) has not changed. These data are best explained by the excellent survival rate of the more common types of thyroid carcinoma (papillary and follicular) and by its prolonged natural history, despite lung, bone, or other metastases. From a biologic perspective, little clinical significance is attached to cancer of the thyroid because the aforementioned histopathologic types are only rarely responsible for the death of a patient. In contrast, medullary and anaplastic thyroid carcinoma frequently contributes to the death of the patient.

How Is Thyroid Cancer Diagnosed?

History and Presentation. Although the risk of cancer in a detected thyroid nodule is only 2% to 5%, the following factors enhance the probability of a nodule's being malignant.

Past Medical History. A previous history of low-dose and high-dose (>2000 cGy) cervical, facial, or mediastinal irradiation is significant because more than 75% of children with papillary thyroid carcinoma have such a history. Additionally, after a latency period of 25 years or more, there is an exponential increase in both benign and malignant thyroid nodules up to an equivalent radiotherapeutic dose of approximately 1500 cGy.

For persons with a familial history of thyroid cancer, a detailed evaluation and examination are mandatory. Individuals with a positive pedigree for medullary thyroid carcinoma are at great risk, for the gene for it is autosomal dominant and is transmitted to 50% of the offspring.

Age and Sex. Since approximately one half of all isolated thyroid masses in children are malignant, the detection of an isolated lesion in a child under age 16 warrants aggressive therapy. Although thyroid disease is more common in females, the presence of a solitary nodule in the young male (<40 years) is highly suspicious for cancer.

Age exerts a major role in the behavior of differentiated thyroid carcinoma. The poorer prognosis with increasing age abruptly appears at approximately age 40 years in men and approximately age 50 years in women. The mortality rate is threefold greater for men and tenfold greater for women with presentation of a thyroid neoplasm in the older age categories. These differences between young and old patients are significant for both recurrences and death rates.

The Isolated Nodule. In patients having excision of nodular goiters, the reported incidence of cancer is as high as 15%, whereas this incidence doubles for glands resected with solitary nodules.

Physical Characteristics of the Gland and Related Structures. A sudden increase in size of a solitary nodule, stony, firm masses, palpable lymph nodes, and vocal cord paralysis are signs of malignancy.

Physical Examination

1. A palpable solitary nodule is the cardinal physical finding in the majority of patients with thyroid carcinoma (Figs. 15-6 and 15-7).

2. The reported incidence of malignancy in solitary nodules is 10%. The frequency increases to greater than 20% if the nodule is nonfunctional ("cold") on iodine-uptake scanning.
3. Carcinomatous nodules often present as stony, hard masses, although nodules in patients with papillary carcinoma may be soft or cystic.
4. Large, fixed lesions or those associated with middle- or lower-jugular (levels III and IV) adenopathy strongly suggest carcinoma (Fig. 15-8).
5. Preoperative visualization of the vocal cords by indirect laryngoscopy should be part of the initial evaluation of every thyroidectomy patient. Paralysis of a vocal cord on the ipsilateral side of the thyroid mass suggests a malignancy.

What Is the Laboratory Evidence for Thyroid Cancer?

Most commonly, the patient presenting with thyroid carcinoma has a euthyroid gland. Thus there is preservation of the functional reserve of the parenchyma (see Chapter 10), with normal laboratory values for protein-bound iodine, serum thyroxin ($^{131}T_3$) resin uptake, and the free thyroxin indices. Only with the rare presentation of advanced invasive destruction of the gland by carcinoma will the patient present with a hypothyroid state. Of some value is the radioactive iodine uptake scan of the thyroid that differenti-

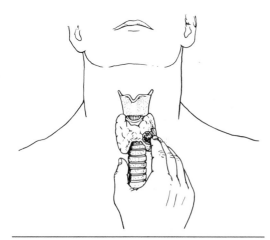

FIGURE 15-6 Inspection and palpation (anterior) of the solitary thyroid lesion.

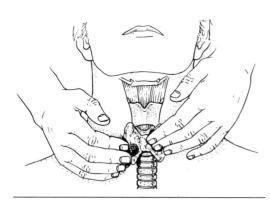

FIGURE 15-7 Thorough evaluation (posterior) with palpation of the solitary thyroid nodule. Evaluate size, location, mobility, fixation, tenderness, consistency, and number.

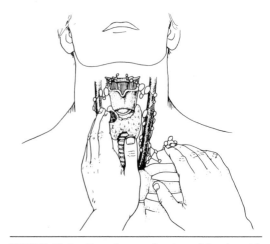

FIGURE 15-8 Complete evaluation of the thyroid and contiguous neck structures. Palpation for regional metastatic disease (levels I-V) of the ipsilateral and contralateral neck is an essential component of the initial examination.

ates the enlarging mass (nodule) from the contiguous thyroid parenchyma. More than 20% of the solitary, cold nodules are malignant and can be distinguished from the adenomatous goiter because they do not pick up the radioactive iodine (nonfunctional area). In contrast, the presence of a hyperfunctional "hot" (toxic) carcinoma is uncommon; finding a cold (nonfunctional) malignant nodule within the diffuse toxic goiter is more common. Although the hot nodule is rarely malignant, it suppresses the normal gland and represents a relative indication for thyroid lobectomy. Functional pulmonary or bony metastases with a proven histopathologic diagnosis of thyroid carcinoma are best evaluated with regional or whole-body radioiodine scans after near-total or subtotal thyroidectomies. Radiographs of the neck and regional anatomic sites are useful to identify any evidence of tracheal compression or displacement. Needle biopsy and fine-needle aspiration are gaining favor as the primary cytologic techniques for evaluation of these masses. These techniques, combined with B-mode ultrasound of the thyroid, allow differentiation of cystic from solid nodules. Most cystic lesions are benign, and most carcinomas are solid lesions. Fine-needle aspiration performed under ultrasound supervision represents an evolving diagnostic parameter. However, false-negative results can be obtained. The clinically or histologically suspicious mass with a negative test result must be reevaluated and, on occasion, will need thyroid lobectomy to identify the problem.

What Are the Pathologic Types of Thyroid Carcinoma?

Carcinoma of the thyroid is derived from the follicle or epithelial cell or the parenchyma. The concept of a two-cell system is the basis for the classification of thyroid epithelial tumors. Mesenchymal stroma tumors are rare. The follicle cell, which is concerned with iodine metabolism, and the C-cell of neuroectodermal origin comprise the cellular origin for most thyroid neoplasms. The C-cell secretes thyrocalcitonin, a calcium homeostatic hormone found exclusively in medullary thyroid carcinoma. Carcinomas of follicular origin are classified as papillary, follicular, Hürthle, or mixed papillary-follicular cell types. The anaplastic, giant cell, and spindle cell variants are considered transformations from the differentiated types, whereas the small-cell carcinoma represents a histiocytic malignant lymphoma. Carcinomas of the thyroid spread intraglandularly from a primary focal point regardless of cellular origin. Metastases occur within the rich capillary and lymphatic networks around the follicles where they can penetrate the capsule to enter the pericapsular and deep cervical lymphatic channels.

The original pathologic classification proposed by Hazard and Smith has been accepted by the American Thyroid Association. Four major classes are recognized on the basis of cell type and biologic behavior: (1) papillary adenocarcinoma, (2) follicular adenocarcinoma, (3) medullary adenocarcinoma (amyloid stroma), and (4) anaplastic (undifferentiated) adenocarcinoma. Additionally, primary lymphoma (lymphosarcoma) or metastatic carcinoma may be present. All four classes originate from different cell types and have variable clinical and metastatic propensity. Thus they require varying treatment approaches and often different guidelines for follow-up.

Papillary Adenocarcinoma. This neoplasm accounts for 60% to 70% of malignant lesions of the thyroid. Females are afflicted two or three times more frequently than males. This tumor comprises 90% of all thyroid cancer in younger persons. Its natural history is characterized by an insidious, slow progression and a short-term survival rate in the absence of therapy. Approximately one fourth of these tumors are pure papillary lesions, whereas the remainder are mixed papillary and follicular. Careful microscopic evaluation confirms multicentricity in as much as 80% of papillary and mixed papillary-follicular lesions. Intrathyroidal microcalcifications (psammoma bodies) are evident radiographically in 50% of the cases. Intraglandular spread is demonstrable in approximately 60%, with metastases to cervical lymphatics evident in 50% to 60% and vascular invasion in 15%. Prognosis is superior for females under age 40 years with small tumors. Over 70% of these neoplasms are functional, demonstrating a selective uptake of iodine 131. Regression of metastases is observed, as is thyroid-stimulating hormone (TSH) suppression after thyroid hormone therapy.

Follicular Adenocarcinoma. Follicular adenocarcinoma accounts for 15% to 20% of thyroid cancers. It has a somewhat more guarded prognosis than the papillary variant. This neoplasm occurs with equal frequency in both sexes and tends to occur after the fourth decade of life. The clear cell and oxyphilic cell (Hürthle cell) forms may be variants of this tumor line. In contrast to papillary carcinoma, its route of dissemination is primarily hematogenous, with both lung and skeletal metastases demonstrable in those cases in which overt capsular and vascular invasion is evident. Those tumors with absent or minimal capsular invasion have a low potential for metastatic dissemination.

Medullary Adenocarcinoma (MCT). Histologic confirmation of amyloid in the stroma is diagnostic of this solid thyroid neoplasm, which was first described in 1959 by Hazard and colleagues. This sporadic and familial tumor of C-cell origin, associated with calcitonin production, is derived from the neuroectoderm and is part of the polypeptide-secreting amine precursor uptake and decarboxylation (APUD) cell series. MCT occurs most commonly as a nonfamilial sporadic neoplasm but is found in the familial multiple endocrine neoplasia (MEN) syndromes. MEN, type IIA (Sipple's syndrome), includes MCT, pheochromocytomas, and hyperparathyroidism. In the common Sipple's syndrome MCT or C-cell hyperplasia is multicentric, and the pheochromocytomata are bilateral in over 70% of patients. The nonfamilial MEN, type IIB, is found in the marfanoid habitus with MCT and pheochromocytomata and with associated mucosal neuromas of the tongue, lips, or conjunctiva and ganglioneuromas of the bowel.

MCT has no sex predilection, and the ages at presentation vary widely. Diarrhea is common in one third of the patients. This is the only thyroid neoplasm in which ACTH production with Cushing's syndrome has been observed. Diagnosis is established readily with basal and pentagastrin-stimulated calcitonin assays. Search for the familial variant, including pedigree screening for pheochromocytomata and hypercalcemia, is appropriate. Assays for serum calcitonin and histaminase provide excellent diagnostic and follow-up tools that can denote residual or progressive disease after total thyroidectomy.

Anaplastic (Undifferentiated) Adenocarcinoma. Approximately 10% to 15% of thyroid cancers are undifferentiated, biologically and clinically aggressive neoplasms. These tumors infiltrate and replace most of the thyroid parenchyma and neck structures and disseminate early to cervical lymphatics, lungs, and visceral organs. The clinical course is rapid, with death usually occurring within a year of diagnosis. The surgeon's role is usually palliative, and often an early tracheostomy is necessary.

How Is Thyroid Cancer Clinically Evaluated?

The previous discussions document the clinical course and natural history of the various histopathologic types of thyroid carcinoma. Indeed, these histopathologic variants correlate well with the cell type and the tumor differentiation (grade) of the presenting thyroid lesion. Very frequently, the well-differentiated papillary-follicular and mixed lesion presents as an asymptomatic mass, with slow, progressive growth of a single lobe or the isthmus of the gland. Conversely, the more undifferentiated (spindle-cell, anaplastic) variants most frequently present with symptoms of infiltration (i.e., hoarseness, dyspnea, dysphagia, tracheal compression symptoms, pain, and infrequently stridor). These observations are observed as part of a constellation of symptoms in approximately 70% of patients presenting with the more aggressive forms of this disease. At least one half of the intermediate-grade (medullary) cancers present with symptoms that are indistinguishable from the more invasive pathologic types. Infrequently, the clinician observes a solitary large cervical lymphatic metastasis from the well-differentiated lesion as the only clinical finding of an occult thyroid primary. In contrast, the invasive follicular, papillary, and medullary pathologic forms may harbor solitary or multicentric lymphatic metastases at cervical level III or IV, which parallels the course of the internal jugular vein. The aggressive anaplastic (spindle-cell) variant is commonly diagnosed clinically by its desmoplastic infiltration of the skin, vessels, and muscles in the region of the thyroid gland. The undifferentiated tumor often presents with extensive nodal disease at levels II, III, and IV and on occasion in contralateral sites.

What Are the Therapeutic Options for Thyroid Carcinoma?

If a patient has symptoms of compression of the trachea or esophagus, neck exploration is indicated. An elective procedure that allows for thyroid lobectomy and isthmusectomy when a solitary nodule presents in an identifiable site of the ipsilateral gland should be planned. Endocrinologic measures using exogenous thyroid hormone that attempt to suppress the thyroid nodule are rarely of value.

Treatment consists of total lobectomy as part of an en bloc resection that includes the regional lymphatics while preserving the recurrent laryngeal nerve if possible. Incisional biopsies and enucleation of suspicious lesions are mentioned only to condemn them because this practice can initiate intraglandular dissemination or wound implantation of neoplastic cells. This technique also may provide for inadequate tissue sampling of remote areas of the gland where an infiltrating neoplastic process may be located. After complete lobectomy with an ipsilateral presentation, frozen section analysis is appropriate. Subsequent therapy is based on the histologic findings. When analysis of the frozen sections cannot differentiate between a benign and malignant process, the neck should be closed while awaiting results of permanent section analysis. Subsequent therapeutic approaches are planned after confirmation of the histopathologic type, tumor grade, and/or evidence of multicentric extension.

When a benign lesion (i.e., follicular adenoma, thyroiditis, adenomatous goiter) is confirmed histologically, future surgery is not indicated. Consideration should be given to supplemental thyroid hormone therapy to aid in involution of the contralateral lobe. If the nodule is a carcinoma, the surgeon and the pathologist should make every attempt to classify the parenchymal neoplasm with regard to its type and grade, for subsequent treatment is dependent on these pathologic features.

The decision to proceed with total or subtotal thyroidectomy for thyroid cancers is related to (1) the histologic grade (well-differentiated versus invasive) and cell type of the neoplasm; (2) the known frequency of bilateral carcinoma for the type of neoplasm present and thus the chance for subsequent recurrence in the contralateral lobe; (3) the probability of permanent hypoparathyroidism; and (4) the necessity for radioactive iodine glandular ablation to augment therapy. Opinions vary about the indications for the more aggressive approach and are related in part to the variations in pathologic classification and follow-up considerations.

Occult sclerosing papillary and encapsulated follicular carcinomas are successfully treated with ipsilateral lobectomy, isthmectomy, and perhaps resection of the medial contralateral lobe. In contrast, the invasive papillary-follicular and all medullary (solid) thyroid neoplasms often extend into the opposite lobe with multifocal involvement, which is best managed by total or near-total thyroidectomy. The latter procedure implies complete lobectomy of the involved site, isthmus resection, and subtotal removal of the contralateral lobe. In both procedures the parathyroids of the contralateral side are identified and preserved with an adequate blood supply to the posterior capsule of the glands. An alternative approach to parathyroid preservation is glandular autotransplantation into muscle compartments of the neck or forearm.

Aside from biopsy, rarely is any operative procedure possible for the aggressive and rapidly lethal undifferentiated (anaplastic) cell type. On occasion, early recognition of this carcinoma,

when it is confined to a single site, warrants an aggressive total thyroidectomy and possible radical neck dissection. Data suggest improved responses to adjuvant irradiation and chemotherapy (doxorubicin, chlorambucil, vincristine) after such cytoreductive measures. The propensity for this neoplasm to invade vital contiguous organs, causing respiratory and esophageal obstruction, often necessitates early tracheostomy and/or esophageal intubation for palliation.

The presence of clinically palpable cervical nodes with any of the thyroid carcinoma types is an indication for nodal dissection. Lymph nodes in the central neck are of particular significance since the biologic potential for metastasis varies with regard to cell type and tumor grade. Well-differentiated lesions tend to remain in nodal arrest for extended periods of time before they invade surrounding structures. This permits nodal dissection without sacrifice of important structures while providing regional control and potential cure of disease. Furthermore, clinicopathologic observation justifies withholding lateral cervical dissections until palpable lymphadenopathy is evident in the well-differentiated primary lesion.

The extent of the nodal dissection depends on the location of the thyroid lesion and the magnitude of nodal dissemination. Extensive node involvement along the internal jugular vein, often found with operable anaplastic and medullary thyroid cancers, requires modified neck dissection. The procedure includes resection of all lymphatic drainage in the central neck compartment from the thyroid cartilage (superior nodes) to the superior mediastinum, with en bloc removal of lateral, inferior, pretracheal, and tracheoesophageal nodal metastases. Removal of the internal jugular vein allows a more thorough extirpation of disease; however, only rarely is removal of the sternocleidomastoid muscle and spinal accessory nerve necessary because these organs are usually spared involvement by invasive tumor.

The anterior superior mediastinal dissection is indicated only for well-differentiated neoplasms with no distant metastases in a patient expected to survive for a long period of time. Mediastinal node dissection for the undifferentiated invasive thyroid lesion is contraindicated because any survival benefit is negated by the high operative morbidity and mortality rates.

How Should the Patient With Thyroid Cancer Be Followed?

Although the method for evaluating recurrent thyroid cancer has varied among clinics throughout the world, the specific interval for follow-up (every 3 to 6 months) is standard. Physical examination should focus on reexamination of the wound and the ipsilateral lobe of involvement. Comprehensive evaluation for recurrent nodal disease in midline and supraclavicular sites is emphasized. Routine interval radiograms of the chest (every 6 to 12 months) are important to document pulmonary metastases. Exogenous thyroid hormone replacement is essential to provide a euthyroid status to the postthyroidectomy patient. The physician may have a strong clue as to the site of dissemination because of the histologic type (e.g., papillary carcinoma commonly has nodal metastases; follicular carcinoma often has pulmonary metastases).

Radioiodine scintiscan is performed in the early postoperative phases to identify functional residual thyroid tissue in the neck and to establish a baseline reference point for evaluation and therapy of recurrent disease.

Recurrent tumors that are nonsuppressible, unresectable, and functionally autonomous are best treated with prophylactic ablation of residual tissue with ^{131}I. This technique has potential radiation hazards, and in no circumstance should it be used as a "prophylactic" measure to prevent recurrence. Only infrequently is extranodal, recurrent, invasive disease resectable; this clinical presentation is best managed by external-beam irradiation and chemotherapy. In contrast, the well-differentiated recurrent or persistent lesion can be treated with either ^{131}I radioiodine therapy or thyrotrophin suppression.

Effective thyrotrophin suppression of unresectable disease may be used in the following circumstances: (1) the neoplasm that fails to demonstrate functional uptake of radioactive iodine; (2) the patient with extensive local, regional, and/or pulmonary disease in whom planned doses of ^{131}I therapy are large and potentially harmful in the amounts required; and (3) the younger patient in whom the radiation risk of ^{131}I therapy is considered great for development of, for example, leukemias and lymphomas and in whom favorable tumor characteristics (low-grade, well-differentiated papillary) are evident. The administration of exogenous thyroid hormone such as L-triiodothyronine (100 to 115 μg daily) will effectively suppress anterior pituitary gland release of thyrotrophin hormone (TSH). Interval reevaluation of the disease response is suggested, with measurement of the serum TSH and thyroxine values, scintillation scan, and radioactive iodine uptake. Medullary carcinoma of the thyroid is a C-cell neoplasm; thus these cancers do not concentrate radioiodine and are nonsuppressible after administration of therapeutic doses of exogenous thyroxine.

Multiple clinical trials have been initiated for use of radioactive iodine in the treatment of cancer of the thyroid. This modality should not be used in children or in the pregnant woman. Applications of radioactive iodine are reserved for (1) autonomously functional and aggressive tumors that are nonresponsive or have diminished responsiveness to suppression with thyrotrophin; (2) functional tumors in middle-aged and elderly patients in whom radiation risks are reduced; and (3) functional thyroid neoplasms in patients who had minimal or no tumor regression after hormonal suppression.

SUMMARY

- Palpable nodules of the thyroid occur in 4% to 5% of the population.
- Fifteen to 30% of palpable nodules are malignant at operation.
- Deaths from thyroid carcinoma are rare (1000 per year in the United States).
- Papillary and follicular carcinomas have higher survival and cure rates than does medullary, anaplastic carcinoma.
- Thyrotrophin suppression is indicated for (1) unresectable disease and/or extensive regional disease; (2) lesions demonstrating lack of radioactive iodine uptake; and (3) young patients.

PITFALLS AND COMMON MYTHS

- A nodule cannot be cancer because the patient is young and the nodule feels so soft.
- Goiters that have been present for a long time never become malignant.
- Laterally located thyroid tissue is a congenital anomaly.
- To cure a cancer, the primary site must always be identified and treated.
- Thyroid cancer runs such an indolent course that treatment by thyroid suppression is sufficient.

BIBLIOGRAPHY

Barrie JR, Knapper WH, Strong EW. Cervical nodal metastasis of unknown origin. Am J Surg 120:466-470, 1970.

Behar R, Arganini M, et al. Graves' disease and thyroid cancer. Surgery 100:1121, 1986.

Bland KI, Klamer TW, et al. Isolated regional lymph node dissection: Morbidity, mortality and economic considerations. Ann Surg 193:372, 1981.

Bland KI, Polk HC Jr. The apudomas: The concept and associated neoplasms. In Copeland EM III (ed). Surgical Oncology. New York, John Wiley & Sons, 1983.

Brunt LM, Wells SA Jr. Advances in the diagnosis and treatment of medullary thyroid carcinoma. Surg Clin North Am 67:263, 1987.

Cady B. Surgery of thyroid cancer. World J Surg 5:3, 1981.

Clark OH, Levin K, et al. Thyroid cancer: The case for total thyroidectomy. Eur J Cancer Clin Oncol 24:305, 1988.

De Vries N, Snow GB. The management of a suspicious lymph node in the neck. Curr Pract Surg 4:31, 1992.

DeGroot LJ, Kaplan EL, et al. Natural history, treatment, and course of papillary thyroid carcinoma. J Clin Endocrinol Metab 71:414, 1990.

Jesse RH, Perez CA, Fletcher GH. Cervical lymph node metastasis: Unknown primary cancer. Cancer 31:854, 1973.

Kaplan EL. Thyroid and parathyroid. In Schwartz SI, Shires GT, et al (eds). Principles of Surgery. New York, McGraw-Hill, 1984.

Leight GS Jr. Nodular goiter and benign and malignant neoplasms of the thyroid. In Sabiston DC Jr (ed). Textbook of Surgery. Philadelphia, WB Saunders, 1991.

Lyerly HK. The thyroid gland. In Sabiston DC Jr (ed). Textbook of Surgery. 1991.

McGuirt WF, McCabe BF. Significance of a neck node biopsy prior to definitive treatment for a metastatic surgical carcinoma. Laryngoscope 88:594, 1978.

Weber CA, Clark OH. Surgery for thyroid disease. Med Clin North Am 69:1097-1115, 1985.

Wells SA Jr, Lairmore TC. The multiple endocrine neoplasias. In Sabiston DC Jr (ed). Textbook of Surgery. 1991.

CHAPTER REVIEW
Questions

1. Common causes for head and neck masses in children include all of the following *except:*
   a. Sarcoma
   b. Carcinoma
   c. Developmental lesions
   d. Inflammatory masses

2. What is the most common malignant neoplasm of the head and neck in children?
   a. Rhabdomyosarcoma
   b. Neuroblastoma
   c. Hodgkin's and nonHodgkin's lymphoma
   d. Thyroid carcinoma
   e. Squamous cell carcinoma

3. A 12-year-old black male presents with a 2-cm soft, palpable, midline infrahyoid mass. Probable cause(s) for this lesion includes which of the following?
   a. Dermoid cyst
   b. Cystic hygroma
   c. Thyroglossal duct cyst
   d. Lymphosarcoma
   e. Thyroid carcinoma

4. Approximately one half of palpable neck masses in *adults* originate where?
   a. Developmental defects
   b. Inflammatory lymphatics
   c. Thyroid gland
   d. Major salivary glands
   e. Metastatic lesions with known primaries

5. Thyrotrophin suppression for recurrent unresectable thyroid cancer is useful in which of the following?
   a. The neoplasm that fails to have demonstrable uptake of radioactive ^{131}I
   b. The patient with extensive pulmonary or regional disease in whom large doses of ^{131}I are required
   c. Younger patients in whom the radiation risk of ^{131}I therapy is excessive
   d. All of the above
   e. None of the above

6. A 63-year-old male carpenter presents with an isolated cervical lesion above the right supraclavicular space at level V (lower posterior cervical nodes). A careful search for the parent neoplasm is nondiagnostic at indirect and direct panendoscopy. All biopsies of visualized mucosal surfaces are negative. What is the appropriate therapy?
   a. Comprehensive irradiation to base of the tongue, larynx, and the right neck
   b. Right radical neck dissection
   c. Bilateral neck irradiation
   d. Comprehensive irradiation of the nasopharynx and the right neck
   e. Multimodal therapy: surgery, irradiation, and cyclic chemotherapy

7. Excluding benign and neoplastic *thyroid* lesions, what are most neck masses?
   a. Congenital cervical masses
   b. Supraclavicular masses
   c. Neoplastic tumors
   d. Inflammatory intraoral lesions
   e. Inflammatory cutaneous infections

8. Common malignant neck masses in children (>2 cm) include each of the following *except:*

a. Hodgkin's lymphoma
b. Non-Hodgkin's lymphoma
c. Soft-part sarcoma
d. Thyroid carcinoma
e. Tuberculous adenitis (scrofula)

9. What is the cardinal physical finding of thyroid carcinoma in most patients?
   a. Multicentric nodal metastases
   b. A palpable solitary nodule
   c. Diffuse symmetric thyroid enlargement
   d. Hypothyroidism
   e. Hyperthyroidism

10. What is the most common histopathologic variant of thyroid carcinoma?
    a. Papillary adenocarcinoma
    b. Follicular adenocarcinoma
    c. Medullary adenocarcinoma
    d. Hürthle cell carcinoma
    e. Anaplastic (undifferentiated) adenocarcinoma

11. Paralysis of a vocal cord on the ipsilateral side of an occult thyroid mass demonstrable on radioactive iodine uptake scan suggests what?

a. Thyroid cyst
b. Functional thyroid nodule
c. A thyroid malignancy
d. Entrapment of the recurrent laryngeal nerve by a remote malignancy
e. A thyroidal metastasis

12. Invasive papillary-follicular and all medullary thyroid neoplasms are best managed by which therapy?
    a. Ipsilateral lobectomy and isthmusectomy
    b. Total or near-total thyroidectomy
    c. Simple ipsilateral lobectomy
    d. External beam irradiation
    e. ^{131}I radioiodine therapy

Answers

1. b	7. c
2. c	8. e
3. a, c	9. b
4. c	10. a
5. d	11. c
6. b	12. b

16 Difficulties in Swallowing

HIRAM C. POLK, Jr.

KEY FEATURES

After reading this chapter you will understand:
- The ease with which most esophageal diseases can be diagnosed.
- The importance of palliation for the esophageal cancer patient.
- The rationale for nonoperative treatment of reflux esophagitis.
- The use and effectiveness of fundoplication.
- The importance of being alert to associated and occult esophageal motility disorders.
- That diverticula are important only with respect to their underlying causes.

HOW DO WE SWALLOW?

Swallowing is initiated in the mouth and pharynx and is completed in the stomach, but the vast majority of clinically significant problems of deglutition are caused by esophageal abnormalities. Because both blood supply and innervation segmentally correspond precisely to the intercostal bundles and dermatomes, the somatic representation of esophageal symptoms correlates closely with the level of disease in the gullet itself.

Familiarity with mechanisms of normal swallowing is essential to the appreciation of all functional esophageal disorders. Swallowing is begun by a complex and integrated response of intraoral and intrinsic and extrinsic pharyngeal muscles, including subtle maneuvers to occlude the nasopharynx and larynx. The pharyngeal peristaltic wave leads to cricopharyngeal relaxation and continues into the upper esophagus as the primary esophageal wave, which moves caudad in an unbroken fashion toward the lower esophageal complex at the rate of 2 to 4 cm per second. Secondary waves originate at sites of local esophageal distention secondary to passage of the bolus and progress in an orderly fashion caudally, emptying the gullet of any retained or regurgitated material.

Physiologically, *lower esophageal complex* describes the distal esophageal ampulla, the fascial insertions arising from the esophageal hiatus in the diaphragm, and the gastric fundus. Although no demonstrable muscular esophageal sphincter exists in humans, the lower esophageal complex normally functions as a sphincter, minimizing reflux of gastric contents into the lower esophagus while allowing orderly esophageal emptying into the stomach (Fig. 16-1). A high-pressure zone in the distal esophagus is largely responsible for such physiologic sphincteric function. The complex relaxes (i.e., the pressure becomes negative) 2 seconds after initiation of swallowing and just before arrival of the primary esophageal wave. The interacting functions of the lower esophageal complex are exceedingly involved and remain imperfectly understood. Present evidence indicates that maintenance of a length of intra-abdominal esophagus responsive to positive intra-abdominal pressure rather than negative intrapleural pressure is particularly important in preserving gastroesophageal competence.

From even such a brief overview of the physiology of deglutition, obvious opportunities become apparent for disorders. Cricopharyngeal

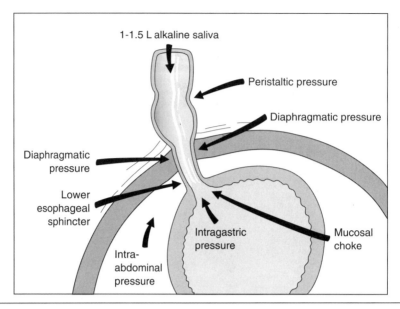

FIGURE 16-1   Pressure relationships at the cardioesophageal junction influence gastroesophageal reflux.

spasm occurs and leads to the familiar cervical pulsion diverticulum. Neoplastic growths may produce mechanical obstruction at any level. When cancer develops, dissemination to the rich network of mediastinal lymphatics is the rule. Furthermore, a multitude of anatomic and functional disorders contrive to alter the intricate functions of the lower esophageal complex.

DIAGNOSIS
Symptoms

Virtually all disorders of the swallowing process are manifested as one of three symptoms (dysphagia, pyrosis, and regurgitation) and share modes of diagnosis (i.e., barium swallow and esophagoscopy), which are definitive for nearly 98% of all patients.

Dysphagia. Dysphagia (difficulty in swallowing) is usually expressed as "My food won't go down," or "My food sticks right here," as the patient points with considerable topographic accuracy to the site of obstruction. The consistency of tolerable foodstuffs often becomes less viscous as the illness progresses.

The common causes of dysphagia are esophageal carcinoma, stricture complicating hiatal hernia, and achalasia, in that order. Dysphagia for both liquids and solids at the outset is typical of motility disturbances such as achalasia or diffuse esophageal spasm, whereas dysphagia for

solids progressing to liquids indicates structural obstruction such as by carcinoma.

Dysphagia developing in a patient with recognized or long-standing heartburn is most commonly due to one of the intrinsic esophageal responses to continued acid injury, as exemplified by the following.

I. Schatzki ring formation, which takes one of two forms
   A. Spastic lower esophageal ring formation caused by irritation of a segment of circular esophageal muscle
   B. Fibrotic ring formation as a response to repeated injury
   The spastic variant outnumbers the fibrotic by 10 to 1 or better.
II. Transmural inflammation resulting in one of two forms of longitudinal esophageal stricture, which may or may not be associated with apparent esophageal shortening
   A. Soft and pliable; amenable to dilation when reflux is surgically controlled
   B. Firm to hard; not amenable to dilation and requiring direct operative repair with major attendant morbidity and mortality
   The pliable variant is far more common in the United States.

Heartburn. Pyrosis (heartburn) is pain produced by reflux of gastric secretions retrograde through the gastroesophageal junction with subsequent esophageal mucosal injury (see Fig. 16-1). It is burning and retrosternal, aggravated by lying supine and by maneuvers that increase intra-abdominal pressure, and ameliorated by antacids. Ninety-five percent of patients with persistent or recurrent heartburn have an associated hiatal hernia. A very few patients may have significant, serious reflux in the absence of a radiographically demonstrable hiatal hernia. Nighttime aspiration of regurgitated gastric contents may produce secondary respiratory symptoms ranging from nocturnal coughing and transient bronchospasm to chronic pneumonitis.

Regurgitation. Regurgitation of recently ingested food or gastric contents, when persistent or recurrent, typically is caused by an esophageal diverticulum or hiatal hernia and gastroesophageal reflux, respectively. Foul or partially digested food products are regurgitated most commonly from diverticula. Aspiration related to a diverticulum occurs more commonly during mealtime than while sleeping.

Peculiarly, infants who have hiatal hernias manifest only effortless regurgitation and its complications, whereas older children present adult symptoms.

Other Variants. Two other symptom complexes are sufficiently common. Some patients with stenoses, large diverticula, or free reflux develop clinical and/or roentgenographic signs of chronic pulmonary infection caused by repeated aspiration. Classically, a sense of strangling or severe coughing while the patient is asleep indicates nocturnal (recumbent) reflux and aspiration.

The other complex is an atypical manifestation of reflux esophagitis. The pain is substernal and crushing and may even radiate to the left shoulder and arm, mimicking angina pectoris. The essential point is to recall that a few patients with reflux esophagitis present as if they have myocardial ischemia and vice versa. Quite a few patients who have had normal coronary arteriograms currently are referred for assessment of whether reflux esophagitis is a feasible cause of their atypical chest pain. The converse is also true (i.e., the "typical heartburn" may be an unusual expression of myocardial ischemia).

What Points in the Patient's History Are Important?

An accurate history alone yields the specific diagnosis in three of four patients. Eight questions are especially useful in reaching a conclusion referable to esophageal symptoms:

1. How long has the symptom been present?
2. Is it intermittent or continuous? Has it been progressive?
3. Do certain foods or exercise aggravate the complaint?
4. Can it be alleviated? If so, how?
5. Is regurgitation or pain part of the problem now, or has it been in the past?
6. Has there been loss of weight indicating likely presence of cancer?
7. Where is the principal symptom manifested?
8. Do other diseases coexist?

The medical history is often erroneously minimized in the diagnosis of esophageal abnormalities, largely because of the great specificity of x-ray contrast studies and endoscopy. The history defines with special clarity those disorders that require urgent treatment, as opposed to the orderly, nonemergent diagnostic and therapeutic measures necessary for the usual chronic esophageal complaint.

Foreign Materials. Ingestion of caustics, exemplified by household lye, can produce direct, immediate, mechanical obstruction caused by intense edema at the site of contact or subsequent, progressive, lengthy esophageal stenoses. Small children and suicidal candidates are the most common victims. The history is often not precise, and most experienced observers recommend early endoscopy down to the level of injury to confirm the diagnosis and the need for therapy. This is especially important since approximately one fourth to one third of suspected victims sustain no injury. Several treatment regimens appear more or less equally successful, but intermittent bougienage (dilation) as warranted by symptoms and confirmed by contrast x-ray studies becomes the keystone of early management. There is no objective evidence of its efficacy, but systemic corticosteroid therapy often is used early, allegedly to reduce acute inflammation. Fibrous strictures unresponsive to this plan often eventually require bypass of the esophagus, preferably with a substernal colon segment.

Solid foreign bodies such as toys or large boluses of food may become lodged in the esophagus. History and contrast studies usually define the problem, and when the patient is stable, endoscopic removal is usually warranted. The physician must subsequently examine the esophagus carefully with additional contrast x-ray studies and endoscopy to exclude an underlying disease process responsible for the obturation of the foreign body and warranting treatment.

Esophageal Rupture (Boerhaave's Syn-

drome). Forceful emesis, often related to acute alcohol abuse, produces a full-thickness tear of the esophagus, usually in and about the esophagogastric junction, with secondary fulminant bacterial mediastinitis. Typically the pain is severe, often associated with shock and cyanosis and minimal hematemesis. Chest films usually show a hydropneumothorax on the left side, and water-soluble contrast x-ray studies of the esophagus confirm the problem. Treatment includes aggressive fluid resuscitation, tube thoracostomy, systemic antibiotics, and early operative closure of the defect.

Table 16-1 gives diagnostic points plus certain characteristic epidemiologic data for four representative illnesses afflicting the esophagus. In typical cases there is little chance to confuse esophageal carcinoma with hiatal hernia. The progressive, slightly painful dysphagia associated with neoplastic occlusion of the esophageal lumen in an emaciated patient is typical of cancer. However, it is totally unlike the transiently incapacitating heartburn of esophagitis attributable to hiatal hernia, which is dramatically relieved by antacids and so regularly aggravated by recumbency—but not by exertion—in a patient who is well nourished.

Physical Signs

The physical signs of diseases of deglutition are usually secondary: (1) weight loss, (2) anemia,

and (3) aspirational pulmonary disease. A cervical esophageal diverticulum may be palpated just anterior to the border of the sternocleidomastoid muscle; compression of the area may evacuate the diverticulum into the oropharynx.

Roentgenography and Endoscopy

For the one patient in four not yielding to the discerning historian, definitive diagnosis in 98% can be made by barium swallow roentgenography and endoscopy with biopsy (Figs. 16-2 through 16-6). Some abnormalities of esophageal motility will not be detected by liquid barium, and the patient may have to swallow a barium-coated marshmallow or other foodstuff to delineate obstruction for solid material. Esophagoscopy allows biopsy documentation of the nature of organic stenoses, and experienced observers approach 100% accuracy in defining gastric acid reflux and esophagitis caused by hiatal hernia. Refined examinations such as intraesophageal manometry and esophageal acid perfusion clarify occasional obscure cases but are infrequently necessary.

Because precise distinction among sources of upper abdominal complaints is highly fallible, patients with heartburn and hiatal hernia require contrast x-ray examinations of the entire gastrointestinal and biliary tracts to discover if other organs are abnormal, possibly contributing to the symptoms initially attributed to esophagitis.

TABLE 16-1   Diagnostic Points in Representative Disorders of Deglutition

Pertinent Characteristic	Carcinoma	Complicated Hiatal Hernia	Achalasia	Cervical Diverticulum
Duration of symptoms	Weeks to months	Months to years	Months to years	Months to years
Characteristics	Rapidly progressive	Intermittent	Persistent	Slowly progressive
Aggravated by	Nothing	Reclining flat	Anxiety	Nothing
Alleviated by	Nothing	Antacids	Antispasmodics	Nothing
Dysphagia	Severe, progressive	Late, if ever	Marked	Uncommon
Regurgitation	Only late	Frequent, acid	Frequent, food	With neck compression
Heartburn	Absent	Prominent	Absent	Absent
Weight loss	Marked	Absent	Mild	None
Anemia	Frequent	Occasional	Uncommon	Rare
Location	Variable	Perixiphoid	Xiphoid	Neck
Comorbidity	Absent	Obesity, pregnancy	Psychologic trauma	Aspiration
Masqueraders	Globus hystericus	Angina pectoris, aspiration	Globus hystericus	None
Typical age (yr)	60+	40+	20+	60+
Predispositions	Black	Female	Asthenia	Distal obstruction

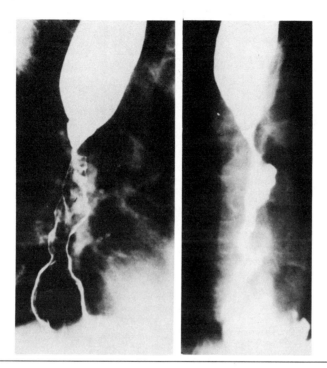

FIGURE 16-2   Benign linear stricture of the esophagus with associated proximal dilation.

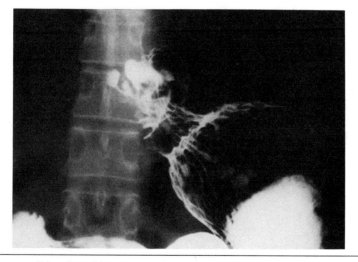

FIGURE 16-3   Sliding hiatal hernia showing gastric folds through the hiatus, a supradiaphragmatic gastric pouch, and a distal esophageal ulcer.

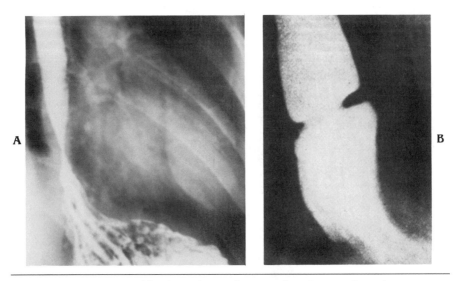

FIGURE 16-4 **A,** A typical benign stricture above a reflux-shortened esophagus associated with a sliding hiatal hernia. **B,** Schatzi ring at junction of squamous and columnar epithelium. A small hiatal hernia is present.

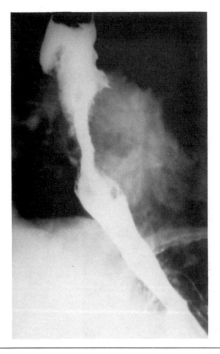

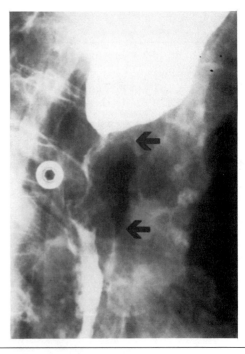

FIGURE 16-5 Carcinoma at lower end of esophagus. This type of lesion may arise from the gastric fundus and involve the esophagus secondarily.

FIGURE 16-6 Carcinoma at the junction of the middle and lower thirds of the esophagus. Note the filling defect with overhanging edge and the marked proximal dilation of the esophagus. The arrows mark the irregular lumen.

WHAT ARE THE RESULTS OF TREATMENT?
Esophageal Cancer

Ninety-eight percent of esophageal cancers are squamous cell type. When adenocarcinoma is discovered in the distal esophagus, it is usually attributable to submucosal esophageal invasion by an upper gastric primary cancer. Regional lymph node metastases or contiguous spread exists in approximately 75% of patients at the time of diagnosis. The local effects of inanition and secondary respiratory complications limit average life expectancy, dated from the onset of symptoms to 8 months. Progressive cachexia occurs until local growth causes tracheoesophageal fistula and respiratory death or until metastatic cancer ablates some vital function. Humane palliation is the goal of treatment.

Nonoperative Management. The following two methods may be used sequentially or in combination:

- *Irradiation.* Regression of the primary carcinoma occurs to such an extent that some patients again swallow effectively for a short while.
- *Esophageal intubation.* Reasonably normal alimentation until the illness runs its course can be achieved in a variable proportion of patients (Fig. 16-7). It may also obturate a neoplastic tracheoesophageal fistula and ameliorate those symptoms effectively.
- Laser restoration of luminal patency for a brief period.

Chemotherapy has not been effective.

Operative Management. The choice of operation depends on the portion of the esophagus involved (Table 16-2). Because the treatments are similarly effective, the actual decision should depend on which method has proved safest and most effective in the particular institution.

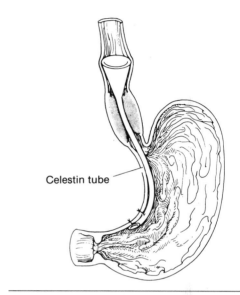

Celestin tube

FIGURE 16-7 Patients with an obstructed esophagus can be fed either by using intubation distal to the obstruction or by passing a catheter or plastic tube through the lesion from above, as shown.

TABLE 16-2 Choice of Therapy: Esophageal Cancer

Site of Primary Neoplasm	Usual Recommended Treatment	Rationale for Choice	Treatment Mortality Rate (%)
Cervical esophagus	Irradiation or en bloc resection and microsurgical jejunal free-graft replacement	High morbidity rate and long delay in restoration of alimentary continuity when operative treatment is used	5
Middle and upper thoracic esophagus	Substernal colon bypass Irradiation/laser Total thoracic esophagectomy	Provides immediate restoration of swallowing, with possible exclusion of patients developing metastatic disease during irradiation	15
Lower thoracic esophagus	Resection and esophagogastric anastomosis	Immediate palliative and definitive therapy available with low morbidity rate but fairly high mortality rate	20

Results of treatment with respect to long-term control of esophageal cancer are uniformly poor, regardless of the method. Approximately 5% of all patients in whom the diagnosis is made survive 5 years; that population base includes many inoperable and unresectable cases. Restoration of normal alimentation with minimal morbidity and mortality is the primary goal of treatment while not denying the occasional curable patient a chance.

Hiatal Hernia and Reflux Esophagitis

Treatment of any sort is required only when esophagitis or some other complication such as stenosis has been objectively identified. Most patients with hiatal hernia do not manifest significant gastroesophageal reflux, and if they do, the esophagus so rapidly and efficiently clears the refluxed acid that no inflammation results. Note that hiatal hernia is unlike most other hernias in several ways:

1. It is usually sliding (i.e., a retroperitoneal structure—in this case the "bare area" of the stomach—makes up part of the wall of the hernia sac).
2. Incarceration and strangulation virtually never occur unless the lesion is the very rare (<1%) rolling or parahiatal variant, in which case mandatory immediate repair is required.

Therefore many asymptomatic hiatal hernias remain so (Fig. 16-8). Most symptomatic but totally untreated hiatal hernias progress to intolerable esophagitis or, less commonly, to stenosis via inflammation leading to fibrosis. Such a stricture, often associated with esophageal shortening secondary to both longitudinal and circumferential fibrosis, occurs in approximately 1% of patients with hiatal hernia, but its prevention is especially important because of the tenfold increase in the mortality rate of patients undergoing subsequent operative treatment for hiatal hernia associated with persistent esophagitis compared to that when stricture resection is required.

Nonoperative Management. An appropriate medical treatment regimen includes the following.

I. Alleviation of factors predisposing to increased intra-abdominal pressure such as:
   a. Tight-fitting garments
   b. Pregnancy (self-limiting)
   c. Obesity
   d. Urinary or alimentary obstruction
   e. Respiratory disease producing chronic cough

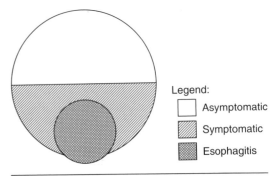

Legend:
□ Asymptomatic
▨ Symptomatic
▩ Esophagitis

FIGURE 16-8 Schematic showing proportion of adult hiatal hernias that are symptomatic. Note that approximately half of patients who are symptomatic have esophagitis. The great majority of patients with esophagitis have hiatal hernias.

II. Promoting the effects of gravity to reduce gastroesophageal reflux by:
   a. Elevation of the head while sleeping (blocks under the head of the bed)
   b. Avoidance of lying down after eating or drinking
III. Dietary restrictions to diminish gastric distention and/or acid secretion:
   a. Abstention from acid-stimulating materials such as alcohol, coffee, tobacco, chocolate, aspirin, and carbonated beverages
   b. Avoidance of liquids for 2 hours after breakfast and lunch and altogether after dinner
   c. Frequent small meals in lieu of fewer larger meals
   d. Dry, bland diet
IV. Frequent ingestion of small amounts of antacid, either liquid or chewable mints
V. Possible use of cimetidine, which may increase lower-esophageal sphincter complex tone

A therapeutic paradox exists: absence of reservoir function in the gullet demands use of antacids frequently and in small doses, but such a regimen tends to increase weight and, hence, intra-abdominal pressure.

Reasonable symptomatic control of esophagitis secondary to hiatal hernia is achieved by such a regimen in approximately two thirds of patients during short follow-up periods (Fig. 16-9). However, it is unclear whether patients will adhere to such regimens over long periods of time and whether control of symptoms will be maintained throughout life once it is achieved.

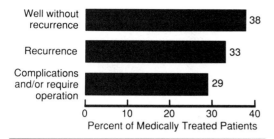

FIGURE 16-9 Results of medical treatment for hiatal hernia.

There is some evidence that omeprazole (Prilosec) may sharply increase the effectiveness of medicinal treatment, but it is presently very expensive and of undetermined long-term value. Esophagitis apparently does not progress to fibrosis when there is consistent medical control of the patient's symptoms of heartburn.

Operative Management. An operation is indicated when:

- Nonoperative measures no longer can be tolerated by the patient.
- Pain persists despite faithful adherence to an effective medical regimen.
- Stenosis appears or progresses under the same conditions.
- Carcinoma cannot reasonably be excluded.

Operative repair should seldom be undertaken unless esophagitis, or a related complication, objectively can be demonstrated, usually via esophagoscopy. The technical goals of operation are twofold: (1) correction of the anatomic disorders (i.e., reduction and repair of the hiatal hernia) and (2) alteration of fundal and esophagogastric anatomy to control the functional abnormality of reflux of gastric secretions into the distal esophagus (fundoplication). Technical measures shown in Fig. 16-10, in addition to suture of the diaphragmatic crural defect, have obtained long-term control of both reflux and hernia in 95% of patients undergoing an operation. These procedures are feasible through transabdominal or transthoracic incisions. Coexisting diseases and the patient's body build, not the surgeon's personal preference, should determine which incision is used. The most common coexistent diseases are cholelithiasis, peptic ulcer, diverticulosis and diverticulitis of the colon, and pulmonary aspiration.

Crural suture alone fails to maintain control of hernia and/or reflux. Procedures to reduce gastric acid secretion such as vagotomy and pyloroplasty have not improved these results, which is as expected because the gastric acidity of patients with hiatal hernia unassociated with duodenal ulcer is in the normal range.

The immediate morbidity rate after operative repair for hiatal hernia approaches 10%. Late and functional morbidity from the procedures is minimal. A broadly based Veterans Administration trial of medical and surgical treatment of severe esophagitis showed somewhat better results in the surgically treated patients. Variable percentages of patients have some early dysphagia, which responds promptly, and only a few are plagued by gaseousness and inability to vomit.

On the other hand, the development of a stricture or stenosis of the esophagus secondary to continued peptic injury represents a therapeutic problem with a much greater risk of death and disability. The key diagnostic factor is the development of dysphagia, usually superimposed on a long history of heartburn. Usual studies readily define the problem, but carcinoma must be excluded. The central component of therapy is termination of reflux. If the stenosis is soft and pliable, hernia repair, an antireflux procedure, and several dilations will correct the problem. If the stricture is unyielding, therapeutic approaches vary, but all are of a higher order of risk. Options include (1) splitting the stricture and patching the defect with gastric fundus (Thal), (2) esophageal lengthening by the method of Collis and dilation, and (3) resection of the stenosis and interposition of isoperistaltic jejunum (Merendino) or colon. The latter works especially well but is an intrinsically risky procedure.

Achalasia

Cardiospasm, or *achalasia,* refers to a failure of the distal esophageal segment to relax with the arrival of the primary peristaltic wave, producing a functional obstruction and marked dilation of the proximal esophagus. Achalasia is regularly symptomatic, although many victims coexist with their illness by subtle, if unconscious, alterations of their diet and eating habits. This illness does not progress in the ordinary sense, although proximal dilation of the obstructed esophagus occurs and accumulation of food in the organ may aggravate the obstructive symptoms and cause notable bad breath.

Nonoperative Treatment. Anticholinergic and antispasmodic medications produce generally unsatisfactory results. There is much current enthusiasm for improvement resulting from use of calcium chemical blockers; however, their real value has not yet been determined. Should obstructive symptoms become intolerable, forceful

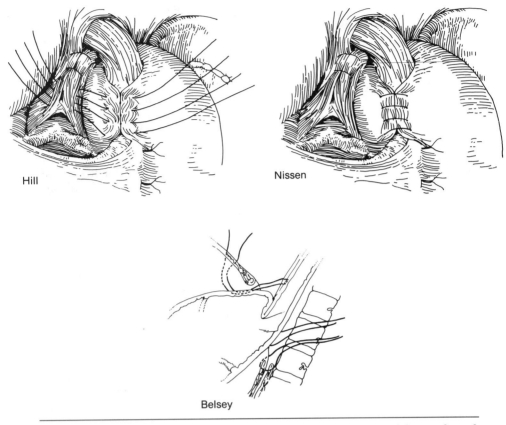

Hill

Nissen

Belsey

FIGURE 16-10   Types of repair for hiatal hernia. Note that tightening of the esophageal hiatus accompanies the wrapping procedures (fundoplication).

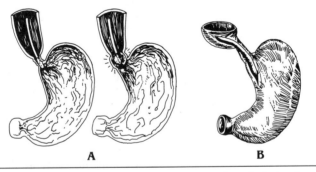

A   **B**

FIGURE 16-11   **A,** Nonoperative hydrostatic bougienage for achalasia of esophagus. **B,** Operative myotomy.

dilation may be accomplished by inflation of an intraesophageal balloon at precisely the cardio-esophageal junction, intentionally producing rupture of the esophageal muscle (myotomy) without damage to the mucosa (Fig. 16-11, **A**). The technique demands considerable precision and experience to achieve long-lasting allevia-tion of esophageal spasm without rupture of the organ, mediastinitis, and death. In the best hands this technique, although requiring repetition in some patients, achieves long-lasting control of dysphagia in 80% of patients. Esophageal rup-ture, which is not necessarily fatal, occurs in 1% of patients undergoing forceful dilation.

Operative Management. Data indicate that operative treatment produces a better control rate with similarly low risk. The goal of treatment is to incise anteriorly the longitudinal and circular muscle of the distal esophagus, extending down onto the stomach (Fig. 16-11, **B**). If particular attention is not paid to additional maneuvers maintaining esophagogastric competence against reflux, postoperative esophagitis will produce poor outcomes in 20% to 25% of otherwise satisfactory results. Operative treatment (cardiomyotomy, modified Heller procedure) can be accomplished by both transthoracic and transabdominal approaches, although the former is preferred. The operative mortality rate is less than 1% and the early morbidity rate is approximately 15%. Late morbidity, assuming control of postoperative gastroesophageal reflux, is absent, and more than 90% of patients who have undergone the operation remain well.

Other Motility Disorders. Dysfunction of the propulsive action of both longitudinal and circular muscles of the esophagus occurs rarely. The illnesses are similarly poorly understood but are often first suspected when an observant diagnostic radiologist describes "tertiary waves" (Fig. 16-12) in the esophagus after barium swallow. Antispasmodics are seldom helpful for long, and dilation of lengthy or multiple segments often fails. If a patient is markedly symptomatic and these symptoms persist to the point of significant alteration of life-style, a very long esophageal myotomy, which usually provides lasting relief, may be considered.

Esophageal Diverticula

Esophageal diverticula are classified as in Fig. 16-13. They are important primarily as a manifestation of an underlying disease. Pulsion lesions have a high frequency of associated distal esophageal abnormalities, which should be regularly sought to preclude recurrence by failure to eliminate predisposing causes. Typically, the lesions and resultant symptoms slowly but steadily worsen. Neck compression will empty the cervical sac characteristically and cause the contents to regurgitate into the mouth. The role of cricopharyngeal muscle spasm in such diverticula and other difficulties in deglutition localized to the neck is now more widely appreciated, especially in elderly patients who are subject to cerebrovascular disease. Traction diverticula in the middle third of the esophagus are seldom symptomatic and are often associated with inactive mediastinal tuberculous lymphadenitis.

Nonoperative Management. No nonoperative treatment for esophageal diverticula exists

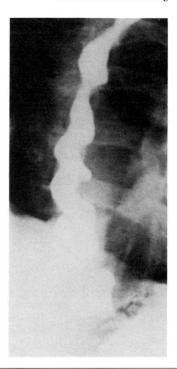

FIGURE 16-12 Disordered motility as a primary lesion in esophagus of an older man.

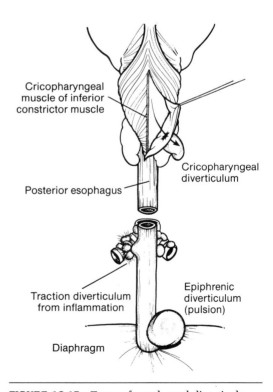

Cricopharyngeal muscle of inferior constrictor muscle

Cricopharyngeal diverticulum

Posterior esophagus

Traction diverticulum from inflammation

Epiphrenic diverticulum (pulsion)

Diaphragm

FIGURE 16-13 Types of esophageal diverticula.

except those directed toward predisposing causes such as distal esophageal obstructions or motility disorders of the gullet. Palliative treatment is also seldom helpful.

Operative Management. Operative treatment entails excision of the diverticulum, with correction of other esophageal abnormalities if present. The operative mortality rate is less than 1%, and

morbidity is minimal. Cervical diverticula may even be excised with the patient under local anesthesia when necessary. Recurrence is very rare unless predisposing causes are allowed to persist. Transection of the cricopharyngeal muscle commonly is being added to such procedures and appears to reduce the failure rate and enhance overall deglutition.

PITFALLS AND COMMON MYTHS

- Multimodality therapy helps the patient with advanced esophageal cancer.
- H$_2$-blockers alone will control reflux esophagitis.
- Dysphagia in the elderly is first managed by getting new dentures.
- The fact that angina-like pain may be caused by esophagitis (and vice versa) is not recognized.
- Crural repair is not a necessary component of the surgical management of refractory esophagitis.

SURGICAL PHARMACOPEIA

Drug	Indications	Dosage
Tums, Rolaids	Heartburn (watch for renal lithiasis)	As needed
Gaviscon	Probably best antacid for reflux esophagitis	1 tablespoon qid and prn
Simethicone (Mylicon-80)	Useful for gas bloating after fundoplication	Chew two tablets prn
Omeprazole (Prilosec)	Severe heartburn	20 mg/day for 4-8 wk

BIBLIOGRAPHY

Bremner CG. Benign strictures of the esophagus. Curr Probl Surg 19:401-492, 1982.

Ellis FH Jr, Crozier RE. Cervical esophageal dysphagia: Indications for and results of cricopharyngeal myotomy. Ann Surg 194:279, 1981.

George FW III. Radiation management of esophageal cancer with review of intraesophageal radioactive iridium treatment in 24 patients. Am J Surg 139:795, 1980.

Giuli R, Sancho-Garnier H. Diagnostic, therapeutic, and prognostic features of cancers of the esophagus: Results of the international prospective study conducted by the OESO group (790 patients). Surgery 99:614, 1986.

Gott JP, Polk HC Jr. Repeat operation for failure of antireflux procedures. Surg Clin North Am 71:13, 1991.

Hobsley M. Oesophagus. In Disorders of the Digestive System. Baltimore, University Park Press, 1982, pp 9-18.

Mannell A. Carcinoma of the esophagus. Curr Probl Surg 19:553-648, 1982.

Meeroff JC, Rogers AJ. Management of gastroesophageal reflux: An algorithm. Hosp Pract 22:165, 1987.

Orringer MB. The esophagus: Historical aspects and anatomy. In Sabiston DC Jr (ed). Textbook of Surgery: The Biological Basis of Modern Surgical Practice. Philadelphia, WB Saunders, 1991, p 655.

Sarr MG, Hamilton SR, Marrone GC, et al. Barrett's esophagus: Its prevalence and association with adenocarcinoma in patients with symptoms of gastroesophageal reflux. Am J Surg 149:187, 1985.

Wald H, Polk HC Jr. Anatomical variations in hiatal hernia and upper gastric areas and their relationship to difficulties experienced in operations for reflux esophagitis. Ann Surg 197:389, 1983.

CHAPTER REVIEW
Questions

1. True or false: Supranormal gastric acidity frequently contributes to reflux esophagitis associated with sliding hiatal hernia.
2. The most frequent causes of dysphagia in middle age and beyond are, in order:
   a. Achalasia
   b. Carcinoma
   c. Stricture secondary to hiatal hernia
3. What is the principal indication for an operation in a symptomatic patient with hiatal hernia?
   a. Incarceration
   b. Anemia
   c. Strangulation
   d. Esophagitis
   e. Dysphagia
4. The treatment of choice for a 60-year-old woman with a soft, pliable esophageal stricture associated with a sliding hiatal hernia is:
   a. Repeated dilation
   b. Resection and replacement with an iso-peristaltic segment of bowel
   c. Dilation and operative hernia repair, including an antireflux procedure

5. Match the patient with the most likely cause of dysphagia.
   1. Elderly black man   a. Hiatal hernia
   2. Middle-aged woman   b. Achalasia
   3. Young adult man   c. Carcinoma
6. What are the underlying causes of a cervical esophageal diverticulum (Zenker)?
   a. Gastroesophageal reflux
   b. Cervical lymphadenitis
   c. Achalasia
   d. Cricopharyngeal dysfunction
7. Which of the following methods of palliation for esophageal cancer are not helpful?
   a. Irradiation
   b. Laser treatments
   c. Diversion
   d. Intubation (Celestin or similar)
   e. Resection

Answers

1. False
2. b, c, a
3. d
4. c
5. 1-c, 2-a, 3-b
6. d
7. c

Hemoptysis, Cough, and Other Symptoms of Pulmonary Lesions

J. DAVID RICHARDSON

KEY FEATURES

After reading this chapter you will understand:
- Why evaluation of a patient with hemoptysis should proceed systematically.
- Emergency treatment of hemoptysis.
- Conditions and diseases in which hemoptysis is a prominent symptom.
- Diagnosis and management of benign and malignant tumors of the lung and mediastinum.

Hemoptysis refers to blood that is coughed from the lungs (Fig. 17-1); it must be carefully distinguished from that originating in the nasopharynx or gastrointestinal tract. It is usually frothy and bright red, whereas blood derived from gastrointestinal bleeding is brown or black and mixed with food particles. Expectorated blood irritates the pulmonary tree, thereby initiating the cough reflex. The afferent part of the reflex arc is in the vagus nerve; the efferent part includes the various nerves supplying the muscles of respiration. Coughing, which consists of inspiration, compression by glottic closure, and expulsion, rids the tracheobronchial tree of foreign material.

The condition is often asymptomatic except for coughing initiated by blood in the tracheobronchial tree. Occasionally, patients are able to point to the approximate area of the lung that is the source of bleeding. Symptoms are usually related to the underlying lesion causing the hemoptysis. The lack of symptoms other than hemoptysis should not preclude a thorough evaluation for an underlying cause, since isolated incidents of hemoptysis may precede other symptoms of carcinoma of the lung by many months. Pleuritic chest pain (pleurisy) may be associated with pneumonia, whereas shortness of breath is common in patients with massive pulmonary neoplasm, causing compression atelectasis.

WHAT ARE THE COMMON CAUSES OF HEMOPTYSIS?

The more common causes of hemoptysis of surgical interest and their underlying mechanisms are listed in Table 17-1. However, hemoptysis may be caused by other conditions, such as mitral stenosis, aortic aneurysms, and arterial hypertension. Rarely, true idiopathic hemoptysis occurs in normal persons, and exhaustive diagnostic studies fail to elucidate the cause. The overwhelming importance of hemoptysis is related to its association with lung carcinoma, and it is this association that demands a careful evaluation of all patients who cough up blood.

DIAGNOSTIC STEPS IN EVALUATING HEMOPTYSIS

A thorough history and physical examination will usually suggest the underlying disease.

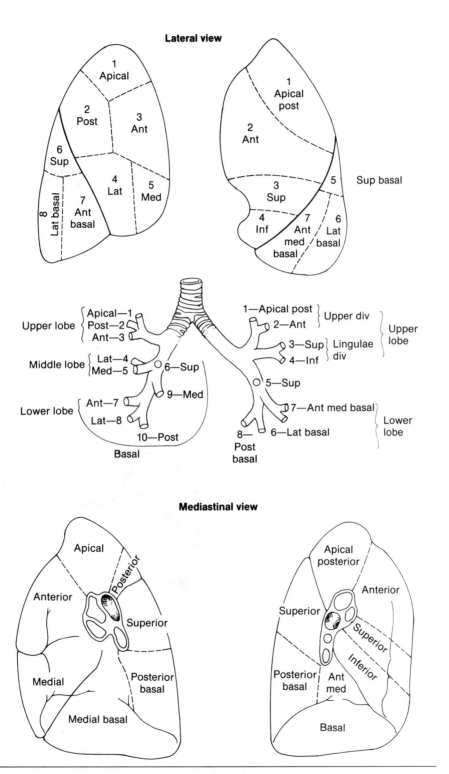

FIGURE 17-1   Diagram of the anatomy of the pulmonary segments.

TABLE 17-1   Causes of Hemoptysis

Cause	Character of Sputum	Etiology
Excessive coughing	Usually blood streaked and on surface of sputum	Trauma to bronchial tree
Pneumonia and abscess	Pink, red, rusty, or dark, depending on organism responsible for pneumonia, and mixed with muco-purulent material	Destruction and erosion of lung tissue by causative organisms
Pulmonary infarction	Dark and mixed with edema fluid	Emboli cause engorgement of capillaries, with eventual necrosis and entry of blood and edema into alveoli
Bronchiectasis	Blood streaked and mixed with purulent material	Erosion of inflamed mucous membranes by infection or trauma of coughing
Pulmonary tuberculosis	Varies from blood streaking to profuse bright red blood	Direct erosion of vessels by tuberculosis organisms
Solitary pulmonary nodules (coin lesions)	Usually blood streaking	Erosion of vessel
Bronchial adenomas	Bright red and profuse	Erosion of surface of tumor
Bronchogenic carcinoma	Initially blood streaking, which may progress to profuse bleeding	Erosion of surface of tumor within lumen of bronchus

Factors that are of particular importance are:

- The character of the blood and associated sputum
- Associated febrile episodes, or symptoms of inflammation
- Chronicity of symptoms
- Associated weight loss or pain
- Smoking habits
- Previous respiratory or cardiac disease

SEQUENCE FOR EVALUATING HEMOPTYSIS

Most patients do not have massive hemoptysis and therefore can have the following orderly work-up to attempt to establish a diagnosis:

1. A chest x-ray examination, including posterior-anterior and lateral views, is performed. A vigorous attempt is made to obtain previous chest x-ray films for comparison, since this may provide invaluable information in determining the need for operation.
2. Computerized tomography (CT) scanning has now assumed a major role in the diagnosis of chest disease and delineation of pul-

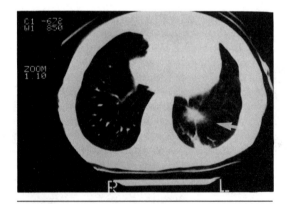

FIGURE 17-2   Arrow shows mass in the lung. A plain radiograph was less helpful because of the retrocardiac position of the mass.

monary nodules (Fig. 17-2). The CT scan is much more effective than standard chest radiographs or even tomograms of the lung. However, CT scans seem to locate small lesions that are benign tumors or granulomas more often than does conventional chest x-ray evaluation, increasing the discovery and necessary evaluation of clinically insignificant nodules.

3. Sputum samples are obtained for cell cytology. Specimens should be collected in the morning and processed in a fresh state.

4. Sputum samples are obtained for smear and culture for bacterial, fungal, and tubercular infection.

5. Direct visualization of the tracheobronchial tree is done to detect the site of bleeding and its cause and in the instance of certain lesions, to determine their resectability. Bronchoscopic examination may be performed with a rigid or flexible bronchoscope. Rigid bronchoscopy permits a larger biopsy to be taken and is also used to remove foreign bodies. Flexible bronchoscopy permits visualization of distal portions of the bronchial tree and allows for "brushing" of peripheral lesions for cytologic examination. Flexible bronchoscopy is used most commonly because it can be performed in an ambulatory setting with topical anesthesia, and it provides better access to more peripheral portions of the lung.

6. Biopsy of all visible lesions is performed. Sputum should be obtained for culture and cytologic studies. Sputum for cytology is obtained following bronchoscopy, since many tumors shed cells after this procedure.

7. *Pleural fluid, if present, is removed by thoracentesis and examined for malignant cells.* This is particularly important because the presence of malignant cells in the pleural effusion means that the patient is not a candidate for operation. However, a straw-colored, nonbloody fluid may occur secondary to an obstruction process and does not rule out a curative operation.

8. If bronchiectasis is suspected, it may be confirmed by a bronchogram (instillation of contrast medium into the bronchial tree of the suspected segment).

9. Cervical, scalene, and mediastinal nodes are biopsied, if present. They are helpful in establishing a diagnosis of malignancy and in staging the disease for treatment purposes. Lung cancer often presents with subcutaneous tumor nodules; therefore a thorough physical examination and inspection of the skin and node-bearing areas is in order.

10. A variety of diagnostic techniques not requiring thoracotomy have been introduced. These include transbronchial needle biopsy and a variety of transpleural biopsy techniques. These types of biopsy have been useful in several specific types of problems. They are useful in diffuse pulmonary infections, such as *Pneumocystis carinii*. Additionally, a diagnosis of malignancy can often be made. If the candidate has other contraindications to operation, this may spare him a thoracotomy. Furthermore, it must be remembered that a *negative result to specimen analysis does not rule out the possibility of a positive diagnosis, since the amount of specimen obtained is fairly small.*

In some patients, even after numerous preoperative studies their bleeding site has not been pinpointed, and they require exploratory thoracotomy if the bleeding can be localized accurately enough to permit operation. Generally this group constitutes 8% to 10% of most series. Both the physician and the patient must be prepared for a major resection if a pathologic examination (frozen section) discloses a malignancy.

PRINCIPLES OF TREATMENT

Fortunately most patients with hemoptysis can be treated initially with bed rest and sedation. Rarely is the hemoptysis of such magnitude that respiratory function is compromised or blood transfusion required. Therefore the physician has the opportunity to carry out diagnostic procedures in an orderly manner. Treatment can be carefully assessed and applied according to reasoned comparisons of risk and reward of therapy. However, in cases in which hemoptysis is massive, early thoracotomy and resection of the involved segment of lung may be necessary.

How Should Life-Threatening Hemoptysis Be Managed?

Occasionally, bleeding will be so massive that it may be life threatening. A patient with significant bleeding, such that operative treatment might be contemplated on an emergency basis, should be placed on bed rest and given codeine in an attempt to suppress his cough mechanism. Often the bleeding will cease long enough so that a work-up can be instituted. When bleeding stops bronchoscopy should be performed promptly, because there will probably still be enough blood present in the affected bronchus to determine its source. Identification of the affected side of the bronchus and, hopefully, the lobe or segment involved, facilitates a limited but definitive resection of pulmonary tissue should there be sudden or massive recurrence of bleeding.

Massive hemoptysis is defined as a blood loss of greater than 600 ml within a 24-hour period. The mortality associated with bleeding at this level is very high.

Although hemorrhagic shock may occur from blood loss alone, the most critical problem with massive hemoptysis is asphyxiation caused by blood in the airway. In this particular instance, it is crucial to determine which lung is bleeding. If the blood is coming from the right lung, a cuffed tube can be advanced into the left mainstem bronchus, and, with the cuff inflated, the left lung is ventilated. Thoracotomy should then be performed to remove the affected portion of the right lung. For bleeding of the left lung, a large Fogarty catheter can be used to occlude the side that is bleeding. Occasionally a Carlens tube can be useful to prevent severe aspiration of blood into the uninvolved side.

During the operation, as much pulmonary tissue as possible should be conserved. Because bronchogenic carcinoma is not the usual cause of hemoptysis, en bloc cancer resections are not warranted. Pulmonary tuberculosis, either active or inactive, and bronchiectasis are the most common causes of life-threatening hemoptysis.

OTHER ENTITIES THAT PRODUCE HEMOPTYSIS
Bacterial Pneumonia

Bacterial pneumonia is usually accompanied by alveolar exudation and bronchitis (which in most instances clears by absorption), bronchial drainage, and coughing. Antimicrobial therapy, postural drainage, and bronchoscopy for aspiration of thick secretions usually produce normal lung tissue with no loss of function.

Complications of Pneumonia. Complications develop in approximately 10% of patients with pneumonia, usually because of delayed or improper treatment. Empyema (infected fluid in the pleural space) is a major complication of pneumonia that requires aggressive intervention. Treatment consists of removal of the infected fluid and reexpansion of the underlying lung. Infected pleural fluid may be removed by (1) thoracentesis, (2) insertion of a chest tube attached to water-seal drainage (closed-tube thoracostomy), (3) rib resection, with insertion of a large-bore tube to establish drainage, or (4) open thoracotomy and decortication, if the process is far advanced and the infection cannot otherwise be controlled.

The procedure used to remove the fluid depends on the length of time the disease process has existed and the nature of the fluid. Early empyema associated with pneumonia may produce thin, watery fluid, which is easily aspirated by needle. Chronic empyema, often seen in neglected or poorly treated individuals, is associated with thick, creamy pus that requires tube drainage to a water-seal bottle. This may be converted to open drainage when scarring and adhesions ensure that the lung is securely adherent to the chest wall so that pneumothorax does not result. Rarely, empyema results in a thick fibrous scar that entraps the lung. If pulmonary function is impaired, the scar must be removed surgically (decortication).

Bronchiectasis is an occasional complication of pneumonia, usually resulting from bronchial obstruction secondary to secretions persisting for a prolonged period. Bronchiectasis, once commonly encountered, is seen with decreasing frequency since the advent of antibiotics.

Some bacterial pneumonias, especially staphylococcal, are prone to causing pneumatoceles—air spaces in the lung tissue due to destruction of alveoli—that may later become lined with bronchial epithelium, forming acquired cysts. Pneumatoceles usually disappear with treatment. Cysts, however, may cause symptoms by compression or may become filled with fluid and/or infected, requiring surgical removal. Occasionally pneumatoceles will rupture and produce a pneumothorax. Tension pneumothorax should always be considered in a patient with staphylococcal pneumonia who has sudden, unexplained cardiorespiratory distress. Insertion of a needle into the affected hemithorax may provide a diagnosis if air escapes under tension and may be lifesaving as well.

Lung Abscess

Lung abscess may occur as a complication of pneumonia, by bronchial obstruction from aspiration of infected material into the bronchi, or by embolism from other infected areas of the body. Positioning the patient for aspiration is determined by the abscess site. The most common locations for abscess in the lung are posterior and anterior segments of the upper lobes and the superior segments of the lower lobes. Fever, localized pleuritic pain, and cough are characteristic symptoms. Chest x-ray films initially may show pneumonitis but later will often disclose cavitation with an air-fluid level (Fig. 17-3). Bronchoscopy is performed to identify an obstructing neoplasm or a foreign body, remove secretions, and promote bronchial drainage.

Treatment of any abscess requires effective drainage. Drainage may be effected by chest percussion and postural drainage. Bronchoscopy is an integral part of treatment by allowing for better drainage. The principle involved is that lung abscesses usually can be managed by internal transbronchial drainage rather than by relying on external drainage through the chest wall. If internal drainage can be established and appropriate antibiotics are used, 90% of pulmonary abscesses heal in a 3- to 4-week period. When abscesses persist, bronchial obstruction is strongly suggested. Uncommonly, large lung abscesses require open drainage by rib resection and insertion of a chest tube. External drainage in such situations is used as a second-line treatment choice. This is because contamination of the pleural space, resulting in empyema and chronic air leaks, requiring pulmonary resection, frequently result from open drainage. Destroyed areas of lung and residual abscess require resection. With effective medical management and operation when indicated, mortality from pulmonary abscess should be less than 5%.

Pulmonary Infarction

Pulmonary infarction will be considered in detail in Chapter 20. Infarcted lung segments or lobes usually become scarred and fibrotic and may require resection if subsequent infection and hemoptysis develop.

Bronchiectasis

Bronchiectasis was once fairly common but is now seen with decreasing frequency in the United States. It occurs secondary to bronchial obstruction with distal infection. Pus fills the bronchi, partially destroying the bronchial wall and causing dilation. According to the degree of dilation, cylindrical, saccular, or cystic bronchiectasis results. The ciliated columnar epithelium lining of the bronchi is destroyed, thus eliminating the ciliary action essential for removal of secretions. The patient's coughing of excessive amounts of purulent, foul-smelling sputum, especially on awakening in the morning, is almost diagnostic. Chest x-ray films may show increased bronchovascular markings. Bronchograms outline the dilated bronchi. Basal segments of the lower lobe are most frequently involved. Upper lobe disease is typical of tuberculosis. One third of patients with bronchiectasis manifest bilateral disease.

Long-term treatment with appropriate antibiotics and postural drainage allows many patients to remain symptom-free. Operation is reserved for disease localized to segments or lobes, and yields excellent results when all involved

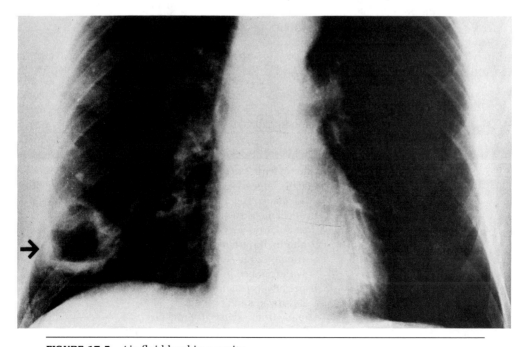

FIGURE 17-3 Air-fluid level in a cavity.

areas can be removed. Bronchiectasis, if not treated effectively, leads to empyema, lung abscess, brain abscess, or emphysema.

Pulmonary Tuberculosis

Although there have been dramatic changes in the treatment of pulmonary tuberculosis over the past 25 years, it still remains an important disease worldwide and one that is far from eradicated in this country. Additionally, pulmonary tuberculosis is being encountered with increasing frequency in this country, particularly in many inner-city settings and in patients who are immunocompromised. Operative treatment is not indicated until medical treatment has proved futile. Only approximately 10% of tuberculosis hospital inpatients require operation, and the vast majority of these procedures are for removal of residual infection. Adequate chemotherapy for 1 year will convert the sputum from positive to negative in 95% of patients. Relapse following adequate treatment is uncommon.

The advisability of operation for each patient is influenced by age, adequacy of drug therapy, patient reliability in following prescribed therapy, chronicity of disease, residual pulmonary function; and social factors, such as danger to contacts, employability, and insurability. The duration of drug therapy depends on the individual situation. For example, a 30-year-old patient, in otherwise good health, with a large cavity and positive sputum culture, may be offered operation after three months of drug therapy failed to convert the sputum. Older patients, or debilitated individuals who are poor surgical risks, may be continued on drug therapy. The standard indications for surgical resection are listed in Table 17-2. However, it should be emphasized that surgery is a seldom-required treatment and that medical treatment remains the predominant mode of therapy.

Prior to chemotherapy, the hospital mortality rate was 25% with lobectomy and 50% with pneumonectomy. With the appropriate use of chemotherapy, properly selected patients are subject to a mortality rate of 1% for segmental resection and lobectomies, with a major complication rate of less than 10%. With pneumonectomy, usually performed in patients with extensive disease and poor pulmonary function, a 10% mortality is the norm.

WHAT SYMPTOMS SHOULD PROMPT CHEST X-RAY EVALUATION?

Chest x-ray examination is a relatively inexpensive and potentially valuable screening tool for patients at high risk for lung cancer, based on smoking history. It has been difficult to show in large-population studies that this type of screening is beneficial; however, it is clear that patients with symptoms of a pathologic condition of the lung should be so screened. These symptoms include the following:

- Hemoptysis
- Persistent cough
- Persistent hoarseness
- Chest pain
- New onset of wheezing

The precise role of CT scan has not been determined in the evaluation of lung cancer, but it

---

TABLE 17-2 Indications for Surgical Resection in Tuberculosis

Lesion	Comment
Residual cavity, positive sputum	After at least 3 months of treatment with drug therapy
Residual cavity, negative sputum	Usually large cavities that show no sign of regression with adequate drug therapy; seen mainly in younger patients
Closed cavity, nodular disease	Bronchial obstruction resulting from caseous necrosis or nodular disease; acid-fast bacilli usually present in cavity, although sputum tests yield negative results
Bronchiectasis	Secondary to healing of tuberculosis process, may be associated with repeated infection or hemoptysis
Unstable nodular disease or destroyed lung	Especially in patients who develop repeated infections in destroyed lobes or lungs
Massive hemorrhage or hemoptysis	Usually from cavities or bronchiectasis
Solitary nodule, granuloma	When carcinoma cannot be ruled out

probably should not be used in the primary survey. CT scan is useful in detecting central lesions that may be difficult to delineate on routine chest x-ray evaluation. CT is also very useful in detecting the presence of multiple lesions and is therefore a good method for determining whether or not a patient with known cancer has a new primary or multiple metastatic lesions.

SOLITARY PULMONARY NODULES

Solitary pulmonary nodules, or *coin lesions,* usually refers to sharply circumscribed peripheral lung nodules less than 5 cm in diameter, with or without evidence of calcification and without cavitation. Hemoptysis is rarely the presenting symptom. More commonly, the lesion is seen on a chest x-ray film ordered for a totally unrelated illness. The majority of preoperative diagnostic studies, such as bronchoscopy, biopsy, sputum studies, and other examinations, are usually unrewarding. Table 17-3 shows the type of previously undiagnosed pulmonary nodule resected in a series of 887 male patients of all ages. Fifty-one percent of patients over age 50 and 46% of those over 45 years of age were found to have malignant nodules. Size of the lesion

TABLE 17-3   Solitary Pulmonary Nodules* in Males, All Ages

Lesion	Percent	
Malignant tumors	36	
Primary carcinoma		(32)
Metastatic carcinoma		(3)
Adenomas		(<1)
Miscellaneous tumors		(<1)
Granulomas	53	
Histoplasmosis		(18)
Tuberculosis		(14)
Coccidioidomycosis		(11)
Unidentified		(9)
Cryptococcoses		(<1)
Actinomycosis		(<1)
Aspergillosis		(<1)
Blastomycosis		(<1)
Miscellaneous lesions	3	
Cysts, nodes, A-V fistula, infarct, etc.		
Pleural or chest wall lesions	1	
Mesothelioma, fibroma, etc.		
Hamartomas	7	

*Total of 887, 6.0 cm or less in diameter.

correlates poorly with malignancy, although most cancers (75%) are over 2.0 cm in diameter. An increase in size on serial roentgenograms is almost diagnostic of a neoplasm. Roentgenographic demonstration of calcification within the lesions indicates a lesser likelihood of malignancy but does not exclude it.

What Is the Treatment for Solitary Pulmonary Nodules?

The vast majority of patients presenting with undiagnosed solitary pulmonary nodules should undergo exploratory thoracotomy. Wedge excision should be performed if the lesion is benign, whereas lobectomy or pneumonectomy should be performed if it is malignant. Mortality in properly selected patients is well under 5%. Moreover, solitary pulmonary nodules are the only form of bronchogenic cancer offering an excellent chance for cure by operation. An exception is the young person who has a solitary nodule that shows no increase in size but that has concentric areas of calcification, which strongly supports its origin as being an old fungal disease. These individuals should be monitored with yearly chest x-ray evaluation.

Bronchial Adenomas. Bronchial adenomas are usually located in the walls of the major bronchi, with a small amount of the tumor visible by bronchoscopy and a much larger mass present outside the bronchus (iceberg effect). The two most common types are carcinoid (85%) and cylindroma or adenoid cystic type (12%). Often those tumors grow slowly for a number of years, producing bronchial obstruction and subsequent hemoptysis. The cylindromatous tumors invade adjacent tissues and more frequently metastasize to nodes. Cylindromas are often slow growing but are prone to local recurrence. They are relatively radioresistant.

The extent of resection is determined by size and location of the tumor. Thus, procedures range from sleeve resection of the bronchus for very small lesions to lobectomy or pneumonectomy. Ninety percent of patients are well after surgical resection of favorable lesions. The results with cylindromatous lesions are not as favorable as with carcinoid lesions for the reasons previously mentioned.

Carcinoma

Bronchogenic carcinoma is now the leading cancer killer because of its dramatic rise in women in the past two decades. It can be said that smoking

TABLE 17-4   Cell Types and Characteristics of Carcinoma of the Lung

	Percent	Sex	Growth Characteristics
Epidermoid	50	75% in men	Occurs in major bronchi, causing distal atelectasis; tends to spread by lymphatics
Undifferentiated large cell	20	38% in women	Located more peripheral from hilus of lung; spreads by lymphatics and bloodstream
Small cell (oat cell)	9	80% in men	Very cellular and largely extrabronchial, causing little or no atelectasis; early lymphatic and hematogenous spread
Adenocarcinoma	20	30% in women	Majority occur in periphery of lung; metastasizes by bloodstream
Bronchiolar or alveolar cell	1	—	Occurs as a diffuse, patchy pneumonia and as a slow-growing, well-circumscribed local lesion

by women has led to true equality with men in terms of the development of lung cancer. Most carcinomas arise from bronchial epithelium, typically in the upper lobes (63%). The various cell types, with frequency and characteristics, are shown in Table 17-4.

The typical patient is a 55-year-old man or woman with a lengthy history of cigarette smoking. Early symptoms of carcinoma are cough, wheeze, hemoptysis, or fever resulting from pneumonitis distal to the tumor. Pain, indicating chest wall extension, and marked weight loss are late symptoms of advanced cancer.

Symptoms remote from the lung may be important presenting features of bronchogenic carcinoma. About 20% of patients with lung cancer present with metastases. Metastases to the liver or brain may herald the presence of a previously unsuspected pulmonary carcinoma.

Other extrapulmonary manifestations are caused by the elaboration of hormonal material from the tumor itself. It is crucial to be aware of these syndromes, since they may be caused by a tumor that is still in the curable stage. Pulmonary osteoarthropathy is commonly associated with carcinoma of the lung. This condition can be distinguished from arthritis because the bones themselves, rather than the joints, are tender, and radiographs of the fingers may show a fine linear deposition of calcium along the periosteum. Clubbing of the fingers also occurs with carcinoma of the lung. The causal mechanisms are unknown.

ACTH-like substances elaborated by oat-cell carcinoma may mimic Cushing's syndrome. Parathyroid hormone–like substances may be produced by some squamous carcinomas, resembling primary hyperparathyroidism. Inappropriate ADH syndrome may occur, with water retention and symptoms of hyponatremia.

CRITERIA FOR OPERATION AND RESECTABILITY

Patients with tumors beyond the limits of surgical resection should be identified to prevent unnecessary exploration, since exploratory thoracotomy for nonresectable lesions carries an operative mortality as high as 20%.

Students are often confused by the terms *operability* and *resectability*. There are certain criteria for operability. This means that if these criteria are met, the patient is a candidate for operation. They are:

- Good general medical condition without major heart or lung disease, such that the patient could withstand a thoracotomy and possible removal of lung tissue
- Absence of specific signs of nonoperability as shown in Table 17-5

While there are no absolute, universally applicable guidelines, a general rule of thumb has been that a patient should have a forced expiratory volume in one second (FEV_1) of greater than 1500 ml to tolerate a lobectomy and an FEV_1 of greater than 2000 ml to tolerate a pneumonectomy. In both of these situations the patients should be left with a postoperative FEV_1 of greater than 1 L/sec.

The term resectability is applied to certain situations where the patient appears operable

TABLE 17-5   Signs of Inoperability in Lung Cancer

Absolute Signs	Relative Signs
Lymphatic spread to cervical axillary, or remote mediastinal nodes	Mediastinal nodes (may be removed at operation)
Distant spread to other organs (brain, bone, kidneys, adrenals, etc.)	Phrenic nerve paralysis
Small cell cancer (some controversy)	Pericardial extension
Superior vena cava syndrome	May be excised but usually will be unresectable at operation
Malignant pleural effusion	Chest wall extension; chest wall can often be excised
Widened carina (with biopsy-proven cancer)	Superior sulcus (pancoast tumor) may be resected after a course of radiation therapy
Paralyzed vocal cord (invasion of recurrent laryngeal nerve)	

but at the time of operation, the tumor cannot be resected. These may include:

- Extension into the mediastinal structures or pericardium, precluding resection
- Extension into both lobes requiring a pneumonectomy when that would not be tolerated
- Unexpected adenopathy precluding curative resection
- Pleural disease limiting curability

In general, the debulking of lung cancer when a cure is not *probable* is not advisable.

Noninvasive methods to examine the patient's tumor short of exploratory thoracotomy also involve CT scanning, which aids in the assessment of mediastinal nodes. However, the presence of mediastinal adenopathy is insufficient for a definitive tissue diagnosis.

Several invasive methods short of exploratory thoracotomy may be used to determine resectability of the tumor and to stage it preoperatively. Mediastinoscopy involves an incision above the suprasternal notch, through which a fiberoptic mediastinoscope is introduced into the superior mediastinum and by which lymph nodes are identified. The surgeon should not biopsy any structure before aspirating it with a long needle to exclude the presence of a vascular structure. By using such careful techniques, serious complications are kept to a minimum; one group reported 300 consecutive mediastinoscopies without an operative death or serious complication.

Mediastinoscopy is extremely valuable in diagnosing central lesions, which prove to be malignant in about 65% of cases, but it is of less value in diagnosing peripheral lesions. Since lesions involving the left hilum and left upper lobe

are difficult to evaluate by standard mediastinoscopy, a small interspace lateral incision may improve visualization of the subaortic area.

Controversy still remains about the procedure of choice for treatment of mediastinal lymph nodes that have tested positive for cancer. Because a 2% 5-year survival occurs in patients with positive mediastinal nodes, radiation therapy alone may be warranted for this stage of the disease. Some investigators recommend surgical treatment combined with radiotherapy for squamous cell carcinoma that has positive mediastinal lymph nodes on the same side of the trachea, with a projected 5-year survival of 20%.

The surgical procedure may be scaled to the nature and extent of the tumor, ranging from segmental resection to pneumonectomy. Fifty percent of patients entering the physician's office with carcinoma of the lung will be found to be inoperable on initial history and physical examination because of distant metastases. Another 25% will be explored and discovered to have nonresectable tumors because of extension of the tumor into the mediastinum or carina. The remaining 25% of the patients will have tumors amenable to surgical excision, and of this latter group only about 8% (2 of the initial 100 patients) will be alive at 5 years.

The prognosis for special groups in which one is able to surgically excise the tumor is better, however. Resection of a malignant solitary pulmonary nodule without lymph node involvement carries about a 50% 5-year survival rate. Squamous cell carcinoma without nodal metastases, treated by lobectomy or pneumonectomy, yields a 30% to 35% 5-year survival. If nodal involvement is present, 5-year survival drops to 8% to 10%. Adenocarcinoma and undifferentiated large-cell lung cancers have a much lower survival rate.

Hospital mortality for pneumonectomy (8% to 10%) results largely from pulmonary insufficiency and heart failure. Segmental resection and lobectomy are associated with a hospital mortality of half that of pneumonectomy. Thus every effort should be made to eliminate all patients with nonresectable lesions from surgery. Accordingly, each patient is evaluated individually, and the risks of surgery, along with the chances of cure, are carefully considered before the surgeon selects a procedure that may lead to the patient's premature death.

Although radiation has a place in the palliative management of some patients (prevention of hemoptysis or bronchial obstruction by reducing tumor mass), it has limited value for patients who are not candidates for surgery. Recent successes with multiple-drug chemotherapy to treat oat-cell carcinoma of the lung have been extremely encouraging, resulting in an objective response rate, i.e., measurable decrease in tumor size, in one third to one fourth of the patients treated. The survival rate for this group has thus been extended from less than 6 months a few years ago to up to 2 years if the patient responds to chemotherapy.

Palliation may be achieved in certain patients by the mechanical means that open an obstructed bronchus. The use of laser therapy to core a channel through the tumor often relieves distal atelectasis and pneumonia and may significantly improve the patient's quality of life, although it does not ultimately affect long-term survival. We usually follow such endoscopic procedures with radiation therapy.

DIAGNOSIS OF THE SPECIFIC CELL TYPE OF LUNG CANCER

In a broad sense, the surgeon or pulmonary medicine specialist needs to answer three questions when evaluating a patient with possible lung cancer:

- Is it cancer? Can a diagnosis of malignancy definitely be established?
- Is the tumor a small-cell or oat-cell cancer, or a non-small-cell cancer?
- Can the tumor be resected for potential cure?

The need to establish the diagnosis of cancer is obvious. However, the mere fact that a sputum cytologic study or bronchoscopy does not establish a diagnosis should not be interpreted to mean that cancer is not present. In patients with

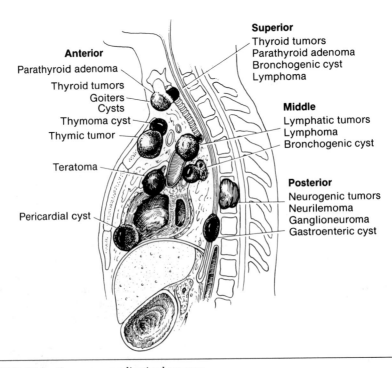

FIGURE 17-4 Common mediastinal tumors.

a definite lesion, a thoracotomy may be the appropriate maneuver if the patient is an acceptable candidate. The second important step is to determine whether the patient has small-cell or non-small-cell cancer; then operation is clearly indicated if all acceptable criteria are met. Since patients with small-cell cancer respond favorably to chemotherapy and radiation therapy protocols, surgery may not be warranted. Studies regarding operation plus adjuvant treatment for small-cell cancer are being reviewed, but it appears at present that nonoperative therapy is the mainstay of treatment. Although the response rate of small-cell cancer to this protocol is high, this response does not often translate into a meaningful, long-term survival advantage.

Mediastinal Tumors

Mediastinal tumors rarely cause symptoms, except those of compression because of size, and almost never cause hemoptysis. They are usually discovered when reviewing a routine chest x-ray film and present a diagnostic problem. A lateral chest film is vital in order to accurately assess the location of the mass (Fig. 17-4).

It is helpful to consider the various organs in the mediastinal compartments. Since the anterior mediastinum contains thyroid, thymus, and pericardium, tumors in this location arise from these structures. The posterior mediastinum contains sympathetic ganglia, nerves, and the esophagus, whereas the major bronchi and lymphatic tissue are located in the middle compartment. Fig. 17-4 shows the tumors arising in the various locations.

Surgical excision of the tumor is recommended in almost every instance, since a malignant process cannot be excluded. Operative mortality is low (1%), with complete cure to be expected, except in the case of the most malignant tumors.

PITFALLS AND COMMON MYTHS

- The presence of pulmonary nodule in a patient who is a good risk for operation requires complete evaluation including a potential thoracotomy. Failure to obtain a positive diagnosis by bronchoscopy or sputum cytology does not mean the patient does not have cancer or obviate the need for a thoracotomy.
- If pneumonia fails to resolve in a patient at risk for cancer, this should suggest the possibility of an obstructing lesion and prompt investigation with CT or bronchoscopy.
- Although it is difficult to show an improved survival in a population using screening chest radiographs, the presence of symptoms such as hemoptysis, persistent cough, new onset of wheezing, or chest wall pain should prompt a chest x-ray evaluation.

BIBLIOGRAPHY

Aronchick JM. Lung cancer: Epidemiology and risk factors. Semin Roentgenol 25:5, 1990.

Grippi M. Clinical aspects of lung cancer. Semin Roentgenol 25:12, 1990.

Jackson CV. Preoperative pulmonary evaluation. Arch Int Med 148:2120, 1988.

Lederle FA, Nichol KL, Parenti CM. Bronchoscopy to evaluate hemoptysis in older men with nonsuspicious chest roentgenograms. Chest 95:1043, 1989.

Mullen B, Richardson JD. Primary anterior mediastinal tumors in children and adults. Ann Thorac Surg 42:338, 1986.

Sankila RJ, Karjalainen ES. Relationship between occupation and lung cancer as analyzed by age and histologic type. Cancer 65:1651, 1990.

Steele JD. The solitary pulmonary nodule. J Thorac Cardiovasc Surg 46:21, 1963.

CHAPTER REVIEW
Questions

1. Which one of the following procedures is the most important for diagnosis in patients with hemoptysis?
   a. Skin test
   b. Scalene node biopsy
   c. Bronchoscopy
   d. Sputum culture

2. Combination chemotherapy has been most useful in the management of which type of pulmonary neoplasm?
   a. Small cell carcinoma
   b. Squamous cell carcinoma
   c. Alveolar cell carcinoma
   d. Adenocarcinoma

3. The most important pathologic finding in predicting prognosis in patients with squamous carcinoma of the lung is:
   a. Vascular invasion
   b. Lymph node involvement
   c. Bronchial metaplasia
   d. Histologic differentiation

4. The most common cause of a coin lesion of the lung is:
   a. Primary carcinoma
   b. Granuloma
   c. Hamartoma
   d. Metastatic carcinoma

5. Unresectability in lung cancer is determined by:
   a. Positive scalene nodes
   b. Positive bone roentgenogram
   c. Malignant pleural effusion
   d. None of the above
   e. All of the above

6. Which of the following are *not* commonly found in the anterior mediastinum?
   a. Ganglioneuroma
   b. Thyroid tumors
   c. Teratomas
   d. Thymomas

7. A patient has a persistent cough with one episode of hemoptysis. The chest x-ray films do not reveal demonstrable lesions. At bronchoscopy a slightly rounded lesion is found in the mainstream bronchus. It is smooth except for a slight erosion. This most likely represents what lesion?
   a. Small-cell lung cancer
   b. Tuberculosis
   c. Sarcoid
   d. Bronchial adenoma
   e. Hamartoma of the lung

8. Which of the following statements about lung cancer is false?
   a. Lung cancer is much less common in women.
   b. The incidence of lung cancer is nearly equal in the sexes.
   c. The lung cancer incidence in women is increasing rapidly.
   d. Lung cancer now represents our largest cancer killer in the United States.

9. Which of the following is *not* a sign of inoperability for lung cancer?
   a. Vocal cord paralysis
   b. Positive cervical lymph node
   c. Straw-colored pleural effusion
   d. Superior vena cava obstruction
   e. 6 cm solid adrenal mass on CT scan

10. Which of the following rarely causes hemoptysis?
    a. Bronchial adenoma
    b. Large-cell cancer
    c. Small-cell cancer
    d. Cavity tuberculosis
    e. Mediastinal lymphoma

Answers

1. c	6. a
2. a	7. d
3. b	8. c
4. a	9. c
5. e	10. e

18 Heart Murmurs: Acquired Valvular Heart Disease

LAWRENCE H. COHN

KEY FEATURES

After reading this chapter you will understand:
- The pathophysiology of congestive heart failure and valvular heart disease.
- Diagnosis and treatment of diseases of the cardiac valves.
- The systemic derangements associated with acquired valvular heart disease.

Heart murmurs are produced by turbulent blood flow. Under normal conditions, the flow through the blood vessels and cardiac valves is smooth, laminar, and silent. If flow becomes excessive, the walls of a vessel become uneven as a result of disease, or if there is any irregularity on the surface of a valve, flow becomes turbulent, and a murmur is audible. Normal heart valves open completely and allow laminar flow. If a valve is thickened from disease and becomes obstructive, turbulent flow causing a murmur will result. Functional murmurs may be heard in children and adults when the flow is excessive, such as after exercise or with hyperthyroidism, and must be distinguished from murmurs that are associated with intrinsic, pathologically deformed cardiac valves. Murmurs are graded I through VI, according to the intensity of the sound. They may be high or low pitched, musical or harsh, and occur during systole or diastole. Grade I is a murmur that is barely audible, whereas grade VI is a murmur that is audible without placing the stethoscope on the patient's chest. Murmurs may indicate valvular heart disease. Despite the pres-

ence of murmurs and the underlying pathoanatomy that produces these sounds, many patients with valvular heart disease may be asymptomatic and function normally for decades, with the only abnormality an auscultatory one. These patients may have normal heart size and normal exercise capacity. Usually, however, murmurs result from mechanical and physiologic deviations from normal cardiac function (Fig. 18-1).

Most cardiac valvular defects eventually lead to heart failure as a result of obstruction of outflow from the atria or ventricle or regurgitation back into the atria or ventricle. Myocardial failure is the inability of the heart to pump an adequate supply of blood throughout the body to accommodate the metabolic requirements asso-

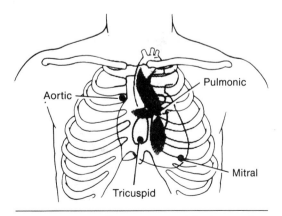

FIGURE 18-1 Surface anatomy of the heart valves and the location of murmurs.

315

ciated with normal organ function and exercise. Patients in varying stages of valvular disease may exhibit abnormalities in cardiac output only during exercise, when increased demands require increased cardiac output or, eventually, at rest during terminal stages of their disease. Valvular lesions on the left side of the heart produce congestive heart failure, a backup of blood into the pulmonary circulation producing shortness of breath, exercise intolerance, and fatigue. Patients who have primarily right-sided cardiac failure from severe pulmonic stenosis, tricuspid valve disease, or right ventricular infarction have peripheral venous stasis, congestion in the liver, anasarca, and peripheral edema. Most commonly, a combination of left- and right-sided heart failure in patients in the United States results from left-sided valve lesions, such as mitral stenosis or regurgitation.

A classification of the various pathophysiologic mechanisms producing left- and right-sided congestive heart failure is listed in the box below.

Compensatory mechanisms develop when congestive heart failure ensues. There is a dilation of the heart; pulmonary vascular resistance rises; sodium retention increases; sodium clearance decreases; sympathetic tone increases, manifested by increased heart rate; myocardial contractility decreases; and systemic valvular resistance and venous tone increase. In some patients there may be massive dilation of cardiac chambers, yet pressures within the heart are low. In other patients, chamber size may remain normal, but chamber pressures behind the valvular obstruction or regurgitation may become extremely high.

This chapter will investigate the pathophysiology, diagnosis, and treatment of the most commonly encountered acquired cardiac valvular lesions that produce congestive heart failure (Table 18-1).

TABLE 18-1   Cardiac Valvular Diseases: Diagnosis and Management

	Mitral Stenosis	**Mitral Regurgitation**
Cause	Usually rheumatic fever; rarely, congenital	Rheumatic fever, myxomatous degeneration, rupture of chordae tendineae or papillary muscles, myocardiopathy, infective endocarditis
History	Congestive heart failure, predominant in females	Thromboemboli, fatigue, congestive heart failure; may be asymptomatic
Cardiac examination	Accentuated mitral first sound, loud opening snap, increased P_2, low-pitched diastolic murmur with presystolic accentuation; TR in advanced cases	Left ventricular heave, apical systolic murmur widely referred LV enlargement
ECG	Atrial fibrillation, left atrial hypertrophy, RVH	Atrial fibrillation, left atrial enlargement, LVH
Chest x-ray evaluation	Prominent left atrial appendage and pulmonary artery, calcific deposits on valve, Kerley B lines (lymphatic engorgement in lung periphery) ↑ Pulmonary plethora	Prominent left atrium, left ventricular hypertrophy, Kerley B lines, pulmonary congestion
Cardiac catheterization	Increased pulmonary artery and wedge pressures, rising with exercise	Increased left atrial pressure, high V wave, regurgitation of contrast on LV angiography

DOE = dyspnea on exertion; SOB = shortness of breath; LVH = left ventricular hypertrophy; RVH = right ventricular

PHYSIOLOGIC CLASSIFICATION OF HEART FAILURE

Mechanical abnormalities
  Resistance load (hypertension, aortic stenosis, pulmonary stenosis)
  Flow load (aortic or mitral regurgitation, left-to-right shunts)
  Primary
  Secondary (dilation of the valve ring in heart failure)
  Resistance to inflow
    Constrictive pericarditis
    Tamponade
    Restrictive myocardial disease (scleroderma amyloidosis)
    Mitral stenosis
  Primary myocardial (muscle) failure
    Cardiomyopathy (hereditary, alcoholic, ischemic)
    Ischemia (coronary heart disease)

Inflammation (rheumatic or viral myocarditis)
  Metabolic (metal poisons, myxedema)
Venous congestive states (high output failure)
  Renal failure with fluid retention
  Intravenous fluid or blood overload
  Chronic severe anemia
  Arterio-venous fistula
  Cirrhosis
Arrhythmia
  Severe prolonged tachycardia
    Metabolic failure (exhaustion)
    Greatly decreased time for filling
  Severe bradycardia: usually associated with other disease when it causes failure
    Congenital heart block (rates 35 to 50) are tolerated in children, but in older adults rates of 40 to 45 cause symptoms.
  Asystole, ventricular tachycardia, or fibrillation

Aortic Stenosis	Aortic Regurgitation	Tricuspid Disease
Rheumatic fever, congenital bicuspid valve, rheumatic senile calcification	Rheumatic fever, infective endocarditis dissecting aneurysm, Marfan's syndrome	Usually associated with mitral or aortic disease; exceptions: infective endocarditis with narcotic addiction or tumor; rheumatic fever in Third World countries
SOB, DOE, syncope, angina on exertion	Cardiac failure that may occur late, especially if the disease develops slowly	Usually minimal, since even complete tricuspid excision is well tolerated
Diamond-shaped systolic ejection murmur in the right second interspace, radiating to the neck; diminished peripheral pulses $\downarrow A_2$, $\downarrow$ pulse pressure	Diminished arterial diastolic pressure, increasing as disease worsens; blowing systolic murmur at left sternal border	Edema, ascites, elevated venous pressure, peripheral edema, pulsatile liver
Left ventricular hypertrophy; atrial fibrillation in late stages	Left ventricular hypertrophy	Right atrial hypertrophy
Left ventricular hypertrophy in long-standing disease; calcified valve on fluoroscopy; occasional poststenotic dilation	Left ventricular hypertrophy, pulmonary congestion, LV dilation	Right atrial hypertrophy
Left ventricular pressure > aortic pressure; increased left ventricular end-diastolic pressure, slow upstroke LV pressure	Increased LVEDP, wedge pressure, regurgitation of contrast on aortography	Increased right atrial pressure with high V wave

hypertrophy; LVEDP = left ventricular end-diastolic pressure; A_2 = aortic second sound; P_2 = pulmonic second sound.

MITRAL VALVE DISEASE
Mitral Stenosis

Etiology and Pathology. The cause of acquired mitral stenosis is rheumatic fever, but the differential diagnosis may include congenital mitral stenosis, carcinoid syndrome, left atrial myxoma, cor triatriatum, or congenital webs. Rheumatic mitral valve disease results from four types of fusion of the mitral valve apparatus that leads to stenosis: (1) commissural, (2) cuspal, (3) chordal, and (4) combined.

Pathophysiology. In patients with mitral stenosis there is obstruction of blood flow in the left atrium at the mitral valve, slowing the flow of blood into the left ventricle. The left atrial pressure increases and there are concomitant increases in the pulmonary venous and arterial circulation. Reduction of the mitral orifice results in a pressure gradient between the left atrium and the left ventricle, usually in excess of 15 mm Hg at end-diastole. With a stenotic mitral valve, higher pressures in the left atrium are required to maintain a normal cardiac output at rest, which in turn elevates pulmonary venous and capillary pressures. This results in exertional dyspnea, fatigue, and a gradual reduction in physical capabilities. In longstanding cases, pulmonary hypertension may become fixed, with increasing systemic arterial desaturation. Left atrial contraction, which normally augments left ventricular end-diastolic volume by about 20% in patients with mitral stenosis, is lost when atrial fibrillation develops, a common sequela.

Signs and Symptoms. Patients complain of weakness, shortness of breath, dyspnea on exertion, and, eventually, nocturnal dyspnea and orthopnea as they progress to functional class IV. Physical examination of a mitral stenosis reveals a loud first heart sound followed by an opening snap that is caused by billowing of the fibrotic anterior mitral leaflet. The pulmonary second sound is often accentuated, because patients usually have some degree of pulmonary hypertension. At the apex, one usually hears a low-pitched, rumbling, diastolic murmur, intensified just before systole, if the patient is in sinus rhythm but without change in intensity in patients with atrial fibrillation.

Noninvasive Diagnosis. The ECG will show left atrial enlargement if the patient is in sinus rhythm, whereas the QRS and T waves are normal. Otherwise, atrial fibrillation is commonly diagnosed by ECG. Chest x-ray films will show enlargement of the left atrium and left atrial appendage, enlargement of the main and branch pulmonary arteries, and pulmonary plethora as a result of pulmonary venous congestion. On barium swallow, the esophagus may be displaced posteriorly by the enlarged left atrium. In addition to pulmonary plethora, Kerley B lines and engorged lymphatics will be found at the base of both lungs. In advanced cases, generalized hemosiderosis of the lungs may also be noted.

Echocardiography has become extremely important in all diagnoses of valvular disease, particularly in the diagnosis of disease of the mitral valve. In most instances conventional M-mode echocardiography can be used to clarify the extent of the pathologic state without cardiac catheterization. The classic finding in mitral stenosis is a reduced descent of the diastolic E-F slope. The use of 2-D echocardiography has become routine because it can yield very clear, dynamic images of the obstructed mitral valve and is diagnostic for mitral stenosis, showing reduced leaflet motion, calcification, and left atrial thrombus.

Cardiac Catheterization. The most accurate method of diagnosing acquired valvular heart disease, which is still the traditional "gold standard" of diagnosis, is cardiac catheterization and angiography. This is done by inserting catheters (no. 4 to no. 6 French) into the heart via a peripheral vein or artery. Cardiac chamber pressures are measured by strain gauge manometers. Samples of blood are taken to measure the oxygen saturation and content of the blood in each chamber. From these data abnormal pressure gradients are noted, step-up or step-down in oxygen saturation resulting from intracardiac shunt is found, and pulmonary and systemic resistances are calculated. Fig. 18-2 shows the nor-

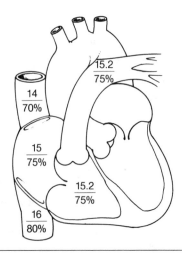

FIGURE 18-2 Schematic of normal oxygen content and saturation in heart chambers and vessels. Oxygen content (vol %)/O_2 saturation.

mal oxygen content in volume percent and oxygen saturation by percentage for each right- and left-sided cardiac chamber and great vessel. Normal intracardiac pressures, in millimeters of mercury, systole over diastole, are seen in Fig. 18-3.

Cardiac catheterization in moderate to severe cases of mitral stenosis shows a marked discrepancy between the left ventricular end-diastolic pressure and the left atrial pressure during diastole (Fig. 18-4). The left ventricular end-dia-

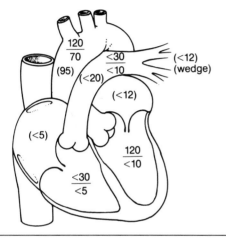

FIGURE 18-3 Schematic of normal intracardiac pressure in mm Hg systole/diastole (mean).

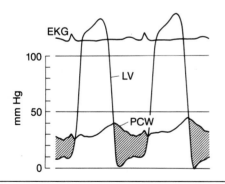

FIGURE 18-4 Pressure tracing from a 50-year-old woman with progressive fatigue and dyspnea on exertion and a history of childhood acute rheumatic fever. The pulmonary capillary wedge *(PCW)* pressure is elevated, and there is a mean gradient (cross-hatched area) of 22 mm Hg between pulmonary capillary wedge (PCW) and left ventricular *(LV)* pressures throughout diastole. The calculated mitral valve area was reduced to 0.8 cm². (From Braunwald EB. Valvular heart disease. In Braunwald EB [ed]. Heart Disease: A Textbook of Cardiovascular Medicine. Philadelphia, WB Saunders, 1980, p 1097.)

stolic pressure is normal in most cases, pulmonary pressure and right ventricular pressures are elevated, and right atrial pressure is elevated if there is functional tricuspid regurgitation. The valve area by calculation is narrowed, usually less than 1.0 cm², whereas the ejection fraction of the left ventricle may be reduced only slightly or not at all.

Natural History and Medical Therapy. Patients with mitral stenosis will inexorably become incapacitatingly dyspneic, although the time course of the disease is considerably longer than in most other forms of valvular heart disease. Episodic pulmonary edema or atrial fibrillation in symptomatic patients may be improved by restricting sodium intake and prescribing a course of diuretics and digitalis. The onset of chronic atrial fibrillation usually signals the final phase of the disease. Anticoagulants are necessary for patients who have sustained systemic emboli or who are in atrial fibrillation. Bacterial endocarditis may develop in a patient with severe mitral stenosis, but it is uncommon. The natural history of mitral stenosis is long, and there is approximately a 60% 10-year survival rate in patients in functional class III and a 40% 10-year rate in patients who are functional class IV.

Operative Treatment. Surgical treatment will be indicated in virtually all patients with mitral stenosis who are functional class III or IV (Table 18-2). Occasionally some patients who are functional class II are operated on, depending on the patient's age and degree of limitation, because of systemic arterial emboli. Transfemoral/transatrial mitral valve balloon dilation, an interventional cardiologic procedure, is being used with increasing frequency. This procedure is now very widely used for noncalcific mitral stenosis and early results seem encouraging, although there are no good studies as yet reporting on long-term results.

There are three main operations that are performed for calcific valves or for patients in whom a thrombus is detected preoperatively. They are (1) closed mitral commissurotomy, (2) open commissurotomy, and (3) mitral valve replacement. A closed mitral commissurotomy involves the restoration of flexibility to the leaflets without producing insufficiency, and is done transatrially by the surgeon's fingers, through the ventricle with a mechanical dilator, or by a combination of the two techniques. This operation was performed extensively prior to the development of the heart-lung machine since there was little else that could be done in terms of operative therapy. It is used very little in North America at

TABLE 18-2   Classification of Patients With Diseases of the Heart (New York Heart Association)

Class	Capacity
Functional	
I	Patients with cardiac disease but without resulting limitation of physical activity. Ordinary physical activity does not cause undue fatigue, palpitation, dyspnea, or anginal pain.
II	Patients with cardiac disease resulting in slight limitation of physical activity. They are comfortable at rest. Ordinary physical activity results in fatigue, palpitation, dyspnea, or anginal pain.
III	Patients with cardiac disease resulting in marked limitation of physical activity. They are comfortable at rest. Less than ordinary activity causes fatigue, palpitation, dyspnea, or anginal pain.
IV	Patients with cardiac disease resulting in inability to carry on any physical activity without discomfort. Symptoms of cardiac discomfort. Symptoms of cardiac insufficiency or of the anginal syndrome are present even at rest. If any physical activity is undertaken, discomfort is increased.
Therapeutic	
A	Patients with a cardiac disease whose ordinary physical activity need not be restricted.
B	Patients with cardiac disease whose ordinary physical activity need not be restricted, but who should be advised against severe or competitive physical efforts.
C	Patients with cardiac disease whose ordinary physical activity should be moderately restricted and whose more strenuous efforts should be discontinued.
D	Patients with cardiac disease who should be at complete rest, confined to bed or chair.

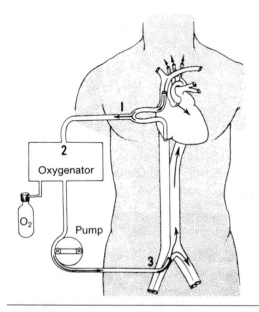

FIGURE 18-5   Diagram of cardiopulmonary bypass: *(1)* Venous blood removed from superior vena cava and inferior vena cava; *(2)* passed through chamber rich in concentrated oxygen; *(3)* oxygenated blood is pumped back into systemic circulation via femoral artery or via cannula in aortic arch.

present. The open reconstructive operation has the advantage of thorough inspection of the valve, commissures, and fused chordae (which may be incised and the valves debrided of calcium). If a thrombus is present, it can be safely removed. Mortality for open mitral valve commissurotomy is less than 2%. Cardiopulmonary bypass required for this operation is diagrammed in Fig. 18-5. The long-term results of reparative techniques indicate that the restenosis rate is low. The probability that a repeat operation will be necessary at 10 years is about 10%.

Mitral Regurgitation

Etiology and Pathology. The etiologic factors in mitral regurgitation (MR) are diverse and are associated with a number of cardiac and noncardiac diseases, such as endocrinopathies, autoimmune diseases, and connective tissue disorder. Mitral regurgitation may be caused by dilation of the mitral annulus; pathologic changes in the valve leaflets, the chordae tendineae, or the papillary muscles; or a combination of these. The most common causes of mitral regurgitation in North America are myxomatous degeneration, rheumatic valve disease, calcification of the mitral annulus, chordal rupture or papillary muscle infarction secondary to ischemic heart disease, or bacterial endocarditis.

Pathophysiology. The primary event in mitral regurgitation is backward displacement of the blood during ventricular systole into the left atrium from the left ventricle. The primary early effects are reduction of the left ventricular volume and reduction of systolic ventricular pressure and radius. With mitral regurgitation there is reduction of left ventricular tension, the left ventricle may increase its total output, and, for many patients, enormous regurgitant volumes may be sustained for prolonged periods, maintaining a forward cardiac output at normal levels despite regurgitation. In chronic, advanced cases, left ventricular end-diastolic volume increases, there is dilation of the left ventricle, elevations in the left atrial pressure, and pulmonary resistance. Adaptation to the chronic pressure load on the left atrium is achieved by dilation of the atrium, with maintenance of relatively low atrial pressures and the transmission of pressures to the right heart chamber, or by the thickening of the left atrial wall and maintenance of high atrial pressures with symptoms of pulmonary congestion.

Signs and Symptoms. The clinical history is quite variable in patients with mitral regurgitation, and the clinical course of some patients with MR may be very prolonged. Congestion and shortness of breath are late symptoms. The most common early symptom is chronic fatigue secondary to reduced cardiac output, while patients with acute mitral regurgitation from a ruptured papillary muscle will have pulmonary edema, cardiogenic shock, and advanced cardiovascular collapse. Physical examination shows a brisk carotid pulse and hyperdynamic precordium, a pansystolic or late systolic murmur at the apex, with referral to the axilla. The pulmonary second sound is split and is usually increased by pulmonary hypertension. The first sound is usually soft, and a third heart sound is not uncommon.

Noninvasive Diagnosis. An ECG usually exhibits left atrial enlargement if there is sinus rhythm, left ventricular enlargement, and, occasionally, left ventricular hypertrophy. Radiologic findings demonstrate a large left atrium, right ventricle, and main pulmonary artery. In late cases, the left ventricle may be hugely enlarged, often touching the left lateral thoracic wall. Calcification of the mitral annulus, a common cause of MR in the elderly, may be seen on fluoroscopy. An echocardiogram is diagnostic and demonstrates left atrial and left ventricular enlargement. The valvular pathology causing regurgitation can usually be determined by left ventricular ejection fraction. Left ventricular end-systolic and diastolic dimensions can be determined from 2-D echocardiograms and are used as prognostic indicators for the timing of surgical intervention.

Cardiac Catheterization. Cardiac output is decreased, left atrial pressure with predominant V wave is markedly increased (Fig. 18-6), left ventricular end-diastolic pressure is normal or markedly elevated, depending on the functional state of the left ventricle. The ejection fraction may be normal or depressed, depending on the stage of the disease. MR is diagnosed by observing the prompt appearance of radiopaque dye in the left atrium and pulmonary veins following injection of dye into the ventricle (left ventricular angiocardiogram).

Natural History and Medical Treatment. Medical treatment includes pharmacologic therapy for congestive heart failure, especially after afterload reduction. Salt restriction and diuretic therapy are also cornerstones of therapy for this condition. The natural history of mitral regurgitation is quite variable and depends on the extent

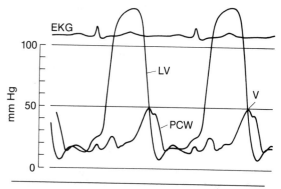

FIGURE 18-6 Pressure tracings from a 59-year-old man with SOB on exertion, a loud systolic murmur, and evidence of ruptured chordae tendineae on echocardiogram. The pulmonary capillary wedge *(PCW)* pressure is elevated (mean = 25 mm Hg), with a markedly increased regurgitant V-wave peaking at 50 mm Hg. In addition, left ventricular end-diastolic pressure is elevated to 27 mm Hg. These findings are consistent with severe mitral regurgitation. (From Braunwald EB. Valvular heart disease. In Braunwald EB [ed]. Heart Disease: A Textbook of Cardiovascular Medicine. Philadelphia, WB Saunders, 1980, p 1112.)

of the volume of regurgitation and the chronicity of the condition. At one end of the spectrum, acute mitral regurgitation with rupture of a papillary muscle in a previously healthy individual may result in sudden cardiogenic shock, requiring operative intervention within hours of onset. At the other end of the spectrum, patients with moderate mitral regurgitation may be stable for decades, but as the left ventricle fails, regurgitation may progress, and at this point an elective valve operation may be required. In general, about 80% of patients with chronic mitral regurgitation survive 5 years and 60% survive 10 years.

Operative Therapy. All procedures for mitral regurgitation must be done with cardiopulmonary bypass. Most patients are functional class III and IV, but increasingly, in patients who are functional class II, who may show marked enlargement of their cardiac silhouette indicating left ventricular decompensation, or who present with intermittent atrial fibrillation, early operation may be indicated.

Mitral Valve Reconstruction. Reproducible reconstructive plastic procedures on the valve are now possible and have been advocated by a number of surgeons. The results have been excellent in a large group of patients, where the local pathologic condition has been repaired, precluding valve replacement. The annulus is narrowed with sutures or, most commonly, a semiflexible prosthetic ring is sutured around the annulus, which restores the valve to its original anatomic curvature after resection of portions of valve leaflets or chordoplasty. Operative mortality in these procedures is less than 3%.

Mitral Valve Replacement. For patients with severe valvar calcification or severe anatomic distortion of the valve, replacement is necessary. Mitral valve replacement is performed on total cardiopulmonary bypass. After the heart is made ischemic and the blood emptied from the heart, the left atrium is opened and the valve carefully excised. Sutures are placed around the annulus and then are passed through the prosthesis that will be placed in the mitral annulus. Valves are basically of two types: *prosthetic,* which includes ball and cage or bileaflet disc valves, or *bioprosthetic,* which includes porcine or pericardial valves treated with glutaraldehyde. The operative mortality for uncomplicated mitral valve replacement is about 5% in most large centers throughout the world. Morbidity and mortality appear to be greater in those who have enlarged hearts with chronic atrial fibrillation, regardless of the type of valve used. Operative mortality also

varies, depending on the clinical presentation and the functional state of the patient. Patients in functional class III have a risk of less than 2%, whereas those who are functional class IV may have a risk of 5% to 10%. Operative survival is similar for both types of valves, but the major difference between these valves in the long term is the incidence of thromboembolus and the need for long-term anticoagulation therapy. Patients with prosthetic heart valves must take warfarin for long-term anticoagulation; however, there is still a persistent thromboembolic rate. Patients with porcine valves do not need warfarin unless they are in chronic atrial fibrillation. Death of patients at an extended time after mitral valve replacement usually results from progression of myocardial disease, irrespective of the correction of the mechanical problem, complications of arteriosclerotic heart disease, or thromboembolism.

AORTIC VALVE DISEASE
Aortic Stenosis

Etiology and Pathology. Valvular aortic stenosis may be the result of a congenital malformation, rheumatic fever, or calcific degeneration. The most common cause of aortic stenosis is calcific congenital bicuspid valve disease. Bicuspid valves may not be stenotic at birth, but valvular aortic stenosis increases, since any abnormal architecture chronically induces turbulent flow. Although unusual, bacterial endocarditis may develop on congenitally calcific bicuspid valves.

Pathophysiology. The primary hemodynamic abnormality resulting from aortic stenosis is obstruction to left ventricular outflow, resulting in the development of left ventricular hypertrophy. A peak systolic pressure gradient exceeding 40 mm Hg with a normal cardiac output or an effective orifice area of less than 0.8 cm^2 represents critical obstruction of left ventricular outflow. As obstruction progresses, left ventricular compliance is reduced, and left ventricular end-diastolic pressure rises to maintain normal cardiac output. Late in the course of aortic stenosis there is dilation of the left ventricle, increase in left ventricular end-diastolic volume, pulmonary hypertension, and chronic atrial fibrillation.

Signs and Symptoms. The primary symptoms of a stenotic aortic valve are angina pectoris, syncope, and congestive heart failure. Once these symptoms appear, the prognosis is poor, and the survival curve shows a marked increase in mortality. The time from the onset of symptoms until death is approximately 2 years for patients with heart failure, 3 years for patients with syncope, and 5 years for patients with angina. Angina pectoris in a patient with aortic stenosis and normal coronary arteries results from the combination of increased oxygen demands of the hypertrophied myocardium and the reduction of oxygen delivery to the myocardium due to compression of the coronary vessels by the hypertrophied muscle. Syncope is orthostatic and related to reduced cerebral perfusion. Congestive heart failure is related to pulmonary congestion and pulmonary venous hypertension.

Physical examination shows a slow upstroke of the arterial pulse and a precordial systolic thrill in the second right intercostal space. The first sound may be normal, the second sound is either single or may show reverse splitting. The pulmonic second sound is always louder than the aortic second sound. The murmur of aortic stenosis is a diamond-shaped, harsh ejection murmur. With severe left ventricular failure, the murmur may become softer and actually disappear, while the slowly rising pulse becomes even more difficult to palpate.

Noninvasive Examination. The principal ECG finding is that of left ventricular hypertrophy in more than 80% of patients. There may be S-T segment depression and T-wave inversion, indicative of the "strain" pattern of severe left ventricular hypertrophy. Calcium infiltrates into the electrical bundles from the annulus may cause bundle-branch block or even complete heart block. Chest x-ray films show a heart of normal or slightly enlarged size, with occasional poststenotic dilation of the ascending aorta. Calcification in the aortic valve is virtually diagnostic in younger patients, but in elderly patients calcification may indicate only mild obstruction. The echocardiogram demonstrates decreased mobility of the aortic valve leaflets, a reduced aortic orifice, and decreased indices of left ventricular function. Late in the course of the disease, an echocardiogram may show depression of the left ventricular ejection fraction and increased end-systolic volume of the left ventricle.

Cardiac Catheterization. There is a marked increase in left ventricular pressure with a peak systolic pressure gradient between the left systolic pressure gradient between the left ventricular pulse and the aortic pulse (Fig. 18-7). The end-diastolic pressure may be elevated in patients with severe heart failure and reduced cardiac output. Angiography demonstrates rigid, calcified leaflets that fail to open. Coronary arteriography should be performed in patients with

aortic stenosis, if they have angina or if they are over 40 years of age.

Natural History and Medical Treatment. The medical management of aortic stenosis should include prompt treatment of atrial dysrhythmias, reduction in exercise, and treatment of congestive heart failure. The natural history of this disease is quite well documented, and a very poor prognosis is indicated with the onset of even one of these three classes of symptoms. Forty percent of patients treated medically survive only 5 years, and 10% survive 10 years.

Operative Treatment. The appearance of any of the previously described symptoms and documentation of a peak gradient in excess of 30 to 40 mm Hg are indications for operation. There is an incidence of sudden death in addition to the other major symptomatic problems. Occasionally even an asymptomatic patient, particularly a child or teenager, will require operation, since there may be documentation of increasing left ventricular hypertrophy with "strain." The primary operation for calcific aortic stenosis is aortic valve replacement. The results have improved dramatically so that the risk of isolated aortic valve replacement is now less than 5%. These data reflect increased surgical skills, better valve devices, and improved myocardial protection

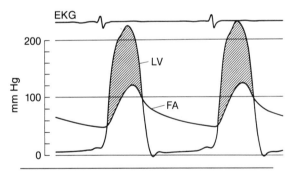

FIGURE 18-7 Pressure tracings from a 77-year-old man with a history of recent syncopal attacks. A mean pressure gradient of 90 mm Hg (cross-hatched area) between left ventricular (*LV*) pressure and arterial pressure measured at the right femoral artery (*FA*) is demonstrated. In addition, the arterial pressure curve has a markedly delayed upstroke with a reduced rate of rise. The calculated aortic valve area was narrowed to 0.5 cm². (From Braunwald EB. Valvular heart disease. In Braunwald EB [ed]. Heart Disease: A Textbook of Cardiovascular Medicine. Philadelphia, WB Saunders, 1980, p 1130.)

during the period of time the heart is ischemic and the valve is being replaced. The patient is placed on cardiopulmonary bypass, the heart is arrested, and the aorta is cross-clamped and opened in its proximal portion. The valve is sharply excised, all of the calcium is carefully debrided from the annulus, and a series of non-absorbable, plastic-coated sutures are placed around the annulus and then through the sewing ring of a prosthetic or bioprosthetic valve. The aorta is closed, the heart reperfused, and the patient weaned off the bypass.

Patients who have associated coronary disease have a slightly higher overall operative mortality. The functional classification of the patient is critical in determining long-term survival. When dealing with the aortic valve, it is important to consider the type of replacement valve to use (prosthetic or bioprosthetic), since thromboembolism is not a common finding in the natural history of aortic stenosis, and most patients are in normal sinus rhythm. There is a clear difference between the rates of long-term thromboembolic and bleeding complications in patients receiving prosthetic versus bioprosthetic valves. Since a majority of patients with this disease are 70 years old or older, a porcine valve is often chosen.

Aortic Regurgitation

Etiology and Pathology. The etiology of aortic regurgitation falls under two main categories: primary valve disease or primary aortic root disease. Bicuspid aortic valve disease, infective endocarditis, and rheumatic valve disease are the most common acquired causes of primary valve disease. The most common pathologic forms of aortic root disease are annular aortic ectasia, Marfan's syndrome, or dissection of the aorta. In these conditions the aortic leaflets may be perfectly normal, but they separate and fail to coapt as a result of massive stretching of the annulus. As with mitral regurgitation, a myriad of systemic diseases may have an effect on the aortic valve, causing it to regurgitate.

Pathophysiology. In aortic regurgitation, blood leaks into the left ventricle from the aorta during diastole, while during systole the entire left ventricular stroke volume is ejected into the high-pressure aorta. With aortic regurgitation, the increase of left ventricular end-diastolic volume is the major hemodynamic compensating mechanism. Dilation of the left ventricle increases with time, which leads to hypertrophy of the left ventricle and enormous increases in left ventricular volume. As the end-diastolic volume

increases, the elevation of the aortic regurgitant volume–ejection fraction and forward-stroke volume may decline, and with advanced regurgitation there may be left atrial and pulmonary hypertension, or even right-sided heart failure. Since the major portion of coronary blood flow occurs during diastole, when arterial diastolic pressure is low in aortic regurgitation, normal coronary perfusion pressure may be low and, consequently, effective coronary blood flow may be reduced. The result is an increased demand of oxygen since the hypertrophied dilated heart, with its increased systolic wall tension and reduced coronary blood supply, sets the stage for myocardial ischemia in the absence of obstructive coronary disease.

Signs and Symptoms. Some patients with chronic aortic regurgitation may be virtually asymptomatic, even with 4 + regurgitation. The onset of symptoms of congestive heart failure and myocardial ischemia develop only after a considerable period. Orthopnea, paroxysmal nocturnal dyspnea, and fatigue are the most common symptoms of late congestive heart failure associated with a valve lesion. Patients with acute aortic regurgitation from either endocarditis or an aortic dissection, however, when initially seen usually have advanced cardiovascular collapse and often require emergency therapy because of extremely low cardiac output. Physical exam shows an increased pulse pressure, a low diastolic pressure, hyperdynamic circulation, and cardiomegaly. The diastolic blood pressure is usually below 70 mm Hg and the pulse pressure is in excess of 70 mm Hg. A high-pitched decrescendo diastolic murmur is best heard at the midsternal border. This is a high-pitched, blowing murmur that begins immediately after the second heart sound. A midsystolic ejection murmur is usually heard secondary to a large volume of blood flow ejected across the aortic valve. A low, rumbling presystolic murmur (Austin-Flint) may be heard at the apex, when the regurgitant jet displaces the anterior leaflet of the mitral valve, causing it to vibrate during inflow from the left atrium.

Noninvasive Diagnosis. The ECG shows left ventricular diastolic volume overload and left ventricular hypertrophy. X-ray films show a large cardiac silhouette; the aortic arch may be widened, and aneurysmal dilation of the aorta suggests aortic root disease. Echocardiography is extremely important in the diagnosis and management of aortic regurgitation. The echocardiogram shows increased motion of the septum in the posterior wall, the left ventricular end-diastolic diameter is increased, the aortic root is dilated, and the left atrium may be enlarged. Fluttering of the anterior leaflet of the mitral valve can be shown by both echo modes.

Cardiac Catheterization. The left ventricular end-diastolic, left atrial, and pulmonary artery pressures are usually elevated (Fig. 18-8). The left ventricular end-diastolic pressure (LVEDP) may be so elevated (because of free aortic regurgitation [AR]) that it approximates the systemic diastolic blood pressure and actually reduces the amount of AR. In severe cases contrast media injected above the aortic valve regurgitates into the left ventricle (LV) during the first diastole, and usually completely opacifies the ventricle. Gradations of AR (1+ to 4+) have been well codified by angiographers, related to rapidity of visualization of the dye in the LV and rapidity of ejection of dye from the LV.

Natural History and Medical Treatment. Chronic aortic regurgitation has a long natural history. Seventy-five percent of patients with chronic AR survive for about 5 years, and 50% for 10 years after diagnosis. Once the patient becomes symptomatic the condition deteriorates rapidly, and without surgical treatment death may occur within 2 years. Congestive heart fail-

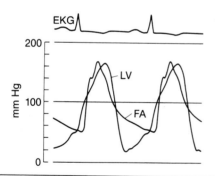

FIGURE 18-8 Pressure curves obtained from a 63-year-old man with symptoms of left ventricular failure and a loud decrescendo diastolic murmur. The femoral arterial (*FA*) pressure tracing demonstrates a widened pulse pressure of 115 mm Hg and equalization with left ventricular (*LV*) pressure late in diastole. The LV pressure curve exhibits a steady pressure increase throughout diastole, culminating in a markedly elevated end-diastolic pressure of 44 mm Hg. These findings are indicative of severe aortic regurgitation. (From Braunwald EB. Valvular heart disease. In Braunwald EB [ed]. Heart Disease: A Textbook of Cardiovascular Medicine. Philadelphia, WB Saunders, 1980, p 1140.)

ure should be treated, even in the absence of symptoms. Atrial dysrhythmias are poorly tolerated by patients and should be prevented or reversed. In addition to taking digitalis, patients who adhere to dietary salt restriction, diuretics, and vasodilator therapy for afterload reduction often exhibit impressive improvement.

Operative Treatment. Indications for operation vary from emergency surgery, related to aortic dissection or acute bacterial endocarditis, to prolonged observation of a patient with asymptomatic aortic regurgitation. One operates only when there are signs of cardiac enlargement. If there are symptoms, such as objective enlargement of heart size as shown on chest x-ray examination, and especially by LV, operation is indicated. Newer LV volume indices determined by echocardiogram are precise in indicating operation for the asymptomatic patient.

Valve replacement is the usual treatment for patients with aortic valve insufficiency, as it is for those with aortic stenosis. Patients with an aortic dissection or annular dilation of the ascending aorta may require reconstructive surgery, with reimplantation of the coronaries and a composite valve conduit graft. Endocarditis of the aortic root provides a surgical challenge for reconstruction if there are annular abscesses, or detachment of the anterior leaflet or mitral valve. The cryopreserved homograft aortic valve is the valve of choice in patients with endocarditis because there is no prosthetic material in these valves. Bioprosthetic or prosthetic valves have a similar incidence of postoperative endocarditis. In some selected cases, patients with AR and no valvar calcification may be candidates for leaflet reconstruction.

Operative mortality in aortic valve replacement is slightly higher in patients with aortic regurgitation than with aortic stenosis because of the severe left ventricular dysfunction often present in aortic regurgitation. Late survival results, particularly in the functional class IV patient, are poor despite correction of the regurgitation, and these patients should be referred earlier for surgery, before reaching this level of impairment.

TRICUSPID VALVE DISEASE
Tricuspid Stenosis

Etiology and Pathology. Stenosis of the tricuspid valve is of rheumatic origin. Tricuspid atresia, right atrial tumor, or the carcinoid syndrome may also simulate functional tricuspid stenosis. Rheumatic tricuspid disease almost always appears with mitral valve disease and is reported to be found in about 14% of autopsies of patients with rheumatic heart disease. Isolated tricuspid stenosis is virtually unknown in the United States but is relatively common in India and Middle and Far Eastern countries.

Pathophysiology. A diastolic pressure gradient exists in the right atrium and the right ventricle that is augmented when the transvalvular blood flow increases during inspiration and reduces when blood flow declines during expiration. A diastolic pressure gradient of more than 5 mm Hg often is enough to elevate the mean right atrial pressure and the systemic venous pressure, which may cause liver distension, ascites, and peripheral edema of the legs and arms.

Signs and Symptoms. The main symptom in tricuspid valve disease is that of fatigue and peripheral edema, usually out of proportion to the dyspnea of mitral valve disease. Anasarca and liver distension may also be found.

The physical examination is the same as that for patients with multivalvular rheumatic disease. Physical findings that suggest tricuspid stenosis are a prominent jugular venous pulse, ascites, and peripheral edema. The lung fields are clear. On auscultation there is a tricuspid opening snap, which is located centrally, at the right lower sternal border. A diastolic rumbling murmur is best heard over the lower left sternal border augmented by inspiration, or any activity that increases venous return.

Noninvasive Diagnosis. The ECG shows right ventricular hypertrophy, with right atrial enlargement out of proportion to the right ventricular hypertrophy. Atrial fibrillation is quite common. Chest x-ray films show marked cardiomegaly with enlargement of the right atrium without dilation of the pulmonary artery and with minimal changes in the lung. An echocardiogram generally shows a reduction in the E-F slope of the anterior leaflet of the tricuspid valve and paradoxical motion of the septal leaflet in diastole. Two-dimensional echocardiography is extremely valuable in visualizing the stenotic valve and its results are diagnostic without other modalities.

Cardiac Catheterization. There is a pressure differential between the right atrial and right ventricular end-diastolic pressure measurements. Patients in sinus rhythm show a very large "a" wave, indicating a strong atrial contraction.

Natural History and Medical Treatment. The basic approach to management of these patients is repair or replacement of the almost invariably associated left-sided valve lesions. Medical preparation for surgery includes dietary salt restriction, diuretic therapy, and bed rest to improve hepatic function and diminish edema. There are no satisfactory studies of the natural history of this lesion, because it is commonly associated with left-sided rheumatic valve lesions.

Operative Treatment. If there is true organic tricuspid stenosis without regurgitation, a commissurotomy may suffice. If commissurotomy does not restore reasonable normal valve function, tricuspid valve repair should be performed. If the tricuspid valve is calcific, replacement of the tricuspid valve with a bioprosthetic one is the preferred approach. Prosthetic valves have a tendency to thrombose; therefore they are used less frequently.

Tricuspid Regurgitation

Etiology and Pathology. The most common cause of tricuspid regurgitation (TR) is dilation of the right ventricle and the tricuspid valve annulus (which are complications of right ventricular failure and pulmonary hypertension secondary to mitral valve disease) or a number of other congenital and acquired cardiac problems. In addition, endocarditis is an important isolated valve lesion, particularly in narcotics addicts and in hospitalized patients.

Pathophysiology. In functional tricuspid regurgitation, severely elevated pulmonary artery pressure causes dilation of the right ventricle and the tricuspid annulus and regurgitation into the right atrium. If the valve is affected by an infectious process, regurgitation occurs with lower pulmonary artery pressures (<60 mm Hg systolic).

Signs and Symptoms. Most patients with tricuspid regurgitation have advanced mitral valve disease, pulmonary hypertension, and chronic low cardiac output. Chronic fatigue and the symptoms related to increased abdominal distension, ascites, hepatomegaly, and possibly even cardiac cirrhosis may be prominent.

Physical examination will reveal a prominent jugular venous pulse. The right ventricular impulse is prominent, and there is a right ventricular heave. Systolic pulsation or an enlarged liver are commonly present. A third heart sound may be heard and a pansystolic murmur of tricuspid regurgitation is noted in the subxyphoid or peristernal area. Any maneuver that increases venous return will cause an increase in the intensity of the murmur.

Noninvasive Diagnosis. An ECG may show right atrial enlargement and right ventricular enlargement with the other findings of left-sided valvular heart disease. The major changes seen on chest x-ray evaluation are cardiomegaly, dilation of the right ventricle and the right atrium, enlarged pulmonary artery, and changes of pulmonary hypertension. An echocardiogram will demonstrate a dilated right ventricle and right ventricular diastolic overload with paradoxical motion of the ventricular septum. Prolapse of the valve may be present, the right atrium will be enlarged, and there will be systolic pulsations.

Cardiac Catheterization. There is an elevated right ventricular end-diastolic and right atrial pressure, whether the TR is the result of primary or secondary causes. If it is secondary, there is usually pulmonary hypertension and probably a concomitant pathologic condition of the mitral valve. A pulmonary artery pressure less than 40 mm Hg suggests a primary cause, while a pressure greater than 60 mm Hg suggests that the regurgitation is secondary to right ventricular dilation and pulmonary hypertension. Dye injected in the right ventricle will appear very early in the right atrium.

Medical Treatment. Dietary salt restriction and diuretic therapy are cornerstones of therapy for this disease. Mild tricuspid regurgitation in the absence of severe pulmonary hypertension does not usually require surgical treatment.

Operative Treatment. Surgical management of functional tricuspid regurgitation may be accomplished almost always by the annuloplasty techniques previously described to stabilize the base of the septal cusp. Organic tricuspid valve disease may be repaired by annuloplasty techniques but may occasionally require tricuspid valve replacement with a low-profile tissue valve device.

BIBLIOGRAPHY

Akins CW. Mechanical cardiac valvular prostheses. Ann Thorac Surg 52:161, 1991.

Carpentier A. Cardiac valve surgery—the "French correction." J Thorac Cardiovasc Surg 86:323, 1983.

Cohn LH, Allred EN, Cohn LA, et al. Long-term results of open mitral valve reconstruction for mitral stenosis. Am J Cardiol 55:731, 1985.

Cohn LH, Allred EN, Cohn LA, et al. Early and late risk of mitral valve replacement: A 12-year concomitant comparison of porcine bioprosthetic and prosthetic tilting disc mitral valves. J Thorac Cardiovasc Surg 90:872, 1985.

Cohn LH, Allred EN, DiSesa VJ, et al. Early and late risk of aortic valve replacement: A 12-year concomitant comparison of the porcine bioprosthetic and tilting disc prosthetic aortic valves. J Thorac Cardiovasc Surg 88:695, 1984.

Cohn LH, Couper GS, Kinchla NM, et al. Decreased operative risk of surgical treatment of mitral regurgitation with or without coronary artery disease. J Am Coll Cardiol 16:1575, 1990.

Culliford AT, Galloway AC, Colvin SB, et al. Aortic valve replacement for aortic stenosis in persons aged 80 years and over. Am J Cardiol 67:1256, 1991.

Hammermeister KE, Henderson WG, Burchfiel CM, et al. Comparison of outcome after valve replacement with a bioprosthesis versus a mechanical prosthesis: Initial 5 year results of a randomized trial. J Am Coll Cardiol 10:719, 1987.

Hickey MSJ, Blackstone EH, Kirklin JW, et al. Outcome probabilities and life history after surgical mitral commissurotomy: Implications for balloon commissurotomy. J Am Coll Cardiol 17:29, 1991.

Rahimtoola SH. Valvular heart disease: A perspective. J Am Coll Cardiol 1:199, 1983.

CHAPTER REVIEW
Questions

1. Replacement of heart valves should be reserved for patients who are functional class III or IV because:
   a. Long-term results of valve replacement are not known.
   b. Prostheses tend to thrombose.
   c. Patients require anticoagulant therapy postoperatively.

2. A 50-year-old person with a history of rheumatic fever during childhood, who presents with dyspnea on exertion, ankle edema, a systolic murmur heard best along the upper right sternal border, and a diastolic murmur heard best along the lower left sternal border, probably has:
   a. Pressure gradient across the aortic valve
   b. Increased left ventricular end-diastolic pressure
   c. Both a and b

3. Symptomatic valvular heart disease is associated with a history of rheumatic fever in what percentage of patients?
   a. 95
   b. 75
   c. 50
   d. 25

4. Aortic stenosis is associated with a _____ murmur.
   a. Diastolic
   b. Systolic
   c. Both

5. The most ominous development in aortic stenosis is:
   a. Coexistence of a diastolic murmur
   b. Syncopal attacks
   c. Valve leaflet calcification
   d. Congestive heart failure

6. A wide pulse pressure is suggestive of:
   a. Tricuspid stenosis
   b. Aortic stenosis
   c. Mitral regurgitation
   d. Aortic regurgitation

7. The most common cause of tricuspid regurgitation in North America is:
   a. Prolapse
   b. Functional, secondary to mitral valve disease
   c. Endocarditis

8. Long-term negative risk factors in patients with AR who are undergoing active valve replacement include:
   a. Cardiomegaly
   b. Decreased LV ejection fraction
   c. Congestive heart failure
   d. All of the above

9. The valve of choice for aortic valve endocarditis is the:
   a. St. Jude valve
   b. Hancock porcine valve
   c. Cryopreserved homograft valve

10. Catheterization findings in mitral stenosis usually include:
    a. Increased pulmonary artery wedge pressure
    b. Increased intraventricular end-diastolic pressure
    c. Increased pulse pressure

11. Operations for mitral regurgitation may be reparative rather than for replacement when:
    a. The valve is not calcified.
    b. There is a segmental local pathologic condition such as a ruptured chordae.
    c. The annulus is dilated.
    d. All of the above.

12. The auscultatory findings in mitral regurgitation include:
    a. Holosystolic apical murmur
    b. Loud pulmonary second sound
    c. Mid-systolic click
    d. All of the above

Answers

1. a	7. b
2. c	8. d
3. c	9. c
4. b	10. a
5. d	11. d
6. d	12. d

19 Heart Murmurs: Congenital Heart Disease

JOHN A. WALDHAUSEN
JOHN L. MYERS

KEY FEATURES

After reading this chapter you will understand:

- What clinical and physiologic considerations are important in evaluating congenital heart defects.
- The importance and treatment of left-to-right shunts.
- Characteristics of specific lesions.
- What congenital defects are associated with obstruction.
- The management of patients with congenital heart disease.

Estimates are that of each 1000 live births in the United States, approximately 8 to 10 infants will be born with congenital heart disease. Half of these patients will have serious defects, most of which can be either totally corrected or effectively palliated if diagnosed and treated promptly.

PHYSIOLOGIC CONSIDERATIONS

Congenital heart defects are often either obstructive to blood flow (aortic stenosis, pulmonic stenosis, coarctation of the aorta) or are abnormal communications between the systemic and pulmonary circulations (ventricular septal defect, patent ductus arteriosus, atrial septal defect). In the latter case, the direction of flow across the defect, particularly in a ventricular septal defect and a patent ductus arteriosus, is dependent upon the relationship between the pulmonary vascular resistance (R_p) and the systemic vascular resistance (R_s). As long as the R_p is less than R_s, the flow across the defect is left-to-right, or from the systemic side to the pulmonary side.

When a ventricular septal defect is equal to or larger than the orifice of the aorta or pulmonary artery, the pressure between the right and left ventricles is equal. However, flow is still left-to-right as long as R_p is less than R_s. In patients with progressive pulmonary vascular obstructive disease, R_p can exceed the R_s, resulting in a right-to-left shunt.

In an atrial septal defect the shunt is from left-to-right, because the right ventricle has a thinner wall and thus is more compliant than the left ventricle. Since the right ventricle is more compliant than the left, it receives more blood during diastole from the atria when there is an interatrial communication.

In patients with a ventricular septal defect or a patent ductus arteriosus, the left ventricle must pump not only systemic flow but also shunt flow. This volume overload can readily result in congestive heart failure. In obstructive lesions, hypertrophy of the ventricles occurs and initially compensates for the increased work. Congestive heart failure, in general, is a late manifestation and is related to the degree of obstruction.

In patients with tetralogy of Fallot, the large ventricular septal defect is proximal to the obstruction, which is the result of infundibular and/or pulmonic stenosis and causes a right-to-left shunt and peripheral arterial desaturation. Heart failure is not usually a factor since the heart is not pumping excessive volumes. Because pulmonary blood flow is decreased ($Q_p < Q_s$), the amount of blood that is oxygenated in the lungs is limited and significant hypoxia will occur if bodily demands exceed this limit.

In transposition of the great arteries (TGA) the aorta arises from the right ventricle and the pulmonary artery arises from the left ventricle. Thus the pulmonary and systemic circulations are in parallel rather than in series. Without any communication between the two circulations, death at birth is prompt, since no oxygen is delivered to the body and, in turn, no carbon dioxide is delivered to the lungs. A patent foramen ovale, patent ductus arteriosus, or ventricular septal defect allows some mixing of the two circulations.

WHAT ARE THE CLINICAL CHARACTERISTICS OF CONGENITAL HEART DEFECTS?

Infants and children manifest heart disease primarily by congestive heart failure and/or hypoxemia. One or both of these disorders account for the high frequency of morbidity and mortality associated with congenital heart disease. The box below lists the physical features of common congenital defects.

Congestive heart failure is expressed differently in infants than it is in older children and adults. Early manifestations in infants are failure to thrive, sweating, tachycardia, tachypnea, and weak suck or anorexia. Late signs of failure in-

---

PHYSICAL FEATURES OF NINE COMMON CONGENITAL CARDIAC DEFECTS WITH NORMAL PULMONARY VASCULAR RESISTANCE

Atrial Septal Defects (ASD)
(Fig. 19-2)

S_2 split widened and "fixed"
  RVI normal or hyperdynamic
  Systolic murmur
    Grade 1-4
    Early or midsystolic
    Middle frequency crescendo-decrescendo
    Loudest at 2 ICS LSB
    Transmitted posterior chest wall
  Diastolic murmur
    Grade 1-3
    Mid- or late diastolic
    Midfrequency crescendic
    Localized to xiphoid
    Loudness varies with ventilatory cycle

Ventricular Septal Defects (VSD)
(Fig. 19-5)

LVI, hyperdynamic
Systolic thrill mid-LSB
P_2 normal to ↑, increased volume L-R
Heart failure signs and symptoms (1-6 months old)
Systolic murmur
  Pansystolic (moderate to large VSD)
  Early systolic (small VSD)
  Grade 1-6
  Midfrequency or highfrequency (small VSD)
  Loudest 3 ICS LSB
  Transmitted posterior chest wall, L-R

Diastolic mitral flow murmur (moderate to large VSD)
  Mid-diastolic
  Grade 1-3
  Low frequency (rumble)
  Localized at apex

Transposition of the Great Arteries (TGA)
(Fig. 19-13)

Cyanosis moderate to severe degree

Patent Ductus Arteriosus (PDA)
(Fig. 19-7)

Accentuated extremity pulses; wide pulse pressure
LVI, hyperdynamic
Hyperemic finger- and toetips
Heart failure signs and symptoms (2-6 months old)
Thrill 2 ICS LMCL
Continuous murmur
  Grade 2-5
  High frequency (blowing) crescendo-decrescendo
Loudest 2 ICS LMCL
Transmitted posterior chest wall

Aortic Coarctation (Fig. 19-17)

Femoral pulses absent or weak and delayed
LVI normal or heaving
Systolic murmur
  Grade 1-3
  Midfrequency crescendo-decrescendo

clude hepatomegaly, edema, gallop rhythm, and diminished murmurs and arterial pulse. Heart failure is associated with defects having large arteriovenous (left-to-right) shunts, such as truncus arteriosus, ventricular septal defects, and patent ductus arteriosus. It may also be seen in such critical obstructive lesions as aortic stenosis, pulmonic stenosis, and coarctation of the aorta. Chest x-ray films show cardiomegaly with increased pulmonary vascular markings. Large-volume left-to-right shunts are identified by a left parasternal bulge, hyperemia of the fingers and toes, sweating, a loud pulmonary second sound, and increased frequency of respiratory infections.

Hypoxemia is defined as subnormal arterial oxygen tension and accompanies defects in which unoxygenated venous blood is shunted away from the lung directly into the systemic arterial system. Examples are transposition of the great arteries, tetralogy of Fallot, truncus arteriosus, and total anomalous pulmonary venous connection. The entity is represented by cyanosis, the clubbing of fingers and toes, and the distension of superficial veins. In tetralogy of Fallot with inadequate blood flow to the lung, dangerous and recurrent spells of severe hypoxemia may occur as a result of spasm of the infundibulum and further decrease pulmonary blood flow. These are called *cerebral hypoxic spells;* they consist of increased cyanosis, hyperpnea, and staring. The attacks usually occur in the

---

Aortic Coarctation—cont'd

Loudest 2 ICS LSB or over posterior chest wall to left of thoracic spine

Continuous murmur occasionally over posterior chest wall (pericoarctation collaterals)

Pulmonic Stenosis (PS)
(Fig. 19-4)

RVI, heaving

Systolic thrill 2 ICS LSB

Widened S_2 split ~ severity

Diminished P_2

Early systolic ejection click in expiration

Systolic murmur

    Grade 1-5

    Midfrequency (coarse) crescendo-decrescendo

    Loudest 2 ICS LSB

Transmitted posterior chest wall R > L

Cyanosis with severe PS from RA-LA shunt (infants)

Heart failure signs and symptoms (1-8 weeks old)

RVI normal or heave

Aortic Stenosis (AS) (Fig. 19-19)

LVI, normal or heaving

Systolic thrill 2 ICS LSB, suprasternal notch, or carotid arteries

Early systolic ejection click

Systolic murmur

    Grade 1-5

    Midfrequency (coarse) crescendo-decrescendo

    Loudest 2 ICS RSB or 3 ICS LSB

Transmitted neck

Reversed (paradoxical) splitting S_2

Tricuspid Atresia

Cyanosis mild, moderate, or severe

LVI heave

S_2 apparently single

Systolic murmur (VSD)

    Grade 1-5

    Pansystolic to early systolic

    Midfrequency

    Loudest 3 and 4 ICS LSB

    Transmitted posterior chest wall

Continuous murmur (PDA)

    Grade 1-3

    High frequency crescendo-decrescendo

    Loudest 2 ICS LMCL

    Transmitted posterior chest wall

Tetralogy of Fallot (TlF) (Fig. 19-12)

Cyanosis mild, moderate, or severe

RVI heave

S_2 apparently single

Systolic murmur

    Grade 2-5

    Long to short early systolic ~ severity PS

    Midfrequency crescendo-decrescendo

    Loudest 3 ICS LSB

    Transmitted posterior chest wall

Murmur absent or nonspecific at 2 or 3 ICS LSB

early morning, after eating or after bowel movements, and may either end spontaneously or progress to death.

The use of two-dimensional echocardiography and Doppler imaging is very effective in delineating most congenital cardiac lesions and frequently eliminates the need for invasive catheterization. Cardiac catheterization is still required in some cases to measure pressures and resistance, to identify the source(s) of collateral pulmonary blood flow, and to delineate the pulmonary arteries.

DEFECTS ASSOCIATED WITH LEFT-TO-RIGHT SHUNTS
Atrial Septal Defects (ASD)

Pathophysiology and Diagnosis. Defects in the atrial septum occur at three locations, the most common being the ostium secundum (Fig. 19-1). High defects (sinus venosus type) are associated with anomalous pulmonary venous connections of the right superior pulmonary vein to the junction of the superior vena cava with the right atrium. Ostium primum defects (low defects) are frequently accompanied by a cleft in the anterior leaflet of the mitral or the septal leaflet and the tricuspid valve. An ostium primum defect is a partial form of endocardial cushion defect.

Blood is shunted from the left atrium to the right as a result of increased compliance of the right ventricle, causing an increased right ventricular diastolic volume and thus an increased pulmonary flow as compared with systemic flow. This increased pulmonary blood flow may result in the late development (in 20 to 30 years) of pulmonary vascular obstructive disease. Once the pulmonary-to-systemic resistance ratio is greater than 0.75, closure of the defect is contraindicated, since operative mortality is high and little is accomplished, even if the minimal residual shunt associated with a very high R_p is abolished.

Diagnosis is established by the presence of a systolic murmur in the second left interspace and fixed splitting of the second heart sound at the base (Fig. 19-2). A chest x-ray examination shows right atrial and ventricular enlargement with increased pulmonary vascular markings. If two-dimensional echocardiography demonstrates the atrial septal defect and shows the enlarged right ventricle, cardiac catheterization is not required. If cardiac catheterization is performed, a step-up in oxygen saturation is present

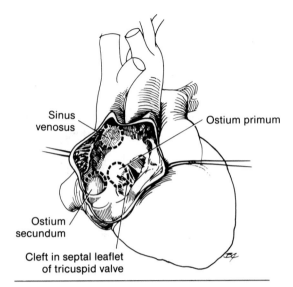

FIGURE 19-1 Location of the three types of atrial septal defects.

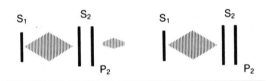

FIGURE 19-2 Murmur and heart sounds in atrial septal defect.

in the right atrium. A pulmonary to systemic (P/S) flow ratio of more than 1.5 : 1 is the usual indication for operation.

Operative Treatment. Basically, the problem is one of too much blood flow to the lungs because of shunting from the left to the right atrium. The operation is designed to close this defect and prevent the onset of pulmonary hypertension. The ideal age for correction is 2 to 4 years. Some atrial septal defects can be closed by direct suture. Larger defects and ones associated with anomalous pulmonary venous drainage and ostium primum defects require a pericardial patch. In an ostium primum defect, repair of the cleft of the anterior leaflet of the mitral valve is required if there is valve insufficiency. Cardiopulmonary bypass is used. Mortality associated with this procedure is less than 1%, and late results are excellent.

Endocardial Cushion Defects (Common Atrioventricular Canal)

Pathophysiology and Diagnosis. Endocardial cushion defects compose 2% to 7% of all cases of congenital heart anomalies, and nearly 50% are in patients with Down's syndrome. Four lesions may occur: (1) a defect in the lower part of the atrial septum (ostium primum), (2) a ventricular septal defect, (3) a cleft in the anterior leaflet of the mitral valve, and (4) a cleft in the septal leaflet of the tricuspid valve. These may occur either alone or in combination, the most common combinations being an ostium primum defect with a cleft in the anterior mitral leaflet or a complete atrioventricular (A-V) canal in which central fusion of the endocardial cushion has not occurred (Fig. 19-3). In the latter, there is an ostium primum and a ventricular septal defect (A-V communis and complete A-V canal as well as mitral and tricuspid valve abnormalities).

Operative Treatment. Again, the basic problem is excessive pulmonary blood flow, and the operation is designed to prevent this. To correct the complete form of common A-V canal, a pericardial or prosthetic patch is used to repair the atrial and ventricular defects; careful suturing in the region of the conduction bundle is necessary to avoid heart block. The mitral and tricuspid valves are attached to the septal patch.

Operative mortality for repair of the complete form of A-V canal is 5%. Frequently symptoms of pulmonary hypertension in infants are so severe that early repair is indicated, although operative mortality is higher (10%).

Ventricular Septal Defects (VSD)

Pathophysiology and Diagnosis. A defect in the ventricular septum is the most common congenital cardiac anomaly encountered at the time of birth. Blood flow across the defect is usually from left to right. The amount of blood shunted depends on the size of the defect and the resistance of the pulmonary vasculature. When excessive blood is shunted, as with large defects, the pulmonary vasculature responds by developing intimal hyperplasia and medial hypertrophy. Resistance increases and therefore reduces the amount of blood being shunted. If uncorrected, pulmonary vascular disease may progress to the point of complete arterial obliteration, and pulmonary vascular resistance may equal or exceed systemic vascular resistance ($R_p/R_s > 1$), at which point the problem becomes inoperable.

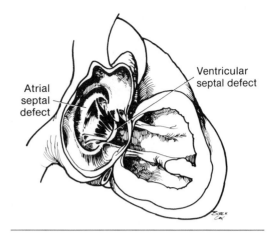

FIGURE 19-3   Common atrioventricular canal.

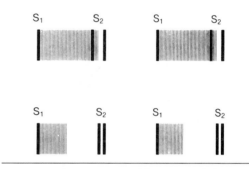

FIGURE 19-4   Murmur and heart sounds in ventricular septal defect. *Above:* Pansystolic regurgitant murmur (mitral insufficiency, tricuspid insufficiency; ventricular septal defect). *Below:* Early systolic murmur (small ventricular septal defect).

When the ventricular septal defect is large, the marked increase in pulmonary blood flow usually becomes evident between the ages of 3 and 12 months, and the patient has clinical signs of pulmonary congestion and failure to thrive.

Examination will reveal a pansystolic murmur heard best at the third left intercostal space (Fig. 19-4). Chest x-ray examination demonstrates left atrial and biventricular hypertrophy with increased pulmonary vascularity. Cardiac catheterization and angiocardiography show a step-up in oxygen content in the right ventricle and the shunting of contrast medium from the left to the right ventricle.

Patients with large defects are prone to developing pulmonary hypertension, so their defects should be closed early. Many smaller defects close spontaneously in infants.

Operative Treatment. Operative closure of the ventricular septal defect is the treatment of choice, and pulmonary artery banding is reserved for special problems such as multiple muscular defects. Pulmonary artery banding increases the resistance to flow across the lung, thus reducing pulmonary blood flow, and protects the pulmonary vasculature. Total correction is then carried out when the patient is 1 to 2 years of age. Total correction in infants usually involves cardiopulmonary bypass and deep hypothermia (20° C).

Anatomically there are essentially four types of ventricular septal defects (Fig. 19-5): (1) high defect under the pulmonary valve (subarterial defect), (2) perimembranous defect just beneath the aortic valve (most common), (3) A-V canal defect or inlet (behind the septal leaflet of the tricuspid valve), and (4) defects in the muscular septum. Large defects are repaired with a prosthetic patch, and care is taken to avoid injury to the bundle of His. If dysrhythmia or heart block occurs, pacing wires are attached to the myocardium to be used with a pacemaker in the postoperative period.

Mortality following the repair of small and moderately sized defects is about 1%. In infants mortality is approximately 5%. Pulmonary hypertension significantly increases the risk of operation. Patients with defects in which the ratio of pulmonary resistance to systemic resistance (R_p/R_s) is 0.75 or more experience a 17% mortality with total correction. In addition to this high mortality there is a high morbidity rate. Furthermore, pulmonary vascular resistance rarely decreases and often continues to rise, leading to early death. Therefore operation for these patients is not indicated.

Patent Ductus Arteriosus (PDA)

Pathophysiology and Diagnosis. The second most common congenital heart defect is a connection between the aortic isthmus and the bifurcation of the pulmonary artery. This allows left-to-right shunting of blood and increased pulmonary flow. The ductus usually closes at birth and closure may still close during the first year of life, but thereafter closure is quite rare. Examination reveals a continuous machinelike murmur heard best at the second left intercostal space (Fig. 19-6). Chest x-ray examination shows increased pulmonary vascularity. Catheterization, which may be performed in complicated cases,

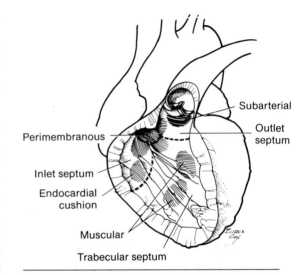

FIGURE 19-5 Location of ventricular septal defects. Perimembranous defect can extend into the inlet septum, the trabecular septum or the outlet septum.

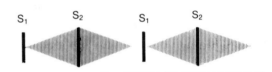

FIGURE 19-6 Continuous murmur as found in patent ductus arteriosus.

will show contrast medium, injected into the aorta, enter the pulmonary artery. Patients not treated surgically may develop fixed pulmonary hypertension, although this may take years and requires a large patent ductus arteriosus. The risk of subacute bacterial endocarditis is high in patients with a patent ductus arteriosus.

Operative Treatment. Since operative mortality is close to zero, the surgical division is advised once the diagnosis has been made (Fig. 19-7). Patients with a P/S resistance ratio of more than 1:1 do not benefit from surgical intervention, since the majority die within 2 years of operation.

Aortopulmonary Window

Pathophysiology and Diagnosis. This defect is a communication between the aorta and the pulmonary artery, just above their valves. Signs

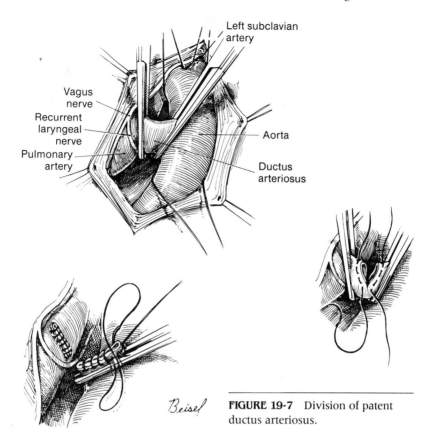

Left subclavian artery

Vagus nerve

Recurrent laryngeal nerve

Pulmonary artery

Aorta

Ductus arteriosus

Beisel

FIGURE 19-7 Division of patent ductus arteriosus.

and symptoms are similar to those found in patent ductus arteriosus but are greatly exaggerated. Pulmonary hypertension almost invariably develops early if the defect is not corrected.

Operative Treatment. Using cardiopulmonary bypass, the defect is closed through the pulmonary artery by direct suture or a patch graft. Mortality ranges from 5% to 10% and is attributable to the high incidence of pulmonary vascular disease present in these patients.

DEFECTS ASSOCIATED WITH CYANOSIS
Total Anomalous Pulmonary Venous Connection

Pathophysiology and Diagnosis. Anatomically, the pulmonary veins converge to form a common pulmonary venous trunk (Fig. 19-8). This trunk may connect to the left innominate vein (supracardiac), to the right atrium or coronary sinus (intracardiac), or to the portal system or inferior vena cava (infracardiac). An interatrial communication is the only route by which pulmonary venous blood enters the left atrium and left ventricle. The prognosis is directly affected by the degree of obstruction to these pulmonary veins and is commonly most severe in the infracardiac type.

Blood volume in the right side of the heart is increased, since systemic and venous blood both return to the right atrium.

Examination shows cyanosis, especially with pulmonary venous obstruction, pulmonary edema, and, usually, congestive failure before the patient is 6 months of age. Without surgical treatment, the prognosis is poor (80% mortality in infancy).

Operative Treatment. Total repair using cardiopulmonary bypass should be performed when the diagnosis is made, usually in early infancy. The common pulmonary vein is anastomosed to the left atrium and the persistent vertical vein is tied off. If an atrial communication exists, it is closed. Intracardiac types of anomalous drainage are corrected by closing the septal

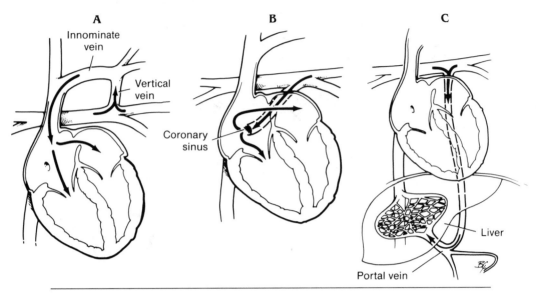

FIGURE 19-8 Total anomalous pulmonary venous connection. **A**, Supracardiac type. **B**, Intracardiac type. **C**, Infracardiac type.

defect, usually with a pericardial patch, in such a way as to direct the anomalous flow of blood to the right atrium through the atrial defect to the left atrium. In patients beyond 1 year of age, mortality is low (5%) and results are excellent. Mortality in infants under 6 months of age is about 10%, especially in those with pulmonary obstruction. The use of deep hypothermia (20° C) and circulatory arrest have lowered these mortality figures.

Origin of Both Great Arteries From the Right Ventricle (Double Outlet– Right Ventricle)

Pathophysiology and Diagnosis. The aorta arises from the right ventricle, as does the pulmonary artery. Blood courses from the left ventricle through a ventricular septal defect that is either subaortic, subpulmonic (Taussig-Bing syndrome), or not related to either vessel to gain access to the aorta and pulmonary artery. Symptoms and clinical findings are quite similar to those of patients with large ventricular septal defects. Occasionally pulmonary stenosis is present and some patients have been mistakenly diagnosed as having tetralogy of Fallot.

Operative Treatment. When the defect is related to the aorta, repair is accomplished with an intraventricular baffle of Dacron that channels blood from the left ventricle through the ventricular septal defect into the aorta. When the

septal defect is related to the pulmonary artery, the baffle channels blood from the left ventricle to the pulmonary artery creating a transposition of the great arteries. In the latter case, an arterial switch operation will permit blood from the left ventricle to reach the aorta and blood from the right ventricle to reach the pulmonary arteries. Alternatively, an intra-atrial repair by transposing the venous return (Mustard or Senning operation) may be performed. The arterial switch operation is now preferred. Mortality has varied but in most centers is 5% to 10%.

Truncus Arteriosus

Pathophysiology and Diagnosis. One large vessel emerges from the heart, which also has a subarterial ventricular septal defect (Fig. 19-9, **A**). The pulmonary blood flow may be (1) through a common artery that branches into the left and right pulmonary arteries after leaving the single arterial trunk, (2) through two pulmonary arteries that branch directly from the main trunk, or (3) from several vessels arising from the descending aorta. The defect usually causes markedly increased pulmonary blood flow, and congestive failure is common in infants. If pulmonary flow is decreased, cyanosis may be present.

Examination often reveals a continuous murmur and increased pulmonary vasculature. The latter may be diminished when small arteries exist. Cardiac catheterization is necessary to de-

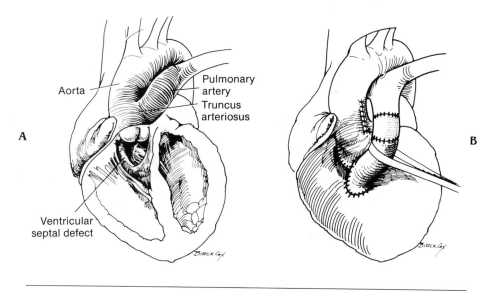

FIGURE 19-9   A, Truncus arteriosus. B, Repair of truncus arteriosus using a conduit.

fine the anatomy. Without operation, death from congestive heart failure usually occurs within the first 6 months.

Operative Treatment. Total correction has been accomplished in a number of patients, especially in those whose pulmonary arteries arise from the ascending aorta. Correction consists of removing the pulmonary arteries from the single arterial trunk, closing the ventricular septal defect, and suturing a valved homograft or a prosthetic conduit containing a xenograft valve from the right ventricle to the pulmonary arteries (Fig. 19-9, **B**). When the procedure is performed in infants, the conduit must be replaced as the child outgrows the prosthesis. Operative mortality is 5% to 10%.

Tricuspid Atresia

Pathophysiology and Diagnosis. The tricuspid valve is atretic and prevents blood from entering the right ventricle, which is small and usually consists of only an outlet chamber. Blood flows through an atrial communication to the left atrium and left ventricle and then to pulmonary arteries through a ventricular septal defect or a patent ductus arteriosus. Pulmonary blood flow is usually decreased but, in some patients, may be excessive. Many patients also have transposition of the great arteries. Cyanosis is usually early and marked. Without operation, mortality is 80% before the age of 3 years.

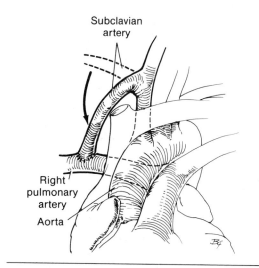

FIGURE 19-10   Blalock-Taussig subclavian artery to pulmonary artery anastomosis.

Operative Treatment. Palliative operations are indicated in infants and small children. Enlargement of the atrial septal defect, if small, should be performed by balloon septostomy. A systemic-to-pulmonary artery anastomosis (Blalock-Taussig) is then performed to increase pulmonary blood flow (Fig. 19-10). Good palliation has been achieved in the majority of patients. In infants with excessive pulmonary flow, pulmonary artery banding should be done. A definitive operation is usually performed between 1 and 4 years of age. The Fontan operation channels all systemic venous blood directly to the pulmonary arteries. For the Fontan operation to be successful, the pulmonary arteries must be of adequate size and the pulmonary resistance low so that systemic venous return can flow through the lungs without an excessive venous pressure (<15 mm Hg). Normal arterial oxygen saturations are obtained and, with restoration of the normal "series" circulation, the volume load on the left ventricle is alleviated.

Pulmonary Atresia With Intact Ventricular Septum

Pathophysiology and Diagnosis. The pulmonary valve is atretic and the right ventricle is usually small (type I) but occasionally is of normal size with marked tricuspid insufficiency (type II). An atrial septal opening is present to allow blood to enter the left ventricle, which then supplies blood to the lungs through a patent ductus arteriosus. Cyanosis is usually present at birth and increases as the ductus closes, often in the first few weeks of life; death soon follows. If not treated, the majority of these infants die within 3 months.

Operative Treatment. Treatment consists of increasing the interatrial mixing of blood by balloon septostomy followed by inserting a systemic-to-pulmonary artery shunt to enhance pulmonary blood flow. A transventricular opening into the pulmonary artery is done in addition to the anastomosis to reduce right ventricular pressure and to increase flow through the right ventricle and thus ventricular growth. Later, in childhood, reconstruction of the right ventricular outflow tract should be done and may require the insertion of a right ventricle-to-pulmonary artery conduit. In some patients, the small right ventricle does not grow and a Fontan operation, as described for the treatment of tricuspid atresia, will be needed for definitive palliation.

Tetralogy of Fallot

Pathophysiology and Diagnosis. This complex defect consists of pulmonary valvular and/or infundibular stenosis and a ventricular septal defect (Fig. 19-11). The stenosis is of such severity and the ventricular septal defect so large that pressures in the two ventricles are equal. Shunting of venous blood from the right to the left ventricle along with decreased pulmonary blood flow due to the stenosis accounts for the cyanosis

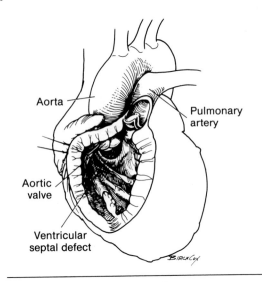

FIGURE 19-11 Tetralogy of Fallot.

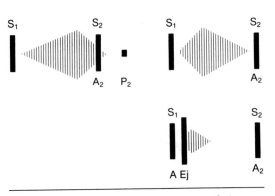

FIGURE 19-12 Murmur and heart sounds in tetralogy of Fallot. *Above, left:* Mild. *Above, right:* Moderate. *Opposite:* Severe. *AEj* = Aortic ejection.

seen in most infants. If the degree of stenosis is mild to moderate, shunting may actually be left-to-right and cyanosis may not occur (acyanotic tetralogy). These patients may live for years without developing symptoms. If the stenosis is moderate to severe, right-to-left shunting is present and cyanosis usually develops within 6 months and progresses. In addition, in older children, squatting, a natural maneuver that increases venous return from the lower extremities and increases systemic resistance and thus more pulmonary blood flow as a result of a relatively lower resistance, may become pronounced. Severe hypoxic episodes resulting from spasm of the infundibulum may develop, which in some cases may be lethal. A systolic murmur is usually heard at the left of the sternum (Fig. 19-12). Chest x-ray films show a "boot-shaped" heart with hypovascular lung fields. Cardiac catheterization and angiography outline the anatomy of the right ventricular infundibulum and ventricular septal defect. Approximately 20% of patients have a right descending aorta and the cranial vessels are reversed, that is, the innominate artery arises from the left side of a right aortic arch. Untreated patients with severe defects experience hypoxic episodes, cerebral infarction, and abscesses, which lead to death.

Operative Treatment. Total correction is recommended for all patients with this anomaly. The ideal age at which to do this is during the first 2 years of life, but infants who are considered too small for total correction and who require palliative surgery undergo either a subclavian-to-pulmonary artery anastomosis called the Blalock-Taussig procedure (see Fig. 19-10) or a modified Blalock-Taussig procedure, in which a prosthetic tube graft of Impra or Gortex is inserted. These palliative procedures increase pulmonary blood flow and arterial oxygenation and allow patients to grow to a size safe for total correction while almost symptom free.

Total correction is performed during cardiopulmonary bypass. The hypertrophied infundibular muscle (parietal and septal bands) is excised and the pulmonary valvular stenosis is relieved. This corrects the obstruction to pulmonary blood flow. The ventricular septal defect is then closed with a patch. At time, the outflow tract of the right ventricle is further enlarged with a gusset of pericardium or prosthetic material. Mortality has ranged from 5% to 10% for total correction with or without previous shunts and long-term results after repair have been excellent.

Transposition of the Great Arteries

Pathophysiology and Diagnosis. The aorta with its coronary arteries arises from the right ventricle, and the pulmonary artery arises from the left ventricle. Venous blood enters the right side of the heart and is immediately ejected into the aorta and systemic circulation (Fig. 19-13). Blood from the pulmonary veins enters the left atrium in the usual fashion and is pumped from the left ventricle into the pulmonary artery and lungs. An atrial septal defect, ventricular septal defect, or patent ductus arteriosus must be present to permit intracardiac mixing; otherwise, death results.

Cyanosis is usually marked, and a chest x-ray film shows varying degrees of pulmonary vascular congestion and an enlarged heart. Pulmonary

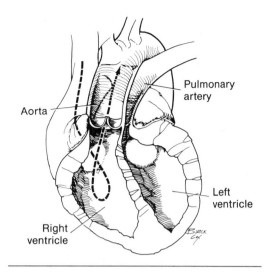

FIGURE 19-13 Transposition of the great arteries.

stenosis is present in approximately 5% of cases, and lung markings may be decreased when this is present. A murmur may not be heard, but, in some patients, it is short and harsh over the precordium. Cardiac catheterization and angiocardiography show marked desaturation and the immediate ejection of contrast medium through the aorta when it is injected into the right ventricle. Mortality is high (80%) in the first months of life, especially in infants with only a patent foramen ovale. Fifty percent of the patients die within 6 months if untreated, congestive heart failure being the most common cause.

Operative Treatment. In the past palliation in infancy was designed to ensure adequate atrial mixing, by either balloon atrial septostomy or the Blalock-Hanlon procedure if the atrial defect is small. In the balloon atrial septostomy, a balloon on a catheter is inflated in the left atrium and pulled across the foramen ovale, leaving the septum primum. In the Blalock-Hanlon operation, the septum is excised. These procedures were designed to allow the child to reach approximately 6 months of age, at which time a total repair can be performed. Infants with ventricular septal defects are prone to develop early pulmonary hypertension, so total correction must be performed before this occurs. Recatheterization at 4 to 6 months is indicated to monitor pulmonary artery pressure.

Total correction by an atrial switch operation is designed to transpose the venous return to the heart. A piece of pericardium is used as an intraatrial baffle to divert blood from the superior vena cava and the inferior vena cava to the mitral valve orifice (Mustard procedure). In the Senning procedure a similar result is achieved by the use of atrial flaps. Vena caval blood is thus rerouted through the mitral valve to the left ventricle, pulmonary arteries, lungs, pulmonary veins, left atrium, over the pericardial baffle to the right atrium, right ventricle, and aorta. Mortality is about 5% for total repair and 10% for patients with large ventricular septal defects. Late results, although it is too soon (15 to 20 years) to be sure, have been fair. Significant atrial dysrhythmias secondary to the removal of the atrial system have been troublesome.

Patients with ventricular septal defects (to allow adequate mixing) and pulmonary stenosis (to protect the lungs from pulmonary hypertension) have survived the longest. These infants may have decreased pulmonary blood flow and thus may require a systemic-to-pulmonary artery shunt. Total correction is done in childhood by placing a baffle in the right ventricle to allow the left ventricle to empty through the ventricu-

lar septal defect into the pulmonary artery. The pulmonary artery is ligated and reconstructed by placing a conduit between the right ventricle and the pulmonary artery (Rastelli procedure).

Today transposition of the great arteries is corrected by an arterial switch operation in which the aorta is transferred to the pulmonary root and the pulmonary artery is transferred to the aortic root (Fig. 19-14). The coronary ostia, including a button of aortic wall, are also reimplanted into the new aortic root (Jatene operation). This operation requires that the left ventricle remain thick-walled (e.g., at birth; with pulmonary artery hypertension with a ventricular septal defect; after preliminary pulmonary artery banding) so that it can sustain systemic pressure. This operation is now performed in neonates and infants, with a mortality of 5% to 10%. Long-term follow-up is not available as yet, although intermediate-length follow-up (10 years) data are excellent.

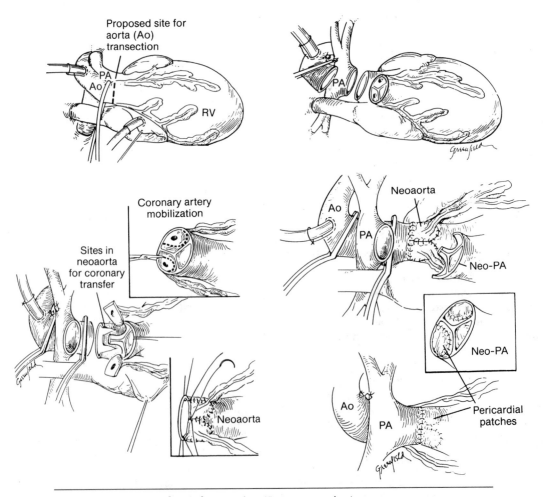

FIGURE 19-14   Arterial switch operation (Jatene operation).

Ebstein's Malformation

Pathophysiology and Diagnosis. The posterior and septal leaflets of the tricuspid valve are displaced downward in the right ventricle. A part of the ventricle becomes thin walled and "atrialized." The valve is usually incompetent.

Patients may live asymptomatically for years but eventually develop cyanosis as a result of a right-to-left shunt across an ostium secundum atrial septal defect, or they develop symptoms of tricuspid insufficiency (right-sided heart failure).

Operative Treatment. Closure of the atrial septal defect and plication of the atrialized portion of the right ventricle is the operation of choice, especially in combination with an annuloplasty of the tricuspid valve to establish valve competence. In some patients replacement of the abnormal valve with a prosthesis is required.

Hypoplastic Left Heart Syndrome

Pathophysiology and Diagnosis. HLHS consists of a number of defects that result in left-sided heart hypoplasia and/or severe obstruction of output on the left side of the heart. The typical patient with hypoplastic left heart syndrome has severe hypoplasia of the mitral valve, left ventricle, and aortic valve. Systemic flow is maintained by right-to-left shunting at the ductus arteriosus. Blood flows retrograde into the aortic arch and down the hypoplastic ascending aorta to supply the coronary arteries. Pulmonary venous return shunts from left to right at the atrial level through the foramen ovale (Fig. 19-15).

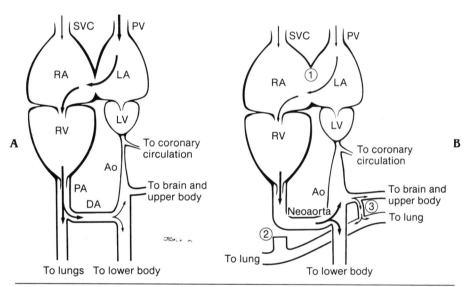

FIGURE 19-15 Physiologic schematic of the heart and central circulation in hypoplastic left heart syndrome (HLHS). **A,** Unoperated: Branched arrows, their thickness approximately proportional to the volume of blood flow, indicate division of flow into parallel circulations in which perfusion depends on relative resistances. Pulmonary veins *(PV),* left atrium *(LA),* left ventricle *(LV),* superior vena cava *(SVC),* right atrium *(RA),* right ventricle *(RV),* pulmonary artery *(PA),* ductus arteriosus *(DA),* and aorta *(Ao)* are depicted schematically as labeled. **B,** After Norwood stage I palliation: As in A, arrow thickness is approximately proportional to the usual blood flow; PA and DA have been replaced by neoaorta (Neo-Ao). The three components of the procedure are as follows: *(1)* an atrial septectomy, which ensures unrestricted PV return, thereby protecting the pulmonary vasculature from high venous pressure, which would prevent its normal development. *(2)* Division of the main PA with anastomosis of proximal PA to Ao (addition of pulmonary homograft material augments the native tissue; the appropriately sized neoaortic arch provides the unobstructed ventricular outflow necessary for good ventricular function and systemic perfusion). *(3)* Construction of a (modified Blalock-Taussig) systemic to PA shunt, which establishes the controlled pulmonary blood flow essential for adequate oxygenation and normal maturation of the pulmonary vasculature. (From Karl D. Anesthesiology 74(4), 1990. With permission.)

After birth the ductus arteriosus usually begins to close. This severely limits systemic flow and causes hypoperfusion and acidosis which leads to death. Administration of prostaglandin E_1 to maintain ductal patency and sodium bicarbonate to reverse acidosis are required to resuscitate the patient.

Diagnosis of the syndrome is made using two-dimensional echocardiography.

Operative Treatment. The three objectives of surgical palliation of hypoplastic left heart syndrome are (1) resection of the atrial septum to allow unrestricted flow for pulmonary venous return from the left atrium to the right atrium, (2) reconstruction of the aortic arch and incorporation of the divided proximal main pulmonary artery into the ascending aorta, and (3) control of pulmonary blood flow by the creation of a modified Blalock-Taussig systemic to pulmonary artery shunt with a 3.5 mm to 4 mm Gortex tube graft (see Fig. 19-15). This procedure, the Norwood operation, is performed using deep

hypothermia and total circulatory arrest (Fig. 19-16). Mortality varies from 30% to 50%.

These patients have single-ventricle physiology and need a Fontan operation for definitive palliation, usually at 1 to 2 years of age.

DEFECTS ASSOCIATED WITH OBSTRUCTION
Coarctation of the Aorta

Pathophysiology and Diagnosis. Coarctation of the aorta is usually caused by a localized narrowing distal to the origin of the left subclavian artery and occurs at the insertion of the ductus (juxtaductal coarctation). The majority of coarctations are discrete diaphragmatic types of obstructions, but a small percentage are long hypoplastic segments. The obstruction to blood flow encourages the development of collateral circulation to convey blood around the obstruction to the lower part of the body (Fig. 19-17). In some infants this collateral circulation does not

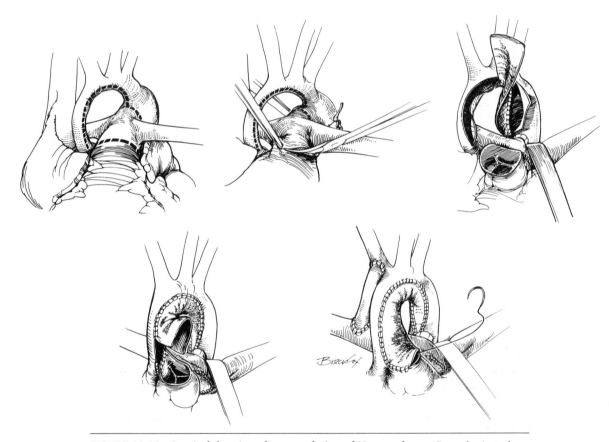

FIGURE 19-16 Surgical drawing after completion of Norwood stage I repair. Anterior view of the heart with hypoplastic aortic root, divided main PA, neoaorta and shunt between the brachiocephalic and right pulmonary arteries.

develop and flow past the coarctation; however, it is maintained by flow through the mouth of a patent ductus arteriosis. Ductal closure results in hypoperfusion of the lower body, acidosis, and congestive heart failure.

A harsh systolic murmur is best heard at the angle of the scapula. The patient will have upper extremity hypertension and weak or absent femoral pulses. In older children, chest x-ray films may show rib notches caused by enlarged collateral intercostal arteries. Catheterization and angiocardiography show increased pressure proximal to the coarctation and a discrete area of narrowing. Approximately 20% of patients have a congenital bicuspid aortic valve. Many patients are asymptomatic for years, but the ideal age for operation is in infancy or before congestive heart failure and hypertension occur.

Preductal coarctations are located proximal to the entrance of the ductus into the aorta and are usually associated with isthmus narrowing. When the ductus is patent, blood from the pulmonary artery empties directly into the descending aorta and may cause lower body cyanosis. Pulmonary hypertension develops with progressive congestive failure. Closure of the ductus will cause decreased blood flow to the kidneys and lower body, resulting in acidosis and a further increase in congestive heart failure. There is a 70% incidence of associated cardiac anomalies in patients with coarctation who develop symptoms in the first few months of life.

Operative Treatment. The basic problem in children with isolated coarctation is obstruction to the outflow path of blood from the left ventricle. Surgical repair is designed to remove this obstruction. The operation of choice is resection of the coarcted segment of aorta and end-to-end anastomosis. Mortality is about 2%. Approximately 5% of patients require replacement of the resected area with a prosthesis (tubular graft).

For the repair of coarctations in infants with congestive heart failure, mortality has been high. This is attributable to the small size and ex-

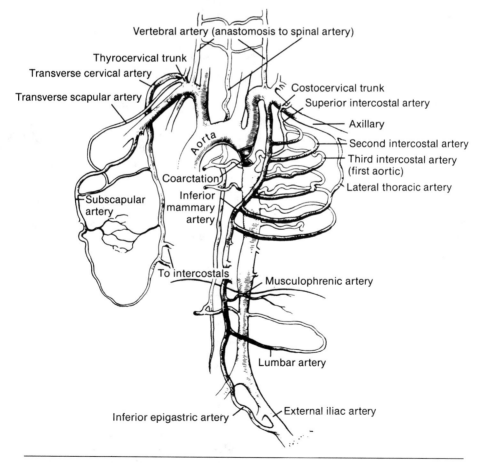

FIGURE 19-17 The collateral circulation in coarctation of the aorta. (From Claget D. Surg Gyn Obstet 98:103, 1954. By permission of Surgery, Gynecology, and Obstetrics.)

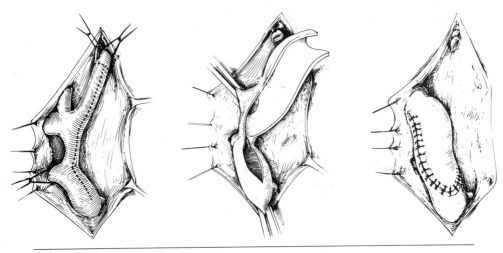

FIGURE 19-18 Repair of the coarctation using a subclavian flap.

tremely poor condition of these infants as well as to associated lesions. Infusion of prostaglandins to maintain preoperative patency of the ductus and thus distal aortic perfusion has drastically reduced the operative mortality in these infants. Resection and end-to-end anastomosis has incurred a 30% incidence of restenosis at the suture line. Alternatively, the subclavian flap procedure, in which the divided proximal subclavian artery is turned down and sutured into the widely opened isthmus of the aorta, including the area of coarctation, has excellent immediate and long-term results with few recurrences of stenosis (Fig. 19-18).

Aortic Stenosis

Pathophysiology and Diagnosis. The defect may occur (1) in the ascending aorta as a hypoplastic segment (supravalvular), (2) at the valve level with fusion of the commissures (valvular), (3) below the valve as a discrete fibrous membrane (subvalvular), and (4) as a diffuse muscular hypertrophy of the left ventricular chamber (idiopathic hypertrophic subaortic stenosis) (Fig. 19-19). The basic defect is obstruction to flow of blood with an increase in pressure and hypertrophy of the left ventricle.

A loud systolic murmur is heard at the right of the sternum in the second interspace (Fig. 19-20). The chest x-ray film and electrocardiogram show left ventricular hypertrophy. Symptoms may occur in infancy and progress, requiring immediate operation. More commonly, signs of left ventricular failure are gradual and take years to develop, even though a small number

of patients die suddenly, probably from ventricular fibrillation. Operation is indicated once angina, syncope, or left ventricular failure occurs, but in children these symptoms are rare. T-wave changes in the electrocardiogram and evidence of high left ventricular pressure are the most common indications for surgical intervention.

Operative Treatment. Infants who are in a state of severe failure are considered surgical emergencies and are operated on immediately. In general, older children with gradients above 50 mm Hg across the obstruction are operated on with the use of cardiopulmonary bypass. Valvular stenosis is corrected by incising the fused commissure, while being careful not to incise any partially formed commissure and thus prevent the occurrence of postoperative aortic valve incompetence. For the long term, many of these patients will require an aortic valve replacement. Subvalvular stenoses are corrected by resecting the discrete membrane or muscle causing the obstruction. Supravalvular narrowings are enlarged by inserting patch grafts of prosthetic material. Mortality is about 2% for all repairs, but it is much higher in small infants in whom the aortic valve is often poorly developed. In patients with diffuse idiopathic hypertrophic subaortic stenosis, two parallel septal myotomies and an excision of the intervening muscle have given good results.

Pulmonary Stenosis

Pathophysiology and Diagnosis. Obstruction may occur (1) at the valve level with fusion

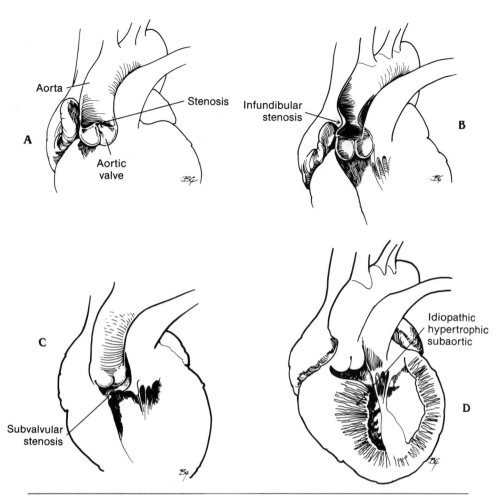

FIGURE 19-19 Aortic stenosis. **A,** Supravalvular. **B,** Valvular. **C,** Membranous subvalvular. **D,** Idiopathic hypertrophic subaortic. (From Johnson's Surgery of the Chest, 5th ed. Chicago, Year Book Medical Publishers, 1985.)

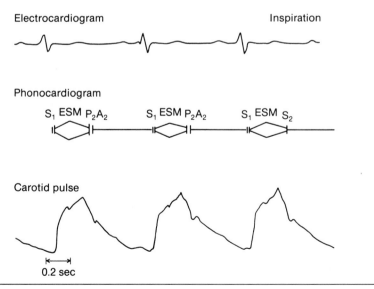

FIGURE 19-20 Phonocardiogram and carotid pulse pressure changes in severe aortic stenosis.

of the commissures (Fig. 19-21), (2) distal to the valve in the main pulmonary artery or its branches, or (3) in the right ventricle by hypertrophied muscle in the infundibulum. The latter form of stenosis is almost always associated with a ventricular septal defect. The resulting effect is increased right ventricular pressure with right ventricular hypertrophy. When the pressure becomes extremely high, blood may shunt from the right to left atrium through a patent foramen ovale, with resulting cyanosis. A prominent systolic murmur is heard in the left second intercostal space near the sternum (Fig. 19-22). In valvular stenosis, poststenotic dilation of the pulmonary artery (resulting from turbulent flow through the deformed valve) may be seen on the chest x-ray film. Cardiac catheterization and angiography demonstrate high right ventricular pressure and the location of the obstruction.

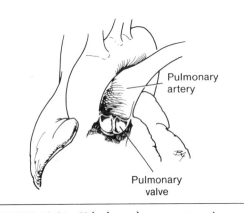

FIGURE 19-21   Valvular pulmonary stenosis.

Operative Treatment. Patients with right ventricular pressures of 70 mm Hg or higher are advised to have surgery. Most procedures are performed with the patient on cardiopulmonary bypass and consist of incising the fused commissures (pure valvular stenosis) or resecting muscle from the right ventricle (infundibular stenosis). Mortality is 1% to 2%. Associated atrial or ventricular septal defects are closed at the time of correction. Occasionally valvular pulmonary stenosis causes severe symptoms, especially of congestive heart failure in infancy, and emergency operation is required. A closed transventricular valvotomy is performed. More recently, patients with valvular pulmonary stenosis undergo pulmonary valvuloplasty using balloon dilation in the cardiac catheterization laboratory.

Congenital Mitral Valve Disease

Pathophysiology and Diagnosis. Congenital lesions are rare and are commonly associated with endocardial fibroelastosis. A leaflet may be thickened, the commissures fused, and the chordae tendinae thickened and short. Either stenosis or insufficiency or a combination of the two may result. Symptoms and findings are similar to those found in adults with mitral valve disease.

Operative Treatment. Annuloplasty with narrowing of the annulus of the mural leaflet is the operation of choice for mitral insufficiency. Valve replacement similar to that used in adults is resorted to only if valvuloplasty fails. Xenograft valves rapidly calcify in children and are not used in the mitral position. Surgical intervention should not be considered unless symptoms are

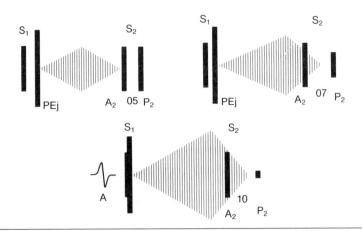

FIGURE 19-22   Characteristics of murmurs in pulmonic stenosis. *Above, left:* Mild. *Above, right:* Moderate. *Center:* Severe. *PEj* = Pulmonary ejection.

significant, at which point most small children have large enough hearts to accept the small prosthetic valves used in adults.

Heart Block

Occasionally, during the repair of such congenital defects as ventricular septal defect or tetralogy of Fallot, the bundle of His, which conducts the impulse that causes the heart to beat, is injured. When this occurs, temporary mechanical pacing is necessary. An electrode is placed in the right ventricle or sutured to the anterior wall of the heart and is attached to an external battery-operated pulse generator to stimulate the heart. If the heart block persists, the pacemaker battery is inserted subcutaneously for permanent pacing.

Aneurysms of Sinus of Valsalva

Pathophysiology and Diagnosis. These defects occur in the sinus that is formed by the attachment of the aortic annulus to the wall of the aorta. When there is a separation of the annulus from the aortic wall, the resulting aneurysm may rupture into either the right atrium, the right ventricle, or, rarely, the left side of the heart. Rapid runoff of blood occurs during systole and diastole, with a resultant increased pulmonary flow. A continuous murmur can be heard, and cardiac catheterization reveals a step-up in the oxygenation of blood in the chamber into which the fistula empties. If the tract is large, progressive symptoms of congestive failure occur.

Operative Treatment. Once the diagnosis is established, operative intervention is indicated, since operative mortality is less than 5%. Correction is undertaken using cardiopulmonary bypass. The site of rupture of the aneurysm (right atrium or ventricle) is identified, the aneurysm excised, and the tract is closed by direct suture or patch graft.

Coronary Arteriovenous Fistula

Pathophysiology and Diagnosis. A branch of the coronary artery empties directly into the pulmonary artery, right ventricle, right atrium, left atrium, or vena cava. Thus a tract from high to low pressure is formed, producing a left-to-right shunt. A continuous murmur is present, and catheterization shows a step-up in oxygen saturation in the chamber into which the artery enters. In addition to symptoms of a left-to-right shunt, patients may have evidence of myocardial ischemia as a result of poor blood supply to the ventricle because of the rapid runoff of blood through the fistula.

Operative Treatment. The fistula should be ligated as close as possible to the low-pressure chamber.

Origin of Left Coronary Artery From Pulmonary Artery

Pathophysiology and Diagnosis. The left coronary artery arises from the pulmonary artery, which is in a low-pressure system. Accordingly, blood supplied by the right coronary artery flows from the coronary artery into the pulmonary artery. Symptoms occur in the first few months of life and consist of heart failure with electrocardiographic findings of ischemia or myocardial infarction.

Operative Treatment. Traditional treatment consists of ligating the vessel at its entrance into the pulmonary artery. However, now the preferred method is reconstruction by implanting the left coronary artery directly into the aorta.

Arch Anomalies: Vascular Rings

Pathophysiology and Diagnosis. The aortic arch may develop abnormally and produce vessels that encircle the trachea and esophagus. Double aortic arch, one developing anterior to the trachea and one posterior to the esophagus, may connect and form a ring around these structures. A right aortic arch with a segment behind the esophagus may attach to the ligamentum arteriosum (remnant of ductus) to form a circle. Dysphagia, obstructed respiratory sounds, and recurrent pulmonary infections are frequent findings. Diagnosis is most readily made with a barium esophagogram that shows the indentation of the esophagus by the abnormal artery. Injection of a contrast medium into the aorta aids in identifying the anatomy and is occasionally necessary before operation.

Operative Treatment. Many patients with vascular rings are asymptomatic and require no operation. If symptoms are present, operative division of the ring is indicated at a site that will not compromise blood flow to a vital structure.

Corrected Transposition of the Great Arteries

Pathophysiology and Diagnosis. The aorta originates from a posterior ventricle that has a tricuspid valve (morphology of the normal right ventricle). The pulmonary artery originates from an anterior ventricle with a mitral valve (morphology of the normal left ventricle). Systemic and pulmonary venous drainage is normal. The anatomic situation is not hemodynamically abnormal, but additional lesions, such as ventricular septal defect and pulmonary stenosis, are common. Insufficiency of the systemic atrioventricular valve is also common, probably because the tricuspid valve is less able to withstand the systemic ventricular pressure than is a mitral valve. Associated lesions determine symptoms. There is a tendency for the onset of A-V dissociation, leading to heart block and syncope. Fatal episodes have occurred.

Operative Treatment. Repair of septal defects and pulmonary stenosis in these patients has been accompanied by a high incidence of complete heart block. Placement of a valve prosthesis to replace the systemic atrioventricular valve is often required for valve insufficiency.

BIBLIOGRAPHY

Bane AE, Geha AS, Hammond GL, et al. Glenn's Thoracic and Cardiovascular Surgery, 5th ed. Norwalk, CT, Appleton & Lange, 1991.

Keith JD, Rowe RD, Vlad P. Heart Disease in Infancy and Childhood, 3rd ed. New York, Macmillan, 1978.

Kirklin JW, Barratt-Boyes BG. Cardiac Surgery. New York, John Wiley & Sons, 1986.

Sabiston DC Jr, Spencer FC. Gibbon's Surgery of the Chest, 5th ed. Philadelphia, WB Saunders, 1991.

Stark J, deLeval M. Surgery for Congenital Heart Defects. London, Grune & Stratton, 1983.

Waldhausen JA, Pierce WS. Johnson's Surgery of the Chest, 5th ed. Chicago, Year Book Medical Publishers, 1985.

CHAPTER REVIEW
Questions

1. Congenital heart disease in infants often presents with one or more of the following symptoms or findings except:
   a. Cyanosis
   b. Shortness of breath
   c. Hemoptysis
   d. Hepatomegaly
   e. Failure to thrive

2. All of the following lesions but one have a right-to-left shunt in the presence of normal pulmonary vascular resistance:
   a. Tetralogy of Fallot
   b. Ventricular septal defect
   c. Tricuspid atresia
   d. Pulmonic stenosis and atrial septal defect
   e. Complete atrioventricular canal

3. The basic hemodynamic disturbance in congenital lesions with a left-to-right shunt is:
   a. Increased pulmonary blood flow
   b. Right ventricular failure
   c. Left ventricular failure

4. A 1-week-old, severely cyanotic infant presenting to the emergency room is likely to have:
   a. Aortic stenosis or partial anomalous pulmonary venous drainage with atrial septal defect
   b. Transposition of the great vessels, tetralogy of Fallot, or truncus arteriosus
   c. Coronary A-V fistula or pulmonary stenosis

5. Tetralogy of Fallot includes all but one of the following lesions:
   a. Ventricular septal defect
   b. Pulmonic stenosis
   c. Hypoplastic left ventricle
   d. Overriding aorta
   e. Right ventricular hypertrophy

6. Usual signs of congestive heart failure in the infant include all but:
   a. Sweating
   b. Tachycardia
   c. Hepatomegaly
   d. Tachypnea
   e. Pulmonary rales

7. Respiratory obstruction commonly attends:
   a. Pulmonic stenosis
   b. Pulmonary hypertension
   c. Tricuspid atresia
   d. Double aortic arch

Answers

1. c
2. b
3. a
4. b
5. c
6. e
7. d

20 Acute and Chronic Chest Pain of Cardiovascular Origin

BRIAN L. GANZEL
LAMAN A. GRAY, Jr.

KEY FEATURES

After reading this chapter you will understand:
- Angina and coronary artery disease, including origin, diagnosis, and treatment.
- The operative treatment for coronary artery disease and the results.
- Treatment for an acute myocardial infarction.
- The use of ventricular assist devices.
- Diseases of the pericardium.
- Aortic aneurysms and dissections, including operative and nonoperative management.
- Diagnosis and treatment of a pulmonary embolus.

ISCHEMIC HEART DISEASE
What Are the Symptoms of Ischemic Heart Disease?

Ischemic heart disease is the leading cause of death in the United States. More than 600,000 deaths result from myocardial infarction (MI) each year. The disease is most prevalent in men over 40, and more than half of the men affected with the disease die before the age of 65. *Angina pectoris (chest pain) is the hallmark symptom of ischemic heart disease.*

Angina occurs when the blood supply to the heart does not provide adequate oxygen to the myocardium. Lactic acid and other metabolites accumulate within the myocardium until their concentrations are significant enough to stimulate sympathetic nerves and produce pain. The most common cause of decreased blood supply to the myocardium is obstruction of one or more of the coronary arteries with atheromatous plaques. Coronary arteriosclerosis develops principally in the proximal portions of the major vessels. Distally the vessels are almost always patent. This segmental localization of disease is the pathophysiologic basis for bypass grafting.

Chest pain from myocardial ischemia usually begins retrosternally and frequently spreads across the front of the left side of the chest. It is described as a tight, bandlike, heavy, or crushing feeling and may radiate to the jaw, through to the back, or to one or both arms. The pain is provoked by exertion or emotional strain that increases the work of the heart and thus increases the oxygen demand of the myocardium. When the blood supply is compromised to a greater degree, angina may occur while the patient is at rest or terminate in a myocardial infarction. Angina generally subsides within 3 to 5 minutes following cessation of work or even more promptly with the use of sublingual nitroglycerin. Patients with angina are at risk for a myocardial infarction or sudden death. Myocardial infarction may occur during periods of increased exercise, at rest, or even during sleep, which illustrates the very complex nature of the disease.

Natural History

The natural history of coronary artery disease (CAD) can be followed by studying either its signs or symptoms, such as angina or myocardial infarction, or by studying the angiographic appearance of the coronary arteries. The non-

349

angiographic investigation in the well-known Framingham study showed that angina in men resulted in a 4% yearly mortality, whether it arose de novo or in conjunction with a myocardial infarction. Age did not influence survival in this group of patients. The study showed that 1 in 4 men with angina could expect a coronary attack within 5 years; the risk for women was half that. The probability of a coronary attack within 8 years after the onset of angina was about 50% in men over age 45, a risk twice that of the general population. The annual mortality of those patients in the Framingham study who suffered a nonfatal myocardial infarction was 5%. A similar noninvasive study in Sweden showed that 13% of men with a first infarction and 37% of men with recurrent infarctions died within 2 years.

A number of studies of the natural history of CAD, based on the angiographic findings at cardiac catheterization from such centers as the University of Alabama, the Johns Hopkins Hospital, the Cleveland Clinic, and Kingston (Ontario) Hospital, showed that if only one of the three major coronary arteries had more than a 50% stenosis, the annual mortality rate was approximately 3%. If two of the three major arteries were involved, the mortality rate increased to approximately 7%; if all three major vessels were stenotic, mortality rate was 12% per year. High-grade stenosis of the left main coronary artery is much more ominous; the mortality rate rose to approximately 70% at 42 months. In patients with left main lesions, survival rates varied inversely with degree of stenosis. Survival rates were higher for patients with between 50% and 70% stenosis compared with those having over 70% stenosis.

How Is Angina Pectoris Diagnosed?

The physical examination of the patient with angina frequently shows no abnormalities; however, the examination can help to rule out causes of cardiac chest pain other than arteriosclerotic, such as aortic stenosis, severe anemia, cardiac dysrhythmias, or pulmonary hypertension. Since 50% of patients with angina have had no previous infarctions, the ECG may be normal at rest or show nonspecific T-wave depressions, indicating myocardial ischemia. An ECG performed during exercise will show ST depression in 80% of these patients. A radionuclide thallium scan during exercise will be positive in approximately 80% of people with coronary artery disease. Based on the combined studies, a correct

diagnosis of coronary artery disease can be made in 90% of patients (Fig. 20-1).

The only definitive diagnostic procedure is cardiac catheterization, which typically includes selective coronary arteriography and left ventriculography. Cardiac catheterization is performed in a catheterization laboratory. A catheter is introduced into the systemic arterial circuit either percutaneously into the femoral artery or using a cut-down into the brachial artery. The catheter is positioned so that contrast can be injected into the ostia of the coronary arteries (Fig. 20-2). The images are recorded either on photographic film or videotape. Left ventricular function is assessed by passing the catheter retrograde across the aortic valve and injecting contrast into the left ventricular cavity (Fig. 20-3). Multiple views of the coronary arteries and the left ventricle are recorded.

Treatment for Angina Pectoris

In the past few years many advances have been made in the medical management of angina pectoris (see the box on p. 351). Patients are warned to avoid activities that produce angina but are encouraged to perform exercise that does not produce pain to promote collateral coronary blood flow. Important factors in controlling angina are eliminating smoking, maintaining ideal body weight, controlling lipids and cholesterol in the diet, and controlling hypertension and diabetes. Glycerol trinitrate (nitroglycerin, 1/150 of a grain) taken sublingually will rapidly relieve the pain of angina. The drug reduces the cardiac output and the systemic blood pressure and thus the work of the heart for approximately 20 minutes. Nitroglycerin, which should be used liberally before a pain-producing activity is begun, is not addictive and does not lose its efficacy with prolonged use. Long-acting nitrates, such as Isordil, 2.5 mg sublingually three times a day, effectively employ the same mechanisms as nitroglycerin. Nitrol paste strips, 0.5 to 2 inches every 4 hours placed on the skin, may be effective in controlling more progressive angina.

Beta-adrenergic drugs are extremely effective in controlling angina by reducing the oxygen demand of the heart and decreasing the force of myocardial contraction. There are two types of beta blockers, selective and nonselective. The nonselective beta blockers, such as propranolol hydrochloride, inhibit both beta-1 and beta-2 adrenoreceptors. The beta-1 receptors are primarily located in the cardiac muscle and the beta-2 receptors are located in the bronchial and vascular

CANDIDATE SELECTION GUIDELINES FOR PATIENTS WITH ISCHEMIC HEART DISEASE

Medical Therapy Candidates

Patients with nondisabling angina pectoris who are not felt to be candidates for PTCA or CABG

PTCA Candidates

Patients with single- or double-vessel disease with limiting angina pectoris with discrete stenosis amenable to PTCA

or

Significant angina pectoris with lesions amenable to PTCA with a high degree of success

or

Large areas of myocardium at risk with or without significant symptoms

CABG Candidates

Patients with disabling angina pectoris despite medical treatment who are not candidates for PTCA

or

Significant angina pectoris with triple-vessel disease with impaired ventricular function

or

Significant angina pectoris with large areas of potential myocardial jeopardy

or

Critical left main coronary artery stenosis (70% cross-sectional area reduction)

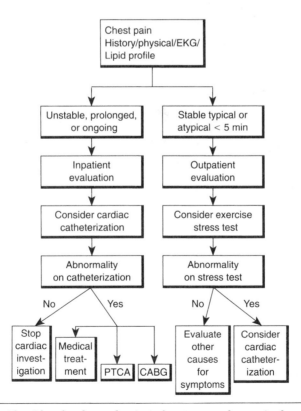

FIGURE 20-1   Algorithm for the evaluation of new onset chest pain thought to be cardiac in origin without evidence of myocardial infarction.

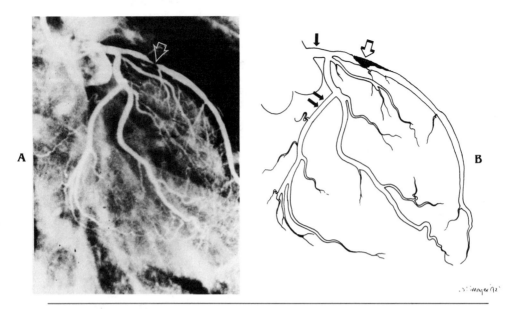

FIGURE 20-2 A, Selective coronary angiogram of the left coronary artery demonstrating a severe stenosis in the left anterior descending coronary artery *(hollow arrow)*. B, Diagram of the angiogram demonstrating a stenosis in the left anterior descending coronary artery *(hollow arrow);* left main coronary artery *(solid arrow);* circumflex artery *(double arrow)*.

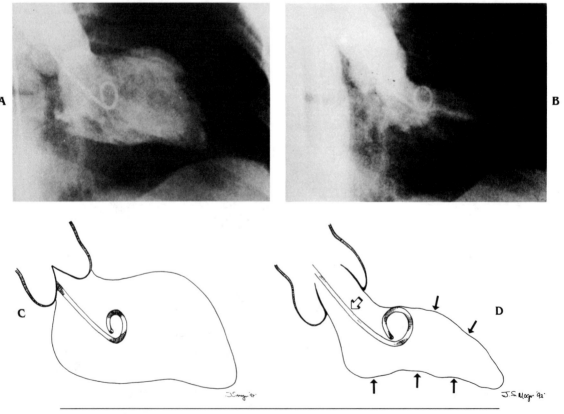

FIGURE 20-3 A, Normal left ventriculogram in the right anterior oblique position with the heart in diastole. B, Left ventriculogram of the same patient with the heart in systole. C, Diagram of the left ventriculogram with the heart in diastole. D, Diagram of the left ventriculogram with the heart in systole. Note the uniform wall motion *(arrows)* and the catheter passing retrograde across the aortic valve *(hollow arrow)*.

musculature. Drugs such as propranolol hydrochloride, given four times a day with a stepwise increase in dosage up to 80 mg four times a day, are very effective in controlling angina. There are side effects, however, which include congestive heart failure and bronchial asthma. The newer selective beta-blocking agents, such as metoprolol tartrate, have a preferential effect on the beta-1 adrenoreceptors located in the cardiac muscle. This preferential effect is not absolute, however, and at higher doses these drugs will also inhibit the beta-2 receptors. The selective beta blockers can be used in patients with compromised pulmonary function because of decreased beta-2 effects.

Calcium channel blockers, such as nifedipine, have become very important in the treatment of angina over the past few years. The calcium channel blockers inhibit the transmembrane influx of calcium ions into cardiac muscle and smooth muscle. The contractile process of these muscles depends on the movement of extracellular calcium ions into the cells through specific ion channels. Calcium channel blockers selectively inhibit calcium ion influx across the cell membrane of cardiac muscle and smooth muscle without changing the serum calcium concentrations. The mechanism of action of this group of drugs is by relaxation and prevention of coronary artery spasm and by reducing oxygen utilization of the cardiac muscle. Nifedipine dilates the main coronary arteries and arterioles both in normal and ischemic regions of the heart muscle and is a potent inhibitor of coronary artery spasm. In addition, it reduces arterial pressure at rest by dilating the peripheral arterioles and reducing the total peripheral vascular resistance against which the heart must beat. This afterload reduction of the heart decreases myocardial oxygen consumption and probably accounts for the effectiveness of the calcium channel blockers in chronic stable angina.

Long-term anticoagulation therapy with warfarin provides no benefit in angina pectoris or myocardial infarction; however, drugs that inhibit platelet function, such as aspirin, do appear to decrease the risk of myocardial infarction in patients with known coronary artery disease.

Percutaneous Transluminal Coronary Angioplasty. In 1976 Gruentzig performed the first coronary angioplasty in Switzerland. Since that time, percutaneous transluminal coronary angioplasty (PTCA) has gained widespread acceptance as a modality for treatment in selected cases. The technique is performed in the catheterization laboratory, where a sterile guidewire is placed in the coronary artery to be dilated. The dilating catheter is then threaded over the guidewire and positioned in the middle of the lesion in the coronary artery. An initial gradient across the stenosis in the coronary artery is measured, then the balloon catheter is inflated one or more times to an inflation pressure ranging from 2 to 12 atmospheres. Once the lesion has been dilated, the gradient across the lesion is remeasured and a contrast medium is again injected into the coronary artery to assess the result. If the post-balloon angiogram is satisfactory, the patient can be discharged from the hospital approximately 2 days later.

The primary indication for percutaneous transluminal angioplasty is angina pectoris causing significant disability to warrant bypass surgery (see the box). The original anatomic indication for selection for an angioplasty was a high-grade discrete stenosis in one dominant vessel. The criteria have been expanded to include two-vessel disease in selected patients. Very rarely, patients with multiple-vessel lesions are candidates for angioplasty.

The primary success rate of performing a balloon angioplasty is approximately 90%. Success is defined as more than a 20% reduction in the stenosis and a reduction of the pressure gradient. Failures usually occur because of intimal dissection or from thrombosis and require emergency surgery. This occurs in less than 5% of angioplasties performed by cardiologists experienced in PTCA. Mortality from performing an angioplasty is approximately 1%. Unfortunately, one third of the people undergoing percutaneous transluminal angioplasty develop recurrent symptoms during the first 3 months. These patients then require either a second balloon angioplasty or surgery.

PTCA is associated with a favorable return-to-work pattern with 98% of patients returning to work following the procedure. The long-term results of balloon angioplasties are not known at this time, but it appears that 30% of patients with coronary artery disease who previously would have been candidates for bypass surgery can now be treated with PTCA.

Surgical Treatment of Angina Pectoris. The indication for coronary artery revascularization is angina that is unresponsive to medical treatment (see the box). The definition of unresponsive to medical management varies with the patient. Obviously there is a difference in the management of a 50-year-old man in his prime working years compared with a man who is 75 and retired. The ideal patient for revascularization is one who has a significant narrowing in the proximal coronary arteries with normal distal vessels and a normal ventricle. More than 90% of all patients with diseased hearts are acceptable for bypass surgery.

A relative contraindication to revascularization is chronic congestive heart failure without associated angina. In this situation, revascularization will not significantly improve ventricular function. The patient has to have angina, or objective evidence of myocardial ischemia, for coronary artery bypass surgery to be beneficial. The operative mortality rate is directly proportional to the left ventricular function and is approximately 2% in patients with normal or slightly impaired ventricles. In patients with a severely impaired left ventricle, however, the risk may increase 6% to 8%.

The selection of the vessels to be bypassed depends on the angiographic findings at the time of catheterization. All vessels with more than a 50% luminal narrowing are bypassed if the distal vessel is adequate to accept a graft. If the vessel bypassed has less than a 50% luminal narrowing, the graft may occlude because of the competition of flow between the bypass and the native vessel. A vessel less than 1.5 mm in diameter cannot support enough flow to keep the graft patent. Therefore, only vessels 1.5 mm or larger are bypassed at the time of surgery. Occasionally the arteriosclerotic process may involve the entire length of the vessel and make it unacceptable for bypass grafting.

Aortocoronary artery bypass grafting is currently the procedure of choice for multivessel ischemic heart disease (Fig. 20-4). A saphenous vein is carefully removed from the leg, dilated under pressure control, and its branches ligated. The patient is then placed on cardiopulmonary bypass, the aorta is cross-clamped, and the heart is arrested with a cold preservative solution in a process known as **cardioplegia.** The use of cardioplegia allows the surgeon to operate on a still, nonbeating heart in a bloodless field. The saphenous vein is then reversed and sutured to the coronary artery distal to the obstruction. Because the vessels are usually 1.5 to 2 mm in diameter, intraoperative magnification is used to facilitate the anastomosis. The proximal end of the vein is then anastomosed to the ascending aorta. The right coronary artery, left anterior descending coronary artery, and circumflex coronary artery are the vessels most commonly bypassed, along with their major branches. It is very common practice to perform four and occasionally five bypasses. When multiple bypasses

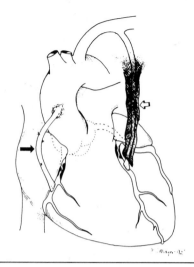

FIGURE 20-4   Coronary artery bypass surgery. *Solid arrow* demonstrates a reversed saphenous vein graft from the aorta inserted distal to an obstruction in the right coronary artery. *Hollow arrow* demonstrates the left internal mammary artery used to bypass a lesion in the left anterior descending coronary artery.

are performed, sequential grafts may be used. In this instance, the end of the saphenous vein is anastomosed end-to-side to a coronary artery, and a second side-to-side anastomosis is performed between the vein graft and a second coronary artery. The proximal vein graft is then sewed to the aorta.

A left internal mammary artery graft to bypass the left anterior descending coronary artery is the conduit of choice (see Fig. 20-4). The patency rate with the use of the left internal mammary artery is 95% at 5 years, whereas the patency rate of vein grafts is only 75% at 5 years. Because of this increased patency rate of the left internal mammary artery, the long-term survival rates are greater in patients who have received this conduit. Therefore the internal mammary artery bypass should be used whenever feasible. Occasionally the internal mammary is significantly smaller than the left anterior descending coronary artery and does not have adequate flow to supply the myocardium, in which case it is not used.

Relief of angina after this procedure is usually dramatic, prompt, and complete in most patients. Approximately 50% of patients are totally asymptomatic and another 40% are dramatically improved following the surgery; 10% of patients are not significantly helped. The degree of postoperative symptoms relates directly to the degree of total myocardial revascularization. If all of the vessels can be revascularized, angina is virtually eliminated. The return of angina suggests occlusion of one or more of the grafts or progression of the disease in the native vessels. The early patency rate of the saphenous vein grafts at 1 year is 85% to 90%. Most of the grafts that close do so within the first 3 to 4 months after surgery. In patients with favorable anatomy, a patency rate of 75% can be expected 5 years after grafting.

One of the major intraoperative complications is myocardial infarction. A major infarction is extremely rare but may result in death during surgery. Small infarctions, however, occur in from 5% to 8% of patients during bypass surgery. These patients are usually asymptomatic and the small infarctions are of no long-term consequence to the patient. They are rarely from intraoperative occlusion of the grafts; rather, they are related to segmental coronary ischemia during cardiopulmonary bypass or areas of the myocardium that could not be revascularized.

Does Coronary Artery Revascularization Prolong Life? Some very impressive figures have become available that indicate that it definitely prolongs life in two- and three-vessel coronary disease. In reviewing a collected series from the literature, the average mortality is 5.9% per year in all patients with angina that is managed medically. A similar review of the surgical literature reveals that the average attrition or mortality is 3% per year following bypass surgery. In six comparable series contrasting the medical versus the surgical attrition rates at the same institution, the annual attrition rate was 6.3% for medically treated patients and 2.8% for surgically treated patients. A composite of several series in the current literature, which gives surgical survival rates after bypass grafting, shows that the annual attrition rate of one-vessel disease following surgery is 1.2%; two-vessel bypasses, 2.3%; and three vessel bypasses, 3.3%. The incidence rate of late myocardial infarction following revascularization is 3% to 4% per year. In a group of 2000 patients randomized between surgical and medical therapy, a definite benefit from surgical intervention was shown in the patients who either had severe left ventricular dysfunction or severe angina with one or two proximal stenoses. Six-year survival was 78% in the surgically treated group and 49% in the medically treated group. With the increasing use of the internal mammary artery graft with its 95% 10-year patency rate, the long-term results for coronary bypass surgery continue to improve.

The evidence that life is prolonged following coronary artery bypass surgery for left main occlusions is unquestionable. Loop and colleagues studied 300 patients with left main coronary artery lesions treated both surgically and medically and found that there is a 5-year survival rate of 88.2% of surgically treated patients, whereas only 51% of the medically treated patients survived 5 years. The 5-year survival rate of 88% in the surgical groups is the same as that expected for 5-year survivals in the life expectancy tables matched for age and sex.

There is excellent presumptive evidence that life is prolonged following coronary artery bypass surgery. If present trends continue, future data will prove that coronary artery bypass in selected patients does indeed prolong life.

What Are the Symptoms of Acute Myocardial Infarction?

Ninety percent of patients suffering an acute MI have chest pain lasting from one half hour to several hours. Ten percent of acute infarctions, especially in elderly persons, are painless. Fifty percent of patients have a past history of progressive or preinfarction angina before the acute infarction. Electrocardiographic abnormalities are present in most patients during an acute myocardial infarction. ST elevation occurs in 95% of patients with the onset of pain and is followed by Q waves in the first few hours. Over the ensuing days, the T waves invert and the ST segments return to the isoelectric line. Laboratory tests are helpful in diagnosing an acute myocardial infarction. They include, in order of increasing specificity, serum glutamate oxaloacetate transaminase (SGOT), serum lactic dehydrogenase (LDH), and serum creatinine phosphokinase (CPK). SGOT increases within the first 12 hours, peaks within 18 to 28 hours, and returns to normal levels within 4 days. Serum LDH increases in 24 to 48 hours, reaches a peak in 3 to 6 days, and returns to normal levels by 8 to 14 days. The LDH isoenzymes are more specific. When fraction one is greater than fraction two, it is highly suggestive of myocardial damage. The CPK becomes elevated within the first 6 to 8 hours, peaks within 24 hours, and returns to normal in 3 to 4 days. Three isoenzymes of CPK have been identified, which include BB isoenzyme primarily in the brain and kidneys, MM isoenzyme primarily in skeletal muscle, and MB isoenzyme primarily in cardiac muscle. An elevation of CPK-MB isoenzyme of greater than 4% is indicative of acute myocardial damage. This will usually become positive 6 to 12 hours after infarction. An isoform of the MM isoenzyme has recently been identified that becomes positive as early as 1 hour following an infarction, which permits early identification of patients with an acute myocardial infarction. The combination of CPK isoenzymes and LDH isoenzymes is more than 90% accurate in the diagnosis of acute MI.

Natural History of Myocardial Infarction

Mortality in patients with an acute myocardial infarction treated in a coronary care unit has declined from approximately 30% to 15% to 20% (Fig. 20-5). The reduction in mortality has resulted from the elimination of primary dysrhythmias as a cause of death. More than 60% of deaths associated with acute infarction occur within the first hour of the event and are attributed to malignant dysrhythmias. The overwhelming majority of these patients do not reach the hospital alive. Careful monitoring of cardiac rhythm and the prompt treatment of dysrhythmias have sharply reduced the instance of in-hospital deaths from dysrhythmias. Today most patients who reach the coronary care units alive but who die later do so from left ventricular failure and shock that occurs within the first 96 hours of the infarction. Ventricular aneurysms occur in up to 13% of patients following infarction; however, clinically significant aneurysms occur much less often. Abnormal papillary muscle function is commonly associated with acute infarction, but rupture of a papillary muscle occurs in only 1% of patients and results in acute

mitral regurgitation. An acute ventricular septal defect occurs in approximately 0.5% of patients. Both papillary muscle rupture and interventricular septal defect are associated with a very high mortality.

Treatment for Myocardial Infarction

The treatment for an acute myocardial infarction has changed over the past few years. After an acute MI there is an area of reversible injured myocardium that surrounds the infarct zone. This area of stunned myocardium depends on the duration and the extent of decreased myocardial blood flow to the area. The peri-infarction zone will regain contractility over a period of several weeks following the infarct. The less severely injured regions may totally regain their peri-ischemic level of function. The prompt reperfusion of the peri-infarction zone is the most important factor related to limiting the size of the infarct and accelerating the recovery of the reversibly injured myocardium. The most severely injured myocardium can benefit from reperfusion if it is performed within the first 2 hours of the infarction. Less severely injured myocardium may have some recovery up to 6 hours after infarction.

Because the peri-infarction zone can recover cardiac function if reperfused within the first 6 hours after infarction, there is great impetus to treat acute MIs very aggressively. This is accomplished by intravenous administration of thrombolytic agents, such as streptokinase or tissue plasminogen activating factor (TPA), within the first 6 hours after infarction. This modality will improve global left ventricular function and reduce mortality from myocardial infarction. Patients who receive systemic thrombolytic therapy should remain on intravenous heparin until coronary angiography is performed within 1 week to identify the underlying coronary anatomy. Percutaneous transluminal balloon angioplasty (PTCA) (see p. 351) or coronary revascularization should be performed at this time to reduce the chance of recurrent myocardial infarctions.

If a skilled cardiac catheterization team is immediately available, the patient with an acute MI of less than 4 hours' duration should be immediately taken to the catheterization laboratory, where the coronary anatomy can be visualized. Depending on the anatomy, either an acute angioplasty can be performed or the patient can be given intracoronary streptokinase or TPA. Results in attaining myocardial reperfusion are more successful when TPA is given by the intracoronary route than when given systemically. If a

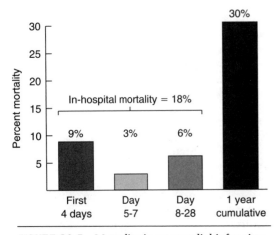

FIGURE 20-5 Mortality in myocardial infarction.

thrombolytic agent is given, the patient should then undergo coronary revascularization approximately 1 week later. Emergency coronary artery revascularization can be performed successfully in patients following a myocardial infarction if done within the first 4 to 6 hours of the onset of pain. It is logistically difficult to bring these patients to the hospital, carry out clinical evaluation, perform coronary angiography, assemble the surgical team, and place the patient on cardiopulmonary bypass in less than 4 hours. Coronary revascularization should be avoided unless the patient is unstable between 6 and 48 hours after infarction because of increased operative mortality.

In addition to these invasive procedures, medical therapy with nitrates, calcium antagonists, beta blockers, and antiplatelet agents should routinely be employed for patients following acute myocardial infarction.

Not all patients are candidates for thrombolytic therapy. Either they are seen by the physician for medical care too late in the course of their infarction, or they have a contraindication to the use of thrombolytic therapy. Bleeding is the most common complication of thrombolytic therapy and patients at risk for bleeding (i.e., by age, prior history of stroke, peptic ulcer disease,

or recent trauma or surgery) are not candidates. Such patients are treated medically with nitrates, calcium antagonists, beta blockers, and antiplatelet drugs. Further investigation and treatment are determined by the presence or absence of symptoms and the results of noninvasive and invasive testing (Fig. 20-6).

VENTRICULAR ANEURYSMS
Etiology and Diagnosis

Ventricular aneurysms occur subsequent to transmural myocardial infarction in 8% to 15% of patients. The aneurysm is first an acute akinetic area of the myocardium. This area can develop a mixed fibrosis and muscle pattern or evolve into a chronic fibrous aneurysm. The mixed pattern of myocardial fibrosis is usually diffuse, is rarely found in an isolated area, and is seen as an area of akinesis on the left ventriculogram. Chronic fibrotic aneurysms are the type most often treated by surgery. They are usually large and consist of thin-walled scar tissue, which causes a paradoxical expansion of the aneurysmal sac during systole. This drastically reduces the efficiency of the left ventricular contraction, not only by the loss of actively contracting muscle but also because of the ventricular

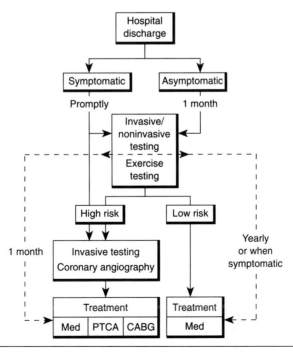

FIGURE 20-6 Guidelines for treatment of patients who have had uncomplicated myocardial infarctions and who are not thought to be candidates for thrombolytic therapy.

volume, which is lost to systemic ejection. The heart incurs severe mechanical disadvantages with the paradox. When 20% of the surface area of the left ventricle is involved in aneurysmal formation, adequate stroke volume and cardiac output cannot be maintained, resulting in congestive heart failure. Ventricular aneurysms occur 20 times more frequently in the left ventricle than in the right ventricle. Approximately two thirds occur in the left ventricular anteroseptal region. The next most common location is the posterior or diaphragmatic segment. This area is involved in from 15% to 30% of patients with aneurysms.

Complications of ventricular aneurysms include recurrent congestive heart failure, angina pectoris, arrhythmias, and episodes of peripheral emboli from clots formed from mural thrombus within the aneurysm.

Chest x-ray evaluation may show cardiac enlargement. Cardiac catheterization discloses segmental enlargement in the left ventricular cavity with dyskinetic movement (Fig. 20-7). Left ventricular end-diastolic pressure will be elevated. Because of the frequency of significant multivessel coronary artery disease, it is essential to study the coronary artery anatomy in these patients using selective coronary arteriography.

The 5-year survival rate of patients with large, untreated left ventricular aneurysms, secondary to myocardial infarction, is only 25%.

Operative Treatment for Ventricular Aneurysms

Current indications for surgery include recurrent congestive heart failure, angina pectoris, intract-

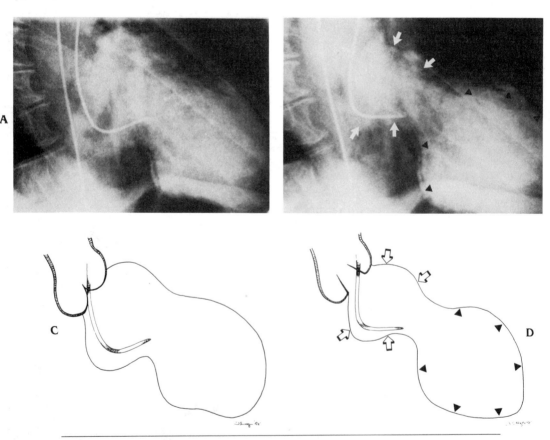

FIGURE 20-7   **A,** Left ventriculogram of a patient with a large anteroapical left ventricular aneurysm with the heart in diastole. **B,** Left ventriculogram in the same patient with the heart in systole. ***Black arrows*** demonstrate the area of dyskinesia. ***White arrows*** point to the normally contracting segments of myocardium. **C,** Diagram of the left ventriculogram with the heart in diastole. **D,** Diagram of the left ventriculogram with the heart in systole. ***Black arrows*** outline the area of dyskinesia. ***Hollow arrows*** point to the normally contracting segments of myocardium.

able ventricular dysrhythmias, and recurrent episodes of peripheral emboli. Operation is deferred for 6 weeks after the acute infarction to allow as much healing as possible. If an operation is performed too soon after an acute infarction, the myocardium is very friable and does not hold sutures well. The goal of surgery for ventricular aneurysms is to excise the area of scar tissue and to approximate the viable areas of myocardium, thereby obliterating the paradox. If there is any significant coronary artery disease in an area of myocardium not involved in the aneurysm, these vessels are bypassed. Mortality for excision of a ventricular aneurysm, with or without coronary artery revascularization, is less than 10%. The long-term results reported have been excellent.

LEFT VENTRICULAR ASSIST DEVICES

During the past few decades the use of mechanical support of the failing heart has moved from the experimental laboratory to clinical practice. All types of ventricular assist devices serve to improve the myocardial oxygen supply versus demand ratio while supporting the systemic circulation.

The Intra-Aortic Balloon Pump

The most common left ventricular assist device used is the intra-aortic balloon pump (Fig. 20-8). A dual-chambered balloon catheter is inserted into the femoral artery and positioned in the descending aorta, just distal to the left subclavian artery. The balloon is then triggered by the electrocardiogram to inflate during diastole and deflate during systole. The balloon is timed to inflate just after the closing of the aortic valve. This inflation displaces approximately 35 ml of blood toward the closed aortic valve, increasing the mean diastolic perfusion pressure and coronary blood flow. The balloon is then deflated just before systole, allowing the blood to return to the space previously occupied by the inflated balloon. This decreases the afterload on the heart and decreases the pressure the ventricle has to exert on the aortic valve to initiate ejection, thus reducing left ventricular work (Fig. 20-9).

Present indications for the insertion of an intra-aortic balloon pump include patients with postmyocardial infarction cardiogenic shock; postmyocardial infarction ventricular irritability refractory to medical management; postmyocardial infarction ventricular septal defects or mitral regurgitation that require hemodynamic stabilization before surgery; ongoing myocardial ischemia refractory to maximum medical management; and left ventricular failure following cardiopulmonary bypass.

Other Ventricular Assist Devices

Over the past few years ventricular assist devices (VAD) that can completely support the circulation of a patient in cardiogenic shock have been developed and are under experimental investigation in a number of centers in the United States. There are currently two indications for the use of such devices. The first is for postcardiotomy cardiogenic shock following cardiac operations on patients who cannot be weaned from cardiopulmonary bypass because of left ventricular failure. Temporary ventricular assistance may allow for the recovery of the native heart. The second indication is as a bridge to transplantation in patients who have already been accepted as heart transplant candidates but who suffer progressive left ventricular deterioration refractory to maximal medical therapy. These patients benefit from ventricular support until a donor organ can be found.

The criteria for insertion of ventricular assist devices include failure of maximum medical therapy of cardiogenic shock including volume infusion, pharmacological support, and counterpulsation using the intra-aortic balloon pump

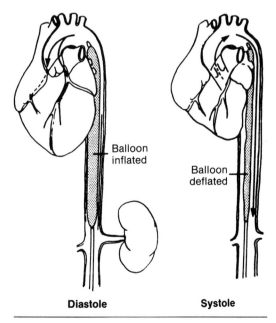

Diastole   **Systole**

FIGURE 20-8 Diagram of the intra-aortic balloon pump positioned in the descending thoracic aorta. (From J Cardiovasc Anes 2:365-373, 1988.)

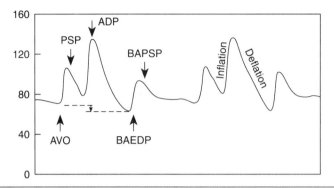

FIGURE 20-9   Diagram of the arterial pressure tracing of a patient with an IABP functioning in the 2:1 mode. **AVO** = aortic valve opening; **PSP** = peak systolic pressure; **ADP** = augmented diastolic pressure; **BAEDP** = balloon assisted end-diastolic pressure; **BAPSP** = balloon assisted peak-systolic pressure. Note balloon inflation occurs on the dicrotic notch and deflation occurs before the opening of the aortic valve.

with the hemodynamic criteria or left atrial or pulmonary artery wedge pressure greater than 25 mm Hg, systolic arterial blood pressure less than 90 mm Hg, and cardiac index less than 1.8 L/min/m².

A number of systems are currently under investigation under clinical trials restricted by the Food and Drug Administration (FDA). These systems include pneumatic devices such as the Pierce-Donachy pump manufactured by the Thoratec Corporation, and electrical devices such as the Novacor left ventricular assist system manufactured by Baxter Corporation.

The Pierce-Donachy pump can take over the entire function of the left, the right, or both ventricles on a temporary basis (Fig. 20-10). The VAD employs the rhythmic compression of a polyurethane, seam-free, highly polished blood sac within the rigid case and is driven by an external air source. The VAD contains inlet and outlet mechanical valves that provide for unidirectional blood flow through the VAD. The VAD is capable of sustaining the total cardiac output of the heart. The device itself is placed on the abdominal wall and cannulas lead through the skin. A large cannula is placed in the left atrial appendage or left ventricular apex and is used for return of blood to the left ventricular assist device. The output cannula of the device is then tunneled back through the skin and attached to the ascending aorta. A right ventricular assist device can be used simultaneously for biventricular assist or used alone for treatment of pure right ventricular failure. The cannulas are connected to the right atrium and to the pulmonary artery and connected to the VAD for right

ventricular assist. The VADs are powered by a pneumatic drive console containing two drive modules that can operate independently of each other. The console can be used to drive one VAD, the second remaining in reserve, or to pump two VADs at the same time as would occur in a biventricular assist.

The Novacor left ventricular system consists of an electrically driven blood pump and a microprocessor control and monitoring console. The blood pump is implanted anteriorly within the left upper quadrant of the abdomen and contains a seamless polyurethane sac that is compressed by dual opposed pusher plates. Tissue valves provide for the unidirectional flow of blood. The pump inflow conduit attaches to the left ventricular apex and pierces the diaphragm to connect to the blood pump. The outflow cannula passes from the pump and is connected to the aorta. Left ventricular assist only is possible with this system.

Results using ventricular assist devices for a bridge to transplantation have been encouraging. For patients who can be stabilized with the devices and then undergo transplantation, the survival rates following transplantation are similar to those patients who undergo transplantation without the need for circulatory support. The results for support following postcardiotomy cardiogenic shock have been less encouraging. Typically only 25% to 30% of patients who are supported have been weaned from the devices and discharged from the hospital. While these results may seem discouraging, this is a group of patients who would otherwise not have survived surgery.

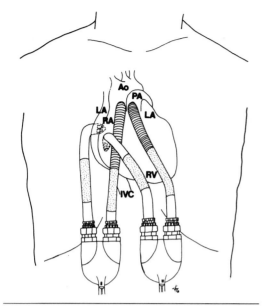

FIGURE 20-10   Diagrams of biventricular assist devices. The pumps are located on the abdominal wall. Inflow to the left VAD is from the left atrium *(LA)* and outflow to the aorta *(Ao)*. Inflow to the right VAD is from the right atrium *(RA)* and outflow to the main pulmonary artery *(PA)*. *RV* = right ventricle; *IVC* = inferior vena cava. (From Ann Thorac Surg 48:222-227, 1989.)

ORTHOTOPIC CARDIAC TRANSPLANTATION
When Is Cardiac Transplantation Considered?

The success in cardiac transplantation over the last 10 years has merited its increasing use (Fig. 20-11). Patients with end-stage cardiomyopathy, whether idiopathic, viral, or ischemic, who have reached a functional class IV status have a less than 10% chance of survival of more than 6 months. These are the patients who are considered for cardiac transplantation.

Patients who are candidates for cardiac transplantation must have terminal heart disease with an estimated life expectancy of less than 12 months. They should be under 60 years old, have normal or reversible hepatic and renal function, be free of acute infection, and have no history of pulmonary infarction within the preceding 2 months. They must be psychologically stable and have a supportive social milieu. The patient should have no systemic illness that would limit life expectancy or compromise a recovery from cardiac transplantation. Contraindications to cardiac transplantation include insulin-dependent diabetics or patients who have pulmonary hypertension with fixed pulmonary vascular resistance.

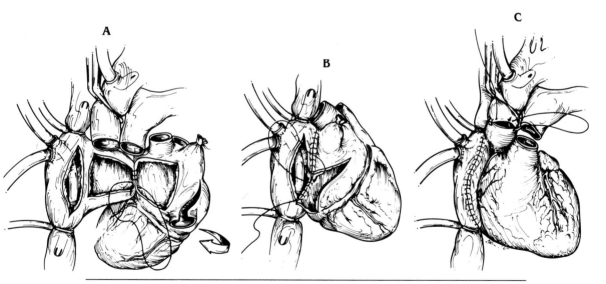

FIGURE 20-11   Cardiac transplantation. **A,** The new heart is placed in the pericardial cavity, and the suture line is begun connecting the donor and the recipient atriums. **B,** After completing the suture line of the left atriums, the donor and recipient right atriums are then approximated. **C,** After the two atriums are connected, the great vessels are connected with running sutures. Following this, air is evacuated from the heart and the cross-clamp is removed. The heart is then reperfused, and the patient is weaned from cardiopulmonary bypass.

What Is Rejection?

The results of cardiac transplantation have dramatically improved with the combined immunosuppression therapy of cyclosporine, prednisolone, and azathioprine. Cyclosporine is initially given in doses of 10 mg/kg. Since many of the major side effects of cyclosporine, such as renal failure, are dose dependent, it is extremely important to monitor serum cyclosporine levels to determine the dose. Prednisolone is initially given at 2 mg/kg and gradually tapered to approximately 0.2 mg/kg over the first 3 months of therapy. Azathioprine is begun at a dose of 2 mg/kg and the dose adjusted according to the white blood cell and platelet counts.

One of the leading causes of mortality following transplantation continues to be acute and chronic rejection. There are few, if any, physical signs or symptoms of rejection until the episode of rejection has become severe. There are no reliable laboratory methods to detect early rejection. For these reasons an endomyocardial biopsy is done at varied intervals after transplantation for histologic monitoring of rejection. The presence of lymphocytic interstitial infiltrate, myocyte necrosis, and hemorrhage determines the severity. Episodes of mild rejection are treated with pulse steroids of 500 mg of methylprednisolone sodium succinate daily for 3 days. Moderate or severe episodes of rejection are treated with cytolytic therapy using murine monoclonal antibody (OKT3), horse antithymocyte globulin (AT-GAM), or rabbit antithymocyte globulin (ATG).

With combined immunosuppressive therapy, the 1-year survival rate is 90% to 95% and the 2-year survival rate is approximately 90%.

PERICARDIUM
What Is Pericarditis?

Pericarditis may occur as a primary process with systemic disease (idiopathic, bacterial, tuberculous, or fungal) or occur secondary to myocardial infarction, cardiac surgery, rheumatoid disease, or uremia. Pericarditis is usually an acute, self-limiting, inflammatory process resulting from a variety of etiologic agents. Commonly, such viruses as Coxsackie virus A and B and influenza virus A and B have been identified as causative agents in acute pericarditis. The disease may occur at any age but is frequently found in younger, otherwise healthy individuals and is characterized by fever, chest pain, marked ST-segment elevation on the electrocardiogram with absence of T waves, and the presence of a pericardial friction rub. Pain associated with pericardial disease probably originates in the adjacent diaphragmatic pleura, since only the lower part of the external surface of the parietal layer of pericardium contains pain fibers. Pain is likely to be referred to the neck and shoulders because of secondary involvement of the diaphragm. Frequently the chest pain is reduced when the patient sits erect and leans forward. The patient may develop acute tamponade, chronic pericardial effusion, or constrictive pericarditis.

Treatment of pericarditis depends on the cause of the disease. In nonspecific types of pericarditis, treatment consists of bed rest for 2 to 3 weeks and analgesics. Salicylates are quite effective in relieving the pain. Occasionally patients will not respond to conservative management, and steroids are used to help control the inflammation process.

Recognizing and Treating Acute Pericardial Tamponade

Normal amounts of fluid in the pericardial sac range from 20 to 50 ml. When amounts of 100 to 250 ml of fluid appear, as when secondary to penetrating heart injury, the heart is prevented from filling in diastole by the increased pressure from the pericardium or the fluid in the pericardial sac. To maintain adequate cardiac output, however, the diastolic filling of the ventricles requires greater venous pressure to overcome the force applied against the heart's surface. Systolic contraction is not limited. Since the pericardium cannot expand, cardiac function is severely compromised.

In acute cardiac tamponade, clinical shock is usually the presenting symptom. The patient is cool and diaphoretic. The heart sounds are distant and the pulse rate is rapid and thready. A pulsus paradoxus can exist and is defined as a decrease in systemic arterial pressure exceeding 10 mm Hg with inspiration. While other signs suggest circulatory collapse, venous distention is characteristic. *The venous pressure rather than the systemic arterial pressure is the most important clue in making the diagnosis.* There is rarely time to perform a sophisticated examination, such as an echocardiogram, and the diagnosis must be made on a clinical basis.

Treatment of acute tamponade must be immediate and is aimed at removing fluid in the pericardium. This may be done by pericardiocentesis, subxiphoid exploration of the pericardium, or thoracotomy.

In acute tamponade, pericardiocentesis is performed as an emergency measure. A needle attached to a syringe is inserted to the left of the xiphoid and directed toward the middle of the right clavicle at a 45-degree downward angle. The pericardial cavity is entered and the fluid is aspirated (Fig. 20-12). The aspiration needle is connected to the electrocardiogram chest lead. When the needle contacts the heart, an energy current will be seen on the electrocardiogram. The needle is then withdrawn slightly and fluid is aspirated from the pericardial cavity. A standard electrocardiogram should be monitored during the procedure to detect dysrhythmias. As the fluid is removed, the signs of shock instantaneously disappear. If the patient has received a thoracic injury resulting in a hemopericardium, a thoracotomy with direct repair of the cardiac injury is preferable to repeated pericardial aspirations.

Chronic Pericardial Effusions

Chronic effusions develop over a long period, allowing the pericardium to stretch. These effusions may contain 1 to 2 L of fluid, with little impairment of cardiac function. Ultimately the volume of fluid around the heart exceeds the elasticity of the pericardium, such that the addition of even a small increase in volume will impair cardiac function, as in acute tamponade.

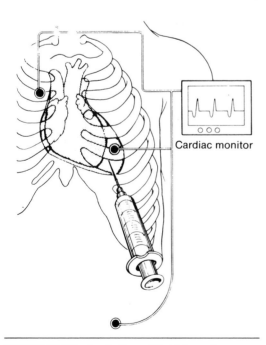

Cardiac monitor

FIGURE 20-12 Aspiration of fluid from the pericardial sac. Note that the ECG monitor should always be in place.

The diagnosis of chronic effusion may be suggested by a chest x-ray examination. The heart shadow is usually enlarged and globular. This is distinct from acute tamponade, in which the heart size shown on x-ray film is normal. The ECG may show low-voltage ST-segment elevation, and QRS abnormalities. Echocardiography is the most effective method used to confirm the diagnosis of a chronic pericardial effusion.

A chronic effusion is aspirated in a fashion similar to pericardiocentesis for acute tamponade and initially can be managed by catheter drainage. Recurrent chronic effusions may require an open drainage procedure and resection of a portion of the pericardium to create a pleuropericardial or abdominopericardial window.

What Is Constrictive Pericarditis?

Chronic constrictive pericarditis results when an inflammatory process causes thick fibrous tissue to constrict the heart, with a decrease in diastolic filling, elevation in venous pressure, and decreased cardiac output. Causes include infections such as tuberculosis or viral, therapeutic irradiation, metabolic and connective tissue disorders, and trauma; the condition may also be idiopathic. A high index of suspicion is important to make the diagnosis of constrictive pericarditis. Evidence of right-sided heart failure, pericardial "knock," and pericardial calcification with small cardiac silhouette on the chest x-ray film are classic findings. Cardiac catheterization, two-dimensional echocardiography, and computed tomography of the chest helps in confirming the diagnosis. Right-sided heart catheterization will reveal equalization of the right side of the heart filling pressures and the "square root" sign on the right ventricular pressure tracing. Two-dimensional echocardiography and CT scan will demonstrate a thickened pericardium. Treatment consists of surgical excision of the thick pericardium, being careful to free all scar tissue from the vena cava and to protect the coronary arteries during dissection. The mortality rate is low, and long-term outcome reflects the underlying disease process.

AORTA
How Are Aortic Aneurysms Diagnosed and Treated?

Atherosclerosis, bacterial infections, cystic medial necrosis, and syphilis may cause destruction, necrosis, and scarring of the wall of the aorta. The vessel then dilates and an aneurysm is formed. It may be saccular, with a narrow neck forming the orifice from the side of the aorta, or fusiform, with involvement of the entire circumference of the vessel (Fig. 20-13).

Patients with aortic aneurysm may be asymptomatic or may have pain. Pain from saccular or fusiform aneurysms is usually secondary to pressure on neighboring structures, such as bone or nerves. It has been described as pressing, boring, or throbbing, and occasionally as sharp and shooting. Cough and wheezing as a result of compression of the trachea or bronchi may be present, and occasional hoarseness is seen from compression of the left recurrent laryngeal nerve. Often there are no signs or symptoms of the aneurysm. It is usually discovered by routine chest x-ray evaluation, which reveals a mediastinal mass. Definitive diagnosis is made by a CT scan of the chest and by aortography.

The natural history of thoracic aortic aneurysms is not well defined. Most of the information on aortic aneurysms comes from studies of the infrarenal aorta and may not apply to the thoracic aorta. It has been shown that the risk of rupture increases with significant pulmonary obstructive disease, severe hypertension, and increased size of the aneurysm. The rate of growth of infrarenal aortic aneurysms is approximately 0.4 cm per year. Most authors recommend repair of infrarenal aneurysms of 5 to 6 cm or greater. For thoracic aneurysms the existing data parallel the infrarenal aneurysm data. In patients with aneurysms greater than 6 cm who were not treated surgically, the 5-year survival was less than 20%, with half of the deaths resulting from rupture of the aneurysms.

Current recommendations for surgery include all symptomatic patients, regardless of size of the aneurysm; all patients whose aneurysms have increased in size during a brief period, regardless of the presence or absence of symptoms; and in asymptomatic patients when the aneurysm is greater than 6 cm.

The techniques used to repair thoracic aortic aneurysms depend on the segment of aorta involved. Aneurysms of the ascending and arch segments are considered together, since the operations are frequently performed at the same setting and the techniques used are similar. Excision

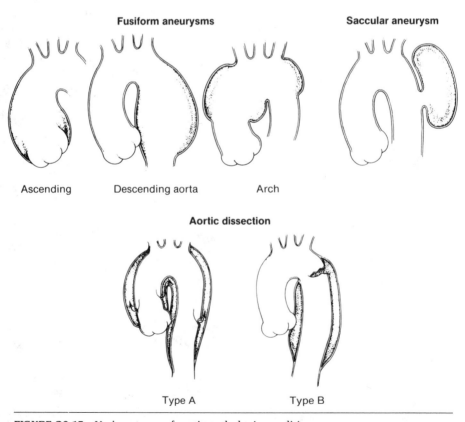

FIGURE 20-13   Various types of aortic pathologic conditions.

and replacement of the ascending aorta is performed for aneurysms involving the tubular segment of the ascending aorta in patients with normal aortic valves. Separate aortic valve replacement and graft replacement is performed for patients with diseased aortic valves and normal sinus segments of aorta. Composite valve grafts are used when the sinus segment of the ascending aorta is involved. When a composite valve graft is used, the coronary arteries are reattached by either direct reimplantation or interposition of small grafts using a modified Cabrol technique. Brachiocephalic vessels are attached to the graft by suturing an island of aorta from which they arise to an opening made in the side of the graft. Cardiopulmonary bypass is required for all of these operations. Profound hypothermia and circulatory arrest is employed for cerebral protection in patients requiring replacement of the aortic arch.

Aneurysms of the descending thoracic aorta are exposed through a left thoracotomy incision using a double-lumen endotracheal tube to allow for collapse of the left lung. The aorta is controlled proximal to the aneurysm, usually between the left common carotid artery and the left subclavian artery. Distal control is obtained at the level of the diaphragm. The aorta is cross-clamped, the aneurysm opened longitudinally, and bleeding intercostal arteries are oversewn. The aorta is transected proximally and distally and a graft inserted using continuous suture techniques. The body may be perfused distally, while the aorta is cross-clamped, by using one of a variety of techniques, including partial cardiopulmonary bypass.

Thoracoabdominal aortic aneurysms are approached through a combined thoracic and abdominal approach. The left thoracotomy incision is extended across the costal margin and down to the pubis in the midline. The descending thoracic aorta is exposed as previously described. The abdominal aorta is exposed retroperitoneally by incising the peritoneum in the left gutter and mobilizing the viscera including the left kidney, spleen, pancreas, and left hemicolon to the right. The aorta is clamped proximally and distally, depending on the extent of the aneurysm. If the origins of the visceral arteries are involved in the aneurysm, they are reimplanted as an island of aorta to the side of the graft. Typically the celiac axis, the superior mesenteric artery, and the right renal artery are reimplanted as a single unit and the left renal artery reimplanted separately or using a short interposition graft. Stenoses at the origins of the visceral arteries are repaired using

endarterectomy techniques. Pairs of intercostal and lumbar arteries that may be routes of spinal cord blood supply are also reattached to the graft in an effort to prevent paralysis. Whether using partial cardiopulmonary bypass prevents the complications of renal failure or paralysis is debatable.

The morbidity associated with surgery for aortic aneurysms can be significant. Complication rates vary according to the segment of the aorta involved. These complications include myocardial infarction, cerebrovascular accidents, renal failure, paraplegia, visceral ischemia, hemorrhage, infection, respiratory insufficiency, and left recurrent laryngeal nerve paralysis. Mortality rates depend on the segment of aorta replaced and typically vary between 5% and 25%.

Aortic Dissection

Aortic dissection is the most common catastrophic illness involving the aorta, with a frequency of more than 2000 new cases per year in the United States. The incidence is highest in men between 50 and 70 years of age. Aortic dissection is rare in patients under 40 years of age, except in those with familial predisposition, Marfan's syndrome, or congenital heart lesions such as coarctation of the aorta. There is an association with pregnancy, and approximately half of all dissections in women under the age of 40 occur during pregnancy.

Classification of aortic dissection is based on the fact that more than 90% of all dissections arise in one of two locations, either in the ascending aorta a few centimeters from the aortic valve or in the descending thoracic aorta just beyond the left subclavian artery at the site of the ligamentum arteriosum. The Stanford classification recognizes two types: type A or proximal aortic dissections, which begin in the ascending aorta, and type B or distal aortic dissections, which begin in the descending thoracic aorta (see Fig. 20-13). The classification carries clinical and prognostic implications. Almost 75% of untreated patients with type A dissection die within the first two weeks after onset, while the mortality for type B is less than half that during the same interval.

The process of aortic dissection involves an initial phase in which the intimal tear occurs, and a subsequent phase in which the dissection propagates. Primary intimal tears, which serve as entry points for the dissection, are located in the ascending aorta in about 60% of all cases of aortic dissection, in the descending thoracic aorta in about 35%, and in the abdominal aorta in the remainder. Aortic dissection has been associated with degenerative changes in the collagen, elastin, and smooth muscle cells of the aortic media. Two main hemodynamic forces are responsible for the propagation of the dissection: dP/dt, or pulsatile load, and the blood pressure.

The diagnosis of aortic dissection should always be considered in a patient who has chest pain. The pain is sudden in onset, severe, and described as ripping or tearing in quality. The pain usually begins in the chest and radiates to the back if the dissection progresses distally. The patient often appears pale and diaphoretic, but may have profound hypertension. Variable symptoms attributable to occlusion or malperfusion of vessels arising from the dissected segment of aorta may be present. Diminution or absence of pulses in one or more extremities is present in almost half of patients with type A dissections and one sixth of those with type B dissections. New cardiac murmurs may also be heard and may be either systolic or diastolic in origin. A diastolic murmur of aortic regurgitation is present in two thirds of the cases with type A dissections and implies disruption of the supporting attachments of the aortic valve with prolapse of the aortic cusps. In 40% of patients, there are neurologic findings as a result of interruption of circulation to the brain or spinal cord. The most common mode of death in a patient who presents with aortic dissection is aortic rupture. The site of rupture is typically opposite the site of intimal tear. In type A dissections this rupture leads to bleeding into the pericardium and death from acute cardiac tamponade. In type B dissections the rupture is into the left pleural space and results in exsanguination.

Computed tomographic scanning is the most accurate simple screening test for determining the presence and extent of aortic dissection; however, CT scanning is limited by its inability to demonstrate the site of intimal tear and not documenting aortic insufficiency. Aortography remains the most definitive method for confirming the diagnosis of aortic dissection. In addition, aortography yields information regarding the site of intimal tear, the extent of dissection, the degree of aortic insufficiency, and patency of the aortic branches, such as renal and visceral arteries. Recently transesophageal echocardiography has emerged as a promising noninvasive method for the diagnosis of aortic dissection.

Medical Management. The goals of medical management are to stabilize the dissection, prevent rupture, and prevent the complications of dissection. It is generally agreed that results with surgical therapy are better than those with medical therapy in type A dissection, and immediate operation is recommended in those patients. In type B dissections, medical treatment may be equal to the results with surgical therapy, although opinions differ about the indication for and the timing of operation in type B dissections. All type B dissections with evidence of expansion, rupture, or distal malperfusion are considered for emergent surgery.

Regardless of the location of the dissection, prompt medical therapy should be instituted in all patients. For initial treatment, intravenous administration of vasodilating agents is recommended. Sodium nitroprusside is very effective, and the dose is varied according to the blood pressure. Sodium nitroprusside can cause an increase in dP/dt that may contribute to the propagation of the dissection; therefore simultaneous administration of beta-adrenergic blockage is essential. Long-term pharmacologic therapy is advised for patients with type B dissection who are stabilized and for patients with type A dissections after they have undergone surgical repair. Follow-up of the patients is essential and should include regular physical examinations, chest x-ray evaluations, and CT scanning.

Surgical Management. The principles of surgical management include resection of the aorta in the region of the intimal tear, obliteration of the false lumen with redirection of blood flow into the true lumen, restoration of aortic valvular competency in type A dissections, and prevention of the complications of the dissection, including rupture and malperfusion syndromes.

Treatment of type A dissections is directed to the ascending aorta, regardless of the presence of distal aortic or aortic branch vessel occlusion. Appropriate early proximal operation usually decompresses the distal false lumen and restores distal circulation. The operation is performed through a median sternotomy using cardiopulmonary bypass. The procedure involves replacement of the ascending aorta, reinforcement of the distal dissected aorta with restoration of flow into the true lumen, and resuspension of the aortic valve to restore aortic competency. Patients with Marfan's syndrome require placement of a valved conduit to eliminate all of the abnormal aorta.

The prognosis and treatment of type B dissections depend on the complications present at the time of hospital admission. The operation, performed through a left lateral thoracotomy, consists of graft replacement of the segment of aorta containing the intimal tear, reinforcement of the distal aorta with obliteration of the false lumen, and restoration of flow down the true lumen.

The results following surgery for either type A or type B dissections are excellent, with mortality rates ranging from 10% to 30%, depending on the clinical status of the patient at the time of operation.

PULMONARY EMBOLISM
What Causes a Pulmonary Embolus?

Pulmonary embolism continues to produce considerable morbidity and mortality, and it has been estimated to be responsible for 3% to 5% of in-hospital deaths in the United States. Classic signs of a pulmonary embolus include tachycardia, tachypnea, pleuritic chest pain, hemoptysis, cyanosis, and elevated venous pressure. However, most patients have nonspecific signs and symptoms and only one third have evidence of deep venous thrombosis. The emboli originate from thrombi in the iliofemoral venous system in two thirds of the patients and from the calf veins in the remaining one third. Other sources of pulmonary emboli include thrombi in the right atrium, septic thrombi in the pelvis, and from tumor thrombi associated with the endovascular invasion of the inferior vena cava by retroperitoneal tumors, such as renal cell carcinoma.

Diagnosis

Pulmonary angiography remains the definitive study for the diagnosis of pulmonary embolism. However, it is an invasive procedure that carries a small but finite risk and logistically may be difficult to obtain in the critically ill patient. The ventilation-perfusion (V/Q) scan using radioactively tagged macroalbumin aggregates shows the distribution of pulmonary arterial blood flow and is compared with the distribution of inhaled radioactive gases to detect areas of ventilation-perfusion mismatching. The V/Q scan is used as a noninvasive screening tool which carries little risk and is readily obtained. Patients with low- or intermediate-probability interpretations on V/Q scan should be studied with angiography if the clinical suspicion is high. A high-probability scan interpretation is usually adequate to establish the diagnosis. Other less specific studies that can be helpful in excluding other diagnoses include electrocardiography, chest x-ray evaluation, and arterial blood gas studies. In 20% of cases the electrocardiogram may show abnor-

malities in rhythm, ST depression, and T wave inversion. There may be evidence of right-sided heart strain with rightward shifting of the QRS axis. The chest x-ray film may show decreased vascularity of the lung fields in the area of the obstruction and a pleural effusion may develop as the result of a pulmonary infarction. Typically, the arterial blood gases show evidence of hypoxia and hypocarbia. When the Po_2 is normal, a major pulmonary embolus can be excluded.

Medical Treatment

Ideally, the treatment of pulmonary embolus should be directed toward the prevention of the primary risk factor of deep venous thrombophlebitis. This is accomplished by maintaining high venous blood flow with elevation of the legs, elastic support stockings, muscular exercises; the patient should avoid keeping the legs in a dependent position. Minidose heparin (5000 units subcutaneously every 12 hours) is recommended as prophylaxis for some high-risk patients.

Once the diagnosis has been made based on objective signs, approximately 90% of patients with pulmonary emboli are effectively treated with intravenous heparin (Fig. 20-14). Heparin

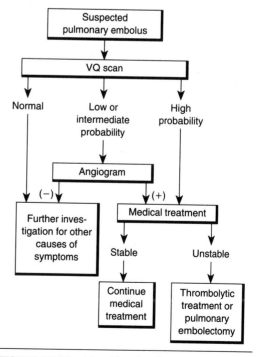

FIGURE 20-14 Algorithm for the treatment of pulmonary embolus.

prevents additional thrombi from developing in systemic veins and prevents the propagation of clots distal to the embolus in the pulmonary artery. Heparin may also aid in the lysis of the embolus. Continuous intravenous administration of heparin is the most reliable method of obtaining and controlling adequate anticoagulation. A loading dose of 7500 to 10,000 units is given, followed by 800 to 1000 units/hr to achieve the desired effect. The activated partial thromboplastin time is maintained at approximately two times control. Symptomatic improvement usually occurs within a few days. Heparin-induced thrombocytopenia and thrombosis is a rare but serious complication of heparin therapy. The platelet count should be closely followed while the patient is receiving heparin therapy, and if the platelet count should begin to fall, the patient's therapy should be converted to oral coagulation using sodium warfarin. Normally warfarin is begun when the patient is asymptomatic and the heparin discontinued when the prothrombin time reaches 1.5 to 2 times control. Warfarin is continued for 3 to 6 months.

The role of thrombolytic therapy is increasing in the treatment of pulmonary emboli. Studies indicate that the rate of resolution of emboli can be accelerated by the use of streptokinase or urokinase, with normalization of hemodynamic disturbances and reperfusion of the lung. Best results are obtained when thrombolytic agents are administered within 72 hours of the onset of pulmonary emboli. Contraindications to the use of thrombolytic therapy include an active site of gastrointestinal bleeding, recent surgery or trauma, or a recent stroke. The single most serious complication of thrombolytic therapy is bleeding. Because of the risk for bleeding complications, the use of thrombolytic therapy should be reserved for patients who have sustained major pulmonary emboli with significant pulmonary or cardiac decompensation.

When Is Surgery Indicated?

Surgical management of pulmonary embolism is considered for three specific conditions: (1) caval interruption or filtration for prevention of recurrent emboli, (2) pulmonary embolectomy for acute embolus with cardiopulmonary decompensation unresponsive to medical management, and (3) pulmonary embolectomy for chronic pulmonary embolus associated with dyspnea, hypoxemia, and pulmonary hypertension caused by organized thrombi obstructing the main branches of the pulmonary artery.

Vena caval interruption or filtration may be associated with serious sequelae and may not completely prevent subsequent embolism. These procedures should therefore not be performed without objective documentation of deep venous thrombotic disease involving the inferior vena cava or iliofemoral system. Only patients who develop recurrent pulmonary emboli while receiving adequate anticoagulation or who have a strong contraindication to anticoagulation should be considered as candidates. Filtration procedures are preferable to caval ligation or clips because of the severe leg edema and venous stasis that occurs with ligation. Placement of the filters can be accomplished percutaneously under fluoroscopy with little morbidity.

Pulmonary embolectomy is indicated in patients with acute pulmonary emboli who have not responded to medical therapy including oxygen, heparinization, or thrombolytic therapy and inotropic support and who exhibit refractory hypotension and hypoxemia. A median sternotomy is employed and cardiopulmonary bypass with hypothermic circulatory arrest is used, that allows the removal of embolic material from the pulmonary arteries under direct vision. The improvement in oxygenation and hemodynamic stability can be dramatic, and the major cause of morbidity is cardiac in origin. Mortality is approximately 25% in carefully selected patients.

In most patients with pulmonary emboli, the embolus resolves and the lung reperfuses. In a small group of patients, however, persistent, chronic obstruction of the pulmonary arteries develops. This results in cor pulmonale with symptoms of dyspnea, cyanosis, and exercise intolerance associated with low arterial PO_2, pulmonary hypertension, and right ventricular hypertrophy. Evaluation includes pulmonary angiography, arterial blood gases, and an assessment of right ventricular function. Bronchial arteriography is also necessary to demonstrate patency of the pulmonary artery distal to the embolus. The ideal candidate is a patient with angiographically documented pulmonary emboli with good distal pulmonary arteries demonstrated by collateral flow from the bronchial arteries. The surgical approach will depend on the location of the thrombus, and cardiopulmonary bypass is usually required. It is necessary to perform extensive and complete embolectomies, including the primary and secondary branches of the pulmonary artery to obtain optimal improvement. Mortality rates approximate 15% to 20%, and significant functional improvement can be seen in up to 80% of patients.

BIBLIOGRAPHY

Baumgartner WA, Reitz GA, Achuff SC (eds). Heart and Heart-Lung Transplantation. Philadelphia, WB Saunders, 1990.

Braunwald E (ed). Heart Disease: A Textbook of Cardiovascular Medicine, 3rd ed. Philadelphia, WB Saunders, 1988.

Crawford ES, Crawford JL (eds). Diseases of the Aorta. Baltimore, Williams & Wilkins, 1984.

Sabiston DC, Spencer FC (eds). Surgery of the Chest, 5th ed. Philadelphia, WB Saunders, 1990.

CHAPTER REVIEW
Questions

1. Ventricular aneurysms result in which of the following physiologic derangements?
   a. Slow heart rate
   b. Decreased stroke volume
   c. Decreased cardiac output
2. Cardiac tamponade is a surgical emergency and should be treated by immediate:
   a. Surgical exploration
   b. Pericardiocentesis
   c. Infusion of fluid
3. Which of the following chest x-ray findings are suggestive of pulmonary emboli?
   a. Atelectasis
   b. Emphysema
   c. Hypovascular segment
4. The most common cause of death after myocardial infarction is:
   a. Shock
   b. Rupture of the heart
   c. Ventricular fibrillation
   d. Aneurysm
5. Symptoms of thoracic aortic aneurysms include:
   a. Pain
   b. Hoarseness
   c. Cough
   d. All of the above
6. Severity of rejection after cardiac transplantation can be determined by:
   a. Symptoms
   b. Electrocardiogram
   c. Endomyocardial biopsy
7. The intra-aortic balloon pump:
   a. Decreases diastolic filling of the coronary arteries
   b. Decreases left ventricular afterload
   c. Is triggered asynchronously
8. Angina pectoris:
   a. Is caused by an imbalance between myocardial blood supply and demand
   b. Is always treated medically
   c. Always precedes a myocardial infarction

Answers

1. b and c	5. d
2. b	6. c
3. c	7. b
4. c	8. a

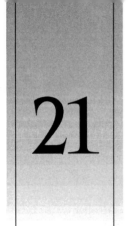

21

Hypertension

G. RAINEY WILLIAMS

KEY FEATURES

After reading this chapter you will understand:
- The pathogenesis of hypertension.
- How to determine which hypertensive patients are amenable to surgical correction.

One of six Americans is hypertensive, but approximately half of those affected are unaware they have the disease. Hypertension is significantly more common among African-Americans, in whom hypertension begins at an earlier age, tends to be more severe, and more often progresses to end-organ disease than in other groups. This high incidence in African-Americans is of particular interest, because hypertension is relatively uncommon among Africans living in Africa. Surgeons are interested in hypertension because it is a significant risk factor when considering surgical treatment of diseases unrelated to hypertension and because it can be caused by surgically treatable lesions. Identifying patients whose conditions fall into the latter group is obviously important; unfortunately, this continues to be difficult to do.

HOW DO HYPERTENSIVE PATIENTS PRESENT?

Hypertension does not produce a characteristic complex of symptoms, and many hypertensive patients are totally asymptomatic. A dull occipi-

tal headache is commonly described and, because it is often relieved by control of the hypertension, cause and effect are assumed. When the hypertensive process results in functional and structural changes in other organ systems, a variety of symptom complexes develop. The most common end-organ systems affected by hypertension are the cardiovascular system, kidneys, and brain. Hypertension is a leading cause of stroke, as well as the catastrophe of massive intracranial bleeding.

PATHOPHYSIOLOGY OF HYPERTENSION

Arterial blood pressure is determined by the interrelationship among blood volume, cardiac output, peripheral vascular resistance, and blood viscosity. Blood pressure is controlled by a highly complex system (which has neural, chemical, and hormonal components), the mechanism of which is not completely understood. The four principal control systems are:

1. *The arterial baroreflex.* Impulses from pressure sensors in the carotid sinus, aorta, and left ventricle are relayed through neural pathways to the brainstem. The efferent arc also involves the sympathetic adrenergic nerves and vagal cholinergic nerves.
2. *Regulation of fluid volume.* This is a slowly responding system that results in loss of fluid with elevated blood pressure and retention of fluid when blood pressure falls.

3. ***Renin and angiotensin.*** The initiating enzyme renin, released from the kidney, splits angiotensin I from plasma globulin, which is then converted to angiotensin II. Angiotensin II also stimulates aldosterone secretion (Fig. 21-1).

4. ***Vascular autoregulation.*** In several organ systems, changes in perfusion pressure result in local changes in vascular resistance to keep perfusion volume constant.

A schematic of the various feedback loops is shown in Fig. 21-2.

DIAGNOSIS

The diagnosis of hypertension is established simply by measuring blood pressure. The clinical significance of hypertension increases with increased levels of blood pressure, but even moderate elevations are associated with decreased life expectancy. For this reason, determining the cause of the hypertension is important in all patients whose diastolic pressure consistently exceeds 90 mm Hg. Causes of hypertension are listed and illustrated in the box on p. 372 and Fig. 21-3, respectively. An algorithm for the investiga-

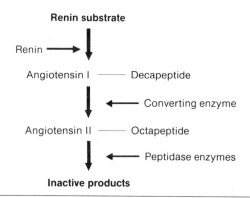

FIGURE 21-1 Renin-angiotensin cascade. (From Fry WJ, Fry RE. Surgically correctable hypertension. In Schwartz SI [ed]. Principles of Surgery, 5th ed. New York, McGraw-Hill, 1989.)

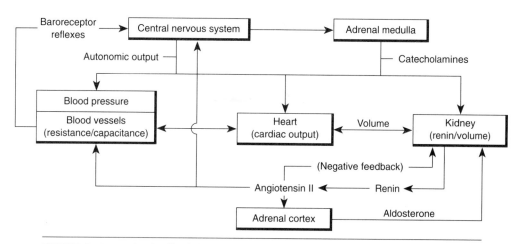

FIGURE 21-2 Major feedback loops regulating blood pressure. (From Haber E, Slater EE. High blood pressure. In Rubenstein E, Federman DD [eds]. Scientific American Medicine, Section 1, Subsection VII. © 1988 Scientific American, Inc. All rights reserved.)

tion of hypertensive patients devised by Fry is reproduced in Fig. 21-4. As with all schemata, this should not be followed slavishly, and, because of cost, tests should rarely be ordered in batteries.

CAUSES OF COMBINED SYSTOLIC AND DIASTOLIC HYPERTENSION

Adrenal hyperactivity
   Cushing's syndrome
   Hyperaldosteronism
   Pheochromocytoma
Renal disease
   Renal artery stenosis
   Fibromuscular hyperplasia
   Dissecting aneurysm (involving renal artery)
   Intrinsic disease: chronic pyelonephritis, glomerulosclerosis
Mechanical
   Coarctation
Other causes
   Idiopathic essential hypertension

WHAT IS ESSENTIAL HYPERTENSION?

In approximately 95% of hypertensive patients, no specific cause for hypertension can be determined; these patients are considered to have essential hypertension. Patients with mild, untreated hypertension are probably not at increased risk at operation, but patients with diastolic pressures exceeding 100 mm Hg should be treated prior to undergoing elective operations. The treatment of essential hypertension is a combination of restriction of dietary salt and administration of a variety of drugs. These are listed by type of action and drug name on pp. 376-377. The side effects of common drugs are also listed. Adequate control of hypertension by a single drug is frequently difficult; therefore combinations of agents are commonly employed. The out-of-pocket cost for a lifetime is considerable. There is, however, good evidence that control of hypertension significantly lessens the incidence of end-organ damage. Because many drugs used in the treatment of hypertension significantly alter the patient's response to various anesthetic agents, this becomes an important factor in the surgical management of hypertensive patients.

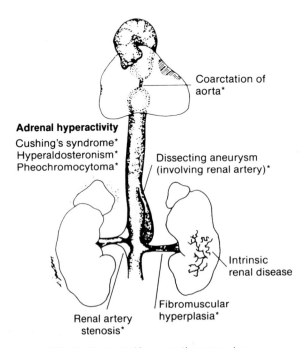

*Effectively treated by operative procedure.

FIGURE 21-3 Causes of some forms of hypertension. Note that many of the causes can be treated by operation.

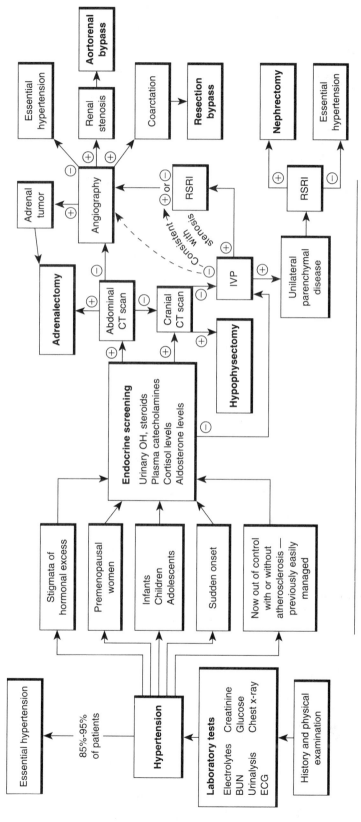

FIGURE 21-4   Algorithm for surgically correctable hypertension. (From Fry WJ, Fry RE. Surgically correctable hypertension. In Schwartz SI [ed]. Principles of Surgery, 5th ed. New York, McGraw-Hill, 1989.)

Early consultation with an anesthesiologist is advisable before operating on patients who are hypertensive.

SURGICALLY CORRECTABLE FORMS OF HYPERTENSION

From 1% to 10% of hypertensive patients have a surgically correctable cause for their condition. This is a highly significant group of patients, and the importance of making a correct diagnosis is obvious. The algorithm outlined in Fig. 21-4 includes surgical options for such patients.

Coarctation of the Aorta

Congenital aortic coarctation is one of the most common causes of hypertension in children but may be encountered at any age. Patients with significant coarctation have diminished or absent femoral pulses; a combination of hypertension and diminished femoral pulses should instantly suggest the diagnosis. Additional findings that suggest increased collateral flow, such as interscapular pulsations or rib notching as seen on chest x-ray evaluation, corroborate the diagnosis.

The mechanism by which coarctation of the aorta produces hypertension has been debated for years. Evidence suggests that both a mechanical factor (increased vascular resistance) and the renin-angiotensin mechanism are involved.

Patients suspected of having coarctation of the aorta should have the diagnosis confirmed by angiography and, when significant coarctation is present, it should be corrected surgically. It is clear that the earlier coarctation is surgically treated, the better the chance for blood pressure reduction. The likelihood of significant control of hypertension becomes so small over time that coarctation probably should not be routinely repaired in patients older than 50 years of age.

Renal Artery Stenosis

Several disease processes may produce extrarenal narrowing of the renal arteries of a sufficient degree to activate the renin-angiotensin pressor system. These lesions include arteriosclerosis, fibromuscular dysplasia, dissecting aneurysm of the aorta, and trauma. The clinical picture produced by all of these entities is hypertension, with or without its cardiac, pulmonary, cerebral, or renal manifestations. The stimulus for increased renin production in renal artery stenosis is probably damping of the pulse pressure in the renal artery distal to the stenotic lesion. Details of the renin-angiotensin I and angiotensin II systems will not be reviewed here.

Hypertension produced by renal artery stenosis has no clinically distinguishing features but, because it is highly amenable to surgical treatment, the diagnosis is very important. It is estimated to occur in up to 5% of the hypertensive population. Any patient with moderate to severe diastolic hypertension who would be considered a candidate for surgical correction if a renovascular lesion were present should have an intravenous pyelogram (IVP). The rapid-sequence excretory urogram is a relatively simple variation that gives additional information. Digital subtraction angiography of the renal vessels has been suggested as a method of screening for renovascular hypertension, but it is probably no more accurate than IVP and is certainly more expensive. If renovascular hypertension is suggested by the preliminary screening, renal vein renin levels should be measured. In unilateral renal artery obstruction, the involved kidney produces excessive amounts of renin, which is detected in the renal vein assay. When the level of renin is 1.5 times or greater than that of the uninvolved side, a significant lesion is almost certainly present. Renal systemic renin indices (RSRI) may be of additional help. This is calculated as follows:

$$RSRI = \frac{\begin{array}{c} \text{Individual renal} \quad - \quad \text{Systemic renin} \\ \text{renin activity} \qquad \text{activity} \end{array}}{\text{Systemic renin activity}}$$

Arteriography is the most accurate method of demonstrating renal artery stenosis. While complications of arteriography have been reduced, it is an invasive procedure and may be replaced by digital subtraction angiography when techniques for that examination are refined.

Surgical revascularization of a kidney with significant arterial lesions results in significant reduction of blood pressure in 90% of patients. Aortorenal bypass grafting is employed in most instances. Endarterectomy, with or without patch angioplasty, and reconstruction using the splenic artery may be preferable in some situations. Transluminal dilation of renal artery lesions is of great interest, but in our experience it has been disappointing so far.

Unilateral Renal Parenchymal Disease

Occasionally a patient is seen who has hypertension, a contracted kidney, and arteriographic findings indicating no extrarenal stenotic lesions. Historically, removal of the involved kidney has not resulted in reduction of blood pressure in most patients. Recently it has been observed that when the atrophic kidney behaves physiologically like an ischemic kidney, as determined by split renal function or renin vein assays, nephrectomy will result in blood pressure reduction.

Cushing's Syndrome

The principal features of Cushing's syndrome are the "moon" face, central obesity, cutaneous striae, and hypertension. The syndrome is produced by excess circulating glucocorticoids. Excessive glucocorticoid levels may result from iatrogenic administration, pituitary or adrenal lesions, or nonadrenal sources of ACTH production, principally malignant neoplasms.

The diagnosis of Cushing's syndrome usually begins with clinical observation of the distinctive physical changes. The most widely used screening test is measurement of the urinary excretion of 17-hydroxycorticosteroids. The plasma cortisol level can be determined, and, like the urinary 17-hydroxycorticosteroids, it is usually elevated in Cushing's syndrome. Measurement of ACTH levels and its response to dexamethasone suppression may be helpful in differentiating pituitary disease from adrenal disease. Cranial and abdominal CT scans and/or magnetic resonance imaging are currently the most accurate methods of demonstrating the lesions anatomically.

The most satisfactory treatment of Cushing's syndrome is surgical removal of the lesion responsible for the syndrome. This is more completely discussed in Chapter 10.

Hyperaldosteronism

Hyperaldosteronism is a condition that occurs less commonly than was once thought. It is caused by hypersecretion of aldosterone, a mineralocorticoid, by an adrenal adenoma or adrenal hyperplasia. Hypertension is present but is usually not severe in adults. The diagnosis is suspected when persistent hypokalemia and metabolic alkalosis are detected in hypertensive patients who are not receiving diuretic therapy. Plasma renin activity is usually low and urinary aldosterone levels are elevated.

Treatment of this condition is discussed in Chapter 10.

Pheochromocytoma

Pheochromocytoma is a rare neoplasm arising in the adrenal medulla and producing norepinephrine and/or epinephrine. The tumor may be unilateral or bilateral, benign or malignant. Patients with pheochromocytomas have episodic or sustained hypertension. Determination of urinary catecholamine and vanillylmandelic acid (VMA) secretions are probably the best screening tests for pheochromocytoma. Confirming tests include measurement of plasma epinephrine and norepinephrine levels. When biochemical evidence for pheochromocytoma exists, it becomes important to localize the responsible neoplasm. Intravenous pyelography may show downward displacement of the kidneys. A CT scan of the abdomen appears to be the most valuable diagnostic tool for locating adrenal lesions as well as other retroperitoneal mass lesions, superseding conventional tomography, arteriography, and retroperitoneal gas insufflation.

Operations on patients with unsuspected pheochromocytoma can be disastrous because anesthesia and operative manipulation of the tumor may result in uncontrollable hypertension or hypotension. Preoperative preparation of patients with pheochromocytoma with alpha-adrenergic and beta-adrenergic blocking agents has decreased surgical risk. Conduct of anesthesia is extremely important.

The surgical treatment of pheochromocytoma is discussed in Chapter 10.

SURGICAL PHARMACOPEIA

Drug	Indication/Complications	Dosage
FOR TREATMENT OF CHRONIC HYPERTENSION		
Diuretics		
1. Benzothiadiazine diuretics		
Chlorothiazide (Diuril)	May require potassium supplementation	250-1000 mg/day
Hydrochlorothiazide (Hydrodiuril, Esidrix, Oretic)	Same	25-50 mg/day
2. Loop diuretics		
Furosemide (Lasix)	Dehydration and electrolyte depletion possible	20-1000 mg/day
Ethacrynic acid (Edecrin)	Same	50-400 mg/day
3. Potassium-sparing diuretics		
Spironolactone (Aldactone)	Relatively contraindicated in the setting of renal insufficiency; watch for hypervolemia	50-100 mg/day
Sympatholytic Agents		
1. Centrally acting alpha-adrenergic agents		
Methyldopa (Aldomet)	Rarely: anemia, liver dysfunction, and mental depression	250-2000 mg/day
Clonidine (Catapres)	Sedative effect, drug interactions; rebound hypertension on discontinuation	0.2-0.8 mg/day
Reserpine	Mental depression (uncommon)	0.1-0.25 mg/day
2. Beta-adrenergic-blocking agents		
Propranolol (Inderal)	Contraindicated in setting of A-V conduction delay; may accelerate cardiac failure or cause bronchospasm	40-640 mg/day
Metoprolol (Lopressor)	Same; less risk of bronchospasm	100-450 mg/day
Labetalol (Normodyne, Trandate)	Oral and intravenous forms available, so it is useful for converting patient from a controlled hypertensive crisis to oral medication; may cause nausea and diarrhea	200-1200 mg/day
3. Alpha-adrenergic-blocking agent		
Prazosin (Minipress)	Syncope, particularly with the initial dose; alcohol intolerance	2-20 mg/day
4. Peripherally acting sympatholytic		
Guanethidine (Ismelin sulfate)	Used in severe hypertension; orthostatic hypotension; sexual dysfunction in men; discontinue 2 weeks before operation	10-300 mg/day
Direct Vasodilators		
Hydralazine (Apresoline)	May precipitate angina or lead to retention of fluid; occasionally implicated concomitant rheumatoid syndrome	20-300 mg/day

Drug	Indication/Complications	Dosage
Converting Enzyme Inhibitors		
Captopril (Capoten)	Rash; may cause hyperkalemia in renal-insufficient patients	75-450 mg/day
Calcium Channel-Blocking Agents		
Nifedipine (Procardia, Adalat)	Sublingual dosage quickly lowers blood pressure; contraindicated in patients with aortic stenosis and heart failure or A-V conduction delay	30-120 mg/day
Verapamil (Calan, Isoptin)	Same; no sublingual form; may cause constipation	240-480 mg/day
FOR CONTROL OF ACUTE HYPERTENSION		
Nitroprusside (Nipride, Nitropress)	Most rapidly acting and consistently effective agent for treating hypertensive emergencies; may cause rebound tachycardia, nausea, emesis, or headache	0.5 to 10 μg/kg/min drip or continuous infusion
Nitroglycerine (Nitro-bid, Nitrostat, Tridil)	Useful in controlling hypertension in the patient with known coronary artery disease	5 to 200 μg/min drip
Labetalol (Normodyne, Trandate)	Oral and intravenous forms available, so it is useful for converting a patient from a controlled hypertensive crisis to oral therapy; may cause nausea and diarrhea	20 mg IV slowly; may repeat up to 80 mg IV q10min or 2 mg/min continuous or drip infusion
Hydralazine (Apresoline)	May precipitate angina or fluid retention	20-300 mg orally q day

BIBLIOGRAPHY

Doyle AE, Donnan GA. Stroke as a clinical problem in hypertension. J Cardiovasc Pharmacol 15:S34, 1990.

Ernst CB, Bookstein JJ, Montie J, et al. Renal renin ratios and collateral vessels in renovascular hypertension. Arch Surg 104:496, 1972.

Francis CK. Hypertension and cardiac disease in minorities. Am J Med 88:3B-3S, 1990.

Fry WJ, Fry RE. Surgically correctable hypertension. In Schwartz SI (ed). Principles of Surgery, 5th ed. New York, McGraw-Hill, 1989, p 1002.

Haber E, Slater EE. High blood pressure. In Rubenstein E, Federman DD (eds). Scientific American Medicine, Vol 1. New York, Scientific American, 1988.

Havey RJ, Krumlovsky F, et al. Screening for hypertension. JAMA 254:388, 1985.

Oparil S. Arterial hypertension. In Wyngaarden JB, Smith LH Jr (eds). Textbook of Medicine, 18th ed. Philadelphia, WB Saunders, 1988, p 276.

CHAPTER REVIEW
Questions

1. Physical findings are suggestive of which types of surgically treatable hypertension?
2. Persistent hypokalemia in a patient with hypertension suggests what condition?
3. What pathologic lesions are responsible for most instances of renovascular hypertension?
4. How are patients with pheochromocytoma pharmacologically prepared for operation?
5. List the lesions responsible for development of Cushing's syndrome.
6. What levels of hypertension should be controlled by medication before operation?
7. Why is surgical correction of coarctation of the aorta not routinely advised after the age of 50?
8. When is the measurement of plasma renin levels of clinical significance?
9. What organ systems are commonly affected by severe hypertension?

Answers

1. Coarctation
   Cushing's disease
2. Hyperaldosteronism
3. Atherosclerosis
   Fibromuscular hyperplasia
4. Alpha-adrenergic and beta-adrenergic blockers
5. Excessive intake of exogenous corticosteroids
   Pituitary adenoma
   Adrenal adenoma
   Adrenal hyperplasia
6. A sustained diastolic pressure of 100 or above
7. The likelihood of relief of hypertension is much diminished in patients older than 50 years of age.
8. Principally in the determination of significant renal artery stenosis
9. Cardiovascular, kidney, and central nervous system

22 Stroke

RONALD J. STONEY
LINDA M. REILLY

KEY FEATURES

After reading this chapter you will understand:
- The causes of stroke.
- The anatomy of the cerebral circulation, including the extracranial carotid arteries.
- A wide spectrum of neurologic presentations.
- The clinical and laboratory (x-ray) evaluation of cerebrovascular disease.

The word *stroke* usually suggests a functionally and psychologically crippled individual who may have an associated speech impairment. The term serves as a graphic reminder of the profound effect that symptomatic cerebrovascular disease has on an individual who *survives* the event. This chapter deals with cerebrovascular disease from a vascular surgeon's perspective. Clinical manifestations of cerebrovascular disease are more intriguing, and the successful management more challenging, than any other vascular bed in the human body.

WHAT ARE THE CAUSES OF STROKE?

There are many causes of cerebrovascular disease, beginning with the heart and ending with arterioles and capillaries within the brain paren-

Supported in part by the Pacific Vascular Research Foundation, San Francisco, California.

chyma. Proximally, lesions within the left-sided chambers of the heart or the valves themselves may accumulate adherent material or degenerate and ulcerate, leaving exposed particulate matter in contact with the flowing blood. These products may embolize through the patent extracranial vasculature to lodge in distal intracranial vessels. These diagnoses may be suspected when prior heart disease, ischemic or valvular, is identified. Surgical correction and/or anticoagulation therapy are therapeutic options, depending on the underlying lesion, yet a cardiac source of stroke is rarely identified.

Beginning with the arch branches and continuing to the skull base, the extracranial arteries contain more than three quarters of the arterial lesions in the predictable locations from which symptoms of cerebrovascular disease originate. These include the innominate, common carotid, subclavian, and vertebral arteries (Fig. 22-1), and *the most important single site of extracranial cerebrovascular disease, the carotid bifurcation and the cervical internal carotid artery* (Fig. 22-2).

The intracranial arteries are the usual site where emboli lodge, having originated in more proximal portions of the extracranial arteries. There are other discrete uncommon events that affect the intracranial arteries, often resulting in a devastating stroke. They include spontaneous thromboses, dissection, and rupture with hemorrhage. Importantly, the intracranial arterial connections between the carotid and vertebral arteries at the skull base, the circle of Willis, provide an anatomic basis that explains the toler-

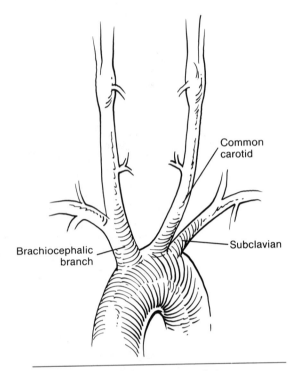

FIGURE 22-1 Extracranial arterial sites represent the predictable locations from which symptoms of cerebrovascular disease originate.

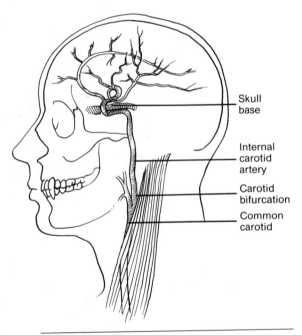

FIGURE 22-2 The carotid bifurcation and internal carotid artery.

ance of the human brain to occlusion of certain major extracranial arteries that supply specific portions of the brain (Fig. 22-3).

Cerebrovascular disease is perverse. Atherosclerosis, the major pathologic process, is preferentially located at the carotid bifurcation but is found in predictable sites in all extracranial arteries. Nonatherosclerotic extracranial diseases that cause cerebrovascular ischemia are uncommon, but for completeness, are listed below:

- Carotid fibromuscular dysplasia
- Internal carotid artery dissection
- Extrinsic carotid compression
- Takayasu's arteritis
- Radiation arteritis
- Aneurysm

This chapter emphasizes atherosclerosis and its extracranial locations, because it is the cerebrovascular disease that most frequently produces cerebrovascular symptoms. Mechanisms for production of ischemic cerebral symptoms are (1) *release of various microembolic fragments* from the plaque itself or thrombus adherent to it, or (2) *hypoperfusion resulting from critical flow reduction* because of the degree of luminal obstruction caused by the disease itself.

THE CLINICAL SPECTRUM OF CEREBROVASCULAR DISEASE

Patients who develop cerebrovascular disease can be grouped into five clinical categories:

1. Patients without symptoms (asymptomatic)
2. Patients with transient neurologic episodes
3. Patients with prolonged neurologic deficits
4. Patients with unstable neurologic deficits
5. Patients with completed stroke

Asymptomatic. These patients are usually discovered because a carotid bruit is detected. Although the bruit is a marker for vascular disease, it is an insensitive indicator of the extent and significance of the disease that may be suspected by its presence. Management of such patients is not standardized, since we lack a clear knowledge of the natural history of asymptomatic cerebrovascular disease. The employment of prospective studies can clarify this dilemma.

Transient Neurologic Episodes. The term *transient neurologic dysfunction* describes episodic, brief, focal neurologic dysfunction second-

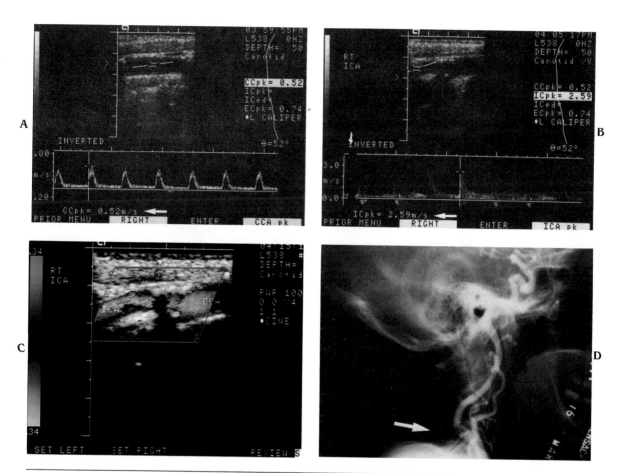

PLATE 22-1 Standard duplex images of **A,** the common carotid artery with a flow of 0.52 M/s *(arrow)* and **B,** the right internal carotid artery with a flow of 2.59 M/s. The higher flow is indicative of an obstructive lesion through which the velocity of the blood is increased. **C,** A color flow duplex scan showing the obstructed internal carotid artery takeoff. Color map at left shows higher velocities graded from red to orange to yellow. Blue signifies retrograde (turbulent) flow. **D,** A carotid arteriogram in the same patient visualizing the stenotic area in the right internal carotid artery. This two-dimensional assessment is augmented by the flow data to improve the estimation of the significance of the lesion.

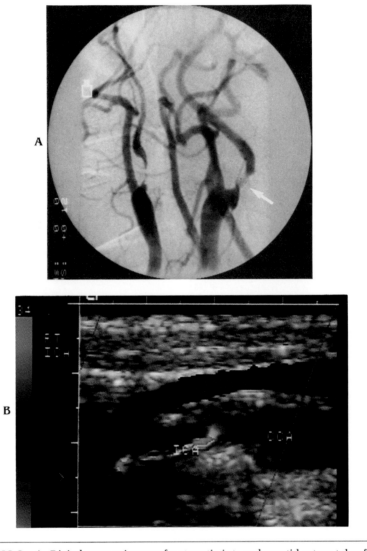

PLATE 22-2 **A,** Digital venous image of a stenotic internal carotid artery takeoff, also seen on the color flow image, **B.** Note the color changes as blood flows through the stenotic area *(ICA).*

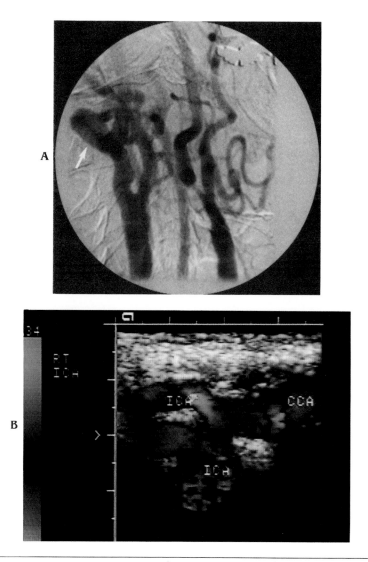

PLATE 22-3 A tortuous internal carotid artery with normal flow seen on **A,** digital venous imaging and **B,** color flow duplex scan.

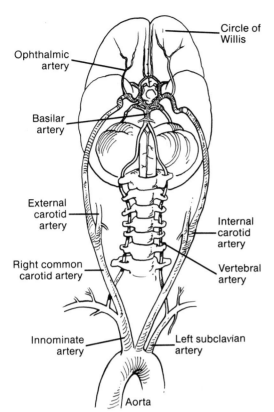

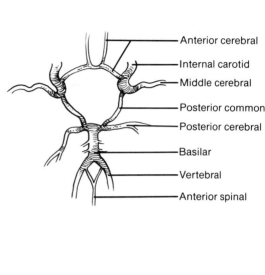

FIGURE 22-3   Anatomy of the intracranial arteries.

ary to ischemia. This includes the classic transient hemispheric ischemic attack (TIA), transient monocular blindness (amaurosis fujax), and transient localized neurologic dysfunction. TIA and amaurosis fujax are brief episodes (usually of minutes' duration) of neurologic or ocular dysfunction involving the hemisphere or retina; these usually completely resolve. There is no permanent ischemic damage and no residual effect at 24 hours.

Prolonged Neurologic Deficit. A transient ischemic episode that produces a focal neurologic dysfunction persisting more than 6 and less than 24 hours includes patients with the clinical categories of *reversible ischemic neurologic deficit (RIND).*

Acute Unstable Neurologic Deficit. This term describes crescendo TIAs, stroke and evolution, waxing and waning neurologic deficits, and, less commonly, progressive stroke. Those patients with unstable neurologic deficits, which include impaired conscious levels or coma, are not urgently investigated for treatment because cerebral infarction has already occurred. *In the symptomatic patient who does not have a significantly depressed level of consciousness, urgent investigation and removal or exclusion of the causative lesion will achieve a much-improved patient outcome when compared with medical treatment, including anticoagulation therapy.*

Completed Stroke. An acute completed stroke is the end-stage of symptomatic cerebrovascular disease, unless the affected patient succumbs to the cerebral infarction itself. The initial objective of treatment is supportive. Later the cause of stroke can be determined by using modern imaging technology: MRI and CT scans can detect intracranial hemorrhage, tumor, lacunar infarction, or primary thrombosis. Other causes of stroke can be detected in the extracranial vessels, although this information is usually gained through duplex scanning or arteriography. Arteriography is not safe to perform in the acute, early phase following a stroke, since the contrast study, as well as any operative intervention that may be indicated, have a significantly higher mortality in this setting in an unstable patient.

CLINICAL EVALUATION

History. History-taking involves personal questioning of the patient and accurate recording of the pertinent history. This should be verified with reliable observers, such as family members or friends. The clinician must understand the sequence of events, the time course, the clinical manifestations, and the resolution so that the most likely sites of extracranial arterial disease causing the dysfunction in the brain or eye can be identified. In this way, unstable lesions can be treated and neurologic tissue at risk can be minimized.

Physical Examination. Physical examination should be focused on the extracranial arterial system. After bilateral brachial blood pressures are determined, the carotid, subclavian, and upper-extremity pulses should be palpated and their pulse volume recorded. Thoughtful auscultation over the subclavian arteries and along the course of the carotid arteries from the clavicle to the angle of the jaw are carried out (Fig. 22-4). If the clinician finds that pulse volume is absent or significantly reduced or identifies a harsh bruit along the course of a major artery or over the carotid bifurcation, this may indicate significant arterial lesions.

Laboratory Investigation. The three objectives of the laboratory investigation of cerebrovascular disease are ensured by the use of specific techniques *(see color Plates 22-1 through 22-3 following p. 380).*

Objectives	Assessment
Arterial lesion	Duplex scanning
Target organ (brain or eye)	CT and/or MRI
Arterial flow channel	Arteriography

The lesions identified may cause symptoms by impairing perfusion or releasing microemboli. The local plaque may be smooth, ulcerated, or contain a hemorrhage within its walls. This hemorrhage may disrupt the plaque surface, allowing the discharge of blood and products of the plaque into the bloodstream.

WHAT ARE THE OPTIONS IN SURGICAL THERAPY?

The objectives of all forms of surgical therapy for patients harboring cerebrovascular disease are the prevention of stroke and the relief or alleviation of existing symptoms.

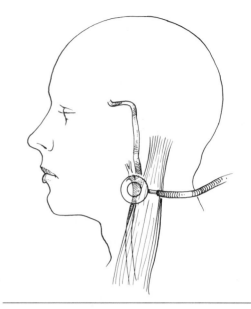

FIGURE 22-4 Auscultation should be carried out over the subclavian arteries and along the course of the carotid arteries from the clavicle to the angle of the jaw.

The clinical assessment and investigation will predictably identify a carotid bifurcation atheroma as the most likely lesion responsible for cerebral ischemia or infarction. Carotid endarterectomy, the most common surgical treatment, when precisely performed by a skilled vascular surgeon for appropriate indications, removes the lesion and provides an optimal environment for arterial healing.

The carotid bifurcation represents the site of symptomatic atherosclerotic lesions in 90% of patients. In the remaining 10% of symptomatic patients, the investigation will uncover the responsible lesion in the brachiocephalic (aortic arch branches) or proximal vertebral arteries. The surgical objectives when treating these uncommon lesions are to restore pulsatile flow to hypoperfused vascular beds, remove or exclude embolic lesions, and repair the lesion or lesion combinations that predispose to the stroke.

There are a number of reconstructive techniques because of the distribution of the proximal brachiocephalic lesions and the anatomy of the aortic branches themselves. These techniques include endarterectomy, grafting, transposition, and reimplantation.

PITFALLS AND COMMON MYTHS

- Imprecise history-taking in characterizing the neurologic or ocular event.
- Failure to identify flow-reducing or turbulence-producing extracranial lesions.
- Reluctance to apply appropriate laboratory investigations to characterize the lesion, target organ, and flow channel.

- Attempting to rely on antiplatelet drugs to control symptomatic cerebrovascular disease rather than targeted laboratory investigations.
- Attempting carotid endarterectomy in patients with an acute stroke and coma.
- Ignoring the stroke potential of TIAs.

BIBLIOGRAPHY

Byer JA, Easton JD. Transient cerebral ischemia: Review of surgical results. Prague Cardiovasc Dis 22: 389-396, 1980.

Dennis M, Bamford J, Sandercock P, Warlow C. Prognosis of transient ischemic attacks in the Oxfordshire community stroke project. Stroke 21:848-853, 1990.

DeWeese JA, Robb CG, Satran R, et al. Results of carotid endarterectomy for transient ischemic attacks five years later. Ann Surg 178:258-264, 1973.

Imparato AM, Riles TS, Mintzer R, Baumann FG. The importance of hemorrhage in the relationship between gross morphologic characteristics and cerebral symptoms in 376 carotid artery plaques. Ann Surg 197:195-203, 1983.

Lusby RJ, Ferrell LD, Ehrenfeld WK, et al. Carotid plaque hemorrhage: Its role in the production of cerebral ischemia. Arch Surg 117:1479-1488, 1982.

Nicolaides AN, Papadakis K, Grigg M, et al. Data from CT scans: The significance of silent cerebral infarctions and atrophy. In Bernstein EF (ed). Amaurosis Fugax. New York, Springer-Verlag, 1988, pp 200-227.

North American Symptomatic Carotid Endarterectomy Trial (NASCET) Investigators. Clinical alert: Benefit of carotid endarterectomy for patients with high-grade stenosis of the internal carotid artery. Stroke 22:816-817, 1991.

Roederer GO, Langlois YE, Jaeger KA, et al. The natural history of carotid arterial disease in asymptomatic patients with cervical bruits. Stroke 15:605, 1984.

Thompson JE. Carotid endarterectomy for asymptomatic carotid stenosis: An update. J Vasc Surg 13: 669-676, 1991.

CHAPTER REVIEW
Questions

1. What extracranial arterial site accounts for the majority of remedial causes of stroke?
2. What basic mechanisms underlie most symptomatic cerebrovascular disease?
3. True or false: Clinical examination for carotid bifurcation atherosclerosis begins with auscultation.
   a. True
   b. False
4. Name three investigative modalities for patients with suspected cerebrovascular disease:
5. True or false: Lesions of the proximal brachiocephalic arteries may produce upper extremity as well as brain or ocular symptoms.
   a. True
   b. False

Answers

1. Carotid bifurcation
2. Microemboli, hypoperfusion
3. a
4. Duplex scan—lesion
   CT or MRI scan—brain
   Arteriogram—flow channel
5. a

23 Lump in the Breast

BERNARD GARDNER

KEY FEATURES

After reading this chapter you will understand:
- The elements of good physical examination of the breast.
- The role of mammography in diagnosis and treatment.
- That biopsy of breast masses is the only certain way of making a diagnosis.
- Treatment of benign lesions.
- The staging of breast cancer, its importance, and criteria for treatment selection.
- How risk factors affect treatment plans.
- The treatment of advanced breast cancer.

DIAGNOSIS
History

Although an adequate history should be obtained concerning onset, trauma to the breast, nipple discharge, previous breast diseases or operations, associated pain, family history of breast cancer, parity, menstrual status, use of exogenous hormones, and nursing status, these factors actually play little role in the initial management of patients with a lump in the breast.

What Are the Key Elements in Physical Examination?

With the patient sitting and facing the examiner, *inspect* for the following:

- Symmetry of breasts
- Position of the nipples and of deformities
- Bulges or dimpling of the skin of the breast
- Pattern of venous drainage

Ask the patient to (1) *raise her arms,* since this will accentuate lesions fixed to the skin by producing dimpling or retraction (Fig. 23-1); (2) *place her hands on her hips and squeeze,* to produce pectoral muscle contraction leading to dimpling if lesions are present that are fixed to the pectoral fascia (see Fig. 23-1); and (3) *lean forward* to produce retraction signs (dimpling) in lesions of the lower half of the breast fixed to the skin or chest wall (Figs. 23-2 and 23-3).

Systematically *palpate* the supraclavicular region, infraclavicular region, and the breast in all quadrants. Some lesions are best felt with gentle fingertip pressure and others by grasping and palpating large areas of the breast. Both methods should be used. Ask the patient to point out the lesion, since she may be aware of one not detected by the examiner. Have the patient lie down and place a pillow under her back so that the breast lies flat on the chest wall (Fig. 23-4). *Palpation in two positions is necessary to discover some lesions.*

Palpate the axillae with the patient sitting and facing you by placing the fingers high in the axilla and compressing the contents against the chest wall (Fig. 23-5).

Normally the female breast has a lobular architecture and may be nodular in some women. The nodules are multiple and blend with the surrounding breast tissue. *A dominant mass is a nodule or lump that is distinctly harder or larger than other nodules that may be present or can be separated on palpation from the surrounding breast tissue.* Such a mass warrants a biopsy (Fig. 23-6). On occasion, several clusters of nodules may appear in one location (usually the upper outer quadrant) in an otherwise soft

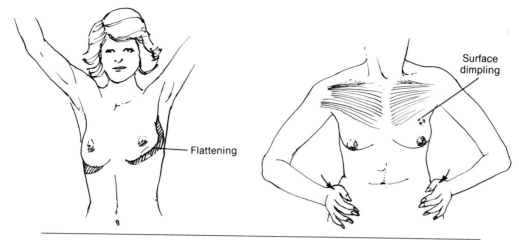

Flattening

Surface dimpling

FIGURE 23-1 Physical examination. Arm movements will frequently reveal areas of flattening of the normal breast contour when an underlying malignancy exists.

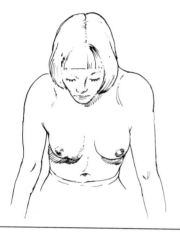

FIGURE 23-2 Having the patient lean forward will occasionally accentuate changes in breast contour when there is an underlying malignancy.

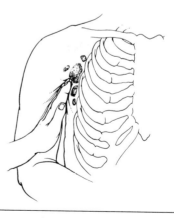

FIGURE 23-3 Skin retraction over a breast cancer.

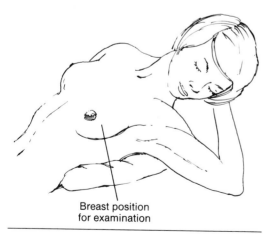

Breast position for examination

FIGURE 23-4 Examination in the supine position as well as sitting up may reveal an underlying lesion. With support under the patient the breast should lie flat on the chest wall.

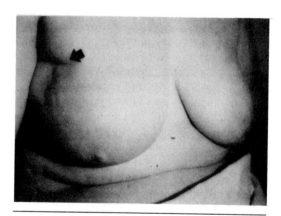

FIGURE 23-5 The axilla should be palpated by rolling the contents against the chest wall. Note that the patient's arm is relaxed and the elbow is flexed.

breast. This is a frequent finding in cystic breast disease, where it is usually associated with breast tenderness.

Clinical Approach

The woman with a breast mass is usually convinced that she has cancer and is in a state approaching panic. A thoughtful and reassuring approach is vital so that preliminary tests can be performed, and if indicated, elective biopsy can be scheduled. There is strong clinical evidence that if the mass is at least 1 cm, it has usually been present for a year or more; therefore a delay of a week for full assessment will not influence the ultimate prognosis.

Mammography and Xerography. Mammography and xerography are discussed together because they are equally effective in detecting a mass (approximately 90%) and have the same radiation exposure. Either test may be ordered, depending on the experience of the available radiologist. These tests are indicated to evaluate both breasts as well as the normal areas of the involved side, so that additional tissue may be removed if a suspicious area is visualized. While they sharply increase the accuracy of the clinical diagnosis of the mass in question, *under no circumstances do these tests obviate the need for histologic confirmation of the lesion.*

Figs. 23-7 through 23-9 demonstrate cancers of the breast as seen on mammography and xerography. Fig. 23-10 demonstrates a benign lesion similar in appearance to Fig. 23-9. Fig. 23-11 shows an inadequate mammogram that was read as negative. This patient had a carcinoma of the breast, demonstrating the importance of the surgeon's seeing the x-ray films for himself or herself.

Special techniques using magnification, squash, and so on have been developed to enhance the value of these radiographic approaches.

Mass Screening. Because of publicity concerning the risk of radiation from cumulative exposures over several years, it has been suggested that routine radiographic screening be limited to patients over age 50 or those with strong family histories of breast cancer. This fear of radiation has also caused a reduction in the use of these techniques in patients under age 35 who are undergoing biopsy or who have clinically obvious benign lesions. In fact, since there have been few studies demonstrating radiation-induced breast cancer after mammographic screening, many physicians still *recommend the procedure regularly for women over age 40 and in all patients with suspicious lesions.*

An interesting observation is that use of *interval mammography in screening programs tends to pick up lesions of worse prognosis.* This is

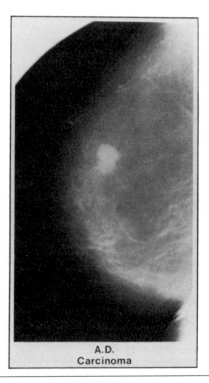

A.D.
Carcinoma

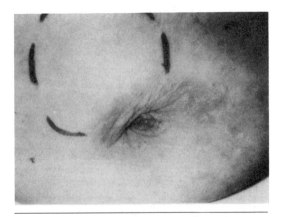

FIGURE 23-6 Retraction of the nipple associated with a breast mass. Usually a sign of malignancy.

FIGURE 23-7 Mammogram demonstrating a small breast cancer. Note the irregular margins and appearance of infiltration.

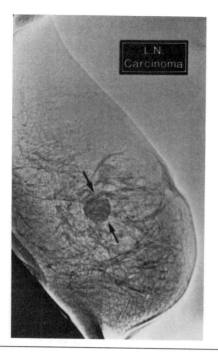

FIGURE 23-8 Xeroradiograph showing a cystic lesion that proved on biopsy to be a breast cancer.

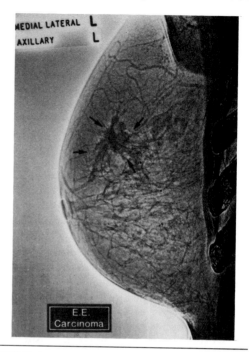

FIGURE 23-9 Xeroradiograph showing an irregular mass that proved to be malignant. (Compare this with Fig. 23-10.)

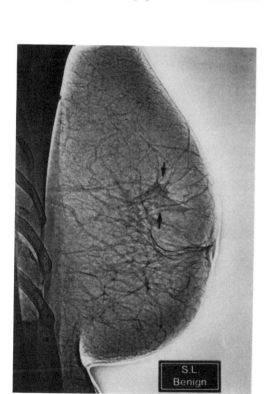

FIGURE 23-10 Xeroradiograph of an isolated benign breast mass.

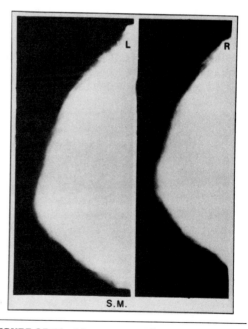

FIGURE 23-11 Mammogram that was read as benign, performed by an inexperienced radiologist. This patient had a breast cancer. No delay in treatment ensued, however, because the surgeon insisted on seeing the films since a mass had been palpated clinically.

explainable if we assume that in a population of women with breast cancer some will have rapidly growing cancers and some slowly growing cancers. At a particular time, mammograms will pick up all breast cancers with a long natural history. Repeat mammograms made 8 to 12 months later will pick up those lesions with rapid growth rates developing or becoming clinically evident during the interval—hence the poor prognosis.

Thermography. Thermography measures the temperature of the breast projected onto a special film. No radiation is involved. Because cancers are warmer than the surrounding tissue, the patterns projected can be diagnostic. However, the accuracy in detecting lesions is under 70%, and false-positive results have been reported, thereby sharply limiting the usefulness of the test.

Sonography. Recently several evaluations of sonographic differentiation of solid or cystic breast masses have been made. While the accuracy of sonography in confirming the presence of small nodules has been demonstrated, its role in clinical management is not clear. Biopsy confirmation is still essential in the evaluation of breast masses, whether they were detected by palpation or by mammography. Cystic lesions may be aspirated, but disappearance of the mass should be demonstrated if biopsy is to be avoided.

Fig. 23-12 shows a sonogram of a mass diagnosed as a cyst, but which was subsequently found to be a fibroadenoma. However, further experience with ultrasonography is warranted, since in the hands of skilled radiologists lesions can be identified that are not evidenced by other techniques.

What Is the Value of Breast Self-Examination? A number of recent studies have confirmed an improved prognosis of breast cancers found in women who regularly practice breast self-examination (BSE), because the lesion is discovered at an earlier clinical stage. The method should be taught in the physician's office and encouraged uniformly.

Aspiration of the Mass. Some physicians routinely aspirate lesions to differentiate cystic from solid masses. If fluid is obtained, it can be cytologically examined. If the mass disappears with aspiration, one may be assured it is benign, although several additional follow-up visits are necessary to be certain that an associated solid tumor has not been missed. Recurrence of a breast mass in a patient previously biopsied for a benign cyst is a good indication for aspiration, since these cysts are often multiple and may reappear in other segments of the breasts.

Cytologic Examination. Cytologic examination can be performed on aspirated material or if a discharge is present. The yield is extremely low, and if the discharge is bloody or associated with a mass, biopsy is indicated regardless of a negative cytology report.

Fine-needle aspiration of breast masses has been used in some centers to avoid unnecessary biopsy or to facilitate rapid treatment. Variable results have limited the usefulness of the procedure, since false-negative reports may reach over 15% in some institutions and indeterminate results average 4% to 18%.

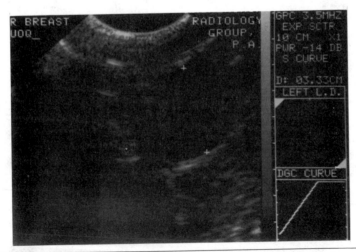

FIGURE 23-12 Sonogram demonstrating a large cystic-appearing tumor that subsequently proved to be a fibroadenoma. Results of aspiration were negative, so a biopsy was performed.

Biopsy. As indicated, biopsy is the only definitive method for diagnosing cancer of the breast. The exact method used is related to the experience and preference of the individual surgeon. Outpatient biopsy with local anesthesia is being used more and more frequently, since it is very safe and can be done with minimal disruption of the patient's schedule and without the necessity of obtaining consent for a possible mastectomy. If cancer is diagnosed, the choice of operation can be discussed with the patient and subsequently scheduled. However, some surgeons still biopsy highly suspicious lesions with the patient under general anesthesia, with frozen section pathologic examination and appropriate further surgery of the lesion if it is positive.

What Is Specimen Mammography? When a *nonpalpable lesion* is operated on, a careful routine is followed to be certain that the lesion has been removed. The patient is admitted and taken to the x-ray department on the morning of surgery. Needles are placed in the breast and a mammogram is performed. With the lesion localized in relation to the needles, the patient is brought to the operating room and under anesthesia the involved segment is removed. Mammography is repeated on the excised breast tissue—carefully labeling all quadrants of the specimen. If the lesion is in the resected specimen, it is brought to the pathology department where careful sectioning and frozen sections are made. Appropriate treatment is then carried out. Follow-up mammograms are suggested to be certain the abnormal tissue has been removed.

TREATMENT
How Do You Diagnose and Treat Benign Breast Lesions?

Breast Abscess. *Unlike abscesses elsewhere, those in the breast may not be fluctuant.* The decision to drain an abscess is based on clinical assessment of the fever, leukocytosis, and failure to respond to antibiotic treatment. Some malignant lesions may present as abscesses. Therefore, at the time of incision and drainage, a generous biopsy of the wall is made for pathologic examination.

A particular abscess located under the areola is associated with a retention cyst of the breast. It is important to identify such a lesion, because it may often demonstrate clinical signs of malignancy, such as firmness and nipple retraction. *Treatment is to resect the lesion and disconnect the subareolar tissue (ducts) to avoid the recurrence that may follow simple drainage.*

Lactation should be suppressed when an abscess occurs in a lactating female.

Fibroadenoma. Fibroadenoma is commonly seen in younger women and is frightening to the patient because of its firmness to palpation. The lesion may be any size and is occasionally nodular, although the usual fibroadenoma is round, smooth, and freely movable. It gives the sensation of a marble in the breast and rarely demonstrates retraction of the skin or dimpling. *Treatment is excision.* In some patients, multiple lesions occur synchronously or metachronously, but careful dissection and reapproximation of the breast tissue will avoid permanent deformity after excision.

Cysts. Cysts are common lesions of the breast that cannot be clinically differentiated from fibroadenomas unless aspiration is done preoperatively. They may occasionally be found after a negative aspiration if they are multiloculated or missed by the aspirating needle. *If they do not completely disappear after aspiration, excision should be made to differentiate them from a cancer.*

Fibrocystic Disease. The term *fibrocystic disease* or *fibrocystic breast condition* has been applied to a variety of breast lesions, which vary from the association of several cysts to a hard, tender, nodular area associated with erythema and heat. In some reports, fibrocystic disease is associated with an increased incidence of breast cancer ranging from 1.5- to 4-fold. This confusion results from imprecise histologic description of the lesion. *Some cystic changes are associated with marked evidence of proliferative breast disease.* It is in these cases that a premalignant potential may exist. Other cystic changes have no proliferative changes or, in fact, *may show involutional changes (fibrosis), and these cases clearly have no premalignant potential.*

When cancer is suspected, mammography or xerography should be performed, followed by a period of observation to see if the lesion will regress. Biopsy is indicated if one area of involvement appears firmer or more distinct than the surrounding areas of the breast, *but in most cases supportive treatment, including local heat, a firm brassiere, and occasionally diuretic tablets,* may be of value. Unfortunately, these patients may have exquisitely tender breasts that are refractory to most treatment regimens. Frequent reassurance that no cancer is present may be necessary.

Fibrous Disease of the Breast. A host of lesions manifested by dense deposits of collagen, ranging from fibrous mastopathy to sclerosing adenosis, are categorized under this poorly understood heading. The lesions may be diffuse or highly localized, simulating a malignancy. Characteristically, the breast has the feeling of firmness, and its margins can be clearly felt. *When the lesion is solitary, a biopsy to confirm the diagnosis must be made.*

Fat Necrosis. Trauma to the breast may lead to a fibrous scar in the fat that may be associated with skin retraction. Since malignancy cannot be ruled out, *a biopsy is necessary.*

Giant Fibroadenoma (Benign Cystosarcoma). Rarely, a fibroadenoma may occupy a major portion of the breast. Rapid growth may be in evidence clinically, and because of the firmness of the mass and bulging margins, it cannot be differentiated from a malignant lesion. *Excision and meticulous reconstruction of the breast* will lead to a satisfactory result, since metastases do not occur. Recurrence of the disease in the involved breast is usually the result of inadequate excision.

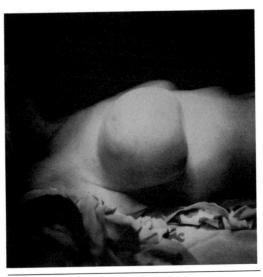

FIGURE 23-13   Cystosarcoma phylloides at operation.

Malignant Lesions

Sarcoma. Cystosarcoma phylloides of the breast represents a spectrum of lesions that range from local microscopic malignancy in small fibroadenomas or benign lesions to highly malignant metastasizing lesions. Thus it is *imperative that the surgeon and pathologist completely understand the clinical significance of the diagnosis and that clear communication exists when the diagnosis is made.* Differentiation should be established between giant fibroadenomas, benign cystosarcoma, focal cystosarcoma, or malignant cystosarcoma phylloides (Fig. 23-13).

In all cases that are not malignant, wide segmental resection is all that is required, with a margin of normal breast tissue around the lesion. Reconstruction will lead to a normal-appearing breast. Even giant fibroadenomas can be resected with minimal deformity by mobilizing breast tissue from the base of the lesion on the pectoral muscle and sliding it to fill the dead space. When a fibroadenoma is resected *that contains focal malignant change identified on permanent sections, the patient is brought back to the operating room for a resection of the involved quadrant* to ensure adequate removal, since extensions of the lesion can be cut across by dissection close to the apparent capsule of the lesion.

Frankly malignant lesions are treated by modified radical mastectomy. Removal of the entire breast is mandated by the high incidence of local recurrence (30%) after lesser procedures. Strictly

speaking, *the potential of these lesions metastasizing to regional nodes is very low,* but the minimal morbidity of added axillary nodal dissection in our hands has led to a more aggressive attitude in the management of this condition. When associated carcinoma is found, the treatment is directed at this ominous lesion and depends on the precise diagnosis.

Cancers Metastatic to the Breast. Cancers from other sites may metastasize to the breast. The most common are lymphomas and malignant melanoma. Careful histologic evaluation will avoid unnecessary radical surgery.

Carcinoma. Cancer of the breast represents 27% of all female cancers, accounting for 19% of cancer deaths in American women. In 1991, 175,000 cases were reported with 44,500 deaths leading to the conclusion that 1 of every 9 American women will have the disease at some time in her life.

The incidence of breast cancer increases with advancing age, being less than 80 per 100,000 between the ages of 35 and 39 and rising to 300 and over 400 per 100,000 for ages 80 and 85, respectively. *The most common occurrence is between 40 and 60 years of age.*

Tumor Markers. In an attempt to predict which patients are likely to develop breast cancer, an enormous research effort has been launched to identify blood or tissue factors that are associated with increased risk.

Clinical tumor markers associated with increased risk are (1) an immediate family member (or members) with breast cancer or (2) a previous history of breast cancer; less frequently predisposing factors include (3) nulliparity, (4) early onset of menses, and (5) failure to nurse after childbirth. There is no proven relationship between breast cancer and previous use of exogenous estrogens.

Recent developments of techniques to identify specific genes in breast cancer tissue have indicated that specific gene expression, amplification, or deletion *may be associated* with the risk of breast cancer or its ability to invade and metastasize. More than 30 polypeptide growth factors and more than 40 distinct oncogenes have been identified, some of which are found in increased levels in breast cancer tissue. Correlation with clinical behavior is presently under active investigation; conclusions must await completion and verification of these studies. Other tumor markers are discussed next.

A number of recent studies have implicated *dietary factors* in the predisposition to breast cancer development. These studies suffer from the fact that dietary analysis during the clinical onset of the disease may not accurately reflect the dietary habits at the inception of the disease many years earlier. While the promotional effects of dietary fat, particularly unsaturated fats and some milk products, on mammary tumors in rodents is well established, only epidemiologic suspicion exists regarding human breast cancer.

Geographic incidence of the disease has been under intensive epidemiologic study with the countries of highest predilection being England and Wales (death rate = 34/100,000 population); Denmark, New Zealand, Scotland, and the Netherlands (31/100,000 population); and the United States and Switzerland (27 to 29/100,000 population), all reported in 1979. Japan, with one of the lowest death rates from the disease (6/100,000 population), represents an unusual opportunity to study the effects of geographic mobility on the incidence of disease. Japanese women living in Hawaii or the mainland United States have in several generations been found to have an increasing death rate from breast cancer, *indicating a strong environmental relationship to the disease.* Within mainland United States, the highest risk is in the northeastern section and the lowest incidence is in the southern states.

Staging and Prognosis. Biopsy is essential for diagnostic confirmation, and *treatment depends on the clinical stage of the disease.* No single staging system for cancer of the breast is fully satisfactory, nor have definitive uniform criteria of inoperability been established. The most commonly used staging system is shown in Table 23-1. Survivals at 5 and 10 years are shown in the following percentages.

	5 Years (%)	10 Years (%)
Stage I	80	70
Stage II	50	30
Stage III	30	15
Untreated	20	<1

The two most constant factors determining prognosis in operable cases are the size of the primary lesion and the involvement of the axillary nodes. The actual number of positive nodes is more significant than the incidence of involved nodes, i.e., 1 positive node of 5 nodes examined is more favorable than 3 positive nodes of 100 examined (Tables 23-2 and 23-3).

A positive bone scan result may determine the presence of metastases in the operable patient. Evidence of metastases on chest or bone x-ray examination is an absolute indication of inoperability. Other such criteria include the presence of histologically confirmed positive supraclavicular nodes, ulceration of the mass, satellite nodules in the skin, arm edema, massive *peau d'orange* (skin edema over the breast), and fixed axillary nodes. Classification into stage III is a relative contraindication to operation as sole treatment.

What Treatment Options Exist for Breast Cancer? Wide excision of the primary tumor plus eradication of the accessible regional lymph nodes of primary drainage (i.e., radical mastectomy) has been most widely employed. *Reports of similar survival rates with widely varying treatment regimens* have led to much controversy about optimal treatment. This is largely because of the difficulties of evaluating retrospective studies of populations that may not have been similar.

Although data on growth rates of cancer are difficult to apply in clinical situations, it is apparent that breast cancer qualifies *as a tumor of moderately slow growth rate that metastasizes relatively early* in its natural history (see Chapter 12). These two factors account for most of the misunderstandings relevant to its treatment. The early metastatic potential of the disease leads, in large series of operable cases, to 40% to 50% 10-year cures (stages I and II). This fact has led to a nihilistic approach on the part of some physicians, which is thoroughly unjustified in the individual case. Furthermore, since all recurrences of breast cancer after mastectomy are caused by metastatic deposits (micrometastases) present before the breast removal, *the slow growth rate*

TABLE 23-1   TNM Classification of Breast Cancer

Primary Tumor (T)
Clinical-Diagnostic Classification

TX	Primary tumor cannot be assessed
T0	No evidence of primary tumor
T1S	Carcinoma in situ: Intraductal carcinoma, lobular carcinoma in situ, or Paget's disease of the nipple with no demonstrable tumor
T1	Tumor 2 cm or less in greatest dimension
T1a	0.5 cm or less in greatest dimension
T1b	More than 0.5 cm but not more than 1 cm in greatest dimension
T1c	More than 1 cm but not more than 2 cm in greatest dimension
T2	Tumor more than 2 cm but not more than 5 cm in greatest dimension
T3	Tumor more than 5 cm in greatest dimension
T4	Tumor of any size with direct extension to chest wall or skin
T4a	Extension to chest wall
T4b	Edema (including peau d'orange) or ulceration of the skin of the breast or satellite skin nodules confined to the same breast
T4c	Both (T4a and T4b)
T4d	Inflammatory carcinoma

Nodal Involvement (N)

NX	Regional lymph nodes cannot be assessed (e.g., previously removed)
N0	No regional lymph node metastasis
N1	Metastasis to movable ipsilateral axillary lymph node(s)
N2	Metastasis to ipsilateral axillary lymph node(s) fixed to one another or to other structures
N3	Metastasis to ipsilateral internal mammary lymph node(s)

Distant Metastasis (M)

MX	Presence of distant metastasis cannot be assessed
M0	No distant metastasis
M1	Distant metastasis (includes metastasis to ipsilateral supraclavicular lymph nodes)

These descriptions are then combined to define four stages:

Stage 0	T1S	N0	M0
Stage I	T1	N0	M0
Stage IIA	T0	N1	M0
	T1	N1	M0
	T2	N0	M0
Stage IIB	T2	N1	M0
	T3	N0	M0
Stage IIIA	T0	N2	M0
	T1	N2	M0
	T2	N2	M0
	T3	N1, N2	M0
Stage IIIB	T4	Any N	M0
	Any T	N3	M0
Stage IV	Any T	Any N	M1

From American Joint Committee for Cancer Staging and End-Results Reporting. Manual for Staging Cancer, 1988.

TABLE 23-2 Number of Negative Nodes
Examined Related to Survival and Recurrence

No. of Nodes	5-Year Recurrence Rate (%)	5-Year Survival Rate (%)
1-5	23	74
16-20	18	74
≥30	20	81

TABLE 23-3 Number of Positive Nodes
Examined Related to Survival and Recurrence

No. of Nodes	5-Year Recurrence Rate (%)	5-Year Survival Rate (%)
1-5	40	60
16-20	42	61
≥30	44	61

plays a significant role in the fact that recurrences may not appear for 8 to 10 years after operation. This being the case, new or nonstandard approaches to treatment evaluated at the end of 5 years may be encouraging, but after 8 years may be disappointing when compared with standard treatment. Therefore *new treatments for primary breast cancer that have not been evaluated prospectively in large randomized trials followed for 10 years should be considered experimental.* The large experience with radical mastectomy over many years, yielding survival rates of 70% for stage I and 30% for stage II at 10 years, must be used as the "gold standard" with which all other treatments should be compared. Results of treatments yielding significantly lower survival rates should be questioned.

From an evaluation of survival data, it appears that a population of 100 women with operable breast cancer can be divided into three main groups. About 50 are incurable when first seen (already metastasized), and 35 to 40 can be cured with a wide local excision. Only a small number (10 to 15) whose lesions have just begun to metastasize to the regional nodes represent the actual population at risk for various treatments. Unfortunately, no current test clearly defines the group into which any individual patient will fall, and therefore all 100 are treated alike. This illustration is useful because it explains why different treatments yield survival data that do not differ

by more than 15%. In fact, *the actual survival rate will vary, depending on the number of patients with early metastases in the total group.* It also emphasizes the *importance of using randomized prospective studies* to evaluate the results of treatment, since those patients operated on will have been staged on the basis of clinical data (physical and x-ray examination) regardless of the actual spread of the disease.

Some recent reports indicate that breast cancer does not spread to regional nodes until it has already metastasized. This theory would not account for the marked differences in survival between groups treated by local excision alone versus those treated by radical mastectomy.

Because of the wide choice of operations and radiotherapy currently being offered to the patient with operable breast cancer, a treatment scheme based on current consensus is illustrated in Fig. 23-14. Reference to this flow sheet during the following discussion will be helpful. Data from the National Surgical Adjuvant Breast Project (NSABP) study of partial mastectomy indicate satisfactory 5-year survival rates using this treatment regimen. However, additional follow-up, use of comparable staging systems, and evaluation of the significance of the high incidence of local recurrence need to be assessed before firm recommendations can be made.

Stage 0

IN SITU LOBULAR CARCINOMA. In situ lobular carcinoma of the breast is treated by wide local excision if only one or two lobules are involved. Rarely, when more lobules are involved, mastectomy may be performed. Reexcision is not done when one lobule is involved microscopically and coincident with breast excision of another lesion (i.e., cyst). Lymph node ablation is not indicated unless coincident invasive carcinoma is present. Baseline mammography or xerography is done and close follow-up is indicated, since 20% of these patients will develop invasive carcinoma on close long-term follow-up. Mirror-image biopsy will yield 20% positive specimens for in situ lobular carcinoma in the opposite breast.

IN SITU DUCT CARCINOMA. Microscopic coincident discovery of in situ duct carcinoma should be treated by segmental mastectomy with breast reconstruction. *A mastectomy is not required as long as the lesion is localized to a few microscopic sections.* Multiple sections are taken to ensure that there is no invasion of breast stroma beyond the duct wall. No adjuvant chemotherapy or radiotherapy is necessary. Mirror-image biopsy is not done, but baseline mammography and close follow-up are undertaken, because ipsilateral in-

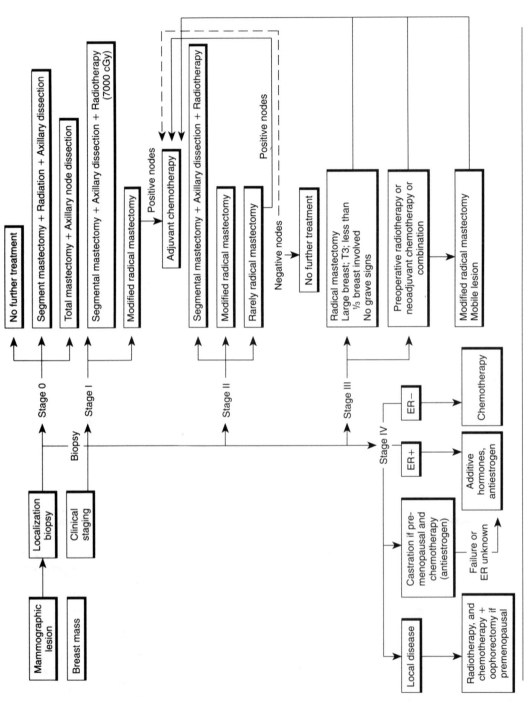

FIGURE 23-14 Algorithm for the management of breast cancer. (Modified from Alfonso A, Gardner B. Principles of Cancer Surgery. New York, 1981. Appleton-Century-Crofts. Used by permission.)

vasive cancer has been reported in 10% to 25% of cases. Occasionally breast radiation is used. If the lesion is not localized but part of a generalized process in the breast with malignant or atypical changes in multiple microscopic sections, mastectomy is carried out. This is particularly used if the lesion is of the comedo type.

INVASIVE LOBULAR CARCINOMA. This is treated exactly as invasive duct carcinoma except that mirror-image biopsy is always done, yielding 60% positive findings in the opposite breast (see below).

Stage I Infiltrating Ductal Carcinoma. Segmental quadrant excision plus axillary node resection is done for stage I carcinoma of the breast if the lesion is peripherally located and the breast is of adequate size. The biopsy scar plus skin measuring 3 cm around the margins of the lesion is included in the resection. If the lesion is in the upper outer quadrant, axillary node dissection is made through the same incision. Postoperative radiation therapy to the reconstructed breast (5000 cGy over 6 to 7 weeks) is included as part of the treatment schedule to avoid local recurrence. Contraindications to this approach include subareolar lesions and patients with relatively small breasts that preclude adequate margins without significant deformity. The excellent results obtainable with standard radical mastectomy or modified radical mastectomy must be presented to the patient, and it should be made clear that the ultimate results with lesser procedures are still under investigation. Some women prefer mastectomy followed in 6 to 12 months by breast reconstruction. In addition the procedure may be useful in resection of nonpalpable (mammography defined) breast cancer. **Since up to 40% of clinically stage I cancer may have axillary node involvement** in pathologic staging, it is imperative to review the pathology of the axillary nodes. Positive-node patients are treated routinely with adjuvant chemotherapy or a hormonal therapy, depending on levels of estrogen binding in the tumor and the menopausal status. Chemotherapy is occasionally recommended for negative-node patients when certain **pathologic markers** for aggressive disease may be present. These include high nuclear grade, vascular or neural invasion, and multiple areas of invasive disease.

In addition, evaluation of DNA synthesis (S-phase) by flow cytometry may be warranted to assess prognosis. **Flow cytometry** involves a system of passing particles (cells) through a measuring apparatus in a fluid stream. This enables certain parameters of the particles to be charac-

terized using an electronic or optical sensor. Results vary, depending on the accuracy and experience of the personnel and the equipment involved. DNA content of cells when compared with a standard for diploid cells will identify any abnormal DNA content (aneuploidy). Identification of the percentage of cells in S-phase (DNA synthesis) is also reported. In breast cancer patients recent studies demonstrate a correlation of prognosis with S-phase (higher S-phase = poorer prognosis), but not with ploidy. This may indicate another group of patients who may benefit from adjuvant chemotherapy.

The levels of circulating growth factors or tissue levels of oncogenes have not been clinically correlated with prognosis in sufficient numbers of patients to make recommendations at this time.

Stage II Infiltrating Ductal Carcinoma. The treatment choices for this stage have led to considerable confusion among patients and surgeons. Modified radical mastectomy is recommended by a majority of practicing surgeons but a plethora of studies now indicate that segmental mastectomy with axillary node dissection and postoperative radiation to the breast may yield equally good results. The necessity of obtaining adequate margins with resection requires that the pathologist mark the specimen carefully. Recurrence of cancer in the ipsilateral breast is 10% to 20% after this treatment, but it is much higher if the margins are involved at the time of resection. Subsequent mastectomy may still be curative.

It therefore appears that the size of tumor relative to the size of breast may play a significant role in the choice of procedure. Since the segmental mastectomy is offered as a cosmetically acceptable treatment for breast cancer (but not because of superior results), the patient's age and social and psychologic setting are all factors in making the decision. The patient should be fully informed of her options concerning breast reconstruction either primarily or secondarily as they affect the ultimate outcome.

Breast reconstruction can be done at the time of the primary operation or electively later. Techniques involve the use of tissue expanders to enlarge the skin flap and space available for a prosthetic implant. Pedicled or free muscle and/ or muscle and skin (myocutaneous) flaps can be used to simulate breast tissue. In a second (or third) procedure the nipple and areolar complex can be reconstructed. When performed by competent plastic surgeons, results of these procedures have been excellent. Patients whose reconstructions are successful express a high level of satisfaction with the result; however, when delayed reconstruction is offered, fewer than 20% of patients avail themselves of the procedure.

Stage III. A modified approach to stage III tumors can be followed. If the patient has a large breast, so that the tumor occupies less than one third of the breast (even if larger than 5 cm) and there are no other signs of inoperability such as metastases, arm edema, satellite nodules, peau d'orange, or ulceration, the patient receives a standard mastectomy and adjuvant chemotherapy.

All other stage III lesions are treated by radiotherapy to the chest wall, breast, axilla, supraclavicular, and mediastinal areas to 6000 cGy over 6 weeks. If, after radiotherapy is completed, the tumor has shrunk significantly and is mobile, a modified radical mastectomy should be carried out, followed by chemotherapy.

ADJUVANT AND NEOADJUVANT CHEMOTHERAPY. It should be stressed that current recommendations for use of chemotherapy after standard treatment for stage I and II breast cancer include all positive-node patients (Table 23-4) and those negative-node patients with pathologic markers indicating aggressive disease (discussed earlier). Preoperative chemotherapy (neoadjuvant) has also been recommended for locally advanced stage III lesions, since reduction in size of the cancer may facilitate a cosmetic resection of the breast. Cures are extremely rare in stage III disease and, at present, nonexistent in stage IV disease.

The use of adjuvant chemotherapy has been extensively investigated and a consensus for its use has been reached (Table 23-5). When adju-

TABLE 23-4 Benefits of Early Clinical Trials (Adjuvant Therapy in Positive-Node Patients)

Author	No. of Patients	Adjuvant Therapy	Follow-Up (Years)	Greatest Subgroup Benefit
Fisher NSABP-B-05	380	L-PAM Placebo	10	Premenopausal women with 1-3 positive nodes
Bonnadonna	386	CMF control	10	Premenopausal patients
Bonnadonna	459	CMF—6 mo CMF—12 mo	7	No difference

L-PAM = L phenylalanine mustard; C = cytoxan; M = methotrexate; F = 5-fluorouracil.

TABLE 23-5 Adjuvant Chemotherapy

Patient	Recommendation for Adjuvant Therapy
Premenopausal Positive lymph nodes	Treatment with established chemotherapy
Premenopausal Negative lymph nodes	No adjuvant therapy recommended, except for high-risk patients (see tumor markers)
Postmenopausal Positive lymph nodes ER +	Chemotherapy should be considered; tamoxifen should be used
Postmenopausal Positive lymph nodes ER −	Chemotherapy ± tamoxifen
Postmenopausal Negative lymph nodes ER ±	No treatment (ER ± tamoxifen)

vant chemotherapy is employed, there is a prolonged disease-free survival in certain subgroups as well as a decrease in 5-year mortality. Whether this will translate into an overall increase in survival is still in doubt. The following conclusions, however, can be made: (1) Polychemotherapy is better than single-drug chemotherapy, (2) prolonged chemotherapy (18 to 24 months) provides no advantage over shorter courses (6 to 10 months), (3) tamoxifen should be added to the regimens of postmenopausal patients regardless of results of estrogen-binding studies, and (4) tamoxifen should not be used alone in estrogen-negative premenopausal patients.

Stage IV. Treatment for stage IV lesions or recurrent breast cancer is by a combination chemotherapy regimen and hormones, with or without radiation therapy. Treatment depends on the extent of disease, status of hormone receptors (necessitating biopsy of accessible lesions), and menopausal status of the patient.

Table 23-6 outlines some commonly used chemotherapy and hormonal regimens for advanced breast cancer. The use of antiestrogens in estrogen receptor (ER)–positive patients has become widespread because of effective results and minimal toxicity. Most other hormonal treatments have given way to early effective chemotherapy, which has uniformly yielded higher response rates. Although castration is still used occasionally, it is rare for adrenalectomy to be used as additional treatment. The current progression now involves chemotherapy in conjunction with bone marrow transplantation when previous treatment has failed to control the cancer. However, results have not yet yielded sufficient cause for enthusiasm for use of this regimen in the treatment of this disease.

Follow-up is conducted at 4- to 6-week intervals. Progression of the disease is an indication for a change of regimen.

Male Breast Cancer. The standard treatment for operable male breast cancer is radical mastectomy. Modifications are not used so that adequate margins are achieved. Skin grafting must be done in all patients to ensure adequate removal of skin with the primary tumor. Failure of treatment may be related to long delays in treatment because of inaccurate diagnosis or failure to perform an early biopsy.

Recurrent or inoperable disease is treated with castration and aminoglutethimide. Chemotherapy is used if these subsequently fail.

TABLE 23-6   Commonly Used Regimens for Advanced Breast Cancer

	Average Response Rate (%)	Comments
Single Agents		
Hormones		Related to estrogen-binding protein
Estrogens	26	Positive patients (>3 fm) respond in >50%
Androgens	21	Negative patients respond in <10%
Progestins	25	
Corticosteroids	23	
Ablation		
Oophorectomy	33	
Adrenalectomy	32	
Hypophysectomy	36	
Antiestrogens	35	
Combination Agents		Duration of responses averaged 5-10 months, which is lower than with single-agent hormones
CMP*	43	
CMF-VP	49	
CMF	57 (48)	
CMF-P	63	
AF; AFC; AFCM	42-49	
CAF-VP	57	

*P = prednisone; C = cyclophosphamide; A = doxorubicin (Adriamycin); M = methotrexate; F = 5-fluorouracil; V = vincristine.

Postoperative Irradiation. Postoperative radiation is not indicated in stage I or II disease that has been treated by mastectomy and axillary node dissection (radical or modified radical mastectomy). *It is, however, essential when segmental mastectomy is performed,* since recurrence of the tumor is inordinately high without it (>40%). Radiation does not replace the need for adequate surgical margins. Recent studies have indicated that when large areas of noninvasive cancer are found in the breast (on multiple microscopic sections) or when histologic studies reveal a comedo-type structure, radiation may not be successful in preventing recurrence. The recommended dose is 5000 cGy given externally to the breast and boosted by implantation to a level of 2000 cGy (total = 7000 cGy). *The axilla must not be irradiated if an axillary dissection has been made.*

Prophylactic Oophorectomy (Castration). Controlled randomized studies have failed to demonstrate that oophorectomy performed concomitantly with mastectomy in cases of operable primary breast cancer alters survival. Castration is reserved for menstruating females with recurrent or inoperable breast cancer. Recent data on estrogen-binding receptors, however, may necessitate a reevaluation of this treatment.

SPECIFIC PROBLEMS IN BREAST DISEASES
Pregnancy

Pregnancy per se does not alter the survival rate for women with breast cancer compared with survival rates for nonpregnant women of similar age. *Reported poor results in these patients were traced to delay in definitive treatment by allowing the pregnancy to proceed normally before breast biopsy.* Early biopsy is recommended in all women with breast masses, under local anesthesia if necessary.

Whether the patient who has undergone treatment for breast cancer should consider further pregnancies depends on the psychologic and social particulars of the patient and her spouse. We usually advise against it in patients with stage II lesions, but a uniform policy is unwise. There is no evidence that another pregnancy is detrimental to the patient with breast cancer, and our advice is based on the prognosis of the primary disease.

Bilateral Disease

Synchronous bilateral breast cancer has been reported in 10% or more of women undergoing routine contralateral breast biopsy at the time of radical mastectomy. The development of a cancer in the second breast has been the subject of much study. The risk varies according to the age of the patient at the time of the first primary lesion. The overall relative risk is 2.9, varying from 9.9 in patients under 50 years of age when first diagnosed to 1.9 in those over 50. The cumulative risk figures were 13% for women under 50 years and 3.5% for women older than 50 years. This implies that occasional cases of histologically diagnosed breast cancer, in a clinically negative breast, lie dormant for long periods or do not develop into clinical cancer. *Synchronous or metachronous breast cancer without evidence of dissemination is treated as a primary disease in each breast.*

Lobular in situ carcinoma of the breast is bilateral in 20% of cases and warrants a contralateral mirror-image breast biopsy. If lobular carcinoma is infiltrating or invasive, up to 60% bilaterality has been reported. For the in situ lesion, wide excision is usually sufficient, although the associated higher incidence of synchronous infiltrating duct cancer in these women has prompted some surgeons to recommend total mastectomy.

Inflammatory Carcinoma

Inflammatory carcinoma must be differentiated histologically from carcinoma with inflammation. The former represents a rare type of breast cancer with a poor prognosis, which is usually treated by primary radiotherapy and chemotherapy. Studies involving adjuvant surgery (mastectomy) to a regimen of preoperative and postoperative chemotherapy have yielded less discouraging results.

Nipple Discharge

Occasionally patients present with nipple discharge and no palpable mass (Fig. 23-15). Every effort at diagnosis should be made, including cytologic examination of the discharge, mammography, and so on. If no lesion is found, the quadrant of the breast that produces the discharge on compression or corresponds to the quadrant of the nipple from which the discharge appears is biopsied. Bloody discharges are often caused by intraductal (benign) papilloma of the breast but may be associated with cancer or tuberculosis. Clear or greenish discharges may be associated with fibrocystic disease or cancer. White discharges may be caused by abscess or secretion of milk and are almost always benign.

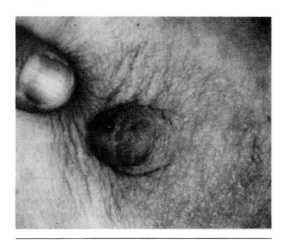

FIGURE 23-15 Example of a bloody nipple discharge.

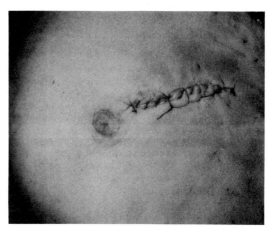

FIGURE 23-16 Paget's disease of the nipple associated with a large duct carcinoma.

Hormone Binding

Determination of estrogen and progesterone receptors should be made on samples of all resected carcinomas, either primary or recurrent. This will be of value should additional additive or ablative hormone treatment become necessary, since up to 60% of estrogen-positive tumors will respond to such treatment, whereas less than 10% of estrogen-negative tumors will respond.

Adjunctive Chemotherapy

Adjuvant studies have shown that estrogen binding correlates more directly with results than progesterone binding. Specimens are also analyzed routinely (see above) for flow cytometric analysis of ploidy and S-phase. Current research of prognosis related to gene expression or amplification will lead to additional studies on the resected tumor in the near future.

Paget's disease of the breast refers to a specific lesion of the nipple and areola marked histologically by the presence of abnormal cells (Paget's cells) and clinically by the appearance of an erosive dermatitis (Fig. 23-16). A high index of suspicion is necessary, and misdiagnosis is common. When the condition is suspected, a biopsy of the nipple is made and pathologic confirmation is sought. The disease is always associated with duct carcinoma, usually arising near the nipple. Appropriate treatment of this underlying lesion is required.

PITFALLS AND COMMON MYTHS

- Underestimating the significance of a positive supraclavicular node. This represents advanced disease and should be treated by a *systemic* approach.
- Delay in biopsy and appropriate treatment of a pregnant woman. Waiting for the patient to deliver can be disastrous, since many of these cancers have short doubling times (in young women).
- Reliance on the mammogram reading. A reading of benign disease or probable benign disease should not lead to a passive approach if a mass can be palpated. A negative mammogram reading should not obviate the need for an otherwise indicated biopsy. Even more important is the necessity of reviewing the mammogram, since in an occasional case the quality may be so poor that *no reasonable conclusion can be reached.*
- Failure to offer the patient adjuvant treatment. Since most studies clearly underscore the advantages of disease-free survival for adjuvant therapy in patients with stage II disease, this should be offered to the patient. A frank discussion of adjuvant therapy should also be held with some patients with stage I disease.
- Any significant delay in the biopsy of a dominant breast mass.

BIBLIOGRAPHY

Adams HO, Bergstrom R, Hansen J. Age at first primary as a determinant of the incidence of bilateral breast cancer, cumulative and relative risks in a population based case-control study. Cancer 55:643, 1985.

Alfonso A, Gardner B. Principles of Cancer Surgery. New York, Appleton-Century-Crofts, 1981.

Atkins SH, Hayward JL, et al. Treatment of early breast cancer: A report after ten years of clinical trial. Br Med J 2:423, 1972.

Dennis C, Gardner B, Lion B. Analysis of survival and recurrence versus patient and doctor delay in treatment of breast cancer. Cancer 35:3, 1975.

Dupont WD, Page DL. Risk factors for breast cancer in women with proliferative breast disease. N Engl J Med 312:146, 1985.

Early breast cancer trialists' collaborative group effects of adjuvant tamoxifen and of cytotoxic therapy on mortality in early breast cancer. An overview of 61 randomized trials among 28,896 women. N Engl J Med 319:1681, 1988.

Edeiken S. Mammography and palpable cancer of the breast. Cancer 61:263-265, 1988.

Faig SA. Assessment of the hypothetical risk from mammography and evaluation of the potential benefit. Radiol Clin North Am 21:173, 1983.

Faig SA. The role of ultrasound in a breast imaging center. Semin Ultrasound CT MR 10:90, 1989.

Fisher B, Baias M, Margolese R, et al. Five year results of a randomized clinical trial comparing total mastectomy and segmental mastectomy with or without radiation in the treatment of breast cancer. N Engl J Med 312:665, 1985.

Fisher B, Redmond C, Fisher ER, Caplan R, and other contributing National Surgical Adjuvant Breast and Bowel Project investigators. Relative worth of estrogen or progesterone receptor and pathologic characteristics of differentiation as indicators of prognosis in node negative breast cancer patients: Findings from the National Surgical Adjuvant Breast and Bowel Project Protocol B-06. J Clin Oncol 6:1076, 1988.

Fisher B, Redmond C, Legault-Poisson S, et al. Postoperative chemotherapy and tamoxifen compared with tamoxifen alone in the treatment of positive-node breast cancer patients aged 50 years and older with tumors responsive to tamoxifen: Results from the National Surgical Adjuvant Breast and Bowel Project B-16. J Clin Oncol 8:1005, 1990.

Forrest APM. Advances in the management of carcinoma of the breast. Surg Gyn and Obstet 163:89, 1986.

Gardner B. The Relationship of Delay in Treatment to Prognosis in Clinical Cancer, Vol VII. New York, Grune & Stratton, 1978.

Hajdu SI, Urban JA. Cancers metastatic to the breast. Cancer 29:1691, 1972.

Kinime-Smith C, Gold RH, Bassett LW, et al. Diagnosis of Breast Calcifications: Comparison of Contact, Magnified, and Television Enhanced Images. Am J Radiol 153:963, 1989.

Leathem AJC. Biological, biochemical and morphological markers of breast disorders and of breast cancer. Acta Histochemica (Suppl-Band XL) 51, 1990.

Margolese R, Poisson R, Shibata H, et al. The technique of segmental mastectomy (lumpectomy) and axillary dissection. A syllabus from the National Surgical Adjuvant Breast Project Workshops. Surg 102: 828, 1987.

Mettlin C. Diet and the epidemiology of human breast cancer. Cancer 53(Suppl):605, 1984.

Meyer JE, Kopans DB, et al. Occult breast abnormalities: Percutaneous preoperative needle localization. Radiology 150:355, 1984.

Nielsen M. Autopsy studies of the occurrence of cancerous, atypical and benign epithelial lesions in the female breast. APMIS 10(Suppl):1, 1989.

Norton LW, Zeligman BE, Pearlman NW. Accuracy and cost of needle localization breast biopsy. Arch Surg 123:947, 1988.

Petrak JA, Dukoff R, Rogatko A. Prognosis of pregnancy-associated breast cancer. Cancer 67:869, 1991.

Polk HC Jr. Improved understanding of mammary cancer. Cancer 57:411, 1986.

Sheldon T, Hayes DF, Cady B, et al. Primary radiation therapy for locally advanced breast cancer. Cancer 60:1219, 1987.

Solin LJ, Fowble BL, Troupin RH, Goodman RL. Biopsy results of new calcifications in the postirradiated breast. Cancer 63:1956, 1989.

Wilkinson EJ, Bland KI. Techniques and results of aspiration cytology for diagnosis of benign and malignant diseases of the breast. Surg Clin North Am 70:801, 1990.

Winchester DJ, Duda RB, August CZ, et al. The importance of DNA flow cytometry in node-negative breast cancer. Arch Surg 125:886, 1990.

CHAPTER REVIEW
Questions

1. A 24-year-old woman with a solitary non-tender movable mass in the breast is seen during her sixth month of pregnancy. The proper management is:
   a. Perform a mammogram. If negative for malignancy, observe carefully until the pregnancy is completed, then biopsy.
   b. Perform an excisional biopsy at once to confirm the diagnosis.
   c. Perform a mammogram and complete bone survey to rule out malignancy, and if negative examine periodically until delivery to see if the lesion will regress.

2. Match the age range with the most common pathology for a breast mass.
   (1) 18-25 years a. Fibrocystic disease
   (2) 35-40 years b. Adenocarcinoma
   (3) 55-60 years c. Fibroadenoma

3. Initial management of metastatic breast cancer in a 42-year-old woman should involve:
   a. Radiation therapy
   b. Modified radical mastectomy
   c. Biopsy and determination of hormone binding
   d. Oophorectomy and adrenalectomy

4. All but which of the following are poor prognostic factors in mammary cancer?
   a. Regional lymph node metastases
   b. Large size of tumor
   c. Intraductal (comedo) carcinoma
   d. Skin fixation

5. Which of the following factors relates best to prognosis in primary breast cancer?
   a. Percentage of involved nodes
   b. Location of cancer in breast
   c. Age of patient
   d. Size of primary mass

6. A patient has a large chest wall recurrence and pulmonary metastases after mastectomy. Why would a biopsy of the recurrence be necessary?
   a. To establish histologic diagnosis
   b. To obtain tissue for hormone binding (ER) determination
   c. To consider alternative forms of chemotherapy

7. List three pathologic markers for a poor prognosis in primary breast cancer.
   a. High nuclear grade
   b. Vascular invasion
   c. Neural invasion
   d. Multiple areas of breast involvement
   e. Positive lymph nodes

8. A patient has a breast mass that tested positive for carcinoma on needle biopsy and an ipsilateral supraclavicular palpable node. What is the correct approach?
   a. Biopsy supraclavicular node; if positive treat with chemotherapy.
   b. Perform modified radical mastectomy, removing supraclavicular node.
   c. Perform modified radical mastectomy and watch supraclavicular node for progression.
   d. Perform modified radical mastectomy and irradiate supraclavicular node.

9. A 32-year-old woman has bilateral breast masses; both have tested positive for carcinoma. The proper treatment is:
   a. Oophorectomy
   b. Chemotherapy
   c. Bilateral definitive operations
   d. Radiation to both lesions

10. A mammogram reveals a unilateral area of stippled calcification. The proper approach is:
    a. Repeat mammogram in 6 months
    b. Needle localization biopsy
    c. Modified radical mastectomy
    d. Segmental mastectomy and breast irradiation

11. A 57-year-old woman had a modified radical mastectomy showing one positive node. The primary tumor was ER positive. Adjuvant treatment should be:
    a. Oophorectomy
    b. Chemotherapy
    c. Estrogens
    d. Chemotherapy with tamoxifen

12. A breast segmental resection reveals a single focus of in situ lobular carcinoma. The proper treatment is:
    a. No further treatment
    b. Breast irradiation
    c. Modified radical mastectomy
    d. Radical mastectomy
    e. Axillary dissection

13. In question 12, a single focus of in situ duct carcinoma is found. The proper treatment is:
    a. No further treatment
    b. Axillary dissection and breast irradiation
    c. Modified radical mastectomy
    d. Any of the above

14. On a breast biopsy, multiple areas of in situ comedo carcinoma are found. The proper treatment is:

a. Breast irradiation
b. Axillary dissection followed by irradiation
c. Modified radical mastectomy
d. Total mastectomy
e. Radical mastectomy

Answers

1. b
2. (1)-c, (2)-a, (3)-b
3. c
4. c
5. d
6. a, b, c
7. a
8. a
9. c
10. b
11. d
12. a
13. d but a is to be preferred
14. d (c is rarely indicated for in situ cancer)

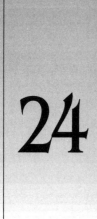

24 Gastrointestinal Bleeding

J. DAVID RICHARDSON
BERNARD GARDNER

KEY FEATURES

After reading this chapter you will understand:
- The general approach to the patient with gastrointestinal bleeding.
- What circumstances should be considered emergent.
- Specific bleeding conditions.
- The current approach to the patient with variceal bleeding.
- Disease entities that cause lower GI bleeding.
- Why diagnosis of occult bleeding may be difficult.

Gastrointestinal (GI) bleeding may result from a variety of conditions occurring from the esophagus to the anus. The more common sites of bleeding are the upper GI tract and the colon, while small bowel blood loss is relatively less common. Specific causes of GI blood loss are listed in Table 24-1. Fig. 24-1 is an algorithm that is helpful in the management of GI bleeding from different sites.

ACUTE BLOOD LOSS OF THE UPPER GASTROINTESTINAL TRACT
Etiology

Although many specific diseases cause acute blood loss from the upper gastrointestinal (UGI) tract, more than 80% of episodes of acute blood loss are attributable to one or more of six specific

pathologic alterations of the upper GI tract (Table 24-2). Acute hemorrhagic gastritis or duodenal ulcers account for almost half of such episodes of blood loss, as determined by endoscopic findings in more than 2000 patients examined during or shortly after cessation of hemorrhage from the upper GI tract. The incidence of various bleeding sites will differ between series in which endoscopy was used and older series that relied on barium contrast studies alone. The diagnosis of bleeding from gastritis in particular can be made with much greater accuracy by endoscopy than by contrast studies alone.

The incidence of a specific cause for GI hemorrhage will vary with the institution and the patient population. In teaching institutions and metropolitan hospitals clinicians encounter gastritis and esophageal variceal hemorrhage more frequently than is found in community hospitals, where the incidence of peptic ulcer disease responsible for bleeding is greater than 50%.

Physiology of Gastrointestinal Bleeding

Massive blood loss is defined as an acute loss of 40% of the circulating blood volume and often results in a hematocrit level below 24% or a hemoglobin below 8 g. With the onset of acute hemorrhage, refilling of the vascular compartment by translocated albumin and interstitial fluid commences (accounting for the fall in hematocrit) and may take up to 24 to 36 hours for completion. In the earliest stages, therefore, *the hematocrit level may not truly reflect the extent*

TABLE 24-1   Common Causes of Bleeding

Upper Gastrointestinal	Lower Gastrointestinal	Small Bowel
Ulcer disease of the GI tract	Neoplasms	Meckel's diverticulum
Gastritis	Inflammatory bowel disease	Inflammatory bowel disease
Pancreatitis	Bacterial enterocolitis	Bacterial enterocolitis
Mallory-Weiss' tears	Hemorrhoids	Hemangiomas, myomas
Hematobilia	Fissures	Sarcomas
Neoplasms	Telangiectasias	
Esophagogastric varices	Diverticulitis	
Aortointestinal fistulas	Blood dyscrasias	
Hemangiomas	Polyps	
Rendu-Osler-Weber's syndrome	Mesenteric thrombosis	
Banti's syndrome		
Collagen diseases		

TABLE 24-2   Etiology of Acute UGI Hemorrhage, Determined Endoscopically*

Cause	Percent
Duodenal ulcer	24
Acute gastritis	20
Gastric ulcer	15
Esophageal varices	14
Esophagitis	6
Mallory-Weiss' syndrome	5
All other causes	10
Undiagnosed	6
TOTAL	100

*Data collected from multiple sources. Total cases: 2205.

of the hemorrhage. Hypovolemia and subsequent decrease in tissue perfusion produce a plethora of homeostatic responses, the most important of which involve stimulation of alpha and beta receptors by adrenal hormones, leading to peripheral vasoconstriction and increased heart rate. Pallor and tachycardia are prominent findings in such a patient. Decreased tissue perfusion is reflected in a fall in urine output and hypovolemia by a fall in filling pressure of the left side of the heart that may be measured as the pulmonary capillary wedge pressure (PCWP). *Adequate resuscitation is therefore monitored by a slowing of the pulse, return of urine output to a range of 30 ml/hr, and a rise in PCWP.* This does not imply that wedge pressures should be obtained in all bleeding patients. It is, however, specifically indicated in patients with other high-risk associated problems, such as congestive heart failure or coronary artery disease, or cases in which large volumes of fluid are required for resuscitation.

What Is the Initial Clinical Approach?

In the majority of patients with active UGI tract hemorrhage, the condition *can be controlled with aggressive nonoperative measures.* The need for subsequent operation can then be considered electively. When confronted with a patient with massive gastrointestinal tract hemorrhaging, however, one must have some criteria to determine when nonoperative treatment should stop and an operation be scheduled.

The most important determinant of the overall approach is the rate of hemorrhage, since this will reflect the size of the vessel involved and the likelihood of spontaneous cessation. After the initial resuscitation (Fig. 24-2) is completed, as determined by a rise in blood pressure, reduction in tachycardia, and increase in urinary output, *the rate of continued bleeding is determined by estimating the rate of blood replacement needed to maintain the vital signs in a stable range.* If more than 4 units of blood per 24 hours or 2 units per 8 hours are needed to maintain blood pressure and tissue perfusion, an operation is indicated. Of course, there are exceptions, and one must not adhere too rigidly to a set policy if the patient's condition is obviously deteriorating at a more rapid rate. The amount of blood transfused before operative therapy is performed may also vary, depending on the cause of the bleeding. *If endoscopic evaluation demonstrates that the bleeding is from gastritis or varices, then a*

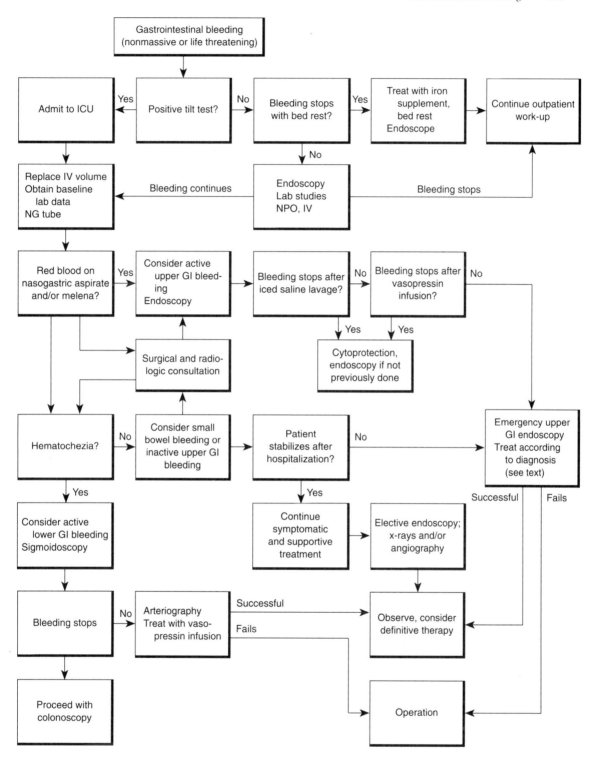

FIGURE 24-1 Algorithm of the management of gastrointestinal bleeding from different sites. (Modified from Meerhoff JC. Managing patients with severe GI hemorrhage. Hosp Pract 186, 1984.)

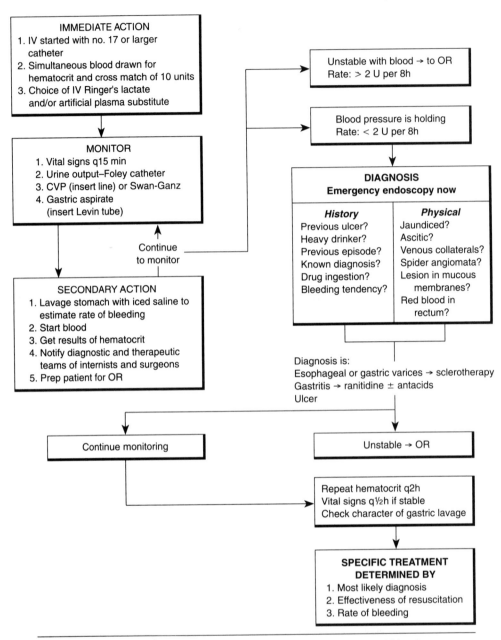

FIGURE 24-2 Sequential flow sheet of massive upper gastrointestinal bleeding. (Modified from Meerhoff JC. Managing patients with severe GI hemorrhage. Hosp Pract 186, 1984.)

greater attempt at nonoperative therapy may be made, because operative treatments for these situations are not as satisfactory as for duodenal ulcers that are bleeding.

Placement of a nasogastric tube allows for assessment of the rate of bleeding. All blood in the stomach should be thoroughly aspirated and clots should be removed. This can be facilitated by using a large-bore tube, such as an Ewald tube, for lavage of the stomach. If profuse bleeding continues, this may prompt an early operation, although every effort should be made to control the hemorrhage nonoperatively. We prefer to leave a tube in place for a day or two to monitor bleeding.

Several factors should be considered in addition to pertinent initial laboratory results. Each patient admitted with a diagnosis of acute upper GI tract bleeding, based either on the patient's history or on presenting symptoms, *should be considered a candidate for a further episode of sudden or massive blood loss.* Appropriate measures should be taken to prepare for that possibility. Ideally, consideration should be given to the following:

1. Admit the patient to the intensive care unit
2. Type and cross-match for 4 to 6 units of packed red blood cells
3. Initiate at least one large-bore no. 16 intravenous line for the rapid infusion of fluids
4. Place an indwelling urinary catheter
5. Monitor input and output and vital signs every half hour
6. Irrigate nasogastric tube with saline at least hourly
7. Frequently determine hemoglobin levels
8. Place a Swan-Ganz catheter if dictated by the clinical situation (elderly patient, associated heart disease, uncertain fluid status, etc.)

The clinician may be lulled into a false sense of security and underestimate the significance of the patient's history of recent hematemesis if the patient does not have signs of active bleeding and/or shock when admitted. Subsequently, if the patient has massive hematemesis and/or the blood pressure falls significantly, coupled with preexisting relative hypovolemia secondary to the patient's first (prehospital) hemorrhage, the entire situation becomes one of frantic activity to initiate large-bore intravenous lines in an anxious and hypotensive patient. *It is far better to have prepared for this possibility than to try to correct the situation after the fact.* If the patient is actively bleeding, gastric lavage with a balanced salt solution through a large nasogastric tube should be initiated and continued until the gastric aspirate clears. This provides an estimate of continued or recurrent bleeding. Occasionally, when the blood in the stomach has clotted, even large nasogastric tubes are ineffective in removing this cast of clotted blood, and the irrigant will appear relatively clear or pink. If other signs of hemorrhage persist, operation must be performed. *As soon as the patient's condition stabilizes, one should proceed with the most effective diagnostic modalities* to determine the specific source of blood loss. Although currently there is no evidence to support or refute the concept that an early, aggressive diagnostic approach to the patient with hematemesis using fiberoptic endoscopy offers a greater probability of survival or

reduction of blood replacement, we still feel this is appropriate. Delineation of the specific bleeding site or sites by flexible esophagogastroduodenoscopy may provide useful information for the operating surgeon in the event that the patient's bleeding does not stop with nonoperative measures or if the patient rebleeds following an interval of quiescence.

How Do You Diagnose the Cause of GI Bleeding?

History. Patients with massive UGI bleeding may present with hematemesis of red blood, or, if gastric acid has acted on the blood, "coffee grounds" vomitus may be the most prominent symptom. Red blood from the rectum caused by upper GI lesion is rare unless there is rapid transit time as a result of preexisting anomalies or the bleeding is massive. *In the latter case there will always be associated symptoms of acute hypovolemia, such as syncope.* More usually, the rectal blood loss is black or tarry because of the action of gastric acid on the blood. It may be explosive, associated with dizziness or syncope, or may occur in several repeated bouts over 12 to 36 hours.

It is always vital to elicit a history of previous episodes, particularly if a diagnosis has been made in the past (i.e., at a previous hospitalization). Symptoms of preexisting ulcer disease, such as persistent pain or ingestion of large amounts of antacids, can obviate or make simpler further diagnostic work-up. Absence of pain, however, does not rule out ulcer disease.

A history of chronic alcohol ingestion may suggest a diagnosis of cirrhosis or portal hypertension; however, one cannot assume that GI bleeding in such a patient results from esophageal varices. Series of endoscopic evaluations in such patients often show gastritis as the most common bleeding source, with esophageal varices and peptic ulcer disease occurring with equal frequency.

The patient should always be asked about bleeding tendencies or known clotting factor deficiencies. *It is essential to obtain an accurate history of the medication the patient is taking* with specific reference to aspirin and other over-the-counter agents that may be gastric irritants, particularly nonsteroidal anti-inflammatory agents.

Physical Examination. Signs of hypovolemia will be present with massive hemorrhage; *signs include pallor, tachycardia, hypotension, sweating, and often an anxious-appearing patient.* Associated signs of cirrhosis, such as liver enlargement, spider angiomata in the skin, and external evidence of venous collateral formation (caput medusa) on the abdominal wall should be noted. Jaundice and ascites clearly point to esophageal varices as a more likely cause of bleeding.

Mucous membranes should be checked for the presence of telangiectasia or other vascular lesions, which may suggest that similar lesions are present in the mucosa of the intestines.

A rectal examination is important to detect the presence of red blood, tarry stools, or brown stools. This may help to clarify the size of the hemorrhage as well as to verify the location.

Use of Indwelling Tubes. The use of nasogastric tubes is valuable as a diagnostic as well as a therapeutic modality, since it delineates the presence of active bleeding in the UGI tract and can be used to gauge continued or repeated hemorrhage. Occasionally a massively bleeding duodenal ulcer may be present although no blood is in the stomach, because pylorospasm prevents reflux of blood into the stomach.

The Blakemore-Sengstaken tube has been used to treat patients with bleeding esophageal varices but can also be used for diagnosis of the site of upper GI bleeding. It is a triple-lumen tube with a gastric and esophageal balloon that can be inflated separately. The continued presence of blood aspirated through the distal lumen with adequate inflation of the gastric balloon implies that the bleeding is from a duodenal or gastric ulcer rather than esophageal or gastric varices. *The tube has several inherent dangers, however, related to its large size, which may produce esophageal or gastric erosions, and to the fact that esophageal obstruction occurs whenever either balloon is inflated,* leading to the possibility of aspiration. Therefore its use should be reserved for specific instances of esophageal or gastric variceal bleeding to be treated nonoperatively, and a proximal nasogastric tube should be used to aspirate saliva or blood from the obstructed esophagus. The patient should also have an endotracheal tube placed to protect the airway from aspiration, which is very common with the use of this type of tube.

Radiology and Endoscopy. Because of the high incidence of upper GI tract hemorrhage from superficial mucosal lesions, *UGI barium contrast studies have limited diagnostic value.* Less than 40% of the specific lesions responsible for the hemorrhage can be detected radiographically.

At present, esophagogastroduodenoscopy with a flexible, manipulable-tipped, fiberoptic instrument appears to represent the most effective method of establishing the specific source of blood loss. A diagnosis can usually be established endoscopically in three of four patients with UGI tract hemorrhage *(see color Plates 24-1 through 24-4 following p. 412).* Through the endoscope successful diagnosis can be augmented by successful treatment. Laser or electrical coagulation of bleeding ulcers as well as emergency sclerotherapy for esophageal varices have been successfully used to stem hemorrhages (see below). Occasionally selective angiography is useful for the diagnosis of upper GI bleeding, but this technique has a much greater role for lower GI hemorrhage. Optimism arising from the initial encouraging results of control of bleeding with selective intra-arterial infusions of pitressin has been tempered by subsequent experience. However, selective angiography has led to numerous other methods of hemorrhage control. These include a wide variety of agents that can be infused, including vasodilators for treatment of bleeding varices to other vasoactive mediators currently under investigation. Additionally, embolization of bleeding vessels using fibrin clots, muscle fragments, or coils has been used to stop hemorrhage from the upper and lower GI tract. While such measures are effective in lower GI hemorrhage, rebleeding is common with most upper GI hemorrhages. The best indications for these modalities are therefore in patients who represent formidable risks for operation. The use of intra-arterial clotting agents needs critical scrutiny.

Specific Bleeding Entities

Duodenal Ulcer. Duodenal ulcers account for one of the two most frequent sources of upper GI tract hemorrhage, the other being acute hemorrhagic gastritis (see Table 24-2). The significance of the hemorrhage may vary greatly. Clinically, the presenting signs may be hematemesis followed by or in conjunction with melena, melena as the only clinical sign, or rarely, the presence only of dark red blood passed by rectum. Massive hemorrhage from duodenal ulcer represents one of the classic indications for surgical correction. A reasonable set of criteria for surgical intervention might include an uncontrolled massive hemorrhage (patient remains unstable), hemorrhage in the presence of persistent ulcer symptoms in a treated patient, a second massive hemorrhage in the hospital under the most favorable treatment conditions, and continued bleeding after aggressive nonoperative attempts at control (i.e., sclerotherapy, laser cauterization) have failed.

Nonoperative Treatment. Since the underlying pathophysiology of duodenal ulcer includes hyperacidity, which is also responsible for the redissolution of the blood clots formed in the bleeding vessels at the base of the ulcer, *the treatment is directed at reduction of all phases of gastric secretion.* The cephalic phase of gastric secretion may need to be treated by careful sedation to avoid the anxiety associated with in-hospital management of acute hemorrhage in certain patients. Anticholinergics have been used in the past but are not used on our services now. A functioning nasogastric tube is used to continually aspirate any acid from the stomach. As soon as evidence of cessation of bleeding has occurred (clear gastric aspirate), neutralization of gastric acid by a continuous drip of antacids is started. The patient should not eat until hemodynamic stability is attained and the threat of emergency operation has abated. One of the H_2 receptor blockers, such as cimetidine or ranitidine, is then started. Although these may be no more effective in a patient with an acutely bleeding episode than would the use of antacids, they have the advantage that they can be given immediately parenterally, whereas antacids are usually withheld until a clear gastric aspirate is obtained. In a patient who has stopped bleeding, H_2-blockers appear to be more effective than antacids in preventing subsequent hemorrhage.

Successful treatment is measured by return of the vital signs to normal, gradual reduction in blood present with successive bowel movements (stool guaiac returns to negative over 2 to 3 days), and maintenance of or improvement in hematocrit levels.

The use of endoscopy to control bleeding duodenal ulcers has progressed in the past few years to where it can be offered early in the patient's course. The use of cautery has yielded to laser in producing coagulation of the bleeding vessel when visualized.

Obviously, restriction of the use of any possible causative drugs is indicated.

Operative Treatment. No consensus exists among surgeons regarding the best operation for bleeding duodenal ulcers. The choice of vagotomy and partial gastrectomy with gastroduodenal or gastrojejunal anastomosis (VGR) or vagotomy and pyloroplasty combined with ligation of the offending vessel (VPL) largely depends on the surgeon's training and the patient's age and general state of health. The majority of operative deaths from bleeding duodenal ulcers occur in patients 70 years of age or older. It does not necessarily follow, however, that the least extensive procedure (VPL) is best suited for the elderly patient. Although the operative mortality for VPL is less than for VGR, the frequency of rebleeding is significantly higher following a VPL than for a VGR. Elderly patients cannot be expected to tolerate a second surgical procedure well, and often the more conservative approach is to proceed with a VGR and accept a slightly increased initial operative mortality with a lower probability of the need for a second operative procedure to control secondary hemorrhage. In situations of this nature the type of operative procedure and its magnitude must be carefully weighed against the risk of mortality or recurrence of hemorrhage. The anatomic disposition of the ulcer at operation may affect the decision. The most important factor is the surgeon, who should be skilled in all techniques and aware of all the clinical considerations in selecting the best procedure for a particular patient at a particular time (Table 24-3).

Currently there are three different approaches to vagotomy. Truncal vagotomy, which is performed by dividing the major branches of the

TABLE 24-3 Comparison of Elective Operative Mortality and Ulcer Recurrence Rates Between Standard Procedures for Duodenal Ulcers*

Primary Procedure	No. of Patients	Elective Operative Mortality (%)	Ulcer Recurrence (%)
Vagotomy and pyloroplasty	1146	1.4	6.5
Vagotomy and partial gastrectomy	4485	1.8	0.7
Vagotomy and gastroenterostomy	185	0.5	13.5
Parietal cell vagotomy	438	0.5	7.3
Subtotal gastrectomy	937	1.8	3.8

*Data collected from multiple sources.

nerve just below the esophageal hiatus, has been the standard technique for many years. However, truncal vagotomy is associated with several problems: incomplete vagotomy, postvagotomy diarrhea, dumping, and increased incidence of gallstones as a result of increased stasis of the gallbladder. In response to this variable dissatisfaction with truncal vagotomy, two modifications of total truncal vagotomy have emerged: the selective vagotomy and the highly selective (parietal cell) vagotomy. Theoretically, selective vagotomy denervates the stomach but leaves the celiac vagal fibers intact, achieving more consistently complete gastric vagotomy without increasing the GI tract transit time. The highly selective or parietal cell vagotomy denervates the gastric parietal cell mass and leaves the antral innervation intact. Both variations were designed to reduce the incidence of recurrent ulceration and avoid postoperative diarrhea. Their long-term value is the subject of ongoing studies. Both the selective vagotomy and the highly selected vagotomy require meticulous dissection of the gastric branches of the vagus nerve and an increased operating time. At the moment, this mitigates against its use in an unstable patient with acute blood loss.

Hemorrhagic Gastritis. Diffuse hemorrhagic gastritis (DHG) accounts for the second of the two most frequent sources of massive upper GI tract hemorrhage. Many chemical agents have been incriminated including alcohol, aspirin, and a variety of drugs used in the treatment of arthritis, including phenylbutazone, indomethacin, steroids, and many of the newer antiarthritic agents. These agents, grouped under the acronym NSAID (nonsteroidal anti-inflammatory drugs), actually often produce frank gastric ulcers as well as gastritis. Additionally, gastritis has been recognized with increasing frequency as a form of "organ failure" (i.e., mucosal barrier failure) in patients who are septic.

The specific pathophysiology of gastritis is not understood, but a variety of insults lead to alteration of the gastric mucosal barrier, thus permitting back-diffusion of hydrogen ions. These hydrogen ions and other toxic substances, such as oxygen-free radicals, which they induce, lead to direct capillary damage with rupture of these vessels and subsequent hemorrhage.

Nonoperative Treatment. After an unequivocal diagnosis of DHG with the exclusion of other potential bleeding sources, treatment as for duodenal ulcer (as described earlier) will usually arrest the bleeding. Avoidance of the offending agent will prevent its recurrence. However, there are situations in which such measures do not arrest the hemorrhage, and an operation must be considered.

Current investigations have indicated the success of H_2-blockers in preventing bleeding in patients at risk for gastritis. While antacids are also effective, the potential for use as parenteral treatment has favored the H_2-blockers (particularly in ICU patients, with whom parenteral therapy does not require the rigorous nursing activities involved with intragastric instillation of antacids). In the ICU the treatment must be combined with pH measurements of the gastric aspirate, so levels are maintained above 3.5. With high gastric pH there is a tendency for bacterial growth (particularly gram-negative organisms) to increase, with resultant aspiration and increased incidence of pneumonia. Ranitidine has been found superior to cimetidine in several studies because of a lower incidence of side effects (particularly in elderly patients). This has been attributed to a lower binding of ranitidine to the cytochrome P-450 system than cimetidine. These enzymes metabolize drugs such as metronidazole, diazepam, propranolol, theophylline, lidocaine, verapamil, and warfarin; thus H_2-blockers should be used with caution in patients receiving these medications. Randomized studies of sucralfate in preventing bleeding from stress ulceration or gastritis has indicated that it is not as effective in raising the pH above 4 as H_2-blockers or antacids, which may account for a lower incidence of pneumonia. However, no definitive recommendation as to its use can be made at this time.

Operative Treatment. Again, there is no consensus among surgeons regarding the most effective procedure to minimize mortality, morbidity, and incidence of rebleeding. Each procedure has its advantages and disadvantages, and unfortunately no procedure is completely effective for the treatment of DHG. It is generally felt that the addition of a vagotomy to any other operative procedure aids in the control of bleeding with DHG (Table 24-4). Occasionally the bleeding will involve the entire mucosal surface of the stomach, and attempts to control the bleeding with less than a total gastrectomy will prove futile. This procedure obviously carries a significant long-term disability; therefore it is truly used as a last resort. The best overall surgical results are probably achieved by a nearly 80% gastrectomy and vagotomy, although the relative merits of the pyloroplasty and vagotomy have not been adequately studied prospectively to exclude this form of therapy as an acceptable alternative.

TABLE 24-4 Incidence of Rebleeding and Mortality Associated With Specific Surgical Procedures for Massively Bleeding Gastritis*

Procedure	No. of Patients	Rebleed (%)	Mortality (%)
Vagotomy and pyloroplasty	392	30	20-30
Vagotomy—resection	150	5-15	20-30
Resection alone	204	40-50	30-45
Total gastrectomy	21	0	0-15

*Data collected from multiple sources.

Gastric Ulcers. The etiologic factors responsible for chronic gastric ulcers are less well understood than those related to peptic ulcerations for the duodenum and pylorus. Experimental evidence suggests a breakdown of the mucosal barrier as the initial pathologic alteration. Usually chronic gastric ulcers are located on the lesser curvature in the proximal two thirds of the stomach. Endoscopically they have been seen on the distal one third of the lesser curvature, particularly when drug induced. Because of their frequent location in proximity to the left gastric artery, bleeding, although not common, may be severe, leading to a patient mortality of 20% to 25%. Gastric ulcers occur most commonly in older patients, a group plagued by other related chronic diseases that contribute significantly to the high mortality associated with surgical correction.

Nonoperative Treatment. Bleeding gastric ulcers are relatively unresponsive to nonoperative management, and an operation is the usual recommendation. The possibility of cancer is always present, and elderly patients cannot tolerate repeated episodes of significant acute blood loss. Both considerations support early operation. A short course of treatment, however, as outlined for duodenal ulcers, may be tried to stop the bleeding so that definitive operation, if indicated, may be performed under optimal conditions.

Operative Treatment. Excision of the ulcer as part of a gastrectomy or combined with distal gastrectomy is the preferred approach when feasible. In cases of high lesser-curvature ulcers a plausible alternative is distal gastrectomy, ligation of the left gastric artery, and plication of the ulcer. If the ulcer is not excised, adequate biopsies must be obtained to rule out the possibility of cancer. Of clinically benign ulcers, 8% to 10% are, in fact, malignant.

Although vagotomy, pyloroplasty, and over-sewing the ulcer have been recommended by some surgeons, the rationale for the use of this operation is less attractive than for duodenal ulcer disease. Patients with gastric ulcer often have little or no acid production, obviating the need for vagotomy. This fact, coupled with the complication of vagotomy, makes vagotomy and pyloroplasty a poor alternative for the treatment of gastric ulcer.

Esophageal Variceal Hemorrhage. Esophageal varices are the result of physiologic venous collateralization circumventing the normal portal venous flow to the liver because of increased portal venous pressure produced by obstruction to portal blood flow through the liver. Obstruction may occur at three levels: (1) the hepatic veins that drain the liver (Budd-Chiari syndrome), (2) intrahepatic obstruction secondary to parenchymal cell and/or regeneration damage (any form of cirrhosis), or (3) occlusion of the portal vein (congenital atresia or stenosis, thrombosis resulting from trauma or infection, or extrinsic pressure). Intrahepatic obstructive disease accounts for at least 90% of all cases of portal hypertension in the United States, by far the most frequent cause being alcoholic (Laënnec's) cirrhosis. Bleeding esophageal varices represents the fourth most frequent cause of massive upper gastrointestinal tract hemorrhage (see Table 24-2), but the greatest number of deaths occur in that group of patients, ***primarily because of*** the extensive underlying liver disease, which is made worse by hypovolemia (hemorrhage), operation, and decompression of the portal vein— ***reducing total hepatic blood flow.*** Mortality for patients hospitalized with cirrhosis and bleeding esophageal varices approaches 70%. The 10% of patients with non-alcohol-induced portal hypertension have essentially normal hepatic function, tolerate surgical decompression of the portal venous circulation well, and have a relatively good prognosis. It is important to remember that

GI bleeding in patients with esophageal varices may come from the varices themselves or from duodenal ulcers, gastritis, or esophagitis. The latter problems tend to present as slower bleeding in some patients.

In years past, elective portal decompression was the most accepted approach to patients with bleeding varices, yielding an average hospital mortality rate of 12%, 5-year survival of 50%, and a 10% incidence of rebleeding. However, very few patients survived attempts at initial control of the variceal hemorrhage, and less than 20% of the patients became candidates for an elective procedure. For this reason, recent attention has been focused on emergency decompression of the portal system, because the frequency of control of the hemorrhage is in the range of 90% despite the high mortality. In a prospective study of emergency shunts in apparently unselected patients who were bleeding from esophageal varices, operative (hospital) mortality occurred in 50%, with late or posthospitalization mortality in 60% of those surviving operation, but almost uniform control of hemorrhage from varices was obtained. This overall improved long-term survival rate was noted in a group in which three fourths of patients who survived the surgical procedure abstained from alcohol intake postoperatively. *Those who resume drinking do not fare as well.* This is reflected by *a late mortality rate of 50% in patients surviving shunting procedures* who resume their drinking, compared with a late mortality of less than 10% for those who do not resume drinking.

An operative mortality, however, may be anticipated if the patient has associated jaundice and ascites and an uncorrectable prolonged prothrombin time. The standard measure of assessing risk for portal decompression operation is through the use of the Child's classification (Table 24-5). In such patients any attempt at nonoperative treatment may be preferable.

Patients who are good operative risks should be seriously considered for elective portal decompression. For all of the above reasons, nonoperative therapy is the preferred treatment in bleeding esophageal varices. Sclerotherapy using a flexible endoscope through which sodium morrhuate (sclerosing solution) is injected into the varices can be expected to yield 90% control of bleeding in one or two attempts. The unresponsive 10% of patients will be candidates for emergency shunt. Some complications have been reported with sclerotherapy; as always, the treatment requires an experienced endoscopist for lowest morbidity.

Vasopressin injection has been used by many investigators either intravenously or into the superior mesenteric artery. There is no advantage to an intra-arterial injection. The treatment is based on the observation that a minimum portal pressure of 12 mm Hg is required for variceal bleeding to occur. The pharmacologic effects of high-dose vasopressin therapy shown in the box below will reduce portal pressure. Although favorable results of up to 75% control of variceal bleeding have been reported, a careful review of controlled studies failed to reveal a clear benefit for use of vasopressin. If used, continuous infusion intravenously is preferred over bolus injection (which allows intermittent return of portal pressure). Again, several controlled randomized studies failed to show a difference from use of a placebo.

Administration of vasopressin plus nitroglycerin (or nitroprusside) has been used to obviate some of the detrimental effects of vasopressin alone. This results from nitroglycerin's ability to counter the increased cardiac afterload and coronary artery resistance induced by vasopressin.

PHARMACOLOGIC EFFECTS OF VASOPRESSIN

Gastrointestinal

Reduction in portal venous pressure
Reduction in splanchnic blood flow
Increased peristaltic activity
Reduction in gastric secretions
Contraction of gallbladder
Reduction in hepatic blood flow
Decreased liver metabolic function

Cardiovascular

Vasoconstriction of vascular smooth muscle
Reduction in coronary blood flow
Elevated systemic and pulmonary blood pressure
Decreased cardiac output
Decreased heart rate

Other

Antidiuresis
Reduction in skin perfusion
Contraction of urinary bladder
Elevation of circulating factor VIII
Increasing circulating plasminogen activator
Contraction of uterus

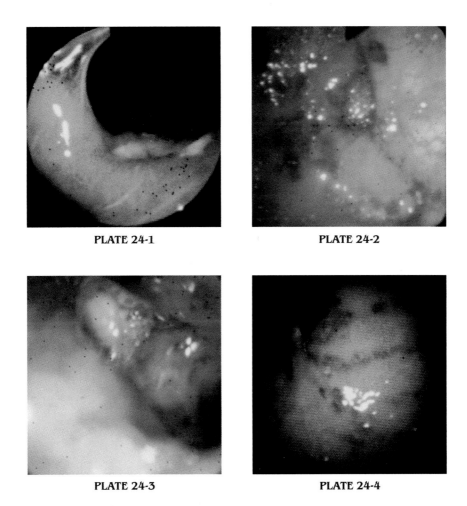

PLATE 24-1

PLATE 24-2

PLATE 24-3

PLATE 24-4

PLATE 24-1 Endoscopic view of the stomach. In the foreground one sees the lesser curve and angularis of the stomach in which there is a 2 cm gastric ulcer. The ulcer appears as a white crater. In the distance the endoscope is seen coming through the gastroesophageal junction.

PLATE 24-2 Endoscopic view of the stomach of a trauma patient who has multiple injuries and has been in the intensive care unit for several days. In the center of the picture is a 5 mm gastric ulcer with a white lining. Adjacent to this small ulcer are several red mucosal erosions that are also part of the spectrum of stress gastritis.

PLATE 24-3 This 30-year-old man entered the hospital with a 2-day history of stomachache and 1 day of GI bleeding. He was hypotensive and required transfusion of 6 units of blood for stabilization. Top of the picture, a 1 cm ulcer crater in the duodenal bulb that was the cause of bleeding.

PLATE 24-4 Endoscopic view of the fundus of the stomach in a patient who suffered a severe head injury and is comatose. It demonstrates multiple red erosions that appear as linear streaks. Such red erosions are caused by mucosal injury and hemorrhage as part of the stress gastritis syndrome.

Reduction in morbidity with use of this combination over vasopressin alone has been reported. Although hemorrhage may be controlled, studies have failed to show a decrease in mortality with the use of this combination of drugs.

Terlipressin, a compound having fewer cardiac effects than vasopressin, has not demonstrated clear superiority in the treatment of variceal hemorrhage. Somatostatin or its analogs have yielded good results in uncontrolled studies and await further clinical evaluation.

Balloon Tamponade. As mentioned earlier, this technique may yield temporary control of bleeding esophageal or gastric varices by compression, but the rate of rebleeding is high when the balloons are decompressed. It is hoped that in the coming decade balloon tamponade will be replaced by sclerotherapy or vasoactive treatment.

Beta blockers such as propranolol have been demonstrated to reduce portal pressure in the majority of studied patients. This effect is independent of the cause of the portal hypertension. Its use is best demonstrated in decreasing the risk of recurrent hemorrhage in compliant patients. It is not currently recommended in a patient with acute GI bleeding.

Laser therapy has also recently been used on a variety of types of GI bleeding. The precise indications for laser therapy and the results that can be expected from its use are not currently known; results of further trials are awaited.

Diagnosis. Frequent flexible endoscopy of the upper gastrointestinal tract has disclosed that fewer than half of patients presenting with UGI tract hemorrhage and a history and clinical picture compatible with alcoholic cirrhosis are actually bleeding from esophageal varices. Therefore, in the absence of massive hemorrhage, intractable shock, alcohol intoxication, and hepatic coma, *endoscopy should probably be performed routinely when the patient is admitted to the hospital or soon thereafter.* In patients bleeding too massively to permit endoscopy, *selective arteriographic studies may be helpful.* Although these usually will not establish esophageal varices as the bleeding site, exclusion of other sources of massive upper gastrointestinal tract hemorrhage can be quite helpful. Other initial studies pertinent to the diagnosis of cirrhosis and documentation of varices include *liver function tests, upper gastrointestinal tract barium contrast studies, selective mesenteric arteriography, splenoportography with direct measurement of portal pressure, and hepatic vein catheterization.* With these examinations the majority of diagnoses can be established conclusively. Other hemodynamic information can be obtained from angiography of the visceral mesenteric arteries as well as radioisotopic estimates of hepatic blood flow. Yet many debate the prognostic value of these measurements in relation to a patient's ability to survive surgical shunt procedures and avoid hepatic encephalopathy.

Physiologic Sequelae of Portal-Systemic Shunts. Hemodynamically the pressure in the portal system is higher than that of the systemic veins if significant cirrhosis is present. Normal venous pressure varies from 5 to 9 cm of water but will frequently exceed 30 cm of water in the portal system in patients bleeding from esophageal varices. Therefore a significant shunt will be created by a portal systemic venous anastomosis. *Any connection of the portal and systemic venous systems that leaves the portal vein to the liver uninterrupted will act physiologically as a side-to-side shunt.* This includes the splenorenal, mesocaval, H-graft, distal splenorenal, and side-to side portacaval shunts. Since the flow will then be from the high-pressure (portal) system to the low-pressure (systemic) veins, the portal vein will act as an outflow conduit. This may be helpful if there is significant ascites secondary to postsinusoidal obstruction (cirrhosis), because it leaves a vent through which the high sinusoidal pressure can be relieved.

TABLE 24-5   Child's Classification of Hepatic Reserve

Criteria	Good A	Moderate B	Poor C
Serum bilirubin (mg%)	<2.0	2.0-3.0	>3.0
Serum albumin (g%)	>3.5	3.0-3.5	<3.0
Ascites	None	Easily controlled	Poorly controlled
Encephalopathy	None	Minimal	Advanced, "coma"
Nutrition	Excellent	Good	Poor, muscle wasting

All shunts decrease the total volume of blood flow to the liver, thereby reducing perfusion of hepatic cells. This effect may be accentuated if significant connections (shunts) between intrahepatic arterioles (hepatic artery supply) and portal venules exist. The decrease in hepatic perfusion is closely related to the anatomic size of the shunt, being smaller in splenorenal shunts than in the portacaval shunts. *This fall in liver perfusion accounts for the development of hepatic encephalopathy that usually accompanies shunting procedures.*

The results of shunting procedures, therefore, depend on a host of factors that have to be balanced by the surgeon at the operating table. These include:

- Anatomic ease of performance
- Choice of shunt
- Presence of ascites
- Extent of cirrhosis
- Experience of the surgeon

Treatment. Following hemodynamic stabilization of the patient, documentation of cirrhosis, and localization of the bleeding to the esophageal varices, surgical decompression of the portal venous system may be considered. It must be stressed that much of the following discussion of shunt surgery is dependent on the failure of alternative treatment methods. The use of sclerotherapy to prevent recurrent bleeding or even as prophylaxis against bleeding in patients with demonstrated varices is now the treatment of choice. The efficacy of beta blockers in preventing recurrent variceal bleeding has also been demonstrated in compliant patients. Direct anastomosis of the portal vein to the inferior vena cava with either an end-to-side or side-to-side anastomosis represents the two most common methods. Neither has any significant advantage over the other, except that the side-to-side portacaval shunt decreases the hepatic sinusoidal pressure, and the end-to-side portacaval shunt does not because of ligation of the hepatic side of the portal vein (Fig. 24-3, *A* and *B*). Both procedures provide maximal decompression of the portal hypertension and esophageal varices. Portal venous perfusion is abolished by both procedures, and total hepatic blood flow is usually decreased. The incidences of hepatic coma and encephalopathy are similar with both procedures. The end-to-side (or conventional) splenorenal shunt (Fig. 24-3, *C*) carries a low incidence of encephalopathy because the shunt is smaller and slightly more peripheral than a portacaval shunt. However, the splanchnic decompression is less effective, and there is a high incidence of anastomotic thrombosis and varix rebleeding. *Its primary use is in patients with associated severe hypersplenism, requiring splenectomy.* The mesocaval shunt (Fig. 24-3, *D*) has hemodynamic effects similar to the end-to-side splenorenal shunt and is useful in situations in which the portal vein is thrombosed; it is also used to avoid intraoperative bleeding from massive retroperitoneal collateral veins. The interposition shunt (H-graft), a modification of the mesocaval shunt, uses a vascular prosthesis between the superior mesenteric vein and the inferior vena cava (Fig. 24-3, *E*). The long-term patency rate for H-grafts is unknown, but technically it is easier than other shunting procedures and carries a lower mortality than do some other types of shunts.

Shunting blood away from the liver in patients with near-normal or normal hepatic function induces progression of the liver damage, presumably secondary to deprivation of hepatic portal flow. The distal splenorenal shunt (Fig. 24-3, *F*) was devised to decompress the esophageal varices selectively, for the most part through the short gastric vessels and the splenic parenchyma. It allows a reasonable rate of patency and is associated with minimal encephalopathy, maintaining liver perfusion with portal venous blood. This is accomplished by diverting the distal splenic vein into the left renal vein and isolating the gastrosplenic venous channels by ligation of the coronary vein, right gastric vein, right gastroepiploic vein, and splenocolic ligaments. More data are needed to assess the long-term results of distal splenorenal shunt. Although technically this shunt procedure is one of the most difficult to perform, current information suggests that it may be hemodynamically superior to other methods. It is probably the shunt of choice in an elective case. Direct portacaval or mesocaval H-graft is preferred in an emergency situation.

Esophagitis. Esophagitis alone is rarely responsible for significant acute UGI tract blood loss. Typically bleeding secondary to esophagitis is slow, presenting as chronic blood loss. Its association with hiatal hernias and the possibility of esophageal intrathoracic gastric ulcerations or gastritis, however, make it a significant source of acute blood loss (see Table 24-2).

Surgical correction is usually indicated, and the choice of procedures largely depends on the anatomic location of the ulcer. Emergency procedures required to control bleeding esophageal or gastric ulcers must always encompass appropriate repair of the sliding hiatal hernia and construction of a valvular mechanism to preclude further gastroesophageal reflux.

Large bleeding ulcers occurring in the herniated portion of the stomach should be approached in a similar fashion to that described above. Smaller ulcers and gastritis occurring in the herniated portion of the stomach should be treated by standard antireflux, valvuloplasty, and hiatal herniorrhaphy repair.

Mallory-Weiss' Syndrome. More frequent attainment of precise diagnosis of upper gastrointestinal tract bleeding has demonstrated a high

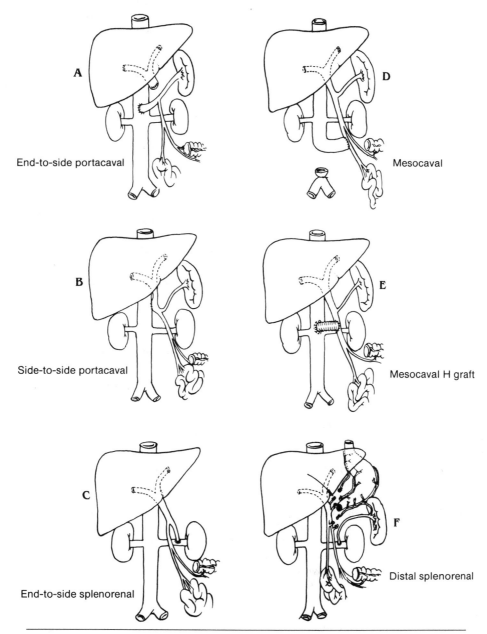

FIGURE 24-3 Some of the common shunts performed for the treatment of bleeding esophageal varices. (Modified from Orloff MJ. The liver and biliary system. In Sabiston DC Jr [ed]. Davis-Christopher Textbook of Surgery, 12th ed. Philadelphia, WB Saunders, 1981.)

proportion of emetogenically induced injury to the distal esophagus. Most commonly associated with alcoholic overindulgence, explosive retching and vomiting produce a sudden increased intra-abdominal pressure that may result in mucosal tears at the esophagogastric junction. Although the ensuing painless hemorrhage may arrest spontaneously, other methods of control often must be employed. If the bleeding is not massive, endoscopic application of vasoconstrictors or balloon tamponade may be tried. Continuous bleeding, however, usually requires laparotomy, large proximal gastrostomy, and oversewing of the bleeding points. Immediate correction of the problem can be expected, with uneventful recovery.

Other Causes. It is beyond the scope of this chapter to describe individually and in detail all the less frequent sources of acute bleeding from the upper GI tract. Together they represent approximately 20% of all sources of upper GI acute blood loss, some of which are quite common in particular clinical situations (e.g., the postoperative period) but overall represent only a small proportion. Given a particular clinical setting, awareness of the possible causes of acute blood loss pertinent to that situation will improve the diagnostic accuracy (see the box at right).

SOME POSSIBLE CAUSES OF ACUTE BLOOD LOSS

Postoperative causes
  Anastomotic suture line
  Marginal ulcer
  Stress ulcer
  Aortoenteric fistula
Curling's ulcer (postthermal burn)
Hemorrhagic duodenitis
Biliary tract
  Hemobilia
  Erosion of pancreatic pseudocyst into
    stomach
  Pancreatic carcinoma with invasion into
    the third or fourth portion of the
    duodenum
  Metastatic tumors
Diverticula of esophagus or duodenum
Vascular abnormalities
  Cirsoid aneurysm
  Telangiectasia
  Hemangioma
  Kaposi's sarcoma
Ischemic bowel disease
Blood dyscrasias

BLOOD LOSS FROM THE SMALL INTESTINE

Small bowel tumors represent 1% to 2% of all GI tract tumors. Primary neoplasms are the most common source of bleeding from the small bowel, which occurs in approximately half of these cases. In fact, the majority of symptomatic small bowel tumors are malignant. Other sources of small bowel hemorrhage include intussusception, Meckel's diverticulum, regional enteritis, nonspecific ulcerations, and aortoenteric fistula. Vascular abnormalities such as cavernous hemangiomata, phlebectasia, hemangiomata, multiple diffuse telangiectasia, and hereditary hemorrhagic telangiectasia may occur.

The ability to establish the diagnosis of these much less common sources of blood loss depends on the exclusion of diseases involving the gastrointestinal tract above the ligament of Treitz and beyond the ileocecal valve. In the majority of cases, this can be accomplished by combinations of endoscopy and contrast x-ray examinations, including angiography.

Therapy usually entails abdominal exploration and resection of the offending portion of the gut if the lesion or lesions can be detected and are sufficiently localized to permit removal without creating a gastrointestinal cripple.

ACUTE BLOOD LOSS OF THE LOWER GASTROINTESTINAL TRACT
Specific Bleeding Entities

Diverticular Disease of the Colon. Bleeding from diverticular disease most frequently is seen in the elderly, arteriosclerotic, hypertensive patient. *It is estimated that some bleeding occurs in up to 42% of patients with diverticular disease, with an overall incidence of massive hemorrhage of 5%.* Diverticular bleeding accounts for approximately 30% of all causes of melena and 70% of causes of massive colonic hemorrhage. However, it does not necessarily follow that patients who have rectal bleeding with radiographically documented diverticula are bleeding from the diverticula. One large group of patients with diverticular disease and rectal bleeding showed a 50% incidence of associated disease and a 30% incidence of associated malignant lesions.

Diagnosis. The pitfalls of assuming a cause and effect relationship between the presence of diverticular disease and rectal bleeding can now be circumvented, in most cases, by thorough endoscopic examination of the colon to the ileocecal valve to exclude other bleeding sources. However, colonoscopy currently has little to offer in localizing the specific source in the presence of active bleeding. *Selective arteriography in the actively bleeding patient is the most efficient method of localizing the site of hemorrhage.* The barium contrast study will not pinpoint areas of diverticular bleeding, but larger lesions may be excluded from consideration, and, not infrequently, barium lodged in the bleeding diverticulum may tamponade the feeding vessel.

Treatment. Bleeding from diverticular disease often stops spontaneously. Therefore adequate blood replacement and other usual supportive measures should be instituted initially, and elective resection should then be considered. If the bleeding is massive and/or relentless, emergency operation is necessary. If the specific bleeding site has been localized preoperatively, that portion of the colon should be resected. If the bleeding site was not localized preoperatively, however, *a subtotal colectomy with ileosigmoid anastomosis is the best overall choice for most patients.* The operative mortality rate for an emergency procedure in patients of this type is significant. Use of operative procedures of lesser magnitude may not control the hemorrhage, hence creating the need for a second major anesthetic and operation, which may be lethal.

Arteriovenous Malformation or Angiodysplasia. Angiodysplasia of the gastrointestinal tract may be encountered from the stomach to the colon. *It is typically seen in elderly patients who have cardiac disease resulting in a low cardiac output.* The association with aortic stenosis is striking but as yet unexplained. The most common site of bleeding is from the right colon. The bleeding pattern is often different from diverticular bleeding in that patients are less likely to bleed massively and often present with iron deficiency anemia and guaiac positive stools rather than with hematochezia.

The diagnosis depends on its consideration by an alert physician. All too commonly a barium enema is obtained *(which will never be diagnostic in this entity)* and, after it is negative, the work-up is halted. An experienced colonoscopist can often recognize vascular lesions in the wall of the colon (usually on the right side). *However, the visceral angiogram remains the primary diagnostic tool.* The strategy for diagnosis of an-

giodysplasia by arteriography is different from the diagnosis of diverticular bleeding. *In the latter group of patients, the angiogram is valuable only while the patient is actively bleeding,* since it depends on extravasation of contrast material into the bowel lumen. In angiodysplasia, the patient is rarely bleeding actively enough to demonstrate extravasation. Rather, *this technique aims to outline abnormal vascular anatomy that is accounting for the blood loss.* It is important that the radiologist be aware of what lesion is suspected and be familiar with the differences between it and diverticular bleeding. The angiogram should include selective arterial studies of all major vessels with delayed films that include the venous outflow. Angiodysplastic lesions have the following criteria on arteriography:

- Early filling of the veins indicating A-V fistula type of physiology
- Vascular tufts
- Persistent filling of the veins

Ulcerative Colitis. Incrimination of ulcerative colitis as the underlying cause for hemorrhage is not difficult. Although infrequent, massive bleeding most commonly occurs in a late stage of the disease. Occasionally it may represent the initial sign of acute idiopathic ulcerative colitis. Patients are usually very ill, and nonoperative therapy has little to offer these patients. The surgical procedure of choice is a total colectomy, proctectomy, and ileostomy. Many surgeons favor delaying the proctectomy in patients with severe metabolic depletion. However, the probability of recurrent hemorrhage from the retained rectum is high and would require a subsequent surgical procedure. As always, this risk must be balanced against the choice of an entirely intraabdominal operation.

Colonic Underperfusion (Vascular Insufficiency). *In elderly patients or those with decreased intestinal blood flow, a syndrome of hypoperfusion occurs, often manifested by acute hemorrhage.* The mucosa of the left colon is most often involved, with bleb formation leading to necrosis that may be seen on sigmoidoscopic examination. A barium enema evaluation reveals a characteristic picture of spasm and minute ulcerations (thumb-printing), which may be confused with ulcerative colitis. *Since the full thickness of the wall of the colon is not involved, the disease is self-limited, and an operation is not indicated.* Barium enema findings will return to normal during the ensuing weeks. If an operation is performed, the serosal surface of the colon may appear normal, but the stress of an operation on a patient suffering from underperfusion may lead to significant morbidity and should be undertaken only when other measures have failed.

Hemorrhoids. External hemorrhoids are obvious by physical examination, and characteristically the patient gives a history of bright red blood per rectum only with irritation or abrasion of the external aspect of the anal orifice.

Internal hemorrhoids may cause bright red rectal bleeding following constipation or straining, or they may produce significant rectal bleeding, while being totally silent clinically and documented only during or immediately following a bleeding episode. Careful examination of the anal canal and distal rectal ampulla should be performed before initiating more expensive and elaborate diagnostic methods in search of a bleeding source. *Sigmoidoscopy and barium enema or colonoscopic examination should always be done to rule out a more proximal lesion coincidentally associated with the hemorrhoids.* Hemorrhoidectomy is the treatment of choice if justified by symptoms or annoying frequent bleeding.

Rarely, patients with advanced cirrhosis of the liver may present with severe rectal bleeding resulting from colonic or rectal varices. Colonoscopy is usually diagnostic.

Polyps. Rectal bleeding is the most frequent sign of the presence of a colon polyp. The presence of rectal bleeding mandates that the patient have a digital rectal examination, proctosigmoidoscopy, and a barium enema or colonoscopy. Discovery of a potential bleeding lesion by one of the first two examinations in no way excludes the need for further investigation. If a lesion is discovered within 25 cm of the anus, it should be excised through the proctosigmoidoscope and delivered to the pathology laboratory for histologic study. If a polyp is found by barium enema, it should be confirmed by a subsequent air contrast barium enema after a good mechanical colon preparation to demonstrate other polyps, which occur in up to 20% of cases. If the second study confirms the presence of the lesion, the patient should then be prepared for colonoscopic polypectomy. Laparotomy and colotomy procedures are no longer necessary for removing polypoid lesions less than 5 cm in diameter unless the endoscopic approach fails or the patient refuses the lesser procedure.

Postirradiated Bowel. Radiation proctitis following therapeutic irradiation for pelvic malignancies frequently can cause moderate rectal bleeding, and occasionally the blood loss may be massive, intermittent, and frequent. *Its diagnosis depends on the history, proctosigmoidoscopic documentation, and biopsy.* In the majority of cases it can be controlled by avoiding high-residue foods coupled with periodic steroid enemas. However, if the bleeding persists or is massive, a left-sided, totally diverting, end colostomy and distal mucous fistula is recommended. Steroid enemas should be continued through the defunctionalized lower colorectal segment. Rarely, even this definitive treatment will not control the bleeding from a radiation-damaged lower colon. Total excision of the remaining rectum and colon is one therapeutic alternative. The operation by definition must be done on irradiated tissue, however, which makes the postoperative complications more significant in number and magnitude. An alternative radical extirpative pelvic operation is a bilateral retroperitoneal dissection of the external and internal iliac arteries, with ligation of the latter bilaterally. Hemorrhage is usually arrested, and collateral circulation preserves the viability of the pelvic colon and rectum.

Miscellaneous. Angiomas, leiomyomas, and rare vascular anomalies can also produce rectal hemorrhage but will not be considered further in this chapter.

CHRONIC (OCCULT) GASTROINTESTINAL TRACT BLOOD LOSS
Etiology

Chronic, slow blood loss from the gastrointestinal tract may occur for extended periods of time without significant specific symptoms. A patient with chronic occult blood loss may sustain a hemoglobin level below 5 g/100 ml without symptoms other than generalized weakness and chronic fatigue. In fact, this vague symptom complex may often be the only stimulus that precipitates the patient's seeking medical advice. Likewise, a patient may seek medical advice because of melena or intermittent small amounts of red blood passed via the rectum. The specific source of blood loss may elude the most thorough, sophisticated diagnostic effort, or it may herald an occult gastrointestinal tumor detectable by the most primitive diagnostic modality—the index finger.

The following is a partial list of various specific lesions responsible for chronic intestinal blood loss, which are often missed radiographically:

- Esophagitis
- Gastritis
- Duodenitis
- Stomal ulcers
- Drug-induced ulcers
- Neoplasms (early)
- Vascular malformations (e.g., hemangioma, telangiectasia)
- Polyp (small)
- Ectopic gastric mucosa in the esophagus
- Diverticula (small intestinal)
- Circular stricture (small intestinal)
- Enteric cysts (duplication)
- Internal hemorrhoids
- Nonspecific ulcers (small intestinal)

The clinician should also consider drug-induced chronic blood loss in patients who have ingested antibiotics, anticoagulants, arsenic compounds, DDT, phenylbutazone, quinine, quinidine, and adrenocortical steroids. Cessation of the agent in question for a short period will often delineate its significance and may possibly avoid the need for further, more elaborate examinations.

Diagnosis

Documentation of a microcytic, iron-deficiency anemia in the absence of known blood loss calls for thorough evaluation of the gastrointestinal tract. Although the time-honored upper GI tract series will detect a great number of significant lesions, no information can be obtained that will indict the observed lesion as the source of bleeding. Therefore fiberoptic endoscopy of the upper GI tract complements traditional x-ray examinations. Biopsies and cytologic washings can be obtained during the same examination. Among patients undergoing esophagogastroduodenoscopy because of iron-deficiency anemia, melena, or both, the cause can be established in 40%. Furthermore, normal findings on examination significantly reduce the possibility that the blood loss originated from the esophagus, stomach, or first half of the duodenum.

However, the same reasoning does not hold true for the colon. Barium enema examination remains the initial diagnostic procedure. In patients with rectal bleeding, colonoscopy should be reserved for those who have had a negative result to a double-contrast study or those with questionable radiographic findings. By this approach, most of the patients with radiographically obvious colon disease will be spared the need for colonoscopy. Yet a negative result to a barium study does not exclude the possibility of significant colon disease, and, in that setting, persisting clinical signs mandate that a thorough colonoscopic examination be performed.

Endoscopic examinations of the upper and lower GI tracts, the antegrade small bowel series, and the barium contrast studies of the colon are currently the most productive examinations for detecting sources of chronic gastrointestinal blood loss. Selective arteriography occasionally will establish the diagnosis and is particularly suited for detection of various vascular anomalies, such as hemangiomas, arteriovenous fistulas, and diffuse telangiectasia. Obviously, angiographic demonstration of these types of lesions is contingent on their size and the presence of active bleeding.

A negative, comprehensive, gastrointestinal tract evaluation in a patient who continues to manifest signs of blood loss represents a frustrating dilemma to both the patient and physician. If the blood loss is minimal and iron replacement maintains a relatively normal hematologic picture, the patient may be restudied periodically. This approach is particularly applicable to elderly patients who represent poor surgical risks. If repeated blood transfusions are required to maintain hemoglobin levels in a physiologically acceptable range, surgical exploration of the gastrointestinal tract should be considered. Unfortunately, the yield in diagnostic findings from such endeavors is only about 10%, and the results in the majority of cases are unrewarding. Based on this low yield, surgical exploration should not be considered until all less invasive diagnostic methods have been exhausted.

BIBLIOGRAPHY

Bray SJ, DiBiase A, et al. Lower intestinal bleeding in the elderly. Am J Surg 137:57, 1979.

Church JM. Analysis of the colonoscopic findings in patients with rectal bleeding according to the pattern of their presenting symptoms. Dis Colon Rectum 34:391-395, 1991.

Dores GM, Miller ME, Kaufman DG. A herald bleed: A case of aorto-esophageal fistula and a review of the literature. RI Med J 74:123-126, 1991.

Geus WP, Lamers CBHW. Presentation of stress ulcer bleeding: A review. Scand J Gastroenterol 25(suppl 178):32-41, 1990.

Helmrich GA, Stillworth JR, Brown JJ. Angiodysplasia: Characterization, diagnosis, advances in treatment. South Med J 83:1450-1453, 1990.

Lang EV, Picus D, Marx NV, Hicks ME. Massive arterial hemorrhage from the stomach and lower esophagus: Impact of embolotherapy on survival. Radiology 177:249-252, 1990.

Lebrec D. β blockers and portal hypertension, hemodynamic effects and prevention of recurrent gastrointestinal bleeding. Hepatogastroenterology 37: 556-560, 1990.

Lewis BS, Wenger JS, Waye JD. Small bowel enteroscopy and intraoperative enteroscopy for obscure gastrointestinal bleeding. Am J Gastroenterol 86: 171-174, 1991.

MacDougall BRD, Bailey RJ, Williams R. H$_2$-receptor antagonists and antacids in the prevention of acute gastrointestinal hemorrhage in fulminant hepatic failure: Two controlled trials. Lancet 1:617, 1977.

MacMathuna P, Westaby D, Williams R. Taking the tension out of the portal system: An approach to the management of portal hypertension in the 1990s. Scand J Gastroenterol 25(suppl 175):131-145, 1990.

Martin LF, Max NH, Polk HC Jr. Failure of gastric pH control by antacids or cimetidine in the critically ill: A valid sign of sepsis. Surgery 88:59, 1980.

Mazzaferro V, Todo S, Tzakis AG, et al. Liver transplantation in patients with previous portasystemic shunt. Am J Surg 160:111-116, 1990.

Meerhoff JC. Algorithm for managing patients with severe GI hemorrhage. Hosp Pract 186, 1984.

Richardson JD, McInnis WD, et al. Occult gastrointestinal bleeding: An evaluation of available diagnostic methods. Arch Surg 110:661, 1975.

Rooney PJ, Hunt RH. The risk of upper gastrointestinal hemorrhage during steroidal and non-steroidal anti-inflammatory therapy. Ballieres Clin Rheumatol 4:207-217, 1990.

Stump DL, Hardin TC. The use of vasopressin in the treatment of upper gastrointestinal hemorrhage. Drugs 39:38-53, 1990.

Sugawa C. Endoscopic diagnosis and treatment of upper gastrointestinal bleeding. Surg Clin North Am 69:1167-1183, 1989.

Terblanche J, Kriage JEJ, Burman PC. Endoscopic sclerotherapy. Surg Clin North Am 70:341-359, 1990.

Warren WD. Control of variceal bleeding. Am J Surg 145:8, 1983.

Westaby D, Polson RJ, Gerison AES, et al. A controlled trial of oral propranolol compared with injection sclerotherapy for the long term management of variceal bleeding. Hepatology 11:353-359, 1990.

Wood RP, Shaw BW Jr, Rikkers LF. Liver transplantation for variceal hemorrhage. Surg Clin North Am 70:449-461, 1990.

CHAPTER REVIEW
Questions

1. What are the two most frequent causes of acute UGI tract blood loss?
2. Of the following, which is the single most effective diagnostic procedure for detecting a UGI source of blood loss?
   a. UGI series
   b. Endoscopy
   c. Arteriography
   d. Blakemore-Sengstaken tube
   e. Laparoscopy
3. What are the two most common causes of massive blood loss from the rectum?
4. A 65-year-old woman is admitted with massive lower GI bleeding that persists after 4 units of whole blood replacement. Outline your diagnostic approach (order of performing the requisite tests).
5. What is the most important single criterion for emergency operation for bleeding duodenal ulcer?
6. List four criteria for classifying a cirrhotic patient into the high-risk category for emergency operation.
7. Which of the following shunts are physiologic side-to-side shunts?
   a. End portal-to-side vena cava
   b. Mesocaval
   c. End splenic to side renal
   d. H-graft
   e. Side portal to side vena cava
8. What is the most likely diagnosis of the following symptoms?
   a. Vomiting of clear material followed by UGI bleeding
   b. Preceding long history of severe heartburn
   c. Lower GI bleeding in an elderly patient with no previous history or current other symptoms
   d. Spots of red blood on a normal brown stool
9. Early operation is indicated for which of the following?
   a. A duodenal ulcer patient who vomits red blood 4 days after stabilization from a previous massive hemorrhage
   b. An 80-year-old woman with bright rectal bleeding and thumb-printing of the left colon on barium enema
   c. An icteric young man with massive ascites who vomits large amounts of blood
   d. A 60-year-old man with an aortic bifemoral bypass (done 3 years previously) who has massive hematemesis
10. Which of the following causes of bleeding are ***not*** commonly found in patients with known esophageal varices?
    a. Gastric cancer
    b. Duodenal ulcer

c. Gastritis

d. Esophageal varices

e. Gastric varices

11. Which of the following statements regarding resuscitation and early care of patients with GI bleeding is *not* true?

a. Patients should be admitted to a unit where they can be closely monitored.

b. A large-bore IV line should be started.

c. A nasogastric tube should be avoided if possible to prevent disturbing clots over potentially bleeding vessels.

d. Hemoglobin levels should be monitored to detect occult blood loss.

e. Urine output should be frequently checked to monitor perfusion and hydration.

12. Which of the following vessels is the likely cause of massive bleeding from a posterior duodenal ulcer?

a. Right hepatic artery

b. Pancreaticoduodenal artery

c. Right gastroepiploic artery

d. Left gastric artery

e. Gastroduodenal artery

13. A patient presents with melena and gives a history of heavy use of antiarthritic agents. An NG tube has some blood present that clears quickly with lavage. What is the most likely diagnosis?

a. Erosive esophagitis

b. Esophageal varices

c. Erosive gastritis

d. Gastric cancer

e. Angiodysplasia

14. A patient is being considered for a shunt operation for bleeding varices. The serum bilirubin is 2.3 and albumin is 3.3. The patient has reasonable nutrition and mentation appears normal. Mild ascites is present. This patient represents what class of risk based on hepatic reserve?

a. World Health Organization poor risk

b. Child's A

c. Child's B

d. Child's C

e. Not classifiable without hepatic angiogram

15. Which procedure currently represents the most widely used maneuver to control variceal bleeding in the United States?

a. Angiographic embolization

b. Devascularization of G-E junction including varices

c. End-to-side shunt

d. Side-to-side shunt

e. Endoscopic sclerotherapy

16. Which of the following statements about bleeding from the small bowel is true?

a. Primary small bowel neoplasms are the most common source of small bowel bleeding.

b. Enteroscopy using a fiberoptic scope passed orally is the most common means of establishing a diagnosis.

c. Benign tumors of the small bowel are more likely to cause symptoms than malignant ones.

d. Small bowel bleeding accounts for 10% to 15% of all patients with GI bleeding who require operation.

e. Small bowel bleeding is easier to diagnose than either gastric or colonic bleeding.

Answers

1. Acute hemorrhagic gastritis and duodenal peptic ulcerations

2. b

3. Diverticulosis and angiodysplasia

4. After an adequate history and physical examination:

a. Rectal examination

b. Sigmoidoscopy

c. Superior and inferior mesenteric artery angiogram

d. Barium enema

e. Colonoscopy

5. After stabilization, the rate of bleeding exceeds a present limit (e.g., 4 units/24 hours)

6. a. Jaundice

b. Massive ascites

c. Prolonged prothrombin time unresponsive to vitamin K

d. Serum albumin below 3.0 g% per 100 ml

7. b, c, d, e

8. a. Mallory-Weiss' syndrome (esophageal or gastric mucosal rupture)

b. Esophagitis (hiatal hernia)

c. Diverticulosis

d. Hemorrhoids

9. a, d

10. a

11. c

12. e

13. c

14. c

15. e

16. a

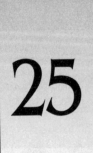

25 Acute Abdominal Pain

BERNARD GARDNER
H. HARLAN STONE

KEY FEATURES

After reading this chapter you will understand:
- The physiology of abdominal pain.
- How to differentiate between visceral and somatic abdominal pain.
- How to analyze the history and physical examination to make a diagnosis.
- Acute abdominal visceral inflammations: appendicitis, cholecystitis, pancreatitis, diverticulitis.
- The diagnosis and treatment of perforations of a viscus.
- How to diagnose ischemic bowel disease.
- The elements in diagnosing intestinal obstruction.
- Why it is important to differentiate small from large bowel obstruction.

In the evaluation of the patient with abdominal pain, a clear and orderly history and physical examination, a synthesis of facts gleaned from a knowledge of anatomy, embryology, and physiology, and an understanding of the pathogenesis of abdominal diseases will lead to the correct diagnosis in nearly every case. On occasion, reliance is placed on radiographs or laboratory tests that diagnostically augment examination of the patient. In the exceptional case in which the diagnosis is still in doubt, special procedures must be undertaken early because **undiagnosed acute abdominal pain represents a medical emergency.** The highest accuracy must be sought;

therefore a diagnosis such as "abdominal pain, rule out . . . , and so on," is **unacceptable.** Such a diagnosis is often a sign of an incomplete history and/or physical examination or muddled thought on the part of the physician.

PHYSIOLOGY OF ABDOMINAL PAIN
What Is the Origin of Abdominal Pain?

Pain arising from intra-abdominal conditions originates from nerve stimulation that travels via the splanchnic nerves to the central nervous system for interpretation. Afferent nerves are divided into visceral (within the wall of the intestine and all of its derivatives) and parietal (present in the parietal peritoneum). *The visceral afferent nerves respond primarily to the stimulus of stretch or sudden distention,* which results from an acute increase in tension on the wall of a viscus such as is present when contraction occurs against a resistance. The parietal afferent nerves are somatic and can be stimulated by sudden pressure (e.g., such as occurs in an incision) and by acute changes in pH or temperature (e.g., in bacterial or chemical inflammation). In the presence of such inflammation, the neural receptors in the peritoneum become acutely sensitive to even the slightest pressure, which explains many of the physical signs of peritonitis. The patient, as always, helps differentiate the sources of his or her pain by describing the pain as "crampy" (visceral) or "constant" (parietal). Additional terms often used to characterize visceral pain are *gas pains* and *colic,* which are forms of intermittent cramp. Parietal pain, often constant, may be sharp or dull depending on its chronicity and intensity.

What Is the Distribution of Abdominal Pain?

Intra-abdominal pain, in general, is referred to the area of the body supplied by the appropriate spinal segments from which the sensory nerves are derived, roughly corresponding to the appropriate dermatomes. The gastrointestinal tract is embryologically divided into three segments of midline origin; therefore *visceral pain is referred to the midline of the abdomen.* Stimuli originating from the foregut below the diaphragm are referred to the epigastrium, stimuli from the midgut are referred to the periumbilical (mid-abdominal) area, and stimuli from the hindgut are referred to the lower abdomen (hypogastrium). The lines of demarcation of these three segments of the gastrointestinal tract are distinct and can be easily recalled if one thinks of the arterial blood supply to the intestine (Fig. 25-1). Anatomically the foregut ends close to the ligament of Treitz, and the midgut ends at the splenic flexure of the colon.

Parietal pain is simpler to understand, since being somatic in origin, it *is referred directly to the area of location of the involved nerves* (e.g., inflammation of the peritoneum in the right lower quadrant is referred to the right lower quadrant). In certain special circumstances somatic branches of other spinal segments supply afferent fibers to a particular viscus. For example, the gallbladder receives a small afferent branch from the right phrenic nerve (C3–5), stimulation of which by inflammation will produce constant pain referred to the right shoulder and scapula. Specific application of this knowledge is described in the following sections.

Diagnosis

History. The characteristics of the original pain, its distribution, its change in character, and associated symptoms must be carefully elicited to

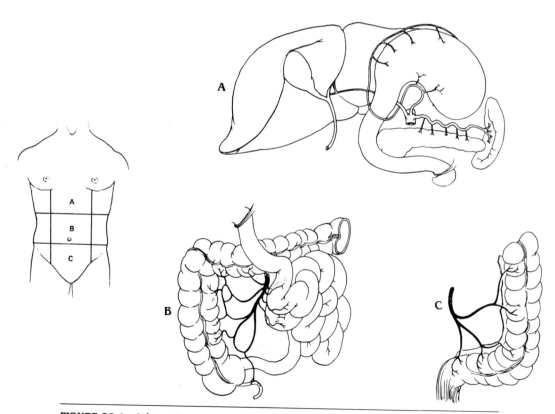

FIGURE 25-1   Schematic representation of referral of visceral pain. **A,** Foregut (celiac axis). **B,** Midgut (superior mesenteric) artery. **C,** Hindgut (inferior mesenteric) artery.

understand the nature of the disease. A correct diagnosis is then established by fitting the natural history of the development of symptoms into a recognizable pattern.

Associated Symptoms. Visceral pain may be accompanied by associated symptoms. *Sudden stretch produces vomiting in addition to cramps.* Such reflex vomiting has two distinguishing characteristics: (1) it does not relieve the pain, and (2) it is not accompanied by nausea. This vomiting is secondary to increased tension within a viscus and does not represent overflow from obstruction of the gastrointestinal tract. *Therefore it also occurs with distention of organs out of continuity with the main flow of food and secretions* in the gastrointestinal tract such as the gallbladder and pancreas.

Visceral pain and vomiting are characteristically manifestations of a mechanical difficulty such as obstruction of the intestine or a stone blocking the flow of bile or urine. The pain is caused by contraction against a resistance (i.e., peristalsis in an obstructed intestine). *In the majority of instances the visceral components of pain represent an early phase of disease, and no systemic signs or symptoms such as fever, leukocytosis, malaise, anorexia, weight loss, weakness, and anemia are present.* If these systemic components of the clinical picture do occur, they may be due to infection, neoplasms, metabolic derangement, or toxemia rather than a purely mechanical cause.

Sequence of Mechanical Versus Systemic Symptoms. The sequence in which the mechanical and systemic components develop (Fig. 25-2) is very important in establishing the nature of the underlying pathology. *The clinical setting in which the earliest symptom of pain occurred is vital in establishing whether the problem is systemic or mechanical.* For example, when a patient with purely visceral pain and vomiting subsequently develops leukocytosis, fever, anorexia, or weakness, the presence of such complicating factors as peritonitis or intestinal gangrene, conditions demanding the immediate attention of a surgeon, should be suspected. In such cases somatic pain is often also present but always follows the development of visceral pain. On the other hand, if a patient with clearly established systemic symptoms such as fever, weakness, malaise, anorexia, or weight loss should then develop the visceral pain pointing to a mechanical problem, a preexisting underlying systemic illness (e.g., inflammation or neoplasm) that may have produced secondary obstruction should be sought.

Therefore close questioning of the patient should center on his or her condition and when the pain first occurred and carefully follow the subsequent course up to the present.

Physical Examination. The patient with *uncomplicated colic (visceral)* will often move around in bed in an attempt to find a comfortable position, maneuvers that usually prove unrewarding. *Peritoneal signs are absent in these cases.*

By contrast, the *inflamed peritoneum (somatic) is tender, and the patient avoids all movement.* Coughing is painful, and flexion of the thighs helps to relax the peritoneum. By the same token, any attempt to stretch the inflamed peritoneum produces pain and may clearly be used to point to the site of the inflammation. Peritoneum over the psoas muscle, for example, can be stretched by extension of the thigh at the hip (Fig. 25-3, *A*). Therefore infections involving the psoas sheath (psoas abscess) or those extending from nearby organs (ureter or pelvic appendix) elicit pain by this maneuver. Internal rotation of the thigh produces stretching of the obturator fascia and therefore pain in ureteral or appendiceal inflammation (Fig. 25-3, *B*). Differential tenderness between the right and left sides of the rectum may be an important sign of a retrocecal or pelvic appendicitis (Fig. 25-4).

All attempts at eliciting signs of peritonitis should be made by examining the seemingly uninvolved areas of the abdomen first. This helps relax the patient, which may be difficult once pain is elicited. *Tenderness in more than one quadrant of the abdomen implies that localization of the inflammation has been lost* and a generalized peritonitis is likely, possibly secondary to perforation of a viscus.

In general, involuntary contraction of the abdominal muscles *(guarding or rigidity)* is a highly reliable sign of intraperitoneal inflammation (e.g., perforated ulcer). *Rebound tenderness* is a form of peritoneal stretching by sudden release of pressure and indicates underlying peritonitis. Both the sign and accompanying peritonitis may be localized or generalized. Since visceral pain is related to the periodic contraction against a resistance, when the small bowel is involved, the *pain produced by peristaltic activity will coincide with the bowel sounds.* Since peristalsis does not occur in the colon, visceral pain and vomiting will be late concomitants of colonic obstruction. *Peritoneal inflammation is associated with reflex intestinal inhibition so that the bowel sounds are lost,* and this represents another sign of peritonitis. The onset of peritonitis can be clearly suggested by both history and physical examination and represents an ominous development in abdominal disease.

Deviations in the Reliability of the Physical Examination. Some conditions may occur in which the physical signs of acute peritonitis may be difficult to elicit.

With **marked obesity,** a significant visceral inflammation may be protected from the overlying peritoneum by a greatly thickened omentum. Palpation of the peritoneum will therefore ap-

pear negative. On occasion perforation of a viscus may occur with protection by omentum and minimal direct signs of peritonitis. A similar situation occurs when **normal intestine overlies the seat of a severe inflammation** and is not involved in the disease process (e.g., the occasional lack of anterior peritoneal signs accompanying acute retrocecal appendicitis).

Patients who have had **multiple full-term pregnancies** or **multiple operations** on the abdomen may be unable to contract their abdominal

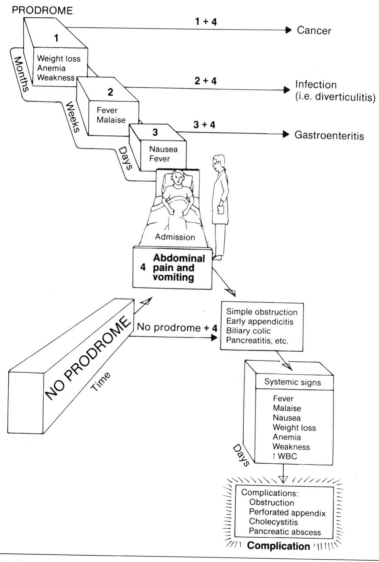

FIGURE 25-2   Schema to illustrate how the proper sequencing of events in the history and physical examination can suggest the right diagnosis. Symptoms caused by mechanical problems must be separated from those secondary to systemic disease. The diagnosis often depends on whether the systemic symptoms preceded or followed the mechanical symptoms.

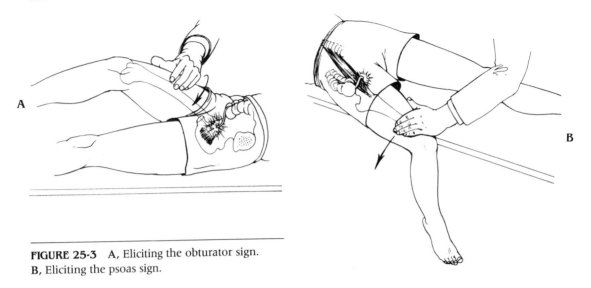

FIGURE 25-3 A, Eliciting the obturator sign.
B, Eliciting the psoas sign.

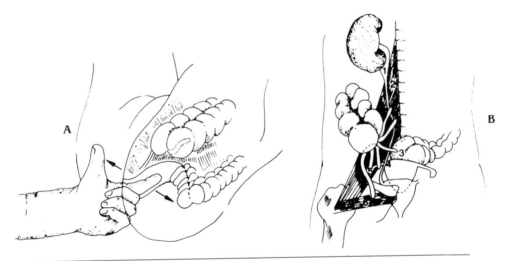

FIGURE 25-4 A, Rectal examination in retrocecal appendicitis. B, Physical signs of appendicitis depend on the location of the organ in relation to neighboring viscera.

muscles. Guarding or rigidity in the presence of peritonitis is impossible for these patients. Therefore palpation may elicit pain, but the lack of muscular rigidity may mislead the examining physician.

A more subtle and infinitely more dangerous situation is the *use of antibiotics,* which may mask the signs of peritonitis by reducing the inflammation of the peritoneum without treating the underlying pathology. Perforation of the gallbladder or appendix has occurred in patients receiving antibiotic therapy when this factor was unrecognized. Patients *treated by analgesics*

may not respond appropriately during physical examination.

Approach to the Patient. As the physician stands in the emergency room faced with a patient having acute abdominal pain, he or she must learn to ask himself or herself several questions in rapid order.

- What is the likely diagnosis?
- What is the pathogenesis of this condition?
- How can the underlying physiologic problem be relieved?
- Is an operation necessary and, if so, how soon?

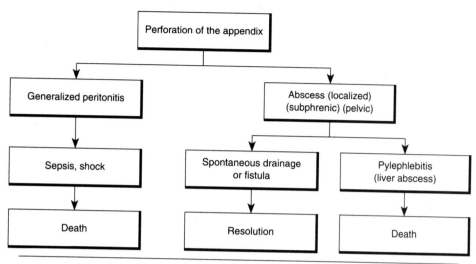

FIGURE 25-5   Perforation of the appendix.

- If no operation is performed, what will happen to the patient?
- How can I recognize an error in judgment?

ACUTE APPENDICITIS

Pathogenesis and Diagnosis. The relatively small size of the appendix accounts for the rapid development of symptoms but in no way should lead to underestimating the lethal nature of untreated appendicitis. *This accounts for one of the best clinical signs of this disease—rapid development of peritonitis without treatment.*

Stage 1. Obstruction of the appendix may be caused by a fecalith, mucous plug, foreign body, parasite, or tumor, accounting for the early signs of periumbilical cramp and vomiting due to distention of the appendix.

Stage 2. Rapid invasion of the wall of the organ by bacteria, with secondary inflammation, leads to the gradual onset of systemic signs of anorexia and malaise associated with a low-grade fever and leukocytosis.

Stage 3. The inflammation spreads to involve the whole wall of the organ and neighboring peritoneum, leading to a change in character of the pain to constant and localized. *Peritoneal signs and symptoms develop according to the location of the organ* (see Fig. 25-4, *B*). The patient at this stage may mimic one with acute pyelonephritis, cholecystitis, or tuboovarian abscess but can be differentiated by eliciting the history of the early stages and therefore the sequence of development of the symptoms.

Young women with right-sided ovarian disease present with a particularly perplexing problem. Often the pain in the latter condition began in the lower right quadrant (no shift). *The point of maximal tenderness in appendicitis (McBurney's point) is two thirds of the distance from the umbilicus to the anterior superior iliac spine* and is 2 to 3 cm above the maximal tenderness found in ovarian disease.

The pelvic and rectal examination (see Fig. 25-4, *A*) *are vital in making the diagnosis,* since the appendix may be protected from the anterior peritoneum and fail to give appropriate palpatory findings. Such protection by omentum and bowel serves to modify the subsequent generalized peritonitis should perforation of the organ ensue—*a factor that makes the disease more lethal in children, whose omentum may be poorly developed.*

Stage 4. The last stage is perforation (Fig. 25-5). All four stages may develop within a 48-hour period.

Diagnosis of acute appendicitis has been enhanced by current radiologic techniques using ultrasound, computed tomography (CT), or barium enema. *None of these tests* should delay operation in the clear-cut case but should be reserved for those cases in which the diagnosis is distinctly in doubt. A barium enema examination is seldom used clinically because of fear that the pressure of the barium may cause perforation of the weakened appendix. Sonograms may rule in or out the presence of significant ovarian disease or demonstrate the fluid-filled area in the right lower quadrant representing the inflamed appendiceal phlegmon. By far the most accurate diagnostic radiologic procedure is CT with oral contrast, which can demonstrate the inflamed area around the cecum or appendix.

In recent years surgeons have investigated the use of laparoscopy to diagnose acute appendicitis under direct vision and rarely to remove the inflamed organ through the laparoscope. Instrumentation and techniques for this procedure are still being developed and therefore are not in widespread use.

Treatment. If the diagnosis is in doubt, antibiotics should be withheld, since they may mask the signs of a developing peritonitis but not prevent perforation. The patient should be observed with nothing by mouth, maintenance intravenous fluids, and frequent physical and laboratory examinations over several hours. If appendicitis is present, development of peritoneal signs will establish the diagnosis.

Perforation increases the mortality rate tenfold, whereas the risk of a negative exploration approaches zero. These facts have inclined surgeons to operate when the disease is reasonably suspected after a careful history and physical examination. Once the decision to operate has been made and if perforation is suspected, antibiotics are in order.

Since the first physician evaluating a patient with appendicitis likely will not be a surgeon, early consultation should be sought. When these consultations are controlled or discouraged (e.g., by certain health maintenance organizations [HMOs]), there may be a tendency to delay the diagnosis, subsequently resulting in a higher rate of perforation.

What Are the Postoperative Complications of Appendicitis?

Wound Infection. This complication occurs in less than 1% of patients with unperforated appendicitis, but rises to 20% with perforation. Infection may be avoided in these cases by *delayed primary closure of the wound planned at the primary operation.* Treatment is directed at drainage of the wound when diagnosed and administration of appropriate antibiotics.

Subphrenic Abscess. The persistence of spiking temperatures starting 4 or 5 days postoperatively without obvious cause should suggest an intra-abdominal collection of pus. *Diagnosis is established by physical examination demonstrating a fixed diaphragm and pleural effusion, tenderness over the seventh or eighth rib later-*

ally, and edema or erythema of the lower lateral chest wall. Additional aids include sonogram, liver lung scan, gallium scan, or CT scan demonstrating the collection. Extraperitoneal drainage depends on appropriate timing and is best done when the clinical signs point to the development of a synthesis between the abscess wall and peritoneum. Transperitoneal drainage is associated with a mortality rate over 10%. The recent increase in successful drainage percutaneously under sonographic or CT scan control indicates that this technique should be tried initially in many cases.

Pelvic Abscess. *Recurrent fever and diarrhea after appendectomy* should suggest the formation of a pelvic abscess. *Diagnosis is made by rectal examination* and is confirmed by sonography or CT (Fig. 25-6). Drainage is never made transrectally until the abscess shows evidence of maturation by failure to descend further on repeated rectal examinations and the thinness of the wall. Drainage is performed in the operating room after needle aspiration has confirmed the presence of pus. If no synthesis between the rectum and abscess wall is certain, a lateral extraperitoneal drainage is performed. Antibiotic treatment may obviate drainage in some cases. Percutaneous drainage by catheter under sonographic or CT scan control should be tried first because it yields excellent results.

Pylephlebitis. This rare complication represents the formation of microabscesses in the liver and usually is found in patients with untreated

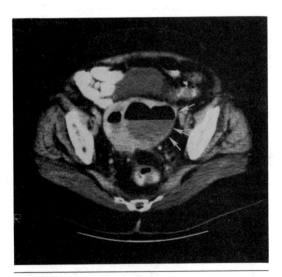

FIGURE 25-6 CT scan demonstrating large pelvic abscess *(arrow)* with air-fluid levels. It was drained percutaneously.

appendicitis. The mortality rate is high in spite of adequate antibiotic treatment. Rarely is drainage successful, since the abscesses are diffuse and quite small.

Appendiceal Abscess. A few patients seek treatment *after the process is clearly walled off,* and under these circumstances antibiotics and elective (interval) appendectomy may be preferred. This is dangerous unless the following criteria are clearly met:

- History is longer than 72 hours.
- A mass is palpable in the right lower quadrant.
- No signs of peritonitis are present elsewhere in the abdomen.

When antimicrobial therapy is begun, the patient is followed at least every 2 hours, and progress should include:

- Fall in temperature
- Fall in white blood cell count
- Reduction in tenderness over the mass
- Decrease in size of the mass over 24 to 48 hours
- Absence of peritoneal signs in other quadrants of the abdomen

If the criteria are met and the patient continues to improve, an interval appendectomy is carried out at 4 to 6 weeks to prevent recurrent appendicitis.

Postoperative complications, depending on the degree of contamination, include wound infection and intraperitoneal abscess (subdiaphragmatic or pelvic).

Summary of Treatment of Appendicitis

Object. *Early operation before perforation.*
Specific Treatment

- No antibiotic therapy if diagnosis is doubtful; prophylactic (short course) antibiotics in unperforated appendicitis; therapeutic (full course) antibiotics in perforated appendicitis
- Preparation for operation by evacuating the stomach, administering intravenous fluids, and evaluating other unrelated problems with electrocardiogram (ECG) and x-ray studies

Supportive Treatment

- Fluids intravenously—maintenance only is needed unless the patient has been ill for several days, then according to urinary output and serum electrolytes

- Nothing by mouth
- Nasogastric suction if patient has vomited

Time of Preparation. Less than 2 hours.

CHOLECYSTITIS
What Is Acute Cholecystitis?

Pathogenesis and Diagnosis. The primary underlying event in acute cholecystitis is obstruction (Fig. 25-7). Less than 5% of acutely inflamed gallbladders are acalculous, and of them, obstruction of the common bile duct by cancer, stone, fibrosis of the ampulla of Vater, or other lesions must be sought before obstruction can be ruled out. *In the vast majority of cases of acute cholecystitis, stones are present in the gallbladder.*

Stage 1 (Fig. 25-8). *The gallbladder is stimulated by certain foods to contract, at which time a stone is forced into the cystic duct* (Fig. 25-9), producing sudden tension on the wall and stimulation of stretch receptors. *Pain is felt in the epigastrium, since the gallbladder is derived from the foregut. Reflex vomiting occurs.*

At this stage the symptoms are similar to those of peptic ulceration except that (1) the pain occurs within 15 to 30 minutes of eating in cholecystitis (gallbladder colic) rather than 1 to 1½ hours as in ulcer disease and (2) the vomiting does not relieve the pain, as it often does in ulcer disease (neutralization of acid) in which it may be induced by the patient for this purpose.

Prognosis. The prognosis at this stage is excellent. There are no systemic sequelae, and the majority of patients are relieved after several hours. This is understandable, since at this stage the stone is not impacted and no specific treat-

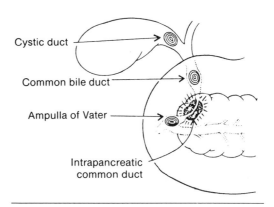

FIGURE 25-7   Diagram of the biliary tract showing common sites of obstruction.

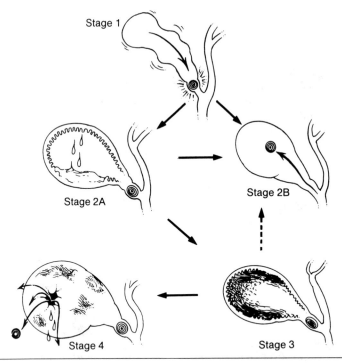

FIGURE 25-8 Schematic representation of the stages in acute cholecystitis. Stage 1: contraction with impaction of stone in cystic duct. Stage 2A: progressive distention (hydrops). Stage 2B: relief (end of attack). Stage 3: infection. Stage 4: perforation. Note that relief of the attack can occur after colic (stage 1) or distention (stage 2A) or on rare occasions after infection has supervened (stage 3).

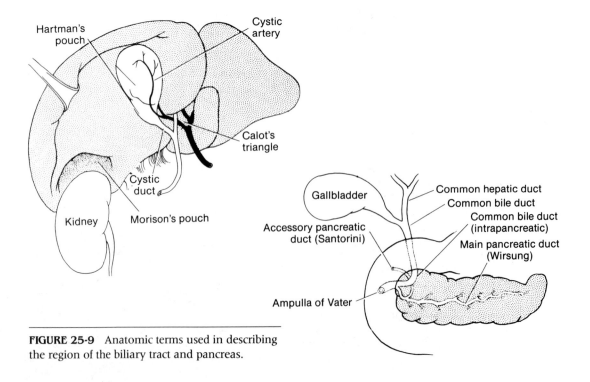

FIGURE 25-9 Anatomic terms used in describing the region of the biliary tract and pancreas.

ment is indicated. With rest, the stone will drop back into the gallbladder, tension is relieved, and the attack is over—until the next forceful contraction that leads to stone impaction.

Stage 2. The gallstone becomes impacted in the cystic duct, and the gallbladder cannot be emptied. Mucous secretion occurs, associated with bacterial growth and chemical irritation of the gallbladder wall. As the full thickness of the gallbladder wall becomes inflamed, the pain moves to the right upper quadrant.

The character of the pain changes from colic to continuous, dull, or aching. If the gallbladder is buried deep in the liver or overlies the posterior peritoneum, there may be back pain that is characteristically associated with right upper quadrant pain and often described as traveling around the side to the back. Shoulder pain is due to somatic innervation of the gallbladder by a branch of the right phrenic nerve via the hepatic plexus. Systemic signs such as low-grade fever and leukocytosis may occur. ***Tenderness in the right upper quadrant is characteristic, but mild and frank peritonitis occurs late in this stage.*** The gallbladder may be palpable. The absence of costovertebral angle tenderness should differentiate the condition from acute pyelonephritis or perinephric abscess, both of which occasionally give anterior abdominal wall findings. One should test for this sign gently so as not to disturb the entire right upper quadrant of the abdomen.

Prognosis. Cholecystitis (1) may develop to the third stage or (2) may subside by release of the impacted stone.

Stage 3. Continued distention of the gallbladder occurs due to persistent cystic duct obstruction. Bacterial invasion accompanies this stage, and peritonitis develops. The right upper quadrant is acutely tender, and there are rigidity and guarding with marked rebound tenderness. Fever may be high, and associated leukocytosis occurs. The remainder of the abdomen is normal, but the patient appears ill and toxic.

Prognosis. The condition (1) may subside or (2) may go on to perforation.

Stage 4. Perforation of the gallbladder occurs. Many physicians regard perforation of a viscus as a sudden bursting. This is not actually the case, although it does represent a catastrophe from the view of morbidity and mortality. The gallbladder is supplied by the cystic artery and occasionally by small branches in the liver bed from the hepatic arterial supply. ***The vessels in the wall are end arteries.*** As the gallbladder distends, ***the tension on the wall increases*** markedly so that a stage is reached when the ***critical closing pressure of the arterioles is exceeded,*** and blood supply to some areas diminishes. Patchy areas of gangrene develop through which bile, pus, and bacteria begin to leak. This perforation may occur freely into the peritoneal cavity (in which case peritoneal signs will develop in the involved quadrants) or may be partly sealed by the omentum, liver, or intestine. Intrahepatic perforation may lead to abscess formation. Perforation occurs in 48 to 72 hours in the usual patient, with progressive distention of the gallbladder. If, however, there is intrinsic arterial disease such as occurs in diabetes, some collagen diseases, or arteriosclerosis, perforation may occur much earlier. ***Therefore in the diabetic patient or in the elderly, acute cholecystitis must be treated more aggressively. Perforation cannot be avoided by using antibiotics,*** since they cannot reach the interior of the obstructed gallbladder and prevent the progressive distention.

Diagnostic dilemmas in the early stages may often be resolved by the use of x-ray examination of the gallbladder and bile ducts. The use of oral cholecystography, the iopanoic acid (Telepaque) loading test, or intravenous cholangiography ***has given way to sonography in most cases*** in which the presence of stones in the gallbladder or ducts can be identified (Fig. 25-10). The use of the HIDA scan is occasionally recommended as a preliminary diagnostic procedure.

Technetium 99m dimethyl acetanalide iminodiacetic acid (HIDA) has been developed to be

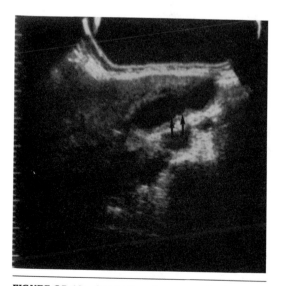

FIGURE 25-10 Sonogram demonstrating layered stones and thick wall *(arrows)* of distended gallbladder in a patient with acute cholecystitis.

excreted by the liver, providing a radioactive scan delineating the extrahepatic biliary tree and gallbladder, even in the jaundiced patient. Stones can be seen, and *visualization of the common duct without seeing the gallbladder is evidence for cystic duct obstruction* (Figs. 25-11 and 25-12). When taken in conjunction with the clinical setting, a diagnosis of acute cholecystitis can be established with a high degree of certainty.

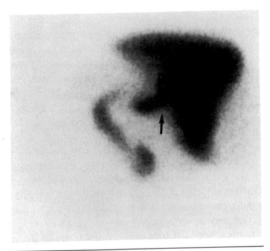

FIGURE 25-11   HIDA scan showing early filling of common hepatic *(arrow)* and bile ducts and no filling of gallbladder (cystic duct obstruction).

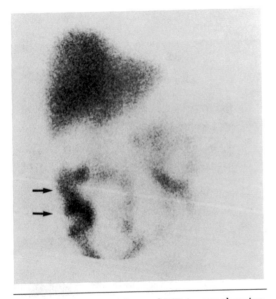

FIGURE 25-12   Late phase of HIDA scan showing dye in liver and small bowel *(arrows)* but not in gallbladder (positive test for cystic duct obstruction).

Treatment
Stages 1 and 2. Treatment is nonoperative and includes:

- Nothing by mouth, to avoid gallbladder stimulation
- Nasogastric suction if the patient is vomiting
- Vagolytic drugs (i.e., atropine or propantheline) to prevent vagal stimulation of acid secretion, leading to contraction of the sphincter of Oddi or direct gallbladder stimulation (not proven)
- Careful monitoring of the development of the patient's signs and symptoms, including (1) leukocyte count every 4 to 6 hours; (2) temperature every 2 hours; and (3) abdominal examination every 2 to 3 hours by the same physician
- *No antibiotics, which may mask the developing signs necessary to diagnose progression of the disease.* Symptoms subside because the stone has dropped back into the gallbladder, and there is no evidence that antibiotic therapy affect this. If the stone remains impacted in the cystic duct, the treatment is directed at the underlying pathology. *Bacterial growth is secondary to the obstruction and is not the primary problem.*

Stage 3. Operation is performed after adequate preparation of the patient, including decompression of the stomach, rehydration with intravenous fluids as necessary, and evaluation of significant associated diseases by appropriate examinations.

The controversy over early versus late operation for acute cholecystitis has been resolved at most institutions so that early operation is performed when the third stage can be diagnosed. The reasons are that (1) there is minimal increase in morbidity in early operation, and (2) disastrous complications such as perforation and intrahepatic abscess are avoided.

Once an operation has been elected, antibiotics are given when serious infection is suspected with *the proviso that the decision to operate not be changed after the institution of antibiotic treatment.* The incidence of postoperative infectious complications is reduced by the systemic use of broad-spectrum antibiotics. However, the organisms cultured from such infections are usually different from those present in the bile, and these complications are most common in patients with diabetes, those who undergo common duct exploration, or those who have other high-risk factors (see the box on p. 433).

What Factors May Complicate the Treatment of Acute Cholecystitis?

Acute Pancreatitis. The coexistence of acute pancreatitis often warrants some delay in operation. *If, however, the third stage of the disease has clearly been reached, early operation is still advised.* A common bile duct exploration is necessary in addition to cholecystectomy. In other words, associated pancreatitis leads toward nonoperative treatment unless signs of inflammation progress. Then early operation is indicated.

Elevation of the serum amylase level does not necessarily indicate pancreatitis. Patients with levels greater than 1000 U/dl associated with acute cholecystitis have common duct stones in over two thirds of the cases. Delay of the operation until an elective time (4 to 6 weeks after the acute attack) leads to a second attack of acute cholecystitis in one third of patients.

Jaundice. Jaundice frequently accompanies acute cholecystitis and may be due to mild pancreatitis, spasm of the sphincter of Oddi, or common duct stone. In general, its presence leads toward earlier rather than later operation. The occurrence of cholecystitis with an accompanying common bile duct obstruction is a serious condition that may lead to cholangitis, septicemia, and shock unless early decompression of the obstruction is performed (see the box at right).

Diagnosis in Doubt. In most cases peritoneal signs are absent, and further diagnostic work-up is indicated. If peritonitis is present, operation usually reveals a condition for which an operation was warranted in any case (e.g., perforated duodenal ulcer or high-lying appendicitis).

Elderly or Debilitated Patient. In most cases these patients cannot withstand the ravages of the underlying disease and *should have earlier operative relief.* The choice of an operation may be modified, however. In those patients for whom general anesthesia is contraindicated,

cholecystostomy with the patient under local anesthesia (Fig. 25-13) is an excellent choice. Recently percutaneous cholecystostomy has been successfully done under sonographic control.

What Is Chronic or Recurrent Cholecystitis?

Once the stones have developed and an acute attack has occurred, recurring attacks are the rule. Some patients may learn to live with the symptoms and avoid foods that produce discomfort, but sooner or later, impaction and a severe attack occur. If the diagnosis can be established in such a patient and no contraindication to an operation exists, elective cholecystectomy should be performed. Stones found incidentally during routine examination (silent stones) eventually lead to symptoms in over half of the patients. The decision to perform cholecystectomy in such patients depends on the status of the patient and the judgment of the supervising physician.

Recurrent acute attacks in patients with chronic cholecystitis may occur in the absence of stones. In some of these patients a small cystic duct may be at fault. Diagnosis is established by cholecystography in which the gallbladder does not fill, assuming the contrast agents have been absorbed and there is no evidence of liver disease. Sonography demonstrating a thickened

---

RISK FACTORS FOR INFECTION IN ELECTIVE BILIARY TRACT OPERATIONS

Age >70 yr
Subsiding acute cholecystitis
Jaundice
Other indications for common duct
   exploration

INDICATIONS FOR COMMON DUCT EXPLORATION AT CHOLECYSTECTOMY

Mandatory

History of jaundice
Common duct >1.2 cm in diameter
Presence of stones in gallbladder smaller
   than diameter of cystic duct
Cholangiogram demonstrating filling defect
   in common duct
Associated pancreatitis
Palpable stone in common duct
Acalculous acute cholecystitis

Suggestive

Common duct 0.9 to 1.2 cm in diameter
History compatible with cholangitis (fever
   and chills, tender liver)
Multiple small stones in gallbladder

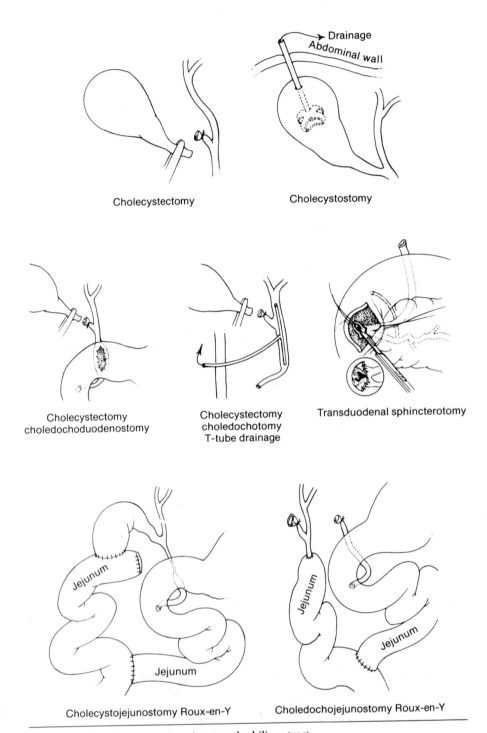

FIGURE 25-13   Common operations on the biliary tract.

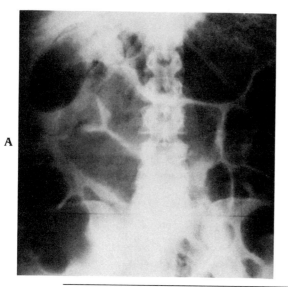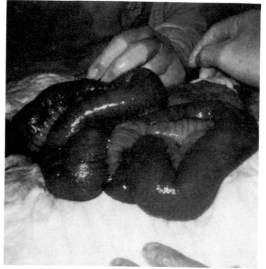

FIGURE 25-14   Gallstone ileus. **A,** X-ray film depicts air in gallbladder and marked ileus pattern. **B,** Dilated bowel at operation, leading to impacted gallstone (at finger).

gallbladder or one containing stones may be diagnostic.

Many attempts at nonoperative management have been made, including the use of a low fat diet, anticholinergic drugs, and weight loss regimens. The patients frequently suppress their recognition of recurring symptoms because of fear of an operation, but the threat of an ensuing severe acute attack is always present. Complications such as pericholecystic abscess, cholecystoduodenal or cholecystocolic fistula (due to stone erosion), or gallstone ileus are seen in such patients (Fig. 25-14). Surgeons who deal with these complications are therefore more prone to recommend elective operation for patients with symptomatic stones.

Fig. 25-15 represents the classic diagram showing the relationships between cholesterol, bile salts, and lecithin concentrations in the bile, leading to instability and formation of gallstones. Attempts to alter these concentrations by use of exogenous bile salts to dissolve existing gallstones have been made. The most commonly used salts are chenodeoxycholic acid (CDCA) and ursodeoxycholic acid (UDCA). Blind studies using these substances have indicated a dissolution rate of 30%, with complete dissolution with UDCA at 12 months and a 7% rate with CDCA. Other studies have shown slightly better results. When bile salt administration is discontinued,

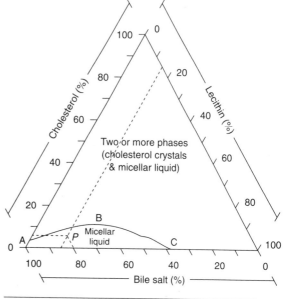

FIGURE 25-15   Method for presenting the three major components of bile on triangular coordinates. Each component is expressed as percentage moles of total bile salt, lecithin, and cholesterol. Line ABC represents maximal solubility of cholesterol in varying mixtures of bile salt and lecithin. Values outside the line represent supersaturation of bile with cholesterol, predisposing to precipitation. (From Small DM. Gallstones. N Engl J Med 279:590, 1968.)

there is a tendency for stones to reform. *The use of lithotripsy* to break up gallstones was introduced recently, but high initial enthusiasm has been tempered by realization that the total volume or size of the stones dictates the success rate and continued use of stone-dissolving bile salt therapy is necessary to assure dissolution and to avoid recurrence. Side effects of bile salt therapy include gastrointestinal upset, diarrhea, and,

with CDCA, changes in liver chemistries. Long-term effects are unknown.

Laparoscopic Cholecystectomy (Fig. 25-16). With marked improvement in the optical system of laparoscopes, techniques involving excision of the gallbladder through the scope have been developed and currently are in widespread use. Complication rates are reduced with experience and have reached acceptable levels of approxi-

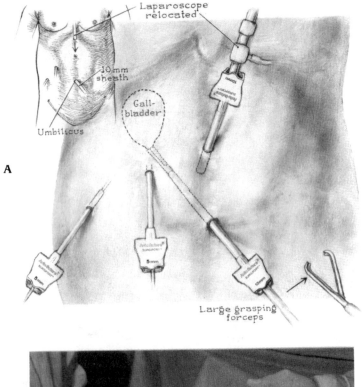

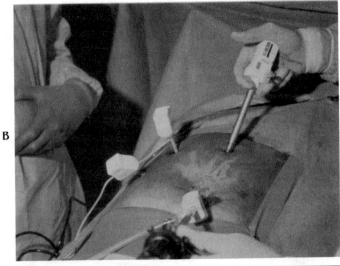

FIGURE 25-16 Laparoscopic cholecystectomy. **A** and **B,** Positions of instrument sheaths and surgeons. (From Flowers JL, et al. Laparoscopic cholecystectomy. Surgical Rds 4(14):271-282, 1991.)

mately 4%. Mortalities are rare when certain guidelines are followed:

- Surgeons performing the procedure should have credentials acquired after taking part in a training period and a period of observation by surgeons experienced in laparoscopic cholecystectomy.
- Selection of patients should exclude those with empyema, hydrops, or gangrenous cholecystitis.
- Pregnant and obese patients are excluded by most centers.
- Jaundice is a relative contraindication, since cholangiography can be done as part of the procedure and common duct stones can be removed by a transduodenal approach (see chapter on Jaundice), avoiding laparotomy.

As instrumentation improves, the procedure can be expected to accomplish a wide variety of other resections and operations. Keeping careful records of complications, however, will be required to determine its ultimate value.

The Role of Cholangiography and Choledochotomy in Common Duct Exploration

At most institutions surgeons recommend the use of operative cholangiography routinely to minimize the problem of retained stones. The box on p. 433 lists the mandatory and suggestive indications for common bile duct exploration. Of the indications for choledochotomy, palpable stones in the ducts are associated with 100% incidence; jaundice or dilation or thickening of the common bile duct is associated with 50% to 60% incidence; and small stones in the gallbladder without other indications are associated with a 30% incidence of choledocholithiasis. The complications of retained stones can be reduced to approximately 3% by a combination of common duct exploration and cholangiography.

Cholangioscopes have been developed that allow the surgeon to see the inside of the common bile and hepatic ducts. Further reduction of retained stones can be expected with the use of all of these combined techniques.

At operation for common duct exploration, a No. 16 T tube should be left in the common duct in case retained stones are found. Through a track of this size (which has taken 2 to 3 weeks to form), a basket for stone extraction can be passed under fluoroscopic control. This method is successful in stone removal in 90% of cases.

PANCREATITIS
What Is Acute Pancreatitis?

Pathogenesis and Diagnosis. Three mechanisms account for the vast majority of cases of

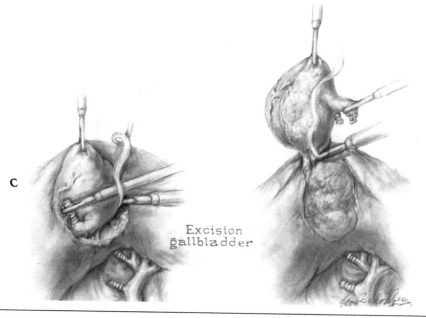

C

Excision
gallbladder

FIGURE 25-16, cont'd   C, Technique of gallbladder excision through the laparoscope.
(From Zucker KA. Surgical Laparoscopy. St Louis, Quality Medical Publishing, 1991.)

acute pancreatitis: duct disruption, duct obstruction, and acinar cell degeneration. Each leads to the escape of pancreatic juice into intrapancreatic interstitial, extrapancreatic areolar, and/or free intraperitoneal spaces. Variable tissue injury is thereby produced, with its severity dependent on the amount of activated digestive enzyme coming into contact with extraductal structures. Accordingly, a progression of pathologic changes can be noted, evolving from mild pancreatic edema through focal or extensive pancreatic and/or peripancreatic necrosis and eventually to a massive retroperitoneal hemorrhage in the most extreme cases (Fig. 25-17).

The attack of pancreatitis may be mild and self-limiting or may advance to extensive pancreatic and peripancreatic tissue destruction. Consequent to this autodigestion of pancreas and intrapancreatic circulating blood components is the production of various vasoactive and coagulopathic peptides. Presenting signs and symptoms depend on (1) whether the disease is at the stage of only local edema or has inflicted more severe pancreatic damage, (2) the amount of associated hemorrhage, (3) whether the peritoneal cavity proper has been involved or all of the pathologic changes are confined to the retroperitoneum, and (4) the prominence of attendant pulmonary and cardiovascular derangements caused by the action of absorbed toxic peptides.

Since the pancreas has a foregut origin, epigastric pain and vomiting are characteristic symptoms. Back pain, caused by stimulation of somatic nerves by inflammation in the retroperitoneum, is a common early finding. The epigastric pain and back pain often occur together and are described as "pain boring straight through to the back" rather than being referred around the flank. Pancreatic ferments and fluid digestants then begin to dissect throughout the retroperitoneum, frequently tracking toward the left diaphragm and pelvis, accounting for the occasional presenting symptoms of left shoulder or left lower quadrant pain. A left pleural effusion, as noted on x-ray film, is a helpful sign in some cases.

With pancreatic necrosis, systemic signs occur early and include fever, tachycardia, leukocytosis, and prostration. These signs reflect absorption of vasoactive amines released from the pancreas during gland autodigestion. Extravascular fluid sequestration and/or hemorrhage due to vessel erosion then lead to hypovolemic shock.

The physical findings in early stages are not too impressive and consist mainly of minor deep

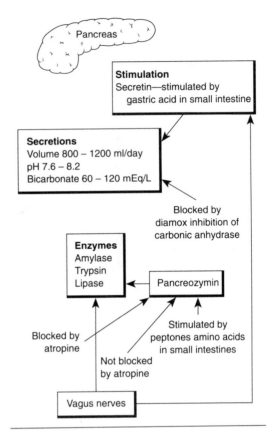

FIGURE 25-17   Some elements in pancreatic physiology.

tenderness in the epigastrium without other overt signs of peritonitis. With hemorrhage and particularly with intraperitoneal escape of pancreatic ferments, however, abdominal guarding and rigidity appear. In these cases differentiation from an acute perforated ulcer may be difficult. Mild jaundice from swelling of the head of the pancreas and thereby compression of the common bile duct occurs in some cases (Fig. 25-18). Nevertheless, bilirubin levels greater than 6 mg/dl are rare and instead suggest some other disease process.

In patients in whom pancreatitis is strongly suspected, the following diagnostic aids are useful:

- Leukocyte count is only modestly increased.
- Serum amylase level is elevated.
- Chest x-ray and decubitus films of the left side of the chest may demonstrate pleural fluid.
- Serum bilirubin level may be mildly elevated.
- Serum calcium level may be depressed.

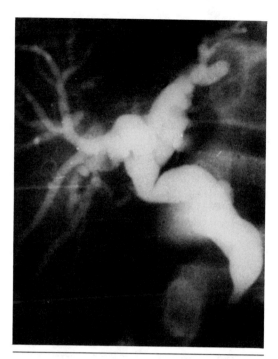

FIGURE 25-18 Narrowed distal common bile duct in acute pancreatitis as demonstrated by transhepatic cholangiography.

- Abdominal x-ray film may reveal dilated jejunum in the midabdomen or generalized dilation of the bowel ending at the splenic flexure.
- Abdominal paracentesis or lavage will yield fluid with a high amylase content.
- Twenty-four-hour urinary amylase level may be markedly elevated in spite of a near-normal serum level.
- Urinary amylase clearance is elevated.

It is important to recognize that elevation of the serum amylase level regularly occurs in other intra-abdominal emergencies such as perforation of the proximal gastrointestinal tract and small bowel gangrene. Some of the highest levels ever seen occur in patients with a perforated duodenal ulcer, whereas, conversely, patients may succumb to severe hemorrhagic pancreatitis with a minimally elevated serum amylase level.

Treatment. The treatment of acute pancreatitis should be based primarily on its underlying cause. Otherwise, problems more life threatening than the original process may follow.

Duct Disruption. Trauma is almost always responsible for duct disruption. Penetrating or blunt abdominal injury, surgical damage to major or minor pancreatic ducts, and forceful operative or endoscopic pancreatography are the usual culprits. Treatment must be directed at obtaining complete control of the extravasating pancreatic secretions, which are responsible for the destructive process. To do so demands immediate operation with either selective resection of the distal gland to include the site of duct injury or continuous evacuation of all escaping pancreatic juice by well-placed closed suction drains.

Duct Obstruction. Pancreatic ducts may become obstructed by suture ligation or more gradually by scar-tissue contracture. However, the usual cause is either lodgment in or, more commonly, passage of a gallstone out through the ampulla of Vater. If the main pancreatic duct empties into the terminal common bile duct (with the ampullary lip by 1 to 3 mm), local edema and/or spasm of the sphincter of Oddi can cause partial to complete obstruction of the pancreatic duct, that is, provided that there is no communication with the accessory duct that might offer an avenue for main duct decompression.

Most episodes of biliary pancreatitis subside spontaneously once the stone has passed. However, unless the biliary tract pathology is corrected, future attacks are almost guaranteed. Accordingly, cholecystectomy with confirmed clearance of the common duct from all stones by operative cholangiography is crucial. If common duct stones are present, they are removed via a standard choledochotomy or transduodenal sphincteroplasty. In the event that the acute attack caused by gallstone lodgment or passage does not subside, either endoscopic papillotomy of the ampulla or operative transduodenal sphincteroplasty should be considered in an effort to relieve any persisting pancreatic duct obstruction. Relief of obstruction offers prompt amelioration of the underlying process, provided that the patient can be made a procedural or operative candidate.

Acinar Cell Degeneration. Various toxins can modify normal acinar production, transport, and/or excretion of enzyme-carrying zymogen granules. Once this secretory mechanism has been damaged, stimulation of the acinar cell to secrete will cause release of activated enzyme directly into the cell itself, followed by cell autodigestion, cell wall disruption, and eventually autolytic injury to adjacent tissues.

Ethyl alcohol is by far the most common responsible toxin. Superimposed on acinar dysfunction (as caused by protracted alcohol abuse or by the briefer ingestion of huge volumes by binge drinking), an acute attack of pancreatitis can be precipitated through maximal stimulation of acinar cells to secrete a juice rich in digestive enzyme as appropriately occurs after ingestion of a large meal. Alcohol administered intravenously consistently fails to initiate an acute attack; only the oral route for alcohol intake appears capable of starting the process.

There is a great propensity for recurrent attacks to occur and for the process eventually to reach a chronic smoldering state. Unfortunately, patient compliance to abstain from all alcohol is seldom achieved, no matter how persuasive the approach taken. Nevertheless, blocking vagal stimulation of the pancreatic acinar cell significantly reduces the likelihood of a future bout of acute pancreatitis, even despite continued heavy alcohol abuse. Thus as a last resort to prevent recurrence, truncal vagotomy with a gastric drainage procedure may be tried in an effort to offset repeated episodes.

For the majority of patients, an acute attack merely requires supportive care. Bed rest, intravenous fluids, and observation are all that is necessary. Nasogastric tube decompression, parenteral antibiotics, H_2-blockers (e.g., cimetidine), aprotinin, and various belladonna alkaloids have never been shown by objective study to be of any true benefit for the uncomplicated case of acute pancreatitis. The patient must not be allowed anything by mouth, must have fluid deficits restored, and similarly must be maintained by intravenous crystalloid solutions.

On admission to the hospital and after 48 hours of therapy, specific clinical signs can be used to assess the severity of the process (see box). By tabulating the total number of positive signs, an eventual outcome can be predicted with a fair degree of accuracy (Fig. 25-19).

The patient must be carefully monitored for evidence of cardiovascular or pulmonary derangements that can be induced by absorbed toxic peptides. Reliable signs that indicate significant quantities of toxic peptides are circulating include:

- Hypocalcemia (serum calcium level <8 mg/dl)
- Overt respiratory distress
- Hypoxemia (blood arterial PO_2 <60 mm Hg while breathing room air)
- Overt shock (blood pressure <90/60 mm Hg)
- Excess intravenous fluid requirements (in addition to daily maintenance of 30 ml/kg body weight; a repletion volume greater than estimated blood volume set at 6% of body weight in kilograms)

SIGNS THAT CORRELATE WITH MORBIDITY AND MORTALITY IN ACUTE PANCREATITIS

At Admission or Diagnosis

Age >55 yr
White blood cell count >16,000/μl
Blood glucose level >200 mg/dl (10 mmol/L)
Serum lactic dehydrogenase concentration >350 IU/L
Aspartate aminotransferase concentration >250 sigma-Frankel U/dl

During Initial 48 Hours

Hematocrit decrease >10 percentage points
Blood urea nitrogen level increase >5 mg/dl
Serum calcium level <8 mg/dl (2 mmol/L)
Arterial PO_2 below 60 mm Hg (8 kPa)
Base deficit >4 mEq/L (4 mmol/L)
Estimated fluid sequestration >6000 ml

Approximately one patient in 15 manifests one or more of these ominous signs and thus needs more specific measures directed at removal or blockage of the production of the toxic peptides. After as optimal a response as possible has been gained through use of intravenous calcium supplements, ventilatory support, infusion of appropriate intravenous fluids, and pharmacologic augmentation of cardiovascular function, standard peritoneal dialysis is carried out. Potassium (4 mEq/L of potassium chloride) must be added to the dialysate if acute renal failure with its attendant hyperkalemia has not complicated the clinical course. A reversal of all ominous signs is generally noted within 12 to 24 hours. Peritoneal dialysis seldom should be done for longer than 5 days because its continued use can lead to significant albumin depletion. Peritoneal dialysis is not uniformly recommended in all centers, however.

Nevertheless, urgent laparotomy is warranted for those patients who:

- Fail to respond to peritoneal dialysis
- Show evidence of massive retroperitoneal hemorrhage (profound and continuing loss of circulating red cell mass, flank ecchymosis, or intraperitoneal bleeding as reflected by the return of gross blood in the dialysis effluent)
- Develop bacterial pancreatitis (persistent high fever, extreme leukocytosis, pancreatic and peripancreatic mass with gaseous emphysema

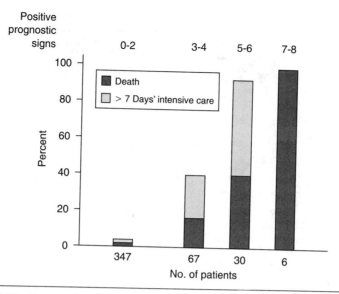

FIGURE 25-19   Prognostic value of "Ranson's criteria" for predicting individual outcome in acute pancreatitis. (From Ranson JH. The role of peritoneal lavage in severe acute pancreatitis. Ann Surg 187:565-575, 1978.)

on CT scan, a purulent effluent when peritoneal dialysis is performed or CT-guided aspiration of peripancreatic fluid, **and** positive blood culture results)
- Have an uncertain cause for their obvious intra-abdominal catastrophe

At laparotomy, debridement of nonviable pancreas is performed, with packing of the pancreatic bed after appropriate debridement of necrotic, infected, and/or ecchymotic adjacent tissues. The head of the pancreas is left intact. The packs are changed on alternate days until sump drainage alone can control the resultant cavity.

What Is the Significance of Developing a Pancreatic Mass?

After an attack of acute pancreatitis, a mass may form in the vicinity of the pancreas or lesser peritoneal sac. It can represent a bacterial abscess, a loculation of blood and necrotic debris referred to as a *pseudocyst,* or pancreatitis persisting as a sterile subacute phlegmon. Some combination of fever, leukocytosis, elevation of both serum and urine amylase, and a palpable, tender epigastric mass may be noted. Treatment for each condition, however, is significantly different.

Pancreatic Abscess. A septic clinical course, often becoming fulminant, characterizes a bacterial pancreatic abscess. Provided that the patient is not receiving antibiotics, blood culture results are routinely positive. On CT scan of the abdomen, the pancreatic and peripancreatic phlegmonous mass is noted to contain multiple radiolucent bubbles (i.e., it appears to have gaseous emphysema). Peripancreatic fluid, obtained by CT-guided needle aspiration, demonstrates bacterial presence on examination of a stained smear. Urgent operation with débridement of necrotic and infected tissues, often resulting in subtotal pancreatectomy, must be done as soon as possible. The resultant wound is managed by open gauze packing. Parenteral antibiotics and energetic supportive measure are likewise required. Despite such efforts, the mortality rate approximates 20%.

Pancreatic Pseudocyst. Chemical pancreatic abscesses, pseudocysts, contain liquefied debris yet do not have a true epithelial wall. Both sonography and CT scan reveal a relatively well-defined cystic mass arising from or adjacent to pancreatic substance. The pseudocyst presents a threat because of (1) its mass effect, obstructing the gastric outlet, (2) its potential to become infected and thereby to progress to bacterial abscess, and (3) its likelihood to rupture and cause a severe chemical peritonitis.

Pseudocysts less than 5 cm in diameter can safely be observed because they often disappear and rarely rupture. However, pseudocysts larger than 8 cm are at risk to burst. Accordingly, for the larger pseudocysts and for those interfering with

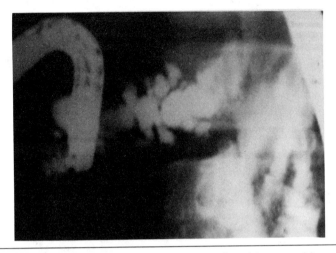

FIGURE 25-20   Irregular pancreatic duct dilations in chronic pancreatitis as demonstrated by endoscopic retrograde cholangiopancreatography. The connection of multiple duct saccules is referred to as a chain of lakes.

gastric emptying, decompression is imperative. Options include CT-guided insertion of a catheter as an external drain or surgical creation of internal drainage into the stomach or into a defunctionalized Roux-en-Y segment of jejunum. If surgical internal drainage is not practical because of immaturity of cyst wall, external drainage with sump suction should be used.

Subacute Pancreatitis. Failure of the pancreatitis to resolve with usual supportive measures can lead to a subacute inflammation. CT scan will show an enlarged pancreas without evidence of other complicating pathology. When an oral diet is begun, there is an immediate exacerbation of the acute process. Accordingly, total parenteral nutrition may be necessary for as long as 3 or 4 months. The process then usually progresses into a chronic state.

Relapsing Pancreatitis. A large proportion of cases of pancreatitis are associated with alcoholism or gallbladder disease. The exact distribution depends on the patient population from which the sample is drawn. Each attack should be addressed according to the principles for treating acute pancreatitis, with efforts later being made to prevent recurrent episodes on the basis of the underlying cause during a subsequent quiescent period.

What Is Chronic Pancreatitis?

Pathogenesis and Diagnosis. Chronic pancreatitis is manifested by the debilitating effects from loss of exocrine function of the pancreas (malabsorption). The gland is fibrosed, and the ducts are irregularly dilated (Fig. 25-20), leading to frequent, almost persistent pain. Many of these patients become addicted to narcotics use.

Clinical findings include:

- Weight loss
- Diarrhea of fatty or bulky stools
- Constant abdominal or back pain
- Soft, variably tender abdomen

Laboratory findings include:

- Low serum carotene levels
- Presence of meat fibers on microscopic examination of stools
- Defective D-xylose absorption
- Defective triolein absorption
- Normal oleic acid absorption
- Diabetic glucose tolerance curve
- Excess fat in stool

Treatment. Nonoperative treatment consists of a high carbohydrate, low fat diet and oral replacement of pancreatic enzymes. Rarely does the patient have any respite from the pain. In some patients operations designed to give pancreatic duct drainage by anastomosis to intestine (Fig. 25-21) have relieved the persistent agony. Pancreatic resection should be avoided whenever possible because the resultant brittle diabetes itself carries a high mortality rate (30%) within the first postoperative year. Instead, pancreatic denervation should be considered via a

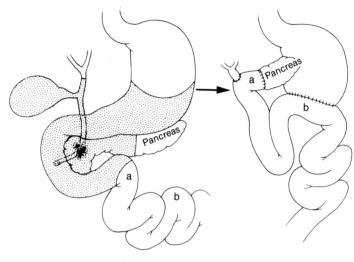

Pancreaticoduodenectomy
(Whipple procedure)

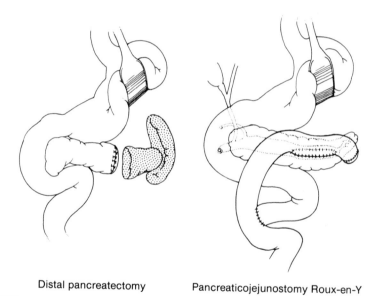

Distal pancreatectomy   Pancreaticojejunostomy Roux-en-Y

FIGURE 25-21   Common operations on the pancreas.

transthoracic splanchnicectomy. However, in some centers pancreatic resections, either partial (Whipple operation; see Fig. 25-21) or total, have yielded acceptable relief of pain.

COLONIC DIVERTICULITIS

Pathogenesis and Diagnosis. An intestinal diverticulum is an outpocketing that may involve all the coats of the intestinal wall (true diverticulum) or only the mucosal layer and possibly serosal layer (false diverticulum) (Fig.

25-22). False diverticula have a propensity for perforation. When inflammation occurs, pain is initially localized to the area involved, since the parietal nerve fibers rather than the visceral are stimulated. In the Western world left-sided (descending or sigmoid colon) diverticulitis is much more common than any other form, and characteristically the diverticula are false. When perforation occurs, it may enter the free peritoneal cavity (Fig. 25-23), or it may be walled off by adjacent small bowel or the retroperitoneum. This latter event is due to the anatomic location

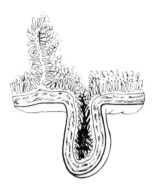 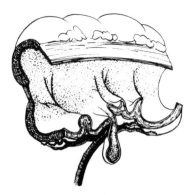

True diverticulum
1. Involves entire bowel wall
2. Antimesenteric
3. Congenital origin
4. Meckel's diverticulum
5. May bleed
6. May perforate (?)
7. May lead to volvulus
8. May become inflamed

False diverticulum
1. Acquired
2. Mesenteric penetration
3. May bleed
4. May perforate
5. May lead to obstruction
6. May become inflamed

FIGURE 25-22 Diverticula of the small and large intestine. *Left,* True diverticulum; *right,* false diverticulum.

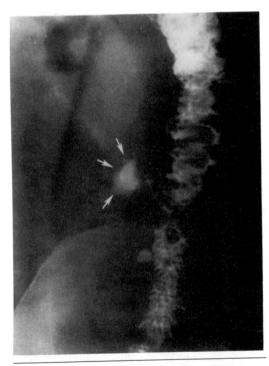

FIGURE 25-23 Barium enema demonstrating perforated diverticulitis of descending colon. (*Arrows* show collection of barium outside of colon with adjacent tract.)

of the descending colon in the retroperitoneum. Inflammation of the colon is often associated with diarrhea, which may occur as a prodrome before signs of peritonitis develop. Rectal bleeding is common but usually small in amount. Systemic signs and symptoms are associated with the onset of pain and consist of fever, leukocytosis, and malaise. Abdominal pain is sharp and localized to the diseased segment unless free perforation or coincident obstruction has occurred.

Treatment. Right-sided colonic perforations cannot be clearly differentiated clinically from appendicitis, and since the latter is far more common, early operation is performed. The tendency for left-sided colonic perforations to wall off early accounts for an approach to treatment different from that for appendicitis. A careful physical examination must be made to determine if the perforation has localized or is free. If it appears localized, the orders should include:

- Nothing by mouth
- Nasogastric suction to prevent distention of the bowel by swallowed air
- Maintenance intravenous fluids to maintain hydration of the patient
- Systemic broad-spectrum antibiotics such as a combination of gentamycin and clindomycin, since infection accompanies all cases of colonic perforation

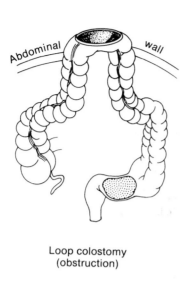

Loop colostomy
(obstruction)

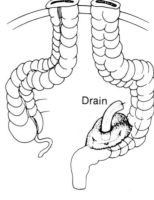

Drain

Double-barrelled colostomy
(perforation)

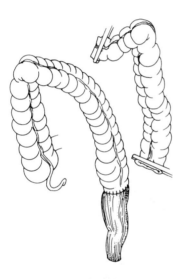

Resection with anastomosis
(colectomy)

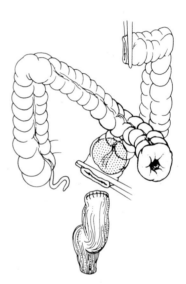

Resection with end colostomy
(Hartmann)

FIGURE 25-24 Common operations on the colon.

- Frequent monitoring of temperature, white blood count, and abdominal findings to confirm that the process has remained localized and is resolving

If the patient remains febrile with leukocytosis after 12 to 24 hours, nonoperative treatment should be abandoned. Similarly, any clinical involvement of the peritoneal cavity outside the primary quadrant or the presence of free intraperitoneal air demonstrated on abdominal or chest x-ray films requires early operation.

The choice of operation in patients with diverticulitis is controversial and depends on the judgment of the operating surgeon (Fig. 25-24). In resolved diverticulitis the choice may be one of the following:

- Elective resection of the involved segment if there is (1) a recurrent attack (less than 15%); (2) persistent deformity revealed by barium enema examination; or (3) difficulty in differentiation from carcinoma
- Nonoperative treatment

In progressing diverticulitis the choice may be:

- Resection of involved segment, with anastomosis
- Resection of involved segment, with colostomy
- Staged procedure: (1) colostomy with drainage of the abscess in the left lower quadrant, (2) resection, and (3) closure of colostomy

Resection of the involved segment with temporary end colostomy is usually performed because the diseased and perforated segment is excised and the complications of an anastomosis in an area of inflammation are avoided. Continuity is usually reestablished within 3 to 12 months.

Operative decisions depend on the acute nature of the attack and the response to treatment. Anastomosis should not be carried out in an unprepared colon when emergency exploration is required. Decisions about resection of the involved segment depend on its fixation to the pelvic wall and the experience of the operating surgeon.

On occasion, associated intestinal obstruction, which may lead to early operation, is a complicating factor. It can be due to abscess obstructing the colon or a small bowel adhesion to the diseased colonic segment with kinking. In general, a barium enema should not be performed as long as signs of peritonitis are present, since extravasation of the barium outside the intestinal lumen would be a serious complication. However, more common use of CT will yield the correct diagnosis, with demonstration of colonic wall thickening or edema, pericolonic inflammatory mass, and abscess.

Another complication occurring with chronic or recurrent diverticulitis is colovesical fistula. The patient usually presents with symptoms of pneumaturia (air bubbles in the urine) or urinary tract infection with colonic organisms. Some patients remain asymptomatic or may only require appropriate antibiotic treatment. Other causes of this condition such as carcinoma, Crohn's disease, or radiation injury to the bowel should be ruled out by diagnostic tests, including barium studies, cystoscopy, colonoscopy, and studies of the urinary tract.

Although nonoperative treatment is successful in many cases, operation consisting of resection of the fistula plus the involved bladder and bowel is usually performed. Primary anastomosis is the rule, since the colonic inflammation is often mild. When severe urinary sepsis is associated or fecaluria is the prominent finding, a staged procedure consisting of a preliminary double-barreled (diverting) colostomy (see Fig. 25-24) is performed, followed by resection, primary anastomosis, and colostomy closure several months later.

FREE INTRAPERITONEAL PERFORATIONS OF THE GASTROINTESTINAL TRACT

Diagnosis and Pathogenesis. The usual causes for gastrointestinal perforations are:

Gastric or duodenal ulcer	80%
Appendicitis	10%
Diverticulitis	5%
Other, including foreign body	5%

The patient often recalls the exact onset of symptoms, even to the minute. The initial pain is sharp, almost as though a blow were struck to the abdomen, and localized to the area of peritoneal contamination. Rapid development of peritonitis follows the extravasation of intestinal contents. If the perforation is based on preexisting inflammatory disease (appendicitis, diverticulitis), systemic symptoms and signs may have preceded the catastrophic event. If the first element of disturbance is the perforation (ulcer, foreign body), the systemic signs will develop with the peritonitis. At the onset in these latter cases, the patients may have been eating or working, there is no vomiting or anorexia, the temperature is close to normal, and no leukocytosis is present.

Physical findings parallel the distribution of intestinal contents in the peritoneal cavity. In those conditions in which rapid sealing of the perforation occurs, the peritoneal signs may be limited to one or two quadrants:

- Guarding and rigidity are marked.
- Rebound tenderness is characteristic.
- The abdomen may be boardlike.
- Bowel sounds are absent (peritoneal intestinal reflex).
- Liver dullness on percussion may be absent as a result of air overlying the liver.

The mesentery of the small bowel runs from the left upper quadrant to the right lower quadrant across the abdomen. *Fluid from a perforated ulcer will occasionally track along the root of the mesentery and collect in the right lower quadrant.* In this case the main peritoneal findings may be in the right lower quadrant, confusing the diagnosis with appendicitis. A careful history of onset, associated symptoms, development, and tenderness in the upper abdomen—which rarely occurs with appendicitis—should clarify the issue.

If, after a history and physical examination,

TABLE 25-1 Treatment of Acute Gastrointestinal Perforations

Treatment	Rationale
Nothing by mouth Nasogastric intubation IV fluids should include colloids and balanced salt.	Bowel function is depressed, and swallowed air will accumulate in intestine. Inflamed peritoneum will respond by weeping fluid into peritoneal cavity, and there may be third-space loss into the greatly dilated arterioles with pooling; therefore hypovolemia may be present.
Monitor urinary output (40 ml/hr before the operation).	As a measure of tissue perfusion
Prepare for surgery by notifying operating room, cross-matching blood, obtaining routine laboratory analysis.	
Order pertinent additional x-ray studies, ECG, determination of serum electrolytes if indicated.	Rule out serious associated disease.
Start antibiotics as soon as decision to operate has been made.	Mortality rate from sepsis is decreased experimentally if good tissue levels of (circulating) antibiotics are present before contamination. Since the operation is often associated with further contamination of peritoneal cavity, antibiotics are best started preoperatively.
Operate as soon as possible.	

there is a doubt as to the diagnosis, x-ray studies of the abdomen and chest and abdominal tap may prove helpful.

X-ray examination of the abdomen and chest with the patient upright for several minutes will reveal free air, usually localized under the diaphragm, in two thirds of patients. This is most easily seen on the upright chest film. Even in those cases with localized peritoneal findings, the tendency for air to rise will make this a worthwhile diagnostic procedure. If doubt as to the diagnosis exists, the instillation of Gastrografin in the stomach may demonstrate the leak. *However, this is unnecessary in patients with peritoneal signs indicating the need for operation.*

Abdominal tap may reveal gastric juice, intestinal contents, bacteria, or white blood cells. A negative result from a tap should be ignored.

Acute abdominal pain, for which an operation is not indicated, may occur in association with lobar pneumonia, myocardial infarction, aortic aneurysm, tabetic or sickle cell crises, spinal root irritation, and so on (Chapter 31). To differentiate clearly between these conditions, a careful history must be obtained. The gentle hand in the physical examination is the physician's best friend in determining the correct diagnosis. Pain often is evident with the softest tap-

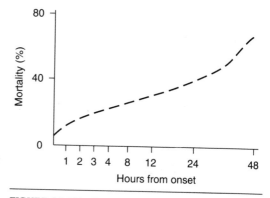

FIGURE 25-25 Representative mortality rates after perforation of the gastrointestinal tract.

ping or percussion and has the same significance as rebound tenderness.

Treatment. For treatment of acute gastrointestinal perforation, see Table 25-1. Fig. 25-25 shows mortality figures.

Operative management depends on the site of perforation. For perforated ulcers simple closure using a pedicle of omentum is preferred. No attempt to close the ulcer primarily is made except under the most favorable circumstances. Rarely, the perforation is an anterior component of a circumferential ulcer, the posterior component of which may bleed postoperatively. If the ulcer is duodenal and extensive, some surgeons have advocated conversion of the perforation to a pyloroplasty with the addition of truncal vagotomy and, if necessary, suture ligation of the ulcer base. The fear of subsequent mediastinitis from the contaminated abdomen is not well founded. A biopsy of perforated gastric ulcers should always be done before treatment to exclude the presence of cancer.

ISCHEMIC SMALL BOWEL DISEASE

The mortality rate of patients with the syndromes listed in Table 25-2 is related directly to the surgeon's ability to diagnose the condition with minimal diagnostic work-up and to operate promptly. Hesitation or delay will almost certainly lead to death of the patient, and even with decisive action, mortality ranges between 40% and 80%.

TABLE 25-2 Ischemic Bowel Disease

Age, Sex	Suggestive History	Physical Examination	Associated Findings	Abdominal Tap	X-ray and Laboratory Findings
Vasculitis (Allergic Inflammatory)					
<50, F	Sudden onset; previous history	Shock, peritonitis	Occasionally an absent pulse, hypertension (renal ischemia), parathesias (nerve ischemias), hematuria (renal infarction)	Blood-tinged fluid	Signs of intestinal gangrene, ileus, air in wall of bowel, marked leukocytosis (occasionally over 35,000)
Arteriosclerosis, Disease of Major Mesenteric Vessels					
>50, ?	Prodrome of mild to moderate pain for several days, then catastrophe; vascular occlusion elsewhere, stroke or myocardial infarction; low-flow state preceding catastrophe	Early mild abdominal tenderness, shock, peritonitis	Previous history, low flow (ischemia) of leg or feet, recent stroke or heart attack, congestive heart failure	Blood-tinged fluid	Signs of intestinal gangrene, ileus, air in wall of bowel, marked leukocytosis (occasionally over 35,000)
Embolism to Major Mesenteric Vessel					
40-60, ?	Sudden onset; previous history of embolism, underlying cardiac disease (e.g., mitral stenosis or auricular fibrillation)	Abdominal tenderness, shock, peritonitis	Murmurs of cardiovascular disease, recent auricular fibrillation, embolism elsewhere, stroke	Blood-tinged fluid	Signs of intestinal gangrene, ileus, air in wall of bowel, marked leukocytosis (occasionally over 35,000)

Suspicion of vascular insufficiency is based on associated vascular or heart disease, previous episodes of embolization, a positive abdominal tap, and other findings (see Table 25-2).

Emergency mesenteric angiography may be diagnostic and allow the passage of a catheter and infusion of papaverine intra-arterially. Relief of the associated spasm may gain time before the operation and avoid bowel necrosis.

Treatment. Immediate operation is the required treatment. Shock in these patients is due to release of toxic material from the gangrenous intestine into the bloodstream and to hypovolemia. This shock may not respond to treatment until the infarcted segment is resected. Therefore hypotension is not a contraindication to immediate operation.

Resection of obviously necrotic bowel is performed, and a complete examination of the arterial supply is made. If mesenteric arterial obstruction is found, relief can sometimes be obtained by embolectomy, bypass, or endarterectomy. *Questionably viable bowel can be evaluated by injecting intravenous fluorescein and using a Wood's lamp to detect viability by fluorescence.* This qualitative method may be improved by the use of quantitative fluorescence or Doppler ultrasound of the mesenteric vasculature. If there is doubt as to the viability of the retained bowel, a mandatory reoperation in 24 to 48 hours settles the issue.

Mesenteric venous occlusion may occur and be difficult or impossible to differentiate from arterial occlusion clinically. Often a history of drug intake, which may be associated with hypercoagulability or evidence of venous occlusion elsewhere (peripheral), may be helpful. These cases must be operated on early and have a more favorable prognosis, since often smaller segments of intestine are involved. Diagnosis and correction of the hypercoagulable state should be performed as an essential part of the intraoperative and postoperative management.

ISCHEMIC COLITIS

A syndrome of colonic ischemia caused by low flow (without arterial occlusion) has been recognized more frequently. It occurs in elderly patients with generalized arteriosclerosis and may follow myocardial infarction, cerebrovascular accident (CVA), or other catastrophes. The patient often presents with rectal bleeding, abdominal tenderness (usually left lower quadrant), and appears ill and toxic. Plain abdominal films may be diagnostic if an air-filled colon can be demonstrated, with characteristic notching or fingerprinting of the border. This diagnosis may be confirmed by barium enema examination.

Treatment is supportive because the condition is self-limited and often resolves after 4 to 5 days, with complete resolution demonstrated by the barium x-ray examination by 3 to 4 weeks.

INTESTINAL OBSTRUCTION

Pathogenesis and Diagnosis. *The cardinal signs of intestinal obstruction are abdominal pain, vomiting, and distention* (see the boxes on p. 450 and Fig. 25-26). In the presence of any two of these signs, obstruction must be assumed and ruled out or treated. The diagnosis can be accurately made by the history and physical examination in nine of every 10 patients. The sequence of appearance of these signs often points to the level of obstruction. *Feculent vomiting is most characteristic of small bowel obstruction* and is related to the length of time that obstruction has been present. *Failure to pass gas or feces by rectum* is usually present in complete small or large bowel obstruction.

Obstruction presents a pure example of bowel distention without involvement of parietal peritoneal nerve fibers; therefore *abdominal tenderness is not found unless the obstruction is due to underlying peritoneal abscess.* In these cases a history compatible with recent intra-abdominal inflammatory disease should be in evidence. Otherwise the presence of abdominal tenderness, guarding, rigidity, or rebound tenderness associated with obstruction is *an indication of interference with intestinal blood flow and demands immediate operation.*

The bowel is hyperactive in attempting to force material past the obstruction, and the bowel sounds are active, high pitched, and intermittent and may *occur in rushes associated with the crampy pain.* As the distention of the bowel progresses, the bowel sounds become less active. Distended intestine does not produce good peristalsis, and the bowel sounds become tinkling and depressed. The patient may have a mild leukocytosis from dehydration and moderate tachycardia from hypovolemia *but does not appear septic.* Hypotension may be present, however, if the hypovolemia is severe (see the box on p. 450).

Flat and upright or decubitus x-ray views of the abdomen will confirm the clinical diagnosis in many cases. The presence of air-fluid levels in

CAUSE OF INTESTINAL OBSTRUCTION

Mechanical: Simple (Partial or Complete) or Strangulated (Almost Always Complete)

Postoperative adhesions
Hernia (internal and external)
Neoplasm
Volvulus
Intussusception
Gallstone ileus
Inflammatory mass with adhesions
Foreign body

Paralytic

Inflammatory disease (intra-abdominal abscess)
Peritonitis
Pancreatitis
Ascites
Hypokalemia
Abdominal trauma
Diseases of other systems
    Spinal collapse
    Pulmonary infarction
    Pneumothorax

SYMPTOMS AND SIGNS OF MECHANICAL OBSTRUCTION

Symptoms

Colicky pain
Vomiting
Lethargy
Lack of flatus or defecation

Signs

Hyperactive bowel sounds
Abdominal distention
Lack of peritoneal signs
Indications of extracellular fluid loss

Look for

Abdominal mass
Groin hernia
Surgical scars

SIGNS OF LOSS OF EXTRACELLULAR FLUID VOLUME

Hypotension
    Orthostatic—early
    Frank—late
Tachycardia
Increased respiratory rate
Dry, cool skin
Poor capillary filling of extremities
Decreased pulse volume
Decreased skin turgor
Decreased urinary output
Hemoconcentration
Increased specific gravity of urine

the small bowel is characteristic but may also occur in patients with severe gastroenteritis and vomiting or in whom enemas have been used.

If obstruction is in doubt, a barium x-ray study should be performed. Barium in small quantities given by mouth or nasogastric tube is safe to use in all cases of small bowel obstruction, since the proximal fluid-filled bowel will dilute small amounts of barium, preventing inspissation. The diagnosis can be made clearly in these cases, and complete small bowel obstruction can be ruled out when barium can be identified as reaching the cecum. Since strangulation or gangrene is rare in partial obstruction, considerable time is gained by such a demonstration. A CT scan with oral contrast can make the same diagnosis. Any demonstration of both dilated and collapsed loops of bowel in the same study indicates obstruction.

In large bowel obstruction, however, barium by mouth is dangerous, since it may convert a partial large bowel obstruction to a complete one by inspissation after water absorption in the colon. Barium enema is, however, quite safe when used in small quantities under fluoroscopic control until the obstructed area is reached.

It is therefore important to evaluate the flat and upright films of the abdomen and the patient's history and physical examination before administering barium. When doubt exists, barium by rectum is safer to use. Clearly, in patients with the appropriate clinical findings and x-ray demonstration of air-fluid levels, a negative barium enema examination will confirm the diagnosis of small bowel obstruction.

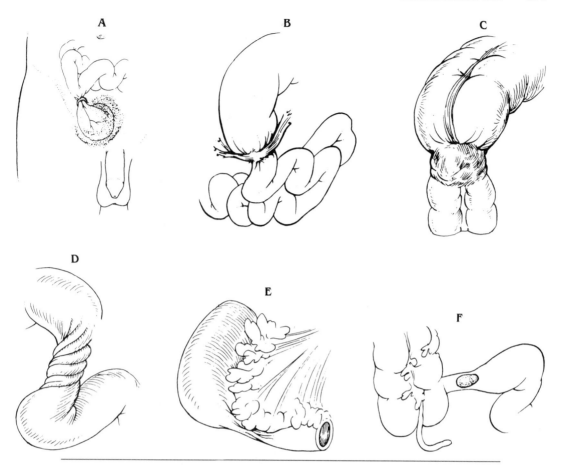

FIGURE 25-26   Some representative causes of intestinal obstruction. A, Hernia. B, Adhesions. C, Tumor. D, Volvulus. E, Stricture. F, Foreign body.

In the rare cases of nonobstructive diseases presenting as clinical obstruction, the demonstration of oral barium entering the colon will gain the time necessary to make the correct diagnosis and avoid unnecessary exploration.

Foregut Obstruction. Occasionally acute gastric dilation may be associated with sharp pain, but foregut obstruction is most often manifested by *early vomiting, little pain, and absence of distention.* The usual cause is obstructing ulcer or neoplasm of the stomach or pancreas. Evaluation of the associated history and systemic signs will point to the correct diagnosis. Since the obstruction is high, vomiting prevents significant acute distention from occurring, although gradual distention of the stomach may lead to marked dilation. The vomitus may contain recognizable food, and the presence of bile indicates obstruction distal to the ampulla of Vater. Feculent vomiting does not occur, since gastric acid-

ity prevents growth of bacteria and residual material is not retained long enough for significant bacterial overgrowth to occur in the achlorhydric patient. *Loss of large amounts of hydrochloric acid from the stomach leads to hypochloremic alkalosis.* The descriptive term *60-40 syndrome* refers to the serum levels of chloride and bicarbonate, respectively, in the most severe form.

Diagnosis is made relatively simple by gastrointestinal series and gastric intubation, yielding residual contents over 1000 ml in most cases, followed by a daily production of 1 to 3 L of gastric suction. Vascular compromise rarely occurs in this condition so that no abdominal tenderness is present.

High Midgut Obstruction. With high midgut obstruction, *vomiting occurs early* and is profuse. *Pain is crampy, midabdominal, and intermittent.* It may be mild if vomiting has relieved the proximal distention. In these cases there is *little or no abdominal distention.* Feculent vomiting occurs only in the presence of stasis of contents in the bowel, with bacterial overgrowth. It takes 48 to 72 hours to develop and is *therefore a sign of the length of time of obstruction rather than the level.* High midgut obstruction can be confused with foregut obstruction except that *small bowel gas may be present on abdominal x-ray film.*

Low Midgut Obstruction. Pain is the earliest sign of low midgut obstruction and is crampy, midabdominal or diffuse, and intermittent. Vomiting occurs after pain and varies from profuse to mild. Distention occurs last and is due mainly to swallowed air. Marked dilation of intestine with air and fluid may be present. Feculent vomiting indicates a long-standing obstruction (over 48 hours). *Strangulation may occur at any time.*

Hindgut Obstruction. With hindgut obstruction, pain is crampy and midabdominal due to onset of small bowel distention and occurs late due to the lack of peristaltic waves in the colon. Vomiting occurs very late or may not occur for the same reason. *Distention is therefore the earliest sign* and may be massive and progressive over many days or weeks.

Strangulating Obstruction. The following clinical findings are important in diagnosing strangulation of the bowel (Tables 25-3 and 25-4):

- Abdominal pain becomes constant instead of intermittent (peritoneal pain instead of stretch).
- Back pain may occur, since ischemic intestinal pain may be referred to the root of the mesentery.
- Bowel sounds disappear (peritoneal intestinal reflex).
- Abdominal tenderness and other signs of peritonitis appear.
- The patient becomes ill. In patients with strangulating obstruction both the toxic products of bacterial growth and bacteria are absorbed into the bloodstream through the bowel wall, which is normally impermeable to these substances. Release of vasoactive amines or other unknown substances from the necrotic bowel leads to toxemia, sepsis, and shock. *Signs to note are leukocytosis (often over 30,000), tachycardia, hypotension (unresponsive to fluids), and prostration.*

Treatment

Foregut Obstruction. This obstruction is not relieved without an operation in most cases.

TABLE 25-3 Differentiation of Simple and Strangulated Obstruction

Signs and Symptoms	Simple	Strangulated
Pain	Colicky	Continuous
Bowel sounds	Always present	Present or absent
Abdominal distention	Present	Present
Tenderness	Absent to mild	Marked
Fever	None	Present
WBC	Normal	Elevated
Left shift	Absent	Present

TABLE 25-4 Differentiating Signs of Peritonitis and Inflammation of Hollow Viscera

Signs and Symptoms	Peritonitis	Hollow Viscera
Bowel sounds	Absent to reduced	Present Hypoactive Normoactive Hyperactive
Pain	Constant	Intermittent (colicky)
Tenderness	Present	Absent
Rebound	Present	Absent
Diarrhea	Usually absent	Absent or present
Vomiting	Variable	Absent or present
Fever	Present	Usually absent*
WBC	Elevated	Normal*
Tachycardia	Present	May be present
Hypotension	Present	May be present
Distention	Present	May be present

*Exceptions are appendix and gallbladder.

Since the patient cannot be satisfactorily maintained on standard intravenous feedings, he or she should be operated on within 5 days of admission. Delay means performing an operation when the patient is in a less optimal condition. Treatment should be directed at early operation after satisfactory diagnosis (Table 25-5). The choice of operation depends on the cause of the obstruction.

Midgut Obstruction. Some cases of intestinal

TABLE 25-5   Treatment of Foregut Obstruction of the Bowel

Treatment	Rationale
1. Nasogastric intubation.	Allows stomach to decompress. Relieves vomiting.
2. IV replacement in a depleted patient, correction of electrolyte abnormalities, replacement of gastric suction.	Presence of depletion and electrolyte abnormalities—aim is to correct patient over 12-36 hours (see Chapter 7).
3. Volume repletion may require colloid solution.	Hypovolemia due to vomiting; hypoalbuminemia from prolonged starvation.
4. Monitor response to 2 and 3 by determining electrolyte levels, urinary output, clinical response.	Control of patient.
5. After 2-3 days of suction, perform GI series; if stomach is distended and obstructed, prepare for operation; continue suction.	Diagnosis should be made. Other diagnostic procedures to perform include overnight gastric analysis with or without betazole (Histalog) stimulation, gastroscopy, stool examination for occult or frank blood, and gastric cytologic examination. *Diagnostic procedures should not delay operation.*

obstruction appear to improve with intestinal intubation. This is due to the removal of accumulated fluid and air, with relief of distention and pain. In those cases in which the obstruction is due to acute inflammatory adhesions such as in the postoperative period, this method of treatment may be successful. In a patient with chronic adhesive obstruction, the release of proximal distention may lead to conversion to a partial obstruction so that the gastrointestinal tract may seem to function adequately. Similarly, in patients with proven far-advanced malignancy, multiple areas of partial obstruction may be impossible to relieve operatively, and long-tube intubation may be indicated.

In most other cases of intestinal obstruction, however, intubation, while relieving distention and therefore making the x-ray film look better, does not relieve the obstruction, and *operative intervention is usually required.* The timing of the operation depends on whether strangulation is present or impending. When strangulation is present, emergency operative intervention is required to salvage the patient. In all other cases the operation is performed as soon as adequate hydration, particularly restoration of normovolemia and normal electrolyte patterns, is obtained and there is evidence of adequate peripheral perfusion as evidenced by urinary output of 30 ml/hr.

A particularly devastating form of strangulating obstruction is due to a volvulus of the small intestine around an adhesive band, *producing an internal hernia and closed loop obstruction.* Gangrene may develop rapidly but be classically difficult to diagnose because the involved loop may be surrounded by normal unobstructed distal small bowel. Persistent high nasogastric output or vomiting may lead to performance of a barium swallow to confirm the diagnosis.

For nonstrangulated mechanical obstruction, the operation should be planned for 8 to 12 hours after admission. This will allow enough time for fluid hydration, volume repletion, and x-ray or other diagnostic procedures. A sample of orders on these patients is:

- Nothing by mouth
- Nasogastric suction
- IV fluid administration, replacement, and maintenance
- Monitor central venous pressure; urinary output, leukocyte count, temperature elevation, abdominal examination, and serum electrolyte levels
- Prepare for operation
- Diagnostic procedures (e.g., x-ray studies)

The use of long- or short-tube intubation has been recommended in some institutions. Although it is true that a certain percentage of patients will resolve by use of nonoperative methods, there is the overriding risk of development of gangrene in some—increasing the mortality rate tenfold. *Additionally, late operation in those who do not respond leads to a higher morbidity rate,* and a number of patients with initial response return within 6 months with the same problem. These concerns have led to adoption of *early operation as the preferred method of treatment of complete small bowel obstruction.*

The exact operative techniques depend on the findings. Obstruction caused by hernia is treated by an operation directly on the hernia. Otherwise, a standard laparotomy is performed. Examination of the bowel is done without manipulation in an attempt to find a collapsed loop, which is used as a guide to the area of obstruction. After release of the obstruction, the bowel is examined for viability, and if there is significant doubt, resection is performed.

Gallstone ileus is an obstruction due to impaction with a large gallstone in the small bowel (see Fig. 25-14). The stone is milked into a normal proximal area and removed by an enterotomy. *The remaining small bowel is examined for any additional stones.* No attempt should be made at this operation to close the fistula from the gallbladder to the small bowel through which the stone passed. The fistulas usually close spontaneously, and reoperation rarely is required.

Preoperative diagnosis can be made by x-ray examinations of the abdomen, demonstrating a small bowel obstruction that appears to proceed down the intestine (progressively involving more small bowel) or the presence of air in the biliary tract.

Persistent dilation of small bowel loops at the operating table is best handled by the passage by the anesthesiologist of a long tube, which is then threaded down the small bowel by the surgeon. Applied suction will usually decompress the bowel for ease of closure. Intraoperative direct bowel puncture should be avoided if possible.

Partial Small Bowel Obstruction. A partial small bowel obstruction should be suspected if, after an acute onset, the patient begins to pass gas per rectum or has diarrhea. *Diagnosis should be clearly established by a thorough barium examination of the upper gastrointestinal tract.* Persistence of a dilated loop may require operation to avoid subsequent development of a complete obstruction.

Hindgut Obstruction. Left colonic obstruction must be diagnosed as a separate entity *because the operative approach is different from obstructions at a higher level.* In hindgut obstruction the cause is frequently neoplasm;

therefore resection is more commonly necessary. Since the blood supply of the colon is more tenuous than that of the small intestine, it is a surgical maxim that anastomosis of a distended colon should not be done. Leakage and infection rates are very high otherwise. A decompressing temporary proximal colostomy or cecostomy is performed to allow the colonic distention to subside. A definitive elective procedure is then carried out after adequate preparation of the patient and bowel. *Such decompressing procedures are best done through small incisions with the patient under local anesthesia* if necessary, because patients with hindgut obstruction are generally in the older age group, have been obstructed for relatively long periods, have other associated diseases, and are therefore poor risks for major operations.

As with all obstructions, nasogastric intubation to prevent further accumulation of swallowed air and intravenous rehydration with a balanced salt solution *should precede diagnostic tests.*

Flat and upright abdominal films will provide evidence of colonic gas in most cases and along with a careful history and physical examination will provide the diagnosis. If the clinical picture points to colonic obstruction but x-ray examination does not confirm the diagnosis, a barium enema examination should be performed as an emergency procedure. It will enable use of the correct operative approach.

Volvulus of the Colon. If a portion of the colon is very mobile between fixed points (retroperitoneal fixation), it may twist and present a closed loop obstruction. Sigmoid and cecum are the most common areas of the colon to produce volvulus. This condition occurs commonly in the elderly or bedridden patients who suffer from chronic constipation.

A characteristic x-ray film pattern is observed, producing a kidney bean–shaped air collection in the left upper quadrant in cases of cecal volvulus and a coffee bean–shaped air collection in the right upper quadrant in cases of sigmoid volvulus. Barium enema examination may be necessary to confirm the diagnosis.

Treatment of volvulus requires early intervention, since a closed loop obstruction is present and vascular compromise may occur early. Cecal volvulus is best treated by laparotomy and right hemicolectomy. Attempts at suturing the cecum to the abdominal wall (cecopexy) have led to recurrences and complications. Most cases of sigmoid volvulus will respond to transrectal intubation or sigmoidoscopy with sudden release of gas and feces, indicating a reversal of the twist. Recurrences of volvulus are the rule, however; therefore definitive treatment usually requires resection of the redundant bowel after adequate preparation.

Strangulated Obstruction. Strangulated obstruction represents an acute emergency that requires immediate operation. There is no requirement for adequate hydration and urinary output in these cases if the patient shows evidence of shock. The following steps should be accomplished within 1 hour of admission:

1. Insert Foley catheter.
2. Insert central venous line or Swan-Ganz catheter.
3. Start IV fluids, consisting of balanced salt solutions while central venous pressure or wedged pressure rises, and measure urinary output.
4. Start broad-spectrum antibiotics.
5. Cross-match blood.
6. Obtain consent and prepare for operation.
7. Notify operating room.
8. Operate within 1 hour.

PITFALLS AND COMMON MYTHS

- Delay in diagnosis is the most common failure leading to malpractice claims in this area. This delay can be caused by failure to order the appropriate x-ray studies in a timely fashion; diagnosing gastroenteritis rather than an acute abdominal emergency; or failure to appreciate the serious nature of the problem.
- Failure to operate in a timely manner—often as a result of waiting for a convenient operating room time rather than emergency time.
- Failure to reassess the problem frequently to determine progression of signs (the "reevaluate in the morning" syndrome).
- Failure to obtain a history of prior antibiotic treatment.
- Failure to insert nasogastric tube before getting x-ray examination. (Aspiration of vomitus in the x-ray department is a major catastrophe.)
- Failure to replete the patient adequately with intravenous fluids.
- Failure to use monitoring catheters.
- Failure to call a surgical consultation early in the patient's course.

SURGICAL PHARMACOPEIA

Drug	Indications/Complications	Dosage
Pain		
Morphine sulfate	Narcotic analgesic	6-10 mg IM q4h or as needed; 2.5-5 mg IV q1-2h
Meperidine (Demerol)	Narcotic analgesic hypersensitivity; contraindicated in persons receiving monoamine oxidase inhibitors; respiratory, central nervous system (CNS), and circulatory depression	50-100 mg IM q4h as needed or 12.5-25 mg IV q1-2h
Antibiotics		
Uncomplicated Appendicitis or Diverticulitis (see the Pharmacopeia section, Chapter 49)		
Cefoxitin sodium (Mefoxin)	Active against gram-positive bacteria except MRSA and enterococci; against gram-negative bacteria except *Pseudomonas*, *Enterobacter*, and *Serratia*; anaerobes hypersensitivity; cross-reaction to penicillin allergy is <2%	1-2 g IV q6h

Continued.

Drug	Indications/Complications	Dosage
Uncomplicated Cholecystitis		
Cefazolin (Kefzol, Ancef)	Active against gram-positive bacteria except enterococci and MRSA; against gram-negative bacteria except indole-positive *Proteus, Enterobacter, Pseudomonas, Serratia*; rash, increased SGOT and alkaline phosphatase levels	1 g IV q6h or q8h
Broad-Spectrum Antibiotics for Perforated Viscus		
Piperacillin (Pipracil)	Penicillin-derivative active against gram-positive bacteria except MRSA; against gram-negative bacteria including *Enterobacter* and *Pseudomonas*; against anaerobes, including *Bacteroides*; hypersensitivity, neutropenia (6%), diarrhea, increased SGOT and bilirubin levels; rarely nephropathy	3 g IV q4h
Cefotaxime (Claforan)	Active against gram-positive bacteria except enterococci and MRSA; against gram-negative bacteria, but many *Pseudomonas* are resistant; against anaerobes but variable *B. fragilis*; hypersensitivity, phlebitis (5%), increased SGOT, diarrhea	1-2 g q6-8h
Ticarcillin disodium and clavulanate potassium (Timentin)	Combination penicillin-derivative and beta-lactamase inhibitor active against gram-positive bacteria except MRSA; against gram-negative bacteria, including *Pseudomonas*; against anaerobes same as penicillin but also may increase prothrombin time, increase SGOT, hypokalemia	3.1 g IV q4-8h
Imipenem-cilaslatin sodium (Primaxin)	Active against gram-positive bacteria except MRSA; against gram-negative bacteria; and against anaerobes; *Nocardia* and *Mycobacterium fortuitum* hypersensitivity, increased aspartate aminotransferase, alanine aminotransferase, and alkaline phosphatase levels, diarrhea, *Pseudomonas* superinfection (9%)	500 mg-1g q6h
Metronidazole (Flagyl)	Active against anaerobes, GI—nausea, vomiting, diarrhea; CNS—headache, paresthesias, rarely ataxia and seizures; disulfiram-like reaction with alcohol; hematologic—neutropenia, thrombocytopenia, mutagenic	500 mg IV q3h or 500 mg suppository
Replacement		
Pancrelipase (Pancrease MT)	Replacement for exocrine pancreatic enzyme deficiency; contraindicated in persons hypersensitive to pork or with acute pancreatitis	Capsules MT 4 and MT 10 with 4000 IU and 10,000 U lipase, respectively; usual dose, 4000-16,000 U with each meal and snack

BIBLIOGRAPHY

Abu-Yousef MM, Phillips ME, Frankel EA Jr, et al. Sonography of acute appendicitis: A clinical review. Crit Rev Diagn Imaging 29:381-408, 1989.

Boyd JB, Bradford B, Watne AL. Operative risk factors of colon resection in the elderly. Ann Surg 192:743, 1980.

Bradley EL, Clements LJ. Spontaneous resolution of pancreatic pseudocysts. Am J Surg 129:23, 1975.

Brewer RJ, Golden GT, Hitch DC, et al. Abdominal pain: An analysis of 1000 consecutive cases in a university hospital emergency room. Am J Surg 131:219, 1976.

Brolin RE. Partial small bowel obstruction. Surgery 95:145, 1984.

Browne DS. Laparoscopic-guided appendectomy: A study of 100 consecutive cases. Aust N Z J Obstet Gynaecol 30:231-233, 1990.

Cacioppo JC, Diettrich NA, Kaplan G, et al. The consequences of current constraints on surgical treatment of appendicitis. Am J Surg 157:276-281, 1989.

Carter MS, Fautini GA, Sanmartano RJ, et al. Qualitative and quantitative fluorescein fluorescence in determining intestinal viability. Am J Surg 147:117, 1984.

Chandhuri TK, Fink S, Mahon CB, et al. Current status of imaging in the diagnosis of acute appendicitis. Am J Physiol Imaging 5:89-96, 1990.

Cox GR, Browne BJ. Acute cholecystitis in the emergency department. J Emerg Med 7:501-511, 1989.

Deck KB, Pettitt BJ, Harrison MR. The length-time correlate in appendicitis. JAMA 244:806, 1980.

Dent TL, Berci G, Ponsky JL. American college of surgeons postgraduate course on interventional laparoscopy. Am J Surg 161:326-409, 1991.

Flowers JL, et al. Laparoscopic cholecystectomy. Surg Rds 14(4):271-282, 1991.

Gardner B, Masur RM, Fujimoto J. Factors influencing the timing of cholecystectomy in acute cholecystitis. Am J Surg 125:730, 1973.

Hoffman J, Rolff M, Lomborg V, et al. Ultraconservative management of appendiceal abscess. J R Coll Surg Edinb 36:18-20, 1991.

Krausz MM, Manny J. Acute superior mesenteric arterial occlusion: A plea for early diagnosis. Surgery 83:482, 1978.

Krukowski ZH, Matheson NA. Emergency surgery for diverticular disease complicated by generalized and fecal peritonitis: A review. Br J Surg 71:921, 1984.

Lewis FR, Holcroft JW, et al. Appendicitis: A critical review of diagnosis and treatment in 1000 cases. Arch Surg 110:677, 1975.

Linder HH, Green RB. Embryology and surgical anatomy of the extrahepatic biliary tract. Surg Clin North Am 44:1273, 1964.

Ness TJ, Gebhart GF. Visceral pain: A review of experimental studies. Pain 41:167-234, 1990.

Orient JM. Evaluation of abdominal pain: Clinicians' performance compared with three protocols. South Med J 79:793-799, 1986.

Pellegrini CA, Thomas MJ, Way LW. Recurrent biliary stricture: Patterns of recurrence and outcome of surgical therapy. Am J Surg 147:175, 1984.

Ranson JHC, Rifkind KM, Roses DF, et al. Prognostic signs and the role of operative management in acute pancreatitis. Surg Gynecol Obstet 139:69, 1974.

Rodkey GY, Welch CE. Changing patterns in the surgical treatment of diverticular disease. Ann Surg 200:466, 1984.

Rothrock SG, Skeoch G, Rush JJ, et al. Clinical features of misdiagnosed appendicitis in children. Ann Emerg Med 20:45-50, 1991.

Sandberg A, Andrew A, et al. Accidental lesions of the common bile duct of cholecystectomy. Pre and perioperative factors of importance. Ann Surg 201:328, 1985.

Sarr MG, Bulkey GB, Zuidema GD. Preoperative recognition of intestinal strangulation obstruction. Prospective evaluation of diagnostic capability. Am J Surg 145:176, 1983.

Stabile BE. Therapeutic options in acute diverticulitis. Compr Ther 17:26-33, 1991.

Stone HH, Fabian TC. Peritoneal dialysis in the treatment of acute alcoholic pancreatitis. Surg Gynecol Obstet 150:878, 1980.

Stone HH, Fabian TC, Dunlop WE. Gallstone pancreatitis: Biliary tract pathology in relation to time of operation. Ann Surg 194:305, 1981.

Stone HH, Mullins RJ, Scovill WA. Vagotomy for prevention of recurrent alcohol induced pancreatitis. Dig Surg 1:136, 1984.

Teplick SK, Harshfield DL, Brandon JC, et al. Percutaneous cholecystostomy in critically ill patients. Gastrointest Radiol 16:154-156, 1991.

Warshaw AL, Lesser PB, et al. The pathogenesis of pulmonary edema in acute pancreatitis. Ann Surg 182:505, 1975.

Weismann H, Frank M, et al. Rapid and accurate diagnosis of acute cholecystitis with 99-m technetium HIDA cholecystography. Am J Roentgenol 132:523, 1979.

Whitworth CM, Whitworth PN, SanFillipo J, et al. Value of diagnostic laparoscopy in young women with possible appendicitis. Surg Gynec Obstet 167:187-190, 1988.

Willis RG, Lawson WC, Hoare EM, et al. Are bile bacteria relevant to septic complications following biliary surgery? Br J Surg 71:845, 1984.

Zeman RK, Garra BS. Gallbladder imaging: The state of the art. Gastroenterol Clin North Am 2:127-155, 1991.

CHAPTER REVIEW
Questions

1. A 45-year-old man is admitted to the emergency room with abdominal pain and vomiting of 1 day's duration. During the previous evening, the patient had imbibed alcoholic beverages heavily. Physical examination reveals a pulse rate of 140, a temperature of 38.3° C (101° F), and abdominal findings consisting of tenderness to deep palpation in the upper abdomen and depressed bowel sounds. The patient is sent to the x-ray department for abdominal films. While there, he becomes diaphoretic, vomits, and dies. What is the likely diagnosis? Why?
2. List the sequence of pathophysiologic events leading to early death in uncomplicated pancreatitis and untreated intestinal obstruction.
3. A 38-year-old woman is admitted with a 2-day history of acute, diffuse cramping, abdominal pain, constant vomiting, and one episode of diarrhea. She had had a gynecologic operation 3 years previously. X-ray films reveal a small amount of bowel gas and are otherwise nonspecific. Abdominal findings reveal no evidence of peritonitis, and leukocyte count is normal. How would you manage this patient?
4. List four findings that differentiate acute cholecystitis from biliary colic.
5. What are the site, source, and character of the fluid loss in acute mechanical complete small bowel obstruction?
6. Why is the pain of left colon obstruction midabdominal rather than in the hypochondrium?
7. What relationship between pain and vomiting may differentiate acute duodenal ulcer from biliary colic?
8. List three reasons why a patient with acute ruptured appendicitis may not have abdominal tenderness to palpation.
9. A patient returns to your office 6 days after an appendectomy, complaining of fever and diarrhea. What is the likely diagnosis? How would you confirm it?
10. A patient with acute cholecystitis has a serum amylase level of 3000 U. What is the most likely cause?
11. What techniques may enhance operative exploration of the common duct?
12. What are three indications for early operation in a patient with acute diverticulitis?
13. Why is a barium enema examination indicated if small and large bowel obstruction cannot be distinguished?
14. List three criteria by which you can determine that strangulation obstruction has occurred.

Answers

1. Acute pancreatitis. The history of alcoholic intake and acute onset are compatible. Intestinal obstruction is unlikely in the presence of depressed bowel sounds this early in the course. Abdominal tenderness is not found in intestinal obstruction unless there is gangrene or perforation, and these events give marked anterior abdominal wall findings—not tenderness to deep palpation. The tachycardia out of proportion to the fever is characteristic of pancreatitis.

2. *Acute pancreatitis*
   a. Necrosis of pancreas
   b. Retroperitoneal hemorrhage and extravasation of fluid
   c. Hypovolemia
   d. Shock
   e. Death

   Intestinal obstruction
   a. Distention of bowel
   b. Intraluminal extravasation of fluid and electrolytes
   c. Hypovolemia
   d. Electrolyte loss
   e. Shock
   f. Death

3. a. The differential diagnosis is intestinal obstruction or gastroenteritis. The acute onset is compatible with either, and the duration rules out a simple staphylococcal gastroenteritis. Treatment should be directed at rehydration, blood examination for electrolyte abnormalities, and then an attempt at quick diagnosis.
   b. Nothing by mouth
   c. Nasogastric tube to suction
   d. Monitor patient response in terms of pulse, blood pressure, urinary output. When the patient is stable (8 to 10 hours), do a limited barium study by mouth with delayed films. If barium can be seen entering the colon, treat nonoperatively until a formal work-up can be evaluated. If dilated small bowel is visualized and no barium enters colon by 24 hours, an operation is indicated.

4. a. Signs of peritonitis in the right upper quadrant
   b. High fever
   c. Persistently elevated white blood count
   d. Tender palpable gallbladder
5. a. Loss into the bowel
   b. Loss from interstitial compartment primarily
   c. Isotonic proteinfree filtrate
6. There is no peristalsis in the colon; therefore the pain will occur when the obstruction has affected the stretch receptors of the peristalting small bowel, which is referred to the midabdominal region.
7. Vomiting in a duodenal ulcer patient usually relieves the pain, since it produces regurgitation of alkaline small bowel contents into the stomach, neutralizing the hyperacidity. In biliary colic, the pain will not disappear with the vomiting, since they are both produced by stimulation of the stretch receptors in the gallbladder.
8. a. The appendix is retrocecal and protected from the anterior abdominal wall by normal bowel.

b. The patient has received antibiotic treatment.
   c. The patient is heavily sedated.
9. Pelvic abscess; rectal examination
10. Common duct stone
11. Cholangiography and choledochoscopy
12. a. Free air seen on x-ray film
    b. Clinical peritonitis outside of left lower quadrant
    c. Failure to respond to nonoperative management
13. The operative approach to the two obstructions is different. Small bowel obstruction requires a laparotomy and exploration, whereas left-sided or transverse colonic obstruction may only require decompression.
14. a. Character of pain changes to constant.
    b. Back pain may occur.
    c. Bowel sounds disappear.
    d. Peritoneal signs appear.
    e. Patient is much sicker.
    f. WBC rises to high levels.

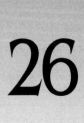

26 Jaundice

A.R. MOOSSA
MARK DEAKIN

KEY FEATURES

After reading this chapter you will understand:
- Bilirubin metabolism.
- The pertinent points in the history and physical examination of a jaundiced patient.
- The value of liver function tests.
- The available imaging techniques and the sequence in which they should be performed.
- The role of surgery in the jaundiced patient.
- The various causes of extrahepatic obstruction and the common operations performed for this condition.

Jaundice is a clinical sign. Derived from the French word *jaune,* meaning yellow, jaundice is defined as the yellow discoloration of the skin and mucous membranes (sclera, conjunctiva, soft palate), resulting from the retention of abnormally large amounts of bile pigments (mainly bilirubin) in the body fluids. Jaundice becomes clinically evident when the serum bilirubin level exceeds 2 mg/dl.

Jaundice results from *excessive production* of bilirubin, such as occurs with increased hemolysis (prehepatic jaundice); from hepatic diseases that lead to the *incomplete uptake, transport, conjugation, or excretion of bile pigments* (hepatic jaundice); or from *extrahepatic biliary tract obstruction* (posthepatic jaundice). Since conjugation of bilirubin with glucuronic acid occurs within the hepatocyte, jaundice can also be classified as unconjugated or conjugated hyperbilirubinemia.

Hemolytic jaundice is defined as the hyperbilirubinemia associated with increased red blood cell destruction. Serum bilirubin is mainly unconjugated. Maximal production of bile pigments is 1500 mg/day, *which should be sufficient to raise serum bilirubin levels by only 3 mg/dl.* Thus serum bilirubin levels in excess of this amount indicate associated parenchymal liver disease and/or bile duct obstruction.

Surgical jaundice describes extrahepatic biliary obstruction in patients who would benefit from biliary decompression either by internal or external biliary drainage, in contrast to nonsurgical jaundice, for which an operation on the bile ducts has nothing to offer. Patients with biliary obstruction can be easily identified by imaging techniques showing dilation of the biliary tree proximal to the obstruction. The patient has *pale stools* and *dark urine* because of the diminished bile secretion into the bowel lumen and the increased urinary excretion of conjugated bilirubin, which is water soluble.

Cholestasis is defined as the *failure of normal amounts of bile to reach the duodenum;* therefore it occurs whenever there is failure of bile flow anywhere between the basolateral membrane of the hepatocyte and the duodenum. Cholestatic jaundice can result from either extrahepatic biliary obstruction (surgical jaundice) or hepatic disease (nonsurgical jaundice), but not from hemolysis unless there is associated hepatocellular damage. In a patient with cholestasis, bile pigment accumulates within the hepatocytes or biliary passages, a condition that can be recognized histologically.

A simplified working classification of jaundice

460

is shown in the box below. *A complete history, physical examination, blood tests, and an examination of the urine and stool for the presence of bile and urobilinogen provide adequate information to provide appropriate management in 80% to 85% of patients with jaundice.* The remaining 15% to 20% of patients can be managed well only if the clinician understands bilirubin production, transport, storage, conjugation, and excretion and knows how to detect various abnormalities in these mechanisms.

WHAT IS NORMAL BILIRUBIN METABOLISM?

Bilirubin is the breakdown product of hemoglobin and myoglobin (80% to 90%) and of other liver enzymes such as catalase, peroxidase, and the cytochromes. Heme, or porphyrin, not used in hemoglobin synthesis and turnover of non-heme-containing proteins, provides the additional 10% to 20% of bilirubin production (Fig. 26-1). The normal adult bilirubin production is 250 to 300 mg/day, mainly from 100- to 120-day-old erythrocytes. Heme is cleaved in reticuloendothelial cells by microsomal oxygenase to produce biliverdin, which is converted to unconjugated bilirubin by biliverdin reductase. Bilirubin is lipid soluble as a result of its tertiary structure maintained by six intramolecular hydrogen bonds. This bonding can be broken down by alcohol in the diazo reaction (van den Bergh), converting unconjugated (indirect) bilirubin to direct-reacting bilirubin. Unconjugated bilirubin is released from the reticuloendothelial system of the bone marrow, liver, and spleen and is trans-

---

CLASSIFICATION OF JAUNDICE

Unconjugated Hyperbilirubinemia

I. Increased destruction of red blood cells (hemolytic jaundice)
  A. Hereditary or congenital
    1. Spherocytosis
    2. Thalassemia
    3. Sickle cell disease
  B. Acquired autoimmune (Coombs-positive anemia)
  C. Infections
  D. Chemical agents
  E. Physical agents (severe burns)
II. Defective transport and storage of bilirubin
  A. Congenital (Gilbert's disease)
  B. Following viral hepatitis
  C. Drugs
    1. Rifamycin
    2. Novobiocin
  D. Metabolic defects (e.g., jaundice of neonates and premature infants)

Conjugated Hyperbilirubinemia

I. Defective excretion of bilirubin
  A. Congenital secretory failure (e.g., Dubin-Johnson syndrome)
  B. Intrahepatic obstruction
    1. Cirrhosis
    2. Hepatitis (alcoholic or viral)
    3. Amyloidosis
    4. Carcinoma
    5. Granulomatous disease

II. Drugs
  A. Chlorpromazine
  B. Sex hormones
  C. Halothane
  D. Others
III. Extrahepatic biliary obstruction
  A. Choledocholithiasis
  B. Bile duct strictures (traumatic)
  C. Pancreatitis
  D. Periampullary carcinoma originating in
    1. Head of pancreas
    2. Ampulla
    3. Duodenum
    4. Lower common bile duct
  E. Sclerosing cholangitis

Combined Unconjugated and Conjugated Hyperbilirubinemia

I. Biliary obstruction with secondary hepatocyte damage
  A. Prolonged biliary stasis with secondary liver injury
  B. Biliary obstruction and ascending cholangitis
II. Severe hepatocyte damage with
  A. Secondary intrahepatic biliary obstruction
  B. Secondary deficiency in bilirubin uptake, conjugation, and excretion
III. Severe hemolysis with secondary liver damage

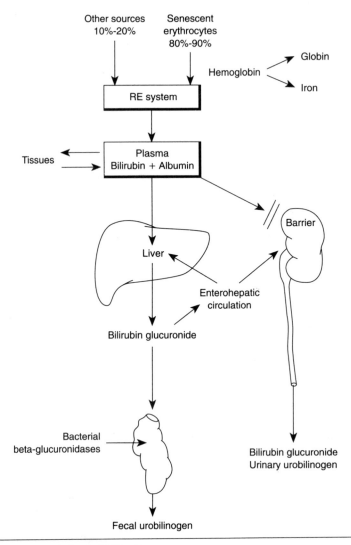

FIGURE 26-1   Metabolism of bilirubin.

ported in the plasma tightly bound to albumin, equilibrating with other body fluids. Fatty acids and organic anions may compete for binding, a competition that is important in the neonate in whom drugs such as salicylates and sulfonamides can facilitate diffusion of bilirubin into the brain and increase the risk of kernicterus.

The bilirubin-albumin complex enters the sinusoidal circulation of the liver where the complex process of changing non-water-soluble, nonpolar, unconjugated bilirubin begins at the plasma membrane of the hepatocyte (Fig. 26-2). Carrier mechanisms at the membrane level probably exist but have not been characterized.

Within the hepatocyte, bilirubin is bound by two basic acceptor proteins, Y and Z, and is stored. Conjugation with glucuronic acid is catalyzed by UDPglucuronyl transferase, producing both monoglucuronides and diglucuronides. Although conjugation with glucuronic acid is the most important mechanism, sulfate, xylose, and glucose conjugation also occurs to a small extent.

The conjugated (direct) bilirubin is transferred against a concentration gradient into the bile canaliculus by an energy-dependent system. At least two independent mechanisms of biliary excretion exist—one for bile acids and the other for bilirubin. In patients with Dubin-Johnson

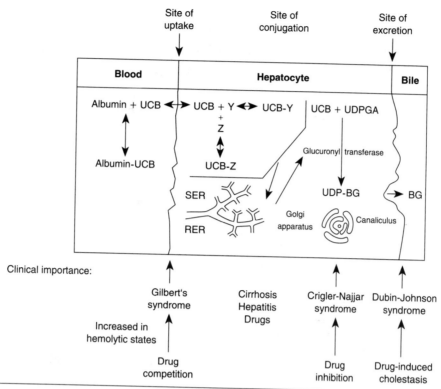

FIGURE 26-2   Role of the hepatocyte in the transfer of bilirubin from blood to bile and the clinical importance of interference with bilirubin metabolism. *SER,* Smooth endoplasmic reticulum; *RER,* rough endoplasmic reticulum; *UDP,* uridine diphosphate; *UDPGA,* uridine diphosphate glucuronic acid; *BG,* bilirubin glucuronide; *Y* and *Z,* acceptor proteins.

syndrome, there is a defect in the excretion of conjugated bilirubin, but bile acid excretion is normal. Conjugated bilirubin produces a direct (aqueous) van den Bergh reaction. Conjugated bilirubin enters biliary channels of progressively increasing caliber to reach the intestine, where bacterial beta-glucuronidases within the terminal ileum and colon hydrolyze the bilirubin, which is then reduced to colorless urobilinogen. Ten percent to 20% of the urobilinogen is absorbed from the terminal ileum and colon and is re-excreted by the liver and kidneys (*entero-hepatic circulation*). Most of the remaining urobilinogen is converted by fecal bacteria into stercobilin, which gives the characteristic brown color to the feces.

The test for urinary and fecal urobilinogen concentration is often ordered and interpreted indiscriminately in the investigation of the jaundiced patient.

Urinary excretion of urobilinogen is a function of multiple variables, including:

- Rate of biliary formation and excretion
- Degree of intestinal absorption of bilirubin, which is increased in patients with diarrhea and after ingestion of broad-spectrum antibiotics
- Renal function and state of hydration; urinary urobilinogen excretion depends on the urinary pH and is increased in alkaline urine

Therefore urinary urobilinogen should be measured under standard conditions of hydration and controlled pH. In the normal adult the range of daily urobilinogen excretion by the kidney is 0 to 4 mg; fecal urobilinogen ranges from 40 to 280 mg/day. The main value of urobilinogen determination is that the total absence of urobilinogen in the urine and feces indicates **complete** biliary obstruction; however, this condition can usually be diagnosed without a urobilinogen determination.

Other Components of Bile

Biliary Cholesterol. Bile is 80% to 95% water. Biliary cholesterol is in the free unesterified form, which is insoluble but is kept in solution by the formation of micelles by molecular aggregation with bile salts and phospholipids. These micelles have a hydrophobic interior and hydrophilic exterior.

Biliary Phospholipids. These components are also insoluble in water and are composed mainly of lecithin (90%) and lysolecithin (3%).

Bile Acids. The primary bile acids are cholic acid and chenodeoxycholic acid, which are converted by colonic bacterial action to the tertiary bile acids, deoxycholic acid, and lithocholic acid.

Gallstones. The three major types of gallstones are (1) cholesterol, (2) black pigment stones associated with hemolytic states and cirrhosis, and (3) brown pigment stones associated with chronic biliary obstruction and cholangitis. Recurrent common bile duct stones that follow cholecystectomy are frequently brown pigment stones. Risk factors for gallstone prevalence are shown in the box at right.

The pathogenesis of cholesterol and pigment stones differs. Bile composition, biliary stasis, and gallbladder function are important factors.

Pigment Stones. Pigment stones are associated with hemolytic states. An increased bilirubin load is important in their etiology, even if the exact mechanism of formation is not clear, because there is also a cholesterol and infective component in the majority of these calculi. In Eastern countries in which infestation with *Ascaris lumbricoides* is endemic, the eggs of the parasite can be found within the stones.

Cholesterol Stones. In the Western world gallstones are composed mainly of cholesterol but may also contain varying amounts of the calcium salts of bilirubin, fatty acids, phospholipids, bile acids, and glycoproteins. Gallstone formation is related to supersaturation of bile with cholesterol, with a lowered proportion of bile acids. The problem is more complex because supersaturated bile is often found in normal individuals, especially during fasting, and other factors that promote or prevent nucleation are of equal importance.

The source of lithogenic bile is the liver, although the exact mechanisms responsible have not been determined. Biliary cholesterol concen-

---

RISK FACTORS FOR GALLSTONE PREVALENCE

Age over 50
Family history
Female
  Sex
  Parity
  Estrogen administration
Obesity
Diet: low fiber intake
Race
  High in American Indians
  Low in black Africans
Hemolytic states
Parasitic infestation
  Clonorchis sinensis
  Ascaris lumbricoides
Cystic fibrosis
Cirrhosis
Interruption of enterohepatic circulation
  of bile
  Ileal resection
  Ileal disease (e.g., Crohn's)
  Biliary fistula
  Cholestyramine
Parenteral nutrition
Somatostatin

---

tration is not related to serum cholesterol levels. The gallbladder plays an important role, as evidenced by the fact that most stones form within the gallbladder. Defective gallbladder contraction leading to stasis, stratification of bile, nucleation factors such as desquamated cells, bacteria, foreign bodies, and changes in the composition of bile in the gallbladder by abnormal resorption of bile constituents are important factors.

DIAGNOSIS OF JAUNDICE

Diagnosis of jaundice is made clinically by observing yellow discoloration of the skin and conjunctiva. It is confirmed by the demonstration of an elevated serum bilirubin level.

Three conditions can imitate mild jaundice:

1. Hypercarotinemia can result from eating large amounts of heavily pigmented vegetables (e.g., carrots, beets, and spinach) and may occur in some patients with myxedema and

panhypopituitarism when the ability to metabolize carotene is impaired. The serum carotene level (normal 40 to 300 μg/ml) is increased in these instances.

2. Lycopenemia may occur in patients who consume large quantities of tomatoes.
3. Addison's disease may be mistaken for mild jaundice by the unwary.

The first steps in diagnosis are to take a careful history and to perform a physical examination that should include *examination of the stool and urine.* The urine is tested for bilirubin and urobilinogen excess, and routine hematologic and biochemistry studies are performed. The place of further investigations such as ultrasonography, CT scan, percutaneous transhepatic cholangiography (PTC), endoscopic retrograde cholangiopancreatography (ERCP), or liver biopsy is determined by the clinician's opinion about the likely cause of the jaundice. Efficient evaluation of the jaundiced patient is vital to avoid injudicious delay of the operation (which may lead to increased morbidity and mortality) for extrahepatic ductal obstruction. Nonetheless, *uncomplicated jaundice should never be treated as an emergency.*

History

The main points to elicit when taking a history from a patient with jaundice include the following.

Age of the patient is often neglected; congenital and inflammatory diseases of the liver are more common in children and young adults. Cirrhosis and neoplastic disease occur in older patients but cannot be totally excluded in the young.

Sex of the patient may be important. Alcoholic cirrhosis occurs more frequently in men, whereas cholelithiasis and oral contraceptive–induced cholestasis occur more commonly in women.

Place of birth may be important, for an African or far Eastern origin suggests exposure to hepatitis B.

Occupation of the patient may be important. Farmers and sewer workers are at risk from leptospirosis (Weil's disease), whereas brucellosis tends to affect farmers, veterinarians, and packing house workers. Employment involving alcohol may suggest the presence of cirrhosis.

Family history is important, and the clinician should particularly note jaundice, hepatitis, gall-stones, or splenectomy in family members. A history of both jaundice and neurologic disease suggests Wilson's disease.

Travel to regions where hepatitis is endemic should be noted, and close *contact* with intravenous drug abusers, other jaundiced individuals, or patients receiving care in renal units should be recorded.

It is important to carefully elicit and document any history of:

- Exposure to drugs, whether prescribed or not
- Parenteral injections (including blood tests), drug abuse, dental treatment, or tattooing, which might confer risk of hepatitis B
- Transfusion of blood or blood products
- Alcohol consumption
- Anesthesia, particularly multiple administrations of halothane
- Previous operations on or around the biliary tree, which might suggest retained stones or a biliary stricture
- Exposure to industrial toxins

In the presence of *abdominal pain,* the history of the onset of illness can differentiate benign obstructive disease from hepatitis. Although both diseases occur acutely, hepatitis is infectious, with the associated prodromal symptoms of systemic disease (i.e., malaise, fever, and anorexia). The patient with hepatitis usually feels better after jaundice appears. *Abdominal pain in patients with hepatitis is caused by distention of the liver capsule.*

Benign extrahepatic obstruction is a mechanical problem, with systemic symptoms developing subsequent to the onset of secondary infection after the appearance of abdominal pain, which may be typical *biliary colic.* Fever is often present in patients with hepatitis, cirrhosis, and neoplastic disorders, but *fever with chills (rigors) is highly suggestive of ascending cholangitis or liver abscess.*

Long-standing systemic symptoms (i.e., weight loss, symptoms of anemia such as lethargy, tiredness, breathlessness) may indicate underlying malignancy, and a history of previous malignancy may point to possible hepatic metastases. *Carcinoma of the lower end of the common bile duct or head of the pancreas is suggested by the gradual onset of painless jaundice.* Weight loss can be masked by the accumulation of ascites.

A history of pruritus is indicative of cholestatic jaundice, mandating evaluation to exclude extrahepatic biliary obstruction. Pruritus is never a feature of hemolytic jaundice.

Physical Examination

Common Physical Signs. By careful examination of a patient in daylight, jaundice can be detected in the bulbar conjunctiva or soft palate when the bilirubin level exceeds 2 mg/dl. The color of the icterus may suggest its cause—obstructive jaundice is characteristically dark green, whereas the hepatocellular type is orange or yellow. A simple and useful diagnostic procedure to perform when the jaundiced patient is first evaluated is visual examination of the stool. The acholic stool characteristic of obstructive jaundice is easily recognized by the gray appearance resulting from increased fat content and decreased bile pigment. In patients with hemolytic jaundice, the stools are well colored. The dark color of the urine in patients with obstructive jaundice results from the presence of significant amounts of bile pigments. This is easily demonstrated by the foam test: if the urine is shaken vigorously in a test tube, a yellow tint appears in the foam. The test results will be positive in patients with cholestatic (hepatic and obstructive) jaundice but negative in patients with hemolytic jaundice.

Does the Patient Have Signs of Parenchymal Liver Disease? Signs of chronic liver disease are important in determining whether there is a long-standing cause such as a primary biliary cirrhosis or an acute pathologic condition such as a gallstone in the common bile duct. Cutaneous spider angiomas (spider nevi) are frequently observed above the diaphragm, especially on the anterosuperior aspect of the upper thorax and on the neck, face, and upper arms; these are indicators of liver disease. Radiating portosystemic venous collaterals (caput medusae) around the umbilicus, splenomegaly, and ascites suggest portal hypertension caused by cirrhosis of the liver. In the male patient feminizing characteristics such as soft skin, loss of pubic hair distribution, gynecomastia, and testicular atrophy commonly appear in patients with advanced liver disease because of their inability to metabolize estrogens. Palmar erythema and Dupuytren's contracture occasionally occur in patients with alcoholic cirrhosis. Flapping tremor, incoordination, confusion, and fetor hepaticus are signs of liver failure.

What Are the Findings During Abdominal Examination? Palpation of a large, hard, nodular liver almost certainly indicates malignant disease. Conversely, if the liver is not palpable, the possibility that there is carcinoma obstructing biliary outflow is remote. An acutely tender liver indicates either inflammation or stretching of the capsule. A palpably enlarged gallbladder associated with long-standing jaundice also suggests carcinoma of the periampullary region (Courvoisier's law), although this sign is considerably less helpful in practice than in theory. In a patient with cholelithiasis the gallbladder may be tender to direct palpation, or Murphy's sign may be positive. Mass lesions of the liver are often palpable and are associated with jaundice. They include hepatoma, amebic or echinococcal cysts, hemangiomas, hamartomas, solitary metastasis, or abscess. Although the spleen is usually palpable in patients with hemolytic anemia, massive splenomegaly is often associated with portal hypertension. Rectal or pelvic examination may reveal peritoneal seedings (Blumer's shelf) in the rectovesical or rectovaginal pouch, which are diagnostic of intra-abdominal carcinomatosis. Palpable supraclavicular nodes (Troisier's sign or Virchow's node) indicate carcinoma until proved otherwise.

SPECIAL TESTS

The multiplicity of the currently available tests makes it necessary to choose carefully those studies needed to solve a given clinical problem. Exploratory laparotomy *should not* be undertaken in a jaundiced patient until the diagnosis is clearly established and the patient's vital functions are returned to as near normal as the underlying disease will allow. *Performing a laparotomy on a patient with undiagnosed jaundice is no longer acceptable.*

Liver function tests help to distinguish between the diseases (Table 26-1), but individual test results may be abnormal in each category or condition. Parenchymal liver damage with abnormal function test results can occur with obstructive jaundice. Conversely, hepatocellular diseases with associated intrahepatic cholestasis occasionally produce an obstructive pattern of blood chemistry results. Liver function tests are usually performed to establish the presence, type, and severity of liver disease as an aid to determining prognosis and management. Liver function tests fall into three categories that indicate the enzymatic, metabolic, or excretory functions of the liver.

Enzymatic Functions of the Liver

Measurement of serum levels of enzymes produced or excreted by the liver can provide a use-

TABLE 26-1 Liver Function Studies in the Diagnosis of Jaundice

| Type of Jaundice | Serum Bilirubin | | Urinary Bilirubin | Urinary Urobilinogen | Serum Alkaline Phosphatase | Serum 5'-Nucleotidase |
	Conjugated (Direct)	Unconjugated (Indirect)				
Prehepatic (hemolytic)	+	+++	0	++	0	0
Intrahepatic hepatocellular	++	++	++	+	+	+
Intrahepatic cholestatic	+++	++	+++	± 0	++	++
Posthepatic cholestatic (biliary obstruction)	+++	++	+++	± 0*	++	++

0, no change; +, mild elevation; ++, moderate elevation; +++, marked elevation.
*Dependent on the degree of mechanical obstruction.

ful index of both hepatocyte injury and bile outflow obstruction. The activity of enzymes found principally within the hepatocyte (transferases) is usually elevated to a greater extent with hepatocyte injury. *Alanine transferase (ALT)* is concentrated principally within the hepatocyte, and increased serum levels usually indicate hepatocyte injury. *Aspartate transferase (AST)* is found in high concentrations in the liver and other organ systems; hence its serum elevation is less specific for liver injury. Transferase elevations are useful in the early diagnosis of viral hepatitis.

Obstructive lesions of the biliary tract can be detected before the appearance of jaundice or other clinical stigmata by measuring the levels of enzymes such as *alkaline phosphatase,* which is elevated with cholestasis and to a lesser extent when liver cells are damaged. The alkaline phosphatase level is also elevated in patients with hepatic cholestasis resulting from other causes such as primary biliary cirrhosis and infiltrative lesions of the liver (e.g., granulomas or metastatic malignant disease, Hodgkin's disease) and in patients with metabolic bone disease. When the serum alkaline phosphatase measurement is combined with that for serum gamma-transpeptidase or 5'-nucleotidase, a more accurate evaluation of liver alkaline phosphatase is possible because neither gamma-transpeptidase nor 5'-nucleotidase is derived from bone. During pregnancy the placental alkaline phosphatase level is elevated. Placental alkaline phosphatase is heat resistant, whereas the isoenzymes derived from bone show marked heat sensitivity. The

effect of heat on liver alkaline phosphatase is intermediate between the other two.

Metabolic Functions of the Liver

The single most useful parameter of hepatic metabolic activity is the albumin-globulin ratio. Serum albumin and globulin levels are little changed in patients with jaundice of short duration. The albumin-globulin ratio is usually normal in patients with uncomplicated prehepatic and posthepatic jaundice but is commonly reversed with hepatocellular disease. Elevations of total serum globulin levels occur in most forms of intrahepatic disease.

Flocculation Tests. These tests are of historical interest only and have largely been replaced by the fractionation of the globulin moiety of the serum. This latter test, however, provides little, if any, increased diagnostic precision. Flocculation tests are based on the observation that sera from patients with hepatic disease react with various substances to produce turbidity or precipitation.

Zinc Sulfite Turbidity Test. A highly accurate measurement of gamma globin levels, this test has the added advantage of being inexpensive.

Thymol Turbidity Test. This test measures the lipoprotein fraction, which is chiefly associated with gamma globulin. This fraction is increased in patients with infectious hepatitis and in patients with subacute and chronic liver atrophy.

Coagulation Studies. Fibrinogen, prothrombin (factor II), and clotting factors V, VII, IX, and

X are synthesized by the liver. Depressed levels of fibrinogen or prothrombin are indicative of hepatic dysfunction. Synthesis of clotting factors II, VII, IX, and X is vitamin K dependent, and changes in these factors alter the prothrombin time (PT). An increase in PT occurs in several clinical situations, including:

- Liver disease
- Diminished absorption of fat-soluble vitamin K because of decreased bile acids in the intestinal lumen
- Prolonged parenteral nutrition
- Sterilization of the gut with antibiotics
- Use of coumarin anticoagulants

Parenteral administration of vitamin K quickly restores the PT to normal except in patients with severe parenchymal liver disease. Hence measurement of the PT before and after vitamin K administration is of prognostic value. Clotting factor VII is synthesized extrahepatically, with elevated levels often observed in association with liver disease. The partial thromboplastin time (PTT) may reflect this association by being either normal or prolonged.

Platelet counts may be depressed in patients with alcoholic liver disease, hypersplenism, or sepsis. *Abnormal bleeding time or hemorrhage during the operation is common in a jaundiced patient;* vitamin K deficiency, impaired hepatic synthesis of clotting factors, primary fibrinolysis, and impaired hepatic clearance of serum proteases and vasoactive factors have all been implicated.

Serum Cholesterol. The liver is largely responsible for much of the synthesis of cholesterol. It also provides the main route for cholesterol esterification, degradation, and excretion. Serum cholesterol levels (normal value, 130 to 250 mg/dl) fall in patients with severe liver damage and rise in patients with cholestatic jaundice.

Excretory Functions of the Liver

Serial serum bilirubin determinations are the most widely used estimations of excretory functions of the liver for bile pigments. The upper limit of normal for total bilirubin is 1.5 mg/dl; for the 1-minute direct fraction, it is 0.3 mg/dl. If the total bilirubin level is elevated and the 1-minute fraction is 0.3 mg/dl or less, the diagnosis is hemolytic jaundice. If the direct fraction is increased and the total bilirubin level is normal or only slightly elevated, partial biliary obstruction

(e.g., with common bile duct obstruction caused by a stone or carcinoma) should be suspected. If the total and direct bilirubin levels are both elevated, the diagnosis probably is extrahepatic biliary obstruction.

The excretory function of the liver can also be estimated by measuring the clearances of substances such as sulfobromophthalein (Bromsulphalein [BSP]), rose bengal–iodine-131, or indocyanine green. These investigations are sometimes useful in selected patients with suspected liver disease, although the sulfobromophthalein test is of little value when the serum bilirubin level exceeds 3 mg/dl. These tests are also influenced by alterations in liver perfusion (i.e., from hemorrhage).

Other Hematologic Tests

Anemia may be present with any one of the three categories of jaundice. The presence of macrocytosis on the peripheral blood smear or an increase in reticulocyte count (reticulocytosis) indicates hemolytic anemia. Further investigations should include blood film, osmotic fragility tests, Coombs' test, and examination of the bone marrow.

Osmotic Fragility Test. In a patient with hereditary spherocytosis, erythrocytes hemolyze in concentrations of saline solution, but erythrocytes from a healthy individual do not.

Mechanical Fragility Test. Increased mechanical fragility occurs in patients with congenital hemolytic anemia or sickle cell anemia and in some cases of atypical hemolytic anemia.

Coombs' Test. Neither the indirect nor the direct Coombs' test is positive with hereditary spherocytosis. In the acquired type of hemolytic jaundice both the direct and the indirect tests are positive when the circulating antibodies are present. Only the direct test is positive when the circulating antibodies are absent.

Tests for Viral Hepatitis. Apart from determining the serum transferase levels, the following tests are available on the sera of patients with suspected hepatitis:

- Hepatitis B surface antigen titer (Australia antigen)
- Hepatitis B surface (IgM or IgG) antibody titer
- Hepatitis B e antigen titer, which correlates with ongoing viral synthesis and infectivity
- Hepatitis core antibody titer, which can be detected after the hepatitis B surface antigen has been cleared from the serum

- Hepatitis C (IgG or IgM) antibody titer
- Cytomegalovirus IgM antibody titer
- IgM antibody titers against Epstein-Barr capsid antigens and the monospot reaction

DIAGNOSTIC IMAGING TECHNIQUES (Fig. 26-3)

The aims of imaging in the jaundiced patient are:

- To confirm or refute a clinical diagnosis of extrahepatic biliary obstruction as evidenced by dilation of the biliary tree proximal to the obstruction
- To identify the cause and the site of extrahepatic biliary obstruction and to select those patients in whom surgical treatment is indicated
- To examine the characteristics of the hepatic parenchyma, which are important in excluding the presence of focal hepatic lesions such as metastases, liver abscess, or hepatoma; this may also aid in the diagnosis of diffuse parenchymal disease

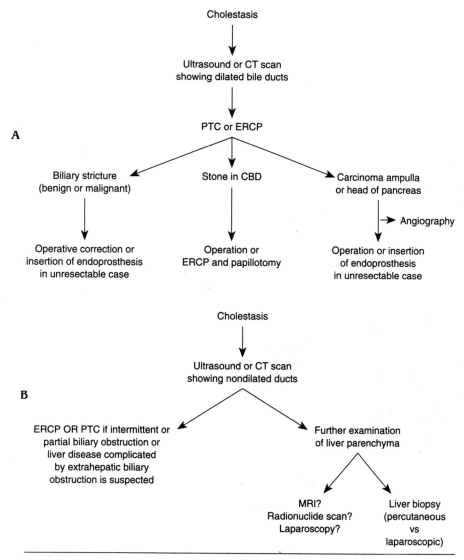

FIGURE 26-3   Management of cholestasis in the patient with a clinical diagnosis of **A,** obstructive jaundice and, **B,** intrahepatic cholestasis.

Ultrasonography (Fig. 26-4) and Computed Tomography (Fig. 26-5)

Two noninvasive techniques, ultrasonography and computed tomography (CT), are complementary and central in the investigation of the jaundiced patient. Dilation of the biliary tree, both intrahepatic and extrahepatic, can be documented in the vast majority of cases. Stones and metastases also can be seen, and solid or cystic masses of the pancreas or at the porta hepatis can be demonstrated. Both tests have a high patient acceptability rate. Ultrasonography has no radiation risk, and it has a 10% to 15% failure rate, usually resulting from the ultrasonographer's inexperience or the presence of ascites, surgically placed hemoclips, obesity, or bowel gas overlying the organ under examination. CT has a small but definite radiation risk, and the patient must be able to avoid moving and to hold his or her breath intermittently during the study.

Contrast Radiology of the Biliary Tract

Percutaneous Transhepatic Cholangiography (Fig. 26-6). Percutaneous transhepatic cholangiography (PTC) or endoscopic cholangiopancreatography (ERCP) are essential for the direct visualization of the biliary tree. These two invasive tests are complementary. One or both should be performed whenever biliary tract obstruction is suspected as the cause of the jaundice.

Endoscopic Retrograde Cholangiopancreatography (Fig. 26-7). ERCP also allows direct endoscopic visualization of the upper gastrointestinal tract and the ampullary region. Mass lesions or varices can be seen. Direct injection of dye into the main pancreatic duct and the main common bile duct delineates any abnormality. Aspirated pancreatic juice or bile with the retrograde cannula may be sent for cytologic examination. Suspicious lesions along the upper gastrointestinal tract can be obtained directly for biopsy, or brush cytology specimens can be taken. The complications of ERCP include injection pancreatitis, pancreatic or biliary sepsis, injury from instruments, and drug-induced reactions. In experienced hands success rates of up to 95% can be achieved.

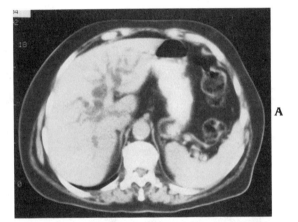

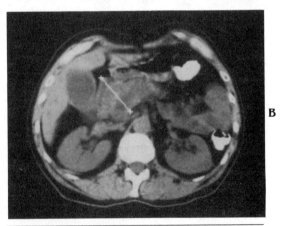

FIGURE 26-5 Computed tomography of the liver and pancreas showing, **A,** dilated intrahepatic ducts and, **B,** carcinoma of the head of the pancreas, causing obstruction of the common bile duct leading to dilation of the gallbladder (Courvoisier's sign).

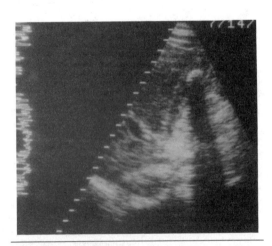

FIGURE 26-4 Ultrasound of the liver and biliary tree, with a solitary gallstone within the gallbladder showing marked echogenicity and acoustic shadowing.

PTC with the fine (Chiba) needle provides an excellent method for visualizing the biliary tree. Success rates of 89% have been reported in the presence of ductal dilation. When the fine-needle technique is used, the incidence of complication (i.e., biliary leak, bleeding, sepsis) after PTC is very low. In view of the inherent risks with either procedure, some precautions must be taken. The patient must be potentially "ready" for an operation whenever PTC or ERCP is performed. It is always safer to plan the procedure with the surgical team alerted, since urgent surgery (within 12 to 24 hours) is indicated if good visualization of dilated ducts is obtained because of the risk of biliary leak into the peritoneal cavity or the introduction of sepsis into an obstructed system.

The main indications for performing ERCP or PTC are:

- To differentiate between extrahepatic and intrahepatic cholestasis when clinical examination, laboratory tests, other imaging techniques, and even a liver biopsy have failed.
- In patients with known obstructive jaundice to provide information about the cause, site, and extent of the obstruction before the operative intervention.
- As a preliminary procedure before the operation to perform temporary drainage of an obstructed biliary system; however, recent prospective randomized studies have failed to demonstrate improved outcome following routine preoperative biliary decompression. Routinely used, the technique increases the duration and cost of the treatment, and the incidence of septic complications is increased once foreign materials (stents) are introduced into the biliary tree. However, in selected severely jaundiced patients (bilirubin level >20 mg/dl) or in those patients unfit for a major operation because of intercurrent disease (e.g., sepsis,

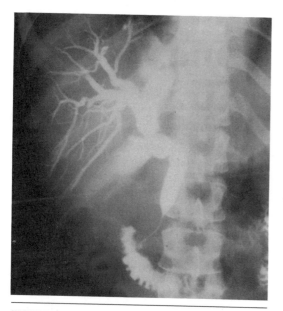

FIGURE 26-6 Percutaneous transhepatic cholangiogram showing a stricture at the lower end of the common bile duct caused by pancreatitis secondary to a small carcinoma of the ampulla of Vater.

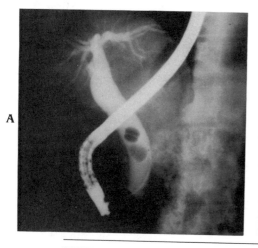

A

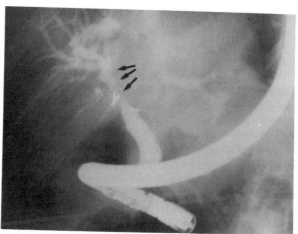

B

FIGURE 26-7 Endoscopic retrograde cholangiopancreatogram showing, **A**, stones within a dilated common bile duct and, **B**, a hilar stricture resulting from injury to the common hepatic duct during cholecystectomy.

cardiopulmonary disease, hepatorenal failure), percutaneous transhepatic drainage, or endoscopic internal stent, drainage of the obstructed biliary tree for several days is a useful adjunctive preoperative measure, but it should not unnecessarily delay definitive surgical treatment.

Oral cholangiography will *not* visualize the biliary tree if the serum bilirubin level is above 2 mg/dl. *Intravenous cholangiography* with tomography can visualize the biliary tree if the serum bilirubin level is less than 4 mg/dl. The test has a high incidence (10%) of anaphylactic reactions, and the quality of the radiographic picture is often poor; therefore both tests are not applicable to the evaluation of the jaundiced patient.

Radionuclide Liver Scans

Radionuclide liver scans are rapidly becoming obsolete, are only occasionally useful, and are often overused and misused in clinical practice. They are based on the uptake and distribution of radioactive material throughout the liver. The material is taken up by parenchymal cells or by reticuloendothelial (Kupffer) cells, and it is excreted through the biliary passages.

Three basic types of nuclear imaging are currently available:

- Technetium-99m sulphur colloid is used for routine liver scans. When injected, it is cleared by the reticuloendothelial system in the liver, spleen, and bone marrow. These scans define the hepatic anatomy and provide the following information: (1) estimation of liver and spleen size; (2) visualization of suspected liver masses (i.e., metastases, hepatomas, cysts, abscesses) that have decreased activity at the involved sites, thus producing "cold" lesions (the mass lesions must be greater than 2 cm in diameter for reliable detection); (3) evaluation of diffuse liver disease (e.g., cirrhosis)—a large area of cellular destruction or replacement fails to take up the radioactive material, and the reliability in distinguishing between the different types of parenchymal disease is low, since they all demonstrate patchy isotope uptake; and (4) assessment of splenic defects (abscesses, hematomas, cysts).
- Technetium-99m–HIDA (Tc-HIDA) and allied compounds are used for hepatobiliary scans to outline bile flow patterns. The radiopharmaceutical agent is taken up by hepatocytes and is excreted in the bile. The scan is helpful in diagnosing acute cholecystitis (nonvisualization of the gallbladder) and evaluating bile flow after biliary-enteric anastomoses (Fig. 26-8). The newer agents are secreted even in the presence of significant jaundice. The usefulness of hepatobiliary scanning for chronic cholecystitis or obstructive jaundice remains limited.
- Technetium-99m–labeled red blood cells are used to obtain blood pool images, since they outline the distribution of sinusoids in the liver. This test is occasionally needed to differentiate hemangiomas (and other highly vascular lesions) from other masses in the liver, all of which produce cold defects on colloid scans. Highly vascular lesions produce hot defects on blood pool images.

Radionuclide liver scans have largely been replaced by ultrasonography and CT with contrast enhancement in the evaluation of hepatobiliary disorders.

Angiography

Celiac and superior mesenteric angiograms visualize the celiac axis, the superior mesenteric artery, and their branches. The application of selective and superselective cannulation of small vessels, injection of drugs and hormones (pharmacoangiography), and magnification radiology have all contributed to the improved accuracy of angiography. Proper delineation of the portal vein and its tributaries is essential in planning portosystemic shunts in patients with portal hypertension. Direct mesenteric arterial infusion of vasopressin is a useful adjunct in the management of variceal hemorrhage. Displacement or encasement of vessels, avascularity, hyperemia, tumor "blush," and venous phase abnormalities can reveal the location of hepatic or pancreatic lesions. Vascular lesions in the liver can be embolized under direct radiologic control. In addition, angiography delineates anatomic variations in the vasculature to the pancreas and to the liver (e.g., identifies the origin of the right hepatic artery from the superior mesenteric artery). This may be essential information for the surgeon in planning a pancreatic or major hepatic resection.

Splenic Portography

Direct puncture of the spleen to measure splenic pulp pressure (which gives an indication of portal venous pressure) and, after injection of contrast material, to delineate the portal circulation is an outmoded method that has been aban-

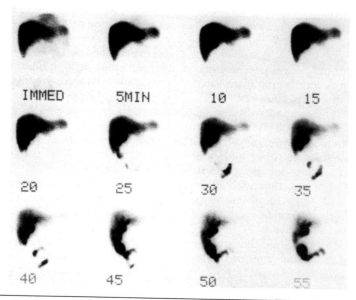

FIGURE 26-8 Biliary scintigraphy with Tc-HIDA showing a functioning hepaticojejunostomy performed to correct a high bile duct stricture.

doned in most countries. It has been totally replaced by the advent of high-quality celiac and mesenteric arteriography, which provides excellent visualization of the portal venous system.

Liver Biopsy

Liver biopsy is an essential step in the evaluation of suspected primary liver disease. Sampling error may occur with percutaneous biopsy of the liver unless diffuse disease is present. CT or ultrasonographic guidance permits accurate biopsy of focal lesions.

There are three contraindications to direct puncture of the liver:

1. A PT that is prolonged more than 3 seconds beyond control
2. A platelet count of less than 40,000/ml
3. The presence of ascites

An alternative method is to perform the liver biopsy through a peritoneoscope, which allows direct visualization of peritoneal surfaces and biopsy of the liver under direct visualization. However, the same contraindications apply. A third option is to use a radiologically controlled transvenous biopsy catheter. In this technique the biopsy catheter is passed via the internal jugular vein, across the hepatic veins, and into the liver substance. This technique avoids the hemor-

rhagic complications; however, it requires a radiologist skilled in the procedure. The advent of sophisticated techniques for investigating the jaundiced patient has rendered the "open" liver biopsy through minilaparotomy an obsolete procedure.

Contrast Studies of the Gastrointestinal Tract

A gastrointestinal series is indicated only if neoplastic disease of the gastrointestinal tract is suspected. Although this series is virtually always performed, it invariably fails to provide useful information.

INDICATIONS FOR SURGICAL INTERVENTION

The indications for an operation in a jaundiced patient can be summarized as follows:

- Surgical intervention is mandatory when biliary obstruction is present to decompress the biliary tree with or without removal of the obstructing lesion.
- Splenectomy is the treatment of choice for patients whose familial hemolytic anemia gives rise to hemolytic crises.
- Selected cases of acquired hemolytic anemia

benefit from splenectomy, although the percentage of good results is decidedly smaller than in the familial group.

Obstructive jaundice rarely necessitates an emergency operation; ample time is usually available for optimal preoperative preparation. Diagnostic laparotomy in the jaundiced patient is an outmoded procedure and is rarely, if ever, indicated. The advent and development of the various diagnostic methods previously described allow the surgeon to make an exact preoperative diagnosis and to plan the operative procedure without resorting to complicated, time-consuming diagnostic maneuvers in the operating room. Thus operations normally should not be recommended until the diagnosis is established and the general condition of the patient is restored to as near normal as circumstances allow.

PREOPERATIVE PREPARATION

The jaundiced patient often has numerous nutritional and metabolic deficiencies. This is especially true of patients with pancreatic or other intra-abdominal cancers. In addition, oral intake may have been curtailed for several days while the patient was undergoing tests. If the patient is in optimal condition, time should *not* be wasted on exhaustive preparations. The following aspects of care are important in the preoperative period.

Nutrition and Hydration. The patient should receive oral alimentation (e.g., Vivonex, Precision, or Ensure) with multivitamin supplements. Grossly malnourished patients usually benefit from a period of intravenous hyperalimentation both before and after the operation. Hydration must be ensured by using additional intravenous fluids. Renal failure due to hypovolemia is a tremendous hazard in the jaundiced patient; continued diuresis must be ensured at all times (before, during, and after the operation). Immediately postoperatively osmotic diuresis can be induced with intravenous mannitol.

Correction of Blood Deficiencies. Anemia should be corrected by blood transfusion as deemed necessary. Since hemorrhage is a common complication of an operation in a jaundiced patient, a preoperative hematocrit value of approximately 40% is advisable. Daily intramuscular injections of vitamin K (10 mg) for at least 5 days before the operation is advisable, whether or not the PT is abnormal. Adequate amounts of blood, platelets, and fresh frozen plasma should be available in the operating room.

Cardiopulmonary Function. Chest x-ray studies, pulmonary tests, and electrocardiograms are essential in the assessment of the patient for the operation. Smoking is prohibited; intensive physiotherapy, active mobilization, and leg exercises are encouraged. Prophylactic digitalization and diuretic therapy are considered in individual cases to achieve maximal cardiovascular compensation.

Bowel Preparation. This procedure is essential, especially in patients who are likely to require an enterotomy at operation. It is provided by supplementing oral alimentation with a clear liquid diet and appropriate amounts of laxatives and enemas as required. Such mechanical bowel preparation may be supplemented with 2 to 3 days of oral nonabsorbable antibiotic therapy.

Prophylactic Systemic Antibiotics. All patients with biliary tract obstruction and those in whom the surgeon expects that intraoperative contamination will occur should be given broad-spectrum antibiotic therapy intravenously for 4 days, starting 6 hours before the operation. Patients undergoing any invasive investigation of the biliary tract such as PTC or ERCP should also receive adequate antibiotic therapy.

Preoperative Biliary Decompression. This procedure may be helpful in some circumstances but is associated with the complications previously described.

SURGICAL APPROACH

The approach to the jaundiced patient must be systematic, and an emergency operation is never indicated. *The only urgent situation occurs when a patient with obstructive jaundice is septic;* acute obstructive cholangitis secondary to biliary tract obstruction demands early (but not emergency) operative, percutaneous transhepatic, or endoscopic biliary decompression after full evaluation, antibiotic therapy, and other resuscitative measures. The diagnostic work-up of the jaundiced patient is summarized in Fig. 26-9. *Not all the investigations outlined are needed in every jaundiced patient.* The physician must use his or her judgment, based on the clinical picture and results from baseline simple noninvasive tests.

The operative treatment of obstructive jaundice depends on the cause and level of the obstruction. Patients with a very high obstructing lesion at the hepatic duct bifurcation are often best decompressed by the radiologist. Laparotomy should be avoided until a preoperative diagnosis is reached. The appropriate operative tech-

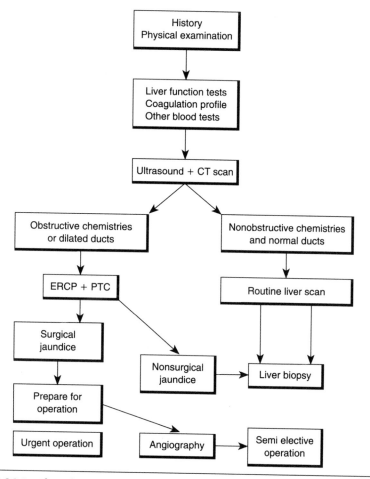

FIGURE 26-9   Flow sheet and diagnostic work-up in the jaundiced patient.

nique ranges from simple exploration of the common bile duct and extraction of stones to resection of a complex bile duct stricture or cancer to pancreatoduodenectomy.

Choledochotomy

Exploration of the common bile duct is performed to relieve obstructive jaundice caused by stones. Cholecystectomy is invariably performed concomitantly, since most common bile duct stones originally form in the gallbladder. The duodenum is mobilized, the common bile duct is incised, and exploration is carried out using stone-grasping forceps, irrigation, and balloon Fogarty catheters. Good operative cholangiography and choledochoscopy are essential to ensure that stones are not left behind. Finally, a T tube is placed in the common bile duct. Postoperatively, the T tube is left to drain freely and acts as a

controlled fistula along which a tract is formed in 7 to 14 days. A follow-up postoperative cholangiogram is then obtained, and if it is normal, the T tube should be removed. The tract will close spontaneously. Prophylactic antibiotics should be given before the T tube is removed because manipulation can induce bacteremia.

Transduodenal Sphincteroplasty

In cases in which a stone is impacted at the ampulla (i.e., the lower end of the common bile duct) or the duct is of small caliber, it may be better to open the duct from below. The duodenum is opened and the sphincter of Oddi incised laterally and sutured in this position by approximating the mucosa of the distal common bile duct to the adjacent duodenal mucosa to provide a permanent widening. The stone can then be extracted by manipulation from above and below. Successful removal is followed by T tube placement (if the common bile duct has also been opened), closure of the duodenum, and operative T tube cholangiography. This procedure often is successfully performed endoscopically, thus avoiding a major laparotomy.

Choledochoduodenostomy

Choledochoduodenostomy has gained wide acceptance as a safe and perhaps simpler means of handling a difficult problem with common bile duct exploration in the presence of an impacted stone in the distal end of the duct, with or without stricture formation. A planned anastomosis is constructed between the common bile duct (diagonal or transverse) and the duodenum, with the final anastomosis at least 2 cm wide. The indications for a side-to-side choledochoduodenostomy vary from surgeon to surgeon but include any of the following situations:

- Multiple stones (more than 10) in the common bile duct, with the implication that they cannot all be removed
- Intrahepatic calculi that cannot be reached
- Reoperation for common duct stones
- Multiple stones in an elderly or frail patient
- Retained impacted stone or stones

One theoretic disadvantage of a side-to-side choledochoduodenostomy is that the blind, undrained part of the duct distal to the anastomosis can act as a sump, and food debris (e.g., vegetable matter) can remain impacted in it (sump syndrome). This possibility is written about more than it is seen clinically.

Some people have advocated complete transection of the duct and its reimplantation into the duodenum—the so-called reimplantation choledochoduodenostomy—but it is rarely indicated. Although reflux of duodenal content into the biliary tree occurs freely from either a sphincteroplasty or any type of choledochoduodenostomy, development of cholangitis is rare unless stenosis of the anastomosis occurs or the anastomosis was too small when constructed. After the establishment of operative or spontaneous biliary enteric communication, air commonly is seen within the biliary tree on plain abdominal radiographs.

Retained Common Duct Stones

After successful removal of common duct stones or after simple cholecystectomy, obstructive jaundice may occur secondary to retained common duct stones. New (primary) common duct stones may also form. Primary stones are soft and crumble easily, whereas retained stones frequently are faceted and quite hard. They may be discovered at the time of postoperative T tube cholangiography or at any time afterward if associated with jaundice or cholangitis.

The first important point is that the problem is best prevented rather than treated. Performing proper operative cholangiography at the time of cholecystectomy and the judicious use of the choledochoscope can reduce the incidence of retained stones to a negligible level. The first attempt at removal of the stone is nonoperative. If a T tube is present, constant irrigation with a heparin solution or sodium taurocholate solution results in crumbling and passage of the stone in some patients. An alternative approach is removal of the T tube and immediate passage under radiologic control of a Dormia stone basket along its tract. With an adequately sized tract (16 French or more), most retained stones can be removed in this manner with minimal morbidity. If a T tube is not present, endoscopic transduodenal sphincterotomy may be attempted, which is 90% successful in experienced hands but is associated with the additional hazard of causing pancreatitis.

Common Duct Stricture

Injury to the common bile duct during routine cholecystectomy may lead to stricture formation and obstructive jaundice. The criteria for successful repair of an injured bile duct are as follows:

- Construction of the widest possible stoma
- Careful mucosa-to-mucosa approximation (duct to duct or duct to small bowel) around 360 degrees
- Good blood supply to the anastomotic line
- No tension on the anastomosis
- Temporary splinting of the anastomosis to ensure that the anastomosis remains patent until healing is achieved and to decompress the proximal biliary tree

If operative injury is recognized at the initial procedure, precise end-to-end anastomosis over a T tube is recommended. In this case the T tube should be brought out through the duct below the anastomosis to preserve valuable upper duct length in case further repair becomes necessary. Unfortunately, most injured bile ducts are recognized at variable times after the injury. Reoperation is difficult and time consuming and must be performed by a surgeon experienced in biliary tract reconstruction. Exploration of the porta hepatis and dissection of the proximal duct must be achieved without injury to the portal vein or hepatic artery. Doing so requires experience and perseverance. Operative repair consists of resection of the fibrous stricture with anastomosis of the proximal duct to a Roux-en-Y loop of small bowel according to the principles outlined previously.

Sclerosing Cholangitis

Sclerosing cholangitis is a rare and difficult condition of unknown etiology. It sometimes is associated with ulcerative colitis or Crohn's disease. The common bile duct is greatly thickened throughout its length, and its lumen is markedly compromised. The condition often is confused with a primary common bile duct carcinoma, and even multiple biopsies do not always confirm the diagnosis. The disease tends to run a long, gradually progressive, and often unpredictable course. The eventual sequelae invariably develop from secondary biliary cirrhosis and portal hypertension. Strictures can occasionally be treated surgically, and once liver disease has become advanced, liver transplantation is indicated in suitable candidates.

Liver Transplantation

Patient selection and timing are crucial to the success of liver transplantation even more than in other surgical areas of endeavor. Patients who might be suitable transplant candidates should be discussed early with the transplant team. The indications for liver replacement in adults can be divided into three groups: those with (1) chronic end-stage liver disease such as primary biliary cirrhosis, chronic active hepatitis, primary sclerosing cholangitis, and cryptogenic cirrhosis; (2) acute hepatic failure such as fulminant hepatitis or that which follows acetaminophen (paracetamol) poisoning; or (3) primary hepatic malignancy. In children additional criteria are (1) inborn errors of metabolism such as tyrosinemia and (2) biliary atresia.

Absolute contraindications for transplantation are active extrahepatic sepsis, human immunodeficiency virus positivity, extrahepatic malignancy, uncorrected hyponatremia, and severe cardiopulmonary dysfunction. Relative contraindications are age above 65 years, portal vein thrombosis, previous upper abdominal surgery, hepatitis B positivity, renal impairment, and biliary sepsis. Postoperatively patients must be maintained on immunosuppressive therapy,

using combinations of prednisolone, azathioprine, and cyclosporine.

Five-year survival rates of up to 90% can be achieved in select patient groups (e.g., those with primary biliary cirrhosis), but overall survival rates are approximately 50% to 60%.

Periampullary Carcinoma (Including Carcinoma of the Head of the Pancreas)

A mass in the ampullary region of the ampulla of Vater may be benign (pancreatitis, pseudocyst) or malignant (primary cancer of the head of the pancreas, ampulla, duodenum, or lower end of the common bile duct). With good preoperative evaluation, obstructive jaundice from any of these causes can be distinguished from one another, and the diagnosis of carcinoma can be established by cytology. In some cases performing operative needle biopsy may be necessary to establish a firm diagnosis. In a small percentage of situations the surgeon may be totally unsure as to whether the mass is benign or malignant and must proceed according to his or her clinical judgment and the patient's general condition. Some surgeons do not recommend obtaining a biopsy specimen from a localized, resectable mass but go directly to resection.

Resectability of a periampullary mass depends on several parameters, including (1) absence of distal spread to the liver or the peritoneal cavity and (2) absence of invasion of the portal vein, superior mesenteric artery, or celiac axis. These conditions should be determined before a surgeon commits to performing a resection. If the lesion is confined to the ampulla, duodenum, or lower end of the common bile duct, the appropriate procedure is a pancreatoduodenectomy (Whipple operation). It entails removal of the head and neck of the pancreas, the lower end of the common bile duct, the gallbladder, the distal half of the stomach, the duodenum, the upper jejunum, and the regional nodes. The body and tail of the pancreas are preserved. If the lesion is a ductal adenocarcinoma of the pancreatic head, some surgeons extend the Whipple operation into a total pancreatoduodenectomy. The risks associated with such major pancreatic resections are unacceptably high worldwide, but a mortality rate under 5% is being achieved in specialized centers where there are experience and expertise in the investigation and treatment of these patients. The 5-year survival rate of patients with true ampullary lesions is 40% to 60%. The 5-year survival rate for patients with cancer of the head of the pancreas is 10% to 25%.

If the periampullary lesion is unresectable or metastatic, palliation is achieved by internal biliary drainage, and a positive biopsy result is mandatory. Palliation is accomplished by anastomosing the gallbladder (if it is distended and the cystic duct is patent) to the jejunum. If the lesion is more extensive and involves the cystic duct, the proximal hepatic duct must be used for the anastomosis. The aim of biliary bypass is to palliate jaundice, pruritus, and impending cholangitis. Gastrojejunostomy should be performed during the same operation to obviate the possibility of later duodenal obstruction (occurs in 35% of patients). The life expectancy of these patients averages 6 to 8 months, although an occasional patient may live as long as 2 years.

NONOPERATIVE RELIEF OF OBSTRUCTIVE JAUNDICE
Papillotomy and ERCP

After ERCP and the identification of common bile duct stones, the cholangiography catheter is replaced by a sphincterotome (Fig. 26-10). By maintaining tension on the cutting wire, the sphincterotome can be bowed within the lower common bile duct and a diathermy current passed along the wire. In a controlled manner the device can be used to divide the papilla and to open the intraduodenal portion of the lower common duct. Any stones within the common duct will either pass spontaneously into the duodenum or can be retrieved using a Dormia stone basket or balloon catheter. Large stones can also be crushed within the duct using a mechanical lithotripsy device or can be fragmented using laser lithotripsy.

ERCP and papillotomy are indicated (1) for patients with retained stones in the common bile duct after cholecystectomy and (2) as a primary treatment for selected patients with choledocholithiasis when associated gallbladder stones are "silent." Suitable patients are elderly or have a coexisting medical disease making them unfit for surgery. In younger, more fit patients, leaving the gallbladder in situ may predispose them to future episodes of cholecystitis, the passage of further stones from the gallbladder to the common duct, and the small associated risk of carcinoma of the gallbladder.

Stenting

To relieve obstructive jaundice caused by malignant biliary obstruction, up to size 10 French stents can be placed across biliary strictures ei-

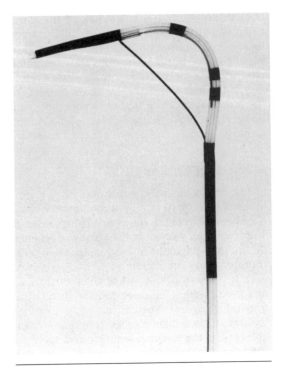

FIGURE 26-10   Wire-guided papillotome.

ther from below after ERCP and access papillotomy or from above after PTC. For either technique, a guidewire is placed across the stricture, and a stent is "railroaded" over the guidewire. The stent thus decompresses the biliary tree. Larger metal stents are available that can be expanded to a greater diameter when in place.

Stenting is an acceptable method of palliation of the symptoms of jaundice in (1) patients with unresectable tumors of the head of the pancreas or ampulla; (2) patients with an extensive tumor at the hilum of the liver that may be difficult to palliate surgically; and (3) patients with coexisting medical problems that make them unfit for surgery.

There is little difference in the overall survival rate between patients with unresectable malignant biliary obstruction whose jaundice is palliated by stenting compared with those with surgical internal drainage. Stenting, however, can require recurrent hospital admissions for catheter replacement (every 8 to 12 weeks), and septic complications are common. Endoscopic stenting is possible only in patients without duodenal obstruction, and in stented patients duodenal obstruction may subsequently develop, requiring gastrojejunostomy.

PITFALLS AND COMMON MYTHS

Several common clinical situations in the management of jaundice result from false assumptions or the misinterpretation of results.

- The presence of gallstones in the gallbladder does not necessarily indicate that gallstones are the cause of the jaundice. Gallstones are common in the general population, and cholelithiasis is only one of the differential diagnoses. Gallstones in the gallbladder alone do not cause jaundice unless accompanied by other complications.

- Conversely, the presence of a pancreatic mass, suggestive of a carcinoma of the head of the pancreas, does not rule out the diagnosis of choledocholithiasis with associated pancreatitis. Direct visualization of the lower end of the bile duct by either ERCP or PTC may be required.

- The absence of bile duct dilation does not exclude choledocholithiasis, especially if (1) the stone has just recently passed from the gallbladder into the common bile duct, (2) the stone is causing intermittent obstruction, or (3) the stone passes into the duodenum before the investigations are performed.

- The diagnosis of carcinoma of the gallbladder is difficult to make preoperatively because of the confusion between the CT and ultrasound appearance of a mass caused by a tumor or inflammation. A tumor at the neck of the gallbladder can be complicated by empyema. An inflammatory mass in the region of the gallbladder can compress the common bile duct to cause jaundice (Mirizzi's syndrome), but it is not uncommon to find an unresectable tumor during laparotomy.

BIBLIOGRAPHY

Cooper AD. Pathogenesis and therapy of gallstone disease. Gastroenterol Clin North Am 20:1, 1991.

Moossa AR. Tumors of the Pancreas. Baltimore, Williams & Wilkins, 1980.

Moossa AR, Schimpff SC, Robson MC. Comprehensive Textbook of Oncology. Baltimore, Williams & Wilkins, 1991.

Schwartz SI, Ellis H, Husser WC. Maingot's Abdominal Operations, 9th ed. Norwalk, Conn, Appleton & Lange, 1989.

Sherlock S. Diseases of the Liver and Biliary System, 8th ed. Boston, Blackwell Scientific Publications, 1989.

CHAPTER REVIEW
Questions

1. A 43-year-old woman is admitted to the hospital with jaundice and mild abdominal pain of 2 days' duration. She had an uneventful cholecystectomy 3 months previously. At admission her temperature is 37.2° C (99° F), and her white blood count (WBC) is 11,700. Outline your management of this patient.

2. List three tests used in the diagnosis of a hepatic mass.

3. A jaundiced patient has an elevated aspartate aminotransferase level, an elevated bilirubin level, and an abnormal prothrombin time. List two methods of differentiating extrahepatic obstruction from intrahepatic cholestasis caused by severe hepatitis.

4. A palpable gallbladder in a patient with extrahepatic obstructive jaundice points to a diagnosis of:
   a. Papillitis of the ampulla of Vater
   b. Common duct stricture
   c. Periampullary carcinoma
   d. Stones
   e. Empyema of the gallbladder

5. List the tests that can be performed in a jaundiced patient within 30 minutes of admission.

6. What is the most important aspect of making a differential diagnosis between hepatocellular and extrahepatic jaundice?

7. Cite the indications for ERCP.

8. List the differences in history and physical examination between a patient with biliary obstruction caused by a stone of the lower end of the common bile duct and a periampullary carcinoma.

Answers

1. If you failed to provide for observation of temperature, WBC, and abdominal findings every 2 to 4 hours, mark yourself *incorrect*. The work-up is incidental to determining that no cholangitis is developing. The differential diagnoses include retained common duct stone, bile duct stricture, and periampullary carcinoma that was missed at cholecystectomy. The recommended investigations include liver chemistries, ultrasonography (or CT

scan), and ERCP (or PTC). If the patient develops obvious cholangitis, urgent biliary decompression by radiologic, endoscopic, or surgical means becomes mandatory.

2. Ultrasonography, hepatic artery angiography, and CT scan.

3. Administer vitamin K; the prothrombin time should respond by returning to normal in the patient with extrahepatic obstruction.

   The alkaline phosphatase level may be normal in a patient with hepatitis but is elevated in a patient with extrahepatic obstruction.

   Ultrasonography or CT scan will demonstrate dilated bile ducts in a patient with extrahepatic biliary obstruction.

   ERCP or PTC will delineate the level of obstruction if present.

4. c

5. Measurement of temperature
   Palpation of the abdomen
   Examination of stool color
   Stool guaiac test for occult blood
   Examination of the urine for bile and urobilinogen

6. Obtaining an accurate history of the onset and development of a patient's symptoms

7. To demonstrate the site of obstruction in a dilated common bile duct
   To visualize the common bile duct when other tests are ambiguous
   To visualize the pancreatic ducts
   To perform a transduodenal papillotomy in the presence of stones retained in the common bile duct or to place a stent in patients with unresectable malignancy (therapeutic)
   (Performing ERCP after gallstone pancreatitis is controversial but may be of benefit in a subgroup of patients.)

8. In a patient with gallstone disease the classic history includes biliary colic, whereas the patient with jaundice associated with periampullary carcinoma is frequently pain free. Jaundice caused by stones is sometimes intermittent, whereas jaundice caused by a tumor is often slowly progressive. On examination, the gallbladder may be palpably enlarged in a patient with a periampullary carcinoma.

27 | Abnormal Bowel Movements

MICHAEL D. TRAYNOR
EDWIN C. JAMES
BERNARD GARDNER

KEY FEATURES

After reading this chapter you will understand:
- How a stool is formed.
- What physiologic abnormalities affect bowel movements.
- Some effective tests for distinguishing the cause of abnormal bowel movements.
- How various diseases affect bowel movements.
- Diagnosis and treatment of inflammatory and malignant bowel conditions.
- The causes of paralytic bowel.

PHYSIOLOGY OF STOOL FORMATION AND TRANSIT
Composition of Stool

The character of a bowel movement depends on several factors: (1) the composition of the ingested food, (2) the integrity of the digestive processes, (3) the absorptive mechanisms in the small and large intestines, and (4) the rate of propulsion along the gastrointestinal tract. For a brief review of the mechanisms of digestion and activities of the enzymes involved in fat, carbohydrate, and protein digestion, see Chapter 10.

In western societies an average stool weight is 200 to 250 g day. Normal stool is composed of nondigested and therefore unabsorbed substances and large numbers of bacteria. The amount of undigested fiber or ash in the diet will control the bulk of the stool, which is composed primarily of normal intestinal flora.

Stools of all consistencies are made up of approximately two thirds water, and stool weight reflects the fecal excretion of water. The absorptive capacity of the colon is critical in the consistency of the stool that is expelled from the rectum. In healthy subjects, the colon absorbs 1 to 2 L of water and up to 200 mEq of sodium and chloride each day. Maximal absorptive capacity of the colon is 5 to 6 L/day, and without this capacity to reabsorb fluid, an overflow state would invariably lead to incapacitating diarrhea.

Absorption in the bowel is affected by several parameters: (1) the state in which the substance is presented to the intestinal mucosa, a factor controlled primarily by the availability and activity of digestive enzymes; (2) the ability of various portions of the intestine to absorb the substance, which relates to the integrity of the intestinal wall and can be altered by disease states; and (3) the rate at which the substance passes along the alimentary canal or bypasses segments of intestine (Fig. 27-1).

Bacterial Flora. Bacteria are normally present in all segments of the intestine, whereas the acidity level of the stomach and duodenum keeps these areas relatively free of bacteria. The number of bacteria increases in samples from distal segments of the gastrointestinal tract, reaching a peak in the left side of the colon. The small number of bacteria in the upper intestine represents an equilibrium, so that significant increases or decreases in bacterial population are associated with well-defined pathologic states (see the box on p. 483).

481

Metabolic Effects of Bacteria on the Host.
Bacteria are responsible for many chemical reactions that can affect the well-being of the host. It can be seen from the box on p. 483 that increases, decreases, or alterations in the bacterial flora can produce changes in stool composition or damage to the intestinal wall that may lead to malabsorption and diarrhea.

How Are Specific Substances Absorbed?

Water. Bidirectional movement of water and electrolytes occurs throughout the intestinal tract. In the duodenum, the movements in each direction are approximately equal, so that the net changes in water movements are not apparent. The bulk of water reabsorption occurs in the distal jejunum and ileum. The fecal contents are liquid as they enter the colon, where an additional 0.5 to 1.5 L/day of water resorption occurs in the colon (Fig. 27-2). Various portions of the colon are important in absorption. A healthy colon absorbs more than 90% of the fluid it receives. If colonic absorption is impaired and subsequently reduced from 90% to 50%, stool volumes will increase from 200 to 750 ml/day. This is enough to constitute a significant diarrhea.

Carbohydrates. Carbohydrates can be absorbed as monosaccharides or disaccharides. Transport is against a concentration gradient and is higher in the jejunum than in the ileum. The preferential absorption of glucose and galactose may be related to the stearic configuration of these molecules.

Fats. Approximately 40% of the calories of an average mixed diet are in the form of fat. Absorption is extremely efficient, so that within a dietary range of 50 to 200 g, the normal upper limit of fat in the stool should be under 8 g/day. Short-chain fatty acids pass directly to the liver via the portal circulation after absorption. The longer-chain fatty acids (over 10 carbon atoms) are resynthesized to triglycerides in the mucosal cells and pass to the lymph channels, from which they enter the bloodstream via the thoracic duct.

Protein. Digestion to amino acids and small-chain peptides is essential for absorption. The proximal segments of intestine absorb these products much more efficiently than do the distal segments. The efficiency of the digestive process is so great that the appearance of intact meat fibers in the stool is an indicator of a malabsorption syndrome.

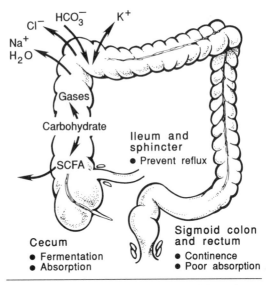

FIGURE 27-1 Absorptive functions of the colon. *SCFA* = short-chain fatty acid. (Modified from Pemberton JH, Phillips SF. Colonic absorption. Perspect Colon Rectal Surg 1:90, 1988.)

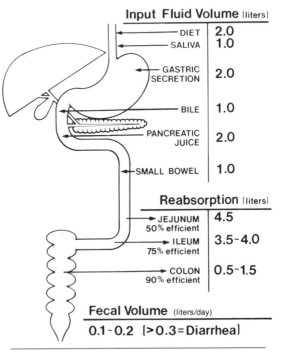

FIGURE 27-2 Intestinal fluid flux. (From James EC, Tolstedt GE, Keller RT, et al. The small intestine. In James EC, Corry RJ, Perry JF Jr [eds]. Principles of Basic Surgical Practice. St Louis, CV Mosby, 1987, p 274.)

METABOLIC EFFECTS OF INTESTINAL BACTERIA

Beneficial

Activation of ingested drugs
Synthesis of vitamin K
Hydrolysis of proteins (provision of essential amino acids)
Production of folic acid (?)
Improvement in efficiency of enterohepatic biliary circulation

Detrimental

Reduction in calories
Uptake of vitamin B_{12}
Destruction of folic acid
Destruction of vitamin C (?)
Consumption of xylose
Lipid hydrolysis (production of abnormal fatty acids)
Formation of carcinogens from ingested drugs (?)
Deconjugation of bile acids
Dehydroxylation of bile acids

Cellulose

Up to 20% of dietary cellulose and hemicellulose that reaches the large bowel is degraded. Sugars can be metabolized in the colon in patients who have a carbohydrate malabsorption problem. However, in a healthy individual, unabsorbed sugars are probably of little significance. The 10% of starch that escapes digestion or absorption by the small intestine is used in the large intestine by the fecal flora for calories and is a major source of volatile fatty acids in the colon.

How Does Transit in the Gastrointestinal Tract Affect Bowel Movements?

To completely understand the definition of transit in the GI tract as it relates to bowel movements, one must have a clear definition of diarrhea and constipation, which represent two ends of a continuum.

Constipation is defined as defecation that occurs less than twice per week, or defecation that requires excessive strain to initiate or complete, is

painful, or feels incomplete. ***Diarrhea is defined as malabsorption or excessive secretion of water (and electrolytes).***

Small Intestine. The speed of transport of food influences the rate of digestion and the time available for absorption to occur.

Segmentation. Rhythmic movements of the small intestine occur at several-centimeter distances that effectively isolate segments of the intestine and lead to improved mixing of food and enzymes as well as better contact with the absorptive surfaces of the villi. The rate of segmentation is higher in the duodenum and slows progressively as the distal ileum is reached.

Peristalsis. It is thought that material progresses along the small intestine by active peristaltic waves that pass from proximal to distal bowel. These last for one to several seconds and are under neurogenic control.

Large Intestine

Segmentation. As with the small bowel, segmentation occurs in the large intestine and is known as ***haustral contractions.*** These movements are more effective for mixing than for forward propulsion. Haustral markings on x-ray films help one to readily differentiate or distinguish colonic gas from that in the small intestine, which can be identified by the valvulae conniventes.

Mass Movements. Since peristalsis does not occur in the colon, propulsion of fecal matter relies primarily on the mass movements of long segments of colon. It has been demonstrated that these are associated with minimal or no rise in intraluminal pressure, thus accounting for the failure of colonic stretch receptors to be stimulated with distal obstructions—thus the late appearance of pain and frequent absence of vomiting in left-colonic obstruction (see Chapter 25).

Rectum and Anus

Defecation. The act of defecation is a complex procedure involving the autonomic and sympathetic nervous systems. When a fecal bolus enters the rectum, the receptor, which is believed to be outside the rectal wall and most likely is located in the pelvic floor, will register a sensation, causing the urge to defecate. Distention of the rectum causes a reflex relaxation of the internal sphincter, which allows the fecal contents to make contact with the anal canal while the external sphincter and puborectalis contract. This in turn allows the sensory epithelium of the anal canal to sense and discriminate the contents, which is known as ***sampling response.*** If rectal distention is maintained for a long time, the rectal musculature adapts to decrease the rectal pressure. This is known as ***accommodation response.*** However, urge and defecation occur when the stimulus from the rectum increases rapidly to overcome the accommodation response, usually when a large amount of liquid stool enters the rectum.

The act of defecation proceeds, with the person assuming a squatting or sitting position to straighten out the angle between the rectum and anal canal. Expulsion of feces is accomplished by contraction of the rectum and by increased intra-abdominal pressure by the Valsalva maneuver. Although any rise in abdominal pressure causes an immediate increase in the reflex tone of the pelvic floor muscles, defecation straining abolishes the reflex tone of the pelvic floor muscles and the anal sphincter muscles. After defecation is completed, the voluntary sphincters contract actively and the normal postural tone is restored.

DIARRHEA
Diagnostic Approach

After a thorough history is taken and a physical examination performed, a diagnosis can be made based on several main objectives: (1) evaluation of the stool, (2) measurement of the absorptive capacity of the bowel, (3) evaluation of transit time, and (4) ancillary tests.

Four major mechanisms can lead to excessive loss of fecal water: osmotic retention of water in the lumen, secretion of solute and water into the lumen, exudation, and disorder contact between chyme and the absorptive surface (see the box below).

Osmotic Diarrhea. Osmotic diarrhea occurs when water-soluble molecules are so poorly absorbed that their presence in the lumen causes retention of excessive water in the bowel. This type of diarrhea can be caused by fecal bacteria forming unabsorbed carbohydrates into organic

---

DIARRHEAL AND STEATORRHEAL STATES

Lesions Affecting Intestinal Wall

Gluten-sensitive enteropathy
Tropical sprue
Crohn's disease
Ulcerative colitis
Radiation (factitious) colitis
Macroglobulinemia
Lymphoma
Amyloidosis

Infection

Bacterial
  Typhoid
  Shigellosis
  Staphylococcal
  Enteritis
  Cholera
Parasitic infestations
  Whipple's disease

Alteration in Bacterial Flora

Blind loop syndrome
Antibacterial drugs (overgrowth of pathogenic organisms)
Gastric hypoacidity (resection)
Gastric hyperacidity

Maldigestion

Bile duct obstruction
Pancreatic duct obstruction (carcinoma)
Pancreatitis, chronic
Pancreatic resection
Cystic fibrosis (pancreas)

Rapid Transit

Bowel fistulas
Short bowel (from extensive or multiple resections)
Tumors
  Intrinsic
  Extrinsic

Vascular Deficiency

Mesenteric occlusion
Polyarteritis

Biochemical (Hormonal)

Thyrotoxicosis
Diabetes mellitus
Carcinoid syndrome
Zollinger-Ellison syndrome
Vagotomy
Villous adenoma
Pancreaticogenic watery diarrhea syndrome

anions or by the overuse of saline laxatives or antacids, which are poorly absorbed polyvalent ions such as magnesium and phosphorus.

Secretory Diarrhea. This occurs when the mucosa of the small or large intestine is stimulated to secrete rather than absorb fluid.

Exudative Diarrhea. Exudative diarrhea occurs as a consequence of the outpouring into the bowel of protein, blood, or mucus from sites of inflammation. Classic examples are found in patients with inflammatory bowel disease (Crohn's colitis, ulcerative colitis) or parasitic and bacterial infections.

Disordered Contact Between Chyme and the Absorptive Surface. Abnormal intestinal transit can be seen after significant intestinal resection or bypass in which patients develop the short bowel syndrome. It can also be seen with motility disorders. Slow transit leads to stasis, the "blind loop" syndrome, resulting in bacterial proliferation, malabsorption, and diarrhea. Drugs can also interfere with intestinal motility and create problems with absorption.

Evaluation of the Stool. Careful microscopic examination of the stool should be made to determine the presence of undigested meat fibers or excess fat to establish the existence of malabsorption. Since diarrhea may be caused by a series of infectious agents, culture studies for pathogens and examination for ova and parasites are fundamental to a complete evaluation. A stool guaiac test may indicate the presence of an intrinsic mucosal lesion (carcinoma). The size, consistency, presence of mucus, blood, and undigested food, and associated fever or weight loss are historical factors that may be of diagnostic value.

Measurement of the Absorptive Capacity of the Bowel. Special diagnostic procedures involving the use of radioactive-labeled substrates to determine the absorptive function of the bowel can differentiate primary from secondary malabsorption states. For example, patients who exhibit normal absorption of oleic acid but defective absorption of triolein clearly have the ability to absorb fats but a defect in fat digestion. Such a condition may be present in chronic pancreatitis, with a failure to produce or excrete pancreatic lipase. Testing for the absorption of D-xylose, decreases in the serum levels of fat-soluble vitamins (A, D, K, and E), and the presence of osteomalacia, indicating a defect in calcium absorption, may elucidate a malabsorption syndrome.

Evaluation of Abnormalities in Transit Time. Fluoroscopic delineation of the passage of barium through the GI tract will indicate the rate of transit, abnormalities of the contour, distensibility, and mucosal lining of the gut, and the presence of short circuits or blind loops. In healthy subjects with normal bowel habits, contents of the colon will be moved, under resting conditions, at a rate of only 1 cm/hour. Another important measurement of transit time is to have the patient ingest radiopaque markers and then take serial x-ray films to monitor their excretion, which provides a mouth-to-anus transit time. It is estimated that it takes 12 hours for markers to leave the stomach, pass through the small intestine, and into the colon. Thereafter transit through the large intestine occurs in 36 to 48 hours. One third of this time is taken up in the right colon, one third in the left colon, and one third in the rectosigmoid region.

Ancillary Tests. The direct visualization and biopsy of segments of the gut provide pathologic evidence for many disease entities associated with diarrhea. Rectal and sigmoidoscopic examinations are essential, and biopsy of appropriate lesions or abnormal-appearing mucosa may yield evidence of parasitic infestations, colitis, or cancer. The extended use of colonoscopy and fiberoptic endoscopy of the upper GI tract has provided significant diagnostic advances, particularly when associated with small intestinal or colonic biopsy. ***Endoscopic retrograde cholangiopancreatography*** (ERCP) has provided direct visualization of the pancreatic ducts and facilitated the diagnosis of chronic pancreatitis and pancreatic carcinoma.

What Causes Malabsorption?

Defective Digestion

Chronic Pancreatitis. Chronic pancreatitis is a disease manifested primarily by weight loss and malabsorption. It is characterized by steatorrhea, which is malabsorption of fat caused by decreased production of pancreatic lipase, and tends to result in large, bulky, greasy stools that may float on the surface of the water in the toilet bowl. If the pancreatic gland is quite scarred, this is usually an end-stage pancreatitis found most frequently in chronic alcoholics. The main pancreatic ducts are dilated as a result of chronic destruction of the gland, leading to persistent or recurrent pain syndromes. The gland may also show calcifications on x-ray examination.

The diagnosis can be confirmed by ERCP that shows the obstructed ducts and a classic "chain-of-lakes" type of appearance (Fig. 27-3). Other diagnostic tests include CT scanning, to assess

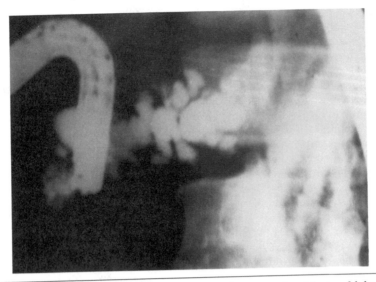

FIGURE 27-3   ERCP in a patient with pancreatitis demonstrating "chain-of-lakes" appearance.

the gland, and duodenal aspiration, which can accurately determine pancreatic insufficiency in advanced cases. Amylase values are usually normal or low. Indirect tests of pancreatic function include pancreatic polypeptide release, radio-immunoassay of trypsin, and measurement of pancreatic isoamylase inhibitor. Patients may be thin and cachectic. Addiction to pain-relieving drugs is common.

Treatment. Supportive treatment with exogenous pancreatic enzymes improves the nutrition of the patient but does not relieve the primary syndrome of chronic pain. Operations that have been described for this disease and that involve some sort of drainage procedure to the pancreatic ductal system include the following:

1. *Retrograde pancreaticojejunostomy* (Duval). The procedure involves resection of the tail of the pancreas with anastomosis of the dilated duct to a Roux-en-Y loop of jejunum. Long-term results have not been good, with recurrent pain appearing months to years after the procedure in most cases.
2. *Side-to-side pancreaticojejunostomy* (Puestow). The dilated pancreatic duct is located and opened for its length throughout the pancreas. A Roux-en-Y loop of jejunum is anastomosed to the duct for drainage. The results have proved more successful than retrograde drainage, with 60% of patients free of pain in long-term follow-up. In some cases the duct is small or attenuated, and the drainage procedure fails.

3. *Subtotal pancreatectomy* (Child). In cases in which drainage is impractical because a duct is small or has failed to provide satisfactory drainage, a subtotal (90% to 95%) resection of the gland has provided relief of pain. This procedure leaves the most proximal portion of the pancreas intact, which avoids some of the complications of duodenal resection and biliary duct anastomosis.
4. *Total pancreatectomy.* Total pancreatectomy is the most drastic procedure and is used in refractory cases when the patient has persistent weight loss and incapacitating pain. This will render the patient diabetic and insulin dependent and will also necessitate exogenous pancreatic enzyme supplementation.

Obstruction of the Pancreatic Duct. Obstruction of the pancreatic ductal system leads to a change in the character and number of stools as a result of inability of the pancreatic digestive enzymes to come in contact with food. Weight loss is characteristic. This combination of symptoms can indicate an early carcinoma of the pancreas (without jaundice) or, on occasion, calculous obstruction at the ampulla of Vater (Chapters 25 and 26). The diagnosis is extremely difficult and may require ERCP or, more rarely, abdominal exploration. Treatment of pancreatic carcinoma is discussed in Chapter 26.

Malabsorption Due to Rapid Transit

Abnormal Substances in the Stool. An irritating substance such as blood in the lumen of the gut may produce diarrhea. In some cases, the action of increased bacterial growth may provide considerable breakdown and metabolism of normal bile acids to products such as deoxycholic acid that produce marked irritation of the bowel lumen and diarrhea. This is thought to be the mechanism involved in diarrhea resulting from bacterial overgrowth of resistant strains when antibiotics are used. In patients receiving oral or systemic antibiotics, pathogens such as *Staphylococcus aureus* may overgrow the normal intestinal flora, leading to the dreaded complication of *staphylococcal enteritis.* Treatment is to restore the normal intestinal flora by using specific antibiotics, Lactobacillus tablets, and, rarely, the administration of stool enemas from a noninfected patient.

Another classic example of pathogen overgrowth is *pseudomembranous colitis,* which usually produces a severe diarrheal syndrome characterized by yellowish pseudomembranes along the colonic and rectal mucosa. The condition, an inflammatory necrosis of the large intestinal mucosa, can follow administration of any broad-spectrum antibiotic but most often occurs with the use of clindamycin, ampicillin, and the cephalosporins. The responsible agent is an enterotoxin produced by an overgrowth of *Clostridium difficile,* an organism normally a part of the regular colonic flora. Diarrhea may not always be a major component of the infection, since some patients may first be seen in an acute surgical emergency situation with perforation or toxic megacolon.

Diagnosis is made by fiberoptic sigmoidoscopy, which demonstrates an inflamed, friable mucosa with yellowish plaques and a grayish membrane, and by stools that are confirmed to contain the *C. difficile* enterotoxin. Treatment is first to discontinue the offending antibiotic. In severe cases, metronidazole, given intravenously, is the drug of choice, which usually results in resolution of symptoms and abdominal signs within a week. In less severe cases of pseudomembranous colitis, vancomycin, 250 mg, can be given orally for 7 days.

A similar mechanism of bacterial overgrowth is present in patients with the *blind loop syndrome.* This is a postsurgical complication occurring after intestinal bypass procedures that exclude segments of the gastrointestinal tract, allowing them to remain outside the main flow of the intestinal contents. In the past it more commonly occurred after a Billroth II gastrojejunostomy than other operations of the small bowel. It is caused by stagnation of intestinal contents that have been excluded from the flow of chyme. The bacterial proliferation interferes with metabolism of folate and vitamin B_{12}, causing megaloblastic anemia. Patients experience abdominal cramping, bloating, diarrhea, steatorrhea (as a result of altered absorption of fats and bile acids), and weight loss. Results of the *Schilling test* (radioactive cobalt 57–labeled vitamin B_{12} absorption) will be abnormal. Treatment is by judicious use of antibiotics and operative correction by taking down or resecting the intestinal bypass and restoring the main continuity of the intestinal canal.

Mechanical Short Circuits

Pathogenesis and Diagnosis. Mechanical short circuits occur when an abnormal connection of one segment of bowel with another leads to bypassing a long segment of the gastrointestinal tract. They may be caused by:

- Ulcer disease, with production of a gastrocolic or gastrojejunocolic fistula—prone to occur after a Billroth II anastomosis or simple gastrojejunostomy if recurrent or marginal ulceration causes perforation into the adjacent transverse colon or small bowel
- Iatrogenic injury of segments of the bowel at operation with subsequent production of fistulas
- Foreign body perforations with fistula
- An abscess resulting from disease in one segment of bowel that erodes into a second segment
- Crohn's disease (noted for the development of internal and external fistulas)
- Carcinomas

The diagnosis is established in patients with severe diarrhea and weight loss by demonstration of the abnormal connection on appropriate contrast studies of the GI tract. A fecal odor to the breath is characteristic of gastrocolic fistula, and the profuse diarrhea may lead to severe prostration because of the large segment of intestine that is short-circuited.

Treatment. Operative treatment is designed to correct the abnormality by resection of the fistulous tract and reestablishment of intestinal continuity. When an abscess is present in a patient with sepsis, drainage and maintenance of nutrition by hyperalimentation may precede operative intervention.

Short Bowel Syndromes. Diseases that have necessitated resection of long segments of intestine may lead to chronic diarrhea. The history of a previous operation will suggest the diagnosis, which can be confirmed by contrast studies of the GI tract. Treatment is difficult, and a large number of procedures have been designed to slow the transit. These include (1) reversal of segments of small intestine (creation of an antiperistaltic segment) and (2) establishment of small bowel loops to recirculate the enteric contents. Neither of these two procedures have been found to be exceptionally beneficial.

Malabsorption Resulting From Intrinsic Bowel Disease

A large number of malabsorption syndromes result from a variety of primary small intestinal conditions such as idiopathic sprue, Whipple's disease, and allergies to food, although patients with such conditions represent relatively infrequent admissions to a surgical service. Granulomatous enteritis (Crohn's disease) and ulcerative colitis are grouped in the same category of nonspecific inflammatory bowel disease, but both diseases manifest many clinical features that are similar. However, contrasting clinical features allow the correct diagnosis on clinical grounds alone in all but about 15% of cases. Clinical overlap in some patients makes the distinction difficult for even experienced pathologists. When surgical intervention is contemplated, it is critical to know the correct diagnosis, because the *continent ileal pouch procedure* is contraindicated in patients with Crohn's colitis because of the risk of pouch involvement with progression of the disease.

Crohn's Disease

Pathogenesis and Diagnosis. The cause of Crohn's disease is unknown, although two broad categories, infectious agents and altered immune mechanisms, have been suggested. Symptoms of Crohn's disease range from single episodes of mild abdominal pain to severe derangement of bowel function, with fistulas, chronic diarrhea, and bowel obstruction. Although some patients have limited disease both anatomically and temporally, Crohn's disease is usually chronic, affecting a significant portion of the small and large bowel in varying patterns and presentations (Fig. 27-4). Any area of the intestine can become involved, from the esophagus to the anus. The disease (Fig. 27-5) is characterized by full-thickness inflammatory thickening of the bowel wall; edematous bowel mesentery—"creeping fat"; intermittent involvement of the bowel (skip areas); lymphatic involvement; granulomatous inflammation with granuloma (sarcoidlike) cells; and ulceration and fissures of the mucosa. After the disease has been present for some time, chronic changes include fibrous stricture, bowel adhesions, fistulas, and abscesses.

Most often fistulas and abscesses occur between segments of small bowel but may involve colon and bladder and colon and vagina. Fistulas

may present externally, either through the abdominal wall or, frequently, as perineal fistulas. The abscesses may drain internally or externally, or, in some patients, remain inadequately drained, necessitating surgical drainage.

Clinically, most patients have acute or chronic symptoms, but a patient may be seen for an abdominal emergency that mimics appendicitis, diverticulitis, or an ill-defined peritonitis, suggestive of bowel perforation. In general, patients usually present with a chronic pain syndrome, persistent diarrhea, malabsorption and malnutrition, weight loss, and complications of intestinal obstruction, fistulas, or abscesses. Patients may manifest clinical features of fever, malaise, vitamin deficiency, anemia, and, at times, clinical signs of sepsis from perforation, fistulas, or abscesses.

The diagnosis of Crohn's disease can be difficult and, in a *chronic case,* ulcerative colitis must be excluded before a definite operation is undertaken. In an *acute case,* the diagnosis may be made by exploratory laparotomy because of a precipitating complication. If the diagnosis is

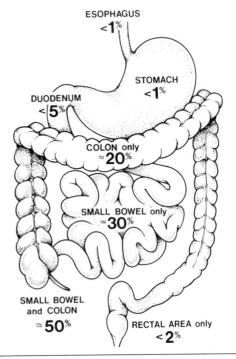

FIGURE 27-4 Incidence of Crohn's disease in GI tract. (From James EC, Tolstedt GE, Keller RT, et al. The small intestine. In James EC, Corry RJ, Perry JF Jr [eds]. Principles of Basic Surgical Practice. St Louis, CV Mosby, 1987, p 280. Reprinted with permission.)

suspected and an operation is avoided, confirmation is usually attained by radiographic examination or biopsy via endoscopic means. *Complete radiographic examination of the entire intestinal tract with an upper gastrointestinal series and small bowel follow-through and a barium enema is important in the overall diagnostic evaluation of these patients.* One should search for the so-called *string sign* (Figs. 27-6 and 27-7) representing marked disease in the terminal ileum.

Treatment. The treatment of Crohn's disease is expectant. Nonoperative management is the mainstay of treatment, with surgical intervention reserved for the correction of serious complications (see the box on p. 490).

Sulfasalazine (Azulfadine) has been the standard treatment for patients with both Crohn's disease and ulcerative colitis. Corticosteroids are widely used in treating active symptomatic Crohn's colitis and are usually the only drugs

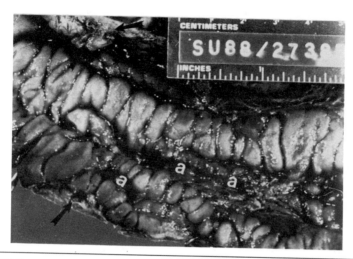

FIGURE 27-5 Rectosigmoid Crohn's disease: *a,* ulcerations and fissures of the mucosa, and full-thickness inflammatory bowel changes *(arrows).*

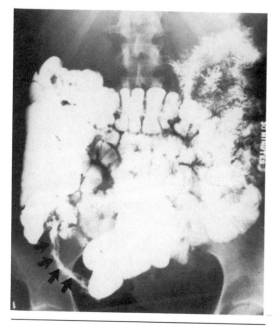

FIGURE 27-6 Upper GI series showing Crohn's ileitis *(arrows).*

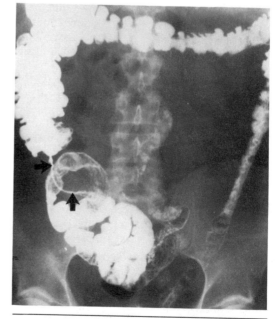

FIGURE 27-7 Upper GI series showing "string sign" in Crohn's disease *(arrows).*

INDICATIONS FOR SURGERY
IN CROHN'S DISEASE

Intractability
Obstruction
Internal fistula
Colo- or enterocutaneous fistula
Intra-abdominal abscess
Massive hemorrhage
Fulminating colitis
Toxic megacolon
Free perforation
Cutaneous and systemic complications
Severe anal and perianal involvement
Severe mucosal dysplasia
Carcinoma

Adapted from Gordon PH, Nivatvongs S. Principles and Practice of Surgery for the Colon, Rectum, and Anus. St Louis, Quality Medical Publishing, 1992, p 726.

used in the acute stage of ulcerative colitis. In patients with chronic disease, sulfasalazine and corticosteroids are often used in combination with one another. Azathioprine and 6-mercaptopurine are useful adjunctive drugs in both diseases because of their immunosuppressive and steroid-sparing characteristics. Indications for the use of immunosuppressive treatment include steroid toxicity, steroid dependence, fistulas (perianal, enterocutaneous, internal), and recurrent Crohn's disease (after previous multiple small bowel resections). Side effects are multiple and include gastrointestinal problems, headache, leukopenia, bone marrow depression and malignancy (non-Hodgkin's lymphoma). The antibiotic metronidazole decreases the inflammatory response in Crohn's colitis and is particularly of benefit in perianal and fistulous disease. The quinoline antibiotics are being used increasingly in the treatment of Crohn's disease.

Operation generally involves resection of diseased segments followed by reanastomosis of grossly normal-appearing bowel. Unfortunately, there is recurrence in about 50% of patients. Occasionally a simple bypass with exclusion of the diseased segment of bowel is indicated rather than resection or a diversion procedure.

Nutritional Support. Crohn's disease is often associated with severe states of malnutrition as a result of loss of the absorptive capacity of large segments of the small intestine and persistent diarrhea. ***Anemia and low serum albumin levels are common.*** In patients who are malnourished, a period of hyperalimentation (3 to 6 weeks) is indicated to avoid complications of poor healing and recurrent infection. Oral hyperalimentation with the elemental diet supplemented with appropriate vitamins and minerals (particularly zinc, phosphates, vitamin B_{12}, calcium, and vitamin D) may be successful. Caloric intake should be over 3000 calories per day in patients with serious infections and fistulas. When diarrhea is severe, antidiarrheal medications such as diphenoxylate (Lomotil) or loperamine (Imodium) are indicated. When diarrhea is refractory, parenteral hyperalimentation with complete bowel rest is preferable. A weight gain of 4 to 6 pounds per week should be the goal of treatment, with a demonstrative rise in the serum albumin levels to over 3 mg/dl.

On occasion a patient with chronic nutritional depletion or one who has had an extensive resection or multiple resections of small bowel may require maintenance on a home parenteral hyperalimentation program. Some patients lead a near-normal life, although they do require long-term indwelling simple catheters that may incur intermittent problems with thrombosis and infection. Some catheters last many months without sequelae if good general catheter technique and care are practiced.

Ulcerative Colitis

Pathogenesis and Diagnosis. Like Crohn's disease, **ulcerative colitis** is a disease of unknown cause, variable manifestations, chronicity, and, at times, major physical disability for the patient. Also as in Crohn's disease, personality disorders or acute psychic trauma may be a predisposing factor. Unlike Crohn's disease, results of operative treatment for ulcerative colitis are quite rewarding. Generally the disease is confined to the colon and primarily to the left side of the colon and the rectum. The distal few inches of the terminal ileum may be inflamed (**backwash ileitis**) from spilling of the diarrheal stool, which is reversible and should not be confused or mistaken for the ileocolitis of Crohn's disease.

Pathologically, ulcerative colitis is characterized by multiple coalescing ulcerations of the colonic mucosa. Inflammatory changes accompany the ulcers in the mucosa—crypts and glands become progressively replaced and microabscesses occur intramurally. As a result of the inflammatory changes and longstanding disease, fibrosis eventually foreshortens the colon with rigidity and loss of the normal haustration (Figs.

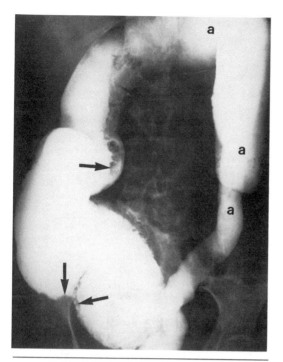

FIGURE 27-8   Barium enema demonstrating ulcerative colitis: *a,* fibrosis, foreshortening, and loss of normal haustration. "Cobblestoning" of the colonic mucosa as a result of pseudopolyposis is shown *(arrows).*

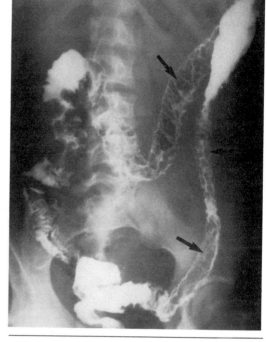

FIGURE 27-9   Barium enema demonstrating ulcerative colitis: marked "cobblestoning" as a result of pseudopolyposis *(arrows).*

27-8 and 27-9). The rectum and sigmoid tend to be more commonly and severely diseased. As opposed to the transmural involvement with Crohn's disease, the primary pathologic defect appears to be at the mucosa level, with *inflammation confined to the mucosa and submucosa* (Figs. 27-10 to 27-12).

The clinical presentation usually consists of crampy abdominal pain associated with bloody diarrhea. The magnitude of the diarrhea may be immense, with patients spending most of the day in defecation. They lose weight, becoming emaciated as well as anemic and dehydrated. *Stool cultures and smears should be taken and examined for bacterial pathogens, ova and parasites, chlamydial infection, and viruses.* Complete radiographic examination of the GI tract is recommended to exclude Crohn's disease and as a baseline for future examinations. Barium enema is not indicated in the acute stage because of risk of perforation or precipitating toxic megacolon. Diagnosis is confirmed by endoscopy (flexible sigmoidoscopy or fiberoptic colonoscopy) and biopsy.

The major complications arising from ulcerative colitis are *intractable disease, anorectal abscesses and fistulas, perforation, massive hemorrhage, toxic megacolon, and propensity to carcinoma.* The incidence of carcinoma of the colon and rectum arises proportional to the chronicity of the disease and the area of colonic mucosal involvement. Multiple carcinomas may develop in the same patient. Early radiologic diagnosis is hampered by the loss of mucosal signs resulting from the ravages of the disease. Accuracy of such radiographic studies has been reported as low as 50%. Cumulative risk of cancer increases with the duration of the ulcerative colitis. The known factors that increase risk are onset in childhood (about 3% develop cancer at 10 years), total large bowel involvement, duration of disease longer than 15 years, and persistent inflammation.

The risk of malignancy is about 25% to 30% at 25 years of age, 35% at 30 years, 45% at 35 years, and 65% at 40 years. Because of the strong inherent risk of malignancy in this disease, the physician must not temporize in the

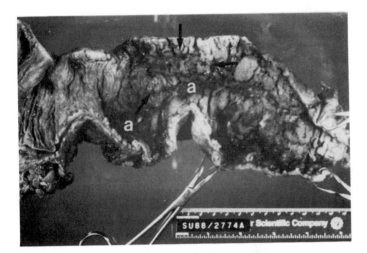

FIGURE 27-10   Resected ulcerative colitis specimen: *a*, mucosal and submucosal inflammation, and pseudopolyposis *(arrows)*.

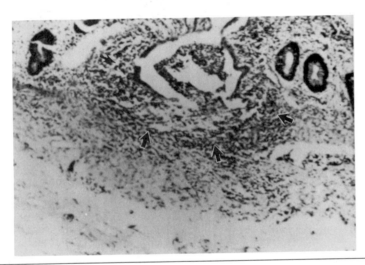

FIGURE 27-11   Photomicrograph showing crypt abscess *(arrows)* in ulcerative colitis.

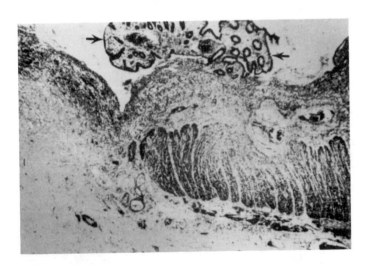

FIGURE 27-12   Photomicrograph showing pseudopolyp *(arrows)* in ulcerative colitis.

management of these patients. Patients who have had the disease for 10 years or more should undergo colonoscopy and multiple biopsies every 6 to 12 months.

Treatment. The initial treatment of ulcerative colitis is nonoperative, involving supportive care of the patient's malnutrition and dehydration, control of the diarrhea, relief of pain, and psychologic support. As previously discussed in the section on Crohn's colitis, the same medications are used in patients with ulcerative colitis. Because of the ever-present risk of malignancy of the colon and rectum, *early total proctocolectomy and ileostomy should be considered.* Other indications for operation include intractability, severe mucosal dysplasia, disease longer than 15 years, fulminating colitis (urgent), massive hemorrhage (emergency), toxic megacolon (emergency), and cutaneous and systemic complications.

Toxic megacolon is a life-threatening complication manifested by *fever, dehydration, and massive colonic distention.* Patients have signs of prostration and peritonitis. The diagnosis is confirmed by abdominal radiographic examination and rectal biopsy. A barium enema is contraindicated because of the risk of perforation. These patients are acutely ill, and an operation must be performed before perforation results, which carries a mortality of 80% or higher.

Preoperative correction of fluid and electrolyte derangements and anemia is desired but must be done expeditiously. Steroid therapy has been reported to modify the disease, but their use creates the risk of masking perforation and peritonitis. Early operation is often more desirable after an initial attempt at treatment (12 to 24 hours) fails. The operation of choice for toxic megacolon is proctocolectomy in one or two stages, depending on the stability of the patient's condition.

Proctocolectomy with a continent ileal reservoir is the preferred operation for the elective treatment of ulcerative colitis. This was initially done by means of a Koch continent ileostomy. However, the procedure that is currently popular is that of Parks et al., which uses Koch's concept of an ileal reservoir applied to the anal sphincter to maintain natural continence. The operation is a proctectomy, anal mucosectomy, and ileal pouch–anal anastomosis. Functional results are excellent and patients live a normal life span with an average of 4 to 6 bowel movements a day. With resection of the colon and rectum, the risk of carcinoma and other complications associated with ulcerative colitis is removed.

Bacterial Enteritis and Parasitic Enteritis. Diarrhea may be a prominent symptom in enteritis from any cause. The most common organisms are the *Salmonella* (typhoid), *Shigella,* and *Staphylococcus* groups. Many strains of toxigenic *Escherichia coli* also cause certain diarrheas, specifically traveler's diarrhea. Depending on the specific organism, the entity may be self-limiting as a result of production of a toxin (*Staphylococcus*) or progressive, leading to ulceration of the bowel and possibly perforation as is occasionally seen in typhoid disease.

A host of parasites may infest the bowel, producing diarrhea. The most devastating is amebic dysentery, produced by *Entamoeba histolytica.* Examination of the stools for ova and parasites and pathogenic organisms will establish the diagnosis. Several blood agglutination tests and skin tests may prove useful.

Treatment is by specific antibiotic therapy, depending on the etiologic organism responsible for the infection. Patients may require bowel rest and intravenous fluid therapy.

Radiation (Factitial) Enteritis. After a patient has received radiation to the abdomen or pelvis, two distinct types of syndromes may occur. Early radiation-induced enteritis may appear within 2 weeks of the start of radiotherapy, resulting in diarrhea and nausea. Changes in the bowel are acute, with inflammation and erythema. Treatment is supportive.

Late radiation enteritis may develop 2 to 10 years after treatment and is manifested by scarring, thickening of the bowel wall, narrowing of the lumen, and persistent diarrhea and anal soilage. The rectum is frequently involved, although any segment of the intestine caught in the radiotherapy beam may be affected. The pathologic injury is ischemic in nature, with occlusion of the microvasculature of the bowel wall.

Treatment by resection is hazardous because of the devascularization produced in the involved segments. Since the rectum is frequently involved, operation will lead to the need for a permanent colostomy in many cases. This should be undertaken only after all supportive measures, including a temporary diverting colostomy, have failed to provide relief.

Decreased Transit Time Due to Neoplasms. Tumors present within the lumen of the small or large bowel can produce diarrhea by intrinsic attempts of the bowel to pass them. Included in this category are small bowel tumors, polyps, cancers, and villous tumors. Carcinoma of the colon or rectum is quite common in North America; however, cancer of the small intestine is relatively rare. Benign and malignant neoplasms can present with no symptoms, hemorrhage, obstruction, perforation, metastases (liver or lung), and intussusception. Common benign and malignant tumors of the small bowel are listed in the box below.

NEOPLASMS OF THE SMALL INTESTINE

Benign

Leiomyoma
Adenomatous polyps
Hamartomas (Peutz-Jeghers syndrome)
Neurofibromas
Angiomas

Malignant

Lymphoma (lymphosarcoma)
Carcinoid
Adenocarcinoma
Metastases from colon, pancreas, ovary, etc.
Sarcoma

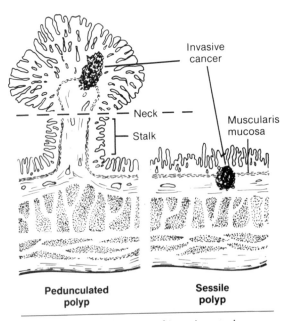

FIGURE 27-13 Definition of invasive carcinoma in polyps: cancer has to invade the muscularis mucosa layer. (From Nivatvongs S, Becker ER. The colon, rectum, and anal canal. In James EC, Corry RJ, Perry JF Jr [eds]. Principles of Basic Surgical Practice. St Louis, CV Mosby, 1987, p 309. Reprinted with permission.)

Adenomatous Polyps

Adenomatous polyps of the colon and rectum are considered neoplastic. Common polyps are the tubular, villous, and tubulovillous adenomas, which are classified according to histologic criteria identified under the microscope. Tubular adenomas are most common (75%), followed by tubulovillous adenomas (15%) and villous adenomas (10%). Malignant potential is related to type and size, with an estimated malignancy rate of 5% for tubular adenomas, 40% for villous adenomas, and 22% for tubulovillous adenomas. *Polyps smaller than 1 cm in diameter rarely have invasive carcinoma;* however, the incidence of carcinoma does increase significantly with increasing size.

Most colorectal polyps can be removed by proctosigmoidoscopy or colonoscopy. Colorectal resections are reserved for patients in whom colonoscopic polypectomy cannot be accomplished because of large size, sessile or flat configuration, or the polyps are unreachable by the colonoscope.

Polyps with invasive carcinoma must be treated like a frank malignancy. Malignancy is defined as the invasion of cancer through the muscularis mucosal layer (Fig. 27-13).

Villous adenomas can produce a secretory diarrhea that causes the patient to lose excessive amounts of electrolytes, specifically sodium, chloride, and potassium. These lesions have a higher malignant potential than other polyps of the gastrointestinal tract. Large villous adenomas manifest an even greater risk of malignancy.

Extrinsic Masses. Diarrhea can be a manifestation of any mass involving the colon or rectum, either neoplastic or inflammatory, that produces enough irritability. Contrast studies of the GI tract may demonstrate displacement of the colon or rectum, and a CT scan is sometimes helpful in the diagnosis.

CARCINOMA OF THE COLON AND RECTUM

Clinically, symptoms of carcinomas of the colon and rectum are nonspecific. A change in bowel habits (constipation, rectal bleeding) may occur initially but does not necessarily imply early disease. Symptoms that probably imply advanced cancer include abdominal pain, bloating, constipation, and diarrhea, usually owing to a partial bowel obstruction. Involvement of the rectosigmoid, sigmoid and descending colon areas, and splenic flexure tends to cause obstruction. Involvement of the transverse and right colon often presents with bleeding, anemia, and weakness. Rectal bleeding by stool can be bright red or dark, with or without clots, if it is from the left side of the colon or rectum. Bleeding from the right side of the colon is usually occult, unless in large amounts, which would be unusual.

Early detection of colon and rectal cancers is the key because symptoms usually mean advanced disease. The mainstay of the diagnostic work-up is a thorough history and physical examination (to include digital rectal examination) and colonoscopy in suspected or at-risk patients. Low rectal carcinomas are often palpable on careful examination. Barium enema (particularly the air contrast study) and colonoscopy compliment each other in the work-up (Fig. 27-14). For low risk individuals (no known risk factors or signs but over age 50), screening for blood in the stools by the Hemoccult or Hemo-Quant tests is practical and effective in identifying patients with early clinical stage cancers.

Operations for carcinomas of the colon are performed based on extent and the site of involvement of the colon (Fig. 27-15). Survival and prognosis for carcinomas of either the colon or rectum depend on the extent of invasion through the bowel wall, extent of lymph node involvement, and whether there are distant metastases. The Dukes staging system has become the time-honored clinical method of predicting prognosis in these patients, and clinical staging depends on a number of factors (Fig. 27-16).

Operations for carcinomas of the rectum depend on the level of the tumor from the anal verge. An anterior resection is the standard operation for a carcinoma of the upper rectum. When treating very low rectal carcinomas, in which a 4 cm in situ distal resective margin is not possible, *abdominoperineal resection* is the operation indicated (Fig. 27-17). This procedure requires removal of the anal canal and rectosigmoid colon, leaving the patient with a permanent descending colostomy.

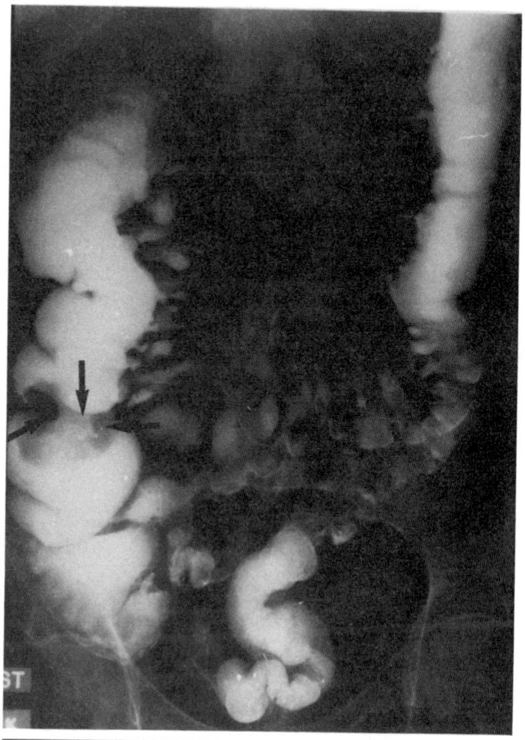

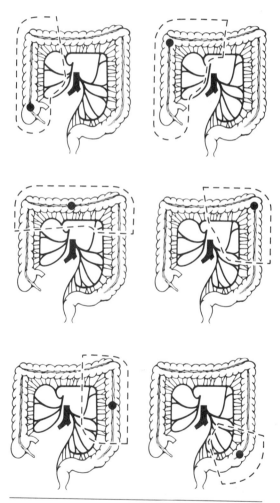

FIGURE 27-15 Operations for carcinomas of the colon. Note that the segments are removed with their major blood supply to ensure a thorough lymphatic removal.

FIGURE 27-14 Barium enema showing "apple core" carcinoma involving ascending colon.

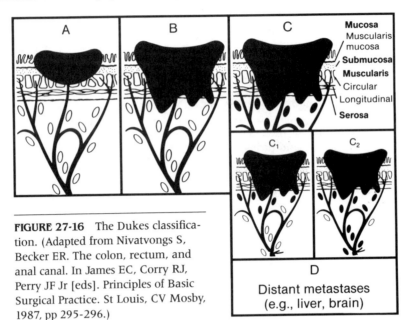

FIGURE 27-16 The Dukes classification. (Adapted from Nivatvongs S, Becker ER. The colon, rectum, and anal canal. In James EC, Corry RJ, Perry JF Jr [eds]. Principles of Basic Surgical Practice. St Louis, CV Mosby, 1987, pp 295-296.)

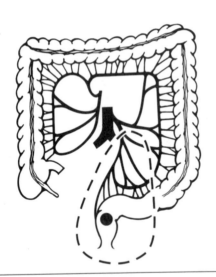

FIGURE 27-17 Abdominoperineal resection for low rectal carcinomas.

Idiopathic Diarrhea

Under this heading are grouped diarrheas of unknown cause. Variably described as mucous colitis, spastic colon, and other conditions, they require supportive medical treatment. Administering bulking agents such as Metamucil may be beneficial.

Neuroendocrine and certain islet cell tumors can be associated with diarrhea. Different tumor types, clinical features, and diagnostic features are outlined in Table 27-1. These tumors are generally found in the pancreas; however, they can also be found in the mucosa of the duodenal area.

WHAT CAUSES ABNORMAL DEFECATION?

Diarrhea may be a prominent symptom of certain anorectal diseases or conditions and needs to be differentiated from incontinence. Diseases of the anorectal area are more thoroughly discussed in Chapter 30. Conditions that are prone to cause abnormal defecation include the following:

Sphincter spasm
A. Anal fissure
B. Inflammatory strictures
   1. Lymphogranuloma venereum
   2. Tuberculosis
C. Postsurgical stricture
Tenesmus
A. Inflammatory disease of the anorectum
B. Tumors of the anorectum
Incontinence
A. Defects in sphincter control
   1. Postsurgical
   2. Tumor invasion
B. Prolapse or procidentia

TABLE 27-1   Non-Insulin-Producing Islet Cell Tumors Associated With Diarrhea

Tumor Syndrome	Clinical Features	Diagnostic Features
Glucagonoma	Necrolytic migratory erythema, mild diabetes, psychiatric disturbances, venous thrombosis	Excessive glucagon release after intravenous administration of tolbutamide
Somatostatinoma	Dyspepsia, diabetes, gallstones, steatorrhea, hypochlorhydria	Hyperglycemia without ketonemia; stool weight and stool fat increased
Calcitoninoma	Diarrhea	Secretory diarrhea while fasting; additional osmotic component while eating (decreased small-bowel transit time)
Gastrinoma	Severe peptic ulcer disease, secretory diarrhea	High acid secretion; secretory diarrhea stops with histamine (H_2) receptor antagonist therapy
Vasoactive intestinal polypeptideoma	Large-volume secretory diarrhea, hypokalemia, metabolic acidosis, hypochlorhydria	Stool electrolytes (sodium + potassium X 2) account for osmolality of stool water without gap; fecal pH as high as 8.0 on fasting (colonic bicarbonate secretion); concomitant elevation of plasma PHM

From Pemberton JH, Phillips SF. Constipation and diarrhea. In Moody FG, Carey LC, Jones RS, et al (eds). Surgical Treatment of Digestive Disease, 2nd ed. Chicago, Year Book Medical Publishers, 1990, p 50. Reprinted with permission.
PHM = Peptide histidine methionine.

CONSTIPATION AND OBSTIPATION

Constipation was defined at the beginning of this chapter. *Obstipation* is present when the patient is unable to have a bowel movement. However, constipation is by far more common, outnumbering all other chronic digestive complaints. It is believed to be three times more common in women than men, and its incidence is markedly increased after the age of 65. Constipation is also common in children and is often the result of psychologic attitudes or unsatisfactory diets that tend to provide inadequate bulk. Important historical data include a recent decrease in the number or frequency of bowel movements and, in some patients, complete failure to have bowel movements.

Acute Constipation

The most frequent cause of acute constipation is obstruction of the small bowel or colon. *Intestinal adhesions* from previous operations are the most common cause of small bowel obstruction (Fig. 27-18) in the United States, followed by (1) incarceration of small bowel in hernias, (2) in-

flammatory bowel disease, (3) strictures (from radiation), (4) intussusception, (5) enteroliths (gallstone ileus), (6) volvulus, and (7) abscesses. Neoplasms are the most common cause of colonic obstruction, followed by (1) incarceration in hernias, (2) inflammatory bowel disease, (3) volvulus, and (4) abscesses.

A more detailed discussion of intestinal obstruction is given in Chapter 25.

Adynamic (Paralytic) Ileus. When the bowel loses its peristaltic, propulsive action, the condition is called an *adynamic* or *paralytic ileus.* However, this condition mimics intestinal obstruction when decreased intestinal mechanical motility moves intestinal contents ineffectively along the gastrointestinal tract and ceases completely. The box on p. 498 lists examples of conditions that cause adynamic intestinal motility and functional obstruction. The best way to establish the diagnosis is with supine and upright or lateral decubitus x-ray examination, which frequently shows significant amounts of air in both the small intestine and colon (Fig. 27-19).

Most cases of adynamic ileus occur after operative manipulation of the small intestine, but the condition is also common after thoracic and ret-

CAUSES OF ADYNAMIC ILEUS

Neurogenic

Postoperative (thoracic or abdominal operations)
Following trauma (abdominal or remote)
   Spinal cord injury
   Head injury
   Abdominal wall or retroperitoneal injury
   Pelvic or lumbar spine fracture
   Long bone fracture
Following painful illness, such as myocardial
   infarction

Metabolic

Potassium deficiency
Sodium deficiency (late)
Diabetic ketoacidosis
Renal failure

Vascular Accidents

Thrombosis of mesenteric vessels
Embolus to mesenteric vessels
Vasculitis of mesenteric vessels
   Hypertension
   Postcoarctation repair polyarteritis
Peritonitis

roperitoneal operations and may be seen following infections of the pelvis and spine. After laparotomy the bowel may remain flaccid for several days. Adynamic ileus occurs in acute inflammatory conditions such as appendicitis, cholecystitis, and pancreatitis. Frequently patients with trauma present without intra-abdominal injury but have absence of bowel sounds and an adynamic ileus. Chemical abnormalities such as low serum potassium, magnesium, or calcium may lead to paralysis of the bowel smooth muscle, producing an adynamic ileus.

Postoperative or postinjury adynamic ileus is usually self-limiting if treated properly. Treatment is by nasogastric decompression, the administration of intravenous fluids, and reversal of electrolyte and metabolic abnormalities. In some patients, resolution of inciting factors will be required. Narcotics should be discontinued if they are a suspected contributing factor. Decompression of large amounts of air from the colon can be accomplished with a rectal tube. The drug metaclopromid can stimulate peristalsis in some patients.

Occlusions of either the bowel venous or arterial systems can bring about *hypoxic paralysis* of the bowel. Atherosclerosis occurs in mesenteric vessels, and some patients develop gangrenous bowel resulting from major vascular occlusions. Sudden occlusion of a normal major mesenteric

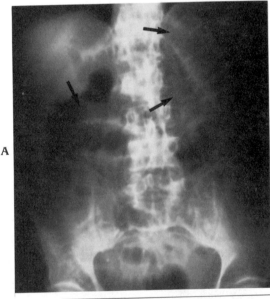
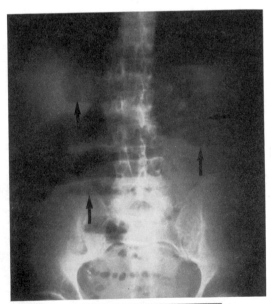

A

B

FIGURE 27-18   Small intestinal obstruction. **A,** Supine flatplate showing dilated loops of small intestine *(arrows)*. **B,** Upright flatplate showing dilated loops of small intestine and multiple air-fluid levels *(arrows)*.

artery from an embolus will produce an immediate adynamic ileus and bowel death if not treated promptly. This occurs with atrial fibrillation or intramural thrombus in the left ventricle.

Adynamic ileus, not accompanied by circulatory impairment of the bowel wall or peritonitis, presents with absent to decreased bowel sounds, distended, nontender abdomen, vomiting, and signs of extracellular fluid loss from secretion of fluid into the lumen of the bowel.

The patient is relatively unconcerned because abdominal pain is usually absent. If bowel wall ischemia causes peritonitis, the patient will have an acute abdomen. In addition to neurogenic reflexes and metabolic aberrations, adynamic ileus can be seen with peritonitis secondary to any cause (peritoneal-intestinal reflex) and thus may be an important sign of intraperitoneal abscess or perforation. It is an ominous sign when it occurs postoperatively after several days of normal alimentation, and usually heralds a serious intra-abdominal complication.

Another cause of acute constipation is *colonic pseudoobstruction (Ogilvie's syndrome).* This is seen in older patients who have been immobilized after a major extra-abdominal operation such as a knee or hip replacement (Fig. 27-20).

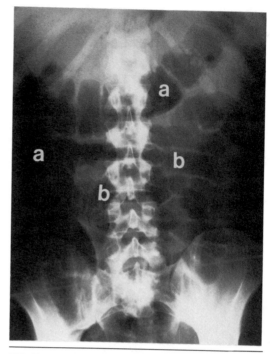

FIGURE 27-19   Adynamic (paralytic) ileus showing *a,* air in the colon and *b,* air in the small intestine.

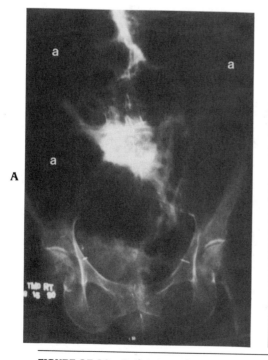

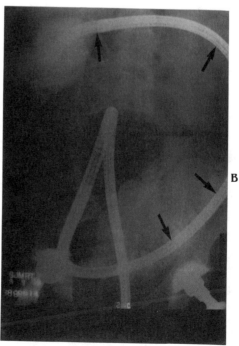

FIGURE 27-20   Ogilvie's syndrome. **A,** Marked colonic dilation *(a).* **B,** Treatment by colonoscopic decompression *(arrows).*

They have marked colonic dilation that progresses slowly over several days and is most prominent in the cecum. This is because the cecum is the thinnest and largest area of the colon in circumference and follows Laplace's law in dilating under pressure.

The treatment for Ogilvie's syndrome is nasogastric decompression, intravenous fluids, correction of electrolyte abnormalities, and decompression by colonoscopy. Patients who have signs of perforation or peritonitis may require operative treatment by tube cecostomy or resection of the colon. Decompression of the colon by colonoscopy should be accomplished, if possible, before more serious consequences ensue.

Acute inflammatory processes such as anal fissure can lead to acute constipation by causing patients to avoid defecation because of severe discomfort and pain. Patients learn that bowel movements exacerbate the pain, causing them to withhold defecation. This makes the stool hard and bulky and further aggravates the inflammatory condition involved. Treatment is with stool softeners or surgery, depending on the condition of the anal area.

Chronic constipation is a more frequent problem than acute constipation in adults (see the box below). It is obvious that there are a multi-

---

CLASSIFICATION OF CONSTIPATION IN ADULTS

No Structural Abnormality

Faulty diet
Poor habits
Pregnancy
Age
Idiopathic slow transit
Irritable bowel syndrome
Pseudoobstruction of the colon

Structural Abnormality

Anal fissure
Stricture of the colon
Colonic or rectal neoplasm
Colonic volvulus
Idiopathic megarectum
Idiopathic megacolon
Aganglionosis
Congenital—Hirschsprung's disease
Acquired—Chagas' disease
Occult renal prolapse
Complete rectal prolapse
Rectocele
Hernias
Endometriosis
Ischemic colitis
Diverticulosis
Puborectalis syndrome

Systemic Abnormality

Endocrine and metabolic
Hyperthyroidism
Hypercalcemia
Porphyria
Pheochromocytoma
Uremia
Multiple endocrine adenomatosis, Type IIB
Scleroderma
Hyperparathyroidism
Amyloidosis
Hypokalemia
Diabetes
Panhypopituitarism

Neurologic

Sacral outflow damage (trauma, surgery)
Cauda equina tumor
CNS (meningocele), paraplegia
Parkinson's disease
Systemic sclerosis (multiple sclerosis)
Collagen vascular diseases

Psychologic

Depression
Anorexia nervosa
Denied bowel action?

Drug Effects

Analgesias (narcotics)
Antacids (aluminum containing)
Anticholinergics
Anticonvulsants
Antidepressives
Ganglion blockers
Psychotherapeutic
Diuretics
Barium sulfate

Modified from Lennard-Jones JE. Constipation: Pathophysiology, clinical features and treatment. In Henry MM, Swash M (eds). Coloproctology and the Pelvic Floor: Pathophysiology and Management. London, Butterworths, 1985, pp 350-375. Reprinted with permission.

tude of causes with which one should be familiar. Treatment depends on the cause, and requires understanding, patience, and concerned care by the physician.

Aganglionic Megacolon (Hirschsprung's Disease). Hirschsprung's disease is usually found in children, but rarely it can occur in adults. Ascending from the anorectal juncture, *congenital* or *acquired absence of myenteric ganglia* may result in a segment of distal bowel without motor activity or function. This dynamic collapse of intestine creates a functional obstruction of the colon. The degree of obstruction, clinical presentation, and treatment depend on the length of involved bowel. *Marked dilation of the normal bowel results proximal to the aganglionic segment.*

Surgical treatment is based on resection of the aganglionic colonic segment and reestablishment of bowel continuity to the anus via a direct pull-through anastomosis to the upper anus (Swenson), longitudinal anastomosis to the posterior rectum (Duhamel), or endorectal pull-through by means of a muscular tube of mucosal stripped rectum (Soave). Great care must be taken not to resect the normal dilated proximal bowel. Protection of the anastomosis with a proximal colostomy is usually recommended. These operations are illustrated in Fig. 27-21.

The *diagnosis* of Hirschsprung's disease is made by endoscopic biopsy of the involved rectal or colonic mucosa that shows *absence of myenteric ganglia.*

The evaluation of severe functional constipation in adults is rather complex, not well understood, and includes the following:

Colonic dysmotility
  Slow transit
  Constipation predominant in irritable bowel syndrome (disorder defecation)
  Animus
  Descending perineum syndrome
  Hirschsprung's disease
  Disturbed rectal sensation
  Occult rectal prolapse
  Predentia (complete prolapse)
  Rectocele
  Posturorectal hernia

Several of these disorders are cured with operation. One must do a complete work-up for extracolonic as well as functional causes of constipa-

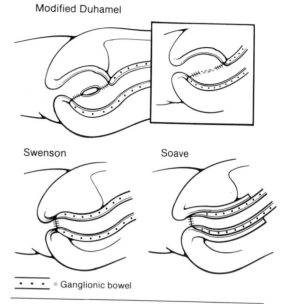

Modified Duhamel

Swenson   Soave

• • • • = Ganglionic bowel

FIGURE 27-21 Three basic operations for aganglionic megacolon. (Adapted from Guzzetta PC, Anderson KD, Altman RP, et al. Pediatric surgery. In Schwartz SI, Shires GT, Spencer FC, Husser WC [eds]. Principles of Surgery, 5th ed. New York, McGraw-Hill, 1989, p 1707. Reprinted with permission.)

tion and be wary of the irritable bowel syndrome. *If the diagnosis is irritable bowel syndrome, operative intervention is fraught with failure.*

Physiologic tests to evaluate chronic constipation include:

Colonic transit
Pelvic floor function
Anorectal manometry
Electromyography
Scintigraphic balloon topography
Scintigraphic evaluation
Balloon expulsion
Defecating proctography
Upper gastrointestinal manometry

These tests should be performed for any patient with severe intractable constipation before an operation is undertaken. Anatomic abnormalities such as rectal prolapse, rectocele, descending perineum syndrome, and posturorectal hernia should be surgically repaired.

PITFALLS AND COMMON MYTHS

- Not performing a thorough history and physical examination.
- Not performing colonoscopy in a patient with occult rectal bleeding.
- Not making the immediate correlation of perianal inflammatory and fistulous disease with Crohn's disease.
- Waiting too long to recommend definitive surgical treatment for ulcerative colitis.
- Incomplete clinical work-up for Crohn's disease and ulcerative colitis (i.e., complete radiologic studies, including the use of colonoscopy and multiple biopsies).
- Underestimating the value of examining the stool appropriately in patients with diarrhea (microscopically for content, ova, and parasites and with cultures for pathogens).
- Not performing routine screening for blood in the stools (Hemoccult or HemoQuant testing) in low-risk individuals for colon and rectal cancer (no known risk factors, age over 50).
- Missing an incarcerated hernia (with colon) in acute colonic obstruction.
- Not looking for synchronous carcinomas in patients with colon and rectal cancer (incidence in the range of 2%).
- "A stricture in diverticulitis" is a carcinoma until proven otherwise.
- Think "ovarian carcinoma" in a woman with extrinsic compression of the colon.

BIBLIOGRAPHY

Alfonso A, Gardner B. Principles of Cancer Surgery. New York, Appleton-Century-Crofts, 1981.

Beart RW Jr, McIlrath DC, Kelly KA, et al. Surgical management of inflammatory bowel disease. Curr Probl Surg 17:10, 1980.

Goldstein F. Current status of medical treatment for inflammatory bowel disease. Am J Gastroenterol 78:871, 1983.

Gordon PH, Nivatvongs S. Principles and Practice of Surgery for the Colon, Rectum, and Anus. St Louis, Quality Medical Publishing, 1992, p 726.

Grant CS, Dozois RR. Toxic megacolon: Ultimate fate of patients after successful medical management. Am J Surg 147:106, 1984.

Hardy JD. Hardy's Textbook of Surgery. Philadelphia, JB Lippincott, 1983.

Hobsley M. Disorders of the digestive system. In Physical Principles in Medicine Series. Baltimore, University Park Press, 1982, pp 133-162.

James EC, Corry RJ, Perry JF. Principles of Basic Surgical Practice. St Louis, CV Mosby, 1987.

Khige RM. Infectious diarrhea: An update. Compr Ther 9:26, 1983.

Kock NG, Darle N, Hulten L, et al. Ileostomy. Curr Probl Surg 14:8, 1977.

Lennard-Jones JE, Morson BC, et al. Cancer in colitis: Assessment of the individual risk by clinical and histological criteria. Gastroenterology 73:1280, 1977.

Pemberton JH, Phillips SF. Colonic absorption. Perspect Colon Rectal Surg 1:90, 1988.

Schwartz SI, Shires GT, et al (eds). Principles of Surgery, 5th ed. New York, McGraw-Hill, 1989.

Triadafilopoulos G, Hallstone AE. Acute abdomen as the first presentation of pseudomembranous colitis. Gastroenterology 101:685, 1991.

CHAPTER REVIEW
Questions

1. Correct statements regarding Crohn's disease include:
   a. There is transmural involvement.
   b. The best treatment is a continent ileal reservoir.
   c. The entire gastrointestinal tract may be involved.
   d. There is mucosal involvement only.
2. Prognosis for carcinoma of the colon and rectum depends on:
   a. Lymph node metastasis
   b. Distant metastasis
   c. Area of the colon involved
   d. Depth of penetration through bowel wall
3. Which of the following choices has the greatest risk of malignancy?
   a. Tubular adenoma
   b. Tubulovillous adenoma
   c. Hamartoma
   d. Villous adenoma
4. Correct statements regarding Hirschsprung's disease include:
   a. It is best to resect an abnormally dilated bowel.
   b. Operations to correct this disorder are described by Duval, Puestow, and Child.
   c. This disorder is the result of acquired or congenital absence of myenteric ganglia.
   d. Hirschsprung's disease commonly occurs in children.
5. Small bowel obstruction is most commonly caused by:

a. Incisional hernias
b. Radiation enteritis
c. Adhesions from previous intra-abdominal operations
d. Malignant tumors of the small bowel

6. Characteristic findings in pseudomembranous colitis include all except:
   a. Recent history of broad-spectrum antibiotic use
   b. Massive rectal bleeding
   c. Diarrhea
   d. Endoscopic colonic yellowish membranes and inflammation

7. The calculated normal transit time through the large bowel is:
   a. 4 hours
   b. 5 days
   c. 12 to 24 hours
   d. 36 to 48 hours

8. List four clinical features characteristic of Crohn's disease.

9. Known clinical factors that increase risk of malignancy in ulcerative colitis are:
   a. Onset in childhood
   b. Total large bowel involvement
   c. Duration longer than 15 years
   d. Persistent inflammation

10. A 70-year-old man has undergone a total hip replacement and develops massive colonic dilation. The most likely diagnosis is:
    a. An obstructing "annular" rectal carcinoma
    b. A mesenteric vascular occlusion
    c. Pseudoobstruction of the colon (Ogilvie's syndrome)
    d. Toxic megacolon

11. Drugs that are effective in treating both Crohn's colitis and ulcerative colitis are:
    a. Metronidazole
    b. Corticosteroids
    c. Azathioprine and 6-mercaptopurine
    d. All of the above

12. Which of the following is/are important in the diagnosis of diarrhea?

a. History and physical examination
b. Examination of the stool, including appropriate cultures
c. Endoscopy and biopsy
d. Contrast x-ray studies of the intestine

13. The best way to diagnose an adynamic (paralytic) ileus is:
    a. Upright and supine abdominal flatplates
    b. Upper GI series and small bowel follow-through
    c. Upper intestinal endoscopy
    d. All of the above

14. The minimum criterion to establish invasive carcinoma in a colon or rectal polyp is involvement of the:
    a. Serosa
    b. Muscularis layers
    c. Regional lymph nodes
    d. Muscularis mucosa

Answers

1. a, c
2. a, b, d
3. d
4. c, d
5. c
6. b
7. d
8. Full-thickness inflammatory thickening of the bowel wall; edematous bowel wall—"creeping fat"; intermittent involvement of the bowel (skip areas); lymphatic involvement; granulomatous inflammation with granuloma (sarcoidlike) cells; and ulceration and fissures of the mucosa.
9. a, b, c, and d
10. c
11. d
12. a, b, c, and d
13. a
14. d

Abdominal Masses

FRANK B. MILLER
JAMES I. HARTY

KEY FEATURES

After reading this chapter you will understand:
- How to distinguish emergency from nonemergency masses of the abdomen.
- Diagnosis, history, and physical examination of abdominal masses.
- Radiologic and endoscopic aids in diagnosis.
- Gastrointestinal cancers, including liver masses and other intraperitoneal disease.
- Retroperitoneal masses, including carcinoma of the pancreas and renal masses.
- Masses involving the major abdominal vessels.
- Pelvic masses.

For an abdominal mass, there are a myriad of possible diagnoses and thus a systematic approach is essential. A good history and physical examination, especially noting the location of the mass (Fig. 28-1), and a knowledge of the surface anatomy of the organs that commonly generate masses (Fig. 28-2) refine the diagnostic process and allow the clinician to select further diagnostic studies cost effectively. An abdominal mass may be classified by cause, anatomic location, tissue or organ system of origin, or clinical implications (see the box at right).

GENERAL APPROACH
Which Takes Priority—Diagnostic Studies or Operative Intervention?

For most mass lesions, an operation is necessary to confirm the diagnosis and to accomplish treat-ment; thus the timing of operative intervention is important, so that the diagnostic tests do not result in a detrimental delay. Indeed, a vital component of clinical judgment is evaluation of the objective symptoms and signs that indicate how quickly an operation must take place.

For the purposes of this chapter, abdominal masses are discussed according to their anatomic location. An orderly approach to diagnosis involves thorough history-taking, physical exam-

---

COMPLEMENTARY METHODS FOR CLASSIFICATION OF ABDOMINAL MASSES

Anatomic Location	Clinical Course
Intraperitoneal	Acute
Retroperitoneal	Chronic
Pelvic	Emergent
	Nonemergent

Cause	Tissue or Organ System
Neoplastic	
Benign	
Malignant	Gastrointestinal
Primary	Hepatic
Metastatic	Pancreatic
Inflammatory	Splenic
Traumatic	Vascular
Congenital	Connective tissue
Degenerative	Neurogenic
Infectious	Gynecologic
	Urologic

Epigastric—RU quadrant

Gallbladder
  Hydrops
  Empyema
  Carcinoma
  Passive dilation of gallbladder
    secondary to carcinoma
Liver
  Primary cancer
  Metastatic cancer

Epigastric—LU quadrant

Pancreas
  Edematous pancreatitis
  Lesser sac collection
  Pseudocyst
  Abscess
  Carcinoma
  True cysts
Splenomegaly
  Traumatic, hematologic
Aortic aneurysm
Carcinoma of stomach

Flank

Kidney
  Cysts
  Abscess
  Hypernephroma
  Wilms' tumor
  Hydronephrosis

Flank

Kidney
  Cysts
  Abscess
  Hypernephroma
  Wilms' tumor
  Hydronephrosis

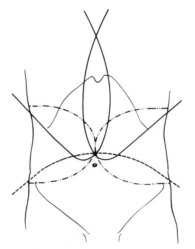

Pelvic—RL quadrant

Appendix (abscess/induration)
Mucocele
Regional enteritis
Colon (cecal carcinoma,
  inflammatory)
Mesenteric panniculitis
Ectopic kidney

Pelvic—LL quadrant

Colon
  (Acute diverticulitis with abscess/
  induration, carcinoma)
Ectopic kidney

Midpelvic

Gynecologic disease (uterus, tubes,
  ovaries, gravid uterus)
Colon/rectal cancer
Intussusception
Pelvic kidney

Retroperitoneal fibrosis/tumors
Mesenteric tumors/cysts
Omentum
Urinary bladder

FIGURE 28-1 Location of abdominal masses according to their organ of origin. Represented are the characteristic areas of the abdominal cavity or flank where these masses typically present.

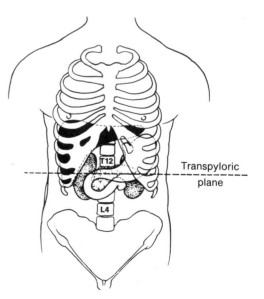

Transpyloric
plane

FIGURE 28-2 Anatomic scheme of location of the upper abdominal viscera and surface anatomy.

ination, and the use of a variety of diagnostic tests, so that within a short time the likely cause, location, and operative approach can be clearly defined (see the box below). Before this can be done, however, *the clinician must establish that the disease does not acutely threaten the patient's life.* Under these circumstances, it may be necessary to operate with only a clinical impression of the diagnosis gathered after a brief history is taken, physical examination is performed, and a few key diagnostic tests are done. If the condition is not emergent, sufficient time can be allotted for safely conducting more-detailed diagnostic studies.

History

A thorough history will include data about the onset of the mass, change in size, and associated symptoms. When the patient is known or thought to have a chronic intestinal disease such as ulcerative colitis, the clinician is alert to the fact that this sharply predisposes the person to development of highly invasive colon cancer, and the typical symptoms of that neoplasm may literally be lost in the chronic milieu of blood,

---

A SYSTEMATIC APPROACH TO ABDOMINAL MASSES

1. Is the lesion symptomatic?
2. Are the onset of the mass and its related disease process sudden (acute) or gradual (nonacute)?
   If onset is acute, proceed to immediate diagnostic evaluation relative to acuteness of process: emergent versus urgent.
3. Are inflammatory or infectious signs present?
   If so, are they local, or local with associated systemic response? Is the inflammatory process primary or secondary to another disease, e.g., neoplastic, metabolic, or vascular?
4. How can the mass be evaluated?
   X-ray examination
   Organ function tests
   Sonography
   Endoscopy
   Aimed at the suspected organ itself or at a neighboring organ that reflects the disease

---

diarrhea, and mucus. Indeed, ulcerative colitis that has been active for longer than 10 years and that involves the entire colon—regardless of the current state—is a reasonable indication for colectomy based on the likelihood of subsequent development of colorectal cancer.

A family history of colonic polyps or tumors is particular grounds for suspecting familial polyposis and the immense likelihood of emergence of carcinoma amid the innumerable polyps. Special follow-up and even elective colectomy may be warranted in many patients.

Onset. The clinical setting in which a mass appears is of paramount importance. Although the discovery of a mass is, by definition, an acute event, it may be superimposed on a preexisting systemic illness that may be manifested by weight loss, anorexia, weakness, anemia, febrile illness, and so on. The duration of such systemic signs and symptoms is often helpful in delineating the cause as neoplastic, vascular, infectious, or inflammatory.

Is the lesion symptomatic? If not, was it casually discovered by the patient, or by a physician in the course of an examination?

The discovery of an asymptomatic mass indicates a significant cause. The acute inflammatory lesions are virtually eliminated as causative factors, and the chronic inflammatory ones become unlikely. Neoplasm, other degenerative diseases (aortic aneurysm), or congenital anomalies are more likely.

Change in Size. Expanding masses or those associated with severe pain imply that rupture or hemorrhage has occurred or may be imminent and therefore are prime indications for urgent work-up and treatment.

Associated Symptoms. A complete system review should concentrate on the gastrointestinal, gynecologic, and urinary systems.

Gastrointestinal System. Is the mass associated with cramps, pain, vomiting, obstipation, constipation, diarrhea, melena, jaundice, inability to eat, or other symptoms? Such symptoms suggest an obstruction, erosion into the gastrointestinal tract, or proximity of the mass to the stomach, small bowel, biliary tract, or colon.

Gynecologic System. The relationship of the abdominal mass to menstrual characteristics may be important to discern the presence of an ectopic pregnancy, endometriosis, or ovarian tumor.

Urinary System. If the mass is associated with urinary tract infection, stones, or other obstructive phenomena, this may indicate the presence of hydronephrosis or perinephric abscess. Hematuria may be a prominent symptom with renal tumors. Pneumaturia may indicate perforation of a sigmoid colon mass into the bladder, which may occur with diverticulitis or colon carcinoma.

General Physical Examination

A complete physical examination may indicate the cause of the mass. Evidence for the presence of a neoplasm includes wasting, lymph node enlargement from metastatic cancer, or an associated nodular liver. Hypertension examination of the eyegrounds for diabetic or hypertensive retinopathy, or of the peripheral arteries for bruits or decreased pulses, may suggest a degenerative disease, such as any one of several manifestations of atherosclerosis. General infectious processes may be evidenced by the presence of fever or may be detected during examination of the lungs, lymph nodes, or spleen.

Examination of the Mass

Palpation. Direct examination of the mass should elicit the following characteristics:

- General location in the abdomen
- Size
- Contour—smooth masses may be cystic, nodular masses neoplastic
- Tenderness—may be a presumptive sign of impending rupture, infection, or recent enlargement
- Texture—soft masses tend to be benign, whereas hard masses tend to be malignant
- Mobility or fixation—fixed masses tend to be attached to fixed structures, particularly retroperitoneal ones, and are more likely malignant or infectious
- Movement with respiration—may indicate that upper abdominal organs under the influence of diaphragmatic motion (liver, spleen, stomach) are involved
- Pulsation—transmitted pulses expand in one plane (usually anteroposterior); direct pulsatile masses (aneurysm) also pulsate laterally
- Fluctuation—fluid within a mass usually implies a cyst or an abscess, rarely a neoplasm, except for ovarian tumors

Percussion and Auscultation. Abdominal masses rarely contain sufficient air to provide a resonant percussion note. Examination of the remaining abdomen, however, may confirm significant displacement of bowel or associated ascites. Occasionally, auscultation of a mass may disclose a bruit, which implies a vascular origin or a highly vascularized neoplasm.

Rectal and Pelvic Examination. A rectal and pelvic examination is vital to delineate pelvic, perirectal, or intrarectal masses and should include bimanual examination of the abdomen and pelvis. A test for occult blood should always be performed.

Diagnostic Tests: What Tests in What Order?

Diagnostic investigations have two principal goals with respect to abdominal masses: to define the responsible organ and to determine the disease process. The surgeon can facilitate the work-up by consulting with the radiologist, who can then provide specific examinations or special views to pinpoint the location of the mass.

An acute abdominal series should be completed as the initial radiographic evaluation. This includes PA and lateral chest x-ray films and flat and upright abdominal films. Frequently the mass can be seen on radiographs, but more importantly one looks for other abnormalities, such as pleural effusions, free intraperitoneal air, dilated bowel loops, calcifications involving vessels, organs, or stones, or retroperitoneal air.

Computed Tomography. Computed tomographic (CT) scanning has further refined the diagnosis of abdominal lesions, as it has intracranial ones. Body scanning has been especially helpful with pancreatic masses (Figs. 28-3 and 28-4) and other obscure or inaccessible masses, with increasing resolution approaching 1 cm. CT scanning has become the initial diagnostic procedure for most abdominal masses after history-taking, physical examination, and abdominal x-ray evaluations have been completed. If a CT scan is contemplated, it should be done before any barium studies of the GI tract are initiated, because any residual barium in the GI tract will cause a scattering of the x-rays, thus resulting in a poor or inadequate CT scan. Abdominal and pelvic CT scans will identify and help differentiate almost all abdominal masses. If not contraindicated, oral and intravenous water-soluble contrast should be administered.

Ultrasonography. Ultrasound is a safe, rapid, noninvasive diagnostic modality that is readily available in most hospitals. It is excellent for evaluating pelvic and biliary tract problems and is the diagnostic test of choice if one suspects an enlarged gallbladder. Acute cholecystitis, hydrops, or an obstructed biliary tract outflow can all present with a palpable gallbladder. Ultrasonography is also an excellent tool for evaluating pelvic masses. It can be especially helpful in

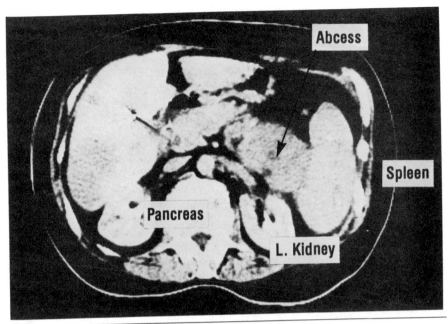

FIGURE 28-3   A lesser sac infected fluid collection (pancreatic abscess) lies anterior to the body and tail of the pancreas and displaces the left kidney posteriorly and an enlarged spleen laterally.

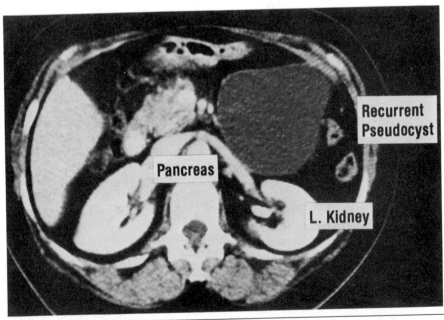

FIGURE 28-4   A recurrent pancreatic pseudocyst is seen to lie anterior to the body and tail of the pancreas, pushing the stomach anteriorly and toward the midline, and to "point" toward the abdominal wall at the site of previous external drainage. Because of its relatively high location under the costal margin, this mass was not palpable.

an obese patient, when examination is difficult and the presence of a mass is in question. It also helps distinguish the mass as solid or cystic.

Ultrasonography is very helpful for retroperitoneal organs such as the pancreas, aorta, and kidney. It is the method of choice for following pancreatic pseudocysts or small abdominal aortic aneurysms. The technology of ultrasonography continues to improve, with better resolution, and the method will be used more frequently as this decade progresses.

Gastrointestinal Contrast X-ray Evaluation. An upper GI series, small bowel follow-through, and barium enema will delineate lesions arising within the GI tract. Mucosal studies will often differentiate carcinomas from lesions arising from the wall of the bowel (e.g., leiomyoma, lymphosarcoma). In addition, masses arising outside the GI tract can be localized by the presence of pressure defects or displacement of the bowel. The direction of displacement may be important to differentiate intraperitoneal from retroperitoneal masses. Pelvic masses can be frequently outlined by the relationship to the sigmoid colon or rectum.

Endoscopy. Sigmoidoscopy, fiberoptic colonoscopy, and gastroduodenoscopy are all used to delineate and biopsy lesions within the gastrointestinal tract, in many cases providing the diagnosis and facilitating the operative treatment of such lesions. Sigmoidoscopy should be performed early to demonstrate rectal displacement or obstruction, which might influence the performance of subsequent contrast studies.

Intravenous Pyelogram. This is an important study used to delineate the location and, frequently, the origin of retroperitoneal masses. Since the ureters are attached to the peritoneum, their anterior displacement is a characteristic finding in retroperitoneal masses that are centrally located. To demonstrate this, a lateral view on the intravenous pyelogram (IVP) must be included. In addition, nonvisualization of a kidney, displacement of the kidney, defects in the collecting system, or indentations of the bladder may indicate the presence, location, and likely origin of a particular mass.

Cystoscopy. This endoscopic technique is useful for defining masses that compress, erode, or invade the urinary bladder.

Conventional Radionuclide Imagery. Scintiscans with a variety of ever-promising isotopes have been useful on occasion in defining some masses. The method is dependent on the specificity of isotope uptake by the tissue forming the mass. Such methods require most careful interpretation and a continuing concern for accuracy. Some isotopes, such as radioactive iodine-131 in the thyroid, have an affinity for a specific organ. Others, such as technetium or strontium, are much less specific, depending on cellular activity and/or blood supply. Gallium, for example, has been used to define inflammatory tissue, including abscesses, with variable reliability.

These methods require special skill and experience and refinement of both by reviewing all correlations (positive and negative) and by continuing observation of the patient to achieve the highest value in the clinical situation. They are supplemented in most situations by ultrasonography and CT scans.

Retrograde Cholangiopancreatography. The ability to cannulate the ampulla of Vater by using the fiberoptic endoscope has led to the infusion of contrast material into the biliary and pancreatic ducts with x-ray delineation. This can be a vital examination for certain pancreatic or biliary masses.

Arteriography. Radiographic visualization of the arterial supply to a mass will usually determine its organ of origin. The multiple sites of arterial supply to a given organ may require catheterization of more than one arterial trunk (e.g., celiac and superior mesenteric arteries to visualize a pancreatic lesion). These studies will demonstrate the displacement of arteries in the vicinity of the mass, the characteristic of the blood supply (vascular masses are usually malignant, avascular masses may be cystic), and invasion of the vessels by tumor (encasement). As a result, arteriography has replaced less-specific studies (e.g., retroperitoneal air insufflation) in delineation of abdominal masses. Frequently, in association with computed tomography, specific characteristics of a mass can be defined to determine the precise operative approach. Arteriography is especially beneficial in planning the operative approach for a mass in the liver. Arteriography is also helpful in diagnosing visceral artery aneurysms; however, its use in abdominal aortic aneurysms is for assessing the extent of involvement of the aneurysm and defining the outflow. *The diagnosis of abdominal aortic aneurysms should be made by physical examination, lateral abdominal x-ray views, ultrasound, or CT scan—not by arteriography.*

The disadvantage of arteriography as a means of refining the diagnosis of abdominal masses is the problem of access. Usually achieved by retrograde cannulation via the femoral or brachial arteries, such access is associated with thrombosis or persistent bleeding at the site in less than 0.5% of studies. *The majority of abdominal masses do not require arteriography for diagnosis or preoperative evaluation.*

WHAT MASSES REQUIRE URGENT OR EMERGENCY TREATMENT?
Masses Associated With Bacteremia

Clinical Setting. Acute onset of fever, tachycardia, and malaise associated with a tender abdominal mass indicate that the mass may contain pus or may represent a frank or impending GI perforation. Leukocytosis, with an increased number of premature neutrophils, is usually present. The location of the mass may indicate the urgent need for drainage or diversion of the fecal stream.

Diagnostic Tests. If gastrointestinal perforation is suspected, barium studies are contraindicated; plain x-ray films of the abdomen and chest are done first. Free intraperitoneal air, best seen on an upright chest x-ray film, is generally diagnostic for a ruptured viscus and requires urgent operative intervention without further diagnostic studies. Retroperitoneal air, masses displacing organs, and calcification in an aneurysm wall are further examples of abnormalities that may be seen on plain x-ray evaluation. If it is not obvious that a patient needs an urgent operation, an abdominal and pelvic CT scan with oral and intravenous contrast media is usually the next step. The CT will almost always show the mass and generally help differentiate the cause. If one suspects the mass to be a distended gallbladder, ultrasonography would be the diagnostic choice after plain x-ray films.

Barium studies, IVP, and arteriography are usually not needed in such patients. Laparoscopy is usually not indicated when a mass is felt. This generally indicates the disease process is further advanced and beyond the realm of the laparoscope. However, some enlarged, infected gallbladders can be removed with use of the laparoscope. An intra-abdominal abscess from a perforated ulcer could be drained and the ulcer closed via a laparoscope and gastroscope. This technology is in its infancy; its use and indications should continue to expand. A CT scan may be helpful to differentiate suspected acute pancreatitis from a process requiring immediate operation (e.g., an alimentary tract perforation). In many instances an operation may be required before any additional examinations are ordered

and without a firm diagnosis in hand.

Treatment. Control of sepsis is essential, and broad-spectrum antibiotics are started in large parenteral doses. Nasogastric intubation, administration of intravenous fluids, and preparation of the patient for operation are simultaneously performed. If the initial treatment clearly provides relief of bacteremia, as manifested by reduction in temperature, leukocytosis, and/or tenderness over the mass, operation may be delayed hour by hour until a clearer definition of the cause can be ascertained (see further discussion in Chapter 25). In diverticulitis or cancer, complete resolution of sepsis over 12 to 24 hours may allow the pertinent gastrointestinal contrast studies to be performed electively. If the condition is not resolving clinically, an operation with drainage, diversion, and/or resection of the intestine must be performed.

Masses With Actual or Impending Rupture

Clinical Setting. Masses that are expanding in size and that are tender, painful, or pulsating may rupture. Masses that rupture usually involve pus, stool, or blood—any of which when released suddenly into the peritoneal cavity can be catastrophic to the patient. Operation before the rupture occurs is mandatory to avoid the patient's death. Ruptured aortic aneurysms carry a 50% to 70% mortality in most centers, compared with rates of 5% to 10% when unruptured.

Diagnostic Tests. Diagnostic tests should be limited according to the severity of the clinical situation. Where a recent increase in size of the mass is demonstrated, immediate operation may be indicated, particularly if tenderness is elicited. A lateral x-ray film of the lumbar spine will delineate the presence of an aortic aneurysm in 50% of cases by demonstration of calcification in its anterior wall. If the patient is stable, a CT scan usually gives the most useful information in patients with an abdominal mass.

Treatment. *In ruptured aortic aneurysm, operation is indicated as soon as possible if the patient's life is to be saved.* The patient's hemodynamic status will dictate the speed with which operative intervention should be initiated. If the patient's condition is stable and the diagnosis is in doubt, a CT scan should be done urgently. Evidence of a ruptured abdominal aortic aneurysm, even in a stable patient, requires immediate operative repair.

Where the size is increasing slowly over a period of days, such diagnostic maneuvers as a CT scan (pancreatic pseudocyst), ultrasonography, or HIDA (hepato-iminodiacetic acid) scan for hydrops of the gallbladder, may be carried out. In all cases the aim of treatment is to operate before a rupture occurs.

Masses Associated With Gastrointestinal Obstruction

Clinical Setting. The cardinal signs of intestinal obstruction will be present (e.g., crampy abdominal pain, vomiting, distension). (This is discussed in Chapter 25 in detail.) The obstruction is usually from a tumor of the intestinal tract itself (e.g., colon carcinoma) or from a mass impinging on the intestine. The latter may be neoplastic, infectious, or cystic.

Diagnostic Tests. The diagnosis of small or large bowel obstruction should be made by appropriate flat and upright abdominal films. If a large bowel obstruction is suspected, a proctosigmoidoscopy and barium enema, if necessary, should be done. This will determine whether an obstruction is present and will help in operative planning to correct the obstruction. For small bowel obstructions, barium studies or upper endoscopy are usually not helpful and may be harmful. If a gastric outlet obstruction is suspected, however, an upper GI series will confirm this. Exact identification of the nature of the mass is not necessary and can usually await relief of the obstruction.

Treatment. The treatment of intestinal obstruction is discussed in Chapter 25. Essentially, the usual plan includes fluid rehydration, intestinal decompression, and operation within 4 to 12 hours. Treatment of the mass must await operative diagnosis. Resection will depend on the surgeon's judgment and, in many cases, will necessitate a second operation after the obstruction is relieved, the patient's condition is stabilized, and an exact diagnosis is established. When infection and obstruction occur simultaneously, the patient is treated first for the sepsis and then for the obstruction. Failure of the infectious process to resolve may necessitate earlier operation, even before the patient is thoroughly evaluated.

SPECIAL ABDOMINAL MASSES
Intraperitoneal Masses

Can a Stomach Carcinoma Present as a Mass? Carcinomas constitute 95% of gastric cancers. Although there is no clear explanation, the incidence of carcinoma of the stomach in the United States has declined by 50% during the past 25 years. It is more common in men than women (2 : 1), in blacks than whites, and in the 50- to 70-year-old age group. This age group has a higher incidence of atrophic gastritis, which may be etiologically significant in the development of gastric cancer. Similarly, patients with achlorhydria have a fourfold increase in stomach cancer compared with those with normal acid production in the same age group. The incidence of gastric carcinoma is significantly increased in patients with achlorhydria and pernicious anemia and those who have undergone previous gastric operations.

Approximately one third of such patients will have an epigastric or left upper quadrant mass. This implies a lower chance of resectability but not necessarily incurability. In most patients, symptoms are vague and long-standing, including indigestion, postprandial fullness, nausea, and vomiting. Often, unexplained weight loss, anorexia, and anemia finally bring the patient to the attention of a physician. Occasionally, free perforation or massive upper gastrointestinal bleeding is the precipitating event.

Signs of incurability are a pelvic mass secondary to ovarian metastases (Krukenberg's tumor), cervical nodes (Virchow's), hepatic or peritoneal metastases manifested by ascites and/or fullness in the cul-de-sac of Douglas (Blumer's shelf) on rectal examination, and distant metastasis (lungs and brain). Clinically demonstrable lung metastases are unusual but have been documented at autopsy in 25% of patients.

The diagnosis can be made by radiographic contrast studies and by endoscopic examination, tissue biopsy, and cytologic studies. Abdominal CT scans are generally done to evaluate the extent of the local tumor and to look for metastatic disease (adjacent lymph nodes, liver). Treatment consists of adequate gastric resection, usually including appropriate regional lymph nodes.

The outlook for patients with gastric carcinoma is poor (Fig. 28-5). Two thirds of patients have physical or operative findings of spread beyond the stomach, and less than one third of the remainder survive 5 years.

What Small Intestinal Masses Are There? Small bowel masses are uncommon but may appear in any part of the abdomen. *Regional enteritis* in the chronic form is characterized by constant aching pain and abdominal soreness, which usually implies an advanced disease state

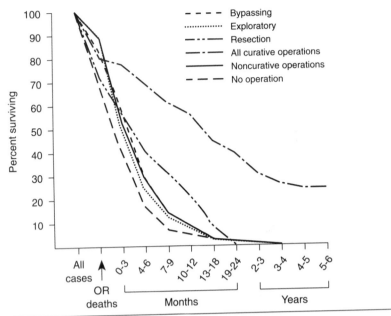

FIGURE 28-5 Graphic representation of survival in carcinoma of the stomach. (From Lawrence W Jr. Carcinoma of the stomach. Ca 23:303, 1973.)

and partial obstruction, and is often associated with a tender, palpable, ballottable right lower quadrant mass. Typically these patients are thin and have a history of bowel irregularity. The diagnosis can be established with small bowel contrast radiographic studies. Treatment is discussed in Chapter 27.

Ileocecal intussusception is characterized by a sausage-shaped abdominal mass, varying in location; it is typically found in an infant or young child (80% occur between 3 months and 2 years) with colicky abdominal pain, distention, and hematochezia. The absence of palpable bowel in the right lower quadrant can be confirmed by plain abdominal x-ray evaluation that discloses an absence of cecal bowel gas and a pattern consistent with intestinal obstruction. The diagnosis is established by cautious use of barium enema, which may also be used to attempt hydrostatic reduction in favorable situations in children. If nonoperative reduction fails or is contraindicated, the intussusception must be reduced operatively or resected in situ. In adults with intussusception, a tumor is usually present and is the cause of the intussusception.

Appendix

What Are the Symptoms and Signs of Appendicitis? The history and physical examina-

tion are the most important diagnostic aids in appendicitis. A white blood count is also valuable; generally no other tests are needed. In an adult with a typical history of anorexia, periumbilical and/or epigastric pain that later settles in the right lower quadrant, and with nausea and subsequent emesis associated with leukocytosis and low-grade fever, *a tender right lower quadrant mass is periappendical induration and edema or abscess until proved otherwise.* Diagnostic maneuvers are limited to exploration. Treatment consists of appendectomy. If a walled-off abscess is present, drainage is instituted (Chapter 25). Occasionally the appendix cannot be identified or safely removed because of intense inflammation. Drainage with subsequent appendectomy (6 weeks) can sometimes be a safer alternative. Perforated cecal carcinomas can mimic appendicitis. Good surgical judgment plus frozen section pathologic examination will help decide whether a right colon resection is indicated.

In an infant with abdominal pain and tenderness, low-grade fever, and leukocytosis, a markedly thickened, acutely inflamed appendix can often be sensed on bimanual rectal examination.

Mucocele. Occasionally an asymptomatic right lower quadrant mass represents a mucocele, which is a cystic dilation of the appendix containing mucoid material. This is typically be-

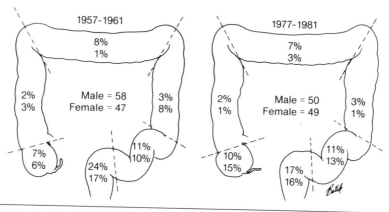

FIGURE 28-6 Distribution of colorectal cancer by sex. (From Netscher DT, Larson GM. Colon cancer: The left to right shift and its implications. Surg Gastroenterol 2:13, 1983. With permission from S. Karger AG, Basel.)

nign but occasionally contains a slowly progressive papillary adenocarcinoma. Appendectomy without rupture of the mucocele is adequate treatment.

Colon

Colon Carcinoma. Colorectal carcinoma is the most common newly diagnosed cancer in North America. One third of patients with right-sided carcinoma present with a palpable mass. Left-sided colon and rectal carcinomas are more likely to present with obstructive symptoms or red blood per rectum. Some 40% to 50% of colonic cancers can be palpated on digital rectal examination or visualized by the sigmoidoscope (Fig. 28-6). Three percent of all patients with large bowel cancers have more than one colorectal carcinoma present; thus a complete evaluation of the colon and rectum should be done. When possible, endoscopy of the large bowel should be done on all these patients. This allows for visualization and biopsy of the tumor. Rigid proctosigmoidoscopy can be easily done to 25 cm and is an excellent way of visualizing the rectum. Flexible sigmoidoscopy can be performed to 60 cm and is preferred by many because of its greater length and better tolerance by the patient. Colonoscopy and/or barium enema are used to examine the rest of the colon. Colonoscopy is more accurate but more expensive, and one is not always able to visualize the complete colon, as compared with use of a barium enema.

Dukes developed a useful classification scheme (Fig. 28-7) that has been repeatedly modified. His original A was limited to the bowel wall, B included extension through the bowel

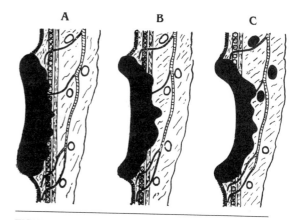

FIGURE 28-7 Classification of cancer of the rectum into three groups (**A, B,** and **C**) according to the depth of spread. (From Dukes C. Proc R Soc Med 30:371, 1936.)

without nodal metastases, and C encompassed regional nodal metastases. This system has been modified several times to include B_1 and B_2, C_1 and C_2, and D stages. Many advocate use of the TNM system, which includes more variables. The future of cancer staging will involve cellular and biologic activity measurements of the tumor.

The clinical manifestations of right and left colon cancer are different (Table 28-1). Right colon malignancies are usually large, fungating, ulcerating lesions that predispose the patient to chronic blood loss because of the large friable surface area of the tumor. Colon obstruction is uncommon because of the large caliber of the right colon, the liquid nature of the stool at this level, and the growth pattern of the cancer, unless it obstructs the ileocecal valve. Therefore, in

TABLE 28-1   Comparison of Symptoms and Signs Associated With Right and Left Large Bowel Cancers

Symptom or Sign	Right Colon Cancer	Left Colon Cancer
Abdominal pain	Frequent	Uncommon
Altered bowel habits	Diarrhea frequent	Obstructive: ↓ stool caliber
Palpable mass	Often present	Usually present
Rectal bleeding	Occult	Visible
Anemia	Frequent	Uncommon

lesions of the right colon, microcytic hypochromic anemia and weakness are typical. The bulky right colon tumor is situated in the right iliac fossa, is ballottable or fixed, and nontender.

Left colon lesions are napkin-ring or annular lesions, which predispose the patient to bowel obstruction because of the constricting nature of the lesion, the smaller caliber of the left colon, and the solid consistency of the stool at this level. A change in bowel habits, such as increasing constipation, decreased caliber of stools, and visible rectal bleeding, is typical of left colon cancers. The bleeding associated with these tumors is seldom profuse. A palpable mass is present in some sigmoid tumors, but much less often than with right-sided lesions. Many rectosigmoidal cancers can be felt on careful rectal examination.

Any change in bowel habits, especially in a person over 40 years of age, supraumbilical abdominal pain in right-sided and infraumbilical pain in left-sided colon lesions, blood in the stools, and anemia are cardinal signs and symptoms of colon cancer and warrant evaluation (Fig. 28-8).

Despite anecdotal data to the contrary, colorectal adenocarcinoma behaves biologically much as do other cancers. While some colon cancers double in size only every 600 days or so, it is their local manifestations that often determine survival, especially lumenal obstruction and, much less commonly, hemorrhage. Half of all colon cancers destined to recur after curative resection do so within 18 months. The mean duration of survival if the recurrence is untreated is but an additional 6 months.

The treatment of choice is adequate surgical resection. Operative mortality should not exceed 5% in skilled hands. The outlook is good when the lesion is detected promptly and properly treated. The importance of resectability and lymph node involvement for long-term survival is shown in Fig. 28-9. The relative 5-year survival rate for lesions confined to the bowel wall is twice as great as for those patients with lymph node involvement following surgical resection.

Does Diverticulitis Require an Operation? Diverticula occur most commonly in the sigmoid and descending colon and are generally not seen in persons under 35 years of age; incidence increases significantly with age. More than one third of people over 65 and two thirds of those over 85 are affected. However, most such lesions never produce symptoms of any sort.

Inflammation is the most frequent complication of diverticulosis. Acute diverticulitis is often referred to clinically as *left-side appendicitis* and occurs in about 40% of patients who experience complications of diverticulosis. More serious complications, such as intestinal obstruction, free perforation with peritonitis, or fistula, occur in about 15% of patients who develop diverticulitis. Acute exacerbations of diverticulitis may be associated with left lower quadrant pain, tenderness, and muscle guarding, along with fever and leukocytosis. A tender, fixed mass may be palpable and may be well defined but is more often sensed as a vague, tender fullness.

Contrast radiographic studies should be deferred until the acute inflammatory signs abate. *Treatment consists of bowel rest and systemic antibiotics, which, in the absence of such complications as abscess, free perforation, or obstruction, are usually successful.* With clinical improvement, the left lower quadrant mass, which is most often induration and edema, gradually subsides. Failure to improve and persistence or presence of a tender mass in a patient with sepsis denote abscess formation and require operative intervention. A CT scan is helpful in establishing the diagnosis and evaluating for an abscess.

All of the serious complications ultimately require surgical attention, the extent and timing of which is a function of the particular complication. Resection of the involved colon and diversion of the fecal stream (diverting colostomy) may be necessary to achieve resolution of the inflammatory process.

Other Inflammatory Masses. Two very un-

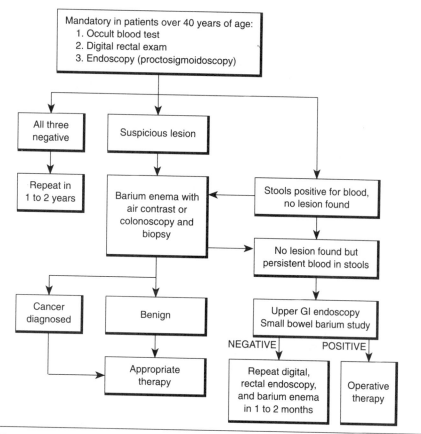

FIGURE 28-8   Algorithm for diagnosis of colorectal cancer.

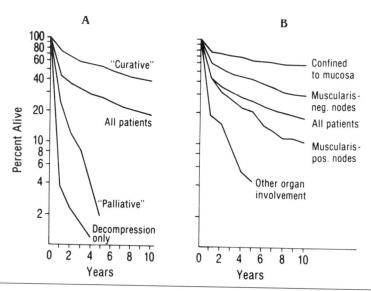

FIGURE 28-9   Colon cancer survival by treatment (**A**) and microscopic extent (**B**) of disease. (From Floyd CE, Stirling CT, Cohn I Jr. Cancer of the colon, rectum and anus: A review of 1,687 cases. Ann Surg 163:835, 1966.)

usual inflammatory masses typically involving the right colon and cecum are caused by *Entamoeba histolytica* and *Actinomyces israelii*. Both usually reflect an especially significant history or clear-cut histologic changes after resection.

Omentum

Torsion of the omentum, whether primary or secondary, may present as an acute abdomen, mimicking acute appendicitis, acute cholecystitis, or twisted ovarian cyst. Depending on the bulk of strangulated omentum involved, a mass may or may not be palpable. Laparotomy is indicated when the surgeon is confronted with an acute abdomen, at which time the omental torsion is resected.

Omental cysts are rare, usually an incidental finding at laparotomy, and are typically small. Occasionally they may be large and, if palpable, are usually smooth, ballottable, nontender mid-abdominal masses. Diagnosis is made at laparotomy, and treatment is complete excision.

Omental tumors are usually metastatic and typically of gastric, colon, or ovarian origin. If palpable, they are firm, ballottable, and nontender. Multiple masses may be palpated that are the result of metastatic disease. Definition of the primary site is essential.

Mesentery

Primary mesenteric tumors, both benign and malignant, are quite rare. Small bowel obstruction may complicate such tumors, depending on their location in the mesentery. Diagnosis is generally made at laparotomy, with surgical resection the treatment of choice. This can only be accomplished when the process is peripheral to the superior mesenteric artery and vein. Metastatic tumor implants into the mesentery are much more common than are primary tumors.

Liver

The normal liver can be outlined on surface anatomy, as shown in Fig. 28-2. Hepatomegaly secondary to hepatitis of variable cause and cirrhosis can usually be readily differentiated from problems requiring exploration. Ultrasonography can usually differentiate obstructive from nonobstructive jaundice based on the size of the biliary ducts.

Carcinoma of the Liver. Primary carcinoma of the liver is unusual in the United States: as determined by postmortem examination, the in-

cidence is 1 in 400. It is much more common among Asians. It occurs predominantly in adult men and typically arises in a patient with a cirrhotic liver. The patient usually complains of dull but persistent upper abdominal pain and a dragging sensation, and a large, nontender, variably nodular liver is found on physical examination. Associated findings often include weight loss and fever.

Liver function test results are variable. Typically the alkaline phosphatase level is abnormal. A CT scan will disclose a space-occupying lesion and may indicate the extent of spread of the tumor. Selective arteriography will localize the lesions by pooling and increased vascularity and aid in preoperative determination of resectability. Percutaneous liver biopsy may provide definitive pathologic information preoperatively, but the final diagnosis and delineation of resectability usually require laparotomy.

Treatment includes resection, if anatomically possible, in the absence of distant metastases, followed by chemotherapy. Radiation therapy is of no value. Transplantation following total hepatectomy has been reported. The prognosis is probably even poorer than is reflected by the collected series shown in Table 28-2.

Metastatic malignancy to the liver is much more common and often presents as solitary or multiple hepatic masses. In most instances, the primary cancer has been diagnosed or is readily detected. Isolated hepatic metastases in the absence of other metastatic or recurrent disease deserve careful consideration, as resection is occasionally followed by long-term survival (see Table 28-2). A CT scan and arteriogram are warranted to determine the possibility of resection of the metastases. If spread to both lobes or distant metastases are discovered on the above studies, then resection would not be indicated.

Miscellaneous Liver Masses. Benign adenomas of the liver have been found to be etiologically related to the use of oral contraceptive medications. Hepatic adenomas are usually solitary, and a typical presentation is that of acute intraperitoneal hemorrhage. Such patients require laparotomy and suture of the bleeding site. Whether resection is essential or whether such lesions regress with discontinuation of the causative agents is not yet known with certainty.

A patient who has pyogenic liver abscess usually presents with systemic signs of sepsis. However, hepatomegaly or a right upper quadrant mass can be the method of presentation. Typically, the lesion is tender. A variable number of patients (20% to 50%, depending on the source)

TABLE 28-2 Surgical Treatment of Liver Cancer

| | Primary Liver Cancer (Adults) (%) | | Metastatic Cancer (%)* | |
	Asian Patients	Nonasian Patients	All	Colon and Rectum
Operative mortality	24	22	—	—
Alive at 2 years	23	59	48	47
Alive at 5 years	6	36	21	21

Reprinted with permission from Foster JH. Survival after liver resection for cancer. Ca 26:493-502, 1970.
*These represent highly selective cases.

display few if any signs of infection. Liver abscess is usually attributable to complications of abdominal trauma and/or inflammatory processes, especially in the biliary tract. Parenteral drug abuse is another important predisposing cause. Liver function derangements and nuclear scans are associated with frequent diagnostic errors. Because the abscesses are often multiple, an abdominal CT scan should precede exploration and drainage. Carefully chosen antibiotics should be initiated before operation, and a long period of therapy after drainage may be necessary. Such treatment in the uncompromised host is regularly effective.

Benign solitary nonparasitic cyst of the liver presents as a painless and asymptomatic right upper quadrant mass. Diagnosis is made on the basis of extrinsic compression of adjacent viscera by a variety of imaging methods. Treatment is surgical, except for small cysts, and depends on the character and location of the cyst. Hydatid (*Echinococcus*) cysts are extremely rare in the United States and are regularly treated successfully with oral metronidazole when recognized as such. Ultrasound or CT scan are both excellent diagnostic studies.

Gallbladder and Extrahepatic Biliary System

Abdominal masses related to this organ system are limited to benign and malignant disease of the gallbladder and choledochal cysts. The gallbladder underlies the paracentral point (Fig. 28-2) and is palpable as an abdominal mass in disease states that include carcinoma, hydrops, empyema, and passive dilation secondary to periampullary carcinoma.

Hydrops of the Gallbladder. A palpable, tender gallbladder may result when calculi obstruct the cystic duct, causing absorption of the bile in the gallbladder. The mucosa of the gallbladder continues to secrete, with resultant distension of the gallbladder with a white mucinous material. Cholecystectomy is indicated to avoid:

- Extrusion of the impacted calculi into the common bile duct, possibly resulting in obstructive jaundice with or without cholangitis
- Empyema of the gallbladder secondary to infection of the hydrops
- Intraperitoneal perforation

Hydrops of the gallbladder is an urgent indication for operation. Preoperative ultrasonography or HIDA scan will help confirm the diagnosis.

Empyema of the Gallbladder. The pathogenesis of empyema or abscess of the gallbladder is described in Chapter 25 and represents an acute surgical emergency. The patient is septic, with a typical chronic cholecystitis-cholelithiasis history and has an exquisitely tender right upper quadrant mass, with marked involuntary muscular guarding. The mass usually is perceived to move with the liver on inspiration and expiration. Cholecystectomy is the treatment of choice. Again, ultrasound or HIDA scan usually confirms the diagnosis.

Carcinoma of the Gallbladder. Carcinoma of the gallbladder is a disease of the elderly; 75% of such patients are over 60 years of age. They are predominantly female, which is consistent with the higher incidence of biliary disease in general in women. Carcinoma of the gallbladder is found in approximately 1% of routine cholecystectomies. However, the incidence increases with age and can be as high as 10% in patients with symptomatic cholelithiasis. Conversely, 90% of patients with carcinoma of the gallbladder have biliary calculi.

The clinical features of this disease are similar to those of benign biliary disease. The diagnosis is seldom made preoperatively. Typically, there is a history of chronic cholecystitis-cholelithiasis, and at the time of hospitalization about half of these patients are jaundiced. A mass is palpable in approximately two thirds of patients and can be differentiated from the liver in about one third of these. Although not documented, one differentiating point, in the absence of cholangitis, may be relative nontenderness of the mass. Laboratory diagnostic support is not helpful. The calcified (porcelain) gallbladder should be removed because of a particularly high incidence of associated carcinoma.

Treatment ranges from cholecystectomy to cholecystectomy with right hepatic lobectomy and lymphadenectomy of the portal triad. Regardless of the stage of the disease or the treatment provided, carcinoma of the gallbladder has a 5-year survival of less than 2%.

Periampullary Carcinoma. The gallbladder that is not chronically inflamed and scarred will become distended in 25% to 50% of patients with obstructive jaundice secondary to periampullary carcinoma (Chapter 26). Passive distension of the gallbladder under these circumstances (Courvoisier's sign) is a nontender, palpable, right upper quadrant mass in patients who have the accompanying signs and symptoms of obstructive jaundice.

Choledochal Cyst. Congenital cystic dilation of the extrahepatic biliary tree is called *choledochal cyst* and takes three common forms: (1) diffuse fusiform dilation of the entire common bile duct, (2) a cyst localized to the distal common bile duct, or (3) cystic dilation of the hepatic and common bile ducts, with the cystic duct entering the choledochal cyst.

Approximately one third of choledochal cysts occur in children. In adult women they occur, rarely, as an epigastric mass associated with pain, tenderness, and jaundice. Percutaneous transhepatic or endoscopic retrograde cholangiography is usually helpful in planning operative correction. Treatment consists of internal drainage modified relative to operative findings.

Spleen

Trauma. "Spontaneous rupture of the spleen" is probably a misnomer, since occult blunt trauma associated with systemic disease that increased the fragility of the spleen is most likely responsible. This complication should be considered whenever a patient presents with an obviously enlarging spleen associated with hemodynamic instability, no cognizant history of trauma, and systemic disease states, such as infectious mononucleosis, malaria, congestive splenomegaly, or hematologic disorders.

Traumatic splenic rupture secondary to blunt trauma, resulting in a splenic mass, is an unusual isolated finding and is commonly associated with left lower rib fractures and variable degrees of intra-abdominal organ injury.

It is difficult to delineate the anatomic position of the normal spleen by surface markings (Fig. 28-10). This organ can best be palpated bimanually with the patient supine in a slight right lateral decubitus position. An enlarged spleen is rarely confused with other masses.

Ninety percent of ruptured spleens bleed intraperitoneally, and the patient presents with hypotension, tachycardia, tachypnea, restlessness, and left upper quadrant and/or generalized abdominal tenderness and ileus. However, vital signs may be stable and minimal abdominal findings elicited. Kehr's sign, or left shoulder pain secondary to left diaphragmatic irritation, is very helpful. Often multiple organ system injury is present, and pure signs and symptoms of splenic rupture are obscured.

Plain radiographic examinations of the abdomen are most useful diagnostically, reflecting an enlarged splenic shadow, medial displacement of the stomach, and caudal displacement of the splenic flexure of the colon secondary to an enlarging splenic or perisplenic hematoma. In patients obtunded as a result of alcoholic or drug intoxication or neurologic injury, or when findings on physical examination are equivocal, diagnostic peritoneal lavage is an efficacious adjunctive test with 98% accuracy when properly administered and interpreted. If the patient is hemodynamically stable, a CT scan is very helpful in evaluating spleen, liver, or kidney injury and may, in the clear absence of other injuries, permit nonoperative management. Leukocytosis is meaningless and not specific for splenic rupture, merely reflecting stress response. In such situations the traditional treatment of choice is splenectomy. Splenic repair or segmental splenic resection to preserve the spleen's role in host defense mechanisms is warranted, especially in infants and young children, and in adults when the patient is stable and the degree of injury will allow repair.

Hematologic Disorders. Numerous hematologic disorders and diseases of the reticuloendothelial system are associated with splenomegaly. The systemic manifestations and diagnostic abnormalities of the underlying disease process easily explain the development of splenomegaly (see the box on p. 519). Splenectomy is viewed as a simple excisional procedure. In the presence of significant hematologic disorders, which affect coagulation and/or response to infection and/or massive splenomegaly, splenectomy becomes a major task with corresponding risk. When splenectomy represents definitive treatment for a process (e.g., congenital spherocytosis) or relative cure, as with idiopathic thrombocytopenic purpura, there is no question of its value. In every instance the physician must weigh the likelihood of benefit from splenectomy against the risk of operation and should usually immunize such patients against pneumococcal infection before splenectomy.

HEMATOLOGIC DISORDERS AMENABLE TO SPLENECTOMY

Hemolytic anemias
Thrombocytopenic purpura—idiopathic and thrombotic
Hypersplenism—primary and secondary
Myeloid metaplasia
Hodgkin's disease, lymphosarcoma, leukemia, and reticulum cell sarcoma
Miscellaneous disorders
    Felty's syndrome
    Sarcoidosis
    Gaucher's disease
    Niemann-Pick's disease
    Fanconi's syndrome
    Porphyria erythropoietica
Spontaneous rupture

Retroperitoneal Masses

Pancreas. The surface anatomy of the pancreas is frequently misjudged. Fig. 28-11 indicates the orientation of the tail of the pancreas toward the left axilla. Pancreatic masses include carcinoma, pseudocysts, true cysts, abscesses, and acute lesser sac collections associated with acute pancreatitis.

Carcinoma. Carcinoma of the pancreas accounts for 2% to 3% of all cancers. Vague left abdominal or back pain, anorexia, and weight loss are symptoms of carcinoma of the body and tail of the pancreas. Only in the advanced stages of the disease will a firm left upper quadrant mass be palpable, at which time it is common to note ascites, metastases to the cul-de-sac of Douglas, or palpable periumbilical, inguinal, or supraclavicular lymph node metastases.

Carcinoma of the pancreas is located in the

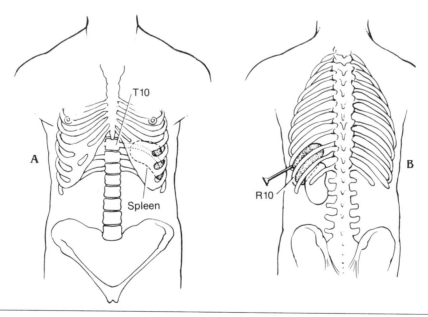

FIGURE 28-10 **A,** Anterior and **B,** posterior surface anatomy in relation to the location of the spleen. Note needle placement for splenic puncture (pulp pressure measurement of splenic portography). This would be incorrect placement if a thoracentesis was intended.

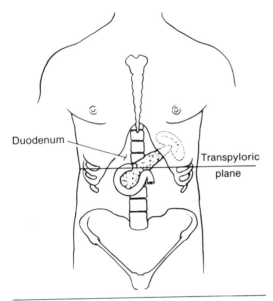

FIGURE 28-11   Relation of the pancreas to surface anatomy and some internal organs.

ELEVEN EARLY OBJECTIVE SIGNS USED TO CLASSIFY THE SEVERITY OF PANCREATITIS

At Admission or Diagnosis

1. Age over 55 years
2. White blood cell count over 16,000/ mm³
3. Blood glucose over 200 mgm/dl
4. Serum lactic dehydrogenase over 350 IU/L
5. Serum glutamic oxaloacetic transaminase over 250 Sigma Frankel Units/dl

During Initial 48 Hours

6. Hematocrit fall greater than 10 percentage points
7. Blood urea nitrogen rise more than 5 mg/dl
8. Serum calcium level below 8 mg/dl
9. Arterial Po_2 below 60 mm Hg
10. Base deficit greater than 4 mEq/L
11. Estimated fluid sequestration more than 6000 ml

From Ranson JHC, Spencer FC. The role of peritoneal lavage in severe acute pancreatitis. Ann Surg 187:566, 1978.

periampullary region in 65% of cases. Typical signs and symptoms include obstructive jaundice and hepatomegaly, with a distended gallbladder in 25% of cases. The tumor itself is seldom associated with a clinically palpable mass (Chapter 26).

Resection of cancers truly confined to the periampullary region by pancreatoduodenectomy (Whipple) yields a 25% 5-year survival rate in selected patients. Biliary and gastric decompression is beneficial for the patient not amenable to resection. Newer methods of biliary decompression such as biliary stents placed endoscopically are used more frequently in unresectable or elderly patients. For pancreatic carcinomas the 5-year survival rate is less than 5%.

Pancreatitis. Acute edematous pancreatitis accounts for approximately 1 of every 400 hospital admissions and is associated with the presence or history of alcoholism, biliary tract disease, trauma, and upper abdominal operations (Fig. 28-12). Objective assessment of the severity of the process is needed (see the box above). These signs correlate closely with risk (Fig. 28-13). Acute pancreatitis may present with a tender, fixed epigastric and/or left upper quadrant mass, and a transmitted aortic pulsation may be present. Associated persistent serum and urinary amylase elevations are present. Acute pleuropulmonary complications frequently supervene. The diagnostic possibilities in the acute

phase include an edematous pancreas and an acute lesser sac collection. The most efficacious diagnostic tool in this circumstance is a CT scan. Treatment includes nasogastric decompression, intravenous fluids, and possibly systemic antibiotics. Therapeutic peritoneal lavage may be helpful if the patient does not respond to standard treatment. Operation is indicated only if perforative ulcer disease and gangrenous intestine (two other common causes of hyperamylasemia) cannot be excluded, or if the patient's condition is rapidly deteriorating (Chapter 25). Again, a CT scan will help differentiate the diagnosis of acute pancreatitis in a very sick patient presenting with an acute abdomen.

If the patient has florid sepsis, the most likely diagnosis is pancreatic abscess, which may follow pancreatitis or result from secondary infection of an acute lesser sac collection or pseudocyst. Pancreatic abscess occurs in 1% to 4% of patients with acute pancreatitis and accounts for 6% to 16% of deaths in acute pancreatitis. These abscesses are known to extend into the sub-

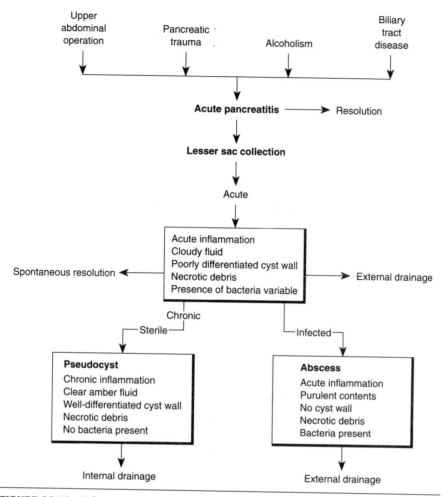

FIGURE 28-12 Schema of potential progression of lesser sac collections and surgical treatment.

hepatic and subphrenic spaces, dissect retroperitoneally, and sometimes present initially as a scrotal mass. Prompt external drainage is the treatment of choice. Uniformly fatal if untreated, the mortality in externally drained cases is approximately 35%. In patients with a necrotic, infected pancreas and retroperitoneum, surgical debridement, packing, and subsequent planned debridements may be necessary.

Lesser Sac Collections. The incidence of acute lesser sac collections is unknown, and a certain number will resolve spontaneously (Fig. 28-12). Others will persist and may become infected, resulting in abscess, the clinical presentation and treatment of which have been discussed. If they persist and remain sterile, pseudocyst formation results.

Pseudocysts and True Cysts. Pseudocysts occur in 10% to 20% of cases of acute pancreatitis as an

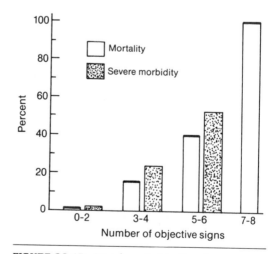

FIGURE 28-13 Number of objective signs present. (From Ranson JHC. Risk factors in acute pancreatitis. Hosp Prac 21(4):68-78, 1985.)

immediate or delayed finding. Such a collection is called a pseudocyst because it occurs in the lesser sac without an epithelium-lined wall. The risk of such a collection is related to infection (Fig. 28-3) or rupture into the free peritoneal cavity, which results in virulent chemical peritonitis. A certain number of pseudocysts resolve spontaneously. If they are persistent, internal drainage should not be undertaken less than 6 weeks after the estimated onset of the pseudocyst. If, at the time of operation, cyst wall substance is insufficient to allow internal drainage, disaster can be avoided by employing external drainage (Chapter 25). True cysts of the pancreas may be congenital or acquired and are most common in older women with no history of pancreatitis.

Kidney. The topographic anatomy of the kidney and ureters is shown in Fig. 28-14. In a thin patient, the kidneys may be palpable with the patient relaxed and supine and the examiner's left hand posteriorly elevating the flank, while the right hand compresses anteriorly and laterally below the costal margin in the anterior axillary line. As the patient breathes slowly and easily, the entire kidney can be outlined. In an obese patient the kidney usually is not palpable.

Abdominal Mass Secondary to Obstructive Disease

Hydronephrosis. Obstruction or stasis of urinary flow results in hydronephrosis. If this is an acute event, the kidney may be palpably enlarged. However, in chronic obstruction, the kidney will atrophy and may no longer be palpable. The process may be secondary to a multitude of pathologic entities (Table 28-3) and be unilateral or bilateral. Flank tenderness may be found if secondary infection has occurred.

Renal function is normal in unilateral hydronephrosis, and laboratory parameters are of little diagnostic value. Excretory and retrograde urograms are usually diagnostic.

Abdominal Mass Secondary to Renal Cystic Disease

Cystic diseases of the kidney are a heterogeneous group of conditions that differ in clinical presen-

TABLE 28-3   Causes of Hydronephrosis

Origin	Cause
Within ureteral lumen	Stones
Within ureteral wall (intrinsic)	Ureteral tumors
	Strictures
	Congenital ureteropelvic junction obstruction
Outside ureteral wall (extrinsic)	Retroperitoneal pelvis
	Extension from local neoplasms (e.g., colon, cervix)

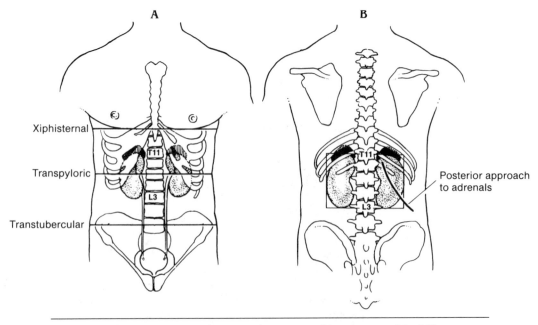

FIGURE 28-14   **A,** Anterior and **B,** posterior topographic anatomy of the kidney.

tation, clinical progression, and prognosis. Those most likely to present as an abdominal mass are simple renal cysts, multilocular cysts, multicystic kidney, and polycystic kidney.

Simple Cysts. The simple cyst is the most common cystic abnormality of the kidney. Simple cysts may be solitary, multiple, unilateral, or bilateral. They are uncommon in children. They are acquired abnormalities of undetermined cause and rarely destroy significant amounts of renal parenchyma unless they are multiple.

Simple cysts are detected most commonly as an incidental finding on excretory urography. Less frequently, they are symptomatic and pre-

sent as either a palpable abdominal mass or flank pain. Hematuria and infection are not commonly found with simple cysts.

A common diagnostic problem is the differentiation of renal cysts from solid renal masses—more specifically, hypernephroma. A systematic approach, as outlined in Fig. 28-15, using nephrotomography, ultrasonography, computed tomography, cyst puncture, and renal arteriography will provide the diagnosis in the vast majority of cases. Abdominal exploration for a simple renal cyst is not indicated unless the cyst is symptomatic or the diagnostic work-up cannot distinguish between cyst and neoplasm.

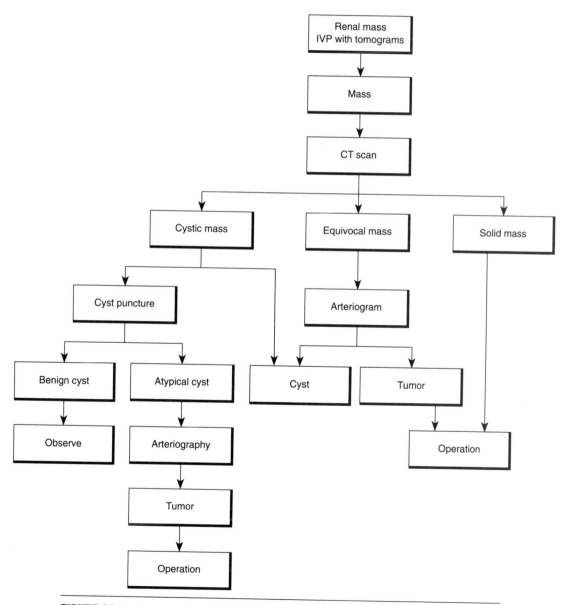

FIGURE 28-15   Systematic evaluation of renal mass.

Multilocular Cysts. Multilocular cysts of the kidney are unusual lesions. They are characterized by septa that divide the cyst into multiple noncommunicating chambers. They are felt to be congenital, although they are usually not discovered until later in life. Some feel they are a benign form of nephroblastoma (Wilms' tumor).

The usual clinical presentation is an asymptomatic mass found incidentally. Excretory urography shows a cystic lesion indistinguishable from a simple cyst. Arteriography usually shows an avascular mass. CT scan will show the characteristic septa. These lesions are often difficult to distinguish accurately from neoplasms, and a diagnostic exploration is sometimes required.

Multilocular cysts are best treated by partial nephrectomy.

Multicystic Kidneys. Multicystic kidney is a nonhereditary disease of the newborn. It is usually unilateral and is invariably associated with ureteral obstruction or atresia. Bilateral multicystic kidneys are much less common and are a cause of neonatal renal failure. Multicystic kidneys are characterized by a large, irregularly lobulated mass of cysts. Excretory urography shows nonfunction of the multicystic kidney. Differentiation between hydronephrosis secondary to congenital ureteropelvic junction obstruction in the newborn may be difficult even after ultrasonography, intravenous pyelogram (IVP), and a renal scan have been performed. Retrograde pyelography and even exploration may be necessary. Therapy for multicystic kidney has been surgical removal. There is a higher incidence of congenital malformations of other organ systems at autopsy.

Polycystic Kidney Disease. There are two forms of polycystic disease—infantile and adult.

Adult Polycystic Kidney Disease. Adult polycystic kidney disease is a hereditary disease transmitted by autosomal dominant inheritance and therefore the patient will be likely to have a family history of the condition. With progressive age, the patient develops multiple cysts on both kidneys. The clinical presentation may include enlarged kidneys on palpation, flank pain, hematuria, hypertension, and azotemia. Excretory urography will demonstrate enlarged renal shadows and bizarre spidery deformity of the calyces. Retrograde pyelography is contraindicated because of the risk of infection. Differential diagnosis includes bilateral hydronephrosis, bilateral renal tumors, and multiple simple cysts. However, the clinical picture and family history are usually sufficiently clear to make the diagnosis.

Treatment of adult polycystic disease is supportive. Infections, hypertension, and uremic complications must be treated as they arise. Nephrectomy is sometimes necessary to control exsanguinating hemorrhage, uncontrollable infection, and refractory hypertension.

Infantile Polycystic Disease. Infantile polycystic disease is a rare hereditary condition transmitted by autosomal recessive inheritance. It may also affect older children in which case the disease is usually less severe. Newborns with the severe form of the disease die within the first few days of life, usually due to respiratory insufficiency secondary to associated pulmonary hypoplasia. Older children develop progressive renal failure, hypertension with congestive heart failure, and portal hypertension secondary to hepatic fibrosis. The differential diagnosis includes bilateral multicystic kidney disease, bilateral hydronephrosis, bilateral renal tumors, and bilateral renal vein thrombosis.

Infantile polycystic disease is usually fatal. However, chronic dialysis and renal transplantation have improved the outcome of these patients. Portacaval shunting may be required for portal hypertension.

Abdominal Mass Secondary to Renal Infections

Nephric and Perinephric Abscess. A perinephric abscess is a collection of pus between the capsule of the kidney and Gerota's fascia. In most cases this is secondary to rupture of a renal parenchymal abscess into the perinephric space. Most of these renal abscesses are secondary to ascending urinary infections that cause pyelonephritis. Therefore the gram-negative enteric bacilli are usually responsible. However, a few are secondary to hematogenous spread of staphylococci, usually from skin infections.

Frequently the diagnosis is not made on admission. Most patients are admitted with a diagnosis of acute pyelonephritis, infected hydronephrosis, fever of unknown origin, or acute abdomen. Perinephric abscess is more common in patients with diabetes, urinary calculi, and repeated urinary tract infections.

Presenting clinical symptoms are most frequently fever, flank pain, and chills. Physical signs are flank tenderness and an abdominal or flank mass.

Acute pyelonephritis may be differentiated from perinephric abscess on clinical grounds, insofar as in patients with acute pyelonephritis there is a shorter duration of symptoms before they come to the hospital and a shorter duration of fever after antimicrobial therapy is initiated.

The diagnosis is usually made with an intravenous pyelogram and nephrotomogram. Retrograde pyelography is usually not helpful. Arteriograms and ultrasonography may help with the diagnosis. A CT scan can be helpful in visualizing the abscess.

Treatment consists of drainage of the abscess. Nephrectomy may be necessary if there is a significant amount of renal damage.

Xanthogranulomatous Pyelonephritis. This is a special kind of inflammatory disease that may present as an abdominal mass. It is characteristically associated with a nonfunctioning kidney on intravenous pyelogram, renal calculi, and infection in the diabetic patient. Invariably it has been associated with pyelonephritis or chronic renal abscess. It may be confused with renal neoplasm when the arteriogram is viewed, because there may be some vascularity of the abscess, suggesting a malignant tumor.

Abdominal Mass Secondary to Renal Neoplasms

Hypernephroma (Adenocarcinoma of Kidney, Renal Cell Carcinoma). Eighty percent of renal neoplasms are adenocarcinoma. The malignant change occurs in the epithelial cells of the proximal convoluted tubule. Two thirds occur in men, and the majority occur in the fifth or sixth decade. Unfortunately, symptoms do not usually commence until late in the course of the disease. The classic triad of symptoms is hematuria (gross or microscopic), flank pain, and flank mass. The latter two symptoms are ominous and usually signify advanced disease. Renal cell carcinoma is capable of mimicking many conditions and can present in several ways other than the triad of symptoms. These may be summarized as follows:

1. Systemic manifestations such as malaise, anorexia, or fever of unknown origin
2. Hormonal manifestations secondary to ectopic production of hormones notably erythropoietin and renin
3. Metastatic disease without genitourinary symptoms

Approximately 50% of patients have metastatic disease at the time of initial diagnosis. These tumors spread by direct extension as well as lymphatic and hematogenous routes. Careful physical and radiologic examination should be per-

formed on the common areas of spread (i.e., liver, lung, and bone).

The diagnosis is readily suspected when the patient presents with hematuria, flank mass, and flank pain. IVP with nephrotomography is the initial test. If the mass is solid, a CT scan should be performed. CT scanning is as accurate as arteriography in the diagnosis of most renal masses. It has the added advantage of helping to stage the extent of disease more accurately than arteriography, since it can define the local extent of the tumor, the presence of lymphadenopathy, liver metastases, and degree of invasion of the renal vein and inferior vena cava. Therefore angiography is less commonly performed on a routine basis and is reserved for those unusual cases where the CT scan is inconclusive or the surgeon wishes to define the vascular supply of the tumor or embolize the kidney preoperatively. Metastatic work-up should include chest x-ray examination, liver, bone, and CT scan. Hepatic dysfunction with abnormal liver function tests is occasionally seen in patients who subsequently are proven to have no liver involvement. Liver function test results return to normal after the kidney has been removed.

The treatment of choice is nephrectomy if the work-up shows that the disease is confined to the kidney. Although spontaneous regression of metastases following nephrectomy has been reported, this is a very rare occurrence, and, unless the patient has severe flank pain or symptomatic hematuria, nephrectomy is not generally indicated in patients with metastatic disease. Radiation therapy may be used to control lung and/or bone metastasis, which may be painful. Hormonal therapy with medroxyprogesterone acetate (Provera), a progesterone agent, may provide some relief to patients with diffuse metastases, but other forms of chemotherapy have yielded disappointing results.

The survival rate in patients with renal cell carcinoma depends on the stage of the disease.

Wilms' Tumor (Nephroblastoma). Wilms' tumor is second to neuroblastoma as the most common intra-abdominal solid malignancy in children. It is a mixed embryonic tumor that forms before differentiation of renal tissue takes place. There is no sex predominance, and most cases are diagnosed before the child is 7 years of age, most commonly at 3 years of age.

The most frequent presenting feature is an abdominal mass, often discovered by the patient's parents. The mass may be smooth or irregular. Gross hematuria is unusual, but microscopic hematuria is usually present. Hypertension is a variable finding, as are associated congenital defects such as hemihypertrophy, aniridia, and genitourinary tract anomalies.

The differential diagnosis usually rests between hydronephrosis, multicystic kidney, and neuroblastoma. Renal vein thrombosis and polycystic kidney are less likely.

If a diagnosis of Wilms' tumor is strongly suspected, inferior vena cava injection of an iodinated contrast medium will provide information about the renal mass and allow visualization of the cava to rule out extension of the tumor to the vena cava. Arteriography is usually not necessary and in very young children carries the risks of vascular injury.

Treatment consists of surgery, radiation therapy, and chemotherapy. Surgery should remove all the intra-abdominal disease, and any unresectable tumor should be marked with clips for future radiation. Radiation is used postoperatively, except in children under 2 years of age whose disease is confined to the kidney. Postoperative chemotherapy consists of administration of actinomycin D and vincristine. Prognosis depends on the age of the patient and the stage and grade of the tumor. Children under 2 years of age generally have the best prognosis.

Neuroblastoma. Neuroblastoma is the most common intra-abdominal solid tumor in children. It is composed of malignant embryonic sympathetic neuroblasts that arise from the neural crest. An unusual feature of neuroblastoma is spontaneous regression and spontaneous maturation from a highly malignant neuroblastoma to a benign ganglioneuroma.

Like Wilms' tumor, the most common presenting symptom is a palpable abdominal mass. Fever, malaise, weight loss, and anemia are less frequent. Metastases tend to go to the bone and bone marrow as well as the liver; the lung is less frequently involved. This helps distinguish neuroblastoma from Wilms' tumor, where bony metastases are uncommon and the lung is the most common site of metastatic disease.

Plain x-ray films may show a punctate calcification in about 30% of tumors. IVP may show typical displacement of kidney; lytic or blastic bone metastasis favors the diagnosis of neuroblastoma. Twenty-four-hour urine collection and evaluation for vanillymandelic acid (VMA) and homovanillic acid (HVA) are required. Bone marrow examination should be performed because of the high rate of involvement.

As for Wilms' tumor, management consists of surgical removal of as much tumor as possible, followed by radiation and chemotherapy. The prognosis is influenced by the patient's age and the stage and grade of disease, together with the presence of metastasis. Overall prognosis, however, is less favorable than with Wilms' tumor.

Aortic Aneurysm. The predominant retroperitoneal vascular mass is the fusiform arteriosclerotic abdominal aortic aneurysm. It represents an asymptomatic and incidental finding on routine physical examination or radiographic study in approximately half of cases. Typically found in men in the fifth to seventh decades of life who have other evidence of arteriosclerotic cardiovascular disease, the aneurysm presents as a pulsatile mass skewed to the left of the midline, located between the xiphoid and umbilicus. A pulsatile, epigastric mass is usually an abdominal aortic aneurysm. Lateral abdominal radiographs document the presence and relative diameter of the aneurysm if calcification is present. If there is still doubt, ultrasonography is near 100% sensitive and is an excellent method for measuring size and extent of the mass. Erosion of the lumbar spine is seldom present in arteriosclerotic abdominal aneurysms; with such a finding, one should suspect a rare syphilitic aneurysm. Aortography is not a necessary adjunctive diagnostic tool. Abdominal aortic aneurysms seldom involve the renal arteries (2%), often extend into the common iliac arteries, but rarely involve the external iliac arteries. Depending on the patient's habitus, these aneurysms are usually palpable when they reach 5 cm in diameter. A normal aortic pulsation in a patient with accentuated lumbar lordosis may be mistaken for an aneurysm. The deceptively high location of abdominal aortic aneurysms can be better understood by referring to Fig. 28-16.

Aneurysms can become symptomatic from rupture, acute expansion, or vessel wall hemorrhage. All require immediate attention and treatment. The patient may have signs of an acute abdomen; back pain of variable severity with occasional bilateral posterior thigh radiation; nausea and vomiting; symptoms and signs of systemic sepsis characterized by fever, leukocytosis, and anemia; or profound shock. Rarely, a leaking aneurysm may dissect retroperitoneally to present as a mass in the left femoral canal under the inguinal ligament.

A leaking or ruptured aneurysm is an obvious indication for emergency resection, depending on the individual circumstances. If the patient's condition is unstable, rapid operative intervention is imperative. In a symptomatic yet stable patient where the diagnosis of rupture may be in doubt, a CT scan can determine whether an aneurysm is present and whether rupture has occurred. If an aneurysm is found but there is no evidence of rupture and no other cause for the patient's pain, an early repair should be done. Asymptomatic abdominal aortic aneurysms greater than 6 to 7 cm should be considered for repair because of a substantially greater risk of rupture (Table 28-4). Smaller aneurysms can also rupture. These should be repaired or followed, depending on the patient's age and associated medical problems and the size of the aneurysm.

A comparison of the survival curves for surgically treated and nontreated patients is shown in Fig. 28-17. The subsequent cause of death in patients with resected aneurysm was related to the complications of generalized arteriosclerosis, especially coronary artery disease. All large aneurysms (6 to 7 cm) should be resected, because the average operative mortality of 5% to 10% compares favorably with an average 1-year mortality rate of 50% in untreated cases. The operative

mortality rate reflects the presence of associated disease states, such as coronary artery disease, peripheral arterial obstruction, cerebrovascular disease, and hypertension, while aneurysmal rupture is the most common cause of death in untreated cases. The data indicate that aneurysms that measure less than 6 cm in diameter should be electively resected only in low-risk patients.

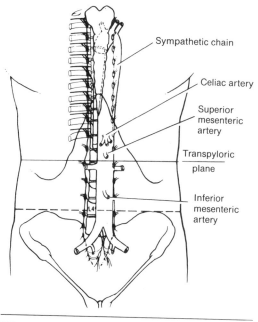

FIGURE 28-16   Topographic anatomy of abdominal aorta.

TABLE 28-4   Importance of Size in Untreated Abdominal Aortic Aneurysm: Death Resulting From Rupture (%)

Authors	<7 cm	>7 cm
Crane	4	82
Gleidman et al.	18	72
Sommerville et al.	10	83
Szilagyi et al.	20	43*

*Based on 6 cm.

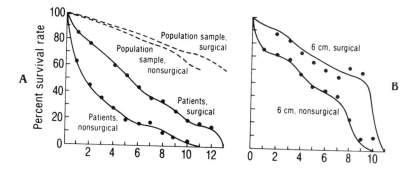

FIGURE 28-17   Comparison of operative and nonoperative treatment of aortic aneurysms in populations standardized for **A,** cardiac and renal function and for **B,** a standard sized aneurysm. (From Szilagyi DE, et al. Abdominal aortic aneurismectomy. Ann Surg 164:684, 1966.)

Other Retroperitoneal Diseases

Idiopathic Retroperitoneal Fibrosis. Idiopathic retroperitoneal fibrosis is more common in men in the fourth and sixth decades of life, although it may occur at any age. One third of patients with this condition will have an abdominal or pelvic mass at some stage of the disease process, which is self-limiting, with the residual depending on the organ system involved. Most commonly found are urinary tract symptoms secondary to ureteral compression or obstruction; leg edema or ischemic symptoms secondary to vascular compression; peripheral neuropathy; and, rarely, symptoms of duodenal, biliary, and sigmoid colon obstruction.

Retroperitoneal Tumors. A multiplicity of tumors arise from the variety of embryonic tissue derivatives occupying the potential retroperitoneal space. These tumors are typically discovered as abdominal masses, because symptoms are usually absent. However, the function of adjacent organs is occasionally compromised as a result of the tumor (e.g., gastrointestinal and/or genitourinary obstruction, lower extremity edema secondary to venous and lymphatic compression, or radicular pain from nerve compression). Evaluation of such symptoms may lead to early discovery of the retroperitoneal tumor.

The majority of retroperitoneal tumors occur in adults, and less than one fifth are found in children. In children over 1 year of age, 50% of palpable abdominal masses represent malignant neoplasms of the retroperitoneum and pelvis. Overall, 75% of retroperitoneal tumors are malignant, most commonly sarcomas.

A preoperative CT scan helps the clinician to determine the operative approach, but diagnosis can be confirmed only by biopsy at laparotomy. Treatment consists of surgical resection and/or radiation or chemotherapy.

PELVIC MASSES
Uterus

The vast majority of pelvic masses are found in the female reproductive system.

Myomata. With the exception of the gravid uterus, uterine myomata (fibroids) are the most common pelvic masses in women, occurring in 20% of women over 30 years of age. They are of exceedingly variable size and are found most often in the corporeal area of the uterus. Myomata are easily diagnosed on bimanual pelvic physical examination, in which case a variably enlarged, irregular uterus ballottable in continuity with the cervix is noted. The normal uterus is triangular in shape, similar to a small pear. Uterine myomata are benign, and sarcomatous degeneration occurs rarely. There is no increased incidence of endometrial carcinoma with myomata.

Myomata may be subdivided into subserous, interstitial, or submucous, depending on their location in the uterus. The submucous variety is least frequently noted and usually presents with vaginal bleeding in the absence of a significantly enlarged uterus. The interstitial variety is usually seen in an enlarged uterus with an altered contour on palpation. The subserous type presents as pedunculated polyps. A laterally situated subserous myoma may extend between the leaves of the broad ligament to present as a retroperitoneal mass palpable on bimanual examination, lying laterally adjacent to and in continuity with the cervix and body of the uterus. Treatment depends on the size of the myomata, symptoms, age, and child-bearing desire of the patient.

Adenomyosis. Adenomyosis uteri, the benign invasion of the uterine musculature by glandular tissue, usually results in a normally contoured, enlarged uterus. The overall incidence of adenomyosis uteri is approximately 25%; in one fourth of such cases there is associated endometriosis and attendant pelvic peritoneal fixation, with symptoms of menorrhagia, colicky dysmenorrhea, referred rectal and sacral pain, and palpable nodules on the uterosacral ligament. Treatment is usually hysterectomy.

Endometrial Carcinoma. Localized endometrial adenocarcinoma is not indicated by an enlarged uterus but by abnormal vaginal bleeding. In unusually advanced cases of diffuse adenocarcinoma with peritoneal metastases and contiguous pelvic fixation, a grossly enlarged nodular uterus will be found on bimanual pelvic examination.

Endometriosis. Extraendometrial implants of uterine lining characteristically cause pelvic and abdominal pain and are associated with infertility. Uncommonly, but not rarely, endometriosis is a cause of a mass in the pelvis or occasionally in the abdomen. The implants may involve the adnexa and pelvic colon and require care in preoperative diagnosis and preparation, because in some cases they may be mistaken for diverticular masses.

In summary, myomatous uterine enlargement presenting as a pelvic mass is generally an asymptomatic process, with those symptoms present usually reflecting the size and position of the uterus, such as a dragging sensation, constipation, urinary frequency, recurrent urinary tract infections, and uterine prolapse. On physical examination, the uterus will be freely mobile, enlarged, and often irregular. Isolated submucous myomata may cause abnormal vaginal bleeding. This sign, regardless of uterine size or contour, may represent a much more ominous process, such as myometritis, carcinoma, sarcomatous degeneration, or endometriosis. Physical findings under these circumstances may include a large, tender, boggy uterus and pelvic and contiguous organ fixation. Diagnostic dilation and curettage (D & C) are indicated in every such patient.

Fallopian Tubes

Inflammatory. Normally the fallopian tubes are palpable on bimanual examination lateral to the uterus as pencil-sized, nontender cords. Acute and subacute endosalpingitis caused by gonococcal infection results in a minimal increase in size of the tubes, but pyogenic infection is associated with noticeable enlargement of the ovarian tubes because of marked interstitial inflammation. Physical examination usually discloses an exquisitely tender cervix and bilaterally tender adnexa with either disease, as well as palpably enlarged tubes on bimanual examination with pyogenic salpingitis. Cervical smear and culture will aid in determining the specific treatment. Chronic enlargement of the fallopian tubes, bilateral or unilateral, may be secondary to pyosalpinx, chronic interstitial salpingitis, or hematosalpinx.

Ectopic Pregnancy. In a woman presenting with an acute abdomen and an adnexal mass, the most important possibilities are tubo-ovarian abscess and ruptured ectopic pregnancy. A history of amenorrhea and signs of hypotension and anemia would favor the latter, whereas foul vaginal discharge and evidence of sepsis are compatible with tubo-ovarian abscess. In each instance, a variably sized adnexal mass together with tenderness to palpation and muscle guarding are present. A helpful differential point on physical examination is that the abscess tends to be fixed and the ectopic pregnancy freely ballottable. Culdocentesis or laparoscopy helps to confirm the diagnosis. Purulent material in the cul-de-sac points to abscess; blood in the cul-de-sac indicates ruptured ectopic pregnancy.

A third and less urgent possibility with a similar clinical presentation and bleeding into the cul-de-sac is a ruptured ovarian cyst with intraperitoneal bleeding. This is usually a corpus luteum cyst that should stop bleeding spontaneously; however, an operation is frequently warranted to rule out other causes of the illness (e.g., appendicitis). Laparoscopy can be diagnostic and therapeutic in all the above.

Carcinoma. Primary carcinoma of the fallopian tubes accounts for less that 1% of malignancies of the genital canal. This occurs in patients from the third to eighth decades, is bilateral in up to half of cases, and is rarely diagnosed preoperatively. A unilateral distal tubular nodule with proximal tubal dilation simulating hydrosalpinx in the absence of adhesions should arouse suspicion of a primary tubal malignancy. Much more common are secondary tubal tumors because of the frequency of ovarian and uterine cancers, which involve the fallopian tubes via lymphatic extension.

Advances in cytology indicate that persistently positive smears in association with biopsy and curettage material are helpful in detecting tubal and ovarian carcinomas before they are clinically palpable. They are rarely diagnosed preoperatively because of the absence of abnormal physical findings.

Ovaries

Cysts. Inflammatory and dysfunctional enlargements of the ovaries commonly produce pain and menstrual irregularities. Neoplastic lesions are less often associated with clinical manifestations, and therefore diagnosis may be delayed. On careful bimanual pelvic examination, the normal ovaries are 2 to 3 cm nodules in the lateral adnexa and can be located by following the fallopian tubes from the lateral aspect of the uterus.

By definition, cystic enlargement of the ovary by more than 3 cm is an ovarian mass. Follicular cysts may attain sizes of 8 to 10 cm and produce pelvic discomfort, menstrual irregularities, or an acute abdomen secondary to rupture, torsion, or infarction. Cases not requiring surgical intervention usually resolve promptly and should be watched initially in young women. Procrastination is unwarranted in older women because of an increasing incidence of cystic cancer. Cysts of the corpus luteum may attain a size of up to 10 cm in diameter. If these cysts rupture and hemorrhage, the clinical picture and physical findings of an acute abdomen and hypotension with a ballottable adnexal mass are similar to that of ruptured ectopic pregnancy.

Bilateral ovarian enlargement associated with oligomenorrhea, anovulation, infertility, mild virilism, hirsutism, and enlarged clitoris is characteristic of the **Stein-Luventhal syndrome** and is successfully treated in 90% of cases by wedge resection of the ovaries. The ovaries are twice the normal size, with a thickened tunica studded with bluish cysts.

Tumors. Three fourths of all ovarian tumors arise from the basic germinal epithelium and are characterized by the serous and mucinous cystadenoma and cystadenocarcinoma. They often attain great size and frequently involve tube, uterus, and contralateral ovary, metastasize to distant organs, including omentum, and, if they are malignant, are associated with a poor prognosis of 20% 5-year survival. Rupture may result in pseudomyxoma peritonei, with subsequent intra-abdominal transformation of peritoneal mesothelium to a mucin-secreting epithelium and gradual recurrent accumulation of gelatinous material in the peritoneal cavity. Therefore every effort should be made to extirpate the cysts intact.

Benign solid tumors, which are far less common than benign cystic tumors, may attain great size. The fibromyoma (fibroma) is associated with Meigs' syndrome, ascites, and hydrothorax. Sarcomatous lesions are rare. Lymphoma of the ovary is usually secondary to gastrointestinal disease.

Cancer that has metastasized to the ovaries is fairly common and usually originates in the genital canal, most commonly the uterine body, or the gastrointestinal tract (Krukenberg's), breast, or kidney.

BIBLIOGRAPHY

Bland KI, McCoy DM, Kinard RE, Copeland EM III. Application of magnetic resonance imaging and computerized tomography as an adjunct to the surgical management of soft tissue sarcomas. Ann Surg 205:5, 473-481, 1987.

Council on Scientific Affairs, AMA. Ultrasonic imaging of the abdomen: Report of the Ultrasonography Task Force. JAMA 265:1726-1731, 1991.

Johnson LB. The importance of early diagnosis of acute acalculus cholecystitis. Surg Gyn Obstet 164: 197-203, 1987.

Mullins RJ, Malangoni MA, Bergamini TM, et al. Controversies in the management of pancreatic pseudocysts. Am J Surg 155:165-172, 1988.

Rattner DW, Warshaw AL. Surgical intervention in acute pancreatitis. Crit Care Med 16:89-95, 1988.

Sharp KW. Acute cholecystitis. Surg Clin North Am 68:269-279, 1988.

Gastrointestinal and hepatobiliary malignancies. Surg Clin North Am 66:4, 1986.

CHAPTER REVIEW
Questions

1. A 60-year-old woman is admitted with a large, centrally located abdominal mass. All the following necessitate an urgent work-up except:
   a. Hypotension
   b. Pain
   c. Tenderness
   d. Size of mass
   e. Fever

2. A 54-year-old man is admitted with a tender mass of the right upper quadrant that is 6 cm in size and that moves with respiration. After history, physical examination, and basic laboratory work, the test most likely to be diagnostic is:
   a. CT scan
   b. Ultrasonography
   c. Arteriogram
   d. Liver scan

3. The most common primary neoplasm that presents as an abdominal mass is located in the:
   a. Stomach
   b. Colon
   c. Ovary
   d. Liver
   e. Pancreas

4. A tender, fixed mass is most typically representative of:
   a. Congenital anomaly
   b. Expanding cancer
   c. An inflammatory process
   d. Remote trauma

5. Relatively common causes of retroperitoneal masses include:
   a. Renal cyst
   b. Pancreatic pseudocyst
   c. Abdominal aortic aneurysm
   d. None of the above
   e. All of the above

6. Rank the following neoplasms from most to least favorable as to 5-year survival rates after surgical treatment.
   a. Liver
   b. Stomach
   c. Colon
   d. Pancreas

7. Significant anemia most frequently complicates:
   a. Adenocarcinoma of the sigmoid colon
   b. Adenocarcinoma of the ascending colon

8. A tender lower abdominal mass in a pre-menopausal woman, associated with fever and leukocytosis, is most likely to be:
   a. Infarcted pedunculated uterine fibroid
   b. Pelvic abscess secondary to diverticulitis
   c. Pyosalpinx
   d. None of the above
9. The classical triad of symptoms for renal cell carcinoma includes:
   a. Fever
   b. Hematuria
   c. Flank mass
   d. Leukocytosis
   e. Pain
10. The best reason to obtain an arteriogram in a patient with an abdominal aortic aneurysm is to:
   a. Establish the diagnosis
   b. Estimate the size
   c. Evaluate arterial runoff
   d. Determine resectability

Answers

1. d
2. b
3. b
4. c
5. e
6. c, b, a, d
7. b
8. c
9. b, c, e
10. c

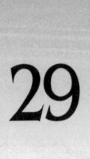

29 Hernia

H. HARLAN STONE

KEY FEATURES

After reading this chapter you will understand:
- The types of hernia.
- The causes and anatomy of congenital hernias.
- The types of repair and the anatomical features of the various repairs.
- How to differentiate an incarcerated hernia from a strangulated hernia.
- Anterior wall hernias and diaphragmatic hernias.

DEFINITION

A hernia develops whenever the lining or contents of one finite anatomic space protrudes abnormally either into a surrounding tissue plane or into some adjacent body cavity. The defective hiatus in supporting structures is generally referred to as a *ring* or *neck,* while an outpocketing from the parent cavity is called the *sac.* Although a sac need not be present, all hernias by definition are associated with a weakness, defect, or dilated hiatus in the confining wall of a primary compartment.

CLASSIFICATION

Hernias are categorized according to whether contents of the hernia sac return spontaneously or physically can be returned to the parent cavity. This manual procedure is called *hernia reduction.* Rarely, both contents and sac are reduced,

yet contained viscera remain trapped within the sac, thereby establishing hernia *reduction en masse.*

Hernias that cannot be reduced are said to be *incarcerated.* Incarceration may be chronic or acute and can threaten viability of contained organs if their blood supply is compromised. With impairment of content vascularity, the hernia is said to be *strangulated.* If circulatory compromise is not relieved by hernia reduction or operation within a short period, the entrapped viscera may progress from ischemia to actual necrosis. Such a hernia has then become *gangrenous.*

The incarceration and subsequent strangulation of only a portion of the circumference of a segment of bowel may fail to obstruct but can lead to localized bowel gangrene, soon followed by intestinal bleeding and eventual perforation. The hernia is then generally referred to as a *Richter's hernia.* Should the hernia contain an intestinal diverticulum, specifically a Meckel's diverticulum, it is called a *hernia of Littre,* even though its clinical behavior is similar to that of a Richter's hernia.

When the lining of the hernia sac is composed in part of the peritoneal surface of an intra-abdominal organ, a *sliding hernia* results. Such a hernia usually occurs in the groin, with the cecum and appendix participating on the right side and the sigmoid colon furnishing a portion of the sac on the left. On hernial protrusion, the involved intra-abdominal organ slides retroperitoneally through the hernial ring, with the anterior peritoneal surface of the viscus representing the posterior wall of the hernia sac.

PATHOGENESIS AND DIAGNOSIS
Congenital Hernias

Congenital hernias are characterized by:

- Persistence of the fetal communication between original cavity and satellite receptacle for some migrated viscus
- Failure of an embryonic canal to obliterate
- Prenatal development of some defect in the confining wall of a body cavity
- Dilation of a physiologic hiatus that normally serves to interconnect various components of a single organ system

The two basic anatomic features of a congenital hernia are:

- A prenatally developed fascial ring
- An established continuity between peritoneal protrusion and abdominal cavity

The diameter of the ring, size of the hernia, distance of sac progression, and viscera contained vary with respect to type and location of the hernia. Some congenital hernias appear with such regularity that their presence almost suggests a normal stage of development, especially since many of these hernias have a propensity for spontaneous resolution.

Acquired Hernias

Acquired hernias result from the dilation of a normally situated hiatus or from local attenuation of mesenchymal derivatives constituting cavity wall. Since the majority of hernias occur in or about the abdomen, the term hernia is often taken to refer only to various forms of peritoneal outpouchings. Although the following discussion is directed almost exclusively toward abdominal hernias, a similar process may evolve elsewhere.

The development of an acquired hernia is favored by the inappropriate stress of increased intra-abdominal pressure. Sites of inherent weakness in the abdominal wall are areas with a normal anatomic hiatus or with inferior fascial composition. Dense collagen offers no guarantee against future attenuation of supporting structures. When the applied force tears or stretches a pure collagen fiber matrix, a return of tissue to its original configuration fails to occur. Unless sufficient elastic fibers are present to provide an effective recoil, any distortion of physical contour

persists. These crucial elastic fibers are reduced in number and/or effectiveness when:

- Extensive scarring follows local infection or trauma
- The proportion of elastic fibers has been reduced by age or some generalized disease
- Elastic fibrils have been overstretched by obesity or abdominal distension
- Poor nutrition prohibits the normal elaboration of collagen in concert with effective replacement or reconstitution of damaged elastic fibrils

The stress of increased intra-abdominal pressure is greater if it is exerted as an intermittent paroxysm rather than as a constant force. Collagen bundles are continually disrupted by repeated insults before definitive repair of the initial injury can be achieved. Without elastic fibers, there is no resiliency. Dilation of the fascial ring and attenuation of local tissues then continue unabated. Such conditions are met in patients with the spasmotic cough of chronic lung disease, in patients with anatomic obstructions of the lower urinary tract (usually caused by benign prostatic hypertrophy, cancer of the prostate, or urethral stricture), and in the occasional patient experiencing tenesmus of anorectal disease. In contrast, more chronic and especially more continuous forms of increased intra-abdominal pressure may thin the supporting structures and may stretch elastic fibers to their extreme, yet when the abnormal force is removed there is a relatively rapid return of the abdominal wall to its original boundaries. Examples of this remarkable ability are found in the regain of previous abdominal girth following pregnancy, correction of mechanical intestinal obstruction, and the elimination of chronic ascites.

Accordingly, the patient with an acquired hernia should be investigated for presence of factors that may have contributed to hernia development through intermittent increases in intra-abdominal pressure, which in turn lead to a weakening of supporting mesenchymal structures. Before undertaking hernia repair, the surgeon must evaluate the severity of preexisting respiratory disease, and attempts should be made to improve overall pulmonary function. A good history and physical examination, plus careful scrutiny of the chest x-ray film, are usually sufficient. Lower urinary tract obstruction can be graded by an accurate history (especially directed at frequency, urgency, nocturia, hesitancy, stranguria, and force of stream) and by volume of residual urine. The latter is determined by having the patient first void in an attempt to empty the bladder and then be catheterized to permit measurement of the volume of residual urine in the bladder. Rectal examination is also performed to assess prostatic size, consistency, and contour, as well as to detect the presence of suspicious nodules. For lower intestinal disease, a careful history is combined with proctosigmoidoscopy and, selectively, a barium enema x-ray study. Among individuals older than 40 years of age when hernia is first noted, almost 15% have significant pathologic conditions of the lower intestine, including an associated colonic cancer in approximately 2%.

Complications of Hernias

Most problems caused by an abdominal hernia result from hernia incarceration. Bowel trapped in a protruding hernia sac may be kinked within or compressed at the neck of the sac and thereby will become obstructed. Acutely incarcerated hernias account for the majority of intestinal obstructions in children and young adults. It is second only to adhesions as the most common cause of intestinal obstruction in middle and late adulthood.

If an acute incarceration persists, circulation to the organs within the sac is compromised, and visceral gangrene may result. The bowel then becomes necrotic, bleeds, and eventually perforates. Should a solid organ (e.g., the ovary, as commonly occurs in little girls) become incarcerated, infarction similarly occurs. Whenever incarceration is of recent onset, there is always risk to organ viability from interruption of its blood supply. Duration of incarceration thus assumes great importance; accordingly, early reduction by either external manipulation or operative repair is mandatory for the acutely incarcerated hernia.

Other complications include local pressure effects on structures in proximity to the hernia sac. They usually occur at the hiatus through which hernia sac and normally situated organ conduit both enter or exit the abdomen. Compression can then lead to partial obstruction of a hollow viscus (such as the esophagus, as it descends into the abdomen) or neurologic deficits from direct pressure on an adjacent nerve trunk (e.g., the sciatic nerve in cases of herniation through the greater sciatic foramen).

Rupture of a hernia, although rare, occurs when both sac and its supporting fascia suddenly give way and permit free communication of the peritoneal cavity with another body cavity, an unrestricted tissue plane, or even the surrounding external environment. Rupture is generally confined to hernias of the anterior abdominal wall in the vicinity of the umbilicus or a prior laparotomy incision. If there has been skin disruption as well, the threat of bacterial peritonitis demands emergency repair. Unfortunately, external hernia rupture usually occurs in patients who are malnourished, afflicted with the intractable ascites of end-stage liver disease, have relatively huge ventral hernias, are obese, or are in a terminal stage of some malignant process.

TREATMENT
Indications for Repair

Not all hernias need to be repaired. Some spontaneously regress and eventually involute; others are seldom associated with any serious complication. Accordingly, the need to repair a given hernia should be based on its natural course as an anatomic entity, seriousness and incidence of present or possible future complications specific to that kind of hernia, chances for achieving a satisfactory and lasting repair, prior and anticipated therapy for those conditions favoring hernia formation, and, finally, the general ability of the individual patient to withstand operation.

Hernia Reduction (Nonoperative)

Since risk of strangulation and gangrene is relatively great in an acutely incarcerated hernia, immediate but gentle efforts should be made at hernia reduction. If this is unsuccessful, emergency operation is almost always indicated.

Manual reduction of the abdominal hernia can usually be accomplished with relative ease if a few simple steps are taken. Without doubt, the most important measures facilitating nonoperative hernia reduction are sedation and relaxation of the patient. After the patient has been placed on a stretcher or bed, morphine sulfate (0.15 mg/kg of body weight) or an equivalent opiate is given intravenously over an interval of a minute or so. The desired drug effect is obtained almost immediately. However, if the agent has been administered intramuscularly, a longer period must elapse (i.e., 20 to 30 minutes). All too often there is a tendency to attempt hernia reduction immediately after the sedative has been given. These efforts not only fail but may inflict additional injury to the entrapped viscera.

Frequently the hernia will spontaneously reduce without manipulation once a satisfactory degree of analgesia and relaxation has been achieved. Otherwise, when the patient appears to be adequately sedated, gentle and continuous pressure is exerted on the dome of the hernia protrusion. After only a few moments of such pressure, the hernia easily reduces in most cases of nonstrangulated incarceration. If the hernia fails to reduce after several minutes of such continuous pressure, further attempts at reduction should be abandoned, and emergency correction, with the patient under adequate anesthesia, should be carried out in the operating room.

Persisting with unsuccessful manual efforts at reduction merely causes untoward injury to the contents of the sac. On the other hand, rarely have gentle efforts ever resulted in reduction of gangrenous bowel, rupture of an incarcerated viscus, or disruption of the hernia sac.

When the incarceration is chronic and is not associated with acute symptoms suggestive of strangulation or obstruction, manual reduction is unnecessary. Repair of the hernia can then be scheduled as an elective procedure—provided there are no contraindications to operation.

Hernia Repair (Herniorrhaphy)

With respect to the quality of local tissues, little can be accomplished other than the correction of obvious nutritional deficiencies. Regional anatomy must dictate the appropriate use of structures available for hernia repair. Fascia of good quality will hold sutures and will not disrupt unless subjected to excess tension. Repositioning of tissue planes is facilitated by sharp division from original adjacent connections, thereby accomplishing what is called a *relaxing incision*. When local structures are of insufficient strength, autogenous fascia from another part of the body (fascia lata) or some fascial substitute (synthetic fabric made of polypropylene or Gortex) offer a reasonable alternative. Any hiatus permitting communication from one body cavity to another or the passage of specific anatomic conduits outside the abdominal cavity proper should be narrowed or even obliterated, if physiologically possible.

The basic principles of hernia repair are:

1. Eliminate or control factors that have favored the evolution of an acquired hernia, hindered the spontaneous resolution of a congenital hernia, or predisposed toward the development of significant complications in either type of hernia.

2. Totally remove the sac or at least interrupt the communication between abdomen proper and hernia pouch.

3. Correct any associated fascial defect by narrowing a normally situated hiatus, by transferring supporting structures to overcome any local fascial weakness, by implanting autogenous fascia or synthetic fabric to buttress an area of tissue attenuation, or some combination of these techniques.

Factors that cause an intermittent increase in intra-abdominal pressure have previously been cited. The result is a progressive weakness or disruption in mesenchymal tissues of the abdominal wall. Whenever possible, treatment of the responsible disease states should be instituted before operative repair of the hernia, because the long-term success of surgical correction is remarkably dependent on control of these predisposing influences.

It is not always necessary to remove the sac. If the hernia ring is broad and the peritoneum protrudes for only a short distance, the sac need merely be inverted and fixed in place by a few sutures. In fact, excision of such a sac may complicate an otherwise simple operation. If the sac is a long and narrow serosal process, however, either it should be excised or the neck of the sac should be divided. In addition, a high ligation of the sac is performed at or above the deepest level of the hernia ring. The distal sac can then be completely excised or left widely open, either procedure obviating the subsequent development of a seroma or its equivalent hydrocele.

Fascial repair is indicated in cases with a true defect or weakness in the abdominal wall. Patency of a peritoneal outpouching may be the basic cause for a given hernia and, once eliminated, may demand no other measure for repair; however, if there is any enlargement of a normally placed hiatus, the abdominal ring should be narrowed appropriately to permit passage only of its important anatomic conduits. Otherwise the canal can be obliterated selectively when its normally contained structures no longer serve a useful purpose.

If the confining fascia is of poor quality, sturdier tissue must be brought into the area as an additional supporting layer or as a replacement for the defective local tissue. Tension on the suture line must not be excessive, or else the hernia repair will almost immediately disrupt once the muscle relaxation achieved by general or spinal anesthesia has passed. Thus the herniorrhaphy should make use of relatively healthy tissues, sutured under minimal tension, based on reliable adjacent structures, and so situated as to provide adequate strength at points of potential weakness. Occasionally local tissues are of such poor quality that they must be augmented by autogenous fascia, usually taken from the fascia lata of the patient's thigh, or by an inert synthetic fabric, such as prolene (polypropylene).

Complications. Most of the major complications following herniorrhaphy are related to the surgical incision. The incidence of wound infection is significantly increased when there has been bacterial contamination of the incision during operation (as occurs when gangrenous bowel must be resected or when the colon is inadvertently entered during sac dissection of a sliding hernia) or when a wound hematoma develops because of incomplete hemostasis. The resulting scar is thick, consists of disorganized collagen bundles, and contains almost no elastic fibrils. Subsequent hernia recurrence is then all too common.

Most of the other complications are direct consequences of a general anesthetic, laparotomy, or bowel resection. These include atelectasis, paralytic ileus, intra-abdominal abscess, and generalized peritonitis.

SPECIFIC TYPES OF HERNIA

Hernias are generally named for their area of origin and occur in almost any part of the body that has a real or potential cavity. Abdominal hernias are usually grouped according to the specific region of the abdominal wall through which they pass. The majority develop in the groin, protrude through the anterior abdominal wall, or pass through muscular defects in the diaphragm. Nevertheless, abdominal hernias may occur on rare occasions in other areas, especially as outpouchings into actual or potential spaces within the abdomen proper.

Groin Hernias

The most common abdominal hernias of clinical significance occur in the groin (Fig. 29-1). These are of three basic types: the indirect inguinal hernia, the direct inguinal hernia, and the femoral hernia. In children, almost all hernias in the groin are of the indirect inguinal variety. In adult women, the development of a direct inguinal hernia is exceedingly rare, whereas the frequencies of indirect inguinal and femoral hernias are approximately equal. Young adult men primarily have indirect inguinal hernias. Older men have a somewhat greater incidence of indirect inguinal hernia over direct inguinal hernia, although femoral hernias do occur. In adults, combinations may be present and should not be overlooked at operation.

Differentiation of a groin hernia is based on whether the hernia:

- Progresses down the inguinal canal through both rings in concert with the cord structures (indirect inguinal in Fig. 29-1, **A**)
- Pushes through an attenuated transversalis fas-

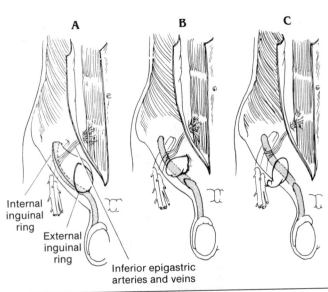

Internal inguinal ring

External inguinal ring

Inferior epigastric arteries and veins

FIGURE 29-1 Anatomic relationships in **A**, indirect inguinal hernia; **B**, direct inguinal hernia; and **C**, femoral hernia.

cia behind and then through the external inguinal ring (direct inguinal in Fig. 29-1, **B**)

- Pushes beneath the inguinal ligament, medial to the femoral vein, and then down into the very proximal anteromedial thigh (femoral in Fig. 29-1, **C**)

By having the patient suddenly increase intra-abdominal pressure with a strain or cough, individual groin hernias can usually be differentiated by area of initial and subsequent bulge in relation to the inguinal ligament and pubic tubercle. A finger can also be used to invert the sac to identify the structures immediately adjacent to the deepest fascial defect. Still, despite careful examination, an exact anatomic diagnosis may be impossible.

Indirect Inguinal Hernia. Indirect inguinal hernias in children develop as a persistence of the peritoneal communication between abdominal cavity and tunica vaginalis of the scrotum (Fig. 29-1, **A**). In adults, there is the protrusion of a new peritoneal process along the same path; that is, the sac progresses through the internal inguinal ring, obliquely down the inguinal canal, out the external inguinal ring, and eventually reaches the scrotum. The hernia sac can descend to any level or, if it is congenital, may be incompletely obliterated for varying depths.

If the neck of the hernia is wide, bowel or any nearby intra-abdominal organ can easily pass back and forth into the sac. However, when the neck of the hernia is narrow in proportion to the length of the sac, there is a propensity for the hernia to become incarcerated. This is especially true when the contained organ is on a pedicle, such as a loop of small intestine, an ovary, or a fallopian tube.

Repair of an indirect inguinal hernia is primarily based on interrupting the communication between peritoneal cavity and hernia sac (Fig. 29-2). The sac is always ligated at its base, that is, flush with the internal abdominal ring. The distal sac need not be removed but can be left open to drain into the soft tissues of the scrotum.

Usually sac division after high ligation is all

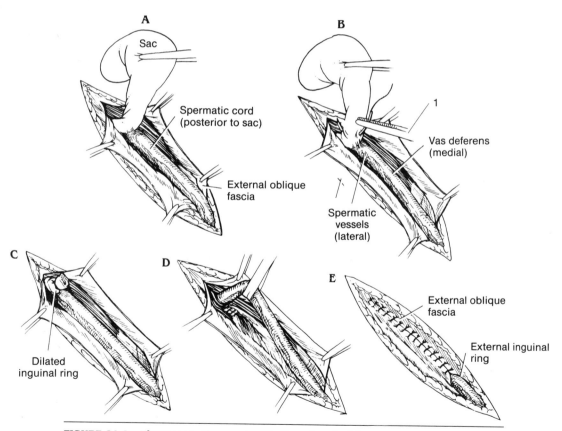

FIGURE 29-2 Elements in the repair of indirect inguinal hernia. **A,** Indirect hernia dissected into internal inguinal ring. **B,** Transfixion suture placed high at level of internal ring. **C,** High ligature of sac performed. **D,** Sac reduced. Sutures placed in transversalis fascia to narrow internal ring. **E,** Deep repair carried out as in Fig. 29-3.

that is required in children. Occasionally, however, the internal ring may be dilated widely by the massiveness of the hernia or its long duration. In these cases, the deep abdominal hiatus must be tightened by several sutures placed in the transversalis fascia (Fig. 29-2). In most young adults and in all of the elderly, when the indirect inguinal hernia is not of congenital origin, the internal ring must be narrowed. Attenuation of fascia medial to the internal ring may not permit adequate repair of the abdominal hiatus or strengthening of the adjacent posterior floor of the inguinal canal. Under these conditions, any residual weakness can be reinforced by interposing a layer of internal oblique fascia, by turning down a flap of anterior rectus sheath, or by repositioning the transversalis fascia (Fig. 29-3).

Direct Inguinal Hernia. Medial and slightly inferior to the internal inguinal ring is a triangular area of abdominal wall made up of but a single layer of transversalis fascia (see Fig. 29-1, **B**). This space, called *Hesselbach's triangle,* is bounded laterally by the inferior epigastric artery, medially by the lateral margin of the rectus sheath, and inferiorly by the inguinal ligament. There is an absence of external supporting fascia in this locale because internal oblique muscle and fascia arch in a horizontal plane to join transversalis fascia and thereby form the conjoined tendon. Superficial to this fascial gap is the external inguinal ring. With repeated stress, the single layer of transversalis fascia can be stretched; it then gradually bulges through superimposed tissue defects in more superficial fascial layers. However, because a definite hiatus is not present in the transversalis fascia, the peritoneal outpouching of the direct inguinal hernia is confined to the general area of the external inguinal ring, and accordingly the sac cannot progress down into the scrotum. Since the hernia neck is wide and the sac is shallow, rarely does a direct inguinal hernia become incarcerated.

Successful repair of the direct inguinal hernia is based on reinforcement or replacement of defective fascia in Hesselbach's triangle. The sac is of little importance and need only be inverted. Adequate fascia for repair can be obtained from the conjoined tendon (Bassini), by pulling fresh transversalis fascia down and suturing it to Cooper's ligament (McVay), through use of external oblique fascia by transposing the external inguinal ring laterally (Halsted), or by turning down a fold of anterior rectus sheath (see Fig. 29-3, **A**). With more meticulous dissection of the inguinal floor, however, adequate fascia can usually be

found to permit a layered and relatively lasting repair of the abdominal wall defect (Shouldice). Whenever fascia used for repair is placed under extreme tension, wound disruption is almost assured. Accordingly, an incision is made in the fascial attachments above and medially to eliminate adverse forces being applied to the newly interposed tissue. General weakness of all local fascial elements may dictate the use of distant autogenous fascia as a free graft of some synthetic fabric or mesh (polypropylene).

Femoral Hernia. A femoral hernia develops as a peritoneal outpouching that passes beneath the inguinal ligament into the potential space of the femoral canal (see Fig. 29-1, **C**). The neck of the hernia is thus situated immediately medial to the femoral vein. The sac usually progresses toward the foramen ovale, where the greater saphenous vein penetrates the enveloping fascia of the anteromedial thigh. Because of a narrow neck, femoral hernias are exceedingly prone to incarcerate, often producing a Richter's type of hernia. Since the bulk of the hernia is beneath the deep fascia, it seldom is obvious unless careful examination demonstrates the bulge to be inferior to the inguinal ligament as well as medial to the femoral vessels.

Femoral hernias arise from an absence of fascial support at the medial end of the femoral canal. Accordingly, correction must include removal or inversion of the sac, as well as obliteration of the superior entrance into the femoral canal (Fig. 29-4). Suture attachment of transversalis fascia to Cooper's ligament will interpose reliable fascia across the abdominal aspect of the femoral ring. Since femoral hernias primarily develop in the elderly and in obese women, a relaxing incision to prevent overstretching of the transversalis fascia is an important adjunct.

Evolving Repair Techniques. During the past decade, two new methods for groin hernia repair have been introduced. Both are based on insertion of synthetic mesh to serve as a buttress against hernia protrusion. With one technique, the plane between transversalis fascia and peritoneum is developed via a suprapubic incision; a sheet of fabric is then inserted over the internal inguinal ring and inguinal canal floor after the hernia sac has been either divided or completely reduced. The other method uses a laparoscopic transabdominal approach to affix patches of mesh over the same area of inguinal ring and canal from within. Only greater experience and longer patient follow-up will reveal the practicality and reliability of these innovations.

Text continued on p. 542.

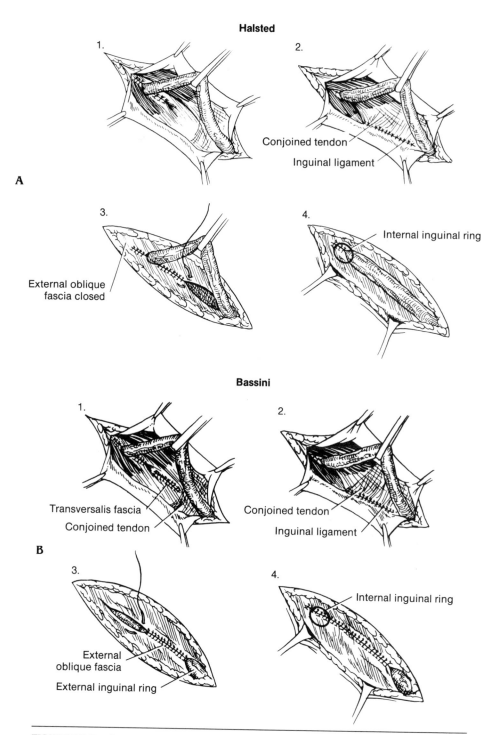

FIGURE 29-3 Common types of hernia repair. **A, Halsted.** This procedure, seldom used now, is primarily for direct inguinal hernias. There is relatively high recurrence rate. *1,* Hernia sac is excised and internal ring narrowed. *2,* Conjoined tendon is sutured to edge of the inguinal ligament. *3,* External inguinal ring is transposed laterally to overlap internal ring. *4,* Obliterated inguinal canal; spermatic cord is subcutaneous. **B, Bassini.** This repair is frequently used for large indirect and some direct inguinal hernias. There is a relatively low recurrence rate with indirect hernias. *1,* Hernia sac is excised or inverted; internal ring is tightened. *2,* Conjoined tendon is sutured to the inguinal ligament. *3,* External oblique fascia is closed *over* spermatic cord. *4,* Completed repair: internal inguinal ring is in normal position.

Continued.

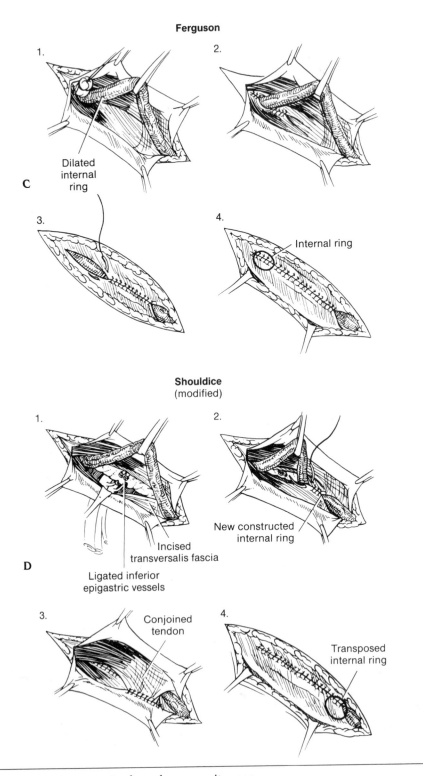

FIGURE 29-3, cont'd   For legend see opposite page.

McVay

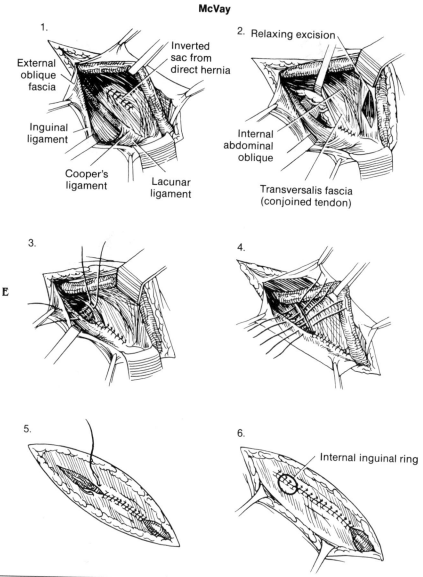

1.

External oblique fascia

Inguinal ligament

Cooper's ligament

Lacunar ligament

Inverted sac from direct hernia

2. Relaxing excision

Internal abdominal oblique

Transversalis fascia (conjoined tendon)

3.

E

4.

5.

6.

Internal inguinal ring

FIGURE 29-3, cont'd   C, Ferguson. This is the preferred method of repair for indirect inguinal hernias in children and young adults. There is no indication for use in any other type of groin hernia. *1,* Hernia sac with purse string suture; high ligation. *2,* Tightened internal ring; closure of transversalis fascia by imbrication. *3,* External oblique fascia is closed. *4,* Inguinal canal is left undisturbed; internal ring is narrowed. **D, Shouldice (modified).** This method is seldom chosen for direct hernia repair, except when performed in conjunction with orchiectomy. There are few, if any, other indications for use. *1,* Transversalis fascia is incised to provide a layered closure of the floor of inguinal canal. *2,* Internal ring is transposed medially as transversalis fascia is closed over the cord. *3,* Conjoined tendon is sutured to the inguinal ligament. *4,* Inguinal canal is obliterated if cord is removed as part of this repair. **E, McVay.** This procedure is primarily selected for direct inguinal hernias, rarely for indirect inguinal hernias; it must be combined with a relaxing incision in the rectus sheath. *1,* Transversalis fascia is closed to reduce direct hernia. *2,* Transversalis fascia and conjoined tendon are sutured to Cooper's ligament medially. *3,* Transversalis fascia is sutured to femoral sheath laterally. *4,* Conjoined tendon is sutured to the inguinal ligament by imbrication. *5,* External oblique fascia is closed over cord. *6,* Completed repair: internal inguinal ring is at normal level.

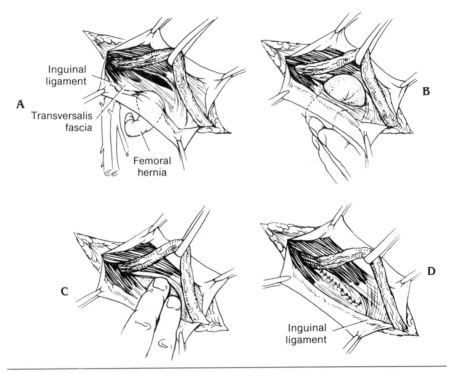

FIGURE 29-4   Repair of femoral hernia. **A,** Femoral hernia. **B,** Hernia sac mobilized and brought out from under inguinal ligament. **C,** Hernia sac reduced. **D,** Remainder of repair identical to McVay repair (Fig. 29-3, **E**).

Hernias of the Anterior Abdominal Wall

Abdominal hernias are most easily recognized when they develop in the groin and through the anterior aspect of the abdominal wall. The latter variety are also referred to as ***ventral hernias***, although such a term is taken to be more specific for herniation in the abdominal midline.

Umbilical Hernia. A true umbilical hernia normally develops in almost 90% of African-Americans and approximately 20% of Caucasians at some time during their first months of life. There appears to be no relationship to infection of the umbilicus or other perinatal event, as its incidence seems to be influenced by race alone. The peritoneal protrusion is through the fascial defect that contains atrophied umbilical vessels and remnants of the yolk stalk. Skin is the only tissue superficial to the sac. Even though the neck of the sac is narrow, incarceration is uncommon.

Between the ages of 1 and 5 years, the majority of umbilical hernias close spontaneously. A few, however, persist into school age and rarely into adulthood. Repair is warranted if the hernia remains beyond the age of 6 or is complicated by episodes of incarceration. Some parents consider the umbilical hernia to represent a blemish and energetically seek repair of the defect. More time is often required to explain to them why the hernia need not be repaired than to carry out correction in the operating room. Nevertheless, unnecessary surgery should always be avoided.

When repair is indicated in children, a curved incision is placed above or below the umbilicus to permit dissection of the hernial sac and its separation from the overlying skin (Fig. 29-5). The hernia ring is then closed in a single layer of interrupted sutures that grasp both fascia and peritoneum. Fascial imbrication is contraindicated, because it overstretches tissues and thereby weakens the final result. The umbilical skin fold is next reattached to the fascia beneath in order to create the appearance of a normal navel. In adults, repair is carried out through a transverse incision, entering the peritoneal cavity to free adherent omentum or intestine, followed by a simple one-layer fascial repair. In very obese patients, reinforcement of the fascial closure with synthetic fabric, such as polypropylene mesh, and excision of the umbilicus may be desirable.

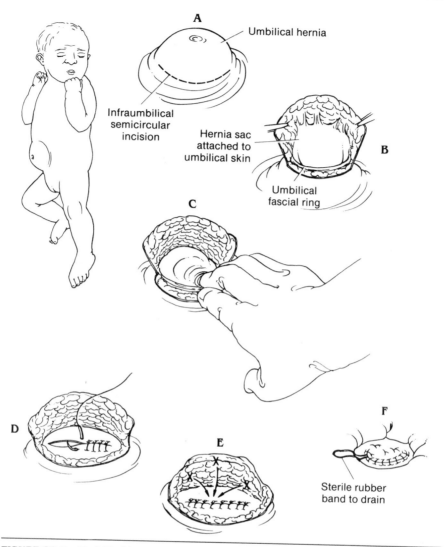

FIGURE 29-5   Umbilical hernia repair in children. **A,** Umbilical hernia incision.
B, Hernia sac. **C,** Umbilical sac peeled from umbilicus and reduced. **D,** Fascial ring
sutured. **E,** Umbilical skin sutured to fascia below. **F,** Umbilical skin closure.

Ventral Hernia. Ventral hernias that arise in or near the abdominal midline are called *epigastric* if above the umbilicus, *paraumbilical* if in the vicinity of the navel, and merely *ventral* if inferior to the umbilicus. Although increases in intra-abdominal pressure do favor the development of these hernias, distraction of midline abdominal fascia as a result of obesity or poor nutrition appears to be of greater importance. The hernia may be established with a sac or merely with properitoneal fat that has pushed through some small fascial defect. If the ventral hernia contains omentum, it is called an *epiplocele.* Ventral hernias tend to be multiple and to occur as a group, with thin fascial bands separating one from the other. Those developing at the umbilicus are rarely in the exact center of the navel, as would be the case with a congenital umbilical hernia. Instead, they are eccentric in location and protrude away from the umbilicus.

Ventral hernias occasionally incarcerate and therefore should be repaired if the patient's general status permits. Unfortunately, the factors that led to the development of the initial hernia also predispose toward a recurrence. Defective fascia, regardless of whether overstretched or of poor quality, will not hold sutures well and usually disrupts as local tissue tension increases.

Therefore repair should generally include a provision for additional fascial support to reinforce the weakened abdominal wall.

Although the hernia sac is usually excised, its inversion is simpler and saves considerable operating time. Small gaps in the fascia are closed with a few well-placed interrupted sutures. Larger and more complicated defects generally demand a basic repair that is fashioned from, or supplemented by, a fold of anterior rectus sheath, the interposition of autogenous fascia, a synthetic fascial prosthesis (polypropylene mesh), or some combination thereof.

Incisional Hernia. A subsequent hernia may develop in any abdominal incision because of poor technical closure at the time of operation, some complication in the abdominal wound itself (especially infection), excessive mechanical stress being placed on the healing incision, or metabolic deficiencies that impair the production of a well-healed wound.

Complications and principles for management of the incisional hernia are generally the same as those for the ventral hernia. A satisfactory repair can often be gained by merely approximating the sides of the hernia ring without the addition of fascial or synthetic mesh reinforcement.

Spigelian Hernia. Abdominal herniation occasionally develops through the weakened area where the semicircular line of Douglas (a horizontal crescent marking the lateral termination of the posterior sheath of the rectus muscle) crosses the semilunar line of Spigelius (the junction of the aponeurotic fibers of the internal oblique and transverse abdominis muscles at the lateral border of the rectus abdominis muscle). Since the neck of the hernia is narrow and the sac may be long, incarceration is common. Because the hernia lies deep to the external oblique fascia, it is rare for any mass to be definitely outlined on palpation of the abdomen. Presence of a hernia is frequently missed until strangulation of incarcerated bowel has developed or an appendiceal abscess has drained spontaneously into the abdominal wall beneath the deep enveloping fascia.

Omphalocele and Gastroschisis. *Omphalocele* is a congenital failure of abdominal viscera to reduce within the abdomen proper following their developmental herniation into the umbilical cord. A separate and distinct rent in the abdominal wall, usually to the right side of the umbilicus, with extrusion of abdominal contents into the amniotic sac is referred to as a *gastroschisis*. Both anomalies are discussed in Chapter 37.

Diaphragmatic Hernias

Hernias in the diaphragm result from a protrusion through one of its muscular foramina, from failure in normal diaphragm development, or from traumatic and inflammatory erosions.

Hiatal Hernia of the Esophagus. Herniation through the esophageal hiatus is caused by a congenitally short esophagus, a sliding of the abdominal esophagus and proximal stomach into the posterior mediastinum, or a displacement of the gastric fundus into the chest without an associated migration of the esophagogastric junction *(paraesophageal hernia)*. Despite minor differences in symptoms, each type of esophageal hiatal hernia produces upper abdominal discomfort, varying difficulties with swallowing (see Chapter 16), and, occasionally, gastrointestinal bleeding. Esophagitis may follow regurgitation of gastric juice whenever the esophagogastric junction has risen into the thorax and there is a resultant loss of normal abdominal pressure on the terminal esophageal segment. Chronic esophagitis leads to scarring and eventual cicatricial obstruction of the esophagus.

Although esophageal hiatal hernias are common, especially in patients beyond the age of 40, repair is seldom indicated unless it is paraesophageal or significant complications develop (e.g., esophagitis, bleeding, or obstruction). Anatomic return and fixation of the esophagogastric junction within the abdomen alone may not be sufficient, because surgical correction must also include some technical maneuver to prevent recurrent acid regurgitation (e.g., by transmitting intra-abdominal pressure against the terminal esophagus).

Hernia Through the Foramen of Morgagni. The *foramina of Morgagni* are located behind the costosternal junction on either side of the sternum and provide the access for internal mammary vessels to pass into the abdomen and then to continue on as the superior epigastric artery and vein. On rare occasions, small bowel, transverse colon, or omentum herniate into the anterior mediastinum through this dilated hiatus. Because the neck is narrow, strangulation is common. Even though the patient presents with mechanical intestinal obstruction, first indication of the true diagnosis all too frequently is mediastinitis or a feculent empyema.

Congenital Diaphragmatic Hernia. During prenatal life, development of the diaphragm may be arrested at any of several stages. Usually this occurs posterolaterally (often referred to as the *foramen of Bochdalek*) or involves the entire central portion of the diaphragm. If on the right, the liver serves as a buttress and prevents organ herniation into the chest. However, if this occurs on the left, abdominal viscera are readily pushed into the left side of the thorax. These infants usually have respiratory distress at birth, although if ventilatory impairment is minimal, subsequent signs may be only those of intestinal obstruction.

Surgical repair should be carried out as soon as the diagnosis has been made. Clinical findings and basic management are given in greater detail in Chapter 37.

Traumatic Diaphragmatic Hernia. Rents can be produced in the diaphragm by external penetrating wounds, surgical injuries, or sudden increases in intra-abdominal pressure as a result of acute abdominal compression. Depending on the size and magnitude of the diaphragmatic tear, abdominal viscera then herniate into the pleural space above. If the hernia is small, contains a solid organ such as the spleen, or does not immediately obstruct the lumen or compromise the blood supply of incarcerated bowel, the onset of symptoms may be delayed for many years. At a later date the usual complication is mechanical intestinal obstruction, often incomplete and intermittent until it eventually progresses to a total mechanical block. The correct preoperative diagnosis can be made by detection of supradiaphragmatic trapped bowel on chest x-ray examination or a gastrointestinal contrast series. Knowledge of the condition before operation will then dictate a transthoracic approach, thereby facilitating hernia reduction and diaphragmatic repair.

If the hernia has resulted from a sudden compressive force to the abdomen, acute respiratory distress is often produced by pulmonary collapse and contusion as intra-abdominal organs crowd into the involved hemithorax. Immediate exploration must be carried out, preferably through the abdomen. The hernia is reduced, the rent in the diaphragm closed, and any injured abdominal viscus appropriately repaired or removed. Since the greatest threat to life is respiratory insufficiency, a nasogastric tube should always be passed as soon as possible to prevent additional pulmonary compression by the inflated gastrointestinal tract.

Other Abdominal Hernias

Although rare, hernias can develop through any aspect of the abdominal wall, especially in the flank, where they are referred to as *lumbar hernias*, into the pelvis, or through any intraabdominal peritoneal defect.

Pelvic Hernias. Bowel can protrude through any of the several fascial or muscular foramina that permit passage of nerves and blood vessels into the buttocks or out the pelvis. More commonly, these are sciatic or obturator. The patient presents with a combination of mechanical intestinal obstruction and either peripheral nerve pain or neurologic deficit corresponding to the nerve trunk involved.

Other pelvic hernias occur wherever a gap exists in the levator sling in the floor of the pelvis and generally occur as bulges just lateral to the midline perineal raphe.

Internal Hernias. Hernias can develop within the abdomen through any real or potential defect in peritoneal lining. Areas with an anatomic predilection are located at sites where bowel mesentery begins and ends (*paraduodenal* and *paracecal*), where peritoneal folds create a normal recess (*foramen of Winslow* into the lesser peritoneal cavity), and where defects, either congenital or acquired, exist in the intestinal mesentery. Bowel obstruction without obvious cause is the usual presenting feature.

PITFALLS AND COMMON MYTHS

- The incidence of persistent or recurrent sliding hernias after initial repair is great because of a failure to appreciate the true nature of the hernia. The sac must be eliminated completely, followed by return of the previously attached viscera to the abdomen and then appropriate repair of the dilated fascial ring.

- Another major error is to mistake the sliding colon for a hernia sac. Inadvertent entry into the bowel contaminates the operative field and almost ensures the development of a wound infection.

BIBLIOGRAPHY

Glassow F. The Shouldice repair of inguinal hernia. In Varco RL, Delaney JP (eds). Controversy in Surgery. Philadelphia, WB Saunders, 1976, pp 375-388.

Morton JH. Abdominal wall hernias. In Schwartz SI, Shires GT, et al (eds). Principles of Surgery, 5th ed. New York, McGraw-Hill, 1989, pp 1525-1544.

Nyhus LM, Bombeck CT, Klein MS. Hernias. In Sabiston DC (ed). Textbook of Surgery: The Biological Basis of Modern Surgical Practice, 14th ed. Philadelphia, WB Saunders, 1991, pp 1134-1148.

Nyhus LM, Condon RE (eds). Hernia, 3rd ed. Philadelphia, JB Lippincott, 1989.

CHAPTER REVIEW

Questions

1. What is the approach to a patient with a tender inguinal mass?
2. Differentiate an incarcerated hernia from a strangulated hernia.
3. Why does infection in a hernia repair predispose to recurrence?
4. List three conditions that predispose to development of hernia.
5. List the most common groin hernias in each of the following categories:
   a. Children
   b. Women
   c. Elderly men
6. What are the three anatomic boundaries of Hesselbach's triangle?
7. Why is small bowel rarely found in a sliding hernia?

Answers

1. Early operation. The tenderness implies the presence of infection, and therefore the differential diagnosis is strangulated hernia, abscess, or infected lymph nodes. It is safer to operate early to preclude complications of strangulation, to drain the abscess if present, and to provide a histologic diagnosis on resected lymph nodes.
2. *Incarceration* implies nonreducibility, whereas *strangulation* refers to a compromise in blood supply to hernia contents.
3. Extensive scarring follows infection, with the formation of collagen. Failure to produce elastic fibers results in a wound that does not provide elastic for appropriate recoil when deformed.
4. Chronic cough, obstruction of the lower urinary tract, tenesmus of anorectal disease
5. a. Indirect inguinal
   b. Femoral or indirect inguinal
   c. Direct inguinal
6. Inferior epigastric artery, lateral margin of the rectus sheath, inguinal ligament
7. A sliding hernia is retroperitoneal, involving organs that can slide in this position (cecum, left colon, and so on). A totally intraperitoneal structure cannot pass via this route.

30 Rectal and Perianal Complaints

TERRY C. HICKS
FRANK G. OPELKA

KEY FEATURES

After reading this chapter you will understand:
- The anatomy of the rectum and anus.
- How to examine the rectum.
- Management of common benign conditions.
- Malignant anal disease including carcinoma and melanoma.

The surgeon frequently encounters patients who have anorectal complaints. Making the correct diagnosis and instituting appropriate therapy can be a challenge, because anorectal symptomatology may arise from a myriad of pathologic causes. The cornerstone of success is use of a systematic approach to the problem and maintaining appropriate follow-up. This ensures that patients who fail to respond to treatment are reevaluated and have their therapy adjusted appropriately and provides a safeguard against missing a potentially life-threatening diagnosis.

ANATOMY

A thorough knowledge of anorectal anatomy is essential to the diagnosis and surgical treatment of anorectal disease. Although it is beyond the scope of this chapter to provide definitive description, we will review the basics of normal anatomy and their relationship to common diseases.

The rectum, measuring 12 to 15 cm in length, is the caudalmost portion of the large bowel. It originates approximately at the S_3 vertebra, courses along the sacral curvature, descends through the levator muscles, and terminates at the anorectal juncture (dentate line, pectinate line). The anal canal extends another 3 to 4 cm and terminates at the anal verge. The critical role of the dentate line, with respect to blood supply, innervation, lymphatic drainage, and tumor-bearing potential, is addressed in Table 30-1.

The rectum is embryologically derived from endoderm. It is lined with glandular mucosa, whereas the anal canal below the dentate line is covered with stratified squamous epithelium (anoderm). The dentate line does not serve as a distinct histologic demarcation between rectal mucosa and anoderm; there is a transitional zone composed of columnar, transitional, and squamous epithelium that extends approximately 1 cm above the dentate line. Thus three areas may bear tumors: the rectum (adenocarcinoma), the anal canal (squamous cell carcinoma), and the transitional zone (cloacogenic carcinoma).

The rectum derives its blood supply from three major sources (Fig. 30-1). The primary source is the superior hemorrhoidal artery, which is the terminal branch of the inferior mesenteric artery. It usually divides into two right branches and a single left branch. The lower rectum is supplied by the paired middle and inferior hemorrhoidal arteries. The middle branch extends from the anterior trunk of the internal iliac artery, and the inferior branch extends from the internal pudendal artery. The rectum has two

TABLE 30-1   Important Characteristics Defined by the Dentate Line

	Above the Dentate Line	Below the Dentate Line
Embryology	Endoderm	Ectoderm
Tissue lining	Rectal glandular mucosa, transitional zone, transitional epithelium	Squamous epithelium
Venous drainage	Vena cava and portal system	Predominantly vena cava
Lymphatic drainage	Inferior mesenteric nodal basin, hypogastric nodal basin	Primarily inguinal nodes; also inferior mesenteric nodal basin and hypogastric nodal basin
Tumor potential	Rectal adenocarcinoma, transitional zone, cloacogenic carcinoma	Squamous cell tumors
Hemorrhoids	Internal hemorrhoids	External hemorrhoids

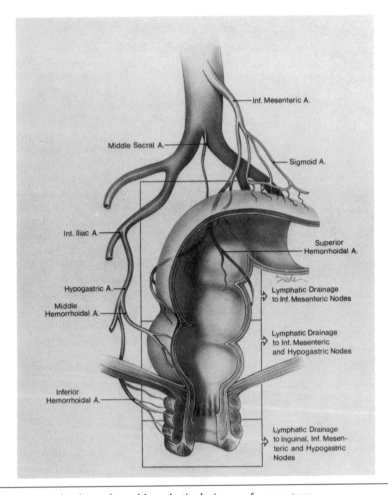

FIGURE 30-1   Blood supply and lymphatic drainage of anorectum.

conduits for venous drainage: the superior hemorrhoidal venous system drains the upper rectum into the portal system via the inferior mesenteric vein, and the inferior hemorrhoidal system, composed of the middle and inferior hemorrhoidal veins, independently drains into the internal iliac vein and ultimately the systemic circulation via the vena cava.

The anal canal derives its blood supply from the inferior hemorrhoidal system. The paired inferior hemorrhoidal arteries penetrate the sphincter muscles to vascularize the subcutaneous tissue of the anal canal. Venous blood drains from the inferior hemorrhoidal veins to the systemic circulation.

The lymphatic drainage of the anorectum is unique and determines the extent of resection necessary for potentially curable cancer (see Fig. 30-1). As occurs elsewhere in the body, the lymphatic system closely follows the arterial blood supply.

The upper and middle rectum drain into the inferior mesenteric nodal basin, following the superior hemorrhoidal artery to the inferior mesenteric artery. The lower rectum may drain to the inferior mesenteric nodal basin or follow the course of the middle hemorrhoidal arteries to the aortic bifurcation to become part of the hypogastric nodal basin. Tumors below the dentate line usually drain directly to the inguinal node; however, if lymphatic obstruction occurs, the inferior mesenteric and hypogastric nodal basins are accessible.

The rectal nerve supply is derived from both the sympathetic and parasympathetic systems. The rectum is therefore insensitive to touch but quite sensitive to stretching. Below the dentate line, somatic innervation makes the anal canal very sensitive to touch. This accounts for the extreme discomfort often associated with pathologic conditions of the anus.

The last pertinent anatomic consideration is the topical morphology of the anal canal. Above the dentate line lie the rectal columns (morgagni), which appear as folds in the mucosa and are formed by the underlying superior hemorrhoidal vessels. At the base of the columns are the anal crypts, the openings for mucus produced by the anal glands. The anal glands usually are located in the anterior and posterior midline. The glands extend from the crypts inward to lie within the submucosa, internal sphincter muscle, and intersphincteric plane. When infected, these glands are the nidus for anal fistulas.

THE RECTAL EXAMINATION

More is missed by not looking than by not knowing.

Thomas McCrae (1870-1935)

When a pathologic condition of the anorectal region is not appropriately identified, it is usually because the physician failed to perform an examination and not because of a lack of clinical acumen. Students and house officers should consistently inspect the anorectum as part of the comprehensive physical examination.

A patient with an anorectal condition will bring to the examination a great deal of anxiety, not only about potential illness but also about the examination itself. Thus it is important for the physician to demonstrate self-confidence, patience, and gentleness in approaching the examination. Informing the patient that the examination is of short duration, involves minimal discomfort, and provides invaluable diagnostic information can alleviate unnecessary anxiety.

A careful history is important for two reasons. First, it aids the physician in determining the correct diagnosis. Second, it protects the examiner and his or her future patients from being unnecessarily exposed to infection (e.g., hepatitis, venereal disease, parasites, or bacterial infections). Before beginning the examination, the examiner should have all of the necessary equipment available, including patient drape, glove, lubricant, Hemoccult testing material, and endoscopy equipment. Good lighting is essential.

For an ambulatory patient, the jackknife position on a tilting table is optimal. For a nonambulatory patient (or if a tilting table is unavailable), the left lateral position is ideal. With the patient's buttocks extended over the edge of the table, the hips are gently flexed, providing adequate exposure for the examination.

A systematic examination is then undertaken. First, the perianal region is surveyed for skin abnormalities, such as pilonidal disease, dermatitis, abscesses, fistula openings, or lesions that may represent potential tumors. The buttocks are spread for better visualization. **Hemorrhoidal tags,** or loose bits of skin arranged around the anus, are often identified. Next, a digital examination is performed with the lubricated glove. It should be explained to the patient that the examination will elicit the urge to defecate and might cause minimal discomfort but that this is a normal sensation. With the pad of the index finger, gentle pressure should be applied to the contracted anus until the sphincter relaxes, which allows the examiner to insert the digit into the canal. Careful evaluation includes testing for sphincter tone and attention to the presence of any tenderness, nodules, or irregularities. Anteriorly, in men, the two-lobed prostate is firm, broad, rubbery, and, in its normal state, nontender and free of discrete nodules. In women, the normal uterine cervix is encountered at a slightly higher level as a smooth, firm, nodular structure.

Posteriorly, the examiner should sweep across the base of the sacrum to detect possible tumors. A careful 360-degree rotation of the examining finger at different levels will often detect other pelvic pathologic conditions, completing this portion of the examination. For completeness, a stool specimen for occult blood should be obtained. To obtain the most accurate results, occult blood specimens should be collected from patients who have adhered to special dietary restrictions (avoidance of red meat, aspirin, excessive vitamin C, and anti-inflammatory drugs) for 48 hours. Although a discussion of endoscopic observations is beyond the scope of this chapter, the student should consult an atlas to appreciate the normal mucosal detail. *A dictum: if in doubt, do a biopsy!*

ANAL FISSURE

An anal fissure is a linear disruption in the lining of the anal canal, usually originating below the dentate line and often extending to the anal verge. This defect represents the most common cause of acute anal pain in adults. Patients describe their discomfort as a cutting, tearing, or burning sensation often associated with bright red bleeding, either streaking the stool or on the toilet paper. The pain is most marked at defecation but often persists to a lesser degree for hours after elimination. It is not uncommon for a severe fissure to cause urinary symptoms such as frequency, dysuria, or retention.

Fissures are usually classified as acute or chronic. An acute lesion represents a tear in the anoderm, whereas a chronic lesion is truly an ulcer. The chronic fissure has a classic morphologic triad of anal ulcer, hypertrophic papilla, and sentinel pile. The sentinel pile represents fibrotic external hemorrhoidal tissue at the distal fissure margin, whereas the hypertrophic papilla is located at the proximal margin (Fig. 30-2).

The cause of anal fissures remains unknown but appears to be multifactorial. Trauma to the anal canal from passage of dry, hard, large-caliber stools appears to be the primary culprit, but persistent diarrhea and internal anal sphincter spasm certainly contribute to the problem. Interestingly, recent manometric studies in patients with anal fissures demonstrated increased resting pressures within the internal sphincter and increased maximal anal pressure.

Although the incidence of fissures is probably similar for both sexes, location differs to some degree. Most fissures are found in the posterior midline in both men and women. However, 10% of women may have anterior fissures, whereas they are seen in less than 1% of men. The clinician should maintain a high level of suspicion for fissures found in the lateral position or for lesions

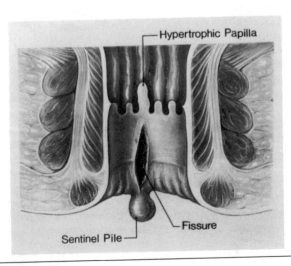

FIGURE 30-2   Classic fissure triad.

with increased induration. These lesions may be manifestations of inflammatory bowel disease, primary syphilis, tuberculosis, leukemia, or anorectal cancer. Diagnostic modalities specific to the diagnosis of each of these conditions should be employed, and if uncertainty still exists, a biopsy is mandated.

The presence of a classic history of anal fissure usually leads to the proper diagnosis, but it is always necessary to gently separate the buttocks and inspect the lower anal canal to confirm the diagnosis clinically. If an acute fissure is identified, examination can be terminated, but if an abscess is suspected a digital examination is necessary. The application of some topical anesthetic cream may make a digital examination tolerable when the presence of an abscess is suspected; if the pain is severe, examination with the patient under anesthesia is necessary.

The initial management of acute fissures is nonoperative. Initial supportive measures include a psyllium stool softener, frequent sitz baths, increased fluid intake, and application of a topical steroidal cream. Suppositories are of no use in the treatment of acute anal fissures, because after their insertion they lie above the levators, preventing contact of the medication with the diseased area.

Patients with fissures that are refractory to nonoperative management or those who complain of unrelenting pain are considered surgical candidates. The lateral internal anal sphincterotomy is currently the surgical procedure of choice, having a cure rate of greater than 97% and a morbidity rate of less than 1%. In this operative procedure, performed with the patient under anesthesia, the intersphincteric groove is identified and the internal sphincter is carefully transected down to the level of the dentate line. The fissure bed itself need not be manipulated. In fissures caused by underlying disease, such as inflammatory bowel disease, leukemia, syphilis, or tuberculosis, the specific disease processes should be addressed primarily.

PILONIDAL DISEASE

Pilonidal literally means "hair nest," and *pilonidal sinus* refers to the presence of a chronic sinus in the intergluteal cleft, often associated with entrapped tufts of hair. Pilonidal disease is an encompassing term to describe the clinical presentation of the pilonidal sinus as a sacrococcygeal mass or cyst, chronic drainage from a sinus or sinuses, phlegmon (cellulitis), or frank abscess.

This disease usually becomes clinically evident between puberty and the third decade, affecting men three times more often than women. It is often, but not always, seen in persons who are obese, have deep gluteal clefts, and possess an overabundance of hair on their buttocks.

The cause of pilonidal disease remains controversial. Some authorities favor the congenital theory, by which a developmental defect results in ectodermal inclusions in the gluteal cleft. The majority, however, support the acquired theory, by which unclean hair becomes traumatically buried subcutaneously into a sinus. This latter theory has gained increasing support because the disease is not seen before puberty, has been noted in other anatomic areas, such as in the finger webs of barbers, and often recurs, even after apparently adequate excision. With continued investigation, it may be concluded that both congenital and acquired factors are contributory.

The treatment of pilonidal disease is governed by the patient's clinical presentation. When pilonidal disease occurs as an acute abscess, it usually responds well to incision and drainage. This procedure is usually performed with the patient under local anesthesia, preferably in an outpatient setting. Results are improved with careful curettage of the cavity and removal of remaining hair or granulation tissue. Once the lesion is reasonably quiescent, a decision for definitive surgery or nonoperative therapy may be made; in either case, however, there is an appreciable rate of recurrence.

If a phlegmon is present, the lesion is best treated by local measures aimed at resolution without incision and drainage. Patients with adult-onset diabetes, heart valve recipients, or individuals who are immunocompromised should be given special consideration for antibiotic therapy.

In treating chronic pilonidal disease, several operative modalities are available, substantiating the fact that no single procedure is universally successful in treating this disease process.

The two most favored techniques are marsupialization, or excision with wound packing. Both procedures utilize elliptical excision of the diseased area. In marsupialization, the skin edges are sewn to the remaining posterior wall of the cyst. The other procedure involves excising the entire cyst wall and packing the wound, allowing it to heal by secondary intention. Some surgeons favor excision of major sinuses through small, separate midline incisions. Then a lateral incision off the midline is used to unroof the branch tracks, with curettage of their linings; this wound heals by secondary intention. With complex or recurrent disease, wide skin excision and a rotation flap procedure may be required.

The cardinal rule in approaching definitive operative treatment of pilonidal disease is to be **conservative.** Excision of only the sinus and the surrounding diseased tissue is necessary. Conservative treatment will prevent the debilitating problems caused by slow wound healing, for which this disease is notorious.

PRURITUS ANI

Pruritus ani is a severe itching sensation of the perianal region. If the process is allowed to progress, it can eventually lead to symptoms of burning and soreness. The causes of pruritus ani are diverse (see the box below). Despite comprehensive work-ups, more than half of cases of pruritus ani are idiopathic in origin. The patient's medical history, including information about diet, systemic disease, and the use of oral and perianal medicines, may identify a nidus. The physical examination should document the severity of skin involvement and identify anatomic causes that may be surgically correctable (i.e., fistulas, fissures, anal papillae, or skin tags).

Treatment is specific for cases with an identifiable cause. Patients with idiopathic pruritus ani should learn the proper techniques for cleansing, drying, and applying medication and should make appropriate dietary adjustments. Keeping the skin clean, dry, and slightly acidic is mandatory. Cleansing with soap should be avoided because it is alkaline and often increases discomfort. Gentle drying with a towel or hair dryer is helpful, because it prevents abrasive trauma. Frequent sitz baths provide relief and promote healing. Incorporating bulk into the diet, along with daily administration of a psyllium seed product, is helpful. Maintaining adequate fluid intake is also beneficial. Steroid creams often give temporary symptomatic relief. For patients whose problems are refractory to treatment, a biopsy is imperative.

CAUSES OF PRURITUS ANI

Personal hygiene: poor cleansing habits, with exposure to residual irritating feces, or, conversely, overmeticulous cleaning, with excessive rubbing and soap use

Diet: coffee, alcohol, citrus, milk, spices, tea, chocolate, colas

Systemic disease: diabetes, leukemia, aplastic anemia, liver disease

Diarrhea states: irritable bowel syndrome, Crohn's disease, chronic ulcerative colitis

Dermatologic problems: contact dermatitis (especially associated with "caine" preparations), psoriasis, lichen planus, reaction to oral antibiotics (especially tetracycline)

Infections: fungal (dermatophytosis, candidiasis), viral, bacterial (erythrasma), parasitic (scabies, pinworms, pediculosis)

Anatomic disorders: fissures, cryptitis, skin tags, ectropion, fistulas, hypertrophied anal papillae, hemorrhoids

Neoplasm: extramammary Paget's disease, intraepidermal carcinoma (Bowen's), other anal tumors

Clothing: tight clothing (underwear and girdles) or clothing materials that fail to allow proper ventilation

Radiation: postirradiation changes

Idiopathic

MALIGNANCIES OF THE ANAL AND PERIANAL REGIONS

Tumors of the anal and perianal regions are rare and represent only 4% of all tumors of the anorectum. Human papilloma viruses, especially subtype 16, have been associated with anal carcinomas. These carcinomas notoriously share the nonspecific symptoms (i.e., pruritus, pain, soilage, bleeding, or the presence of a mass) associated with benign and inflammatory lesions of the region. This makes biopsy essential for any suspicious or nonhealing lesions to prevent misdiagnosis of a potentially fatal tumor.

Epidermoid carcinomas are the tumors most commonly encountered in the anal and perianal region. The natural history of the perianal carcinomas differs from that of anal canal carcinomas. Carcinomas located distal to the anal canal in the perianal region are typically squamous cell carcinomas. These lesions are usually detected before extensive invasion or lymph node involvement occurs and are treated with wide local excision. Anal canal carcinomas may arise anywhere from the proximal transitional zone to the perianal area. Anal canal carcinomas are composed of three major histologic subtypes: squamous cell carcinoma (70%), basaloid or cloacogenic carcinoma (25%), and mucoepidermoid carcinoma (5%). At present the histologic subtypes have no bearing on therapeutic alternatives. Most series consider all three cell types collectively as squamous cell carcinoma and treat them similarly. At the time of detection, most anal canal carcinomas have invaded beyond the mucosa and submucosa into the anal sphincters, and as many as 40% of patients have lymphatic involvement. Therefore wide local excision is reserved only for small anal canal carcinomas confined to the submucosa or mucosa.

To determine the appropriate therapeutic course for a specific cancer of the anal canal, the surgeon must have knowledge of the confirmed histologic diagnosis, the size and location of the tumor, the depth of invasion, and a fundamental understanding of anal and perianal anatomy. (Remember, tumors arising below the dentate line primarily drain to the inguinal nodes but have access to the inferior mesenteric basin and the hypogastric basin, should lymphatic obstruction occur.) Lesions that are small (less than 2 cm) or superficial (mobile without evidence of sphincter invasion) found below the dentate line can be adequately treated by wide local excision. Lesions failing to meet these criteria or arising at or above the dentate line may require radiation therapy, abdominoperineal resection, or combination therapy. Abdominoperineal resection is reserved for patients with fecal incontinence from cancers that have destroyed the anal sphincters or patients with residual cancer after radiation or combination therapy. A posterior vaginectomy should be considered as part of the abdominoperineal resection because of the potential for lymphatic involvement.

Combination therapy with chemotherapy, radiation, and surgical excision in selected series has recently been shown to be effective in the treatment of squamous cell cancers that, in the past, required abdominoperineal resection. Patients receive mitomycin-C and 5-fluorouracil (5-FU) in combination with 3000 to 4500 cGy of radiotherapy in multiple, small fractions to the pelvis over several weeks. Eight to 12 weeks after completion of radiotherapy, the lesion is surgically reevaluated. Nigro et al. noted that in up to 50% of lesions residual tumor was absent, and a large portion of patients demonstrated adequate reduction in the tumor size for local excision, thus avoiding abdominoperineal resection. Using the Nigro protocol, we have confirmed these results. Although similar results have been seen with radiation alone, this technique is not widely accepted.

Patients with squamous cell carcinoma of the anus who have biopsy-proven inguinal metastases may also receive local treatment with radiation therapy. Therapeutic groin dissections serve as an alternative but are associated with significant lower extremity edema. For patients with inguinal metastasis (synchronous) found at the time of diagnosis, the prognosis is poor, with less than 5% surviving 5 years. In patients who develop inguinal metastasis some time after surgery (metachronous) and undergo lymph node dissection, the prognosis for 5-year survival is greatly improved, approaching 75%.

Anorectal melanoma is rare, representing less than 1% of all melanomas. This is the most common site for primary gastrointestinal melanoma. It may appear insidiously as an amelanotic lesion in up to 30% of patients. It also can occur as a bleeding mass, but it is often associated with extremely small lesions that are found incidentally in a specimen taken for another surgical procedure. Anorectal melanoma has devastating consequences. The survival rate is poor (16% to 20% at 5 years), and cure is rare. Careful consideration to avoid either overtreatment or undertreatment is necessary. Currently the optimal surgical treatment is controversial; some investigators recommend wide local excision but most still prefer abdominoperineal resection although it has no proven benefit over limited surgery. Generally, lesions that are small (less than 0.5 cm) or thin (less than 2 mm in depth) may be treated with wide local excision. Large, deep lesions usually require abdominoperineal resection.

The other tumors of this region are rare but deserve brief consideration. Basal cell carcinoma, with its rodent ulcer appearance, responds in a manner similar to lesions in other anatomic areas. It is adequately treated by local excision and, with the exception of one reported case, never metastasizes. Extramammary Paget's disease, a gray, plaquelike lesion, is an intraepithelial adenocarcinoma of apocrine sweat gland origin. Paget's disease of the breast is almost always associated with an underlying invasive carcinoma. Perianal Paget's disease has a 50% incidence of underlying invasion. Intraepithelial lesions are treated with wide local excision. Invasive lesions require an abdominoperineal resection. Bowen's disease (intraepidermal carcinoma) appears as a red plaque or eczematoid lesion, usually appearing in the fifth decade of life. In many patients it may be associated with the subsequent diagnosis of an internal malignancy. It is currently treated with wide excision, 5-FU cream, or dinitrochlorobenzene. Because up to 20% of these lesions recur, close follow-up is vital.

ANORECTAL ABSCESSES AND FISTULAS

Anorectal abscesses and fistulas are a common cause of painful illness requiring costly hospitalization. A variety of abscess-fistulas are caused by infection that originates in anal crypts and glands. Detailed knowledge of the regional anatomy is essential to an understanding of their causes, pathogenesis, and proper treatment.

Cause and Pathogenesis

Small, cryptlike valves are situated around the circumference of the dentate line. Microscopic anal ducts or glands open into the inferior funnels of the crypts. These ducts and glands penetrate by varying distances into the anorectum, internal anal sphincter, or intersphincteric space. Bacteria gain entrance to the ducts and glands and cause suppurative infection, which spreads via the anatomic structures of the area. Diarrhea, hard stools, trauma, or foreign bodies are the main causes of bacterial penetration of the cryptoglandular structures. Infection that penetrates only the anoderm may appear as a very superficial abscess near the anal margin. This type is rare, because the glands usually penetrate more deeply through the internal sphincter into the intersphincteric space, between the internal and external sphincters. From the intersphincteric space, pus may extend in several directions along anatomic lines of least resistance (Fig. 30-3). A transient abscess may remain in the intersphincteric space (high or low), but more frequently infection spreads to other anorectal spaces:

Intermuscular	Anterior anal
High	Superficial
Low	Deep
Perianal	Ischioanal
Postanal	Supralevator
Superficial	
Deep	

Symptoms and Diagnosis of Abscesses

Superficial perianal abscesses are identified by painful, localized, tender swelling. The diagnosis is usually obvious, and immediate simple drainage in the office is indicated. Antibiotic therapy with delay in drainage is contraindicated. Not all acute perianal abscesses are of cryptoglandular origin. The differential diagnosis includes skin furuncles, infected inclusion cysts, hidradenitis, trauma, foreign bodies, and Bartholin cyst abscess. The optimal treatment still may be drainage with follow-up to rule out anal fistula.

Deeper abscesses begin with vague, deep anorectal pain that is not well localized, and initial examination may not reveal an obvious abscess. Tenderness on palpation of the intersphincteric

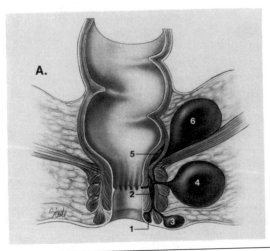
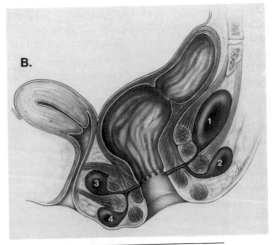

FIGURE 30-3 Anorectal abscesses. **A,** Frontal. *1,* subcutaneous; *2,* low intermuscular; *3,* perianal; *4,* ischioanal; *5,* high intermuscular; *6,* supralevator. **B,** Sagittal. *1,* deep postanal; *2,* superficial postanal; *3,* deep anterior; *4,* superficial anterior.

groove at the anal margin or point tenderness in the anus suggests an intersphincteric abscess. Deep tenderness over one or both ischioanal areas and a posterior tender area on digital examination suggest a deep posterior space abscess with unilateral or bilateral extension to the deep ischioanal spaces (hemi or horseshoe abscesses). The patient who has fever, vague deep rectal pain, and a high, tender rectal mass laterally or posteriorly may have a supralevator abscess. This complicated abscess requires hospitalization, adequate evaluation with the patient under anesthesia, and appropriate drainage. Unfortunately, many of the deeper abscesses go unrecognized, and pus extends along lines of least resistance as the abscess enlarges. At other times an abscess may be suspected and treated with antibiotics, thus delaying surgical treatment and allowing spread of infection. Infection may be recognized, and the skin over the ischioanal area may be red and indurated without fluctuation. Under these circumstances some physicians order antibiotics and hot sitz baths to allow the abscess to "come to a head." However, pus is present and should be drained immediately. Systemic antibiotics and surgical drainage are indicated in complicated situations in which the patient may have septicemia, diabetes, or impaired immunocompetence. Patients who have anorectal abscesses with sepsis secondary to leukemia also need systemic antibiotic treatment.

Symptoms and Diagnosis of Fistulas

Once an anorectal abscess is surgically drained or drains spontaneously, pain and symptoms are dramatically relieved. In more than 50% of cases, as the abscessed cavity contracts, a fistula results that is manifested by a persistent, small, draining opening in the perianal area. This external or secondary opening connects with the primary opening at the dentate line and constitutes a *fistula-in-ano*. A search to identify the origin should be made, and, if it is identified, fistulotomy or fistulectomy should be planned. If the external opening closes and if, after careful examination, the primary opening is not found, nothing further should be done. Recurrence of the fistula at a later date is likely, at which time the primary opening may be more easily identified.

When a persistent chronic fistula is present, there are several ways to identify the primary opening. Statistically, most abscess-fistulas origi-

nate in posterior anal crypts; anterior crypts are the next most common site. However, careful scrutiny of all crypts of the dentate line is necessary.

On inspection of the anal region, location of the external opening can provide a clue as to the primary origin. According to Goodsall's rule (Fig. 30-4), if the opening is anterior to a transverse anal line (coronal plane), the primary opening will be in a direct radial line to the nearest crypt. If the opening is posterior to the coronal line, the primary opening will usually be in a posterior midline crypt, and the tract will connect in a curved direction. Exceptions to Goodsall's rule include anterior openings that are more than 3 cm from the anal margin and multiple openings on one or both sides. In these situations, the primary site is more likely to arise in one of the posterior crypts.

Palpation of the perineal area may reveal an indurated cord beneath the skin, leading in the direction of the primary opening. Digital anal palpation may reveal a suspicious scarred or retracted crypt. Further palpation internally may reveal induration posteriorly, laterally, or circumferentially, indicating fistulas deep in the postanal space or horseshoe fistulas. Endoscopic examinations of the clinically suspected quadrant of the dentate line may reveal the offending crypt, which can be gently probed with a smooth hook. Occasionally a drop of pus can be seen draining from the primary crypt. External prob-

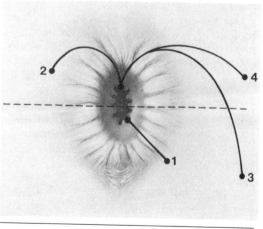

FIGURE 30-4 Goodsall's rule (dotted line is the coronal plane). *1,* Anterior external opening; *2,* posterior external opening; *3,* anterior opening 5 cm from anal margin; *4,* posterior external opening.

ing has limited value because it is painful, and care must be taken to avoid false passage, particularly in fistulous tracts. Radiographic fistulograms are seldom of practical value. A barium enema examination of the colon is indicated in patients with symptoms of inflammatory bowel disease to rule out fistulas related to Crohn's disease.

Fistula Surgery

After the primary opening has been identified, elective surgery is advisable. For simple fistulas, most colorectal surgeons prefer fistulotomy rather than fistulectomy. *Fistulotomy*, incising the fistulous tract from the secondary opening to the primary opening with minor trimming of the wound edges, is definitive treatment. *Fistulectomy* with complete excision of the fistulous tract is unnecessary. When the fistula is deep and goes beneath the entire external sphincter muscle, complete division of the muscle may result in incontinence. This occurs most often in women who have deep anterior fistulas. Under these circumstances, the use of a rubber seton is useful. All of the fistulous tract is divided except for the external sphincter. A rubber band is placed loosely around the muscle, and its ends are tied with silk. At 2-week intervals after surgery, the rubber band is tightened gradually to divide the muscle. The seton principle allows inflammatory reaction and fibrosis to fix the muscle so that the ends do not separate widely after complete division. The resultant smaller defect prevents incontinence.

Complicated deep ischioanal and horseshoe fistulas (Fig. 30-5) have their primary openings in the posterior midline, which communicates with the deep postanal space. They have one or more external openings. Conventional fistulotomy results in marked anal and perianal scarring, dysfunction, and possibly incontinence. Modified fistula surgery, as popularized by Hanley, has replaced conventional fistulotomy in these types of fistulas. Hanley's operation consists of incising from the primary opening and unroofing the deep postanal space. Probes passed from the external openings converge to meet in this space. The external openings are excised, and the intervening fistulous tracts are partially excised or simply curetted. Eliminating the primary origin of the fistula and unroofing the postanal space allows the other tracts to heal, and the resulting healing of the posterior wound

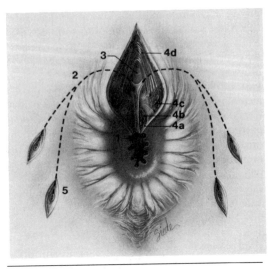

FIGURE 30-5 Horseshoe fistula. *1*, Primary opening in posterior midline; *2*, secondary opening; *3*, deep postanal space, unroofed; *4*, structures incised or separated: *a*, anoderm, *b*, internal anal sphincter, *c*, subcutaneous external anal sphincter, *d*, superficial external limbs, separated; *5*, external openings, excised.

leaves a normal anatomic appearance without deformity or dysfunction.

Postoperative care of fistula wounds includes maintenance of normal, formed stools, hygienic care with hot sitz baths, and periodic office visits to keep the wound edges open.

Rare extrasphincteric supralevator fistulas may be caused by pelvic abscesses, which extend through the levator muscle into the ischiorectal fossa and eventually drain through the overlying perianal skin to exit. These must be differentiated from cryptoglandular transsphincteric abscess-fistulas that extend to the supralevator space or ischioanal spaces. Treatment involves correction of the pelvic septic process seen with resection of sigmoid diverticulitis or inflammatory bowel disease.

Supralevator abscesses and other deep, complicated abscess-fistulas should be treated only after the exact cause, primary opening, and direction and course of the abscess or fistula have been determined. The surgeon should be reluctant to completely divide the entire external anal sphincter, particularly anteriorly in women. Experience and complete knowledge of the anatomy, etiology, and pathogenesis of abscess-fistulas cannot be overemphasized.

RECTAL PROLAPSE (PROCIDENTIA)

By definition, rectal prolapse is intussusception of a full thickness of rectum through the anus. Partial prolapse is a distinct entity involving only eversion of the rectal mucosa for a distance of usually less than 1 cm. The cause of rectal prolapse is multifactorial and reflects failure in one or more of the rectal support mechanisms (i.e., fascia, mesentery, peritoneum, sphincter mechanism, or protective anatomic curvature of the sacrum). This disease is frequently seen in two age-groups—children under 2 years of age and the elderly—especially those who are physically or mentally debilitated.

In children, immature anatomy (weak rectal attachments or incomplete sacral curvature formation) appears to be the cause, and conservative, nonoperative measures are usually successful in treating the prolapse until anatomic maturity is achieved.

Adults with mucosal prolapse may be distinguished from those with true rectal prolapse by identification of the classic radial pattern of the folds separating the mucosa. In rectal prolapse, the mucosal folds have a circumferential appearance.

Adults with complete rectal prolapse may have pain, bleeding, or excessive mucosal discharge. The most debilitating sequela of the disease, however, is incontinence secondary to prolonged dilation of the sphincter and possible nerve injury. Thus it is important to treat this disease before the onset of incontinence because corrective procedures for the prolapse rarely restore sphincter control.

Treatment of rectal prolapse is tailored to the individual patient's general condition and environment. For a feeble patient, circumferential subcutaneous passage of a Silastic loop, steel suture wire (Thiersch), or synthetic loop may achieve sufficient tightening of the anus and preclude further prolapse. This procedure is the simplest and least traumatic to the patient but has a high failure rate secondary to loop breakage, infection, and recurrent fecal impaction.

Patients whose general health permits a definitive procedure may be considered for transabdominal suspension of the rectum, low anterior resection, or excision of redundant bowel through a perineal approach. The most widely used transabdominal procedure is the Ripstein operation. In this procedure, the rectum is mobilized and then secured to the presacral fascia with a synthetic mesh sling. Results of this operation are excellent, and most major series report a recurrence rate of less than 3%. The transanal approach is used by many surgeons who feel that this is a safer procedure than transabdominal suspension and are willing to accept its recurrence rate of 5% to 23%.

HEMORRHOIDS

Hemorrhoids are classified as either internal or external. Internal hemorrhoids arise above the dentate line and are covered by nonsensitive mucosa, whereas external hemorrhoids originate below the dentate line and are covered with well-innervated epithelium (anoderm). Classically, internal hemorrhoids are found in cases of bleeding or prolapse, whereas external hemorrhoids are rarely of clinical significance except when a painful thrombosis occurs in this plexus. The cause of symptomatic hemorrhoids is controversial. Excessive straining for whatever reason (low-bulk diet, excessive exercise, pregnancy, or poor toilet habits) is the primary cause, but other factors such as the erect posture of humans and the lack of venous valves in the hemorrhoidal complexes are certainly contributory. It is important to remember that hemorrhoids are not varicose veins of the anus. Research now shows that hemorrhoids represent discrete vascular cushions or tufts with arterial-venous communications. Degeneration of supporting connective tissue leads to profusion or prolapse during straining or defecation.

The classic symptomatology of hemorrhoids includes bright red rectal bleeding, mucosal prolapse, and occasional perianal itching that is secondary to discharge of mucus. Contrary to many patients' beliefs, anal pain is not a classic symptom of hemorrhoids and is usually present only when subcutaneous edema or thrombosis stretches the anoderm. When a patient complains of anal pain, the practitioner's diagnostic acumen should be directed to other causes, such as abscesses or anal fissure.

Internal Hemorrhoids

For physicians to better classify and treat internal hemorrhoids, a clinical staging system was adopted. First-degree hemorrhoids represent enlarged cushions that do not prolapse. Second-degree hemorrhoids prolapse into the anal canal

TABLE 30-2 Treatment of Internal Hemorrhoids

Clinical Stage	Treatment
First-degree	Conservative treatment with bowel habit education and dietary changes
Second-degree	Dietary and bowel habit education and possible non-operative fixation techniques
Third-degree	Dietary and bowel habit education and possible non-operative fixation techniques (minor third-degree)
Fourth-degree	Hemorrhoidectomy or bowel and dietary changes (for acute strangulated hemorrhoids, urgent surgical intervention may be necessary)

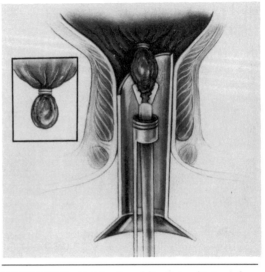

FIGURE 30-6 Rubber band ligation of internal hemorrhoid.

during defecation but spontaneously reduce themselves. Third-degree hemorrhoids prolapse with straining and require manual reduction. Fourth-degree hemorrhoids remain prolapsed continuously.

In treating internal hemorrhoids, the physician should always confirm that the symptoms are truly hemorrhoidal in nature and are not caused by other colorectal pathologic conditions such as rectal prolapse, pruritus, anorectal cancers, or inflammatory bowel disease.

There are currently five major modalities for treating internal hemorrhoids: (1) education in proper dietary and bowel habits, (2) rubber band ligation, (3) photocoagulation, (4) sclerotherapy, and (5) hemorrhoidectomy. These treatments should be individualized according to the degree of the patient's symptomatology (Table 30-2).

All patients should receive education about proper dietary and bowel habits. Consuming a high-fiber diet with adequate liquid intake is essential, and often a psyllium seed product for stool softening is advisable. Patients should also be instructed to avoid straining with bowel movements and to decrease excessive time spent on the toilet.

Nonoperative fixation techniques include rubber band ligation, photocoagulation, and sclerotherapy. The goal of each of these techniques is to fix hemorrhoidal tissue to the under-

lying muscular coat, which results in the reduced likelihood of hemorrhoidal prolapse or bleeding. The banding technique for hemorrhoidectomy is highly successful and may eliminate the risks associated with hemorrhoidectomy, making this an excellent alternative in poor surgical candidates. Adequate exposure of the hemorrhoidal group is obtained with an anoscope; then a special grasping forceps is passed through a channel of the banding ligator in order to grasp the redundant hemorrhoidal tissue (Fig. 30-6). The ligator is then fired, leaving a rubber band around the base of the offending hemorrhoidal group, which will lead to eventual mucosal sloughing. The tissue will usually slough by day 5, and the secondary scarring will fix the residual hemorrhoidal cushion, preventing future prolapse. This treatment is unacceptable for external hemorrhoids, because banding on somatically innervated skin is excruciatingly painful.

Infrared coagulation can be successfully used in treating first-degree, second-degree, and minor third-degree hemorrhoids. The infrared coagulator uses bursts of infrared light that generate enough heat at the apex of the hemorrhoid to cause fixation of the cushion to the underlying muscle. Proponents of this technique point out that the area of trauma can be controlled precisely, allowing the clinician to treat all symptomatic areas in one clinical setting. Proponents of banding suggest that the cost of this instru-

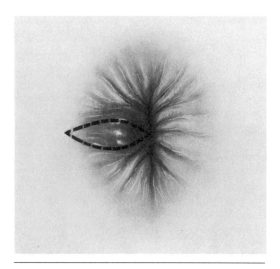

FIGURE 30-7   Excision of thrombosed hemorrhoid.

mentation and the necessity for repeated treatments makes it a second choice for nonoperative treatment.

Sclerotherapy is the oldest form of nonoperative therapy. It involves injection of small amounts of chemical irritants into the mucosal plane at the cephalad end of the hemorrhoid. In skilled hands, sclerotherapy can provide excellent results in primary and secondary hemorrhoids, but it is less popular than the other effective modalities.

Formal hemorrhoidectomy is indicated for patients with severe third-degree, fourth-degree, or strangulated hemorrhoids. This procedure, when performed by an experienced surgeon, offers the most complete and lasting relief of hemorrhoid symptomatology.

External Hemorrhoids

A dramatic source of acute anorectal pain is a thrombosed external hemorrhoid, the subcutaneous rupture or thrombosis of an external hemorrhoidal vein. The onset of pain is acute and is frequently related to exertion or a traumatic bowel movement. The thrombosis is a bluish, subcutaneous nodule that is usually painful. Its natural course is decreasing discomfort over a 3- to 4-day period, with complete resolution within 1 to 3 weeks. Treatment is based on the degree of patient discomfort. If the patient experiences extreme pain after 48 hours, an immediate cure can be obtained by elliptical excision of the overlying skin and clot evacuation performed under local anesthesia (Fig. 30-7). The key is excision and not incision of skin to prevent reformation of the thrombosis. If the symptoms decrease after 48 hours, sitz baths, stool softeners, and reassurance may be sufficient until complete resolution occurs.

SURGICAL PHARMACOPEIA

Drug	Indications/Complications	Dosage
Hydrocortisone acetate 1% and pramoxine hydrochloride 1% (ProctoCream-HC)	Inflammatory and pruritic manifestations of corticosteroid-responsive perianal dermatoses Systemic absorption, producing hypothalamic/pituitary/adrenal axis suppression, is possible	Apply thin film to affected area up to four times daily
Topical aerosol (Proctofoam-HC)		Apply to affected area up to four times daily
Psyllium hydrophilic mucilloid (Metamucil)	Bulking agent that promotes elimination	One teaspoon or tablespoon up to three times per day
Docusate sodium (Colace, Surfak)	Stool softener No known contraindications	50-200 mg daily in capsule, liquid, or syrup
5% Fluorouracil cream (Efudex)	Topical chemotherapy for perianal Bowen's disease	Apply to lesion twice daily for 3-12 weeks

BIBLIOGRAPHY

Boman BM, Moertel CG, O'Connell MJ, et al. Carcinoma of the anal canal. A clinical and pathological study of 188 cases. Cancer 54:114, 1988.

Goligher JC. Surgery of the Anus, Rectum, and Colon, 5th ed. London, Tindall, 1984.

Hanley P. Anorectal abscess fistula. Surg Clin North Am 58:487, 1978.

Hollinshead W. Anatomy for Surgeons, 2nd ed, Vol II: The Thorax, Abdomen and Pelvis. New York, Hoeber, 1956.

Nigro ND. An evaluation of combined therapy for squamous cell carcinoma of the anal canal. Dis Colon Rectum 27:763, 1984.

Nigro ND, Vaitkevicius VK, Buroker T, et al. Combined therapy for cancer of the anal canal. Dis Colon Rectum 24:73, 1981.

Quan S. Anal and perianal tumors. Surg Clin North Am 58:591, 1978.

CHAPTER REVIEW
Questions

1. The most common cause of painful defecation is:
   a. Anal cancer
   b. Abscess
   c. Anal fissure
2. True or false: Pilonidal sinus is most often a congenital lesion.
3. Anal cancer is most commonly:
   a. Basal cell cancer
   b. Adenocarcinoma
   c. Squamous cell cancer
4. Tumors arising below the dentate line may drain to which of the following node basins?
   a. Inguinal
   b. Hypogastric
   c. Inferior mesenteric
   d. All of the above
5. Which of the following is the least acceptable treatment for symptomatic internal hemorrhoids?
   a. Banding
   b. Hemorrhoidectomy
   c. Sclerotherapy
   d. Cryosurgery
6. Rectal prolapse is associated with which of the following complications?
   a. Pain
   b. Bleeding
   c. Incontinence
   d. All of the above
7. Pruritus ani can be caused by:
   a. Chocolate, milk, coffee
   b. Excessive rubbing and overly meticulous hygiene
   c. Erythrasma
   d. All of the above
8. True or false: The Nigro protocol for treatment of anal cell carcinoma includes abdominal perineal resection followed by chemotherapy and radiation therapy.
9. True of false: The lymphatic drainage of the colon and rectum closely follows the venous drainage.
10. Classically, the morphologic triad of an anal fissure is:
    a. Anal ulcer, pain, rectal bleeding
    b. Anal ulcer, hypertrophic papillae, sentinel pile
    c. Anal ulcer, thrombosed hemorrhoid, anal pain
    d. Anal ulcer, sentinel pile, thrombosed hemorrhoid

Answers

1. c	6. d
2. f	7. d
3. c	8. f
4. d	9. f
5. d	10. b

31 Surgical Masqueraders
Abdominal Pain Rarely Requiring Operation

BERNARD GARDNER

KEY FEATURES

After reading this chapter you will understand:
- That evaluation of pain arising from nonoperative sources requires a thorough history and physical examination.
- That the abdominal wall can be a source of pain often confused with hernia or intra-abdominal disease.
- The metabolic disorders that may produce abdominal pain.

A patient may have a disease or condition in which abdominal pain is a prominent symptom, but for which operation is usually not indicated (Table 31-1). The patient with undiagnosed abdominal pain may have any condition from a self-limited gastroenteritis to gangrenous bowel in an internal hernia and therefore represents a potential catastrophe. *Rapid diagnosis is vital and, fortunately, can usually be made by an accurate history and physical examination* (see Chapter 25). *If there is doubt, critical radiologic and laboratory tests should be performed promptly.* In most cases the differential diagnosis will involve the presence or absence of a small intestinal obstruction; therefore, when the diagnosis is unclear, early performance of an upper GI series to rule out complete obstruction by demonstrating barium entering the colon after several hours will gain sufficient time for further and perhaps more definitive studies to be made.

PAIN ARISING FROM THE ABDOMINAL WALL
Localized Processes

Causes. The following may be implicated when undiagnosed abdominal pain is present:

- Trauma to the abdominal muscles, producing contusion
- Hematoma of the abdominal muscles secondary to anticoagulant treatment
- Infection of the abdominal wall with cellulitis or abscess
- Nerve entrapment
- Focal abdominal wall trigger points
- Myofascial pain syndromes
- Rib tip syndrome
- Tumor of the abdominal wall (will require operation in most instances)

These syndromes can frustrate patient and physician when they mimic intra-abdominal disease.

How Do You Diagnose These Conditions?

History and Physical Examination. The diagnosis is indicated by a history of the use of anticoagulants, fever, an enlarging abdominal mass, trauma, location of the mass, localized tenderness, and systemic signs of infection.

Abdominal Wall Test (Carnett's Test). Pain arising from focal abdominal wall syndromes will be accentuated by the tensing of the rectus muscles. This can be accomplished by raising the lower extremities while the patient is lying supine or by raising the head and shoulders. *Pain arising from the abdominal viscera will be di-*

TABLE 31-1 Surgical Masqueraders

Cause	History
Abdominal Wall	
Trauma, hematoma, tumor, infection	Trauma, anticoagulant use, enlarging mass, fever
Viral myositis, toxins	Viral prodrome of malaise, fever, anorexia, spider bite, snake bite
Trigger point, myofascial syndrome, nerve entrapment	Previous operation, parasthesias, no visceral symptoms (e.g., vomiting)
Thorax	
Pneumothorax pleural effusion	Tuberculosis, cancer, trauma
Pneumonia, pulmonary infarction	Exposure, known tuberculosis, preexisting thrombophlebitis, pelvic inflammatory disease, ingestion of drugs, hemoptysis
Constrictive pericarditis, myocardial infarction, embolization	Symptoms of heart failure, anginal prodrome
Central Nervous System	
Cord or nerve root compression or inflammation	Exacerbated by cough or straining, hyperesthesia, causalgia, etc.
Brain, psychogenic, abdominal migraine	Occasional vomiting, abdominal discomfort, cranial nerve symptoms, previous known psychiatric disorder, epilepsy, or migraine headaches
Genitourinary	
Kidney, ureter, bladder	Previous stone or infection, symptoms of infection, back pain, suprapubic pain, pain radiating to thigh or testicle
Ovary, tubes, uterus	Previous infection, exposure to VD, menstrual irregularity, vaginal discharge
Peritoneum	Underlying pneumonia, tuberculosis, cancer, cirrhosis
Metabolic (Exogenous)	
Heavy metal poisoning	Ingestion or close contact with lead, mercury, arsenicals
Food poisoning	Ingestion of contaminated food, epidemic, associated diarrhea common
Metabolic (Endogenous)	
Diabetes, uremia, porphyria, collagen disease, Mediterranean fever, hemolytic diseases, lactose intolerance	Known disease, arthralgias, nerve deficits, anemia, relation to food

Physical Examination	Special Tests
Location of tenderness, mass, presence of fever, cellulitis Fang marks	Biopsy if solid mass is present
Pain exacerbated with rectus muscle tightening, single finger pressure—pain Fascial or muscular cord	Responds to local anesthesia
Hyperresonance to percussion with pneumothorax, flat percussion note, breath sounds ↓↓, egophony over fluid	Chest x-ray film, decubitus film of chest, CT scan
Breath sounds ↓↓, rales, dull percussion note, friction rub	Chest x-ray film, lung scan, pulmonary angiogram
BP ↓↓, thready pulse, pulse pressure ↓↓, venous pressure ↑↑	ECG, chest x-ray film Echocardiography
Duplication of pain by pressure on spine, no abdominal wall rigidity, guarding, or rebound tenderness	X-ray of spine, myelography, MRI, or CT scan
No muscular tenderness, abdominal guarding, etc., neurologic abnormalities	Skull x-ray film, brain scan, EEG, spinal fluid analysis, CT or MRI scan
Suprapubic or CVA tenderness, fever	Urine analysis, leukocytosis, IVP or CT scan, nephrotomography, retrograde pyelography, cystoscopy, arteriography
Pelvic tenderness, mass, vaginal discharge	Smear of discharge, culposcopy, laparoscopy, sonography
Distended abdomen, ascites, tenderness, fever, signs of cirrhosis	Peritoneal tap and smear of fluid, analysis of fluid for protein, culture, chest x-ray film
Lack of peritoneal signs	Smear of peripheral blood, blood or urine levels of offending agent ↑
Fever, lack of signs of peritoneal irritation	Stool culture, blood agglutinins
Lack of signs of peritonitis (unless ischemic bowel necrosis present)	Depending on underlying conditions: blood sugar ↑, BUN ↑, Hb ↓, urine porphyrins ↑, sickled red cells, antinuclear antibody ↑, ESR ↑, CRP ↑, LE prep +, hydrogen breath test +

minished by this maneuver. Single-finger probing of the abdominal wall, flank, and inguinal regions will identify focal trigger points, which can then be injected with local anesthetic agents to break the pain cycle. Relief is frequently obtained.

Nerve entrapment following operations can occur in the surgical scar and may be associated with paresthesias when touched. These can frequently be relieved by local injections of anesthetics. These entrapments have also been described as occurring along the lateral margin of the rectus muscle where the anterior cutaneous branches of the intercostal nerves perforate the rectus sheath.

Myofascial syndromes can be diagnosed by the presence of a taut band of skeletal muscle or fascia that may contain a focal trigger point. The pain may radiate to distant areas. Injection of a local anesthetic provides the best long-term relief, although other treatments involving counterirritants have been used.

The *rib tip syndrome* is caused by hypermotility of the eighth, ninth, and tenth ribs, irritating the intercostal nerves when they shift upward with certain motions. Local anesthetic injection of the involved intercostal nerve may yield relief; in refractory cases rib resection may be required.

Other Tests. Biopsy of a tumor mass is necessary to establish a precise diagnosis.

Systemic Processes

Causes

- Myositis resulting from viral infection (herpetic lesions) or idiopathic causes (primary muscular disease)
- Muscular spasm resulting from toxins

Diagnosis. Generalized malaise, fever, and muscular pains may accompany some viral infections. The onset of the abdominal pain in association with this systemic reaction clearly points to a nonmechanical cause (Chapter 25).

Specific toxins are associated with spasm or contractions of abdominal muscles that may mimic an acute abdomen. The most common is that introduced by the bite of the black widow spider. The history of a bite and/or presence of fang marks may lead to the correct diagnosis. All muscles may become involved, and the severity of pain is greatest in muscle groups closest to the site of envenomation.

Coral snake bites, in contradistinction to pit viper bites, produce little or no reaction at the site of envenomation. Abdominal pains may be an early sign of the potent, nonspecific neurotoxic action and precede peripheral neuromuscular block.

LESIONS LOCALIZED IN THE THORAX
Pleura

Cause. Air or fluid in the pleural space may lead to inspiratory pain referred to the upper abdomen.

Diagnosis
History and Physical Examination. The pain is sharp and usually related to inspiration. There may be a history of a similar episode, trauma, or underlying disease (e.g., tuberculosis, carcinoma) predisposing to the condition. Percussion and auscultation of the chest will most commonly lead to the diagnosis. Eliciting egophony over the fluid is a characteristic finding in pleural effusion.

Other Tests. The chest x-ray evaluation is, of course, the definitive diagnostic test. If the fluid is of minimal quantity (under 250 ml), a decubitus film or a CT scan of the chest may be necessary to demonstrate it.

Lung

Causes

- Lower lobe pneumonic processes may irritate the diaphragm and give rise to referred abdominal pain, which can mimic upper abdominal disease (i.e., cholecystitis).
- Pulmonary infarction may lead to similar circumstances in cases in which the lower pleura or diaphragm is irritated.

Diagnosis
History and Physical Examination. It is very important to distinguish lower lobe infiltrates that are primary from those that are secondary to intra-abdominal disease, with splinting of the diaphragm. Characteristically, primary pneumonia can be clearly distinguished on physical examination by the presence of rales, diminished breath sounds, and dullness to percussion, whereas pulmonary infiltrates secondary to abdominal diseases are usually diagnosed on x-ray examination. A history of intra-abdominal disease should lead to the correct diagnosis. Pulmonary infarction is often associated with preexisting disease of the leg veins or heart, pelvic inflammatory disease, or the ingestion of drugs that predispose to thrombosis. Hemoptysis is an associated symptom pointing to the correct diagnosis.

Other Tests. A chest x-ray evaluation will clarify the presence of pneumonia. Pneumonic processes secondary to intra-abdominal disease are less extensive, appearing as plate atelectasis, with patchy or scattered infiltrates. A complete lobar involvement points strongly to a primary pneumonia.

Pulmonary infarction may be diagnosed on chest x-ray films, by lung scan, or, most definitively, by pulmonary angiography. This latter test is reserved for more severe cases or those in which operative intervention is contemplated (e.g., vena cava ligation) (see Chapter 17).

Heart

Causes. *Constrictive pericarditis* may cause referred abdominal pain by involvement of the diaphragm or by the production of liver swelling, with pain from stretching of Glisson's capsule. This latter condition may occur in any condition that is associated with acute heart failure, leading to tenderness over the liver and abdominal pain.

Myocardial infarction, particularly if the diaphragmatic surface of the heart is involved, may present with acute upper abdominal referred pain. Recurrent angina rarely produces similar symptoms.

Embolization to solid organs (e.g., kidney, spleen) from clots in the heart or diseased valves may mimic acute abdominal disease.

Diagnosis

History and Physical Examination. The presence of preexisting heart disease, symptoms or signs of heart failure, or associated evidence of arteriosclerotic disease in other areas of the body may lead to the correct diagnosis. Constrictive pericarditis and heart failure are always associated with signs and symptoms of increased venous pressure, such as leg or ankle edema, distended or noncollapsing neck veins, shortness of breath, a demonstrable hepatojugular reflux, and so forth. Constrictive pericarditis is also associated with a thready pulse, tachycardia, and narrow pulse pressure.

Other Tests. Electrocardiogram is mandatory whenever acute heart disease is suspected. It will specifically delineate most cases of early myocardial infarction. Chest x-ray films are helpful if pulmonary congestion can be seen or in rare cases of mediastinal widening, an enlarged heart shadow can be visualized. Special views to delineate enlargement of the heart may be helpful. Constrictive disease or small pericardial effusions can be clearly diagnosed by echocardiography, which is also useful in diagnosing valvular disor-

ders or intracardiac clots. Angiography may be definitive in some cases.

LESIONS OF THE CENTRAL NERVOUS SYSTEM
Spinal Cord

Causes. Pain arising from spinal nerves or nerve root levels may be secondary to a variety of primary processes. The gastric crisis of tabes dorsalis, familiar to a past generation of surgeons, once again must be considered in the differential diagnosis of acute abdominal pain because of the increasing incidence of syphilis.

Axial osteomyelitis, herpes zoster neuritis, nerve impingement by arthritis, paraspinal tumors, herniated nucleus pulposus, or spinal collapse may produce abdominal symptoms but not signs.

Diagnosis

History and Physical Examination. Radicular pain from thoracic nerve root irritation is characteristically exacerbated by increase of intrathoracic pressure, such as that created by coughing or straining, and can be associated with hyperesthesias, dysesthesia, or causalgia in the dermatome distribution of the involved nerve. *Eliciting symptoms with manual pressure at the thoracic-axial skeletal articulations is often diagnostic.* Intraspinal cord lesions, such as thoracic spinal cord tumors, should also be considered when nerve root signs are present or accompanied by ascending or descending tract signs. In such a clinical situation or in instances of postoperative thoracic nerve causalgia, rigidity in the abdominal muscles is absent.

Other Tests. X-ray examination of the vertebral column will delineate collapse, interspace narrowing, arthritic changes, or paraspinal masses, which may indicate the correct diagnosis. Myelography may be necessary to demonstrate intraspinal nerve root compression by tumor or herniated disk. Bone tomography of the spine or sonography to indicate the presence of retroperitoneal masses causing root compression may be indicated. These lesions may also be demonstrated by CT scan or magnetic resonance imaging (MRI).

Brain

Causes. Referred abdominal pain is reported to occur as a result of *radiculitis* from *meningeal inflammation* involving afferent sensory neurons from the abdominal viscera. *Posterior fossa tumors* usually present with vomiting but can present as vague abdominal discomfort and may be confused with psychogenic abdominal pain, especially in children.

Psychogenic abdominal pain and symptoms ascribed to *abdominal epilepsy* are different in presentation and mechanism. Cramping abdominal pain of varying intensity and location is seen with psychomotor or temporal lobe epilepsy. Psychogenic pain is basically a hysterical reaction to minor intra-abdominal pain but may be quite difficult to diagnose in the sophisticated conversion reaction.

Abdominal migraine is a syndrome producing episodic severe abdominal pain separated by completely symptom-free periods. In most cases, the syndrome may occur with the typical headache, or, more rarely, may precede the onset of headaches, making the diagnosis difficult.

Diagnosis

History and Physical Examination. The absence of characteristic abdominal somatic nerve involvement is essential to the diagnosis. A careful neurologic examination may demonstrate defects in cranial nerve activity that may point to the CNS origin of the disorder.

Other Tests. X-ray examinations include standard skull films, tomography, angiography, and ventriculography, but they are now often replaced by CT or MRI scans. Other tests include brain scan, electroencephalography, and careful analysis of the spinal fluid with respect to cytology, protein content, and so forth.

LESIONS OF THE GENITOURINARY SYSTEM
Kidney, Ureter, and Bladder

Causes. Obstruction to the flow of urine by stone or tumor may lead to the characteristic renal colic, which may mimic an acute abdominal crisis.

Infection of the bladder (cystitis) or pyelonephritis is often associated with referred abdominal pain resulting from distension of the renal capsule or to associated perinephric abscess (see Chapter 41).

Acute testicular infection may rarely produce pain referred to the lower abdomen; this condition has been confused with acute appendicitis.

Diagnosis

History and Physical Examination. A history of urinary tract disease is helpful in making the diagnosis, particularly when renal stones have previously been passed. The presence of severe infection is associated with the usual findings of fever and leukocytosis. Diseases affecting the kidney produce referred anterior abdominal wall pain and occasionally guarding and rigidity of the anterior upper abdominal muscles. *Characteristically, the presence of costovertebral angle (CVA) tenderness elicited by gentle pressure in the CVA is specific for disease arising in the urinary system.* It is rarely found with acute cholecystitis or appendicitis—the two most common intra-abdominal emergencies confused with primary renal disease. Pain arising from the ureter is often referred to the loin, testicle, or inside of the thigh. Suprapubic pain arising from a distended urinary bladder (e.g., acute urinary retention) is associated with a history of failure to void and tenderness over the bladder.

Other Tests. Urine analysis may lead to the proper diagnosis if microscopic bleeding or white cell casts are found. The presence of protein or scattered white cells does not rule out an intra-abdominal process (e.g., appendicitis). A negative result on urinalysis may, however, be found *where complete obstruction to a ureter is present.* Under these circumstances, an emergency intravenous pyelogram or CT scan with a contrast medium may clearly delineate the blockage or failure of one kidney to excrete the dye. Coincidental intra-abdominal disease is not ruled out by this test but would be extremely unlikely in the presence of a nonfunctioning kidney.

Special studies may be reserved until after the acute emergency is delineated. These include nephrotomography, renal angiography, retrograde pyelography, and cystoscopy.

Ovary, Tubes, and Uterus

Causes. Infection of the tubes and/or ovaries is the primary surgical masquerader necessitating nonoperative treatment. Most other gynecologic disease, such as ovarian tumors or cysts, ectopic pregnancies, or twisted uterine fibroids, may necessitate early operation. Rarely, Mittelschmerz or normal ovulation may produce pain that is confusing in distribution with acute appendicitis.

Diagnosis

History and Physical Examination. A careful menstrual history of every woman is of paramount importance. The relation of the pain to the menstrual cycle, previous occurrences, exposure to venereal disease, a missed period, and so on may point to the correct diagnosis. The physical examination may be helpful if the signs are limited to the pelvic region, associated with or aggravated by cervical motion, or associated with a vaginal discharge.

Other Tests. Microscopic examination of the vaginal discharge may reveal the characteristic intracellular organisms found in gonorrhea.

Where significant suspicion of acute pelvic disease or ectopic pregnancy is present, colposcopy or laparoscopy may be indicated as an emergency. Sonography is routinely done when pelvic disease is suspected.

Lesions of the Peritoneum

Causes. Primary peritonitis may occur as a result of pneumococcal disease (common in children) or tuberculosis. Ascites associated with cancer, liver disease, or heart disease may be a cause of abdominal pain and vomiting.

Diagnosis

History and Physical Examination. Associated bacterial disease or tuberculosis should be carefully discerned. The abdomen may be tender, distended, and frequently contains ascites. A known history of previous carcinoma or cirrhosis may lead to the correct diagnosis. Associated vomiting is frequent.

Other Tests. Smear, culture, and cytologic studies of the peritoneal fluid may immediately demonstrate the cause. Tuberculosis of the gastrointestinal tract or miliary disease is frequently associated with underlying chronic illness, fever and weight loss, and a protein content of the ascitic fluid over 3 g/dl. Demonstration of the acid-fast organisms is diagnostic.

A chest x-ray examination demonstrating the underlying associated infection may be helpful in avoiding unnecessary operation. With the patient under local anesthesia, a sample of peritoneum can be obtained for microscopic evaluation.

METABOLIC ABDOMINAL CRISES
Exogenous Causes

Whenever the cause of abdominal pain is obscure, metabolic origin must be considered. The careful occupational or social history is the route to correct diagnosis in instances of exogenous metabolic poisoning.

Heavy Metal Poisoning. *Acute lead poisoning* is accompanied by headache and myalgia, which usually precede the onset of abdominal pain by days or weeks. Severe hyperperistalsis with cramping abdominal pain appears as the severity of lead intoxication increases. The pains may be episodic and associated with abdominal wall rigidity. Organic lead compounds are capable of producing acute encephalopathy, where blood levels greater than 120 mg/dl are seen. Peripheral neuropathy is predominantly motor and involves the wrist extensors early in the course.

Lead colic may be seen following ingestion of moonshine whiskey that is distilled and condensed in auto radiators containing lead solder. More commonly, lead colic is secondary to industrial uses of lead in paint, storage battery manufacture, and chemical and gasoline production. Because lead inhibits the utilization of iron in hemoglobin synthesis, the hemogram shows hypochromic anemia, with basophilic stippling of the erythrocytes on peripheral smear. Lead inhibits aminolevulinic acid (ALA) dehydrogenase, and there is an increased blood level as well as urinary excretion of both ALA and coproporphyrins. ALA urinary levels greater than 3.5 mg in 24 hours indicate lead intoxication.

Abdominal pain from acute *mercury poisoning* usually follows oral ingestion of mercuric chloride. The pain is of a cramping nature and may be associated with muscle cramps in the extremities. Acute poisoning is characterized by increased salivation, diarrhea, gingivitis, stomatitis, and varying degrees of acute tubular necrosis. The chronically poisoned individual may exhibit erethism, characterized by irritability, timidity, and nervousness. Laboratory confirmation requires examination of 24-hour urine collection. A mercury level greater than 500 μg/day indicates poisoning.

Similar symptoms and abdominal pain occur with *arsenic poisoning.* Arsenic poisoning most often results from suicide or homicide attempts but may occur from the inhalation of organic industrial compounds, insecticides, fungicides, and weed killers. Symptoms of arsenic poisoning are rare with urine levels under 4.0 mg/L.

Food Poisoning. *Salmonella* food poisoning, following the ingestion of contaminated foodstuffs, and botulism, as the result of ingestion or absorption of endotoxin, are characterized by acute febrile illness, with hyperactive gastrointestinal symptoms and particularly abdominal pain.

Staphylococcal food poisoning is self-limited to a short course of cramps, vomiting, and diarrhea, which characteristically subsides after 12 to 24 hours. Fever does not occur.

Snake and Spider Bites. For a discussion of abdominal pain resulting from snake or spider bites, see p. 564.

Endogenous Causes

Diabetes. In diabetic ketoacidosis, acute shifts of potassium ion and sodium ion may cause abdominal pains that closely simulate abdominal emergencies. The diagnosis of diabetic ketoacidosis is made by finding hyperglycemia, ketonemia, and reduction of serum carbon dioxide content. The abdominal pain is usually nonspecific and frequently shifts in location and intensity. If treatment of the ketoacidosis does not bring about resolution of the abdominal pain, *remember intra-abdominal disease and infection can precipitate diabetic acidosis.*

Uremia. Abdominal pain can follow electrolyte imbalance from the vomiting and diarrhea of uremia but may also be caused by uremic pericarditis or uremic pancreatitis. Confirmation of the latter is made difficult because serum amylase levels are high in renal insufficiency. The possibility of primary intra-abdominal disease developing in uremic patients must not be ignored.

Metabolic Errors. C'1-esterase deficiency with angioneurotic edema is often associated with episodes of severe abdominal pain. This hereditary condition is an inborn error of metabolism, whereby biosynthesis of serum inhibitor C'1-esterase, which normally blocks inactivation of complement components, is absent. The colicky abdominal pain is caused by visceral wheals.

Abdominal pain is frequently the presenting complaint with *acute intermittent porphyria.* This hereditary abnormality of pyrrole metabolism is a latent condition provoked into manifest disease by the administration of drugs that induce hepatic ALA synthetase and therefore increase porphobilinogens. Barbiturates, sulfonamides, and estrogenic compounds are known to increase the production of porphyrin precursors. Abdominal pain is severe and colicky and may be associated with spasm without localizing signs but with fever, tachycardia, and leukocytosis. Porphobilinogen in the urine is the diagnostic feature of acute intermittent porphyria.

A similar and interesting syndrome mimicking the acute abdomen is seen with abdominal carcinomatosis, where the mechanism of pain production is believed to be increased prophyrins from neoplastic enzyme induction.

Lactose intolerance is being increasingly recognized as producing a syndrome of abdominal cramps, bloating, and occasional explosive diarrhea, which may be confused with serious intraabdominal disease. It is caused by a lack of the enzyme lactase normally present in the intestine. This enzyme decreases after the age of 5 in the *majority of the world's population* except for persons of northern or central European ancestry, in whom the incidence is lower. Symptoms of this disorder are related to lactose ingestion in the lactase-deficient patient, but why symptoms are sporadic in some people and severe in others

is not known at this time. Lactose is not only present in dairy products, but also in a wide variety of nondairy foods such as breads and cakes, puddings, mayonnaise, some canned meats, weight reduction formulas, and as fillers in certain pills. Diagnosis of the condition is made by a demonstrated elevation in expired hydrogen (from bacterial fermentation of malabsorbed lactose) and correlates well with intestinal lactase activity in mucosal biopsy specimens. The advantage of the hydrogen breath test is its simplicity, ease of repetition, and noninvasiveness.

Treatment of the disease centers around limiting ingestion of lactose-containing foodstuffs, which may be difficult because of dietary dependence on dairy products for intake of calcium, protein, minerals, and vitamins. Strategies to lessen symptoms include increasing the total caloric density and fat content of the diet, substituting foods that do not contain lactose, and using exogenous lactase.

Collagen Diseases. The collagen diseases comprise the group of genetically determined as well as acquired connective tissue disorders believed to be attributable to an autoimmune process. *Although they are surgical masqueraders, complications as described here may demand operation, such as for ischemic small bowel.*

Rheumatoid arthritis, although characterized primarily by diarthrodial joint inflammation, has serious extraarticular features, the most damaging of which is a systemic necrotizing arteritis. This vasculitis can produce abdominal pain when it involves mesenteric vessels, and local ischemia may produce lesions to be treated operatively. The evaluation of abdominal pain in rheumatoid arthritis patients with high titers of rheumatoid factor should suggest this possible cause.

Systemic lupus erythematosus (SLE) is a chronic inflammatory disease with varied manifestations, one of which may be abdominal pain. Such symptoms result from acute intra-abdominal arteritis and organ ischemia. The diagnosis is suggested by the clinical constellation identifying SLE and confirmed by a positive LE cell test, plus a positive assay result for antinuclear antibody.

Scleroderma is also a progressive autoimmune process that when its sclerosis involves the small intestine, can produce abdominal symptoms from either microorganism overgrowth or ischemic vasculitis. Amyloidosis causes abdominal pain by similar mechanisms.

Periarteritis nodosa is a form of necrotizing arteritis that involves the medium-sized muscular arteries by autoimmune process. Abdominal pain is seen if intra-abdominal organ blood supply is affected, and operation may be required for irreversible ischemic changes. Biopsy of involved arteries is diagnostic.

Schönlein-Henoch purpura is a form of allergic hypersensitivity angiitis involving capillaries and small arterioles, which tends to develop within 14 days of an infective process. Abdominal symptoms are caused by nonthrombocytopenic purpuric intestinal lesions, and intussusception may occur. It is accompanied by cutaneous purpura, joint symptoms, and renal involvement, all of which are reversible. In the absence of purpura, this disease is easily confused with acute rheumatic fever.

Giant cell arteritis and *temporal arteritis* are variants of another form of inflammatory arteritis that may occasionally cause abdominal pain.

Dermatomyositis is a diffuse inflammatory disorder of striated muscles of the pectoral girdle and neck that is reported to cause abdominal pain. *It is important to remember that, of patients whose first symptoms began when they were over 40 years of age, 50% will develop malignancies, and abdominal pain may be the first sign of neoplasm.*

Periodic disease is a variety of disorders of unknown cause, characterized by recurrent disease of unusual punctuality over many years in otherwise healthy people.

The hallmark of *familial Mediterranean fever* is abdominal pain from a nonspecific intestinal serositis. The episodes are characterized by chills and high fevers, with severe abdominal pain, often with localized or rebound tenderness and involuntary guarding, rigidity, distension, and diminished bowel sounds. Of these patients, 75% develop pleuritic pain with effusion and friction rubs. Other manifestations include hepatomegaly, splenomegaly, arthralgia, and skin lesions. Laboratory studies reveal neutrophilia of 15,000 to 30,000, elevated erythrocyte sedimentation rate, and elevated serum haptoglobins,

ceruloplasmin, C-reactive protein, serum cholesterol, and triglycerides during attacks. Differentiation from surgical diseases is often impossible.

Hemolytic Diseases. Severe abdominal pain mimicking surgical conditions may be a manifestation of hemolytic crises. This abdominal pain may be colicky or aching in character and presents as a part of the syndrome of fever, chills, malaise, and extremity or back pain, and often an associated hemoglobinuria. Malaria should also be considered when such symptoms are present.

Sickle cell crises are accompanied by abdominal symptoms in 40% of episodes and may mimic perforated peptic ulcers, acute cholecystitis, or appendicitis with right-sided organ involvement or left upper quadrant pain when splenic infarction occurs. They occur in patients with sickle cell anemia, an inherited disorder of the African-American population. Diagnosis is made with the finding of sickle-shaped erythrocytes in the peripheral blood; hemoglobin electrophoresis determines the specific hemoglobinopathy.

Miscellaneous. Peptic ulcer and pancreatitis are known to be caused by hypercalcemia, and consequently the patient with multiple endocrine adenomata or parathyroid adenoma may present with abdominal pain. Pancreatitis may also be caused by primary hyperlipidemias.

Intra-abdominal Hodgkin's disease may be first evidenced by the presence of pain at the site of the lesions when ethanol in any form is ingested.

Severe abdominal pain is a feature of narcotic and barbiturate withdrawal states; in these patients the history may not be offered initially and thus delays diagnosis. Severe vasculitis, sometimes with resultant ischemic injury of visceral organs, is seen in the postoperative patient after correction of coarctation of the aorta. This condition may suggest mesenteric embolism if it is not recognized and systemic blood pressures are not controlled.

PITFALLS AND COMMON MYTHS

- Sometimes, even with maximal utilization of support services and with consummate clinical skill, definitive diagnosis will be unclear initially. In certain of these instances, an experienced and thoughtful surgeon may, on clinical grounds alone, make the decision to operate.

- Careful attention to a detailed history and physical examination most often provides the clues to differentiating the pain of surgical masqueraders from that of diseases that require operative intervention.
- Accurate diagnosis is the basis of appropriate medical or surgical therapy.

BIBLIOGRAPHY

Chutani HK. Intestinal tuberculosis. In Cord WI, Creamer B (eds). Modern Trends in Gastroenterology, 4th ed. London, Butterworths, 1970, p 309.

Cream JS, Gumpel JM, Peachy RDG. Schönlein-Henoch purpura in adults. A study of 77 adults with anaphylactoid of Schönlein-Henoch purpura. Q J Med 39:461, 1970.

Drossman DA. Patients with psychogenic abdominal pain: Six-years' observation in the medical setting. Am J Psychiatry 139:1549, 1982.

Gallegos NC, Hobsley M. Abdominal wall pain: An alternative diagnosis. Br J Surg 77:1167, 1990.

Galler JR, Neustein S, Walker WA. Clinical aspects of recurrent abdominal pain in children. Adv Pediatr 27:31, 1980.

Hanid MA, Levi AJ. Medical causes of pain in the lower abdomen. Clin Obstet Gynecol 8:15, 1981.

Hopper KD, Smazal SF Jr, Ghaed N. CT and ultrasonic evaluation of rectus sheath hematoma: A complication of anticoagulant therapy. Milit Med 148:447, 1983.

Jooma R, Torrens MJ, et al. Spinal disease presenting as acute abdominal pain: Report of two cases. Br Med J 287:117, 1983.

Jorgenson LS, Fossgreen J. Back pain and spinal pathology in patients with functional upper abdominal pain. Scand J Gastroenterol 25:1235, 1990.

Kudsk KA, Tranbaugh RF, Sheldon GF. Acute surgical illness in patients with sickle cell anemia. Am J Surg 142:113, 1981.

Lea AS, Feliciano DV, Gentry LO. Intra-abdominal infections. An update. J Antimicrob Chemother 9(suppl A):107, 1982.

Lee MG. Abdominal pain in sickle cell anemia. Trop Doct 19:177, 1989.

Leguit P Jr, Slot H, Roos C. The acute abdomen in heroin addiction. Br J Surg 69:598, 1982.

Mitchell WG, Greenwood RS, Messenheimer JA. Abdominal epilepsy: Cyclic vomiting as the major symptom of simple partial seizures. Arch Neurol 40:251, 1983.

Montes RG, Perman JA. Lactose intolerance. Postgrad Med 89:175, 1991.

Pattison CW, Haynes IG. Acute intermittent porphyria: A nonsurgical cause of abdominal pain. Br J Surg 69:553, 1982.

Prouse PJ, Thompson EM, Gumpel JM. Systemic lupus erythematosis and abdominal pain. Br J Rheumatol 22:172, 1983.

Reynolds M, Sherman JO, Malone PG. Ventriculoperitoneal shunt infection masquerading as an acute surgical abdomen. J Pediatr Surg 18:951, 1983.

Santoro G, Curzio M, Venco A. Abdominal migraine in adults: Case reports. Funct Neurol 5:61, 1990.

Shepherd HA, Patel C, et al. Upper gastrointestinal endoscopy in systemic vasculitis presenting as an acute abdomen. Endoscopy 15:307, 1983.

Slocum JC. Chronic somatic, myofascial, and neurogenic abdominal pelvic pain. Clin Obstet Gynecol 33:145, 1990.

Wenham PW. Viral and bacterial associations of acute abdominal pain in children. Br J Clin Pract 36:321, 1982.

Zizic TM, Classen JN, Stevens MB. Acute abdominal complications of systemic lupus erythematous and polyarteritis nodosa. Am J Med 73:525, 1982.

CHAPTER REVIEW
Questions

1. How may abdominal pain attributable to heavy metal poisoning be differentiated from the abdominal pain of collagen diseases?
   a. Prompt surgical intervention
   b. Observation and hemoglobin electrophoresis
   c. Selective arteriography
   d. History and physical examination

2. True or false: Operative intervention is never indicated for the acute abdominal pain seen with the collagenoses.
   a. True
   b. False

3. List five extraperitoneal structures that can give rise to referred abdominal pain.

4. Two weeks after an acute myocardial infarction a patient develops acute abdominal pain. List two conditions that may cause this that do not require operation.

5. Describe Carnett's test.

6. What condition is diagnosed by use of the hydrogen breath test?

Answers

1. d
2. b. Frank ischemia from severe vasculitis may produce surgical complications in many of the collagenoses.
3. Intercostal nerve, lung, heart, kidney, testicle
4. Constrictive pericarditis, embolization to a solid organ, pulmonary infarction, heart failure with pulmonary effusion
5. Tensing of rectus muscles causes pain in abdominal wall disease—may relieve pain from abdominal viscera.
6. Lactose intolerance

32 The Ischemic Lower Extremity

RICHARD H. DEAN

KEY FEATURES

After reading this chapter you will understand:
- That a careful clinical evaluation can often pinpoint the problem.
- How knowing the value of invasive and noninvasive tests will improve critical evaluations.
- The strategies for treatment of limb ischemia.

Arterial occlusive disease affecting the lower extremity may either produce no clinical sequelae, cause annoying or disabling claudication, or create such severe ischemia that the limb's viability is threatened. The clinical importance of such occlusive disease depends on the quantity of affected tissue mass and the adequacy of alternate or collateral pathways of arterial inflow to the tissue bed. Similarly, a range of diagnostic studies and therapeutic modalities is available from which appropriate evaluation and management can be chosen. Integration of the clinical importance of the arterial lesion—or its morbidity—with the complexity of the required management is critical to proper decision-making. In this manner the risk of the disease can be compared with the risk and benefit of the treatment options, and the most appropriate plan of management can be determined. To arrive at accurate conclusions and properly treat patients with lower-extremity ischemia, the range of symptoms and physical findings of lower-extremity ischemia and the diagnostic tests most useful for establishing a proper treatment plan must be understood.

WHAT ARE THE SYMPTOMS OF LIMB ISCHEMIA?

In the vast majority of patients, a carefully performed medical history alone can assist the clinician in developing a diagnosis of limb ischemia. Pain is the most common presenting symptom. A clear description of its onset, distribution, and character and the factors that precipitate, aggravate, or relieve it usually will determine or exclude a diagnosis even before the physical examination is performed. For purposes of description, the presenting symptoms are described separately for acute ischemia, chronic ischemia, and rest pain.

Acute Ischemia. Acute limb ischemia, when severe, produces the five *P*'s: pain, pallor, pulselessness, paresthesia, and paralysis. Acute ischemia can be caused either by an embolus or acute thrombosis. The distinct clinical pictures of acute ischemia that differentiate an embolus from a thrombosis are summarized in Table 32-1. An embolus produces the most classic symptom complex of severe ischemia, because it frequently lodges in a vessel previously carrying a relatively normal flow; thus no collateral pathways had been established previously. In this circumstance the patient usually describes a sudden onset of severe "boring" or extreme cramping pain throughout the affected part of the limb, which is rapidly followed by the limb's becoming cool to touch, and pale and losing sensation. The presentation of this entire constellation of symptoms indicates that limb-threatening ischemia is present and that blood flow must be reestablished within only a few hours or the limb will be lost.

TABLE 32-1 Factors Suggesting Embolism Versus Thrombosis

Factor	Embolism	Thrombosis
Identifiable source or risk factor for embolus	Usual, particularly atrial fibrillation or prior history of embolism	Unusual
History of claudication	Rare	Common
Physical findings suggestive of occlusive disease	Few; proximal and contralateral limb pulses normal	Often present; proximal or contralateral limb pulses diminished or absent
Arteriography	Minimal atherosclerosis; sharp cutoff; few collaterals	Diffuse atherosclerosis; tapered, irregular cutoff; well-developed collaterals

On occasion the entire sequence of limb-threatening events does not occur, and the patient may, in retrospect, describe the typical onset of pain and coolness, which then subsided. In this circumstance the limb has developed adequate collateral pathways around the occlusion to interrupt the sequence leading to tissue death, and the patient is seen when symptoms of claudication from chronic ischemia lead to the evaluation.

Chronic Ischemia. Chronic limb ischemia, depending on its severity, produces pain or discomfort only when the patient walks (*claudication*) or ischemic rest pain. Claudication caused by arterial insufficiency is usually characteristic. Depending on the site of arterial occlusion, the pain may be in the buttocks, thigh, calf, or foot (Fig. 32-1). Buttocks and thigh claudication is usually described as an aching pain and fatigue or "weakness" of the affected muscles. The combination of buttocks and thigh claudication, impotence, atrophy of the leg muscles, and diminished or absent femoral pulses is the classic description of terminal aortic occlusion, called the *Leriche syndrome,* which is named after the author of the original complete description of the clinical findings of chronic aortic occlusion. Calf claudication is usually described as a cramping pain in the calf muscles. Foot claudication occurs rarely. In contrast to symptoms in the thigh or calf, chronic foot ischemia usually is described as a coolness, numbness, or paresthesia. The *hallmark* of claudication from arterial insufficiency is that it is absolutely reproducible. Given a reproducible amount of stress or limb use, the patient's symptoms always will be reproduced. Nonarterial causes of pain should be sought when the symptoms vary widely on different occasions. Elderly patients frequently present with the complaint of "night cramps," with the

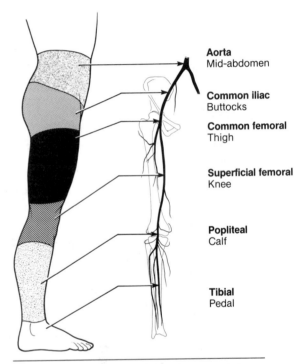

Aorta
Mid-abdomen

Common iliac
Buttocks

Common femoral
Thigh

Superficial femoral
Knee

Popliteal
Calf

Tibial
Pedal

FIGURE 32-1 Site of arterial occlusion and the corresponding site of associated limb ischemia.

presumption that it is caused by "circulation problems." The knowledgeable physician can quickly differentiate this problem from one of a vascular origin. Such night cramps are unrelated to vascular disease and are thought to result from an exaggerated neuromuscular response to stretch.

Rest Pain. Ischemic rest pain when caused by chronic ischemia, is usually limited to the foot. Since the foot is the most distal tissue bed, it is the most ischemic in the presence of proximal arterial occlusive disease. Frequently an elderly debilitated patient will have rest pain in the foot as the presenting symptom. In such circumstances the patient is relatively sedentary and has not been stressing the limb by ambulation. In the absence of such claudication-producing stress, the occlusive disease silently progresses to create an extreme level of limb-threatening ischemia before the patient seeks medical attention. Few sources of pain are as disabling as ischemic rest pain. The patient usually describes it as a "boring, agonizing pain" from which oral analgesics give little relief. Since extreme reductions in perfusion pressure are required to produce rest pain, the effect of gravity may affect the magnitude of the pain. In this circumstance the patient may obtain partial relief from the pain by hanging the foot off the bed or may state that sleeping in a chair is the only way rest can be obtained.

WHAT ARE THE PHYSICAL FINDINGS OF LIMB ISCHEMIA?

Although a thorough medical history may allow rapid confirmation of limb ischemia by physical examination, the physician should perform a complete examination. Unsuspected hypertension, carotid artery disease, cardiac dysrhythmias, and aortic aneurysms are only a few of the important conditions frequently uncovered by the complete "routine" physical examination. In addition, when the ischemia is mild and symptoms are brought on only by prolonged or rapid ambulation, the examiner may find no evidence of vascular disease during a physical examination performed on the resting patient. The arterial lesion may be a moderate stenosis that limits augmented flow only during exercise or may be associated with such rich collateral flow that distal pulses at rest are maintained. For this reason, the clinician should palpate pulses at rest and immediately after reproduction of ambulatory symptoms by exercise. In such a patient with vasculogenic claudication, the pulses will briefly diminish or disappear immediately after exercise.

Palpation of the femoral, popliteal, dorsopedal, and posterior tibial artery pulses and auscultation over the iliac and femoral arteries should be a standard part of the physical examination. Palpation of the femoral pulses may be difficult in an obese patient. To avoid this problem, the examiner should palpate the vessel over the pubicramus of the ilium approximately 3 to 4 cm lateral to the pubic tubercle. Similarly, popliteal pulse palpation may be difficult even for an experienced clinician. Having the patient lie supine and the limb relaxed while the examiner lifts the knee with the proximal portion of both hands cupped under the knee, leaving the fingertips free for gentle palpation in the middle of the popliteal fossa, usually facilitates an accurate examination.

Severe chronic ischemia of the limb may be associated with wasting of the calf muscles, loss of hair growth on the distal aspect of the leg and foot, and atrophy of the skin and subcutaneous tissue. Extreme chronic ischemia of the foot frequently produces a physical appearance best described as the "lobster foot." In such extreme ischemia the foot has cadaveric pallor during elevation and dependent rubor on return to dependency. These findings, called **Buerger's disease,** when combined with the edema of chronic dependency, give the appearance of a lobster's red color. The dependent foot redness is caused by the extreme dermal arteriolar and postcapillary venule dilation associated with extreme ischemia.

Finally, the patient may have skin ulcerations of the ankle or foot or even frank toe gangrene when extreme chronic ischemia is present. A careful history will usually uncover an episode of minor trauma that originally opened the skin in patients with nonhealing ulcers. Similarly, an attempt at cutting the hypertrophic toenails of patients with chronic ischemia is frequently the inciting event that opens the nail bed to bacterial entry and subsequent infection and gangrene. For these reasons, preventive counseling of the patient about protection against trauma and the preferential use of nail files rather than toenail clippers is an important adjunctive measure in treating a patient with extreme foot ischemia.

WHAT ARE THE PITFALLS OF THE HISTORY AND PHYSICAL EXAMINATION?

Several conditions can mimic lower extremity ischemia when approached superficially by an uninformed clinician. Most important among these conditions are neurogenic claudication, venous claudication, and the neuropathy of diabetes.

Neurogenic Claudication. This condition is most commonly caused by stenosis of the lower spinal canal and produces symptoms of leg pain by pressure on the nerve roots. Characteristically, the pain of neurogenic claudication is dermatomal or nerve root in distribution and is described as a paresthesia or numbness. Since assuming an erect posture, not walking per se, increases the lumbar curvature of the spine and increases nerve root compression, the patient can create the symptoms by prolonged standing, without needing to walk. The pain is relieved only by sitting or lying down, not simply by cessation of walking.

Venous Claudication. Like neurogenic claudication, venous claudication may suggest arterial insufficiency on cursory questioning. Since venous claudication is caused by venous hypertension in the lower extremity, the patient will have had a prior history of venous thrombosis and may have associated varicosities. The erect posture initiates the pathophysiology leading to symptoms, and the pain experienced on walking is relieved only by assuming a horizontal posture and leg elevation. Finally, physical examination will usually reveal the lower-leg brawny pigmentation of venous stasis.

Diabetic Neuropathy. The neuropathic pain of *diabetic neuropathy* can at times be confused with symptoms of peripheral vascular disease. The foot pain associated with diabetic neuropathy, however, is usually described as a burning, dysesthetic pain of the plantar surface of the foot and frequently is associated with significant loss of discriminatory sensation. This loss of sensation can lead to unrecognized continuous trauma to pressure points in the foot and breakdown of skin, with formation of a neurotrophic ulcer. This spectrum of clinical problems is commonly referred to as the *diabetic foot.*

WHAT TESTS ARE USEFUL?

Few conditions lend themselves to more accurate diagnosis through use of a complete medical history and physical examination when performed by a knowledgeable physician than does limb ischemia. Nevertheless, refinement in quantifying the magnitude of limb ischemia is available through the use of simple noninvasive tests.

Doppler Ultrasound. The most versatile single such evaluation is provided by use of Doppler ultrasound. Doppler ultrasound is based on the principle that the frequency of an emitted ultrasound beam is shifted when it rebounds from a moving object and that the magnitude of the Doppler shift in frequency is proportionate to the velocity of the moving object (Fig. 32-2). Simple application of this principle to blood vessel examination allows measurement of arterial pressure at respective sites in the extremity and evaluation for the presence of occlusions of the vessel proximal to the site of examination (Fig. 32-3).

Normally lower extremity arterial flow is triphasic, with a rapid upstroke during early systole, a rapid deceleration of velocity during late systole and early diastole, a brief reversal of flow caused by vessel wall elastic rebound during mid-diastole, and then return to a low-velocity forward flow during late diastole. When a proximal occlusion is present, the acceleration and deceleration components have a lower slope, and there is loss of the negative flow component. Through use of these findings, an occlusion can be localized to an arterial segment, and the magnitude of resultant reduction in distal perfusion pressure can be determined (Fig. 32-4). Similarly, resting and postexercise Doppler ultrasound–derived ankle pressures can be used to examine patients with ambulatory symptoms. Exercising muscles induce nutrient vessel vasodilation for augmentation in flow. When there is a fixed amount of flow (F) to the muscle mass caused by a proximal occlusion and exercise induces a reduction in resistance (R), pressure (P) must fall (F = P/R). To perform the exercise test, the patient's ambulatory symptoms are reproduced by exercise. Measurement of the postexercise ankle pressure and demonstration of a drop in pressure when compared to the resting preexercise ankle pressure provides confirmation of the presence of exercise-induced limb ischemia (Fig. 32-5).

The pitfall of using Doppler-derived cuff arterial pressures is that the vessel wall may be noncompliant and may resist external compression by an externally applied cuff. When this is the case, the examiner will not be able to occlude flow through the noncompressible vessel no

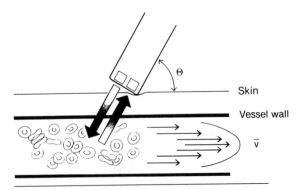

FIGURE 32-2   Schematic representation of the principle of Doppler ultrasound. The shift in frequency of the rebounded beam is proportional to the angle of insonation of the ultrasound beam and the velocity of moving red blood cells from which the ultrasound beam is rebounded.

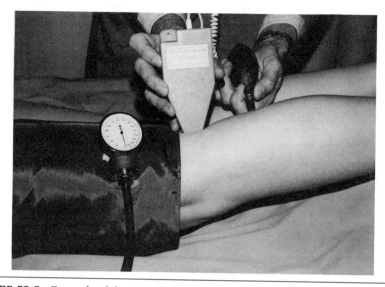

FIGURE 32-3 Example of the use of a handheld Doppler unit in the acquisition of distal thigh arterial pressure. Note that a large cuff is required for thigh pressure measurements. Ankle pressure is similarly obtained with an arm cuff placed just above the ankle and Doppler examination performed over the dorsal pedal or posterior tibial arteries.

FIGURE 32-4 Results of Doppler examination by waveform analysis and acquisition of segmental arterial pressures. Note the triphasic waveform throughout the right limb. In contrast, pulse velocity waveforms obtained over the left femoral and distal vessels are monophasic and have a corresponding drop in arterial pressures at the distal thigh and ankle levels. These findings are consistent with a left iliac artery occlusion.

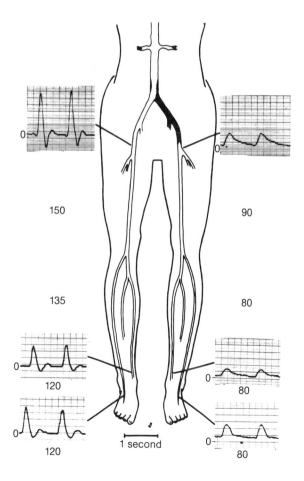

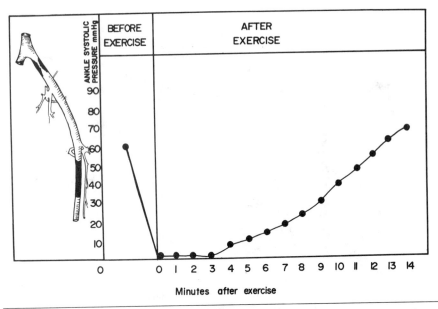

FIGURE 32-5   Graphic display of resting and postexercise ankle pressures in a patient with claudication. The depth of drop in ankle pressure after exercise corresponds to the magnitude of induced ischemia. The duration of time for recovery to preexercise levels is indicative of the magnitude of collateral flow to the involved tissue bed.

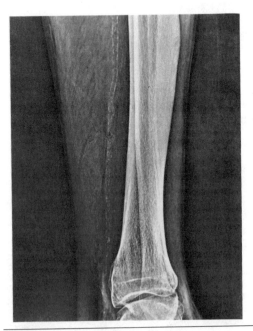

FIGURE 32-6   Xeroradiograph of a diabetic patient with extreme occlusive disease to the extremity. Note the extensive calcifications of the popliteal artery branches. Such vessels are noncompressible with a blood pressure cuff applied to the calf.

matter how high the pressure applied by the cuff. Therefore a very low intra-arterial pressure from very slow-flowing blood may be erroneously recorded as a very high pressure. The clinical situation in which this is common is in the diabetic patient with accelerated calcific atherosclerotic occlusive disease (Fig. 32-6). In this situation the presence of proximal severe occlusive disease is identified by the presence of a monophasic low-velocity pulse waveform. In fact, finding a low-velocity monophasic pulse waveform and a cuff pressure greater than 200 mm Hg is pathognomonic of this variety of diabetic atherosclerotic vascular disease.

Plethysmography. Another method of noninvasive study of pulsatile limb blood flow, plethysmography, measures changes in the volume of the limb throughout the cardiac cycle. To perform the test, a cuff is inflated to either a known pressure or known volume, and pulsatile waveforms are recorded from the cuffs positioned around the thighs, calves, and toes. The resultant changes in volume of the respective cuffs during the cardiac cycle identify the presence or absence of arterial occlusions limiting pulsatile flow at the sites of the respective cuffs.

Arteriography. Arteriography is used as the

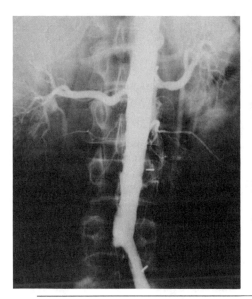
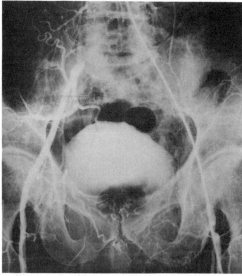

FIGURE 32-7 Arteriogram of the abdominal aorta *(left)* and iliac-femoral segment *(right)* demonstrating a total occlusion of the right common iliac artery. Note the cross-pelvic filling of the distal right common iliac and external iliac arteries.

final diagnostic study in the evaluation of lower-extremity ischemia. The most common technique used for performance of arteriography is the Seldinger technique. In this method the femoral artery is cannulated, and the tip of the catheter is threaded to a position just above the celiac artery. Through multiple injections of contrast media and timed exposure of x-ray films, the entire abdominal aorta, iliac, and femoral arteries and distal vessels are visualized to the feet (Fig. 32-7). In this manner a complete road map of all vessels supplying blood to the lower extremities can be evaluated. The important items of information gained from the arteriogram are the site of the arterial occlusion, the proximal extent of vessel narrowing, and the status of the outflow vessels. The critical issue regarding the status of the outflow vessels is the presence or absence of narrowing or occlusions of the vessels beyond the occlusion. Not only does such "distal disease" limit the likelihood of complete revascularization of the extremity, but it limits the flow through the vascular reconstruction and increases the chances of graft thrombosis during the follow-up period (Fig. 32-8). Arteriography is used to reveal the arterial anatomy to identify the feasibility and most appropriate techniques of revascularization. Alternately stated, arteriography should not be considered a diagnostic study, but instead as a study to plan the strategy of

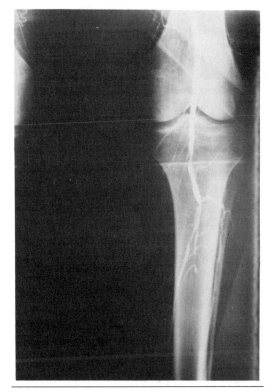

FIGURE 32-8 Leg phase of an arteriogram showing severe occlusive disease in the outflow tract of the popliteal artery.

management. Therefore, unless the patient's symptoms are severe enough to warrant consideration of revascularization, the patient should not be subjected to arteriography.

WHAT ARE THE OPTIONS OF TREATMENT?

Strategies of management of limb ischemia are dependent on the rapidity of onset and the magnitude of ischemia. The options of treatment are more limited when treating acute ischemia. When acute ischemia is total and limb viability is threatened, timely revascularization is imperative. After only 6 to 8 hours of extreme acute ischemia, a limb may not be retrievable; therefore delays in management of acute ischemia must be avoided. The cause of the acute ischemia, whether embolic or thrombotic, is the primary factor that dictates therapy. The techniques that are options for use in treatment of acute ischemia and the factors affecting the choice of therapy for acute ischemia are outlined in Fig. 32-9. Although no perfect algorithm for treatment of all patients is feasible, this outline provides a logical approach to decision-making in patient management.

Certain measures are common to all choices of treatment. The most important of these standard measures is the administration of an anticoagulating dose of intravenous heparin (usually 100 units/kg of body weight) immediately after diagnosing acute ischemia to stop distal propagation of the clot, thereby helping to establish collateral flow around the acute occlusion by maintaining distal vessel patency. Arteriography also is usually a standard part of the management scheme. Nevertheless, if the clinical presentation is classic for a femoral embolus and there are no clinical findings of underlying atherosclerotic occlusive disease, it is appropriate to proceed directly to the operating room for performance of an embolectomy without prior arteriography (Fig. 32-10). When the embolus is not lodged at the femoral artery level and the magnitude of ischemia will allow a delay in revascularization, use of arteriography to localize the embolus and placement of a catheter into the clot for infusion of a thrombolytic agent for 12 to 24 hours may provide revascularization without the need for operation. In most instances, however, the simplicity of embolectomy argues for its preferential use.

When the acute ischemia is from thrombosis rather than embolism, revascularization most commonly requires a standard vascular reconstructive procedure. Depending on the site of occlusion this may require bypass of the occluded aorta-iliac or femoral-popliteal segment.

The treatment of chronic limb ischemia is dictated by the severity of the associated disability and the complexity and site of the occlusive disease (Table 32-2). General considerations such as cessation of smoking and, to the degree feasible, institution of an exercise (walking) program are valuable to essentially all patients. Furthermore, treatment of other risk factors for atherogenesis such as hypertension and hyperlipidemia also is a standard treatment measure. Drug therapy with rheologically active agents (e.g., pentoxifylline) or vasodilators is generally unrewarding. Nevertheless, such agents can be tried in in-

TABLE 32-2   Operations for Treatment of Chronic Lower-Extremity Ischemia

Site of Disease	Procedure Options
Aortic and/or bilateral iliac artery	Aorto-bilateral-femoral bypass Axillo-bilateral-femoral bypass
Unilateral iliac artery stenosis	Percutaneous transluminal angioplasty (PTA) Iliac thromboendarterectomy Femorofemoral bypass Aortofemoral bypass
Profunda femoris artery	Thromboendarterectomy
Superficial femoral or popliteal artery	Femoropopliteal bypass with saphenous vein Femorotibial bypass with saphenous vein

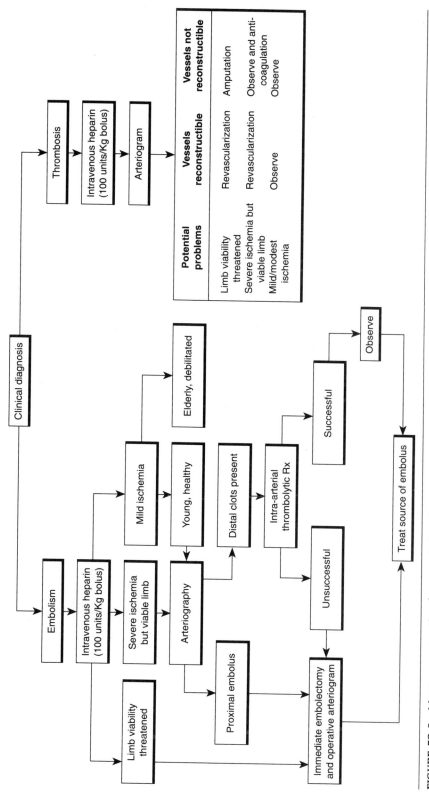

FIGURE 32-9 Management option for acute ischemia.

stances of poor anatomy for reconstruction or borderline indications for intervention or in poor risk patients.

The respective techniques available for revascularization of lower extremity ischemia are summarized in Table 32-2. Results of management are dependent on many variables, including the anatomic location and extent of the disease, the status of the vessels beyond the segment corrected by the intervention, and the type of intervention used for revascularization. (See the reference list for articles that summarize results using the respective modalities.) Some of the principles important in the use of respective techniques are summarized in Figs. 32-10 through 32-13.

CHRONIC LOWER-EXTREMITY ISCHEMIA: FACTORS WEIGHING DECISIONS

	Observation (Medical Treatment)	Intervention (Revascularization)
Severity of symptoms:	Annoying __ Lifestyle-altering __ Disabling __ Limb- or life-threatening ischemia	
Overall life expectancy:	Short ———————————————————— Long	
Risk factors for interventions:	Severe (heart, renal, pulmonary) ——— Absence of risk factors	
Type of intervention required:	Complex ——————————————————— Simple	
Probability of technical success:	Low ———————————————————— High	
Durability of procedure:	Short ——————————————————— Prolonged	

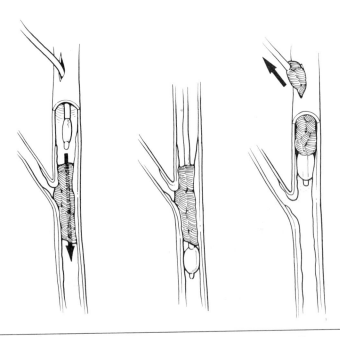

FIGURE 32-10   Balloon embolectomy catheter. Use of this catheter allows exposure of the femoral artery with the patient under local anesthesia and passage of the catheter from this opened vessel to remove the clot from the iliac or distal vessels.

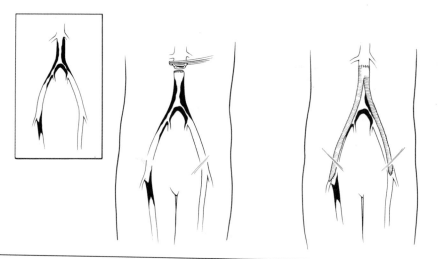

FIGURE 32-11 Placement of an aortofemoral graft to treat aortoiliac occlusive disease. Since the atherosclerotic disease frequently extends up to a level within 2 cm of the renal arteries, the graft should always be attached just below the level of the renal arteries. Likewise, the distal anastomoses should be placed at the bifurcation of the common femoral artery.

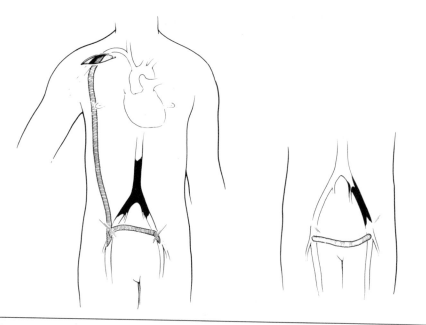

FIGURE 32-12 "Extra-anatomic" grafting techniques to manage aortic or iliac occlusive disease without needing direct interventions. The axillofemoral graft is used when neither iliac artery is suitable as a donor vessel for inflow. The femorofemoral bypass has a durability similar to that of direct reconstructive procedures yet is a procedure that can be performed with the patient under local anesthesia.

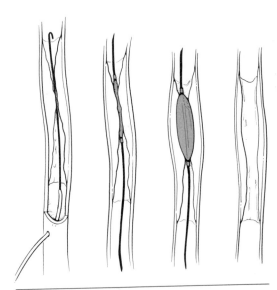

FIGURE 32-13 Use of percutaneous transluminal angioplasty catheter to "dilate" a stenotic vessel. The lesions that are most ideal for use of the balloon angioplasty technique are short (<2 cm) iliac artery stenoses. Although this technique can be used on more distal vessels, the durability of successful balloon angioplasty at these sites is significantly shorter than the results of standard bypass techniques.

In summary, lower-extremity ischemia presents in several characteristic ways. Similarly, there are several methods for interventional management of limb ischemia. Although each modality has advantages in particular circumstances, none of the respective treatment schemes is useful for all instances, and management must be individualized. A surgeon must remember that when revascularizing a limb, he or she is not treating the disease itself but only a side effect of the disease. Therefore the total pa-tient and the general health status must be kept in perspective when recommending complex or new, yet untested, interventional management plans.

BIBLIOGRAPHY

Bergan JJ, Yao JST (eds). Operative Techniques in Vascular Surgery. New York, Grune & Stratton, 1980.

Bernhard VM. Bypass to the popliteal and infrapopliteal arteries. In Rutherford RB (ed). Vascular Surgery. Philadelphia, WB Saunders, 1989, pp 692-704.

Brewster DC. Direct reconstruction for aortoiliac occlusive disease. In Rutherford RB (ed). Vascular Surgery. Philadelphia, WB Saunders, 1989, pp 667-691.

Kumpe DA, Rutherford RB. Percutaneous transluminal angioplasty for lower extremity ischemia. In Rutherford RB (ed). Vascular Surgery. Philadelphia, WB Saunders, 1989, pp 754-763.

Mannick JA, Wittemore AD, Couch NP. Aortoiliac occlusive disease. In Moore W (ed). Vascular Surgery: Comprehensive Review. Orlando, Fla, Grune & Stratton, 1991, pp 350-363.

Perry MO. Acute limb ischemia. In Rutherford RB (ed). Vascular Surgery. Philadelphia, WB Saunders, 1989, pp 541-545.

Quiñones-Baldrich WJ. Thrombolytic therapy for vascular disease. In Moore W (ed). Vascular Surgery: Comprehensive Review. Orlando, Fla, Grune & Stratton, 1991, pp 237-261.

Rutherford RB. The vascular consultation. In Rutherford RB (ed). Vascular Surgery. Philadelphia, WB Saunders, 1989, pp 1-9.

Rutherford RB, Baue AE. Extra-anatomic bypass. In Rutherford RB (ed). Vascular Surgery. Philadelphia, WB Saunders, 1989, pp 705-715.

Taylor LM, Porter JM. Natural history and nonoperative treatment of chronic lower extremity ischemia. In Rutherford RB (ed). Vascular Surgery. Philadelphia, WB Saunders, 1989, pp 653-666.

Veith FJ, Ascer E, Gupta SK, et al. Femoral-popliteal-tibial occlusive disease. In Moore W (ed). Vascular Surgery: Comprehensive Review. Orlando, Fla, Grune & Stratton, 1991, pp 364-389.

CHAPTER REVIEW
Questions

1. The Leriche syndrome includes:
   a. Claudication of the thighs and buttocks
   b. Diminished femoral pulses
   c. Impotence
   d. Atrophy of the leg muscles
   e. All of the above

2. Patients with aortoiliac occlusive disease without associated femoropopliteal disease:
   a. Seldom have resting ischemic pain of the feet
   b. Often have ischemic rest pain in the feet
   c. Seldom have claudication
   d. Often have rubor on dependency
   e. Are usually asymptomatic

3. Percutaneous transluminal angioplasty for peripheral vascular disease:
   a. Yields its best results in patients with segmental iliac artery stenosis
   b. Has long-term success superior to that of aortofemoral bypass
   c. Is contradicted in patients with claudication
   d. Requires general anesthesia
   e. Precludes direct arterial surgery on the same artery(s) in the future

4. True or false: The presence of pedal pulses is evidence of circulation in the foot good enough that a toe amputation for infection is likely to heal.
   a. True
   b. False

5. True or false: The standard arteriogram for femoropopliteal disease should visualize all arteries from the renals to the forefoot.
   a. True
   b. False

6. Risk factors in peripheral arteriosclerosis include (select any or all):
   a. Cigarette smoking
   b. Nervous tension
   c. Hyperlipoproteinemia
   d. Hypertension
   e. Glucose intolerance

7. True or false: The presence of palpable pedal pulses at rest is sufficient evidence to exclude ischemia as a cause of calf claudication.
   a. True
   b. False

8. In the evaluation of lower-extremity ischemia, Doppler ultrasound:
   a. Should only be used in conjunction with arteriography
   b. Helps exclude nonischemic ambulatory symptoms
   c. Decreases the importance or necessity of the nuances of the medical history and physical examination
   d. Provides images of the moving blood and vessel wall
   e. Must be used by a knowledgeable vascular technologist

Answers

1. e
2. a
3. a
4. a
5. a
6. a, c, d, e
7. b
8. b

33 | The Swollen Leg

ANNE E. MISSAVAGE
F. WILLIAM BLAISDELL

KEY FEATURES

After reading this chapter you will understand:
- The pathophysiology of venous disease.
- The distinction between superficial and deep venous thrombosis.
- The criteria for nonoperative or operative management.
- When you should suspect pulmonary embolus, as well as how to diagnose and treat it.
- What preventive measures are important to avoid pulmonary embolus.

Swelling in the legs is usually secondary to an abnormality of the venous or lymphatic system as a result of trauma, involvement of these structures by some primary disease process, a congenital abnormality, or stasis resulting from impaired cardiac function. The underlying process in such disorders often is overloading of the venous or lymphatic system. Subsequent fluid transudation into the tissues occurs, causing tenderness and swelling, the two most common complaints of patients so afflicted.

Unilateral swelling is commonly caused by disease or obstruction of the veins or lymphatics supplying the involved extremity. Bilateral swelling may be secondary to the same diseases or may represent merely one component of a generalized edema (i.e., from hypoproteinemia, fluid overload, congestive heart failure, or excessive sodium retention) (Table 33-1).

DISEASES OF THE VEINS
What Is Thrombophlebitis?

Thrombophlebitis is an obstructive clot in the major (that is, named) veins of the body. Whether thrombosis occurs before inflammation (phlebothrombosis) or inflammation precipitates the thrombus (thrombophlebitis), a relative obstruction to the flow of blood is the result. Stasis, hypercoagulability, and injury to the vein intima were identified by Virchow as the most important etiologic factors for the development of thrombophlebitis. Clinically, advanced age, malignancy, sepsis, cardiovascular disease, major operations or trauma (particularly orthopedic), and immobility all predispose an individual to thrombophlebitis.

The severity of the symptoms is usually governed by the individual veins involved. Superficial veins are not primary channels for the return of blood to the heart. The deep veins, on the other hand, do serve as the principal means for afferent venous flow, because the strategically situated valves allow only unidirectional or centripetal propulsion of venous blood whenever the compressive force of contracting adjacent muscles is applied to the vein walls. Communicating veins, with similar unidirectional valves, connect the superficial system to the deep venous channels, with flow normally permitted only from the subcutaneous veins down into the subfascial deep venous system.

Superficial Thrombophlebitis. Superficial thrombophlebitis is limited to the subcutaneous veins; it most commonly follows intravenous infusions into veins of the arms and legs. With saphenous or any other superficial vein involvement, leg swelling is absent or so minimal it is difficult to detect. There is pain, tenderness, erythema, and induration along the course of the vessel. Because there are many collateral venous channels and because the superficial system is not primarily responsible for venous return, functional impairment is limited except for that caused by tenderness alone.

Deep Thrombophlebitis. Deep thrombophlebitis is clotting that involves the subfascial main channels of the arm or leg. Femoral, iliac, vena cava, or axillary veins produce the most severe symptoms; the involved limb is swollen and engorged with blood because of proximal obstruction to venous return. *Phlegmasia alba dolens* is the usual syndrome that follows major obstruction to venous flow in large proximal veins with phlebitis. The near-complete occlusion causes increased venous and capillary pressure, which eventually leads to extravasation of fluid into the extravascular spaces. Pitting edema then becomes pronounced, accounting for the pale appearance of these limbs. Severe edema results in compression and compromise of capillary flow in the deep fascial compartments; reflex arterial spasm also results. Such a clinical picture is referred to as *phlegmasia cerulea dolens,* because the extremity assumes a bluish mottled hue from cyanosis. Gangrene of the extremity will then develop unless the venous occlusive process is corrected or the pressure impeding capillary flow is relieved (e.g., by fasciotomy).

The clot that forms in the leg veins begins in valve pockets and propagates into the lumen of the vessel. At this point it may irritate the vein wall and elicit an inflammatory response, which, if circumferential, will obstruct flow. It may remain partially occlusive or not occlusive at all, in which instance it is vulnerable to breaking loose and embolizing systemically. Therefore symptoms are variable, depending on whether the clot elicits an inflammatory response and is obstructive (pain and tenderness along the vein involved and swelling distal) or is loose and nonadherent with little inflammation (no local symptoms; may embolize to produce remote symptoms).

Because clinical examination is unreliable, an objective means of diagnosis (i.e., phlebography or noninvasive techniques) must be used before deciding on treatment. A missed diagnosis of deep venous thrombosis can result in death from pulmonary embolism; an erroneous diagnosis of deep venous thrombosis exposes the patient to the very substantial risks of anticoagulation.

The major complications of thrombophlebitis are pulmonary embolism (early) and chronic venous insufficiency (late). Fatal pulmonary embolism occurred in 5% to 10% of patients with iliofemoral thrombophlebitis before anticoagulant therapy was available.

Diagnosis. The gold standard for the diagnosis of deep vein thrombophlebitis is phlebography. It is accomplished by cannulization of a peripheral hand or foot vein, application of a tourniquet is occlude the superficial venous system and to direct blood flow into the deep system, and the injection of radiopaque contrast medium. The demonstration of a clot outlined by the dye or of a complete obstruction of the main channel (demonstrated by seeing collateral flow around a nonvisual segment of deep vein) is diagnostic.

Because phlebography is invasive, uncontrollable, and risky to the patient, alternative noninvasive assessment has become the initial screening maneuver of choice. The most popular and practical technique is *a duplex scan,* which is a combination of Doppler and B-mode ultrasound techniques. An acute obstructive clot can be diagnosed by simple Doppler techniques alone. When the Doppler probe is placed over a major vein, rushes of flow can be heard with each inspiration of the respiratory cycle. If breath holding or a Valsalva maneuver is done, vein flow will stop temporarily, resuming with a rush when the breath is released. Venous obstruction proximal to the Doppler probe will dampen or obliterate this respiratory variation. If there are abundant collaterals and blood flow around a nonobstructing clot, the Doppler examination may not show obstruction. However, B-mode ultrasound can be combined with the Doppler technique to visualize the compromise of the vein lumen by the thrombus. Duplex scanning, when its result is positive, is sufficient to initiate therapy, and phlebography is reserved for patients with equivocal results.

Treatment. Superficial thrombophlebitis produces symptoms that are not severe and are controlled with nonoperative therapy unless infection is present or the clot propagates into the deep venous system.

In almost all instances in which there has not been a break in the integrity of the skin involved with the phlebitis, the process can be considered sterile. Because the morbidity relates only to the local point tenderness, anti-inflammatory agents such as aspirin or ibuprofen provide both pain relief and control of the inflammatory process. Heat and elevation are indicated if pain and ten-

TABLE 33-1 Differential Diagnosis of Lower-Extremity Swelling

Condition	Findings
Cellulitis	Erythema, fever, leukocytosis, tenderness (diffuse) in involved area
Thrombophlebitis	Positive Homans' sign, tenderness in involved vein, calf tenderness, usually unilateral
Lymphangitis	Red streaking of skin, infected focus, no generalized erythema or deep tenderness, unilateral
Superficial varicose veins	Dilated superficial veins, unilateral or bilateral
Deep venous insufficiency	Dilated superficial veins, pigmentation lower leg, ulceration
Lymphatic obstruction (lymph node blockage)	Palpable nodes, diagnosis of carcinoma or lymphoma, usually unilateral, no inflammation
Arteriovenous fistulae	Unilateral enlargement of extremity, bruit, occlusion produces bradycardia
Congenital lymphedema (Milroy's disease)	Unilateral usually, young adult or adolescent, family history
Cardiac decompensation	Bilateral, pitting edema, pulmonary rales, tender liver, edema elsewhere
Hypoproteinemia	Bilateral, generalized anasarca, underlying disease usually
Fluid overload	Usually in-hospital complication, chronic renal disease with uremia, exogenous fluid load

derness prevent ambulation. Because an embolism would require progression of the clot into the deep venous system, it occurs rarely with superficial thrombophlebitis. If thrombosis of the saphenous vein does progress, interruption at the saphenofemoral junction may be indicated.

Bacterial infection of phlebitic veins may occur and is suspected when the vein has been cannulated and local swelling and erythema overlying the vein are noted. Intravenous antibiotic therapy is initiated with either penicillin or cephalosporins active against the usual isolates of gram-positive cocci (*Streptococcus* and *Staphylococcus aureus*) found on blood culture. Purulent drainage from the overlying skin or increasing inflammation suggests the progression to suppurative thrombophlebitis and dictates vein exploration, with excision of all abnormal specified veins, delayed closure of the wound, and continued antibiotic therapy for 3 to 4 weeks to control proximal bacterial seeding of the superficial or deep veins.

By contrast, deep venous thrombosis is potentially morbid and can lead to lethal complica-

tions should embolism occur. Treatment consists of elevation and immobilization of the involved limb and anticoagulation. Lower-limb elevation requires bed rest in Trendelenburg's position with a 20-degree elevation; upper-limb elevation can be accomplished by hanging slings or pillows to limit swelling and discomfort.

Controversy continues regarding optimal anticoagulation therapy, but because acute thrombosis of deep veins in the pelvis and thigh presents such a major risk for embolism and death, vigorous therapy with relatively high doses of heparin administered by continuous intravenous infusion is recommended. After obtaining baseline laboratory studies (hematocrit, platelet count, prothrombin time, partial thromboplastin time), a bolus of heparin (150 units/kg) should be administered intravenously. A dextrose-water solution containing heparin (100 units/ml [25,000 units/250 ml]) is administered by an infusion pump. For the first 48 hours the rate of infusion should approximate 40 units/kg/hr. The key to adequate dosage is obtaining prompt relief of pain and decreased swelling. The dosage can

Special Tests	Treatment
None (occasionally culture of primary focus)	Bed rest, elevation, heat, antibiotics
Phlebography, Doppler ultrasound, plethysmography	Bed rest, elevation, anticoagulants, thrombectomy if iliac veins involved, fibrinolytic agents
None, culture of primary focus	Bed rest, elevation, heat, antibiotics
Brodie-Trendelenburg test, evaluation of deep system	Elastic stockings, avoidance of pressure (crossing legs), elevation, operation if severe or disfiguring, injection sclerotherapy
Brodie-Trendelenburg test, Doppler examination, phlebography	Same as for superficial varicose veins
Lymphangiography, biopsy of palpable nodes	Excision or radiation of nodes, elastic compression
Arteriography	Excision, angiographic occlusion
Lymphangiography not usually successful (hypoplasia of lymphatics)	Supportive, excisional therapy if severe
Central venous pressure (CVP) (elevation), prolonged circulation time	Cardiac glycosides, diuretics, salt restriction
Serum albumin level (decreased)	Depends on underlying disease, protein repletion
CVP (elevated), careful intake-output record	Fluid restriction

then be reduced to 25 units/kg/hr, provided clinical improvement is maintained. Failure to improve within 12 to 24 hours suggests that the clotting stimulus is exceptionally strong; heparin therefore is increased by increments of 10 units/kg/hr every 24 hours until improvement occurs. Because bleeding complications are related more to platelet abnormalities than to the level of anticoagulation reached, heparin therapy is monitored by measuring platelet counts and hematocrit levels daily. Coagulation tests are obtained to ensure that adequate doses of heparin are given. The reason for the arbitrarily high doses of heparin is because antithrombins that act as heparin cofactors are usually depleted in the patient who is clotting and high doses of heparin are required initially to ensure anticoagulation in the obstructed venous outflow.

Oral anticoagulation therapy with warfarin sodium is begun on the second or third day; the heparin is discontinued when the prothrombin time is prolonged to a twice normal control (INR 2-3). Oral anticoagulation therapy is continued for a minimum of 4 months. The patient may

ambulate when the pain and swelling have resolved. Wearing elastic support stockings to control swelling is recommended for at least 6 months, and beyond that time if swelling persists.

When Is Operative Treatment Indicated? In the presence of contraindications to anticoagulation (i.e., active peptic ulcer, gastrointestinal bleeding, gross hematuria or hemoptysis, intracranial or visceral injury, blood dyscrasias, thrombocytopenia) or if pulmonary embolism occurs despite adequate anticoagulation therapy, providing partial or total interruption of the vena cava is advised. This is now possible because filters are available that can be placed percutaneously. If expertise is not available or the patient requires laparotomy to treat a coexisting condition, operative plication or ligation can be used.

The inferior vena cava optimally is interrupted by ligation just below the renal inflow. It can be partially occluded at this level by a clip (Moretz or Miles) that narrows the cava into a single- or multiple-channeled vessel with a diameter reduced to less than 3 mm. Large clots that embolize from the legs are trapped below the kidneys and thus prevented from reaching the lungs.

Massive deep vein thrombosis with edema and compromise of the arterial blood supply has at times been treated by direct removal of the clot (thrombectomy). With the patient under local anesthesia, the femoral vein is exposed, and a catheter with an inflatable balloon on the tip (Fogarty type) is carefully inserted into the thrombosed vein and is pushed through the soft clot into the inferior vena cava. The balloon is then inflated and withdrawn, removing the obstructing thrombus. The distal veins similarly undergo thrombectomy. This procedure is rarely indicated, because most patients improve with limb elevation and anticoagulation. Use of relaxing fascial incisions (fasciotomy) may be important if arterial compromise is a prominent feature.

An alternative to thrombectomy is the use of fibrinolytic agents, streptokinase or urokinase. Proponents of their use claim that functional results are better because venous valvular damage is prevented. Fibrinolytic agents must be used cautiously, especially in surgical patients, because of the increased risk of bleeding and the possibility that the fragmenting clot will be released into the lungs. For all these techniques, therapy with heparin followed by warfarin anticoagulation should be used, unless directly contraindicated, to prevent recurrent thrombosis or embolism.

PULMONARY EMBOLISM
Cause

Venous thrombosis and pulmonary embolism can occur spontaneously as a result of one of the congenital or acquired clotting disorders (Table 33-1). Injury to a limb and major surgery are common precipitating causes, because the soft tissue damage can release thromboplastins, the immobility of the limbs can result in venous stasis, or direct injury to veins can precipitate thrombosis.

Signs and Symptoms

Like venous thrombosis, pulmonary embolism can be silent or catastrophic. When venous clots that embolize are relatively small, they fragment and are trapped in the microcirculation of the lung where they are generally well handled. The pulmonary arterioles are the "catch traps" of the systemic circulation and dispose of the clot readily because the vessels smaller than 0.5 mm have abundant collaterals. Symptoms, when they occur from clots in the small pulmonary vessels, result from release of inflammatory enzymes that tend to constrict adjacent lung units and decrease ventilation, thereby producing a drop in arterial oxygen saturation. Larger or firm pieces of clot that embolize tend to lodge in major segmental pulmonary vessels and cause obstructive symptoms, pulmonary hypertension, and failure of the right side of the heart. Should obstruction to a segment compromise all collateral flow, pulmonary infarction may occur.

Thus the clinical manifestations of pulmonary embolism vary according to the extent and location of the clot. Commonly there are no or minimal symptoms with very small pulmonary emboli. When the volume of clot is larger, transient tachycardia, dysrhythmias, or decreased arterial oxygen saturation and tachypnea occur until the emboli fragment and thereby occlude less of the pulmonary blood flow. Larger emboli produce significant occlusion of major pulmonary vessels, increase pressure in the right side of the heart, and decrease blood pressure by both impeding blood flow and causing dysrhythmia. Patients with these symptoms become tachypneic and apprehensive. Pulmonary infarction occurring after blood flow has been completely obstructed to a pulmonary segment produces the clinical triad of hemoptysis, pleuritic chest pain, and a wedge-shaped density on x-ray film, with the latter corresponding to the infarcted area's spreading distally to the pleura from the point of obstruction. It is estimated that only one episode in ten of pulmonary embolism is significant enough to be recognized clinically; of those that are recognized, only one in 10 results in pulmonary infarction.

Diagnosis

A chest x-ray film, electrocardiogram (ECG), and arterial blood gas studies should be obtained immediately when pulmonary embolism is suspected. The chest x-ray film typically is clear but may demonstrate unexpected conditions such as pneumonia and pneumothorax that can cause similar symptoms. The ECG will document the nature of the dysrhythmia or myocardial ischemia that may be present or provide evidence of strain on the right side of the heart. Blood gas values usually show a fall in arterial PO_2 when pulmonary embolism is present. The PCO_2 is usually consistent with the patient's ventilation.

Specific diagnostic studies consist of a lung

ventilation-perfusion scan and pulmonary angiography. The former is helpful when it is positive or negative but is indeterminate in approximately 75% of cases. Pulmonary arteriography remains the best test and is the definitive study when the lung scan is ambiguous; but because clots can lyse and disappear rapidly, there may be false-negative results from the studies. Pulmonary angiography documents the degree of residual obstruction and helps guide therapy and establish the prognosis.

Treatment

When the possibility of pulmonary embolism is suspected and there is no contraindication to anticoagulation therapy, a bolus of heparin, 10,000 to 20,000 units, should be administered, with the size of the dose related to the severity of symptoms. At this point, time is bought to sort out the problem, and should pulmonary embolism be ruled out subsequently, the dose can be allowed to wear off. An emergent chest x-ray examination, arterial blood gas studies, and an ECG examination should be done to rule out pneumothorax or myocardial infarction. If shock or hypoxemia is present, an endotracheal tube for ventilation and a Swan-Ganz monitoring catheter to guide cardiovascular resuscitation are placed.

If the diagnosis of pulmonary embolism is likely and other probable causes are ruled out, anticoagulation therapy should be continued. As long as the patient's condition is critical, high doses of heparin should be continued at infusion rates of 3000 to 5000 units per hour, an amount sufficient to maintain the partial thromboplastin time above 150 seconds (normal, 15 to 40 seconds). Hematocrit levels should be monitored every 4 to 6 hours and platelets once daily to evaluate the possibility of bleeding.

If the symptoms are minimal, the patient rapidly improves, the diagnosis is questionable, or the risk of anticoagulation is considered high, the diagnosis should be confirmed by pulmonary angiography. Even though indirect assessment such as pulmonary scanning can be done, not more than 25% of the scans will be diagnostic, and angiography will still be necessary to diagnose the pulmonary embolus. Because the therapy for patients with a pulmonary embolus is prolonged, expensive, and potentially dangerous, confirmation of the diagnosis is required. Unless pulmonary embolus is ruled out, heparin therapy, once started, should be continued until the patient is asymptomatic, at which time he or she can be transferred to oral (warfarin) anticoagulation therapy, which is continued until the patient has resumed normal activity.

Should anticoagulants be contraindicated or should a bleeding complication develop, the percutaneous placement of a caval filter is indicated.

Prevention

Pulmonary embolism is one of the most common causes of preventable hospital deaths. Yet measures to prevent postoperative thromboembolism are not commonly used, mostly because of unfamiliarity with effective preventive measures and concern about potential bleeding complications. Physical methods to prevent postoperative thromboembolic complications include leg elevation, wearing elastic stockings, intermittent pneumatic compression, and early ambulation. Only the latter two, however, have been shown effective. Pharmacologic methods include administering low-dose heparin, oral anticoagulation with vitamin K antagonists (warfarin sodium), and low-molecular-weight dextran. The last is ineffective in high-risk situations but may be useful for patients at lower risk.

All patients may benefit from implementation of noninvasive physical methods to prevent stasis and subsequent deep vein thrombosis when surgery is performed. Intermittent pneumatic compression can be initiated during the surgical procedure to control venous stasis and can be continued in the postoperative period until the patient is ambulatory. Patients with a high risk of deep venous thrombosis (>25%) include those more than 40 years old, those with malignancy, those who are obese, and those who have had lower-extremity surgery. In these patients low-dose heparin therapy to decrease the risk of deep vein thrombosis and pulmonary embolus should be considered in addition to noninvasive maneuvers.

VARICOSE VEINS

Varicose veins (varices) are enlarged and tortuous subcutaneous veins that occur in the lower extremities, primarily as the result of a congenital weakness, because of a relative paucity of valves in the superficial or communicating veins, or as a sequel to deep venous thrombophlebitis and insufficiency. Varices lead to further damage because segmental dilation of a vein renders its valves incompetent when the cusps are no longer capable of coapting across the expanded lumen (Fig. 33-1). A longer column of blood is brought

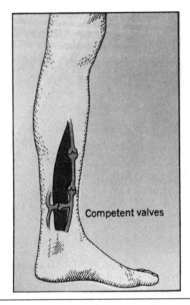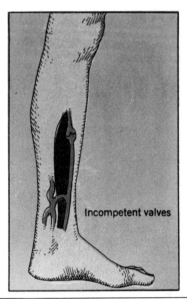

FIGURE 33-1 Perforating veins in the normal and postphlebitic leg.

to rest on the subjacent valve, rendering it similarly incompetent. As this process continues, perforating branches become incompetent and allow blood to flow in reverse direction from the deep to the superficial systems. Only at the points where competency of the perforating veins is maintained can blood be pumped by muscle action from the saphenous system to the deep venous channels and then upward to the heart.

A common complaint is aching and swelling in the legs, especially after long periods of standing. For the most part, however, when venous incompetence is confined to the superficial veins, the primary complaint is cosmetic. Only when superficial venous incompetence results from high pressures in the deep venous system do serious, disabling complications occur.

Diagnosis

A diagnosis of incompetent valves limited to the superficial venous system is made by elevating the patient's leg to empty the veins, applying a tourniquet at the thigh level, and having the patient stand (Brodie-Trendelenburg test). With the tourniquet in place, normally competent veins tend to remain empty and fill gradually from below. If, by a quick removal of the tourniquet, blood does not immediately fill the superficial system below, the response indicates competent valves in the saphenous vein. If there is, instead, a sudden engorgement of the saphenous system on removal of the tourniquet, the saphenous valves are incompetent. Rapid filling of the veins of the superficial system with the tourniquet in place suggests an incompetence of the valves in the perforating veins and the deep venous system. Failure of the varices to empty during rhythmic contraction of leg muscles, such as when the patient is walking, further confirms the abnormal reversal flow in the communicating veins (Perthes' test).

In questionable cases, competence of venous valves can be assessed by using a directional flowmeter.

Treatment

Wearing good-quality elastic stockings to just below the knee is effective in controlling symptoms of aching and swelling caused by superficial venous insufficiency. Full-length stockings are seldom prescribed because the discomfort they cause behind the knees often results in the patients not wearing them. Periodic leg elevation and avoidance of prolonged stationary standing and sitting should be encouraged.

Interruption or complete removal of the incompetent superficial veins is usually beneficial. The saphenous system with its tributaries can be excised by exposing the greater and less saphenous veins at their junctions with the common femoral and popliteal veins, respectively. A wire stripper passed through the vein is forcibly withdrawn from counter incisions at the ankle level, thereby removing the vein in the process.

Smaller incisions are used to ligate and excise communicating tributaries and any incompetent perforating veins. The superficial varicosities increase the load carried by the deep venous system. Although deep vein involvement may be present, excision of these superficial varicosities lightens the burden of this deep system. If stasis ulceration or dermatitis is present secondary to deep venous insufficiency, the perforating veins responsible should also be interrupted. The operative morbidity rate is very low, and results are usually excellent. Nevertheless, patients should be encouraged to wear elastic support hose for the remainder of their lives.

The indications for this operation are severe symptoms of aching, edema, or superficial infection or a cosmetic appearance that is psychologically disturbing to the patient. Because the saphenous vein is used frequently for bypass of atherosclerotic peripheral or cardiac lesions, its early and unjustified removal is discouraged.

Injection sclerotherapy, an alternative to vein stripping, is gaining popularity in the United States. Both major and minor varicosities ("spider" veins) can be satisfactorily treated at considerably savings in cost compared to that for surgery. Multiple injections of a sclerosant solution (sodium tetradecyl sulfate) produce a localized phlebitis that, with repeated injections, ultimately leads to obliteration of the vein segments. Leg compression with elastic bandages for several days after the sclerosant injections is essential for satisfactory long-term results.

DEEP VENOUS INSUFFICIENCY

Incompetence of the deep and perforating veins occurs almost exclusively as a sequela of deep venous thrombosis (postphlebitic syndrome) (Fig. 33-2). The valvular incompetence that follows vein thrombosis alters venous hemodynamics, and the normal reduction of venous pressure with calf muscle contraction does not occur. This persistently elevated pressure is transmitted to capillaries in the subcutaneous tissue and skin in the most dependent nonsupported portion of the limb, usually around the ankle. The capillaries become abnormally permeable and allow extravasation of red blood cells and plasma products. A filtration edema occurs that eventually induces induration and fibrosis of skin and subcutaneous tissue. The damage to the skin and subcutaneous tissue causes a further increase in pressure in small vessels, causing reduced nutritional blood flow. The skin atrophies, and an ulcer may develop spontaneously or may be induced by minor skin trauma (Fig. 33-3).

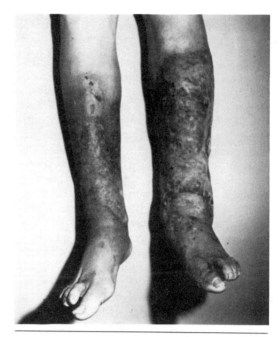

FIGURE 33-2   Chronic stasis dermatitis that has resulted from the chronic leakage of blood and plasma into the subcutaneous tissue.

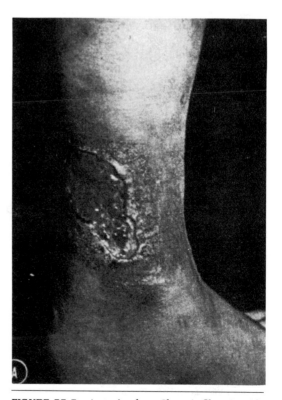

FIGURE 33-3   A stasis ulcer. Chronic fibrosis with progressive scar formation leads to devascularization and ulceration.

Distinguishing Deep Venous Insufficiency From Varicose Veins

Simple varicose veins are not associated with the same high pressures as those associated with deep venous insufficiency. The former has maximal hydrostatic pressure equal to the distance from groin to ankle, whereas deep venous insufficiency is associated with pressure equal to the distance from heart to ankle, to which can be added the force of skeletal muscle compression. Even though direct pressure measurement can be done in a superficial vein in the foot or ankle as previously described, the Brodie-Trendelenburg test can document that the superficial veins are filling from the deep system (rapid engorgement of the superficial veins with the thigh tourniquet in place when the limb is made dependent). Ascending phlebography can distinguish between deep venous obstruction with blood flow through collaterals or patency with lack of valvular function. Dye is injected in a superficial foot vein with an ankle tourniquet in place to ensure the dye enters the deep system.

Treatment

Nonoperative therapy is directed at counteracting and reducing the sustained venous hypertension. This is done by providing good-quality elastic stockings and encouraging leg elevation whenever possible. If an ulcer is present, local care consists of frequent dressing changes or compressive paste dressings (Unna-type boot) if the ulcer is clean and local débridement if the ulcer is heavily contaminated. Systemic antibiotics are used if cellulitis is present. Use of topical ointments is avoided. If edema is marked, diuretics are prescribed.

Operative therapy is indicated if symptoms are not controlled by these conservative measures. Ulcer excision with skin grafting is often the initial procedure. However, our experience indicates that ulceration will recur unless the underlying perforating veins are interrupted. This can be accomplished locally by wide excision of the ulcer to the fascia. It can be accomplished by ligation and stripping of varicose veins, if present, and by extensive subfascial ligation of the incompetent perforating veins. Newer operations are directed at correcting valvular incompetence by venous transposition, valve repair, or transplantation of valve-bearing segments of arm veins. Elastic compression and leg elevation are continued indefinitely, even after operative correction.

ARTERIOVENOUS MALFORMATION
What Is the Role of Arteriovenous Fistulas?

Arteriovenous fistulas are an uncommon cause of swollen legs that may be congenital or acquired. Congenital fistulas represent development anomalies and are present from birth. They range in complexity from single "birthmarks" to complex vascular anomalies (Klippel-Trenaunay syndrome), with various degrees of venous involvement. Acquired arteriovenous fistulas usually result from a penetrating injury to an adjacent artery and vein and generally consist of one abnormal connection. Associated false aneurysms are common.

Signs of chronic venous insufficiency with edema, engorgement of tortuous dilated superficial veins, and occasionally ulceration may develop in either congenital or acquired cases. In congenital cases the involved extremity may be longer than the other. This occurs in children in whom the enhanced bone and muscle growth is due to abnormally brisk extremity blood flow.

Treatment

Arteriography is essential in planning optimal therapy. For a traumatic arteriovenous fistula, a direct approach with division of the fistula and repair of the artery and vein is preferred. For congenital cases, operative therapy is generally less satisfactory. Some relief can be obtained by selective angiographic embolization of arterial branches leading to the fistula. Because it is seldom possible to remove each of the innumerable small abnormal vessels, lifelong treatment with elastic support is necessary.

LYMPHATIC ABNORMALITIES
What Diseases of the Lymphatic System Cause Swelling?

Flow of lymph depends on respiratory movements, muscular contractions, transmitted movements from arterial pulsations, and to some extent, gravity. Water and electrolytes can readily leave and enter capillaries and lymphatics. Protein can exit but cannot reenter these channels. If lymphatic obstruction occurs, local extracellular fluid will gradually assume a high protein content, thereby increasing its oncotic pressure and, accordingly, attracting more water. The result is swelling of the extremity. Because lymphatics are abundant in the dermis, the edema of lymphatic obstruction is prominently manifest in the skin. The skin is pale and thickened with pitting (peau d'orange) changes related to prominence of glandular openings in the edematous skin. Long periods of sitting in a chair can also produce swelling caused by compression of lymphatic channels in apparently normal individuals.

Acute Lymphangitis

Infected areas of the leg routinely permit bacteria to pass into and along lymphatic channels. The resulting lymphangitis is associated with dilation of the small blood vessels along the lymphatics. Redness and tenderness along these channels can easily be seen and at one time were referred to as "blood poisoning."

Differentiation of lymphangitis, cellulitis, and thrombophlebitis should be made early because the treatment for each is varied.

Treatment

Immobilization of the extremity and the administration of an appropriate antibiotic (penicillin, penicillin analog, or cephalosporin) usually controls the infection, which usually is due to *Streptococcus* and/or *S. aureus*. In addition, therapy must also address the primary focus of the infec-

tion, be it a leg ulcer or some other suppurative area.

Bed rest and elevation of the extremity are helpful adjuncts. Mild heat increases vascular dilation and promotes healing and is generally delivered by electric heating pads.

What Causes Lymphatic Obstruction?

The cause of chronic lymphatic obstruction can be primary and congenital (Milroy's disease) or secondary to neoplasm, scar, surgical removal of lymph nodes, or lymphangitis from filariasis, lymphogranuloma venereum, or repeated streptococcal infections that can result in widespread obstruction to the lymphatic drainage of the extremity. Massive edema and limb enlargement may reach major proportions (i.e., elephantiasis).

Treatment

Conservative measures include leg elevation and application of pressure on the extremity by elastic stockings or pneumatic compression. Infections should be treated with an appropriate antibiotic. In patients with massive edema and swelling surgical excision of skin and subcutaneous tissue has been tried, as have attempts to drain the leg by insertion of an omental pedicle graft to serve as a wick. In general, these procedures have not been as satisfactory as the staged excision of all involved subcutaneous tissues.

SURGICAL PHARMACOPEIA

Drug	Indications	Dosage
Heparin	DVT prophylaxis	5000 units subcutaneously bid
Heparin*	DVT/PE (Missavage/Blaisdell therapy)	Bolus: 150 units/kg IV (higher for PE) First 48 hr: 40 units/kg/hr Thereafter: 25 units/kg/hr
Warfarin†	DVT/PE	5 mg PO first day (higher initial dose may be inadvisable because of protein C inactivation)
Urokinase, streptokinase, and tissue plasminogen activator	Controversial	Vary too widely to recommend

*The partial thromboplastin time should be serially measured and kept between 2 and 2½ times the control. Platelet counts should also be monitored, since heparin-induced antibody formation is a recognized complication.
†The prothrombin time should be followed and kept approximately twice normal.

BIBLIOGRAPHY

Blaisdell FW. Acquired and congenital clotting syndromes. World J Surg 14:664, 1990.

Browse NL, Stewart G. Lymphoedema: Pathophysiology and classification. J Cardiovasc Surg 26:91, 1985.

Consensus Conference on Prevention of Venous Thrombosis and Pulmonary Embolism. JAMA 256: 744, 1986.

Criado E, Johnson G. Venous disease. Curr Probl Surg 5:339, 1991.

Dale WA. The swollen leg. Curr Probl Surg 9:3, 1973.

DeWeese JA. Venous and lymphatic diseases. In Schwartz SI, Shires GT, et al. (eds). Principles of Surgery, 4th ed. New York, McGraw-Hill, 1984, p 975.

Gloviczki P, Merrill SW, Bower TC. Femoral vein valve repair under direct vision without venotomy: A modified technique with angioscopy. J Vasc Surg 14:645, 1991.

Greenfield LJ. Results of a multicenter study of the modified hook-titanium Greenfield filter. J Vasc Surg 14:253, 1991.

Hanrahan LM, Araki CT, Rodriguez AA. Distribution of valvular incompetence in patients with venous stasis ulceration. J Vasc Surg 13:805, 1991.

Hobbs JT (ed). The Treatment of Venous Disorders. Philadelphia, JB Lippincott, 1977.

LePage PA, Villavicencio JL, Gomez ER. The valvular anatomy of the iliac venous system and its clinical implications. J Vasc Surg 14:678, 1991.

Nicolaides AN, Sumner DS. Investigation of Patients With Deep Vein Thrombosis and Chronic Venous Insufficiency. Los Angeles, Med Orion, 1971.

(PIUPED). Investigators value of the ventilation/perfusion scan in acute pulmonary embolism: The prospective investigation of pulmonary embolism diagnosis. JAMA 263, 1990, p 2753.

CHAPTER REVIEW
Questions

1. The three most important predisposing factors for thrombophlebitis are:
   a. Hypocoagulability, abnormal vein, and trauma.
   b. Hypercoagulability, stasis, and endothelial injury.
   c. Stasis, arteriovenous (AV) fistula, and congenitally abnormal vein.

2. Varicose veins can be caused by:
   a. Incompetent valves in the superficial system.
   b. Thrombophlebitis in the deep system.
   c. Either of the above.

3. Vena caval ligation is indicated after:
   a. Small pulmonary embolus to right lower lobe.
   b. Major pelvic trauma.
   c. Massive pulmonary embolism in the patient who cannot be given anticoagulant therapy.

4. Deep vein thrombophlebitis is:
   a. Usually treated with 2 weeks of bed rest and heparin.
   b. Rarely associated with pulmonary embolism.
   c. Treated by early ambulation with elastic stockings.
   d. Usually treated with relatively long-term anticoagulation therapy.
   e. Treated by inferior vena caval ligation.

5. Varicose veins:
   a. Should be operated on when diagnosed to avoid embolization.
   b. Usually result in deep thrombophlebitis.
   c. Are due to incompetent perforating veins.
   d. Should be operated on only for severe symptoms or compelling cosmetic reasons.
   e. Should not be removed because they can be used for bypass surgery.

6. Lymphangitis is best treated by:
   a. Antibiotics, immobilization, and elevation.
   b. Hot soaks.
   c. Early motion.
   d. Occlusive dressings.
   e. Drainage.

7. Congenital AV fistulas may be associated with:
   a. Retardation of growth of the involved extremity.
   b. Early epiphyseal closure.
   c. A longer extremity on the involved side.
   d. All of the above.

8. Pulmonary embolism can result in:
   a. Transient dysrhythmias.
   b. Fall in arterial PO_2.
   c. Hemoptysis.
   d. All of the above.
   e. a and b above.

Answers

1. b	5. d
2. c	6. a
3. c	7. c
4. d	8. d

34 Skin and Soft Tissue Lesions

CHARLES M. BALCH
HIRAM C. POLK, Jr.

KEY FEATURES

After reading this chapter you will understand:
- The indications for biopsy of lesions in this location.
- The description of common benign lesions of the skin.
- The management of skin cancers.
- Diagnosis and treatment of melanoma.
- Soft tissue lesions, including sarcoma.

Physicians are asked frequently to render judgments about the clinical significance of various skin and soft tissue lesions. Although the patient's history in regard to the specific lesion in question may play some role in establishing a clinical diagnosis, the details of physical examination and, in selected instances, some form of surgical biopsy more often provide the needed information. Subsequent operative removal of the lesion is usually the optimal primary therapy. The surgeon should know both the appropriate margins to use when excising the various benign and malignant lesions discussed below and the indications for deploying multidisciplinary cancer care when appropriate.

TO BIOPSY OR NOT?

The principles of the diagnosis and subsequent management of skin and soft tissue abnormali-

ties are fairly simple and straightforward. Although most skin lesions and soft tissue masses are benign, the possibility of a malignant process must always be considered in the differential diagnosis. Most skin lesions or soft tissue masses can be diagnosed as malignant or benign on the basis of their characteristics on physical examination. On occasion, however, the decision is equivocal whether the observer is an experienced clinician or a neophyte. In such instances some form of biopsy is appropriate for clarification, but the type of biopsy varies considerably, depending on the size and location of the lesion in question.

There are three key principles relating to the biopsy. First, the surgeon should not undertreat or overtreat the problem before an accurate diagnosis is established. Second, under no circumstances should the chance for an ultimately appropriate treatment be compromised by the biopsy approach if the lesion is not malignant. It is also important to avoid a disfiguring excisional procedure because of a "suspicion" of a malignant process. Third, all removed tissue, even that from a cosmetic excision, must be sent for formal pathologic examination and histologic study.

Performing a small incisional biopsy to establish a diagnosis is usually the first step for all skin and soft tissue lesions unless the lesion is small enough that total excision is possible without jeopardizing possible subsequent therapy if malignancy is proved later. In some instances obtaining cultures of bacteria and fungi is an appropriate initial step or part of the biopsy procedure. Direct consultation with the surgical pathologist examining the biopsy specimen is another vital aspect of the decision-making process to determine the future management of the individual patient. Consideration must be given to special procedures that may be necessary, and the tissue may need appropriate processing for electron microscopy or immunohistochemical stains, both of which require special fixation.

An effort to "stage" the neoplastic process, if it is a malignant one, will assist in developing a meaningful prognosis for the patient and in identifying the most appropriate treatment strategy from a range of treatment options. Staging usually is determined by physical examination, laboratory and radiologic evaluations, and pathologic information. Since the details of this entire diagnostic process differ somewhat with the various skin and soft tissue lesions, the assessment of problems in these two general anatomic sites is discussed separately.

BENIGN SKIN LESIONS

Most localized, solitary skin lesions are benign, and many can be identified clearly as benign processes without proceeding with either incisional or excisional biopsy. However, most skin lesions brought to the physician's attention by a patient will have undergone some discernible, possibly subtle change for the patient to have noticed the problem. This history of a change in the appearance of a skin lesion is usually an indication for a diagnostic biopsy, even when the clinical presentation strongly suggests a clinically insignificant problem.

The presentation may be that of a surface lesion or a lesion that seems to arise in the dermis or superficial subcutaneous tissues. Common epidermal surface lesions include warts (verruca vulgaris), moles or nevi, various forms of keratosis, and angiomas of various kinds. Although all of these lesions are innocuous from the standpoint of their impact on health, some variations in clinical presentation of each of these lesions require differentiation from the major skin cancers: basal cell carcinoma, squamous cell carcinoma and its variations, and cutaneous melanoma. Epidermal inclusion cysts, sebaceous cysts, and keloids often are seen initially with intracutaneous components, but they must be differentiated by clinical examination or biopsy from the rare but locally malignant lesions arising in the dermis and subcutaneous tissues.

Some of the specific features of this group of benign processes are described in more detail.

Warts

Verruca vulgaris is a troublesome lesion that can occur on virtually any skin surface, particularly the fingers, hands, feet, and knees. Warts are caused by an intradermal viral infection and are often multiple. They often vanish spontaneously, giving rise to many folklore treatments described as "successful." Warts on the soles of the feet (plantar warts) can become quite painful because of the development of an underlying bursa.

Moles

Moles, or *nevi*, fall into multiple categories, but they are commonly either intradermal lesions or compound nevi with both epidermal and dermal components. The reason for their removal is often aesthetic; a truly benign nevus has little risk of becoming its malignant counterpart, the malignant melanoma. This is true for the junctional nevus, too, but it is the benign precursor of melanoma when malignant transformation does take place. Most nevi brought to the attention of a physician for other than cosmetic considerations are noted by the patient because of some subtle change in the skin lesions. Since a newly discovered pigmented lesion in an adult or a pigmented lesion with a change in color, shape, or elevation may represent either a new melanoma or melanomatous transformation of a junctional nevus, such lesions should be given careful attention even if they do not have the classic features of a melanoma. These lesions are usually moles but often require diagnostic biopsy.

Keratoses

A keratosis is an epidermal lesion with a hypertrophic change and is classified as senile keratosis, actinic keratosis, arsenical keratosis, or seborrheic keratosis. It may appear as a thickened area in the epidermis and may be yellow, gray, brown, or black. Keratoses are frequently multiple and may be confluent. Although they are often considered precancerous lesions, malignant change in them is quite infrequent. The major problem posed by this group of epidermal skin lesions is differentiating them from squamous carcinoma, basal cell carcinoma, or melanoma, particularly when they are the darker pigmented type of keratosis. Equivocal skin lesions of this type require more thorough evaluation, usually biopsy or excision.

Angiomas

Angiomas are called **hemangiomas** or **lymphangiomas,** and they assume a number of clinical presentations. Those appearing first in early childhood as "strawberry hemangiomas" have a typical red, irregular, and raised appearance and can be expected to regress spontaneously. The port wine stain, a flat, pigmented malformation present from early childhood, is also a classic clinical presentation that can be identified easily. Small, discrete cutaneous hemangiomas or lymphangiomas first noted in adulthood often require biopsy assessment, since they may mimic malignant melanoma or the rare dermal form of sarcoma known as **Kaposi's angiosarcoma.** The clinical presentation and the history of the skin lesion at the time of examination have much to do with the decision to proceed with biopsy for histologic study.

Cysts

The term **sebaceous cyst** includes both cystic enlargement of sebaceous glands caused by plugging of their ducts and the more frequent epidermal inclusion cyst secondary to trapped epithelium resulting from some often previously unrecognized trauma. In this latter lesion the entrapped epidermis continues to grow and desquamate, and it fills the surrounding dermis and adjacent subcutaneous areas with keratin and desquamated cells. These cystic lesions are usually brought to attention because of either gradual enlargement or secondary inflammation in the "cyst." Usually there is an identifiable pit in the surface of the skin at the apex of the raised dermal lesion, and the precise diagnosis can often be made on clinical grounds. Surgical management of this problem is usually for cosmetic reasons or for dealing with the secondary infection in the cyst that brings it to the patient's attention.

Another cystic condition of the skin is chronic suppurative infection of the cutaneous apocrine glands (hidradenitis suppurativa). This process occurs in the axilla, groin, or perineum and is brought to attention by the inflammatory process associated with it. Another classic skin cyst is the pilonidal cyst or sinus that develops in the sacrococcygeal region. Some of these lesions result from penetration of the local skin by growing hairs that set the stage for cyst formation and repeated infections. Repeated trauma and poor hygiene often bring this problem to the clinician's attention. None of these latter cystic processes of the skin raises significant questions about the differential diagnosis of neoplasm, but they often do require therapeutic intervention.

Keloids

Keloids represent hypertrophy of the skin and dermis in the site of a previous injury or surgical scars, and they may develop into large ugly nodules. This process, which occurs more frequently in blacks than whites, is easily recognized on physical examination. The management of keloids is primarily cosmetic. The differential diagnosis of large keloids does include the dermal fibrosarcoma, dermatofibrosarcoma protuberans, but this is a rare condition.

MALIGNANT SKIN LESIONS

Malignant skin lesions, or skin cancers, of major significance, in order of decreasing frequency, are basal cell carcinoma, squamous cell carcinoma and its variants, and melanoma (Table 34-1). Extremely rare malignant skin lesions include sweat gland carcinoma, Merkel cell carcinoma, and sebaceous gland cancer. Skin cancer is by far the most common type of malignant disease in man, and it is estimated that almost half of all individuals who live to be 65 years of age will have at least one skin cancer during their lifetime. Typically these cancers are rather slow growing and, except for melanoma, are usually not very aggressive. Although the differential diagnosis of many of the benign lesions discussed thus far includes a consideration of skin cancer, classic presentations of these malignant lesions are described.

TABLE 34-1 Incidence and Mortality Rates for Cutaneous Cancers

	Incidence	Death
Basal cell carcinoma	1000	5
Squamous cell carcinoma	180	10
Malignant melanoma	50	15

Modified from Emmett AJJ, O'Rourke MGE (eds). Malignant Skin Tumours, 2nd ed. New York, Churchill Livingstone, 1991, pp 6–13.

Basal Cell Carcinoma

Basal cell cancers typically occur on skin areas with chronic exposure to sunlight, chemicals, or trauma. More than 90% appear on the forehead and nose, in the hair margin, and around the eyes in the central portion of the face. Caucasians are most susceptible, particularly those with fair complexions. The predominant types are (1) the more common nodular, ulcerated cancer, which is elevated, with an umbilicated, ulcerated center surrounded by a raised margin and a waxy or pearly border and (2) the superficial variant cancer, which usually is multiple and often occurs on the trunk. It is a plaquelike lesion with a crusted reddened center and a slightly raised pearly border.

The name of this cancer implies an origin from the basal layers of the epidermis. Hematogenous metastases from this lesion are rare, and even metastases through lymphatic channels to regional lymph nodes are extremely uncommon. Most of these lesions are quite small, but local extension and invasion pose a major therapeutic problem in a few unusual basal cell carcinomas, particularly those ignored for a number of months or years. For the usual small lesion, several types of treatment are considered acceptable and effective: excision with small tumorfree margins around the lesion; a more limited excision or electrodesiccation with curettage of the base of the lesion; or radiation therapy for anatomic locations where surgical reconstruction would be difficult or disfiguring. Local surgical removal with a narrow margin is the most practical approach for most patients, since this can be easily accomplished with the patient under local anesthesia. *The surgeon must verify pathologically negative surgical margins to avoid a local recurrence.*

Other treatments have been used but are not so widely accepted. Among these modalities are chemosurgical destruction with zinc chloride paste (Mohs method), topical chemotherapy with 5-fluorouracil, and cryotherapy. Mohs chemosurgery requires extensive histologic mapping and frequent treatment sessions over a long interval of time; therefore it is rarely used except for some local recurrences or in unusually difficult anatomic locations where total surgical excision of the basal cell carcinoma is not feasible without major destruction of adjacent normal structures. Topical chemotherapy is generally considered ineffective with established basal cell carcinoma and is rarely used, although it is useful for extensive keratoses. Excision remains the standard treatment for patients with this form of skin cancer.

Squamous Cell Carcinoma

Squamous cell carcinoma of the skin also develops primarily in areas of the skin exposed to actinic radiation: 75% occur on the head, 15% occur on the hands, and the rest are randomly distributed. The gross clinical appearance of this form of skin cancer is quite variable, ranging from a scaly skin ulcer or grossly punched out ulcerated skin mass to a large, fungating tumor of the skin. Squamous cell carcinomas of the skin are more aggressive than basal cell carcinomas and have a modest tendency to spread through lymphatics to regional lymph nodes, especially those that arise on the arms or hands. This tendency, although infrequent, demands a careful clinical assessment of the regional lymph nodes, and it accounts for the small but significantly increased risk from these lesions as compared with basal cell cancers.

Squamous cell carcinomas of the skin are often treated in a fashion similar to the treatment of basal cell carcinoma. When confirmed by histologic diagnosis, however, surgical excision or primary radiation therapy, rather than electrodesiccation and curettage, which sometimes are used for basal cell cancers, is mandatory. When surgical excision is used, the margin of normal tissue around the lesion should be a little more generous than that considered acceptable for basal cell cancers because of the possibility of lymphatic spread. However, the frequency of lymphatic involvement is too low to warrant elective removal of the regional lymph nodes when they are not clinically enlarged.

Uncommon variants of squamous cancers of the skin are as follows:

- Bowen's disease. This is a superficial intraepidermal carcinoma usually found on the trunk. It has some association with the occurrence of visceral cancers (suggesting a possible carcinogen responsible for both).
- Marjolin's ulcer. This is a squamous cell carcinoma arising at the site of an old or chronically open burn scar; this variant is particularly aggressive in terms of both regional and distant spread if the initial surgical treatment is unsuccessful.
- Cancers arising in long-standing, chronically draining sinus tracts of patients with osteomyelitis or other chronic infections (also can be quite virulent).

- Squamous cell carcinomas developing in the skin at the site of prior radiation therapy. Fortunately, these radiation-induced skin cancers are seen less frequently today than they once were because of refinements in radiation therapy for the treatment of visceral cancers and the fact that x-ray treatment is no longer used indiscriminately for the treatment of benign skin problems.
- Squamous cell carcinoma of the skin caused by prolonged exposure to coal tar derivatives, hydrocarbons, and arsenicals. Pott's description of such cancers' developing on the scrotum of chimney sweeps in 1775 was the first instance of a cancer's being correctly ascribed to a specific carcinogen.

Hereditary Skin Cancers

Basal cell nevus syndrome is an autosomal-dominant disease that demonstrates a propensity for the development of multiple basal cell carcinomas at an early age. In addition, there is variable penetrance of other traits such as jaw cysts, rib and spine defects, calcification of the falx cerebri, and hyperparathyroidism. Another skin cancer problem is xeroderma pigmentosum, also an inherited disease. Multiple basal cell and squamous cell carcinomas and melanomas arise in these patients and may be related to an inability to repair DNA. Fortunately, both of these hereditary syndromes are quite rare.

Cutaneous Melanoma

Melanoma of the skin deserves more concern than the other skin cancers, because the frequency of treatment failure and death from melanoma is in the range expected for some visceral cancers and because its incidence is increasing at an alarming rate. Approximately half of these melanomas arise from preexisting nevi. Intense exposure to ultraviolet radiation from sunlight (especially UV-B rays) is considered the causative or promoter agent for most melanomas. This hypothesis is supported by the greater frequency of this problem among the fair-skinned populations who live closer to the equator (e.g., in Australia) and to a somewhat lesser degree in the sunbelt of North America. Indeed, the incidence of melanoma among fair-skinned individuals in these geographic areas (i.e., those that tend to sunburn rather than suntan) approaches that of common cancers such as colorectal cancer.

Approximately 70% to 80% of melanomas occur in fair-complexioned, sandy-haired, freckled individuals, especially those with red or blond hair. Conversely, melanoma is infrequent among racial groups whose skin has greater pigmentation such as blacks, Hispanics, and Orientals. When melanoma does occur in these latter groups, however, it tends to arise in less pigmented sites such as the palms, soles, subungual areas, or mucous membranes. These forms of melanoma are probably not related to sunlight exposure.

The key word in terms of diagnosis of melanoma of the skin is *change.* Any pigmented skin lesion that is thought to enlarge, alter in pigmentation, or develop any other subjective or visible change should be evaluated by biopsy and histologic examination. A small area of the pigmented lesion may become locally elevated from the surface of the skin, or a portion of the pigmented lesion may become darker or lighter in pigmentation. The observed change deserves further diagnostic study despite the fact that the lesion ultimately may be proved benign. Melanomas can also cause a constant bothersome itching sensation that may bring them to a patient's attention.

Some melanomas present as ulcerating skin lesions, lesions without pigmentation, or lesions with pyogenic features, so the index of suspicion of melanoma must remain high. Other skin lesions often confused with melanoma include pigmented basal cell cancer, hemangiomas, sclerosing angiomas, pigmented keratoses, and pyogenic granulomas, in addition to the more common freckles and benign pigmented nevi. The ABCD mnemonic denotes the clinical features of a mole that suggest biopsy: *A,* asymmetry; *B,* border irregularity; *C,* color variation; and *D,* diameter greater than 6 mm.

Generally it is wise to excise a "suspicious" skin lesion for biopsy if the possibility of melanoma exists on the basis of these described changes. The actual size of the lesion in a few patients might make this impractical, however, and a partial biopsy of the most suspicious area of the lesion is an appropriate approach in this instance. The major problem with a limited biopsy is the possibility that microstaging based on the representative thickness of the melanoma may be uncertain and thus compromise the use of this primary staging factor for determining prognosis and for planning treatment.

The most definitive aspect of staging of malignant melanoma is an accurate determination of the tumor thickness of the melanoma in the skin itself (Fig. 34-1, *A*). The depth on histopathologic staging has been stated in terms of dermal anatomy by Clark's classification. Epidermal involvement, level I, represents only a noninvasive change and is therefore not truly malignant. Level II indicates only papillary dermal involvement, level III the interface between papillary and reticular dermis, level IV the reticular dermis itself, and level V, the subcutaneous fat. For each of these microscopic levels of invasion, the likelihood of metastases and survival can be predicted (Fig. 34-1, *A*).

Another microscopic staging method is the approach described by Breslow in which an optical micrometer on the microscope is used for measuring the tumor thickness in terms of millimeters rather than histologic anatomic landmarks. Thickness has similar prognostic features, as shown in Fig. 34-1, *B*, and now is favored by clinicians because it is more quantitative and reproducible compared with interpreting Clark's level of invasion. Nevertheless, both measures have value and should be included in the pathology report and in staging of the patient using the criteria listed in Table 34-2.

In addition to tumor thickness and level of invasion, other prognostic factors are of great importance, including ulceration of the melanoma (which reflects an invasive property of the malignant cells); the gender of the patient (women do better than men); and the anatomic location (extremity melanomas are less aggressive biologically). Interestingly, there is a prognostic hierarchy for the body parts from which the melanoma arises: the arm is best; then come the leg, head, and neck; and the trunk is worst of all. The presence of regional lymph node metastasis is another particularly adverse prognostic indicator. These factors should also be used to stage the patient, using the criteria listed in Table 34-2.

Surgical excision is the treatment of choice for almost all melanoma. Radiation therapy and chemotherapy are therapeutic tools that have proved useful for palliation of some patients with recurrent melanoma or metastatic melanoma. Classically, very wide and deep excision was recommended, often with a split-thickness skin graft to close a large surgical defect. However, it has been apparent in recent years that a margin of 2 to 3 cm of normal skin around the malignant melanoma is safe and adequate. Guidelines regarding surgical margins are listed in Table 34-3. The depth of the excision should be sufficient to encompass the lesion in its entirety and usually includes the entire subcutaneous tissue under the lesion, but not necessarily the underlying

TABLE 34-2 1988 AJCC-UICC pTNM Staging System

Stage	Criteria*
IA	Primary melanoma ≤0.75 mm thick and/or Clark's level II (pT_1); no nodal or systemic metastases (N_0, M_0)
IB	Primary melanoma 0.76 to 1.5 mm thick and/or Clark's level III (pT_2); N_0, M_0
IIA	Primary melanoma 1.51 to 4 mm thick and/or Clark's level IV (pT_3); N_0, M_0
IIB	Primary melanoma >4 mm thick and/or Clark's level V (pT_4); N_0, M_0
III	Regional lymph node and/or in-transit metastases (any pT, N_1 or N_2, M_0)
IV	Systemic metastases (any pT and N, M_1)

AJCC = American Joint Committee on Cancer;
UICC = Union Internationale Contre le Cancer;
p = pathologic classification.
*The measured thickness takes precedence over Clark's level in the T staging.

TABLE 34-3 Guidelines for Excision of Cutaneous Melanoma

Thickness (mm)	Margin (cm)
In situ (level I)	0.5-1.0
<1	1
1.0-4.0	2*
>4	3-4*

*It may be necessary to reduce these margins in certain anatomic locations in which skin must be preserved such as around the eyelids, the ear, and the fingers.

fascia. The narrower lateral margins now employed usually allow primary closure of the surgical defect.

Chemotherapeutic perfusion of an extremity containing locally advanced forms of melanoma, systemic chemotherapy, and various forms of immunotherapy are being evaluated in clinical trials as adjuvant therapy. Unfortunately, none thus far has improved survival rates sufficiently to warrant its use as standard treatment after surgery.

Melanomas can spread by both hematogenous and lymphatic routes. Although this is well recognized, most questions about the surgical

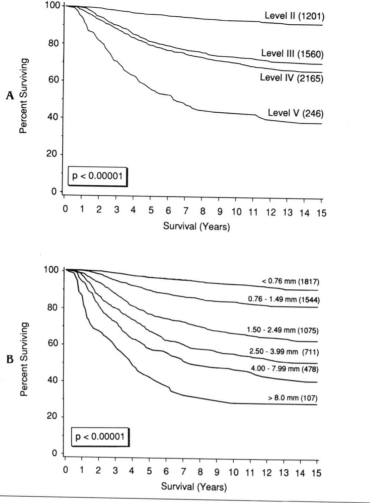

FIGURE 34-1   Survival times for stages I and II melanoma patients according to **A**, level of invasion and **B**, tumor thickness.

management of the more invasive melanomas center around the surgical management of the regional lymphatics, since the control of hematogenous spread is beyond current therapeutic ability. In a patient with a melanoma and clinical evidence of involvement of the regional nodes, it is generally agreed that regional lymph node dissection is an appropriate procedure. In such patients who prove to have histologically involved regional lymph nodes, the prognosis is often poor despite apparently adequate excision of the melanoma and the regional nodes containing metastases (Fig. 34-2). For this reason, there has long been an interest in the possible benefit of removal of the regional lymph nodes in patients

with the more invasive malignant melanomas, even when there is no clinical evidence of lymph node involvement. This approach has been proposed for intermediate thickness lesions (1- to 4-mm thickness [histologic staging]), because these subpopulations of patients have been the ones who have demonstrated subsequent lymphatic spread more frequently. Despite retrospective data suggesting benefit from such "elective" lymph node dissections, clinical trials addressing this question have not yet reported their results. In the meantime, surgeons must follow their own judgment after reviewing the available data but should consider performing elective lymph node dissection in selected patients with inter-

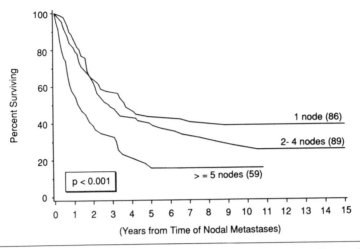

FIGURE 34-2   Survival times for all stage III melanoma patients according to the number of nodal metastases.

mediate thickness melanomas when the potential benefits outweigh the risks and complications.

Cancers of Skin Adnexa

Carcinoma can develop in the skin adnexa. This includes sweat gland carcinoma, a cancer that is quite rare and that can metastasize to both regional lymph nodes and distant sites. It is most commonly seen in the axillae or the anogenital region. Sebaceous gland cancers and carcinomatous degeneration of sebaceous cysts are also rare clinical problems, and many of them occur on the scalp. These rare forms of cancer of the skin adnexa are best treated by the same principles described for squamous carcinoma.

SOFT TISSUE MASSES

Soft tissue masses arising in the subcutaneous tissues most often represent a benign process such as a lipoma, a synovial cyst of "ganglion," or a benign neurofibroma. Soft tissue masses in the deeper tissues are more likely to be malignant lesions of the mesodermal tissues (sarcomas), but benign soft tissue neoplasms or cysts can arise in these locations as well. Although a superficial subcutaneous mass may not always require biopsy and histologic study, if the clinical findings are characteristic of one of the benign disorders listed, deeper masses that are less defined must always be assessed by some form of biopsy procedure.

BENIGN NEOPLASMS OF THE SOFT TISSUES
Lipomas

The most frequent benign soft tissue mass is the lipoma. A lipoma usually arises in the superficial subcutaneous tissues and is initially seen as a discrete, somewhat movable mass that feels almost cystic on palpation. Lipomas are frequently multiple, occurring in several locations, and often are brought to the physician's attention because of a recent increase in size of a mass that the patient has been aware of for a long time. In this circumstance, further questioning often reveals a recent gain in total body weight. Since these masses appear grossly and microscopically identical to normal fat tissue when histologically sectioned, such "growth" probably is not true neoplastic growth.

Most lipomas are excised for cosmetic reasons if they are large enough to be visible. Excision usually can be accomplished by a simple enucleation procedure after exposing the fatty mass through an incision in the overlying skin. For deeper subcutaneous masses clinically considered lipomas, it is wise to expose the mass through a small incision initially and perform only a limited incisional biopsy, unless the lesion is grossly identical to normal fat tissue at the time of operative exposure. This technique avoids compromise of a subsequent resectional procedure if the biopsy result proves the mass to be a malignant lesion (sarcoma).

If the lipomas occur in muscle or within muscle compartments, a simple incisional biopsy, as described for deep subcutaneous masses, first must be performed to confirm the diagnosis. Enucleation of a mass in a muscle compartment on the assumption that it is a lipoma might prejudice a subsequent adequate local limb-sparing resection if the histologic diagnosis confirms some form of sarcoma.

Synovial Cysts

Another benign soft tissue mass requiring differentiation from a sarcomatous process is a cyst arising from synovial tissues. Normal synovial tissues not only line the various joints but also surround moving tendons and occur in the bursas around the body. The most frequent location of a synovial cyst is the dorsal aspect of the wrist, the so-called *ganglion.* These synovial cysts are not really outpouchings of the joint space, but they usually arise from other synovial tissues near the wrist, finger, or foot and ankle. Synovial cysts may be seen initially as a classic cystic ganglion and will not require surgical excision for diagnosis, but chronic discomfort or cosmetic deformity is often an indication for surgical excision.

A history of some trauma before development of a synovial cyst may be revealed, and acute local trauma also can lead to the disappearance of such a mass. Although nonmedical treatment of the wrist ganglion by a direct blow to achieve cyst rupture has often been described, the lesion usually reappears after a short interval. If symptoms from a synovial cyst are present or if there is uncertainty about the actual diagnosis, formal surgical excision is the best course to follow.

Nerve Sheath Tumors

Nerve sheath tumors, which are small, benign, firm, smooth, movable subcutaneous masses, may be either solitary or multiple and are either neurilemomas or neurofibromas. They may or may not arise from an identifiable nerve trunk, but this nerve is often not grossly apparent despite the origin of the lesion from the neural sheath tissues. In patients with more than one of these subcutaneous lesions and a café-au-lait spot somewhere on the trunk, the clinical diagnosis of neurofibromatosis (or von Recklinghausen's disease) can be made with confidence. Occasionally one of these neurilemomas becomes sarcomatous; therefore a history of recent enlargement of such a mass requires a biopsy diagnosis.

Other Benign Soft Tissue Masses

Areas of fat necrosis (usually secondary to trauma), foreign bodies, fasciitis, and chronic abscesses can all present as a soft tissue mass that simulates a neoplasm. An appropriate history and physical examination usually provide correct diagnosis.

MALIGNANT SOFT TISSUE NEOPLASMS

As noted previously, a primary consideration for any new soft tissue mass is the possibility of a cancer arising from one of the mesodermal tissues—a soft tissue sarcoma. These relatively rare lesions comprise only 1% to 2% of all cancers in adults but represent a somewhat larger fraction of childhood cancers. They have been clinically classified on the basis of their presumed histogenesis (Table 34-4), but there are some categories for which the cell of origin is in doubt. Although all of these various categories of sarcomas have been identified as different pathologic entities, the major prognostic feature for any of them is the degree of differentiation of the sarcoma on microscopic study. This histologic differentiation is also a major factor in the currently used staging schemas for soft tissue sarcomas.

Sarcomas have been described in virtually all anatomic locations, although in adults the preponderance of lesions occurs where there is a bulk of mesodermal tissue (e.g., the extremities, particularly the thigh). Also, variations in location and predominant age group seem to occur with differing histologic classifications (e.g., distal extremity locations for synovial sarcoma in young adults). Children with rhabdomyosarcoma, the most frequent soft tissue sarcoma in this age group, have a much different anatomic distribution of lesions than adults, with the genitourinary tissues and the head and neck common locations. The usual clinical presentation of any soft tissue sarcoma is that of a solid mass in the subcutaneous or deeper tissues brought to attention by physical size, local discomfort, or trauma or by a recent increase in size without other symptoms.

Soft tissue sarcomas spread by local invasion, in the lymphatics (rarely), or by hematogenous dissemination (usually to the lungs or pleura). Thus surgical removal with very narrow margins of normal tissue around the sarcoma leads to a high likelihood of local recurrence at the primary site. This is the basis for the general concept of

TABLE 34-4   Cell of Origin of Soft Tissue Sarcomas

Germ Cell Layer	Normal Cell	Sarcoma
Ectoderm	Nerve cell sheath	Malignant neurofibrosarcoma
		Alveolar soft-part sarcoma (?)
Mesoderm	Adipose cell	Liposarcoma
	Fibroblast	Fibrosarcoma
		Dermatofibrosarcoma problems
		Malignant fibrous histiocytoma (?)
	Smooth muscle	Leiomyosarcoma
	Skeletal muscle	Rhabdomyosarcoma
	Tenosynovial cell	Synovial sarcoma
		Epithelioid sarcoma (?)
		Malignant giant cell tumor
	Blood vessel	Angiosarcoma
		Hemangiopericytoma
		Lymphangiosarcoma
		Kaposi's sarcoma
	Miscellaneous	Malignant mesenchymoma
		Malignant granular cell tumor

sarcoma treatment—removing the sarcoma surgically with a generous margin or envelope of normal tissue in all directions. Sarcomas often have the misleading appearance of being encapsulated, and it is important to avoid enucleation of the tumor because this pseudocapsule contains malignant cells that may not be completely removed by the operation. Examination of a frozen section from the surgical margins is important to ensure that the tumor excision was complete. Regional lymph nodes in adults are rarely involved by sarcomas, and this route of regional spread is usually not a treatment consideration unless the regional nodes are enlarged. The major and often the only site of distant spread is the lungs, and this is the basis for effective surgical removal of metastases in some patients.

Another treatment modality for soft tissue sarcomas is radiation therapy. Clearly local disease control is better with a combination of surgery and radiation treatments for certain clinical presentations, particularly those patients with high-grade (i.e., less differentiated) malignancies and those in whom surgical margins were necessarily narrow because of large size (i.e., >5 cm) or anatomic considerations. The radiation therapy is generally administered postoperatively, but some centers advocate giving preoperative radiation therapy. No clinical trials have proved one sequence of treatment better than the other.

Anticancer chemotherapy has been temporarily beneficial in some patients with distant metastases, but none of the currently available drugs has proven value as prophylactic or adjuvant chemotherapy after complete surgical resection. However, chemotherapy programs are clearly beneficial for virtually all children with rhabdomyosarcoma, irrespective of site and stage. Finally, there is a role for surgical excision of pulmonary metastases in selected patients in whom the number of tumors are few (i.e., 5 or less) and slow growing (a tumor doubling time of 30 to 40 days or more) and the surgical risks are minimal. A 5-year survival rate of 30% to 40% has been reported in several surgical series after pulmonary metastectomy in selected patients.

PITFALLS AND COMMON MYTHS

- Famous last words: It is just a mole!
- "Superficial spreading" melanomas are not necessarily superficial.
- A little sun does not hurt; tanning booths are not the same as real sun.

BIBLIOGRAPHY

Balch CM. The role of elective lymph node dissection in melanoma: Rationale, results and controversies. J Clin Oncol 6:163-172, 1988.

Balch CM, Houghton AN, Milton GW, et al. (eds). Cutaneous Melanoma, 2nd ed. Philadelphia, JB Lippincott, 1992.

Caldwell EH, McCormack RN, et al. Skin cancer. In Clinical Oncology, A Multidisciplinary Approach for Medical Students and Physicians. New York, American Cancer Society, 1983, pp 222-229.

Edmonson JH, Fleming TR, Ivins JC, et al. Randomized study of systemic chemotherapy following complete excision of nonosseous sarcomas. J Clin Oncol 2:1390; 1984.

Emmett AJJ, O'Rourke MGE (eds). Malignant Skin Tumours, 2nd ed. New York, Churchill Livingstone, 1991, p 425.

Friedman RJ, Rigel DS, Silverman MK, et al. Malignant melanoma in the 1990s: The continued importance of early detection and the role of physician examination and self-examination of the skin. Cancer 41:201-226, 1991.

Lawrence W Jr, Neifeld JP, Terz JJ. Manual of Soft Tissue Tumor Surgery. New York, Springer-Verlag, 1983.

Mihm MC, Fitzpatrick TB, Lane-Brown MM, et al. Early detection of primary cutaneous malignant melanomas. N Engl J Med 289:989, 1973.

Suit HD, Mankin HJ, et al. Preoperative and postoperative radiation in the treatment of primary soft tissue sarcoma. Cancer 55:2659, 1985.

Veronesi U, Adamus J, Bandiera DC, et al. Delayed regional lymph node dissection in Stage I melanoma of the skin of the lower extremities. Cancer 49:2420, 1982.

Veronesi U, Cascinelli N. Narrow excision (1-cm margin): A safe procedure for thin cutaneous melanoma. Arch Surg 126:438-441, 1991.

CHAPTER REVIEW
Questions

1. Outline the proper approach for treatment in a patient with a firm mass (7 cm in diameter) of the thigh and a negative chest x-ray film.
2. All moles should be:
   a. Excised
   b. Electrocoagulated
   c. Observed for signs of change
   d. Biopsied
   e. Ignored
3. Squamous cell cancer of the skin:
   a. Has the same prognosis as basal cell cancer
   b. Is a natural progression of basal cell cancer
   c. Rarely metastasizes to lymph nodes
   d. Should be electrocoagulated
   e. Should be radiated
4. Outline the management of a 1 cm nevus of the arm that has begun to enlarge and change color.
5. What *clinical* feature is the major prognostic factor for melanoma?
6. List the four major prognostic variables for a localized primary melanoma.

Answers

1. An incisional biopsy is made to obtain tissue for permanent slides and histologic diagnosis. Later treatment will depend on precise diagnosis.
2. c
3. c
4. Excise the nevus with the patient under local anesthesia to obtain a diagnosis, and if it is melanoma, determine the tumor thickness and level of invasion by histologic staging. For some surgeons the decision regarding advisability of regional lymph node dissection depends on the measured tumor thickness (i.e., 1 to 4 mm tumors), whereas other surgeons believe only palpable lymph nodes should be treated by dissection. However, there is general agreement that wide resection of the primary melanoma is appropriate treatment, with a 1 cm margin for this melanoma (<1 mm), a 2 cm margin for an intermediate thickness melanoma (1 to 4 mm), and a 3 to 4 cm margin for a thicker melanoma.
5. Regional lymph node enlargement clinically considered due to metastasis
6. Tumor thickness, location, gender, and ulceration

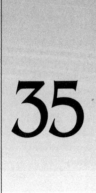

35 Trauma

H. HARLAN STONE
TIMOTHY C. FABIAN

KEY FEATURES

After reading this chapter you will understand:
- What a trauma system consists of and how one functions.
- The various trauma scoring systems and how to use them in evaluating patients.
- The pathophysiology of trauma and the effects of trauma on the organism.
- Management of a multiple-trauma patient.
- The sequence of evaluation and treatment.
- The surgeon's role as trauma team leader.
- Penetrating and blunt abdominal trauma and traumatic injuries of the chest.
- Management of spinal trauma.

Surgeons have always been especially concerned with the effects of trauma—not just because patients who have sustained an injury usually require surgical care, but also because an operative procedure itself entails the creation of one or more wounds.

The modern trauma surgeon should appreciate the social significance of his or her work and actively contribute to accident prevention programs and to organizational efforts to improve systems for care of the injured.

TRAUMA SYSTEMS

A proliferation of trauma systems, spurred by the observation that nearly one in four trauma deaths was preventable, has occurred during the past decade. The prime culprits in the deaths were hemorrhage, tension pneumothorax, and other injuries that are easily managed through an organized approach by immediately available facilities and knowledgeable surgical personnel.

The three basic components of a trauma system are (1) prehospital care and transportation, (2) system-wide communications, and (3) appropriately designated hospitals. System requirements are variable and must be individualized according to regional, geographic, and population differences, since metropolitan and urban areas create quite different demands and challenges.

Sophisticated electronics allow highly effective communication between paramedics at the accident scene and physicians at the base hospital. Care begins immediately in the field, during which time hospital staff are preparing for patient arrival. Helicopter transportation is a key component in both outlying urban and rural trauma systems.

Trauma Center Levels

Trauma centers have been designated *levels I through III*, according to their individual capabilities. Level I and II hospitals are usually the larger facilities with a full array of surgical services, including general surgery, neurosurgery, orthopedics, thoracic surgery, and plastic and maxillofacial surgery. Level III hospitals are the smaller units in which patients with major injuries are resuscitated and stabilized before transfer

TABLE 35-1 Description of Glasgow Coma Scale

Measure	Description	Value
Eye opening	Spontaneous (normal)	4
	To speech: not necessary to request	3
	To pain	2
	None	1
Best motor response	Obeys: moves to command	6
	Localizes: purposeful movement toward stimulus	5
	Withdraws: from painful stimulus	4
	Decorticate posturing (flexion)	3
	Decerebrate posturing (extension)	2
	No movement	1
Verbal response	Oriented: name, age, place	5
	Confused: answers questions	4
	Inappropriate words: recognizable	3
	Incomprehensible sounds	2
	None	1

to a level I or II hospital. Level I and II facilities must have operating rooms available 24 hours a day solely for the care of trauma victims. Level I hospitals, in addition, must have general surgical, neurosurgical, and anesthesia personnel inhouse 24 hours a day; such personnel should be present near the time of patient arrival at a level II facility. An effective system not only demands close coordination of all participating institutions and personnel, but also triage and transfer protocols previously agreed on and formalized in writing.

What Are the Commonly Used Trauma Scoring Systems?

Four trauma scoring systems are widely applied: Glasgow Coma Scale, Revised Trauma Score, Injury Severity Score, and Abdominal Trauma Index. These scoring systems are used for patient management, triage, quality assurance, prediction of outcome, and stratification in clinical research.

Glasgow Coma Scale (GCS). The GCS is a quantitative measure that objectively assesses the degree of neurologic insult and the patient's level of consciousness. It can be rapidly performed by prehospital, nursing, and physician providers. Its three parameters are eye opening, best motor response, and verbal response (Table 35-1). The sum of these components comprises the GCS. All patients with a GCS less than 8 are comatose, whereas those with a score greater than 8 are not

TABLE 35-2 Revised Trauma Score

GCS	Respiratory Rate	Systemic Blood Pressure
13-15 = 4	10-29 = 4	>89 = 4
9-12 = 3	>29 = 3	76-89 = 3
6-8 = 2	6-9 = 2	50-75 = 2
4-5 = 1	1-5 = 1	1-49 = 1
3 = 0	0 = 0	0 = 0

Survival rates for the respective RTS are 12 = 99%; 10 = 88%; 6 = 63%; 5 = 46%; 2 = 29%; 0 = 3%.

in coma. As a general rule, head injury is assessed as:

Severe	GCS less than 8
Moderate	GCS 9 to 12
Minor	GCS 13 to 15

Revised Trauma Score (RTS). This is a combined physiologic and neurologic scoring system over a numerical range of 0 to 12. It correlates well with eventual mortality and accordingly has been used as a prehospital triage tool for delivering patients to the appropriate level trauma center. Its three components are the GCS, respiratory rate, and systolic blood pressure. The values in Table 35-2 are applied to each of the three components; the summed value gives the RTS.

Injury Severity Score (ISS). This score was developed as a predictor of mortality after vehicular accidents. It is calculated by using the Abbreviated Injury Scale (AIS), which assigns a point value (1 to 6) according to the severity of each organ injured. The ISS is calculated by taking the three body systems with the highest AIS values, squaring each of these three AIS scores, and adding them to form the ISS. The following mortality rates correlate with the ISS in bluntly injured patients below age 50 years: 1, <1%; 10, 1%; 20, 15%; 35, 38%; 45, 56%; 75, 93%.

Abdominal Trauma Index (ATI). This index was developed as a means to predict infection after abdominal injury. Abdominal organs are assigned a risk factor number (1 to 5) and a severity of injury number (1 to 5). The products of those numbers for each organ injured are added to determine the ATI. An ATI of less than 25 is associated with less than a 10% chance of infection, whereas ones over 25 have a 30% or greater risk of subsequent infection.

PHYSIOLOGY OF TRAUMA
Local Response to Injury

The area of injury—the wound—represents a physical break in tissue continuity as a consequence of some extraneous source of energy, be it mechanical, thermal, or chemical. The wound can be classified further as internal (closed) or external (open), which is determined by the absence or presence, respectively, of a defect in the protective body surface.

Effect of Wounding

With injury and thus loss of tissue continuity, blood vessels are disrupted and a variable amount of hemorrhage occurs. Bleeding is controlled by (1) vessel retraction, (2) local vasospasm, (3) the coagulation mechanism, and (4) clot retraction. Blood in the wound subsequently forms a clot, which provides the fibrin mesh on which invading cellular elements migrate in an attempt to prevent or control infection and to provide for ultimate repair of tissue.

Inflammation is the body's response to injury, and it initiates the process of healing. It has two components: vascular and cellular.

The *vascular* portion of inflammation is initiated by an exaggeration in the blood supply and thus greater capillary perfusion at the site of injury. This is associated with a local increase in the metabolic rate and an acceleration in foreign-body removal. Increased capillary permeability simultaneously allows plasma to exude into the wound. The result is tissue edema, segmental capillary stasis, and a significantly greater lymph flow. This vascular response accounts for the cardinal signs of inflammation.

The *cellular* component of inflammation includes (1) activation and migration of phagocytes (leukocytes, histiocytes, and tissue macrophages), (2) endothelial proliferation (capillary buds), and (3) fibroblastic proliferation. This migration of fibroblasts along the fibrin matrix and their subsequent deposition of collagen is the cellular response that produces granulation tissue. The immature capillary buds account for the friability and easy bleeding, the fibroblasts for the fresh collagen, and leukocytes for the purulent exudate.

Process of Healing

The area in the immediate vicinity of the wound responds by initiating the reparative process. Healing is the mechanism by which the original cohesion of tissues is regained. The removal of foreign material and the process of repair blend imperceptibly, yet repair can never fully begin until most, if not all, foreign material has been removed.

The *three stages of healing* are:

- *Lag.* Foreign material is removed, and there is proliferation of both endothelial buds and fibroblasts.
- *Fibroplasia.* In this stage there is further proliferation of fibroblasts and deposition of collagen.
- *Contracture.* In the final stage of healing collagen contracts and thereby reduces wound size.

Healing can be classified into one of three types:

- *Primary intention:* Healing progresses without complication or wound disruption.
- *Secondary intention:* Healing is complicated by infection or wound disruption so that ultimate closure is obtained by contracture of granulation tissue alone.
- *Delayed primary intention:* Wound breakdown has previously occurred, yet closure is gained through operative reapproximation of the edges once granulation tissue has appeared.

Delay in Healing. No agent or process has been discovered that will accelerate the normal process of wound healing. Nevertheless, many different factors do delay significantly such repair, and it is only through control of these adverse influences that the healing process can be aided (Table 35-3).

TABLE 35-3   Common Factors in Delayed Healing

Cause	Conditions	Mechanism
Inadequate blood supply	Arteriosclerosis Diabetes mellitus Primary arterial disease Low-flow syndromes	Decreased inflammatory response Metabolic defect Failure to remove foreign material Poor nutrition
Infection	Wound infection from any source	Persistence of foreign proteins Continued destruction of tissue Collagen lysis
Catabolic state (negative nitrogen balance)	Old age Malignant disease Liver disease Debilitating illness Intestinal fistula	Failure to make collagen or new protein

Systemic Response to Injury

Stimuli that initiate the systemic response to injury vary considerably in severity and duration. They can be objective events (e.g., trauma, infection, metabolic aberrations) or mere subjective impressions (the psyche). Patients, likewise, have individual variations in their responses to trauma.

There are five phases in the *systemic response to trauma* (Table 35-4). The magnitude and duration of each phase are determined primarily by similar extremes in the inciting stimuli. Although each stage is a separate entity, there is a progressive continuum from one phase to the next. A significant complication automatically reverts the process to an earlier phase.

Because of the major role played by various hormones, titles for the initial stages reflect the dominance or waning influence of a given endocrine system (see Table 35-4). Such changes in metabolism, fluid and electrolyte balance, wound healing, and even emotional response of the patient are consistently present. Fluid shifts into the wound, altered circulation at the site of injury, preexisting disease, medications, and a multitude of other factors can mask the overall systemic response without altering the character of the response.

PRINCIPLES OF MANAGEMENT
Local Wound Management

All sizable or critically located wounds that communicate with the patient's external environment (i.e., open wound) require surgical attention. Basic steps in management are:

- *Arrest of hemorrhage:* initially by local pressure or a hemostat; subsequently by ligature
- *Cleansing:* removal of all gross contamination, usually followed by irrigation with physiologic solutions, preferably through a pressure jet
- *Debridement:* excision of all nonviable tissue
- *Dressing:* protection of the wound from the outside environment through application of a sterile cover
- *Selective closure:* initial closure only of wounds expected to heal by primary intention; use of healing by delayed primary closure (wound approximation 2 to 4 days after injury) or by secondary intention (spontaneous contracture of granulations) for heavily contaminated wounds, when there has been considerable lapse in time since injury, or if infection already has become established

Management of Systemic Problems

After major trauma, initial management must be directed first toward resuscitation of the patient. This stepwise approach, in decreasing order of priority, includes:

1. *Airway:* establishment of an airway, often requiring insertion of a mouthpiece, endotracheal tube, or, if other measures are ineffective, tracheostomy or cricothyroidotomy
2. *Hemorrhage:* stoppage of exsanguinating bleeding by direct pressure, clamp, or, as a last resort, tourniquet; application of the hemorrhage-controlling clamp within a body cavity may require urgent laparotomy or thoracotomy

TABLE 35-4   Phases of Systemic Response to Injury

	Adrenergic	Corticoid	Corticoid Withdrawal	Anabolic	Fat Gain
Relative duration	1	30	20	150	250
Pituitary gland					
Antidiuretic hormone (ADH)	++++	++	-----	0	0
Adrenocorticotropic hormone (ACTH)	+++	++++	0	0	0
Adrenal gland					
Medulla	++++	+	0	0	0
Cortex	+	++++	0	0	0
Electrolyte balance					
Sodium	+	+++	---	0	0
Potassium	-	---	+++	+	0
Water	+++	++++	----	0	0
Hydrogen				0	0
Nitrogen	-	---	--	++	0
Serum levels					
Sodium	-	---	+++	0	0
Potassium	+	+++	--	0	0
Hydrogen	+	+	--	0	0
Wound	Fresh	Granulations	Beginnings of tensile strength	Strong hyperemic scar	Mature, blanched scar
Psyche	Withdrawn	Short attention span	Fatigues easily	Normal activity	Regain of fat

+ = Positive balance or greater-than-normal value; 0 = zero balance or normal; − = negative balance or less-than-normal value.

3. *Cardiothoracic derangements:* correction of obvious alterations in cardiac or thoracic physiology (pericardiocentesis for cardiac tamponade or tube thoracotomy for tension pneumothorax)

4. *Intravenous management:* establishment of an intravenous line with a large-bore cannula as soon as possible; blood for type and crossmatch and necessary baseline studies (hematocrit, white blood count, and amylase) should be drawn at the same time

5. *Visceral protection:* provision of protection for extruded or exposed vital organs by a sterile dressing

6. *Wounds:* covering open wounds by sterile dressings until more definitive management can be rendered

7. *Fractures:* splinting of obvious fractures appropriately

8. *Urine:* unless contraindicated by suspicion of a urethral injury, catheterization of the bladder to provide fresh urine for assessment of both present and past status of the urinary tract and to begin measurement of hourly urinary output as a guide to fluid therapy

9. *Patient history:* events of the injury plus past medical history of, for example, significant diseases, medications, allergies, operations

10. *Physical examination:* a rapid, yet sufficiently detailed, examination for discovery of other injuries not yet revealed and preexisting disease processes

After the above measures are performed, administration of additional therapy is selective and is based on the severity of the injury and the specific organs involved.

APPROACH TO THE PATIENT WITH MULTIPLE TRAUMA
What Is the Trauma Team Leader's Role?

Significant injury to two or more organ systems qualifies as multiple trauma. For optimal management, each major system with a significant injury must be given care just as expert as if it were the only area to have been damaged. However, it is virtually impossible for more than a single specialist to direct patient management at any given moment. If this is attempted, only chaos results, with one physician's order canceling those prescribed by the other members of the medical team, or, even worse, inflicting harm on an injured organ system about which the physician has limited knowledge.

What is needed under these circumstances is a team leader—an individual with experience in overall management of the trauma patient—even though the injuries sustained are not necessarily in that person's own area of surgical expertise. All orders should be written specifically by the team leader or, at the very least, given the leader's approval before their execution. In this way there can be no undue detriment to the patient because of a conflict of interests between participating specialists. Usually the general surgeon is best qualified to serve as trauma team leader.

Certain priorities must always be kept in mind. They are, in decreasing order of importance:

1. Saving the patient's life
2. Preservation of organ or limb viability
3. Maintenance of useful function of that organ or part
4. Long-term cosmetic results

Often the question arises as to whether an organ or limb can be salvaged or, even though it can be preserved, what useful end can be gained by maintaining viability of that part. Generally, if any three of the five basic components serving a limb or organ require repair, amputation or resection may be the procedure of choice. With four components needing correction, the decision to resect or amputate becomes more certain. The determinants to consider are:

- Skeletal support
- Blood supply
- Nervous system control
- Tissue and/or skin coverage
- Effector mechanism such as the tendon and its muscle motor source

The patient should remain on a single surgical service, specifically that of the team leader, until all systems have stabilized and only one organ or structural injury warrants continued hospitalization. At that juncture, transfer to the service considered most responsible for aftercare can be accomplished without additional risk to the patient.

Organizing Activities

To resuscitate a multiple trauma victim, it is necessary for each member of the team to do his or her job. Performing the following elements is vital, and doing so frequently will necessitate the use of a variety of professional and paraprofessional personnel, who will be working simultaneously.

Preparing the Patient for Examination and Treatment. This necessitates expeditious removal of clothing in the emergency room without aggravating possible existing injuries (i.e., spinal fracture or dislocation).

Monitoring and Recording Vital Signs. A blood pressure cuff should be applied, and blood pressure, pulse, respiration, mental status, and general condition should be recorded on a graph. Blood pressure should be reported frequently to the team leader.

Drawing Blood and Preparing an Intravenous Cannula. One physician should be detailed to a peripheral uninjured extremity to insert a large-bore intravenous cannula for rapid fluid or blood administration. Before starting the IV, blood can be drawn for crossmatch, hematocrit, or other tests. Lactated Ringer's or colloid solutions should be started, depending on the presence or absence of shock, the nature of the injury, and the team leader's preference.

Notifying Other Departments. Other units may need to mobilize personnel for subsequent patient care or diagnostic procedures (e.g., radiology department, OR, blood bank). Specialty services that may be needed (e.g., anesthesiology) should be contacted.

Physical Examination by Team Leader. This systematic physical examination should take a few minutes to perform and may reveal problems needing immediate relief, which can be treated as they are discovered. The approach is to examine those areas that, if abnormal, might "kill the patient first." This sequence is important because as each major catastrophe is ruled out, additional time is gained to go on to the next system.

Cervical Spine. Especially in blunt, decelerating injuries, the cervical spine should always be suspect. It is absolutely crucial to maintain the neck in a fixed anatomic position to avoid additional damage to a cord no longer protected by a stable cervical spine.

Diagnosis. In such an injury there is tenderness to palpation along the cervical spine processes, which may also be abnormal in prominence. An emergency lateral cervical spine x-ray study is of utmost importance, with search on the film for bony displacements, malaligned cervical vertebrae, a posterior indentation to the pharyngeal air column, or other signs indicative of fracture or dislocation.

Treatment. Initially stabilize the area with a collar or sandbags until skeletal traction via skull fixation can be gained.

Upper Airway. Obstruction to the upper airway can be caused by a blood clot, saliva, receded or retroverted tongue, fractured mandible, or direct injury to the trachea.

Diagnosis. Examine the patient's mouth. Lift the jaw and pull the tongue forward if necessary.

Treatment. Suction secretions; turn head to side if necessary to evacuate emesis; secure a reliable airway.

Tension Pneumothorax. This condition can be secondary to either a sucking chest wound or a pulmonary laceration, producing a ball-valve effect so that air enters the chest with inspiration but cannot leave with expiration. Sudden death is produced by mediastinal shift and occlusion of the great veins.

Diagnosis. Diagnosis is made by noting a lateral shift of the trachea away from the hyperresonant involved hemithorax. Decreased breath sounds on the affected side may be difficult to elicit. If a pneumothorax is suspected, do not wait for chest x-ray film confirmation before starting treatment.

Treatment. Insert a large-bore needle into the involved chest and follow with a chest tube connected to an underwater seal. A simple pneumothorax can be converted to one of tension if a positive pressure breathing apparatus is used (e.g., during an operation). Therefore, if pneumothorax ever is suspected, a chest tube must be inserted before use of a ventilator.

Flail Chest. Flail chest is due to direct injury to the chest wall, with multiple fractures of several ribs or the sternum, thereby producing a sizable area of thorax that is free floating and without bony fixation. Inefficiency of respiration is its hallmark. Respiratory distress follows the recirculation of air from the affected side to the unaffected side during inspiration (as the flail collapses) or to mediastinal flutter and venous compression.

Diagnosis. Diagnosis is easily made by palpation of the chest wall, noting the fractures, flail, and crepitus.

Treatment. Flail chest is treated by positive pressure ventilation through an endotracheal conduit after insertion of a chest tube.

Cardiac Tamponade With Heart Failure. This condition is due to direct injury to the great vessels within the pericardium or to the heart itself, with accumulation of blood in the pericardial sac. Death results from inadequate cardiac filling.

Diagnosis. Cardiac tamponade always must be suspected in any patient with a penetrating chest wound, especially over the left anterior thorax. Increased central venous pressure (distended neck veins) indicates a severe form of tamponade. Otherwise, diagnosis is based on shock and a narrowed pulse pressure (difference between systolic and diastolic pressure <20). Muted heart sounds and an enlarged, poorly contracting cardiac shadow seen on x-ray film or fluoroscopy are of value only for more chronic pericardial effusions.

Treatment. Immediate aspiration of pericardial fluid through a long, large-bore needle inserted at the xiphocostal angle and directed toward the left acromioclavicular joint must be done immediately. There is usually insufficient time to attach a cardiac monitor to the patient. Aspiration of nonclotting blood indicates correct placement of the needle and confirms the diagnosis. Prompt operation is then indicated.

Interruption of Blood Flow to an Extremity. This situation occurs secondary to transection or compression of an artery.

Diagnosis. The criteria for determining vascular injury are (1) wound in the vicinity (open or closed), (2) evidence of shed blood (external hemorrhage, local hematoma, bleeding into an adjacent coelom, or acute arteriovenous [AV] fistula), and (3) stocking-glove motor and sensory deficits. Absence of the distal pulse should be considered the result of vessel occlusion or disruption until proven otherwise. True pulse deficits (as shown by physical examination or Doppler method) nearly always indicate injury, but a normal pulse does not rule out a vascular wound (i.e., lateral wall injury or proximal wound with extensive arterial collaterals). A to-and-fro bruit indicates an AV communication, yet some AV fistulae initially will contain an occluding clot that subsequently lyses many hours after the initial evaluation, thus underscoring the importance of follow-up examination. Angiography seldom adds any greater accuracy to the clinical diagnosis except in cases of shotgun wounds with a wide pellet pattern, long-bone fracture with hematoma (especially the femur), and knee dislocation. Although they are invasive, current digital subtraction x-ray techniques permit smaller needle punctures and require less contrast media. Even more practical is the duplex Doppler technique, which is noninvasive and appears highly accurate for peripheral arterial injuries.

Treatment. Treatment consists of eliminating compression (i.e., splinting of a fracture), repair or resection with reanastomosis of the injured vessel, or extraction of the intra-arterial clot with local internal repair or resection as dictated by the pathology noted. Performing a distal extremity fasciotomy is crucial whenever neurologic deficits caused by ischemia were obvious preoperatively or if the popliteal artery was involved.

Hemorrhage. Definitive ligation of bleeding vessels must be accomplished. If hemorrhage may be hidden, certain diagnostic maneuvers such as x-ray studies of the chest, abdomen, and pelvis, cystography, CT abdominal scan, or diagnostic peritoneal lavage are indicated. A change in the hematocrit level is a relatively late indicator of hemorrhage.

Neurologic Examination. An initial evaluation of the neurologic status of the patient is important because changes occurring over the subsequent follow-up period may dictate a need for urgent operation. This evaluation should include observation of:

- *Level of consciousness* (see Table 35-1). Changes in level of consciousness may indicate the presence of intracranial disease or bleeding requiring an operation.
- *Pulse, blood pressure, respirations.* Bradycardia, hypertension, and irregular respirations are signs of increasing intracranial pressure.
- *Pupillary size and reactivity.* Unequal or nonreactive pupils may imply an expanding intracranial hematoma or severe cerebral injury.
- *Eyelids, eardrums, or posterior occipital region for ecchymosis.* This sign may indicate the presence of a basilar skull fracture requiring antibiotic prophylaxis and specific periodic observations.
- *Nose and ears for spinal fluid leak.*
- *Sensory, motor, and reflex status of the cranial nerves, extremities, abdomen, and perianal region.*

ABDOMINAL TRAUMA

Injury of the abdomen and its contained viscera can be caused by either blunt or penetrating trauma. If such major wounds are not corrected within a critical interval of time, death often results from hemorrhage, peritonitis, organ dysfunction, or some combination thereof. Early and appropriate repair is the only reliable means of obviating these lethal complications. The mortality rate approximates 100% if perforation of a hollow viscus or major hemorrhage or both are not corrected within a reasonable time frame. Accordingly, immediate laparotomy is indicated for all patients with known or suspected major intra-abdominal injury.

Penetrating abdominal trauma is commonly associated with gastrointestinal perforation. Delay in exploration and thus delay in closure or resection of any hole in the bowel automatically leads to an expectedly greater incidence of intraperitoneal sepsis. Accordingly, in a hospital that is not a trauma center, it is generally wiser to immediately explore all patients with possible penetrating abdominal trauma rather than to wait for the onset of overt signs of peritoneal irritation (indicating that infection is already established). However, in some institutions a regimen of watchful waiting for abdominal stab wounds has provided excellent results in patients with a negative peritoneal lavage, no signs of peritonitis, stable vital signs, and sufficient personnel to supervise frequent reevaluations. In the case of a patient with a gunshot wound, the halo of contusion around the missile tract may not lead to bowel perforation for several days. Thus rarely, if ever, should the patient with a gunshot wound of the abdomen be observed.

In contrast, blunt abdominal trauma seldom causes intestinal disruption. The usual problem is hemorrhage from a fracture of one or more of the solid viscera—liver, spleen, or kidney. In addition, multiple other nonabdominal organ systems frequently are injured. Unless the hemorrhagic shock resulting from abdominal injury is profound, there is generally time for evaluation of other injuries and for obtaining more accurate determination that a laparotomy is truly warranted.

Evaluation of Patient With Blunt Abdominal Trauma

Assessment of the patient who has sustained blunt abdominal trauma should include a history of how the injury occurred and, in cases of vehicular accidents, whether the patient was the driver (pancreatic and duodenal trauma) or passenger (spleen and kidney wounds). Details about the evacuation of the victim from the scene of injury are also important, for additional tissue damage can easily be inflicted (e.g., moving the leg with an unsplinted fracture).

Other than an assessment of distant injuries that might influence abdominal findings, prime emphasis should be placed on evidence of blood loss (i.e., systemic signs of shock, free intraperitoneal fluid, and definable intra-abdominal hematomas) and signs of peritoneal irritation (i.e., chemical versus bacterial peritonitis and paralytic ileus). Other considerations are obvious contusions, abrasions of the trunk, and clinical fractures.

Useful laboratory data include the hematocrit level as a baseline for later comparison and urinalysis to document both prior renal function and the possibility of urinary tract trauma (gross or microscopic hematuria). The white blood count is also valuable. An immediate leukocytosis is usually noted with splenic or hepatic parenchymal rupture, bleeding into a joint, and, although more delayed in appearance, blood in some other serosal-lined cavity. An elevated serum amylase level raises the possibility that pancreatic, duodenal, or proximal intestinal disruption has occurred.

Radiographic evaluation should routinely include a chest x-ray film and flat and upright films of the abdomen. Insufflation of the stomach with gas, either by having the patient drink a carbonated beverage or by injecting air down the nasogastric tube, often will demonstrate a lateral indentation caused by splenic or perisplenic masses or a fluid collection between the transverse colon and greater curvature of the stomach. X-ray studies used to investigate renal function and urinary tract pathology are intravenous pyelography, cystography, and, particularly in cases of pelvic fracture, retrograde urethrography.

Although physical examination remains the primary modality for evaluation of the abdomen after blunt trauma, associated injuries and an altered mental state often make it unreliable. Approximately 30% of individuals in major auto accidents will have brain injuries (i.e., concussion, contusion, or mass lesion) that prevent satisfactory evaluation. Likewise, cervical and thoracic spinal cord injuries leave the torso insensate below the lesion level. Another problem is the fact that approximately 50% of patients will have an altered mental status caused by substance abuse (i.e., alcohol or illicit drugs).

Diagnostic peritoneal lavage (DPL) and CT scanning have become important components in assessment of the bluntly traumatized abdomen. DPL can be performed by the open, semi-open, or closed techniques. The closed method offers the advantage of being faster, although there are fewer complications with the open technique (cutting down to and visualizing the peritoneum). After insertion of a dialysis-type catheter,

aspiration is attempted; if 10 ml of blood is obtained, the tap is considered grossly positive, and the procedure is terminated. When the minimal amount of blood cannot be aspirated, a liter of saline solution is instilled, and the patient is moved from side to side to mix the added fluid with any blood or intestinal contents that might be present. To be considered a valid test, approximately 700 ml of fluid must return when the empty crystalloid solution bag is placed below the abdomen and the fluid is allowed to drain by gravity. A sample is sent to the laboratory for determination of cell counts, and the result is considered positive with more than 100,000 red blood cells/mm^3 or 500 white blood cells (WBC)/mm^3. An elevated WBC count is usually indicative of small bowel injury; but if the DPL is performed within a few hours after injury, limited peritoneal inflammation will give a falsely negative result. The major criticism against DPL is its unreliability for retroperitoneal injuries and its 50% false-negative rate for diaphragmatic wounds.

CT scanning has an increasingly important role in evaluating blunt abdominal trauma. Its advantage over DPL is not only to detect blood within the abdomen, but also to define the severity of solid-organ injuries and retroperitoneal trauma. Under special circumstances, CT scanning allows observation rather than an immediate operation of minor liver and spleen injuries in hemodynamically stable patients who have small transfusion requirements. Problem areas for CT diagnosis include small bowel wounds (in only approximately 2% of patients with significant blunt abdominal injury), pancreatic trauma when the CT is carried out within the first few hours of injury, and in the diagnosis of diaphragmatic wounds. A major benefit of the CT scan is that it allows the simultaneous evaluation of associated genitourinary injuries, pelvic fractures, and head trauma. A practical resolution to the quandary of which test should be done first is application of CT for evaluation of the hemodynamically stable patient and DPL for the unstable patient with multiple injuries. Fig. 35-1 presents an algorithm for blunt abdominal management that uses both diagnostic techniques. Nevertheless, small bowel and pancreatic injuries remain difficult diagnostic problems and occasionally will be missed during the initial evaluation.

Diagnostic laparoscopy currently is being investigated for use with both penetrating and blunt injuries is an attempt to reduce the rate of

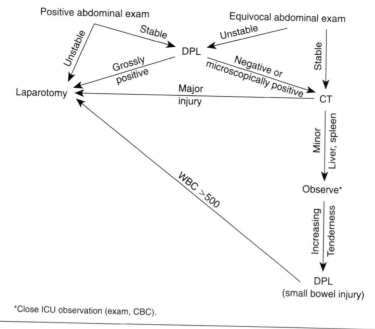

*Close ICU observation (exam, CBC).

FIGURE 35-1   Algorithm for assessment of the bluntly traumatized abdomen.

negative and nontherapeutic laparotomy. Potential applications for penetrating wounds include thoracoabdominal trajectory, tangential gunshot wounds and anterior abdominal stab wounds when peritoneal penetration is questionable. Laparoscopy may also be beneficial in further evaluating some blunt injuries already identified by CT. Potential complications are tension pneumothorax and air embolization.

Visualization of specific areas of the arterial tree, for example, by an aortic arch study, celiac or mesenteric arteriography, or aortography with hypogastric outflow (especially of fractures of the pelvis), is frequently helpful.

Preoperative Preparation

All patients undergoing emergency laparotomy for abdominal trauma should, whenever possible, have certain procedures carried out preoperatively:

- *Placement of an intravenous line:* Initially blood is drawn through a large-bore needle or catheter for baseline studies. Lactated Ringer's solution then is infused until a blood transfusion is available for those patients with trauma below the waist; leg veins are used for injuries above the diaphragm.

- *Administration of antibiotics:* Antibiotics in large doses are given immediately and then repeated every second drug half-life until the operation has been completed or until exploration reveals no intraperitoneal soilage. Cephalosporins are generally chosen because of their wide antibacterial spectrum and low incidence of toxicity and allergy.

- *Insertion of Foley catheter:* Urinary output is monitored at regular intervals as a guide to adequacy of blood and fluid volume replacement.

- *Insertion of nasogastric tube:* A nasogastric tube is passed in an attempt to decompress the stomach and thus lessen chances of aspirating vomitus during induction of anesthesia.

- *X-ray examination:* Routine preoperative studies should include a chest film, x-ray studies of the abdomen, and, selectively, an intravenous pyelogram whenever urgency is not so great as to preclude delay.

Operation

A generous abdominal incision should always be made to allow for a thorough inspection of all potentially injured organs. Most surgeons prefer the full midline approach, although a transverse incision offers almost equal exposure with fewer wound-related postoperative problems.

Immediately after abdominal entry, major bleeding is controlled by direct pressure or pack and then by clamp. Evisceration of the small bowel is generally required for more complete exposure of wounds involving the larger vessels. Once hemorrhage has been controlled and the injured vessels either ligated or repaired, attention can be directed toward examination of the other abdominal viscera, first as a search for co-existent injuries and then for appropriate management of the specific wounds encountered.

TRAUMATIC INJURIES OF OTHER AREAS

Wounds frequently involve more than one organ system and often more than a single body cavity. Immediate attention must always be given to those injuries that impair the cardiorespiratory system, then to those of major vascular structures, and finally to all remaining significant injuries, with priority given to those perforations causing the greatest contamination. The following sections list areas of injury and their appropriate treatment.

Chest

- *Pneumothorax:* If definitely present (plus potential to develop while patient is under anesthesia), requires tube thoracostomy
- *Hemothorax:* Tube thoracostomy, with selective exploration for definite major vascular trauma or continued intrathoracic bleeding
- *Cardiac tamponade:* Pericardiocentesis, then exploratory pericardotomy
- *Esophagus:* Repair after demonstration by radiopaque contrast swallow
- *Diaphragm:* Repair

Skull

- *Wound:* Debridement, primary closure
- *Intracranial bleeding:* Observation (level of consciousness, vital signs, and change in neurologic deficits); selective arrest of hemorrhage and evacuation of hematomas
- *Cerebrospinal fluid leaks:* Closure as soon as possible

Spine

- *Fractures:* Stabilization as soon as possible, preferably at scene of accident
- *Cord injury:* Stabilization of spine, selective laminectomy

Fracture or Dislocation

- *Stabilization:* Maintenance of reduction or, if not reduced, prevention of further tissue damage
- *Hemorrhage:* Replacement of blood volume losses (Table 35-5); selective angiography for suspected major vascular injury
- *Reduction:* Attempt at closed reduction with traction initially, although open reduction may be required
- *Open fracture:* Urgent debridement of wound, followed by closure
- *Ischemia:* Close observation of limbs for development of compartmental swelling and thus ischemia, preferably by direct compartment pressure measurement at frequent intervals for specific high-risk areas (e.g., anterior leg compartment in patients with femoral or popliteal arterial injury); fasciotomy as warranted

Pelvic Fracture or Dislocation

- Evaluate for perforation of bladder (cystography), urethra (retrograde urethrography), or rectum (blood in the rectum on sigmoidoscopy).
- Application of medical anti-shock trousers (MAST) or a G-suit may lessen pelvic bleeding initially.
- To lessen the risk of continued or massive bleeding, especially in Malgaigne open-book fractures, the external pelvic fixator should be applied as soon as possible after the diagnosis of an unstable or displaced pelvic fracture has been made.
- Angiography may be required to identify continued major bleeding from injury to the hypogastric arteries or their branches (especially with Malgaigne's fracture or dislocation of the sacroiliac joint) despite bone stabilization with the external fixator. If major bleeding is present, control is gained best by angiographic em-

TABLE 35-5 Average Blood Loss in Major Fractures of Extremities*

	Closed (Simple)	Open (Compound)
Forearm	5	10
Arm	10	15
Leg	10	20
Thigh	20	40

*In percent of total blood volume.

bolization of both hypogastric arteries. Open operation to ligate the hypogastric arteries should be avoided unless penetrating trauma was the cause.

Extremities

- *Evaluate:* Investigate for skeletal, vascular, and nerve injury
- *Manage:* According to injury

Cervical Spine

- In the neurologically (spinal cord) intact patient with cervical spine injury, it is imperative that diagnosis be made promptly to prevent iatrogenic cord injury. All patients must be assumed to have an injury and accordingly should have cervical immobilization (cervical collar and backboard) beginning at the accident scene and continuing until the injury has been ruled out. In the totally alert patient evaluation begins with palpation of the spine to detect cervical tenderness. With unevaluable patients or those in whom injury is suspected, cross-table lateral x-ray studies should be obtained as soon as the patient is stable. Radiographic evaluation considers both the gentle lordotic curve along the anterior and posterior portions of the vertebral body and the spinous processes. Pedicles, transverse processes, and intervertebral foramina should be symmetric. The prevertebral fat strips should be clear, without widening of the space between the spine and the pharyngotracheal air column (hematoma indicating fracture of ligamentous injury). Anteroposterior and odontoid x-ray films should also be obtained after the initial evaluation. Any tenderness or subtle abnormality demands further investigation by cervical CT scan despite near normal x-ray films.
- Airway management in the patient with documented or suspected cervical spine injury is done with in-line traction maintained by an assistant. When possible, nasotracheal intubation provides the safest technique. However, if it is unsuccessful, orotracheal intubation can be done. Cricothyroidotomy is the preferred approach if these other techniques are unsuccessful. Flexion of the neck should *never* be done, although minor extension is acceptable if emergent access is required to prevent arrest.
- Patients with cervical cord injury often present with hypotension, bradycardia, and warm skin (often incorrectly termed *spinal shock*) as a result of interrupted sympathetic nerve fibers in the cervical and upper thoracic region. If hypotension or bradycardia becomes hemodynamically significant because of inadequate perfusion, low-dose catecholamine support or atropine may be required. Significant improvement in outcome of those patients with cord injury may be achieved by providing large-dose, short-course steroid therapy begun as soon as possible after the injury.

Neck

- *Evaluate:* Investigate for vascular injury, perforation of the pharynx, larynx, trachea, and esophagus; never overlook frequently associated spinal cord, brachial plexus, and intrathoracic injuries
- *Manage:* According to injury

Face

- Stabilize other body systems first, with special attention to the airway. Determine presence of injury to paranasal sinuses and facial bones; control bleeding; protect the eyes; and conserve tissue. Definitive repair can be delayed for as long as 24 to 48 hours.

Other Areas

- Wounds involving other areas of the body are managed according to the extent and type of tissue injury, magnitude of contamination, and urgency of associated trauma.

POSTOPERATIVE COMPLICATIONS

The 10 most common complications after operations for trauma are:

1. *Infection:* Primarily of the wound and/or body cavities explored, but also pneumonia, urinary tract infection, and phlebitis (Fig. 35-2)
2. *Pulmonary insufficiency:* Multiple potential origins (e.g., pulmonary or remote infection, stress, fluid overload or heart failure, pulmonary capillary trapping of particulate matter, retained secretions, pneumonia)
3. *Renal failure:* Caused by gram-negative infection, renal ischemia and/or nephrotoxic drugs, remote infection
4. *Bleeding diathesis:* Multiple transfusions, washout phenomena, overt and masked transfusion reactions, coagulation factor deficits and fibrinolysins, remote infections

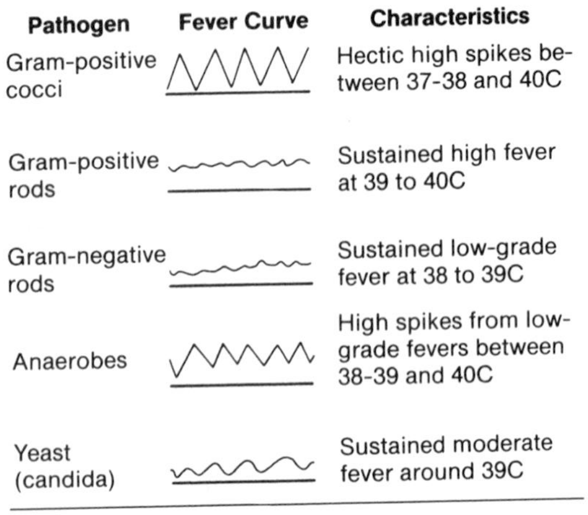

Pathogen	Fever Curve	Characteristics
Gram-positive cocci		Hectic high spikes between 37-38 and 40C
Gram-positive rods		Sustained high fever at 39 to 40C
Gram-negative rods		Sustained low-grade fever at 38 to 39C
Anaerobes		High spikes from low-grade fevers between 38-39 and 40C
Yeast (candida)		Sustained moderate fever around 39C

FIGURE 35-2 Clinical differentiation of type of sepsis by the fever curve.

5. *Wound disruption:* Often caused by wound infection, but favored by profound adynamic ileus, pulmonary problems, and delirium tremens
6. *Paralytic ileus:* If persistent, suspect peritonitis, potassium depletion, and wound dehiscence
7. *Phlebitis:* Can be a septic focus, causing unexplained bacteremia, or can be bland, with a high incidence of pulmonary embolism
8. *Urinary tract obstruction:* Almost always at the level of the bladder neck or in the urethra; usually caused by preexisting disease, although can be caused by periurethral abscess
9. *Allergic reactions:* Common after transfusions of blood or blood products and antibiotic therapy, particularly penicillin and sulfonamides
10. *Pressure necrosis:* Over bony prominences (ischial tuberosities, sacrum, and femoral trochanters); also noted in areas adjacent to any firm, indwelling apparatus (Fig. 35-3)

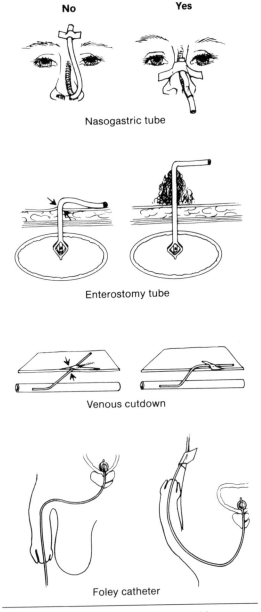

Nasogastric tube

Enterostomy tube

Venous cutdown

Foley catheter

FIGURE 35-3 Pressure necrosis caused by indwelling pieces of medical equipment.

BIBLIOGRAPHY

American College of Surgeons. Early Care of the Injured Patient. Philadelphia, WB Saunders, 1982.

American College of Surgeons, Committee on Trauma. Resources for Optimal Care of the Injured Patient. Chicago, 1990.

Briggs SE, Hendricks D, et al. Penetrating abdominal trauma. Adv Surg (in press).

Martin JD, Haynes CD, Hatcher CR Jr, et al. Trauma to the Thorax and Abdomen. Springfield, Ill, Charles C Thomas, 1969.

Maull KI. Advances in Trauma and Critical Care, Vol 6. St Louis, Mosby–Year Book, 1991.

Moulton RJ, Clifton GL. Injury to the vertebrae and spinal cord. In Moore EE, Mattox KL, Feliciano DV (eds). Trauma. Norwalk, Conn, Appleton & Lange, 1988.

Richardson JD, Polk HC Jr, Flint LM (eds). Trauma: Clinical Care and Pathophysiology. Chicago, Year Book Medical Publishers, 1987.

Shaftan G, Gardner B. Quick Reference to Surgical Emergencies. Philadelphia, JB Lippincott, 1985.

Trunkey DD, Lewis FR Jr. Current Therapy of Trauma. St Louis, CV Mosby, 1984.

Chapter Review Questions

1. A 30-year-old man is struck by a car and sustains multiple injuries. Indicate the order of priority in diagnosis and treatment for the following injuries:
   a. Dislocated cervical spine
   b. Fractured skull
   c. Flail chest
   d. Ruptured spleen
   e. Laceration of the face
2. a. What is the best means of diagnosing a tension pneumothorax quickly?
   b. Why is simple pneumothorax potentially lethal in a multiple trauma victim?
3. Blunt trauma to the right anterior lower rib cage is likely to produce which of the following?
   a. Liver laceration
   b. Hemoperitoneum
   c. Hemopneumothorax
   d. Hematuria
4. Shock associated with long-bone fractures is most commonly due to:
   a. Neural reflexes
   b. Fat embolism
   c. Hypovolemia
   d. Myocardial contusion
5. Rupture of the bladder occurs most commonly in association with:
   a. Lower abdominal gunshot wounds
   b. Blunt seatbelt trauma
   c. Pelvic fracture
   d. Iatrogenic instrumentation
6. For the uncertain cervical spine injury, which method is most reliable at providing the diagnosis?
   a. Flexion-extension x-ray studies of the cervical spine
   b. Vertebral arteriography
   c. CT scan of cervical spine
   d. Cervical myelography
7. Pancreatic injury caused by blunt abdominal trauma is identified best by:
   a. Elevated serum amylase level
   b. Diagnostic peritoneal lavage
   c. Endoscopic retrograde cholangiopancreatography (ERCP)
   d. CT scan of the abdomen

Answers

1. c, a, b, d, e
2. a. Determine tracheal deviation and air under pressure by inserting a needle in the chest.
   b. If the patient will be operated on or placed on a ventilator, the positive pressure ventilation used may convert a simple pneumothorax to a tension pneumothorax. A chest tube should be inserted prophylactically.
3. a
4. c
5. c
6. c
7. d

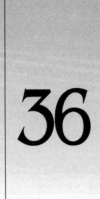

36 Burns

ROGER W. YURT

KEY FEATURES

After reading this chapter you will understand:
- The effect of a burn injury on the organism.
- Measurement of the extent of a burn injury.
- Resuscitation of the burn patient and other emergent measures.
- Wound management.

The disruption of homeostasis that occurs with major burn injury leads to a clinical state that is one of the most challenging in modern medicine. Not only is the clinician faced with the immediate concerns of loss of integrity of body surfaces and fluid but also with the sequelae of activation of mediator cascades that lead to immunocompromise, infection, hypermetabolism, and organ failure. Each patient who sustains major burn injury requires the attention of dedicated surgeons, nursing staff, therapists, and institution-wide support. These individual needs, combined with the number of patients who sustain burn injury (over 12,000 deaths in the United States each year), emphasize the importance of a dedicated approach to the care of the burn injured patient. The regionalization of burn care over the past 20 years has begun to fulfill these needs; nevertheless, all surgeons are challenged with the initial care and resuscitation of these patients and occasionally with long-term care as well.

WHAT PATHOPHYSIOLOGIC CHANGES ARE ASSOCIATED WITH BURN INJURY?

Although burn injury is commonly thought of as a thermal destruction of tissue, it may also be caused by agents that are toxic to tissues. The common denominator of the injury, nevertheless, is destruction of cells and the extracellular matrix. The extent of tissue injury is directly related to the duration of exposure and the intensity of the source, whether this is flame, hot liquid, radiation, or an electrical or caustic source. Current data suggest that tissue destruction associated with burn injury occurs as an immediate, direct denaturation of tissue and a component that evolves in the hours after injury. This dynamic aspect of the wound is related to both the local effects of inflammatory mediators and the circulation to and in the tissue.

Within minutes of large surface burn injury (i.e., greater than 30% of the body surface area) the effects of fluid loss and sequestration are evident clinically. Intravascular fluid shifts to the extracellular space as well as to the external environment as a result of increased capillary permeability. Furthermore, fluid shifts to the intracellular space as a result of the effects of poor tissue perfusion and/or inflammatory mediators and cytokines. These changes occur not only in the injured tissues but also in adjacent and distant tissues as well. All of *these changes combine to form an obligate loss of electrolyte-containing fluid from the intravascular space;* as the changes progress, the loss is manifested as decreased tissue perfusion followed by hypotension. This shift of fluid to the extravascular space continues for the first 24 hours after injury in an appropriately resuscitated patient. However, if resuscitation is delayed more than 1 to 2 hours, the fluid losses are greater and may continue over a prolonged period.

Maintenance of body temperature is a problem in a patient who has sustained burns. The loss of body heat associated with evaporative water loss is compounded in the early period after injury by the administration of large volumes of room-temperature fluids. Within 24 to 48 hours after injury, the patient with surface area burns greater than 25% to 30% becomes hypermetabolic. This increase in metabolism is manifested by increases in cardiac output, renal blood flow, and increased core body temperature. The metabolic rate of patients with large burns approaches twice normal. That at least part of the increased metabolic rate is related to a central resetting of thermoregulatory control is suggested by the fact that patients seek a higher external environmental temperature for comfort. To avoid further increases in metabolic rate that would be driven by a disparity in core temperature and environmental temperature, it is usually necessary to provide an environmental temperature of 33° C (91° F) for these patients. These patients will typically have a core body temperature that is elevated by 1 to 2 degrees, such that *their expected body temperature is 38° to 38.5° C* (100.4° to 101.3° F).

In addition to the cutaneous injury, one must be aware of the possibility of *pulmonary injury* and the dysfunction associated with it. Injury to the respiratory tract occurs when products of combustion enter the airways. It is extremely rare for this injury to be the result of direct heat, with the possible exception of injuries such as those caused by direct steam inhalation. The toxicity of smoke is related to its content of carbon monoxide and noxious chemicals. While carbon monoxide has the systemic effects of displacing oxygen from hemoglobin and interfering with respiratory enzyme function, the other effects of smoke inhalation primarily relate to the direct injury to the airways. These effects are manifested *early after injury as edema of the pharynx, with possible upper airway obstruction and hypoxemia* if the distal bronchial tree is injured. *Delayed effects include progressive pulmonary dysfunction,* structural damage (such as tracheomalacia), and infection.

HOW IS THE EXTENT OF BURN INJURY MEASURED?

Cutaneous burn injury is measured by both depth of injury of tissues and by the amount of surface area injured. While it is quite easy to discriminate a superficial burn from a deep full-thickness burn, an intermediate-depth injury is often difficult to assess. The *partial-thickness* or superficial burn involves the outer layers of the epidermis but leaves the deeper layers intact. Clinically this is seen as a blistered pink and weeping wound that is painful to the touch (i.e., cutaneous nerves are intact). In the absence of infection and with adequate circulation, these wounds will heal within 1 to 2 weeks. The deeper *full-thickness burn* destroys all of the epidermis and the skin appendages. Physical examination reveals a gray leathery appearance, often with thrombosed veins visible, and the skin is inelastic and insensate. These wounds do not heal primarily, but only by contraction and epithelialization from the peripheral uninjured skin. The intermediate-depth burn, often called a *deep partial-thickness* burn, is seen histologically as destruction of the epidermis as well as some of the dermis such that only epidermal elements of skin appendages are spared. On clinical examination the injured skin is intermediate in appearance between deep and superficial injury. Pain sensation may be intact in splotchy areas. Although the skin may be whitish, there is no gross evidence of vascular thrombosis. There is a greater chance that the wound will be deep partial thickness rather than full thickness in those areas of the body where skin is the thickest, such as the back and soles of the feet. However, *the only absolute criterion that can be used to determine this depth of injury is that it will heal within 2 to 3 weeks if infection does not occur.* At least some of the difficulty in evaluating the depth of injury is likely related to the early evolution of the wound. Inadequate or delayed resuscitation may cause such an injury to convert to full-thickness injury, just as infection will. Depth of burn injury is summarized in Fig. 36-1.

Just as depth of injury has implications regarding the potential for the wound to heal, *the amount of surface injury* has implications with regard to resuscitation and prognosis. The area of surface of skin that is injured is estimated by the "rule of nines" (see Fig. 36-2). The upper extremities and head each account for 9% of the *total body surface area (TBSA).* The anterior torso, posterior torso, and lower extremities each can

DEPTH OF BURN

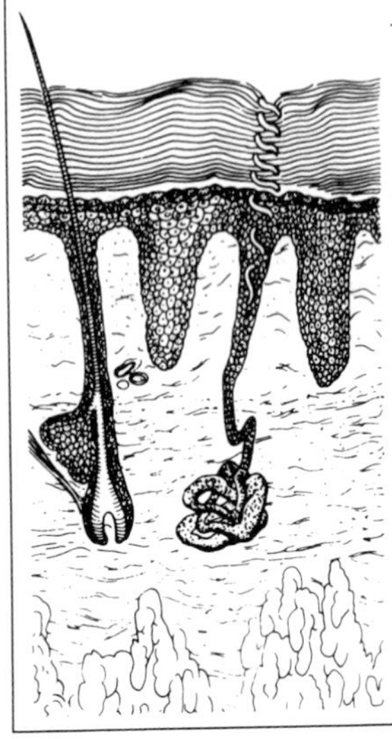

		Usual cause	Gross pathology	Micropathology	Main problems	Uncomplicated healing by
Epidermal		Radiation (sunlight)	Erythema; tiny intra-dermal blebs	Partial epithelial destruction; all rete pegs spared	Pain	Spontaneous epithelial regeneration from skin appendages
Dermal: Partial thickness	Super-ficial	Scald	Erythema; large blebs, bullae	Partial epidermal and dermal destruction; some rete pegs spared	Fluid losses, infection, pain	Spontaneous epithelial regeneration from rete pegs
	Deep	Scald or flame	Patchy erythema; blebs and bullae	Total epidermal and partial dermal destruction; skin appendages spared	Fluid losses, infection, pain	Spontaneous epithelial regeneration from basilar cells
Full thickness		Flame	Charred; blanched	All dermis and epidermis destroyed	Fluid losses, infection, closure	Contracture or skin graft

FIGURE 36-1 The diagram depicts the skin and the layers that are injured on various depths of injury.

be estimated to be 18% of the TBSA. Although this method allows for a good initial estimate of surface area of burn, it is not as accurate as the surface areas listed in Fig. 36-3. Such a chart should be used when evaluating children. In particular, note the relatively large surface area contribution of the head in a child compared with an adult.

ELECTRICAL INJURY

Contact with sources of electrical current can cause injury as a result of the associated flash, which is like any other thermal injury, as well as from the direct effect of the flow of current through body tissues. Current will flow preferentially through the path of least resistance. Muscle, nerve, and vessels are relatively good conductors. High-voltage sources cause denaturation of these tissues, and charring can be seen with these deep injuries. *The primary concern in these injuries is the deep, unseen injury that may occur.* Loss of function in the extremities and/or early increase in muscle compartment pressures indicates muscle damage. Myoglobinuria is a sign of muscle injury. It may present as dark red urine; however, in lower concentrations it is not visible. Life-threatening dysrhythmias can occur at the time of electrical injury or afterward as a result of damage to the conduction system of the heart. Visceral injury may occur

as well. Patients who have sustained electrical shock should have a full radiologic evaluation of the spine and involved extremities, since the *intense muscular contraction associated with electrical injury can cause fractures.*

PULMONARY INJURY

When a patient has been in a fire in a closed space, it should be assumed that he or she has sustained an inhalation injury. Signs of inhalation injury include singed nasal vibrissae, carbonaceous sputum, and hoarseness. Elevated levels of carboxyhemoglobin in the blood will confirm exposure to carbon monoxide. All patients who are suspected of having an inhalation injury should undergo *early fiberoptic bronchoscopy.* Findings of erythema and edema indicate injury to the upper airway. An endotracheal tube should be placed over the endoscope before bronchoscopy is performed so that if there is impending obstruction of the airway the tube may be passed over the scope under direct vision. Delay in controlling the airway can lead to great difficulty in intubating the trachea at a later time when edema becomes extensive.

Injury to the distal airways is difficult to document. Chest x-ray films do not usually show a change in the early period after injury. Xenon-133 ventilation/perfusion lung scan, if done within 72 hours after injury, will confirm paren-

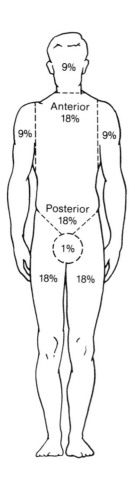

FIGURE 36-2 The percentage of the body surface area that is burned can be estimated by the rule of nines. (From Yurt RW, Pruitt BA. Burns. In Gardner G, Shafton GW [eds]. Quick Reference to Surgical Emergencies. Philadelphia, JB Lippincott, 1986.)

AGE VS AREA

Area	Birth-1 yr	1-4 yr	5-9 yr	10-14 yr	15 yr	Adult	Second-degree	Third-degree	Total	Donor areas
Head	19	17	13	11	9	7				
Neck	2	2	2	2	2	2				
Ant. trunk	13	13	13	13	13	13				
Post. trunk	13	13	13	13	13	13				
R. buttock	2½	2½	2½	2½	2½	2½				
L. buttock	2½	2½	2½	2½	2½	2½				
Genitalia	1	1	1	1	1	1				
R. U. arm	4	4	4	4	4	4				
L. U. arm	4	4	4	4	4	4				
R. L. arm	3	3	3	3	3	3				
L. L. arm	3	3	3	3	3	3				
R. hand	2½	2½	2½	2½	2½	2½				
L. hand	2½	2½	2½	2½	2½	2½				
R. thigh	5½	6½	8	8½	9	9½				
L. thigh	5½	6½	8	8½	9	9½				
R. leg	5	5	5½	6	6½	7				
L. leg	5	5	5½	6	6½	7				
R. foot	3½	3½	3½	3½	3½	3½				
L. foot	3½	3½	3½	3½	3½	3½				
						TOTAL				

FIGURE 36-3 A more exact determination of the surface area of burn can be made using an age-adjusted chart. (From Yurt RW, Pruitt BA. Burns. In Gardner B, Shafton GW [eds]. Quick Reference to Surgical Emergencies. Philadelphia, JB Lippincott, 1986.)

chymal injury when it reveals normal vascular perfusion but localized retention of labeled gas in air spaces. Neither this evaluation nor any other presently available is able to give a quantitative determination of extent of pulmonary injury.

WHAT ARE THE FIRST STEPS IN BURN PATIENT CARE?
Cardiopulmonary Resuscitation

As with all trauma patients, the initial approach to the patient with a burn injury should include evaluation and maintenance of the airway. Intubation in the field or in the emergency room is not necessary immediately unless there is evidence of compromise of the airway (see Pulmonary injury, p. 622). However, anyone who may have an inhalation injury should be administered 100% oxygen. On atmospheric air it takes approximately 4 hours to decrease the carboxyhemoglobin level by one half, whereas this occurs in about 40 minutes on 100% oxygen. Patients with high-voltage electrical injury should have electrocardiographic monitoring continuously for the first 48 hours after injury.

The Burn Wound

All clothing should be removed, especially that which is hot and smoldering. The patient should be covered with a clean sheet and blankets to maintain body temperature. Although application of cold compresses or water to burned areas within 10 minutes of injury will ease the pain of partial-thickness burns and assist in dissipation of the heat in the tissue, this method should be used sparingly in the patient with large burns because of concern for decrease in body temperature.

In patients with chemical burns, all areas of injury are exposed and irrigated with clear water or saline. Immediate and continuous lavage of an injured eye with saline is of utmost importance.

Intravenous Access

If transportation of a patient with a large burn will take 30 minutes or more, a large-bore intravenous catheter should be inserted. Although it is preferable to place the cannula at a site of uninjured skin, if necessary, it is inserted through burned tissue. Early after injury central venous access is not necessary and should not be performed in an uncontrolled situation. Isotonic crystalloid fluids should be administered as estimates of total fluid requirements are being made.

WHERE SHOULD A BURN PATIENT BE CARED FOR?

Once initial care has been administered and the extent of burn estimated either in the prehospital or emergency room phase of care, a determination of where the patient should be cared for is made. The triage criteria and definition of extent of injury, as outlined by the American Burn Association* (ABA), are as follows:

- *Major burn injury.* Second-degree burns of greater than 25% BSA in adults (20% in children), all third-degree burns of 10% BSA or greater; all significant burns involving the hands, face, eyes, ears, feet, perineum; all patients with significant inhalation injury, high voltage electrical burns, and burn injury complicated by fractures, or other major trauma; and all poor-risk patients should be admitted and cared for at a burn unit or burn center.
- *Moderate uncomplicated burn injury.* Patients with second-degree burns of 15% to 25% BSA in adults (10% to 20% in children) with less than 10% BSA third-degree burn should be cared for at a hospital with special expertise in burn care or at a burn unit.
- *Minor burn injury.* Patients with second-degree burn of less than 15% BSA in adults (10% in children) and third-degree burn less than 2% BSA may be treated by primary physicians both on an emergency basis and in a follow-up role.

FLUID RESUSCITATION

Since patients with large surface area burns will require large volumes of fluid, especially during the first 24 hours after injury, it is of value to use guidelines for the administration of fluids. However, it cannot be overemphasized that these *guidelines serve only as an estimate* and that adequacy of resuscitation should be evaluated on the basis of the physiologic state of the patient. Although there are several methods currently in use that give estimates of volume and type of

---

*American Burn Association. Specific optimal criteria for hospital resources for care of patients with burn injury. Birmingham, Ala, 1967.

TABLE 36-1 Estimates of Fluid Requirements for Patients With Burns: The First 24 Hours

	Colloid (ml)	Crystalloid (ml)	Water (ml)
Brooke	0.5 × wt × %	1.5 × wt × %	2000
Modified Brooke	—	3 × wt × %	—
Parkland	—	4 × wt × %	—

wt = weight in kg; % = % of body surface burn.

fluid required (see Table 36-1), the most commonly used formula is that known as the Baxter or Parkland formula. This formula is crystalloid based, as are the others; colloid-containing fluids are not administered during the early period after injury, since they will leak out of the intravascular space and may contribute to sequestration of fluid in the extravascular space after the leak has resolved. Dextrose-containing solutions are not given to avoid hyperglycemia. The Parkland formula is based on the use of isotonic fluid, as is the modified Brooke formula. Others have been successful in resuscitating patients with lower total volumes of fluid (and therefore with less edema) by using hypertonic saline solutions; however, hypernatremia can be a serious complication of this method and must be guarded against.

The Parkland formula as listed in Table 36-1 is used as in the following example: A patient who weighs 70 kg and has a burn that covers 50% of his body surface (only partial or second-degree and full-thickness or third-degree burn area is used) can be estimated to require 70 × 50 × 4 or 14,000 ml of lactated Ringer's solution in the first 24 hours after injury. Seven liters will be required in the first 8 hours after injury (approximately 875 ml/hr) and 7 L in the following 16 hours (approximately 400 ml/hr). Urine output is used as the guide to adjust fluid administration. In an adult the fluids should be regulated such that a urine output of 30 to 50 ml/hr is maintained. The goal in children is to maintain a urine output of 1 to 2 ml/kg/hr. If myoglobinuria is present or there is concern that it may occur (electrical burns and/or increased compartment pressures), fluids should be adjusted to approximately double the hourly output (100 ml/hr in adults; 2 ml/kg/hr in children).

In the following 24 hours after the capillary leak is resolved, patients with large burns should be given colloid to replace those losses. An estimate for replacement is between 0.3 and 0.5 ml per kilogram per percent of burn. In the example

given, the patient would be given 0.5 × 70 × 50 or 1750 ml of plasma during the second 24-hour period along with sufficient water to cover maintenance requirements and evaporative losses.

CONTINUING FLUID REQUIREMENTS

Except for those patients with extremely large burns (>80% BSA) or those who were poorly resuscitated, the capillary leak resolves by approximately 24 hours after injury. Nevertheless, there is an ongoing fluid loss via evaporation from the wounds. These losses have been measured and can be estimated as:

Loss of water (ml/hour) = (25 + % burn) × TBSA

where TBSA is equal to total body surface area in square meters. Fluid loss is replaced with 5% dextrose in water. Once again, this is a guideline or an estimate and must be adjusted based on clinical evaluation. Urinary output should be monitored hourly and plasma sodium concentration should be assessed on a regular basis.

CARE OF THE BURN WOUND
Outpatients

Patients with small areas of burn who do not meet criteria for hospital admission (see ABA criteria) are treated with topical antimicrobials such as silver sulfadiazine. The wound is initially cleared of debris, and blisters that are large enough that they are likely to spontaneously drain (larger than the size of a quarter) are debrided. Smaller blisters can be left intact as a biologic dressing. The wound should be rinsed with clear water twice daily. If the wound is contaminated, silver sulfadiazine is kept on it at all times. The wound need not be covered with a dressing; however, it is often necessary to do so to protect it from additional injury and to keep the topical agent on the wound. Because of the likelihood of infection and the inability to follow the wound regularly, outpatients are usually given systemic prophylaxis against infection with an oral penicillin.

Large Burn Wounds

Once the patient has been initially stabilized, the burn wounds are washed with clean water and loose necrotic tissue and blisters are debrided. This may be done in the operating room but can be done in any area that allows copious rinsing and debridement. Analgesics should be given by the intravenous route, since distribution of drugs is unpredictable in a patient with erratic perfusion of tissue. After the surface area of burn and depth are estimated the wounds are covered with a topical antimicrobial agent such as silver sulfadiazine. In general the open method of wound care is used; that is, wounds are covered with topical antimicrobials but otherwise not covered with gauze or dressings except where necessary to hold splints in position. The advantages of the open method are that the wound can be easily observed, physical therapy is facilitated, and patients can be encouraged to use injured body parts. The disadvantage is that topical agents have to be reapplied frequently.

The primary goal in the patient with large burns is to achieve wound closure as soon as possible. In so doing the chance of burn wound infection is minimized and the duration of the hypermetabolic response is decreased. As soon as the patient is stable, full-thickness burn wounds should be excised and grafted. The extent of excision of wounds at each operative procedure may be limited by the availability of autologous donor skin, the degree of cardiovascular stability, and the availability of alternative methods of wound coverage. In general, excision of 10% to 20% of the body surface area is well tolerated when performed by a team of surgeons and anesthesiologists who are trained in the care of the burned patient. Much larger excisions have been successful and have the advantage of eliminating a majority or all of the potentially infected tissues; however, a well-planned method for coverage of the wound is necessary and often includes use of allograft and cultured autologous skin.

Since the first objective with regard to the wounds of patients with life-threatening burn injury is to reduce the amount of wound as soon as possible, excisions are prioritized to address

closure first and function second. Nevertheless, maintenance and restoration of function should always be addressed through early and continuing physical therapy and surgical intervention as soon as possible.

Circumferential Full-Thickness Burns

The combination of the loss of elasticity of skin that has sustained full-thickness burn and the accumulation of fluid in both injured and uninjured tissue sets the stage for compromise of blood flow in the underlying tissue. Any time a burn encompasses the circumference of an extremity, the circulation must be carefully evaluated at least hourly during the period of resuscitation. If the distal extremity is uninjured, capillary refill can be used to assess perfusion. Blood

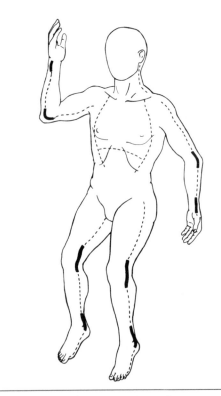

FIGURE 36-4   The correct sites to locate escharotomies are depicted in the figure. If circumferential burns involve the joint space escharotomies should be performed there as well. (From Yurt RW, Pruitt BA. Burns. In Gardner B, Shafton GW [eds]. Quick Reference to Surgical Emergencies. Philadelphia, JB Lippincott, 1986.)

pressure is an unreliable indicator of tissue perfusion and although Doppler blood flow assessment is routinely performed it may not detect significant diminution of muscular blood flow. At the first sign of decrease in perfusion of an extremity, escharotomies should be performed. The incision should be made through the full thickness of the wound on the lateral and medial aspects of the extremity (Fig. 36-4) including joints. It is unusual to have to release the eschar on the torso, but occasionally pressure under eschar can become high enough to compromise expansion of the chest wall, at which time escharotomy may be necessary (see Fig. 36-4).

Infected Burn Wounds

Daily evaluation of burn wounds is the key to early detection of burn wound infection. Signs of infection include softening of the eschar, change in color or hemorrhage in the eschar, and/or erythema at the wound margin. In addition, suspicious wounds should be biopsied for culture. Most burn centers have a routine biopsy protocol for full-thickness biopsy of wounds 2 to 3 times per week. Invasive burn wound infection occurs when 10^6 or greater microorganisms are present in each gram of tissue. Therefore, if wounds begin to approach this level or exceed it, the infection must be eradicated. Although antibiotics can be administered directly into the infected wound by clysis, the preferred approach is surgical excision of the infected wound to the level of viable tissue. If fungal infection is suspected, this can be documented by biopsy with histologic evaluation for presence of hyphae.

CALORIC REQUIREMENTS

As already mentioned, patients become hypermetabolic after major injuries. In patients with large burns the metabolic rate may be double that of normal. If exogenous calories are not sufficient to maintain this increase in metabolic rate, the endogenous stores including protein will be utilized. It is unusual for a patient with a large burn injury to be able to take in sufficient calories to meet his or her needs; therefore, supplemental feeding is provided. This is usually provided as enteral feeding through a soft silastic nasogastric/duodenal tube. During periods when enteral feeding is not tolerated, the caloric requirements are provided via total parenteral nutrition. The daily caloric requirements can be estimated by adding the basal requirements to those required by the excess metabolism. In adults the calculation is:

$$25 \text{ kcal/kg} + 40 \text{ kcal/\% burn}$$

In children the basal requirements are supplemented by 15 kcal/% burn up to 1 year of age, 25 kcal/% burn for ages 1 to 3, and 40 kcal/% burn for ages 3 to 15.

PITFALLS AND COMMON MYTHS

- The formulas used to estimate fluid resuscitation requirements are often used as an absolute determinant for administration of fluid. This approach is incorrect. The adequacy of fluid administration should be evaluated based on the patient's physiologic response.
- There is a tendency to overestimate the extent of surface area burn. Completely disrobe the patient and assess carefully when making an initial "rule of nines" estimate and follow up with a diagram and calculation of the percent of surface area burned.
- Always assume that a patient has had an inhalation injury if he or she is injured in an enclosed space.

SURGICAL PHARMACOPEIA

Drug	Indications	Complications	Dosage
Morphine sulfate	Pain control of the severely burned patient	Use only IV, because IM doses are absorbed erratically in burn patients. Primary side effect is respiratory depression. Maximum respiratory depression may occur up to 30 minutes after receiving an IV dose. Use only in closely monitored situations.	Initial dose 2-10 mg IV/70 kg; may supplement as needed for adequate control
Sodium bicarbonate	Use to alkalinize urine in patients with myoglobinurea to prevent tubular precipitation of this acidic molecule (keep urine pH > 7.0)		1 ampule of sodium bicarbonate (44 mEq/50 ml ampule) as an IV bolus; then add 1 to 2 ampules to each liter of IV fluids for forced diuresis
Topical Antimicrobials			
Silver sulfadiazine (Silvadene)	Second-degree burns or unexcised third-degree burn wounds of the body and scalp	Reversible neutropenia. May not be appropriate to use over large areas in patients with serious infections. Soothing to the burned area. Patients with sulfa allergy may be sensitive to it.	Topical application of cream q8h
Sulfamylon (Mefamide)	Second-degree burns or unexcised third-degree wounds of the nose and ears	Metabolic acidosis. Superior penetration makes it the best for avascular cartilaginous structures. Is often painful when applied to second-degree burns. Patients with sulfa allergy may be sensitive to it.	Topical application of cream q8h
Neosporin or bacitracin ointment	Second-degree burns or unexcised third-degree burn wounds of the face		Topical application of ointment q8h

Drug	Indications	Complications	Dosage
Tetanus toxoid	Indicated for all burn patients if their most recent booster was more than 1 year before injury and they had undergone prior immunization		0.5 ml IM
Antacids			
Alternogel (Mylanta)	Used to prevent Curling's ulcers	Administer through nasogastric tube to all patients with more than 20% TBSA burns to keep gastric aspirate at pH >5.0. If pH is difficult to control or there is a prior history of peptic ulcer disease, one should add parenteral H_2-blocker. Most frequent complication is diarrhea with magnesium- and constipation with aluminum-based antacids.	30-60 ml of antacids per nasogastric tube (clamp ½ h) q3h; may increase dosage up to 90 ml or decrease time interval between doses as needed to maintain pH >5.0

BIBLIOGRAPHY

Cryer HG, Anigian GM, Miller FB, et al. Effects of early tangential excision and grafting on survival after burn injury. Surg Gynecol Obstet 173:449, 1991.

Heimbach D, Engrav L, Grube B, Marvin J. Burn depth: A review. World J Surg 16:10, 1992.

Warden GD. Burn shock resuscitation. World J Surg 16:16, 1992.

Waymack JP, Herndon DN. Nutritional support of the burned patient. World J Surg 16:80, 1992.

CHAPTER REVIEW
Questions

1. A deep partial-thickness burn is most correctly described as an injury that:
   a. Is pink, moist, and painful
   b. Leathery and insensate
   c. Has blanching but delayed capillary refill
   d. Will heal in 2 to 3 weeks
2. The acute risk in the first hours after an inhalation injury is:
   a. Pneumonia
   b. Pneumothorax
   c. Upper airway obstruction
   d. Ventilation/perfusion mismatch
3. The most appropriate care for a patient with a large burn at the scene of injury is:
   a. Wash with cold water and wrap with cold sterile compresses
   b. Remove smoldering garments, cover with a clean sheet and blanket
   c. Start a subclavian intravenous line with Ringer's lactate
   d. Intubate and transport
4. In a patient with a 60% surface area flame burn, the best first operative procedure would be:
   a. Excise the full-thickness burn, which involves all of his right leg
   b. Excise the partial-thickness burn, which involves all of his left leg
   c. Excise the dorsum of both hands and fingers, which have full-thickness burns
   d. Excise the facial injury, which has deep partial and superficial partial-thickness burns
5. A patient who jumped from a second-story window to avoid a fire has a 50% surface area burn but is requiring more fluid than the estimated need. A peritoneal lavage shows gross blood in the aspirate. The best approach would be:
   a. Avoid laparotomy because the patient has a major burn
   b. If a CT scan shows a fractured spleen, treat nonoperatively because of the burn
   c. Perform an exploratory laparotomy
   d. Perform a transverse abdominal incision to avoid making a wound in the burned tissue

Answers

1. d
2. c
3. b
4. a
5. c

37 Pediatric Surgical Emergencies

H. HARLAN STONE

KEY FEATURES

After reading this chapter you will understand:
- The physiologic parameters that influence treatment of infants and newborns.
- A wide variety of conditions that produce a defect in the body mantle.
- How defects in the infant's development result in respiratory distress syndromes.
- The etiology, diagnosis, and treatment of intestinal obstruction in newborns and older infants.

Conditions in the newborn that almost always demand emergency surgical care are (1) defects in body surface mantle, (2) respiratory distress, (3) intestinal obstruction, and (4) peritoneal inflammatory states. In some cases the responsible disease process is quite obvious, whereas a moderately detailed work-up may be required to identify most of the other derangements. Early diagnosis is imperative, since significant delay in treatment uniformly worsens the prognosis.

GENERAL CONSIDERATIONS

Newborns are at the mercy of their environment. In regard to body heat, the temperature control center is immature, there is little subcutaneous fat for insulation, the infant cannot adequately shiver or sweat to generate or transfer heat, and body surface area for heat loss is great in comparison to body weight. The infant must be kept warm in an incubator, folds of blankets, or a wrap of sheet wadding. Unless adequate provision is made to conserve body heat, belladonna drugs should be avoided, since they cause peripheral vasodilation and thereby facilitate additional heat loss. A warming mattress, surgical drapes, and heat lamps aid heat retention. Constant temperature monitoring is essential.

An infant's respirations are primarily diaphragmatic; therefore abdominal distention should be reduced or prevented. A gastrostomy tube inserted at laparotomy offers reliable gastric decompression without the irritation of a nasogastric tube and its consequent occlusion of one of the nares. The airway must be kept clear of mucus by frequent suctioning, use of the prone position, and omission of sedatives. A crying infant is usually a well-ventilated infant.

The function of other organ systems varies, but seldom can adult capacities be equaled. Renal excretion of sodium as well as concentrating and diluting abilities are impaired; similarly the elimination of many drugs is limited by a poorly developed glomerular or tubular mechanism (e.g., penicillin). The liver, likewise, is unable to detoxify or excrete certain drugs or even appropriately handle some normal metabolites (such as bilirubin, thus accounting for physiologic jaundice in the newborn).

A newborn is predisposed toward bacterial infection following operation. There is no acquired resistance. For several days after birth, neutropenia is common, and hypogammaglobulinemia normally persists for several months. Bacteremia is poorly controlled, and thus hema-

631

TABLE 37-1 Maintenance Requirement for Water and Electrolytes

Age	Water (ml/kg/day)	Sodium (mEq/kg/day)	Potassium (mEq/kg/day)
Premature	150-200	2	1.5
Newborn	140-160	3	1.5
4 weeks to 1 year	125-150	3	2.0
1 to 5 years	125-100	3	2.0
5 to 12 years	100-75	2	2.0
12 to 20 years	75-60	2	1.0
Adulthood	50-30	2	0.5

TABLE 37-2 Correction of Dehydration and Electrolyte Deficits

Deficit	Basis	Replacement
Dehydration	(% dehydration) × (body weight)*	Liters of normal saline
Sodium	(1.40 mEq serum Na − patient's serum value) × (ECF)†	mEq sodium
Potassium	(4.5 mEq serum K − patient's serum value) × (TBW)‡	mEq potassium
Acidosis	(24 mEq serum CO_2 − patient's serum value) × (TBW)§	mEq $NaHCO_3$

*Dehydration volume replaced with normal saline according to (% dehydration) × (body weight in kg) = Liters of normal saline; 5% dehydration = Loss of skin turgor, concentrated urine; 10% dehydration = Extreme loss of skin turgor, scant and concentrated urine, sunken eyes, depressed cranial fontanelles.
†Sodium-deficit correction based on extracellular fluid volume (20% of body weight in kilograms): (140 mEq/L serum value) × (ECF in liters) = mEq sodium.
‡Potassium-deficit correction based on total body water (70% body weight in kilograms).
§Acidosis corrected with bicarbonate on the basis of total body water (70% body weight in kilograms).

togenous-origin meningitis is often associated with surgery-related infection during the first 2 years of life. Accordingly, prophylactic systemic antibiotics are usually indicated for sepsis protection during the perioperative period.

At surgery blood loss must be accurately measured and replaced in appropriately small aliquots. The blood volume of a 2000 g newborn is approximately 8% of body weight or 160 ml. A blood loss of 20 ml thus represents almost the same deficit as a 1-unit hemorrhage in the adult.

Infants require a greater volume of free water per kilogram of body weight than do adults; this extra need gradually decreases during infancy (Table 37-1). Although renal function may appear to be normal, sodium and hydrogen ions cannot be excreted as efficiently as in adults through normal tubular exchange mechanisms. Accordingly, maintenance fluid and electrolyte therapy warrants more water and less sodium than in an older child or adult. In addition, close observation for acidosis is a must.

Derangements in fluid and electrolyte balance are mainly those of dehydration (corrected by administration of normal saline) and acidosis (corrected by sodium bicarbonate). Once daily requirements have been calculated, additional water and electrolytes are included in the maintenance schedule as needed to correct measured deficits; these are given continuously in intravenous drips over the ensuing 24-hour period (Table 37-2).

The newborn has an extremely high metabolic rate. Extra calories are needed for growth as well as maintenance (Table 37-3). Endogenous fat stores are not available to the infant, so any delay in oral feedings automatically leads to scavenging of both carbohydrate and protein from developing tissues. All intravenous fluids should therefore contain glucose, preferably at a 10% concentration. Protein hydrolysates are likewise of benefit. Nevertheless, there is no substitute for beginning oral feedings with homogenized formula as soon as possible in a newborn after surgery.

Whenever interruption of normal gastrointes-

TABLE 37-3 Daily Caloric Requirements

Age (months)	Calories (cal/kg)
Newborn	45-50
3-10	60-80
10-15	50-40
15-30	40-35
30-60	35-30
Over 60	30-25

tinal function lasts for longer than 3 or 4 days, intravenous therapy must be modified to provide greater nutritional support as well as standard electrolyte and water supplements. Solutions containing protein hydrolysate, more concentrated glucose, ions other than sodium and potassium, vitamins, trace elements, and fat (e.g., soybean emulsions or intralipid) can be given via peripheral veins provided osmolarity is kept below 600. More concentrated solutions, however, especially those with carbohydrate at 12 g/dl or greater and with a resultant osmolarity of 900 to 1000, must be administered directly into a central venous pool. For such delivery, a cutdown in the neck with a catheter threaded into the superior vena cava or percutaneous cannulation of a subclavian vein have become the preferred procedures.

DEFECTS IN THE BODY MANTLE

Immediately after delivery, an absence of normally protective skin or soft tissue should be easily recognized. These occur over the anterior abdominal wall and along the midline of the back from apex of head to tip of spine. Instead of normal skin, a thin transparent membrane may provide the only protective cover. Drying, with subsequent rupture of the membrane, can then set the stage for fulminant infection.

Omphalocele

During intrauterine life, abdominal viscera enlarge at a rate considerably greater than does the capacity of the peritoneal cavity. To accommodate for this space shortage, there is partial herniation of intra-abdominal organs into the umbilical cord. As prenatal development continues, the abdomen eventually expands sufficiently to allow for the viscera to return. It is during this time that the midgut undergoes its normal 270-degree rotation. If for any reason the contained viscera fail to reduce spontaneously back into the abdomen, a thin membrane of amnion becomes the only protective covering. This form of congenital hernia is referred to as an *omphalocele.*

There are two cell layers to the membranous sac: an outer surface of amnion and an inner lining of peritoneum. Unless kept moist, the omphalocele will become dry and subject to bacterial invasion within a few hours after birth. Rupture of the sac, with evisceration and peritonitis, can then occur. Thus, immediately after the omphalocele surface is cleansed, sterile aqueous compresses should be applied.

Surgical Repair. Treatment is directed toward eventual skin coverage of the defect. The addition of muscle or fascia support is important, but such can be delayed for months to years if other considerations so dictate. Determinants of the specific method for repair include volume of sac contents, diameter of the abdominal wall defect, general status of the infant with respect to other congenital defects, prematurity, and eventual prognosis otherwise.

If the sac is small, if the abdominal defect is 5 cm or less in diameter, and if all herniated viscera can be reduced without undue tension, repair is accomplished in separate layers of skin and midline fascia after sac excision (Fig. 37-1). Larger defects with proportionately larger sacs have permitted visceral development outside of the abdomen, but with resultant loss of organ right of domain within the peritoneal cavity. If these viscera are forced back into the abdomen, the consequent acute increase in intra-abdominal pressure will cause fixed elevations of the diaphragm and a corresponding significant reduction in ventilation capacity. Death from respiratory insufficiency usually follows unless intensive ventilatory support is provided. Increased pressure within the abdomen also obstructs the inferior vena cava, thereby restricting blood return to the heart, which in turn can lead to a state of low-output shock. Either complication may eventuate in death within 12 to 24 hours.

Several methods offer skin cover without risk of a potentially lethal increase in intra-abdominal pressure. One involves application of a caustic agent (mercurochrome) to the omphalocele sac and subsequent creation of a sterile crust, beneath which skin can proliferate from sac margin. Wet dressings of an antiseptic solution (silver nitrate or benzalkonium chloride) can serve the same purpose. Unfortunately, sac rupture and bacterial infection occur in approximately half of these cases, and there is the additional risk of

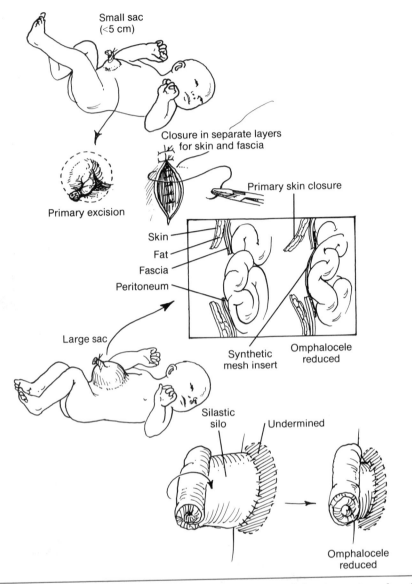

FIGURE 37-1   Steps in repair of the omphalocele. Use of mesh for closure is preferred over the Silastic silo for larger defects. Both techniques are illustrated.

systemic toxicity from absorption of the antiseptic or eschar-inducing chemical. Accordingly, such alternative methods are generally reserved for patients with huge omphaloceles in whom associated major congenital anomalies predict a poor prognosis.

Other methods for repair of a larger omphalocele are based on mobilization of skin and subcutaneous tissue from the lateral abdominal wall (see Fig. 37-1). After excision of the omphalocele sac, any fascial deficit can be bridged by the immediate insertion of synthetic fabric (Prolene mesh) followed by primary skin closure.

There has been considerable interest in the creation of a temporarily expanded abdominal wall through insertion of Silastic sheeting. This material is sutured to the margin of the fascial defect so as to create a silo-like structure protruding from the abdominal midline (see Fig. 37-1). Antiseptic agents are applied to the juncture of the Silastic sheet and abdominal wall. At intervals of several days, the Silastic cone is rolled up like a toothpaste tube. In this way, all displaced viscera are gradually returned to the abdominal cavity proper within a week or two. Following successful reduction, the Silastic silo is removed, and the abdominal wall can then be closed in separate layers of fascia and skin.

When excessive intra-abdominal pressure is avoided, results from the surgical management of omphaloceles are quite good. Nevertheless, the larger the size of sac and defect, the higher the mortality rate. Significant complications and death result primarily from the presence of other major congenital anomalies and/or infections complicating the omphalocele repair.

GASTROSCHISIS

Gastroschisis is a full-thickness defect in the anterior abdominal wall, almost always associated with visceral herniation into the amniotic cavity. Prenatal rupture of an omphalocele creates a similar problem. Bathing of extruded bowel in amniotic fluid causes a chemical peritonitis and leads to the formation of a thick inflammatory peel on the bowel surface. Although its resultant appearance suggests bowel gangrene, rarely is the almost polypoid mass of intestine necrotic. However, local pressure by the hernial ring frequently produces a short segment of intestinal stenosis or atresia at both the sites of bowel exit and re-entrance back into the abdomen.

Surgical Repair. After loose material has been washed from the peritoneal surface, the hernial ring is enlarged to facilitate an attempt at bowel reduction. Rarely can all extruded viscera be returned without significantly increasing intra-abdominal pressure. Accordingly, some form of ventral hernia must then be constructed in a fashion somewhat similar to what has previously been described for large omphalocele repair (Fig. 37-1). Use of the Silastic silo is not routinely advocated, however, because it is associated with a greater incidence of local infection and bowel perforation.

If the infant subsequently demonstrates mechanical obstruction, reoperation is best delayed until after the third postoperative week. By then there usually has been an amazing resolution in the leathery exudative peritonitis. The obstruction is generally caused by a short segmental atresia that was not obvious at initial operation because of the thick inflammatory peel.

Overall results with gastroschisis and ruptured omphalocele were poor in past decades, with mortalities ranging between 30% and 50%.

However, better supportive care, more effective antibiotics, and total parenteral nutrition have now improved survival rates to almost 90%.

Congenital Absence of Abdominal Musculature

Areas devoid of supporting abdominal muscle give infants the unique appearance that has been labeled "prune belly." Functional urinary tract obstruction, present for months before term, leads to congenital hydronephrosis and hydroureter. The upper urinary tract must be decompressed as soon as possible so as to preserve what remains of renal function. Following initial nephrostomy or cutaneous ureterostomy, definitive correction is based on implantation of the ureters into an ileal or colon conduit. The entire extrarenal system for elimination of urine is thereby made up of peristalsing tubules and is no longer influenced by changes in intra-abdominal pressure. Constipation also occurs, leading to long periods of obstipation. Both urinary and intestinal complications are related to the inability to generate sufficient intra-abdominal pressure to facilitate evacuation of waste products from terminal reservoirs, i.e., bladder and rectum. The use of enemas and laxatives, however, can augment bowel function and thus obviate the need for a colostomy in most cases.

Surgical Repair. The lax abdominal wall can be reinforced by an overlap of attenuated fascial layers or by insertion of a synthetic prosthesis. If death from urinary sepsis does not occur at an early age, vertebral deformities appear as the child grows and may progress to extreme degrees of scoliosis because of absent anterior counterbalance to paraspinal muscle pull.

Exstrophy and Epispadias

Direct communication of bladder or urethra with the surface of the ventral midline may occur singly or in combination. With simple *exstrophy* of the bladder there is little or no separation of the symphysis pubis, and thus repair is relatively simple. However, if the external opening is wide and extends down to or even involves the penile urethra, closure must include bilateral pelvic osteotomies. Since there is little likelihood for development of urinary continence despite a meticulous repair of the bladder neck, early resort to an ileal or colon conduit may at times be the safest and most practical approach.

Epispadias, or dorsal fistulization of the penile urethra, presents a problem only in plastic reconstruction. If epispadias alone is present, long-term results are uniformly good. Persistence of any abnormal communication of urinary tract to body surface consistently leads to bacterial colonization of the urine, chronic urinary tract infection, often ureteral reflux with hydronephrosis, and eventually death from urosepsis and/or chronic renal failure.

With *hypospadias,* the terminal urethral opening is abnormally located along the ventral surface of the penis, often as proximal as the perineum. Correction is warranted for adult reproductive function and in rare instances of urethral obstruction. Foreskin provides ideal tissue for elimination of the attendant *chordee* (downward deviation of the distal penis as a result of scarring) as well as plastic urethral construction. It is for this reason that circumcision should never be performed until after hypospadias has been ruled out.

Meningocele and Myelomeningocele

A failure of skin and/or subcutaneous tissues to cover the neural canal causes the spinal cord and its nerves to herniate into a thin membranous sac *(meningocele);* or, if the neural tube has never formed, the cord itself may become both sac and hernia *(myelomeningocele).* This can occur at any level from the apex of the head *(encephalocele)* down the posterior vertebral column to as low as the coccyx, although the thoracolumbar area is the most commonly involved. Inherent to the anomaly is an absence of dorsal bony elements to one or more vertebrae *(rachischisis).* The initial threat to life is infection, since bacterial invasion can follow sac rupture or drying. The application of moist antibiotic compresses offers temporary protection until surgical repair can be accomplished.

With care being taken to preserve all nerves and to minimize trauma to exposed spinal cord, flaps of skin and subcutaneous tissue are mobilized laterally and at oblique angles so as to provide a definitive closure. Several conditions usually coexist and demand careful patient reevaluation during both the immediate and late postoperative periods. Subsequent operations are almost always necessary.

Hydrocephalus occurs in approximately 90% of patients with a meningocele. Whether an inability to absorb cerebrospinal fluid was the initial cause of meningocele is debated. In any event, following closure of the skin defect, hydrocephalus develops in the majority of infants.

Accordingly, head circumference should be measured daily, and if it increases at an excessive rate, decompression of the now-increased intracranial pressure becomes urgent. The ventriculoatrial shunt, established by means of a Silastic tube system, is the procedure of choice; it drains cerebrospinal fluid from one of the lateral cerebral ventricles into the superior vena cava or internal jugular vein. A subcutaneous valve is usually interposed over a prominence of the skull so as to control rate and direction of flow and to permit manual pumping of fluid from the ventricular system if that becomes necessary. A spontaneous arrest of the hydrocephalus usually occurs after several years, but more than half of these children will become mentally retarded unless the hydrocephalus is appropriately controlled at any early age.

Because of the often-associated paraplegia, a cord bladder exists in many of these infants. Functional lower urinary tract obstruction results in reflux into the upper tracts, infection, and consequent damage to renal parenchyma. A drainage procedure is usually required for decompression of the lower urinary tract. The majority of such children eventually come to construction of an ileal or colon conduit to ensure unobstructed ureteral drainage. Appropriate care of the urinary tract is extremely important, since the most common cause of death after the first month of life is urinary sepsis and/or renal failure.

A third component of related anomalies is a direct result of the paraplegia and includes congenital dislocation of the hip, lower extremity spasticity, and decubitus ulceration from pressure on bony prominences. Orthopedic procedures may be required to correct joint contractures and dislocations and to improve joint mobility by muscle or tendon transfer. Physical therapists can aid in the design of supporting braces as well as in supervising the education of the child in use of these appliances.

Thus the meningocele and myelomeningocele herald a group of major problems that severely restrict the child's future. Early recognition and management in harmony with the efforts of other specialists is an absolute necessity if a tolerable life is to be gained for these unfortunate children.

RESPIRATORY DISTRESS SYNDROMES

Although certain derangements in ventilatory exchange may be patently obvious immediately

TABLE 37-4   Diagnosis of Respiratory Distress in the Newborn

	Characteristic History	Obvious to Inspection	Passage of NG Tube	Plain X-ray*
Choanal atresia	✔	—	✔	
Pierre-Robin syndrome	✔	✔	—	—
Cervical teratoma	—	✔	—	—
Congenital goiter	✔	✔	—	✔
Tracheomalacia	—	—	—	—
Pneumothorax	—	—	—	—
Lobar emphysema	—	—	—	✔
Diaphragmatic hernia	—	—	—	✔
Massive pneumoperitoneum	✔	✔	—	✔
Esophageal atresia	✔	—	✔	✔

✔ = Almost diagnostic.
*Nasogastric tube in place.

after birth, many respiratory problems require several days before significant deterioration in pulmonary function is manifest. Irrespective of whether symptoms appear early or late, a few simple diagnostic measures are generally sufficient to give a relatively accurate diagnosis (Table 37-4). First, an attempt is made to pass a nasogastric tube down each nostril. The tube is then left in place while posteroanterior and lateral chest x-ray films are obtained. The abdomen should be included in the same radiographs. Finally, the infant is observed while nursing, because some congenital anomalies may become apparent only when the baby swallows his feedings.

Choanal Atresia

Atresia of the posterior nares may be unilateral or bilateral. When not feeding, the infant has good color and demonstrates no respiratory distress so long as the oral airway is not obstructed—that is, the mouth is open and is not being used to nurse. However, cyanosis develops soon after the baby begins to suckle, usually after he has taken but a few gulps. Likewise, when the baby falls off to sleep and his mouth closes, there can no longer be an adequate exchange of air; the infant immediately becomes cyanotic. Color improves as soon as he awakens with a fretful, angry cry and once again can breathe through his mouth. This same cycle is repeated again and again until fatigue sets in and of itself threatens life.

Symptoms are worse when the atresia is bilateral. The posterior nasal block is membranous in half of the cases, while the remainder have vary-

ing thicknesses of bony occlusion. The diagnosis is made by a characteristic history and the inability to pass a tube through the nares. An oral airway will give temporary respite. Correction is achieved by blunt perforation to create a posterior naris. A plastic tube is then inserted to maintain an open nasal airway during the period of local swelling consequent to the trauma of perforation. Repeated dilations and gradual enlargement of the tube stent are required at weekly intervals for several months.

Pierre-Robin Syndrome

With an arrest in mandibular growth or a failure of primordial elements to migrate into the lower jaw, upper airway obstruction can be caused by a recession of the base of the tongue. Rarely is the tongue larger than normal, even though it seems to be massive when compared with the small jaw. Thus there is micrognathia with apparent macroglossia.

In the first of three clinical categories, there is little difficulty in breathing, except that great care must be taken during feedings. The second category is characterized by only occasional respiratory distress at times other than nursing. However, when feeding, the baby is unable to breathe, sputters, and becomes cyanotic. Such infants can be managed by tube feeding through an intermittently passed nasogastric tube or, when nursing expertise is lacking, a temporary gastrostomy.

The final category includes babies experiencing respiratory distress even when not feeding. Survival after birth is dependent upon the immediate insertion of an oral airway. Subsequently, on an elective basis, the tongue must be fixed anteriorly to prevent obstruction of the hypopharynx. With the Douglas procedure, a large suture attaches the middle third of the tongue anteriorly to the inferior gingival sulcus. Unfortunately, this suture frequently cuts through and thus gives only a brief and unreliable relief from airway obstruction. More lasting success has been obtained by passing a Kirschner wire through the angles of both mandibles so as to push and then hold the base of the tongue forward. Although the pin may be dislodged, a fibrous sling has been established and continues to maintain the tongue in proper position.

Given sufficient time, growth of these babies will overcome the small jaw and receding tongue. Usually by the fourth to sixth month of life there is no longer a functional disability, even though the lower jaw is still remarkably small. Tracheostomy is to be avoided whenever possible; not only are there inherent complications to this procedure, but also it is extremely difficult to wean the child from dependency on a bypassed larynx. Tracheostomy is resorted to only as a last-ditch, lifesaving measure.

Cervical Teratoma

At the time of delivery, dystocia may be caused by a large mass in the anterior aspect of the neck. If the mass contains calcium on x-ray evaluation, it is most likely a benign teratoma. A smaller lesion can be either a teratoma or a congenital goiter. Many of these babies are stillborn or suffocate during the prolonged delivery consequent to a face or brow presentation.

Respiratory distress resulting from airway obstruction develops immediately after birth. An endotracheal tube should then be inserted, and the child is carried directly to the operating room for tumor excision.

Teratomas are usually centered in the midline. Some are so large as to completely obliterate the space between chin and sternum. The tumor is located beneath the deep cervical fascia and is often intimately adherent to the thyroid. Although benign on microscopic examination, an incompletely excised teratoma will recur and rarely may even develop malignant characteristics.

Postoperatively, the endotracheal tube should not be removed for several days. After extubation the child must be observed closely for evidence of respiratory obstruction as a result of tracheal collapse. If such occurs, the endotracheal tube is

reinserted and left in place for several additional days. If airway obstruction returns when the tube is removed a second time, temporary tracheostomy may be required.

Congenital Goiter

During prenatal life, the fetal thyroid may undergo massive hypertrophy in response to maternal stimulation. This occurs when the mother is taking antithyroid medication or is receiving relatively large doses of a compound containing iodine. Because of thyroid inhibition, excess maternal thyroid-stimulating hormone is produced and crosses the placental barrier.

The clinical presentation is similar to that of cervical teratoma. Administration of thyroid hormone and withdrawal of maternal humeral stimulation through delivery will, in time, permit spontaneous regression of the gland. Airway obstruction initially is managed by an endotracheal tube. If after 4 or 5 days the still-sizable goiter is obstructive, operation is generally required. The isthmus, pyramidal lobe, and anterior margin of both lateral lobes are removed.

Tracheomalacia

Absence of tracheal stability may follow prolonged pressure from an external mass (such as cervical teratoma or congenital goiter) or can occur separately. Upper airway obstruction results from tracheal collapse and can be relieved temporarily by insertion of an endotracheal tube. Although bronchoscopy is diagnostic, the true condition is usually unrecognized until tracheostomy is performed. Attempts to discontinue the tracheostomy are begun almost immediately, yet months often pass before the child can tolerate permanent removal of the splinting tracheostomy tube.

Significant complications of tracheostomy in the infant include:

- Iatrogenic pneumothorax
- Erosion of the tracheal cannula into an adjacent major vessel, i.e., innominate artery
- Dependency of the child on a tracheostomy stoma with bypassed larynx
- Aspiration of foreign material
- Occlusion of the lumen of the cannula
- Tracheostomy tube dislodgement

Because of these many dangers, tracheostomy should be avoided whenever possible. If the procedure is performed, however, early removal of the tracheostomy tube must become a priority.

Pneumothorax

Pneumothorax may develop suddenly without any obvious precipitating cause, although usually there has been some antecedent injury from insertion of a tracheostomy, a difficult endotracheal intubation, or necrotizing pneumonia. Its usual onset is a sudden and relatively severe respiratory distress, for there is often a rapid progression to tension pneumothorax.

Although a shift in the mediastinum to one side or the other, increased tympany over the involved hemithorax, and impaired breath sounds may be detected, an immediate evaluation with a portable x-ray machine is the only sure method of diagnosis. Once lung cysts and diaphragmatic hernia have been excluded by chest x-ray examination, a thoracotomy tube is inserted and connected to water-sealed drainage. Seldom is suction required. The thoracotomy tube can usually be removed after several days, when air leaks have sealed and adhesions have developed between parietal and visceral pleura.

Congenital Lobar Emphysema

Although congenital emphysema occurs more commonly in the upper lobes of the lung, it may also occur in other lobes. There can be diffuse lobar involvement or loculation into a single large pneumatocele. Pulmonary deterioration is often rapid and results from compression of the contralateral lung from forces similar to those occurring with tension pneumothorax. The air cyst must be distinguished from pneumothorax, since insertion of a thoracotomy tube not only fails to relieve the respiratory distress but also may cause a massive air leak through rupture of the cyst.

Occasionally lobar emphysema is produced by obstructing extrinsic pressure on a major bronchus by tumor or locally enlarged lymph nodes. However, the usual cause is intrinsic pulmonary disease. After an obstructing mucous plug has been ruled out by bronchoscopy, urgent thoracotomy with resection of the diseased lobe is indicated. Delay is dangerous and may foster a sudden and lethal diminution in pulmonary function.

Diaphragmatic Hernia

Congenital herniation of abdominal viscera into the chest may occur through any of the normally situated diaphragmatic foramina. Although those passing through the esophageal hiatus seldom create any emergency, massive displacement of bowel into the thorax can result from absence of an entire hemidiaphragm or a large muscular defect in the posterolateral aspect of the diaphragm (foramen of Bochdalek). If it is on the right, the liver serves as a protective buttress and thereby prevents herniation of other abdominal viscera. When on the left, however, there is no such interposing viscus, and massive displacement of intra-abdominal organs can freely occur. Although respiratory distress may be delayed, ingested air gradually distends the now partially intrathoracic intestinal tract and progressively diminishes pulmonary function through lung compression and mediastinal shift.

Whenever a diaphragmatic hernia is suspected, a nasogastric tube should be inserted to decompress the stomach as well as to prevent additional gas from passing into more distal portions of the intestine. Physical signs are rarely helpful, except for respiratory distress and the occasional scaphoid-appearing abdomen. A chest x-ray film is then obtained and demonstrates bowel and the nasogastric tube in the ipsilateral thorax. Ventilation with a mask should never be attempted unless an open nasogastric tube can efficiently vent the stomach for escape of insufflated gas. The infant is carried urgently to the operating room, where laparotomy is performed through a midline incision. The viscera are pulled back into the abdomen and the lung is carefully examined through the defect in the diaphragm. If the lung appears hypoplastic, no effort is made to inflate it, since excessive intrabronchial pressure will only damage the contralateral good lung. The defect in the diaphragm is repaired by direct suture, a fascial transfer, or the interposition of a synthetic fabric. A thoracotomy tube should not be inserted, because it will favor a reverse mediastinal shift.

When the defect in the diaphragm is large, then abdominal viscera have developed within the chest, and thus the volume capacity of the abdomen is insufficient to receive them. Accordingly, the abdomen should be stretched manually or an appropriate technique should be used to enlarge the peritoneal cavity (as if managing a large omphalocele). Immediately after operation, a chest x-ray film must be obtained before the child leaves the operating room, since there is a high incidence of contralateral pneumothorax. This would require the insertion of a thoracotomy tube into the opposite pleural space.

The hypoplastic lung can potentially expand and in time will gradually assume near-normal function. If the lung on the involved side has merely been compressed, pulmonary dynamics are unaffected.

In those babies whose severely hypoplastic or damaged lung has necessitated reliance on extremes in mechanical ventilation of the contralateral lung—with its attendant barotrauma—pulmonary function often deteriorates precipitously. Death can occasionally be prevented in these infants by the expeditious use of an extracorporeal membrane oxygenator (ECMO). Although not uniformly successful, ECMO offers the only other option.

Massive Pneumoperitoneum

With rupture of an abdominal segment of the gastrointestinal tract, massive pneumoperitoneum can suddenly develop. As tension becomes extreme, increasing pressure is exerted against the diaphragm; its marked elevation then severely restricts ventilatory exchange. These events are especially prone to occur following more proximal gastrointestinal perforations, specifically those of the stomach.

The usual story is that a premature male does well during his first days of life but then refuses a feeding and, shortly thereafter, is noted to be in extreme respiratory distress from a strikingly distended and tympanitic abdomen. He may vomit small amounts of blood. Passage of a nasogastric tube rarely benefits ventilatory exchange or provides any significant reduction in abdominal distention.

Plain x-ray films reveal the true nature of the problem. On the flat film, intestines are gathered in the midline and resemble the strings of a football (football sign). Even more striking is the upright x-ray film, which demonstrates free intra-abdominal air, both above and below the arc formed by liver and spleen, suggesting a contour somewhat similar to saddlebags (saddlebag sign).

Peritoneal contaminants must be removed as soon as possible and the responsible perforation closed. With the child supine, paracentesis through the anterior abdomen will release sufficient quantities of air to give a dramatic improvement in pulmonary function. Gastric perforations usually occur along the greater curvature as linear necrotic rents and must be debrided before repair. Duodenal perforations are almost always the result of an acute ulcer. Suture closure is ideally reinforced by a patch of omentum or an onlay of hepatic flexure of colon. Bowel perforations are usually caused by necrotizing enterocolitis. Bowel resection is routinely required,

with creation of a terminal enterostomy proximally. Despite appropriate and massive antibiotic therapy, the morality is high (averaging 20%) for any gastrointestinal perforation during infancy.

Esophageal Atresia and Tracheoesophageal Fistula

Because of their related embryonic origins, almost any combination of fistula and/or atresia can develop between the esophagus and trachea (Fig. 37-2). In the most common type representing more than 90% of cases, the proximal esophagus ends as a blind pouch, while the distal esophagus is connected by a fistula to the terminal trachea (Fig. 37-2, *C*). Babies with this condition tend to be premature, have multiple other congenital anomalies, and yet initially have no difficulty with respiration. Later, when they begin to feed, everything ingested is regurgitated without apparent alteration by gastrointestinal secretions. These infants seem to produce an excess of saliva, apparently because swallowed secretions cannot reach the stomach. After repeated frustrations with feeding, the increased intra-abdominal pressure coincident to fretful cries forces gastric contents up the distal esophagus, in a retrograde fashion, directly into the tracheobronchial tree. Aspiration pneumonia from gastric contents, not food, then follows. Unless corrective measures are instituted, starvation and a fulminating pneumonia soon lead to death. The diagnosis is made by:

1. The characteristic feeding pattern
2. Inability to pass a nasogastric tube into the stomach
3. A chest x-ray film demonstrating the tube coiled in the proximal esophageal pouch
4. Varying stages of pneumonia

Steps must immediately be taken to prevent these repeated aspirations of gastric juice. If the baby is otherwise in good condition, urgent thoracotomy is performed, the fistula is divided, and the two ends of the esophagus are anastomosed over a splinting nasogastric tube. A gastrostomy is inserted either before or after the procedure. Occasionally the two ends of the esophagus cannot be approximated without extreme tension and thus predilection for disruption of the suture line. Under these circumstances the fistula is divided and the proximal esophagus is brought out through the neck as a mucous fistula. At some

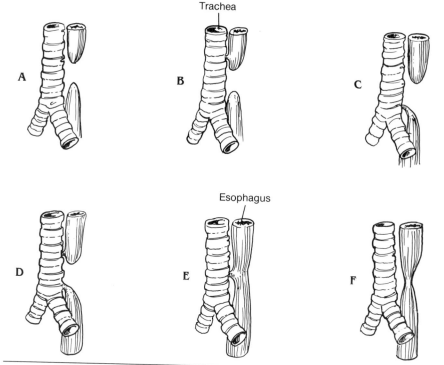

FIGURE 37-2 Types of esophageal atresia. **A,** Esophageal atresia without tracheoesophageal fistula (<8%). This is the usual presentation, with a long gap between the two blind ends. **B,** Esophageal atresia with proximal tracheoesophageal fistula (<1%). **C,** Esophageal atresia with distal tracheoesophageal fistula (>85%). This is the most common type of anomaly associated with esophageal atresia. **D,** Esophageal atresia with proximal and distal tracheoesophageal fistula (<1%). **E,** Isolated tracheoesophageal fistula without esophageal atresia (<5%). **F,** A variant of esophageal atresia without a fistula; much less common than the anatomy depicted in **A.**

time between 6 and 18 months of age, a segment of colon is brought into the chest to serve as an interposing conduit between proximal esophagus and stomach.

If, however, the child's general condition is such as to prohibit any major surgery, a gastrostomy is performed under local anesthesia. This vent ensures a continuous and complete gastric decompression and thereby arrests any gastric acid regurgitation through the distal esophageal fistula. Only then will the pulmonary status improve. *The gastrostomy can never be used for feeding.* If enteral nutrition is planned, then a feeding jejunostomy is installed at the initial operation. After several days or even weeks of tube or intravenous feedings, thoracotomy is carried out, with the goal being fistula division and esophageal repair.

Postoperative care is directed toward continued support of pulmonary function, antibiotic therapy for the ever-present pneumonia, timely administration of proper nutrients, and special attention to the diagnosis and management of commonly associated other anomalies.

INTESTINAL OBSTRUCTION OF THE NEWBORN

The anatomic level of congenital gastrointestinal obstruction varies considerably as to incidence, cause, clinical presentation, and associated anomalies (Table 37-5). Nevertheless, certain factors are common to all.

Maternal Hydramnios. During intrauterine life, fetal ingestion is the main mechanism for removal of amniotic fluid. Obstructions distal to

TABLE 37-5 Relative Incidence of
Gastrointestinal Atresias

Type	Incidence (%)
Esophageal	27
Duodenal	8
Small bowel	14
Colon	1
Anal	50

the ileocecal valve do not exclude sufficient intestinal mucosa to alter the rate of amniotic fluid absorption. More proximal obstructions, however, significantly reduce the absorptive surface and considerably limit the amount of intraluminal fluid that can be removed. For example, approximately 90% of duodenal obstructions are associated with maternal hydramnios.

Bilious Vomiting. With any obstruction, intestinal secretions accumulate, are regurgitated into the stomach, and are then vomited. Since the intestinal tract is relatively free of bacteria during the first few days of life, bile is not degraded and thus retains its characteristic dark green color. With few exceptions, the newborn who vomits bile has a mechanical obstruction.

Abdominal Distention. The degree of abdominal distention is not impressive with proximal obstructions, such as those of the duodenum. However, more distal obstructions eventually lead to quite massive distention.

No Normal Meconium Stool. Although the newborn with mechanical intestinal obstruction may pass material by rectum, seldom does the stool contain bile and almost never does it have the bulky, dark-green appearance of meconium. Rarely, and only when the process is functional, are meconium stools passed by the infant with congenital intestinal obstruction (i.e., adynamic megacolon).

Plain X-ray Evaluation. Since there are no gas shadows distal to the site of obstruction, ingested air provides an excellent contrast and offers a reasonably accurate estimate of the level of obstruction merely on the basis of number of loops of distended bowel. Only if a nasogastric tube has almost completely decompressed the proximal obstruction is there any reason to order a contrast study of the upper intestinal tract.

Barium Enema. With distal obstructions, the cause may be functional or may be caused by a sudden compromise in intestinal blood supply (e.g., midgut volvulus). A barium enema can document the effectiveness of peristalsis as well

as the completeness of colon rotation. If bowel obstruction is not obvious, similar confirmation can be obtained by a small bowel series.

Esophageal Atresia

Esophageal atresia, as mentioned before, is usually associated with a fistula between trachea and distal esophagus. Its clinical presentation thus includes problems with swallowing combined with an ever-worsening respiratory distress resulting from gastric aspiration pneumonia. Both problems demand immediate attention.

Duodenal Obstruction

Congenital obstructions of the duodenum almost always develop distal to the ampulla of Vater and accordingly first present with the vomiting of bile. There are several causes:

- Atresia
- Constriction from an annular pancreas when dorsal and ventral pancreatic anlages have failed to migrate properly
- External compression by the residual ventral mesentery passing from an incompletely rotated cecum to the right peritoneal gutter

In addition to the continued vomiting of dark bilious material, characteristic features include a failure to pass normal meconium stools, minimal abdominal distention, and a double bubble on plain x-ray films, the two large gas shadows clearly defining the stomach and proximal duodenum (Fig. 37-3).

At laparotomy the colon is first inspected to determine the completeness of bowel rotation (see Fig. 37-3). Any obstructing band is divided. Occasionally an atresia lies beneath the site of compression. If one exists, management is similar to that for an isolated atresia or annular pancreas. A segment of proximal jejunum is brought through the transverse mesocolon and a duodenojejunostomy is performed. If technically practical, a duodenostomy is preferred instead. Gastrojejunostomy is contraindicated, for only a more normal progression of food will ensure better mixing with digestive ferments that have been secreted into the proximal duodenum and, accordingly, better absorption of ingested nutrients.

Intestinal Atresia

More distant obstructions are signaled by greater abdominal distention, bilious vomiting, absence

Causes   **Corrections**

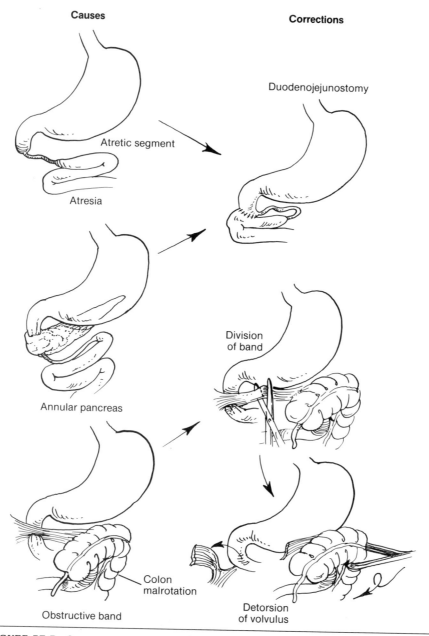

Duodenojejunostomy

Atretic segment

Atresia

Annular pancreas

Division
of band

Colon
malrotation

Obstructive band

Detorsion
of volvulus

FIGURE 37-3   Some common causes of duodenal obstruction and steps in their
correction.

of normal meconium stools, and multiple air-
filled and fluid-filled loops of bowel that can be
seen on plain x-ray film. Small bowel and colon
atresias are usually caused by vascular accidents
during intrauterine life (e.g., volvulus, obstructive adhesive bands, mesenteric thrombosis). The
number of loops of bowel involved is proportionate to the extent of the vascular compromise.
Segments with minor ischemia may have only
become stenotic.

Because of scarring and impairment of intestinal blood supply immediately proximal and distal to the site of atresia, peristalsis is not well
propagated. Unless these segments are resected,
a functional obstruction may result. Any dispro-
portion in bowel size is overcome by placing the
suture line at an angle. Patency of the distal
bowel is ensured by injecting saline to distend
the remaining intestine down to the upper rectum.

Anal Atresia

Almost half of all intestinal obstructions result from anal atresia. Although no lesion is more obvious, it is frequently overlooked because of failure to carry out a thorough examination of the newborn. Clinical findings include massive abdominal distention and vomiting of bile after the first day of life. There is either no apparent anus or an anomalous fistula serves to decompress the rectum into the perineum or genitourinary tract. The sex of the infant and the specific type of atresia determine the site of fistulous opening and the morphologic anatomy of the perineum.

Anal atresias can best be classified into four main groups according to treatment priorities (Fig. 37-4). Types I and IV are probably caused by prenatal ischemia to the developing rectum. With type I there is stenosis of the terminal rectum, whereas type IV is in reality a rectal atresia with the normal anus ending as a blind pouch. The proctodeum has failed to rupture in type II. Type III, comprising the majority of cases, is a true anal atresia and is subdivided according to whether the level of atresia is below (IIIa) or

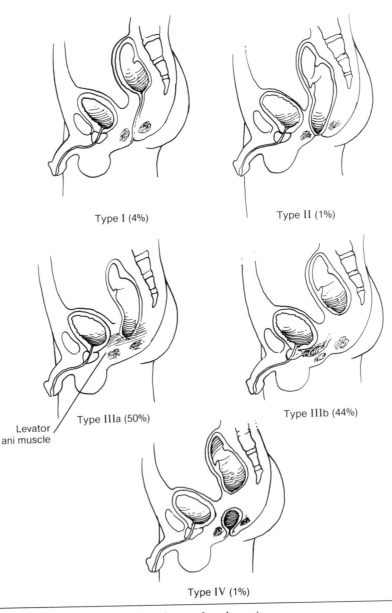

Type I (4%)

Type II (1%)

Levator ani muscle

Type IIIa (50%)

Type IIIb (44%)

Type IV (1%)

FIGURE 37-4   Classification and incidence of anal atresia.

above (IIIb) the levator muscle floor of the pelvis.

With type IIIa, the fact that the blind pouch of rectum has passed through the levator can be demonstrated on x-ray examination by holding the infant upside down while taking a lateral film with a lead marker placed on the perineum. If the distance between the gas-filled blind rectal pouch and marker is less than 2 cm, such children can be managed simply by incising the perineum, dissecting the blind pouch, and suturing its opened end to the perineum. Although an attempt is made to pull the proximal rectum through any identifiable sphincteric structure, continence is primarily guaranteed by the levator sling, in particular the puborectalis, and not by any anal sphincter.

In type IIIb, the length of atresia, as demonstrated on x-ray examination by the gap between marker and gas-filled rectum, is greater than 2 cm. Since the pouch lies above the levator and cannot be reached from a perineal approach, any definitive procedure must place the bowel well anterior in the levator to allow its passage through the puborectalis sling and thus offer a better chance for near-normal control of defecation. A diverting colostomy is first performed, and final repair is delayed until the child has reached an age reasonable for toilet training, i.e., sometime between 18 months and 2 years. By an abdominoperineal approach, with posterior perineal dissection, the mobilized distal bowel is passed through the anterior extent of levator, just posterior to the vagina in the female or prostate and urethra in the male. Guidance for the perineal portion of the operation is provided by electric stimulation of the nerve and muscle to ensure an almost exact passage of terminal bowel within its appropriate sphincteric ring of muscle.

The frequent presence of a rectal fistula must also be considered (Fig. 37-5). Approximately one fourth of infants have no fistula, while another fourth have a perineal fistula that can be dilated to provide a temporary vent if other anomalies make operation too hazardous. One fourth of females have a fistula into the navicular fossa, while the final fourth have a higher fistula that empties into the vagina. Under certain conditions, fistulas even into the vagina can also be used for bowel evacuation.

One fourth of males have a fistula into the urethra, while in another fourth the fistula terminates at the base of the bladder or prostate. It is imperative that any urinary fistula in the male be corrected immediately or a divided colostomy with closure of the distal stump be performed. Otherwise, urinary tract infection can develop and lead to early death from intractable sepsis.

Fistulas of significance occur only in type III anal atresias. A vent for the passage of feces and either division of the fistula or complete bowel diversion by terminal colostomy are required. Best results are obtained when treatment is directed toward providing normal bowel function.

Malrotation of the Colon

When the midgut returns to the fetal abdomen after its herniation into the umbilical cord, the colon normally rotates in a counterclockwise direction 270 degrees on an axis of the superior mesenteric artery. If the rotation is incomplete or abnormal, intestinal obstruction can be caused by residual bands of ventral mesentery or from torsion of abnormally mobile bowel (see Fig. 37-3). Most obstructions caused by persistent bands occur at the junction of second and third portions of the duodenum. Midgut volvulus, on the other hand, not only produces mechanical obstruction but also causes bowel strangulation as a result of torsion at its mesenteric base. If any embarrassment of intestinal blood supply has occurred, the infant may vomit or pass blood in his stool that progressively becomes lighter in color and more profuse. Hypovolemic shock also can develop as a result of blood pooling in the bowel mesentery. Delay in operation increases risk to life as well as to intestinal viability. At operation the bowel is detorted and abnormal bands are divided. Bowel resection is performed as dictated by intestinal viability.

Meconium Ileus

Congenital derangements in exocrine gland function may precipitate the inspissation of intestinal meconium. The resultant obstruction usually occurs in the distal ileum, where rubbery masses of dehydrated meconium plug the bowel lumen. Additional meconium, almost tarlike in consistency, then collects behind the initial concretions. Either before or shortly after birth, bowel perforation can complicate the obstructive process and produce a meconium peritonitis.

Typical clinical features include small-bowel obstruction, dentable masses within the abdomen, unusually tenacious vomitus, granular opacities in the abdomen that can be visualized on x-ray examination, and a colon that is small from lack of use, as noted by barium enema (so-called microcolon). If the ileocecal valve appears incompetent, enemas containing proteolytic enzymes are often successful in relieving the obstruction. However, the majority of babies with competent ileocecal valves require laparotomy.

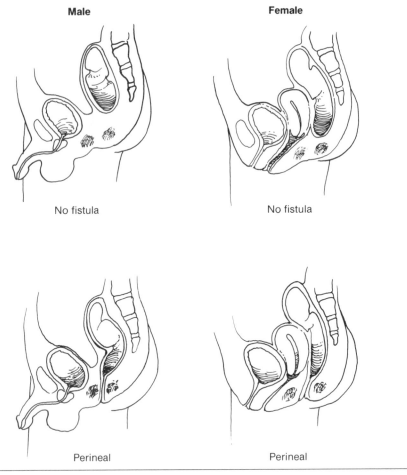

FIGURE 37-5   Rectal fistula associated with anal atresia.

At operation the diagnosis is confirmed by the presence of thick, blackish-green material distending the small intestine and by firm intraluminal masses obstructing the terminal ileum. Dilute solutions of proteolytic enzyme are injected into the bowel lumen to aid dissolution of the obstructing meconium. Although much of the material can be milked down into the distal colon, ileal enterostomy is occasionally necessary. Postoperatively, special formulas and digestive supplements are required to reduce the likelihood of recurrent obstruction from a second episode of inspissation.

Almost all of these children will later manifest other signs of mucoviscidosis, for they subsequently develop cystic fibrosis of the pancreas and chronic obstructive pulmonary disease. A more absolute diagnosis can be made by analysis of the infant's sweat for sodium and chloride content. The overall prognosis is extremely poor, since their crippling lung disease rarely permits survival beyond adolescence.

Hirschsprung's Disease

Congenital absence of autonomic ganglia in the myenteric plexus of bowel produces a functional intestinal obstruction. Usually the disease involves only the rectum and adjacent distal colon, although there may be proximal extension up to and including the cecum or even the terminal ileum. As a general rule, the longer the segment, the earlier symptoms occur, and the more difficult the diagnosis becomes.

With involvement of only the rectum and most distal colon, symptoms of incomplete intes-

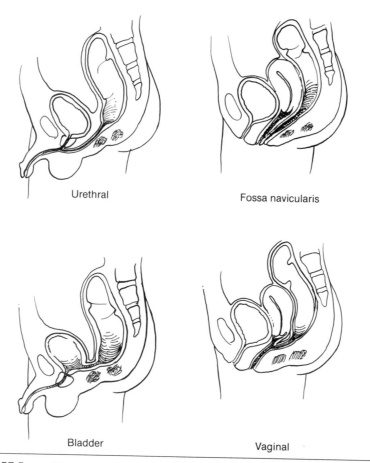

Urethral

Fossa navicularis

Bladder

Vaginal

FIGURE 37-5, cont'd

tinal obstruction may not become significant until late infancy or even early childhood. The aganglionic segment of bowel is collapsed, while proximally there is relatively massive dilation of normally innervated colon. Intermittent yet incomplete decompression has usually been gained by enemas or by occasional episodes of diarrhea. If the condition is neglected, malnutrition results. Enterocolitis is common and occasionally may be fatal. The diagnosis in older children is made on barium enema examination by the typical findings of a narrowed spastic segment of bowel extending distally down to the anus and the atonic appearance of dilated colon normal immediately above. Confirmation is obtained by transanal biopsy of rectal muscularis or suction biopsy of the muscularis mucosa to assess the presence or absence of myenteric gan-

glia. Initial treatment usually demands that a diverting colostomy be performed to relieve the partial intestinal obstruction, to facilitate mechanical cleansing of the colon preoperatively, and protect any subsequent suture line between normal bowel and residual diseased rectum. At a later date functionally innervated bowel is anastomosed to the anus by one of several techniques, with or without resection of the diseased rectum (Fig. 37-6).

In a newborn who has relatively extensive bowel involvement, the obstruction will be almost complete. However, there is no distinguishing zone of transition between a narrowed and adynamic distal colon below and a dilated yet functional intestine above. The clinical picture is one of distal small bowel obstruction on a congenital basis without any discernible interrup-

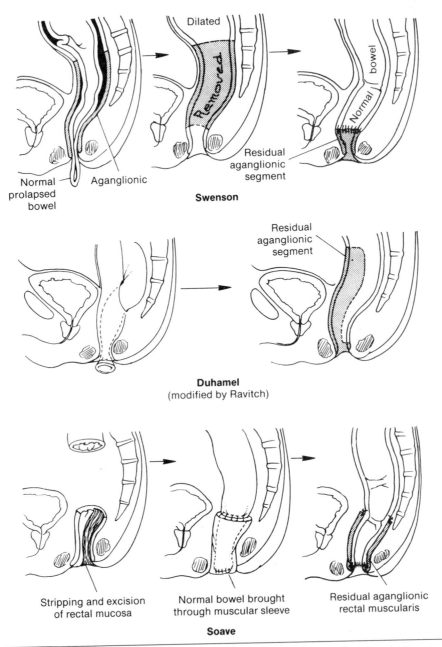

FIGURE 37-6   Some common techniques used in correction of Hirschsprung's disease.

tion in intestinal continuity. Nevertheless, the findings on barium enema are highly suggestive; there is usually a failure of the colon to completely empty, and puddles of barium tend to collect in one or more of the various adynamic segments. Once the diagnosis has been made, an enterostomy or a colostomy is established just proximal to the aganglionic bowel. Frozen section examination of colonic muscularis is extremely important to ensure that the intestinal vent is being placed in functional bowel. Between the sixth month and the second year of life, definitive correction is accomplished by anastomosis of normal bowel to the rectum, with or without total or subtotal excision of the diseased intestine.

WHAT GASTROINTESTINAL OBSTRUCTIONS OCCUR IN LATER INFANCY?

Complications from malrotation of the midgut and Hirschsprung's disease can also produce intestinal obstruction during later infancy and childhood. However, there are other and more frequent causes of mechanical obstruction after the newborn phase, the most common being incarceration of an *inguinal hernia.*

Pyloric Stenosis

During the first 12 weeks of life, gastric outlet obstruction may occur as a result of congenital hypertrophic pyloric stenosis. The incidence is greatest in firstborn males of young parents with a family history of infant difficulty with feeding in prior generations. Initially small volumes of formula are regurgitated, but gradually vomiting becomes strenuous and eventually projectile. Rarely does the vomitus contain bile. Characteristically the baby is hungry and will nurse even immediately after vomiting. Starvation and dehydration gradually ensue.

Examination demonstrates obvious dehydration and failure to gain weight. Gastric peristalsis is vigorous and is easily seen to progress from left to right across the upper abdomen. The mass of an enlarged pylorus can usually be felt in the right upper quadrant and is often referred to as an "olive." When doubt exists, an upper gastrointestinal series shows a failure of the stomach to empty as a result of a stringlike narrowing of the pyloric channel.

Both hydrogen and potassium ions are lost in the vomitus. In an attempt to correct this metabolic alkalosis, renal tubules excrete additional potassium in place of protons, thereby producing an alkaline urine. Thus body depletion of potassium is significant. The dehydration is treated by intravenous administration of normal saline, while three to four times the daily requirement of potassium must be given to provide sufficient potassium for both renal correction of the metabolic alkalosis and repletion of potassium stores.

Once dehydration, alkalosis, and potassium deficits have been reversed, operation can safely be performed. Through a muscle-splitting incision, the enlarged pylorus is incised longitudinally, and its muscle fibers are bluntly separated (Fig. 37-7). The mucosa beneath then bulges as the obstruction is released. Feedings can be restarted within a few hours after operation.

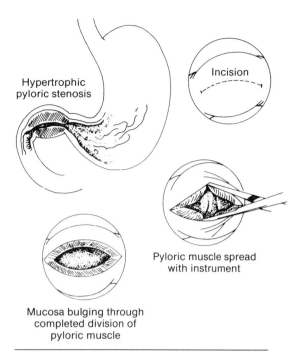

Hypertrophic pyloric stenosis

Incision

Pyloric muscle spread with instrument

Mucosa bulging through completed division of pyloric muscle

FIGURE 37-7   Correction of pyloric stenosis.

Intussusception

Intussusception occurs when proximal intestine (intussusceptum) invaginates into distal bowel (intussuscipiens) and is then propelled by peristalsis down the lumen of adjacent intestine. The mechanical obstruction thereby produced is soon followed by intestinal bleeding when vascularity of the intussusceptum is compromised by this autoingestive form of strangulation. Eventually there is progression to bowel gangrene. Intussusception is usually noted in otherwise healthy male infants at some time between the ages of 3 months and 3 years. The majority of intussusceptions originate in the ileum, though a few begin as a prolapse of ileum into cecum. In approximately 5%, the leading point is either a Meckel's diverticulum or an intestinal polyp. Nevertheless, no obvious cause for the process can be found in the vast majority of patients (Fig. 37-8).

The usual presentation is a sudden onset of symptoms consistent with intestinal obstruction, followed several hours later by the passage per rectum of dark blood mixed with mucus. A mass can often be felt in the right side of the abdomen. Barium enema is diagnostic and demonstrates the coil-spring appearance of an intussusceptum within the intussuscipiens. This same enema will

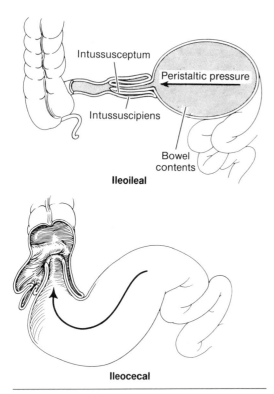

Ileoileal

Ileocecal

FIGURE 37-8   Diagrammatic illustration of intussusception.

also reduce the intussusception in many cases, though care must be taken to avoid exerting excessive intraluminal pressure. If, however, there is no reflux of barium beyond the ileocecal valve and the delicate mucosal pattern of terminal ileum is not displayed, reduction has been incomplete, and emergency operation should be performed. Shock and sepsis promptly ensue if a nonviable intussusception has been reduced or if resection of gangrenous intestine is not soon accomplished.

Surgical Repair. At operation the intussusception is reduced in a retrograde fashion by gentle pressure on the distal bowel. Never should traction be used to extract the intussusceptum, because disruption of gangrenous bowel may cause serious peritoneal contamination. If reduction by this method is impossible, if the bowel obviously is nonviable, or if an intestinal lesion has served as the leading point of the intussusception, bowel resection should be performed. Since in approximately 10% of these children their intussusception will recur, parents should be alerted to its early symptoms.

Meckel's Diverticulum

Meckel's diverticulum, an outpouching on the antimesenteric border of the distal ileum, is a residual of the omphalomesenteric duct or yolk sac. It occurs in 2% of the population, is twice as frequent in males, contains gastric mucosa in half of patients, usually becomes symptomatic within the first two years of life, and causes two major complications: bleeding and obstruction.

If ectopic gastric mucosa is present, acid erosion of the mucosa of the diverticulum or immediately adjacent ileum can produce acute ulceration, intestinal bleeding, and/or bowel perforation. Hemorrhage is common and generally develops without symptoms other than dark red bleeding from the lower intestinal tract. Standard x-ray studies rarely indicate the correct diagnosis. Technetium nucleotide concentrates in gastric mucosa and thus can identify such mucosa, whether in the stomach or at an ectopic locus. Laparotomy thus should be performed whenever bleeding persists or recurs.

The other major complication is obstruction, as caused by the persistence of a portion of ventral mesentery with attachment between ileum and umbilicus or right abdominal gutter. Bowel is trapped beneath or around this band. The resultant mechanical obstruction can be relieved only by division of the fibrous cord.

Rarely, various portions of the omphalomesenteric duct may persist as isolated bowel cysts or as fistulas that communicate with ileum or umbilicus.

What Complications Occur From Duplications of the Intestinal Tract?

Duplications of intestine occur in the bowel mesentery or more posteriorly in the retroperitoneal space and even up into the posterior mediastinum. It has been postulated that these are merely outpouchings from the mesenteric border of intestine. As a result of adhesions between embryonic gut and notochord, a traction diverticulum is created dorsally when the distal foregut or midgut migrates into the abdominal cavity. Such may well explain its frequent association with bifid vertebrae or hemivertebrae of the thoracic spine. Duplications have four major complications:

1. A posterior mediastinal or abdominal mass resulting from distention of a noncommunicating duplication cyst

2. Mechanical intestinal obstruction caused by pressure or torsion
3. Mediastinitis or peritonitis secondary to perforation
4. Intestinal bleeding resulting from contained ectopic gastric mucosa, causing ulceration of the duplicated segment or adjacent intestine with which it often communicates

BOWEL GANGRENE

Intestinal gangrene in the neonate usually results from strangulation of a midgut volvulus, unrelieved congenital bowel obstruction, or necrotizing enterocolitis.

Strangulating Midgut Volvulus

In the infant with a clinical presentation of malrotation of the colon (i.e., midgut volvulus with or without duodenal obstruction), dark blood in vomitus or stool strongly suggests a progression from strangulation to frank bowel gangrene. Shock resulting from some combination of bleeding, fluid sequestration into the bowel lumen, and sepsis is frequently noted.

The urgency of operation cannot be overstressed. Midgut gangrene can destroy so extensive an area for nutrient absorption as to preclude long-term survival. The absolute minimal length necessary for eventual oral maintenance of nutrition is 50 cm of small bowel with an intact colon and 70 cm of small intestine without an ileocecal valve and/or right colon. After detorsion, appendectomy is performed only if all bowel is viable. Otherwise, resection of gangrenous intestine is followed by abdominal stoma construction. Reanastomosis to reestablish bowel continuity is performed electively at a later date.

Gangrenous Intestinal Obstruction

As with adults, failure to provide prompt relief of mechanical intestinal obstruction may result in bowel gangrene. This occurs more commonly in infants with meconium ileus or in total colon aganglionosis. Operation is imperative and demands resection of gangrenous bowel, followed by creation of intestinal vents on the abdominal wall.

Necrotizing Enterocolitis

The newborn gastrointestinal tract is essentially germ free. Bacterial colonization begins immediately after birth, with aerobic gram-negative rods and gram-positive cocci becoming the initial dominant flora. The intestinal mucosa of the neonate is not as impenetrable to microbes as is that of the adult, especially if attended by prematurity, stress, or the hypoxic insult of shock or respiratory distress. Under such conditions, translocation of microorganisms now resident within the intestinal lumen leads to bacterial colonization of the submucosal space. The gases given off by these microbes, principally the gram-negative rods, are poorly absorbed and collect in innumerable tiny bubbles that in turn create a submucosal pneumatosis intestinalis. Accumulation of more gas further separates the mucosa from its nutrient vascular bed, thereby causing mucosal necrosis and slough. The denuded muscularis is then invaded by the same bacteria. Segmental paralytic ileus and full-thickness bowel gangrene ensue, especially in the distal small intestine and proximal colon. Intestinal perforation, bacteremia, septic shock, and death are the natural steps in progression if effective treatment is not soon given.

The diagnosis of necrotizing enterocolitis can be made whenever a preterm or appropriately stressed newborn develops an otherwise unexplained paralytic ileus, produces vomitus or stool that contains degraded bile, blood, or mucosal sloughs, and manifests signs of a more generalized sepsis in addition to overt peritonitis. Plain x-ray evaluation shows these characteristics. There is obvious paralytic ileus of the small bowel and varying lengths of colon, with foamy concentric rings of gas bubbles seen in the walls of these same loops of dilated bowel. Gas bubbles may also be noted in the portal vein. If perforation has occurred, there may be free intraperitoneal gas as well.

Surgical Repair. Surgery is required only for complications of the disease (i.e., bowel gangrene, perforation, and/or persistence of life-threatening sepsis despite otherwise effective antimicrobial measures). Nonoperative as well as preoperative therapy demands energetic extracellular fluid repletion, correction of acidosis, and administration of parenteral antibiotics with proven reliability against aerobic gram-negative rods, such as aminoglycosides. If complications require surgery, all patently gangrenous bowel plus segments of questionable viability must be resected. End stomas are created to decompress intestine proximally and distally as well as to avoid primary anastomosis, a procedure that is rarely if ever secure under these circumstances.

Postoperative care is based on continued parenteral antibiotic therapy, total parenteral nutrition, and ventilatory support as required. Recurrence or persistence of necrotizing enterocolitis is common. Late sequelae include obstructing bowel stricture and various malabsorption syndromes resulting from altered mucosal function and/or the short length of residual bowel.

BIBLIOGRAPHY

Coran AG. Pediatrics: Perioperative problems in care of the surgical patient. Scientific American, 1989.

Holder TM, Ashcraft KW. Pediatric Surgery. Philadelphia, WB Saunders, 1980.

Raffensperger, JG. Swenson's Pediatric Surgery, 4th ed. New York, Appleton-Century-Crofts, 1980.

Ravitch MM, Welch KJ, Benson CD, et al. Pediatric Surgery, 3rd ed. Chicago, Year Book Medical Publishers, 1979.

CHAPTER REVIEW
Questions

1. Primary closure of the fascia in large omphaloceles is potentially lethal because of which two major complications?
2. Absence of abdominal musculature is most commonly associated with which other life-threatening anomaly?
3. After correction of a meningomyelocele, the newborn must be carefully observed for evidences of which additional problems?
4. Which two measures, other than history-taking and physical examination, are most useful in specifying the cause of respiratory distress in the newborn?
5. Diaphragmatic hernias causing respiratory insufficiency shortly after birth are usually on which side?
6. The most common cause of tension pneumoperitoneum, with its dramatic life-threatening implications consequent to acute respiratory distress, is what pathologic lesion in the newborn?
7. The pneumonia associated with tracheoesophageal fistula is caused by what event?
8. What four clinical findings are most useful in the diagnosis of intestinal obstruction in the newborn?

Answers

1. Reduction in vital capacity as a result of forced diaphragm elevation; obstruction to infradiaphragmatic venous return and thus to cardiac output
2. Congenital bilateral hydronephrosis
3. Hydrocephalus, cord bladder with complicating urinary tract infection, and acetabular dysplasia (i.e., congenital dislocation of the hip)
4. Passage of a nasogastric tube and chest x-ray evaluation
5. Left
6. Rupture of the greater curvature of the stomach
7. Gastric acid aspiration
8. Maternal hydramnios, bilious vomiting, abdominal distention, and failure to pass a meconium stool

38 Head Injuries

DONALD W. MARION
PETER J. JANNETTA

KEY FEATURES

After reading this chapter you will understand:
- The effects of massive trauma, including skull fracture, herniation of the brain, and bleeding.
- Direct brain injury and its effects.
- Brain injury in adults and children.
- Grading of head injuries.
- Assessment and emergent care of the patient with a head injury.
- Monitoring and treatment.

Each year more than 2 million people in the United States suffer a head injury. An estimated 150,000 of these people are rendered comatose, and 36% of this group dies. These deaths are related primarily to motor vehicle accidents (MVAs), falls, or assaults. Because head injuries most frequently occur in people in their late teens or early twenties, such injuries account for the loss of more years of potential life than do cancer and cardiovascular disease combined.

Trauma to the head can cause a wide variety of injuries, the mildest being a physiologic disruption of brain function (e.g., a concussion) and the most severe being diffuse contusions and intracranial hemorrhage. Such severe injuries cause increased intracranial pressure (ICP), and elevated ICP is the most common cause of death among head-injured patients who are not brain dead upon arrival at a hospital. Despite recent improvements in both the triage and critical care of those with severe brain injuries, it is unlikely that such patients will ever be able to return to work or school, because brain injury of this magnitude causes permanent cognitive and motor deficits. Even patients with less severe injuries often suffer from subtle memory disturbances, headaches, or dizziness—symptoms that can last for months or even years and that are often refractory to treatment.

Before 1980, a patient's outcome after a head injury was thought to be determined almost entirely at the time of impact. Consequently, either the care given was reactive—the treatment of elevated ICP after it occurred—or the ICP was not monitored at all. However, recent studies have defined mechanisms of secondary brain injury—cellular and biochemical processes that lead to increased ICP—and have demonstrated the existence of an early posttraumatic period during which therapy can intervene to stem the mechanisms that cause secondary brain injury. There is also clinical evidence that secondary brain injury may contribute substantially to the neurologic outcome of patients who experience severe brain injuries; this suggests that prognosis may not necessarily be determined at the time of the initial injury. Thus there is reason to believe that the effective treatment of secondary brain injury will ultimately improve the outcome of many patients who have suffered head injuries.

The appropriate treatment of a victim of head injury depends on the neurologic signs and symptoms exhibited after the injury. Those signs

653

and symptoms can often be related to structural lesions of the skull, meninges, or brain.

WHAT IS THE SIGNIFICANCE OF SKULL FRACTURES?

Skull fractures over the convexity of the head generally are caused by assaults, falls, or MVAs. The most common are *linear fractures* (Fig. 38-1), which usually occur in the lateral skull (parietal bones). Most skull fractures heal spontaneously and do not require surgical repair unless severely depressed. Nonetheless, *the presence of a skull fracture poses a tenfold increase in the risk of an intracranial hematoma.*

Fractures in certain locations of the skull are more likely to cause a hematoma than those in other locations. A fracture through the squamous portion of the temporal bone, for example, probably will tear the middle meningeal artery, which is tethered in a groove in the bone. Disruption of the middle meningeal artery typically causes an epidural hematoma adjacent to the temporal lobe. Fractures overlying the venous sinuses, particularly the superior sagittal sinus, can lead to a subdural hematoma by tearing the sinus. Thus patients who have a fracture of the squamous temporal bone or a fracture that crosses the sagittal midline must undergo computed tomographic (CT) scanning and, in most cases, must be hospitalized for at least 24 to 48 hours.

Skull fractures may also extend along the base of the skull and disrupt the dura mater and the arachnoid on the undersurface of the brain. Consequently a fistula may be created between the subarachnoid space and paranasal sinuses, the nares, or the middle ear, through which cerebrospinal fluid (CSF) may leak. *Basilar skull fractures* are much rarer than linear fractures over the convexity, and anterior basilar skull fractures are more common than posterior basilar skull fractures (Figs. 38-2 and 38-3). Thus patients who have suffered a basilar skull fracture most frequently present with *CSF rhinorrhea,* or leakage of CSF from the nose.

Severe blows to the skull with a blunt object can cause a *depressed skull fracture, wherein fragments of the skull are collapsed into the cranium;* these fragments can tear the dura and penetrate the brain (Figs. 38-4 and 38-5). Neurologic morbidity from depressed skull fractures is caused by the damage to the underlying brain tissue at the time of the fracture, and not by the fragments of bone resting in the brain tissue. If the scalp overlying the fracture is lacerated, the lesion is considered an open depressed skull fracture and poses an increased risk of infection, because contaminated fragments of skin or other debris are likely to have been imbedded in the brain.

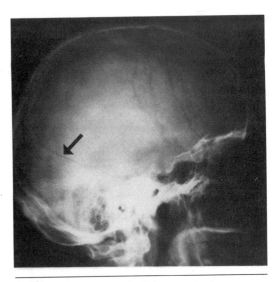

FIGURE 38-1   Linear skull fracture in the posterior convexity of the skull is seen on this lateral skull x-ray film.

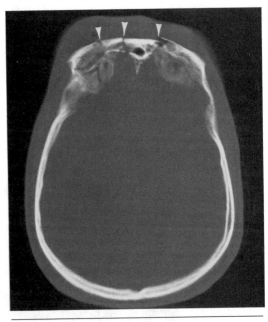

FIGURE 38-2   Axial CT image demonstrating multiple fractures through the superior orbital rims and floor of the anterior cranial fossa on both sides. This patient had a CSF leak from the nose.

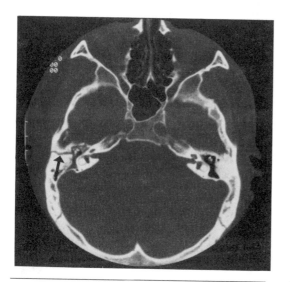

FIGURE 38-3   Axial CT image of a posterior basilar skull fracture. The transverse fracture through the petrous bone *(arrow)* involves the middle ear.

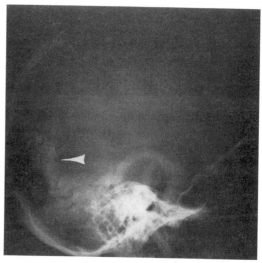

FIGURE 38-4   Lateral skull x-ray film demonstrating an occipital depressed skull fracture *(arrow)*.

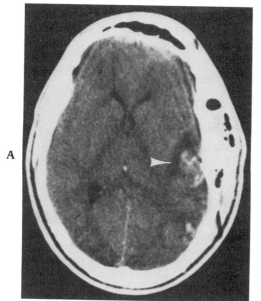

A

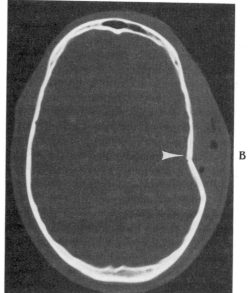

B

FIGURE 38-5   **A,** Axial CT image of a left temporal hemorrhagic contusion underlying a depressed skull fracture. **B,** The skull fracture is more clearly seen when the CT image contrast is adjusted to demonstrate bone rather than soft tissues.

Uncal Herniation

Intracranial hematomas or focal brain swelling following contusions can cause a shift of the hemisphere, and this can, in turn, produce a herniation of medial brain structures through openings in dural partitions of the cranium. The most important of these dural partitions is the foramen of the *tentorium cerebelli (Kernohan's notch)*. The midbrain passes through this foramen and carries incoming and outgoing fibers between the cerebrum and basal ganglia to the cerebellum, lower brainstem, and spinal cord. The third cranial nerve exits the ventral midbrain at the level of the tentorial foramen. Adjacent to the tentorial foramen, in the medial part of the middle cranial fossa, is the *uncinate gyrus (uncus)* of the temporal lobe. A blood clot that forms over the surface of the brain may shift the temporal lobe medially and force the uncus into the tentorial foramen. *The compression of the midbrain caused by the herniated uncus often results in coma,* because the midbrain contains major portions of the reticular activating system that are important in maintaining consciousness. *A fixed and dilated pupil is also a common sign of uncal herniation,* because the distortion of the midbrain caused by the herniated uncus stretches the third cranial nerve, which carries parasympathetic fibers responsible for pupil constriction.

COMMON TYPES OF INTRACRANIAL HEMORRHAGE

The most common form of posttraumatic intracranial hemorrhage is subarachnoid hemorrhage (SAH) (Fig. 38-6). An SAH never requires operative evacuation and is rarely of consequence to the ultimate neurologic outcome of the patient. Recent studies suggest that posttraumatic SAH may cause vasospasm of the larger cerebral arteries, similar to the vasospasm caused by aneurysmal SAH. Nonetheless, there has been no evidence that such vasospasm contributes to neurologic morbidity after a head injury.

The most common surgical hematoma following trauma is the subdural hematoma (Figs. 38-6 and 38-7). This clot results from the tearing of bridging vessels between the dura mater and the surface of the brain, the laceration of brain tissue, or the tearing of a major venous sinus. The blood clot typically is located over the hemisphere and may extend from the frontal lobe to the occipital lobe. If the clot developed as a result

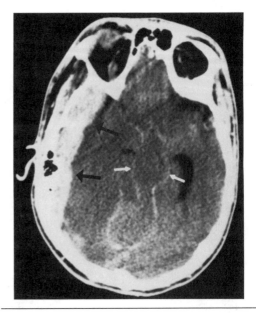

FIGURE 38-6   Axial CT image of a right temporal subdural hematoma *(black arrows)*. The irregular inner border is typical of this type of hematoma, one that follows the convexity of the brain. Also note the subarachnoid hemorrhage in the basal cisterns and observe how the hemorrhage follows the outline of the brainstem *(white arrows)*.

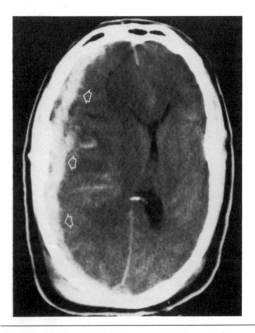

FIGURE 38-7   Axial CT image of a large right convexity subdural hematoma *(arrows)*. The mass of this hematoma causes a shift of the ventricles, which normally lie in the midline.

of contusions and bleeding from the surface of the brain, as is estimated to occur in 40% to 50% of cases, the neurologic deficits caused by the head injury are most likely due to the brain-tissue injury and not the clot. Thus, evacuation of the subdural hematoma in these patients often does not bring immediate improvement in neurologic status.

Although outcome after the evacuation of a subdural hematoma often is not good, it is much worse if the patient has uncal herniation in addition to the clot. Therefore, the presence of a fixed and dilated pupil must always lead to rapid evaluation and surgery if a hematoma is discovered. A study published in 1982 found that mortality after a closed head injury was reduced by 60% when a large intracranial blood clot was removed within 2 hours after injury, compared with cases in which there was a delay of 4 hours or more.

Epidural hematomas occur in 8% of patients who have a severe head injury (Fig. 38-8). They are usually caused by a fracture through the squamous portion of the temporal bone that tears a branch of the middle meningeal artery. As their name indicates, these clots are located between the dura and the inner table of the skull.

Because they tear the dura away from the skull, they have a characteristic smooth and lenticular inner border. Compared with subdural hematomas, epidural hematomas are much less common, but rapid surgical evacuation usually leads to a better outcome. The reason is that these clots rarely damage the underlying brain tissue, and the mass effect that they cause is the only reason for neurologic symptoms and signs. As with subdural hematomas, however, there is a potential for uncal herniation and subsequent brainstem damage. Thus delays in surgical removal can result in a poor outcome.

COMMON BRAIN LESIONS FROM SEVERE HEAD TRAUMA

Severe head trauma also can cause *contusions* of the brain (Figs. 38-5 and 38-9). The slow oozing of blood into the contusion from torn cortical vessels can form intracerebral blood clots that may, depending on their size, require surgical evacuation. The most common sites of cerebral contusions are the tips of the temporal lobes and the inferior frontal gyri, probably because the surfaces of the floor of the anterior and middle cranial fossae are more irregular than other sur-

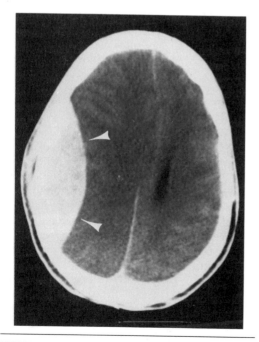

FIGURE 38-8 Axial CT image of a right parietal epidural hematoma. Note the smooth inner border and the typical lenticular shape *(arrows)*.

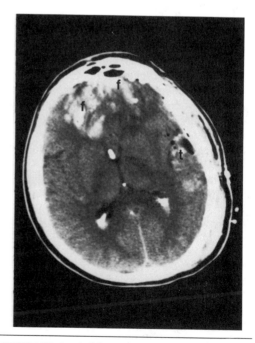

FIGURE 38-9 Axial CT image of bilateral inferior frontal *(f)* and left temporal *(t)* hemorrhagic contusions.

faces of the inside of the skull. The location of cerebral contusions also depends on the motion of the head at impact. If the head is stationary and struck by a blunt object, the contusion is most likely to be located directly under the point of impact. If the head is in motion and strikes a stationary object or surface, as in a fall or MVA, the location of the contusion is more likely to be contralateral to the point of impact—the so-called contrecoup injury.

The neurologic deficits that result from a cerebral contusion depend on the size of the contusion and its location: large contusions that occur in the motor cortex lead to weakness in the contralateral arm or leg, whereas small contusions confined to the inferior frontal lobes or temporal tips may not cause any perceptible neurologic deficits.

A large contusion can also cause uncal herniation. Contusions in the posterior temporal lobes are particularly ominous and need to be watched very closely, because any increase in their size, as might result from hemorrhage into the contusion or swelling, will lead to herniation. Because contused brain tissue almost always swells in the 24 to 48 hours after injury, we advocate the early surgical removal of these lesions before they cause herniation.

WHAT IS SECONDARY BRAIN INJURY?

In addition to contusions, blood clots, and fractures, recent evidence has shown that more subtle, biochemical derangements occur after a head injury. These biochemical processes may be responsible for much of a patient's posttraumatic brain damage. *Ischemia occurring soon after trauma to the brain is believed to initiate a cascade of neurochemical events that ultimately lead to the production of free radicals,* such as the hydroxyl radical, superoxides, and lipid peroxides (Fig. 38-10). A massive influx of ionized calcium into the cell is thought to be a common intermediate step. Free radicals damage cell membranes, thereby causing cytotoxic edema and damage the walls of cerebral vessels, thereby causing vasogenic edema and hyperemia. Because the brain is enclosed in a rigid skull, the swelling caused by edema and hyperemia leads to an increase in ICP that can be severe enough to reduce or stop the blood flow to the brain.

The biochemical processes responsible for early secondary injury may take 6 to 12 hours to develop. Thus there is a therapeutic "window of opportunity" after the primary injury during

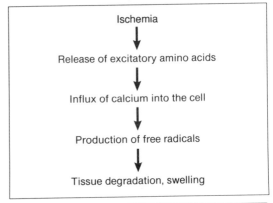

Secondary brain injury

Ischemia

↓

Release of excitatory amino acids

↓

Influx of calcium into the cell

↓

Production of free radicals

↓

Tissue degradation, swelling

FIGURE 38-10 Simplified schematic diagram of one of the cellular and biochemical events associated with secondary brain injury.

which treatment that effectively inhibits some of the reactions might be expected to retard or limit increased ICP.

HOW DO CLOSED HEAD INJURIES DIFFER FROM PENETRATING HEAD INJURIES?

Head injuries can be broadly categorized as closed or penetrating, depending on the mechanism of injury. *Penetrating head injuries* are those in which the skull is pierced by a missile, either with or without penetration of the meninges or brain. Such injuries are different in several ways from *closed head injuries,* which are caused by blunt trauma or by rapid acceleration or deceleration.

Some penetrating head injuries are caused by a low-velocity missile such as a knife or arrow. The type and severity of neurologic deficits sustained from such low-velocity injuries depend on the area of the brain penetrated, the presence or absence of injury to major cerebral arteries or veins, and the development of infection. Thus missiles that penetrate the nondominant anterior frontal lobe may cause no noticeable neurologic impairment; those that penetrate the motor strip may cause a relatively focal weakness of the contralateral arm or leg. If the missile disrupts a major branch of a cerebral artery, the victim may suffer neurologic deficits from either cerebral infarction or a massive intracerebral hemorrhage. Venous injuries are less likely to cause an infarction but can lead to acute subdural hematomas. In addition, because penetrating missiles carry

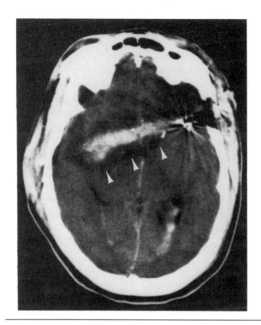

FIGURE 38-11 Axial CT image demonstrating hemorrhage along the tract of a lethal bullet wound *(arrows)* that traversed the basal ganglia of both hemispheres.

contaminated hair and skin fragments into the depths of the brain, *cerebritis* or an abscess can develop. Because the missile may be lodged in the vessel or may have a tamponade effect on a torn vessel, the missile should be removed only after the patient is in the operating room and the surgeon is prepared to repair vascular injuries when the missile has been removed.

The most common cause of high-velocity penetrating injuries is gunshot wounds. In addition to direct tissue injury, vascular injury, and infection, bullets traveling at a high speed through the brain damage a cylinder of brain tissue surrounding the bullet tract that may be 5 to 10 times the diameter of the bullet (Fig. 38-11). A bullet may also ricochet off the inner table of the skull and traverse the brain several times before coming to rest. Thus, high-velocity gunshot wounds usually damage the brain much more extensively than do low-velocity wounds.

Regardless of missile velocity, patients with penetrating head injuries should undergo early operative debridement of the wound. Such debridement should include the involved brain tissue unless this would compromise highly functional areas of the brain such as the motor strip or speech areas of the frontal or parietal lobes. The risk of infection is minimized by copious irriga-

tion of the missile tract with sterile saline, closure of the dura with a pericranial graft, and prophylactic administration of antibiotics for a minimum of 10 to 15 days. These antibiotics should have good central nervous system penetration and offer protection against normal skin flora (staphylococcal and streptococcal species), because these are the organisms most likely to cause an infection.

DIFFERENCES BETWEEN HEAD INJURIES OF CHILDREN AND ADULTS

The most significant difference between head trauma in adults and children is that children tolerate severe head injury much better, particularly compared with elderly persons. Victims of severe head injuries who are under 20 years of age have a 60% chance of making a good recovery, whereas those older than 60 years have an 80% chance of dying. *Intracranial hematomas and contusions are much less common in children than in adults.* However, the diffuse cerebral injuries or diffuse brain swelling associated with head trauma that occurs before puberty has been associated with antisocial behavior, poor performance in school, and a number of other cognitive deficits during the teenage years.

Several signs and symptoms of minor or moderate head injury are seen much more often in children than in adults. Vomiting and generalized seizures are particularly prevalent in infants and young children who sustain relatively minor head injuries. Difficulty in tolerating oral intake is so common after pediatric head injury that, in most cases, children can be safely discharged from the emergency department or hospital if they can eat and drink without difficulty and have no focal neurologic deficits. Early discharge presumes that the victim has reliable caregivers at home who can watch the child closely for at least 24 hours after the injury and are aware of the early signs of neurologic deterioration. Because generalized seizures of brief duration are so common immediately after minor head injuries in infants and young children and rarely indicate a propensity for subsequent seizures, we do not recommend prophylactic anticonvulsants for early posttraumatic seizures in children.

Child abuse often involves trauma to the head, and a severe head injury is the most common cause of death in such cases. Retinal hemorrhages in infants who have sustained a traumatic brain injury are virtually always the result of holding the infant around the abdomen and shaking him or her violently, causing an increase in intrathoracic pressure that is transmitted to the venous system and that ultimately ruptures the fragile retinal veins. If infants or children are suspected of being victims of child abuse, their skin should be well inspected for bruises or lacerations, and an x-ray evaluation of the ribs and long bones should be done to detect fractures in various stages of healing. Social workers or appropriate hospital administrative personnel should be notified if one discovers suspicious signs and symptoms.

SIGNS AND SYMPTOMS OF HEAD INJURIES

The most common manifestation of all head injuries is an alteration in the level of consciousness. Although this can be caused by many conditions including drug or alcohol intoxication, diabetes, and shock, a loss or alteration of consciousness after trauma is most likely the result of a head injury.

Concussion, the least severe form of head injury, is usually manifested as a brief period of confusion or disorientation followed by the return of normal mentation. Traditionally, concussions are considered physiologic injuries that are not associated with brain tissue disruption. They have been graded according to various clinical features:

Grade I: Victim is dazed and temporarily confused but has no memory disturbance

Grade II: In addition to disorientation, victim has anterograde amnesia that may last for several minutes

Grade III: Symptoms of the lower grades are accompanied by an inability to recall a period before the trauma occurred (retrograde amnesia), and victim may lose consciousness for a few seconds to a few minutes

Grade IV: Defined as the loss of consciousness for 5 to 10 minutes after the traumatic incident, with both retrograde and anterograde amnesia

Grade V: Prolonged loss of consciousness

The duration of retrograde amnesia has been correlated with the potential for having an intracranial blood clot: those with retrograde amnesia lasting more than 5 minutes are more likely to have a clot than those with a shorter duration of retrograde amnesia.

The higher the grade of the concussion, the longer it takes the patient to regain normal neu-

rologic function and the more likely there will be permanent or long-lasting neuropsychologic deficits. Although head injuries that do not cause prolonged unconsciousness usually do not cause severe neurologic damage, victims may still have enduring difficulties with both memory and subtle cognitive functions. Studies of athletes who sustained frequent minor head injuries suggest that multiple injuries may lead to persistent short-term memory problems, although such injuries do not affect intelligence. Another effect of even minor concussions is that they predispose the victim to further head injuries. Such factors are important in determining who should be allowed to return to play after head injuries in athletic competition.

Postconcussion syndrome is a constellation of symptoms that occur after minor head injury in an estimated 20% to 30% of persons. It can be very disabling. *Symptoms include headaches, memory loss, dizziness, diplopia, blurring of vision, vertigo, emotional lability, and sleep disturbances.* These symptoms are usually most severe between 4 and 6 weeks after the injury and subside within 2 to 3 months, but the symptoms sometimes persist for years. However, similar symptoms can be caused by hematomas or brain swelling. Therefore, until a thorough neurologic evaluation including a CT scan or magnetic resonance imaging (MRI) of the head has ruled out other possibilities, postconcussion syndrome should never be implicated as the cause of such symptoms. In addition, postconcussion syndrome is never the cause for fixed neurologic deficits such as a hemiparesis, hearing loss, or facial weakness.

Patients with severe head injuries that cause loss of consciousness can be described in terms of the *Glasgow Coma Scale (GCS) score* (see the box on p. 661). The GCS is a codified assessment of the patient's eye-opening, verbal, and motor capabilities in response to verbal or painful stimuli. The composite score ranges from 3 to 15. Because brain injuries of increasing severity cause a stereotypical progression of motor abnormalities, the GCS score bears a close association both with the severity of the brain injury and with the prognosis. The least severe injury leaves the patient able to follow commands. A moderately severe injury may allow the patient to reach for and push away a noxious stimulus—an act that is considered to be a purposeful movement. When a painful stimulus is applied to the finger or toe, patients with more severe brain injuries may not be able to localize the stimulus but will withdraw the extremity. In patients who have uncal herniation, two different types of abnormal upper-extremity posturing may be seen. Each sort of posturing may manifest either spontaneously or only after painful stimuli. The less severe form is a tonic flexion of the elbow and clenching of the fist, commonly referred to as *decorticate posturing.* More severe brainstem injury causes *decerebrate posturing,* characterized by tonic extension and external rotation of the upper extremities. After the most severe head injuries, the extremities will remain flaccid even on painful stimulus. The majority of patients with a high GCS (13 to 15) have a good outcome, and very few die. Those with a GCS of 3 or 4 almost never have a good outcome, and most either die or are left in a persistent vegetative state.

In addition to the GCS, several other signs can help to characterize the severity of the injury. The pupil size, symmetry, and reaction to light can provide important information. *A pupil that is dilated and unreactive to light may indicate uncal herniation.* Oval pupils have been associated with mild or early herniation. Asymmetric pupils in a comatose head-injured patient should always raise the suspicion of herniation. Posttraumatic pupil asymmetry may also occur in an awake patient but then most likely is the result of direct oculomotor nerve injury or is a normal variant; herniation generally does not cause oculomotor nerve injury without affecting consciousness.

Other cranial nerves frequently injured by head trauma include the fourth and sixth nerves, damage of which will cause diplopia. Victims who suffer basilar skull fractures through the floor of the anterior cranial fossa can develop anosmia because of damage to the olfactory nerves. Fractures through the petrous bone can extend through the internal auditory canal and damage the seventh and eighth cranial nerves. Any patient who has radiographic evidence of a basilar skull fracture through the petrous bone or has CSF drainage from the ear should be tested thoroughly for facial nerve and hearing function. The lower cranial nerves (9 through 12) usually are not affected by head injuries.

Very severe head injuries, particularly those associated with uncal herniation, may affect brainstem reflexes. Absence of the corneal reflex, vestibulomotor reflex, or tonic deviation of the eyes following ice-water infusion in the external auditory canal are all ominous signs and are an important clinical accompaniment to the diagnosis of brain death.

INITIAL EVALUATION AND TREATMENT

In the early 1980s several reports documented that early and effective evaluation and treatment of head-injury victims could reduce mortality and morbidity significantly. Since that time, emphasis has been placed on the rapid triage and transport of head-injured patients. Skilled prehospital personnel have been more effectively organized and helicopter evacuation systems developed. As a result of these efforts, the current mortality rate after severe head injury is half that of 20 years ago, and there has been a corresponding improvement in the rate of good recovery.

Appropriate prehospital evaluation of head-injury victims depends to a large extent on the severity of the injury, but several principles apply to all patients:

- *The initial focus must be on the entire patient and not just the head. The ventilatory status and blood pressure of the victim are the first priorities and must be stabilized as rapidly as possible.* Hypoxia and hypotension are more damaging to the injured brain than are blood clots or contusions.
- *The second priority is the cervical spine.* Cervical spine fractures occur in 5% to 10% of pa-

GLASGOW COMA SCALE

Eye Opening

Spontaneously opens eyes	4
To verbal command	3
To painful stimuli	2
None	1

Verbal Response

Oriented and converses	5
Disoriented and converses	4
Inappropriate words	3
Incomprehensible sounds	2
No audible sound	1

Motor Response

Follows verbal commands	6
To painful stimuli:	
Purposeful localization	5
Withdraws from stimulus	4
Flexor posturing	3
Extensor posturing	2
No response	1

Total score equals Eye Opening + Verbal + Motor: 3-15

tients with head injuries. In the comatose patient, the spine should be presumed to be unstable until radiographic evaluation proves otherwise. Neurologic damage from a brain injury is always more successfully treated than is the quadriplegia that can result from the inappropriate manipulation of an unstable cervical spine.

Once these priorities are attended to, treatment can proceed based on the specific type of injury, as follows:

For Concussions

- The patient should be allowed to rest until completely lucid and should resume normal activities slowly.
- If no sequelae of the injury are apparent 10 to 15 minutes after the incident, further medical evaluation probably is not necessary.
- If confusion, headaches, visual disturbances, weakness, or numbness persist, a thorough neurologic evaluation at an emergency department is necessary. If the patient is confused or disoriented for more than 10 minutes after the injury, special care should be taken to ensure adequate breathing and blood pressure before the patient is transported, and the entire spine should be immobilized. When possible, transport should be supervised by trained paramedical personnel; their support is particularly important if the victim is agitated or combative. In such cases, safe transport to the emergency department often requires administration of a short-acting sedative to properly immobilize the patient.

For Patients With Prolonged Unconsciousness

- This condition requires rapid evaluation and transport to a trauma center capable of neurosurgical intervention, because it indicates a high likelihood of an intracranial mass lesion.
- First ensure that the patient's airways are adequate, and that breathing and blood pressure are satisfactory. Then carefully evaluate and record the patient's neurologic status. This examination must include an assessment of the GCS score, the symmetry of the pupils, and their reactivity to direct light.
- Some of these patients, particularly those with irregular or shallow breathing, may benefit from intubation and controlled ventilation while still at the scene of the accident. This must be done only by trained personnel, however, because of the possibility of a cervical spine fracture and injury to the spinal cord if the neck is not kept immobile during intubation. If neuromuscular paralysis is used to facilitate intubation, it is particularly important to document the GCS before the administration of either this or sedative medications.
- Once adequate breathing and blood pressure have been ascertained, the patient should be immobilized on a rigid backboard. The head and neck should be secured in a rigid cervical spine collar.
- A patient who is hemodynamically stable should be transported to a trauma center that is capable of neurosurgical intervention, even if this means bypassing a smaller emergency department that is closer. Severe hypotension, inability to obtain an adequate airway, or other life-threatening problems may require that the patient be taken to the nearest emergency facility for stabilization, but transport to the trauma center should not be delayed to obtain a head CT scan or other diagnostic tests of the head or spine unless the facility is prepared to act immediately on the findings of these studies.
- During initial evaluation and transport, special attention should be given to any deterioration in the patient's neurologic status. Patients who initially can follow commands but then become unresponsive and develop abnormal posturing or a fixed and dilated pupil are at extremely high risk of having an expanding intracranial mass lesion that will require surgical evacuation.

Why Is Historical Information Important?

The temporal association of unconsciousness and head injury does not prove a causal relationship. Thus determining both the victim's medical history and the mechanism of the accident can uncover information important in expediting the patient's diagnosis and treatment. For example, a patient who is unconscious after a motor vehicle accident may first have suffered a syncopal episode that in turn led to the accident. The initial evaluation of the patient should attempt to determine the following:

- Does the patient have a history of diabetes, heart disease, anemia, seizure disorder, paroxysmal syncope, or any other medical condition that carries the risk of loss of consciousness? If the patient is comatose or confused, information should be sought from family, friends, or medical records. The victim's clothes should be searched for medications or prescriptions, and any Medic-Alert jewelry should be identified.

- Could the patient's symptoms be the result of a drug overdose? A documented history of drug use or information from family or friends can help to determine whether this is likely. Other supportive evidence includes needle marks on the arms or legs or the smell of alcohol on the breath. Early recognition and proper treatment of coma secondary to toxic or metabolic causes can significantly reduce subsequent neurologic morbidity and mortality.

- Did the patient experience prolonged hypoxia or hypotension at the scene of the accident? If so, this could be the reason for persistent unconsciousness or neurologic deficits. It is likely that a period of hypoxia or hypotension occurred if a victim was trapped in an automobile or under wreckage for an hour or more.

Knowledge of the mechanism of the injury will also suggest the probability that the patient has a surgical intracranial mass lesion. High-speed MVAs often cause diffuse cerebral swelling and diffuse axonal injury, whereas larger intracranial hematomas are relatively uncommon following such accidents. Low-velocity injuries such as assaults or falls more often cause subdural or epidural hematomas or focal cerebral contusions, all of which may require urgent surgical evacuation. The comatose victim of an assault or fall is approximately four times more likely than the victim of an MVA to require immediate surgery for evacuation of a mass lesion.

In summary, details of the patient's medical history, substance abuse, and circumstances of the traumatic incident can help indicate the most appropriate immediate treatment, suggest the relative risk of the existence of a surgical intracranial mass lesion, and provide important information about the most likely cause of neurologic impairment.

Diagnostic Studies

Evaluation of a head-injured patient in the emergency department must quickly answer two critical questions: *first, does the patient have a large intracranial mass lesion that requires immediate surgical evacuation, and, second, does the patient have a spine fracture?* Because hypotension and hypoxia play a major role in exacerbating brain injury, initial studies must also identify any threat to the patient's hemodynamic stability. We recommend the following sequence of studies for the comatose head-injured patient, all of which should be obtained within 30 minutes after the patient has arrived in the emergency department:

Chest x-ray evaluation
Lateral cervical spine x-ray evaluation (must include all seven cervical vertebrae)
Diagnostic peritoneal lavage
CT scan of the head

Abnormal findings on any of these studies require an immediate response. If a pneumothorax is discovered on the chest x-ray evaluation, a chest tube is inserted while the lateral cervical spine x-ray study is obtained or the diagnostic peritoneal lavage is performed. If there is a low index of suspicion for intra-abdominal hemorrhage, as when the blood pressure is stable and the abdomen soft, an abdominal CT scan may be substituted for peritoneal lavage, but this decision should only be made after the head CT scan has been performed and has established the absence of a surgical intracranial mass lesion. If the diagnostic peritoneal lavage is suggestive or diagnostic of intra-abdominal hemorrhage, the patient is taken to the operating room immediately, without waiting to obtain a CT scan of the head. During surgery on the abdomen, an air ventriculogram of the brain is obtained. If this study reveals a shift of the midline structures, diagnostic burr holes are placed on the appropriate side, and a craniotomy is done if a hematoma is discovered. An ICP monitor should be employed for every comatose head-injured patient who requires extensive abdominal, thoracic, or orthopedic surgery during the first 24 hours after the accident. ICP should be kept below 20 mm Hg during surgery. A CT scan of the head is obtained immediately after life-threatening abdominal or chest injuries are repaired.

Following initial evaluation and stabilization, further x-ray studies should be obtained to rule out the presence of a spine fracture. These should include anteroposterior and lateral views of the entire spine as well as an open-mouth odontoid view of the cervical spine. Axial CT images are obtained through any suspicious areas identified on the plain films. If all of these x-ray studies appear normal, the spine is considered stable, and cervical collars and backboards are removed. If not, appropriate internal or external stabilization techniques are implemented.

The placement of diagnostic or therapeutic burr holes in the emergency department is not recommended, even if the patient is deteriorating neurologically. A common misconception in this circumstance is that the blood clot that causes the deterioration will be liquid and therefore will effectively drain through a burr hole placed on the appropriate side. In fact, virtually all acute hematomas that occur after a head injury are solid clots by the time the patient reaches the emergency department. Thus a burr hole will not be sufficient to remove the majority of the mass lesion. Furthermore, because the emergency department is usually not equipped with adequate suction and cautery instruments, the surgeon does not have the means to achieve hemostasis, and hemorrhage following burr hole placement can be fatal if the superficial temporal or middle meningeal artery is damaged or the patient has a coagulopathy.

Plain skull films are not a routine part of our initial evaluation protocol for patients with severe head injuries. Because the critical issue is whether a contusion or blood clot underlies a skull fracture, a CT scan, which will reveal both a fracture and an underlying lesion, usually obviates the need for a skull x-ray evaluation. There is a subgroup of patients, however, for whom plain skull films still may be appropriate: If the patient has sustained only a minor head injury with or without a brief loss of consciousness, is completely alert and oriented, and has no focal neurologic deficits, plain skull films in both the lateral and anteroposterior views will determine the presence or absence of a skull fracture. *Identification of a skull fracture is important, since the probability of an intracranial blood clot is 10 times greater if there is a skull fracture than if not.* Nonetheless, if there is no tenderness over the scalp on palpation, a skull fracture is very unlikely, and in this situation skull x-ray films probably are not indicated.

Although MRI provides a higher-resolution image of the brain than is possible with CT, several drawbacks characteristic of the current state of the technology make its use impractical for initial evaluation of severely head-injured patients. These include the length of time necessary to obtain an MRI study, the need for the patient to be in a long tubular enclosure that precludes immediate access should cardiopulmonary resuscitation be required, and the impossibility of using conventional ventilators or monitoring equipment, because they contain ferromagnetic parts. Because these problems are not applicable to patients with mild or moderate head injuries, MRI has been used in the evaluation of these patients and has proved to be more sensitive than CT scans in demonstrating subtle lesions located in the gray and white matter of the neocortex. However, the significance of such lesions has yet to be determined, and no study to date has shown an association between them and ultimate neurologic outcome after a head injury.

MANAGEMENT PRIORITIES FOR VICTIMS OF SEVERE HEAD TRAUMA

The most common cause of death in patients with severe head injuries after hospital admission is uncontrolled ICP. An ICP monitor should be placed in all patients who are comatose and have severe traumatic brain injury. The ICP of these patients should be monitored continuously. Elevations above 20 mm Hg must be immediately recognized and treated by medical personnel experienced in the management of patients with head injuries. A systematic approach designed to treat the abnormal physiology of the injured brain is recommended. We use the following protocol in sequence as needed to maintain an ICP below 20 mm Hg:

- Systemic neuromuscular paralysis and narcotic sedation
- Frequent drainage of CSF, a suggestion based on the assumption that a ventriculostomy catheter has been used as the ICP monitor
- Intermittent boluses of mannitol
- Barbiturate therapy
- Moderate hypothermia

In some cases, a sustained increase in ICP requires surgical intervention. During the first several days after the injury, intracranial mass lesions may appear that were not apparent on the initial CT scan. Patients with cerebral contusions are at particularly high risk, because the slow accumulation of blood into the area of damaged brain tissue frequently becomes a large intracerebral hematoma. In addition, severe brain injuries are often associated with a coagulopathy, thought to be due to the release of thromboplastin from damaged brain tissue. The appearance of delayed posttraumatic intracranial hematomas has been associated with abnormal coagulation parameters. Therefore a coagulation profile should be obtained with the initial evaluation of severely head-injured patients and periodically thereafter for the first few days. Abnormalities should be corrected with infusions of fresh-frozen plasma, platelets, or other clotting factors as needed.

Any patient who develops an elevated ICP that is refractory to systemic neuromuscular paralysis, CSF drainage, and mannitol, or who exhibits an abrupt deterioration in neurologic status, should immediately undergo a CT scan to rule out a new intracranial mass lesion that may require surgical evacuation. We routinely obtain a CT scan within 12 to 24 hours after the injury to detect late-onset intracranial hematomas or swelling. In some studies, up to 40% of patients who ultimately required surgery for a traumatic brain injury demonstrated no apparent intracranial mass lesion that would necessitate surgery on the initial CT scan.

Hyperventilation has long been considered a cornerstone in the treatment of increased ICP. Although it remains the most rapid technique to reduce pressure, recent evidence from direct cerebral blood flow measurements suggests that the use of hyperventilation therapy during the first 10 to 24 hours after the injury may be deleterious to the damaged brain. Most studies of the cerebral blood flow soon after head injuries have found that the acutely damaged brain is ischemic and has regions of critically low blood flow. Because hyperventilation lowers the ICP by further reducing cerebral blood flow, it is very possible that the early posttraumatic use of this therapy could worsen preexisting ischemia. This in turn can lead to infarction and can cause ischemia in areas of the brain that previously had normal blood flow. We therefore caution against the prophylactic application of hyperventilation and suggest that its use be reserved for patients whose elevated ICP is refractory to other forms of control. We do not use hyperventilation therapy for comatose head-injured patients during the first 12 to 24 hours after injury, since this is the period during which they are most likely to have cerebral ischemia.

Steroids are currently not considered an effective means of reducing elevated ICP. More than 10 clinical studies have investigated the efficacy of using conventional doses of steroids to treat severe brain injury, and none of these studies has found either a beneficial effect in controlling ICP or a significant improvement in good outcome with any of the various forms of steroids. However, recent laboratory evidence suggests that the doses used in many of those studies may have been too low, and this new information has rekindled clinical interest in the use of steroids. In addition, a group of 21-amino steroid analogs known as *lazaroids* has been found to improve behavioral and histologic outcome following experimental head injuries. These compounds have been shown to retard the production of lipid peroxides, a group of free radicals thought to be important in secondary brain injury. Lazaroids are among the most promising compounds that are currently available for the treatment of sec-

ondary brain injury, and a multicenter clinical study of one of these compounds is now under way.

Comatose head-injured patients also are at risk for a number of systemic complications. Severe head injury causes an increase in the basal metabolic rate, which, in some cases, may reach 170% to 180% of the normal rate. Patients with head injuries are particularly vulnerable to protein caloric malnutrition. Enteral or parenteral caloric supplementation should begin within the first 48 to 72 hours after the injury to limit the degree of protein wasting and weight loss. There is evidence that early nutritional supplementation may also lower the risk of infection in these patients.

Infections are common in patients with severe head injuries; these in large part result from immobility. Some of the more common infections include aspiration pneumonia, urinary tract infections, and meningitis. Aspiration pneumonia often occurs because severe head injury depresses the cough and gag reflexes, making it difficult for the patient to adequately clear oral secretions or the tracheal reflux of gastric contents. The need to closely monitor the fluid balance in patients with a head injury requires the placement of a urinary bladder catheter, but the presence of such catheters is associated with an increased risk of urinary track infections. Meningitis occurs with greatest frequency in patients who have a basilar skull fracture associated with leakage of CSF. However, there is no evidence that prophylactic antibiotic administration reduces the incidence of meningitis, and some studies have found that it actually increases the likelihood of acquiring a more severe and difficult-to-treat infection. Treatment of any infection that develops in these patients should always be preceded by culture sampling of blood, urine, endotracheal secretions, and, when appropriate, CSF. *Antibiotic selection should be guided by the sensitivity of the organisms responsible for the infection, and the use of broad-spectrum antibiotics should be avoided.*

WHAT FACTORS DETERMINE OUTCOME AFTER A HEAD INJURY?

The final results of the Traumatic Coma Data Bank recently were published. This report represents a large group of prospectively studied patients with severe closed head injury and provides the most recent information available on outcome. Among the 780 patients entered into the study, all of whom were unable to follow verbal commands on initial evaluation, several characteristics were shown to be powerful predictors of poor outcome following severe closed head injuries:

- Age > 60 years
- GCS score < 5 on admission
- Presence of a fixed and dilated pupil
- Prolonged hypotension or hypoxia early after injury
- Presence of a surgical intracranial mass lesion

Because the GCS score and large blood clots or contusions are clinical indicators of the severity of injury, and because pupil dilation is associated with uncal herniation, it is no surprise that these features are associated with a poor outcome. However, the study showed that age, hypotension, and hypoxia played a greater role than had previously been recognized. Six months after the injury was sustained, the overall mortality rate was 36% and the rate of good outcome was 27%. Among those who were older than 60 years, who had a GCS score between 3 and 4, had one or both pupils fixed and dilated, and who experienced prolonged hypoxia or hypotension at the scene of the accident, the mortality rate was nearly 100%.

With penetrating head injuries, the prognosis largely depends on the victim's condition during the first few hours after the injury. Those who have a GCS score of 7 or less on initial evaluation have an 80% chance of dying, whereas those with a GCS score of 9 or greater have an 80% chance of making a good recovery. This polarization of outcome can be explained by the path of the missile and whether or not it damages critical brain structures such as the basal ganglia or brainstem. Damage to these structures leads to immediate unconsciousness and flaccidity or abnormal posturing. When these symptoms are present the victim probably will not recover. Conversely, a focal penetration of one or more of the lobes of the brain is often well tolerated, usually does not cause unconsciousness, and may leave the victim either with a focal neurologic deficit that does not cause severe disability or with no deficit at all.

Studies of treatment aimed at retarding or inhibiting the mechanisms that cause secondary brain injury are underway at several head injury centers. Through such studies, it is hoped that mortality following severe head injury can be reduced from its current 36% to between 18% and 20%, and that the rate of good outcome can be correspondingly improved. The recent establishment of high-quality head injury rehabilitation centers is also contributing to long-term neurologic improvement.

PITFALLS AND COMMON MYTHS

- *Concussions never cause long-term disability.*
  On the contrary, several large studies have shown that 20% to 40% of persons who suffer a minor head injury with only a brief loss of consciousness may have short-term memory problems, intermittent headaches, dizziness, and other symptoms that can limit their ability to function at work or in school.
- *All patients who are comatose after a head injury should receive hyperventilation therapy.*
  Recent studies suggest that cerebral blood flow is critically reduced immediately after a severe head injury. Because hyperventilation further reduces cerebral blood flow, it may cause regional cerebral ischemia or infarction in some head-injured patients. One clinical study has demonstrated that patients who received prophylactic hyperventilation for 5 days after their injury had a worse outcome than did patients who did not receive hyperventilation therapy during that time.
- *Burr holes should be placed while the patient is in the emergency department to evacuate a blood clot if the patient is deteriorating neurologically.*
  This practice never has been shown to improve outcome after a head injury. Moreover, placing burr holes in the emergency room can delay more important measures, such as obtaining a CT scan or transporting the patient to the operating room, where an intracranial mass lesion, usually a solid clot, can be treated effectively.

BIBLIOGRAPHY

Cooper PR. Head Injury, 2nd ed. Williams and Wilkins, Baltimore, 1987.

Eisenberg HM and Aldrich EF. Management of head injury. Neurosurg Clin North Am 2:1-506, 1991.

Report on The Traumatic Coma Data Bank. Journal of Neurosurgery 75:S1-S66, 1991.

Bouma GJ, Muizelaar JP, Choi SC, Newlon PG, Young HF. Cerebral circulation and metabolism after severe traumatic brain injury: the elusive role of ischemia. J Neurosurg 75:685-693, 1991.

Hugenholtz H, Stuss DT, Stethem BA, Richard MT. How long does it take to recover from a mild concussion? Neurosurgery 22:853-858, 1988.

Seelig JM, Becker DP, Miller JD, et al. Traumatic acute subdural hematoma. Major morbidity reduction in comatose patients treated within four hours. N Engl J Med 304:1511-1518, 1981.

CHAPTER REVIEW
Questions

1. All of the following diagnostic studies should be obtained in the initial evaluation of the comatose head-injured patient except:
   a. CT scan of the head
   b. Cervical spine radiograph
   c. Chest radiograph
   d. MRI scan of the head
   e. Diagnostic peritoneal lavage

2. The first priority during the initial treatment of a comatose head-injured patient is:
   a. Removal of an intracranial mass lesion
   b. Ensuring an adequate airway and breathing
   c. Stabilizing the cervical spine
   d. Assessing the GCS
   e. Transport to nearest emergency department

3. Which of the following is false?
   a. Subdural hematomas are more common after head trauma in children than in adults.
   b. Subdural hematomas are the most common type of surgical intracranial hematoma after a head injury.
   c. Gunshot wounds to the head may cause few permanent neurologic deficits if they do not damage the brainstem or basal ganglia.
   d. Skull fractures often are associated with intracranial hematomas.

   e. Those who suffer one minor head injury are at greater risk for subsequent head injury.

4. All of the following are associated with an increased risk of central nervous system infection *except:*
   a. Basilar skull fracture
   b. Gunshot wound to the head
   c. Linear skull fracture
   d. Open depressed skull fracture
   e. Knife wound that penetrates the skull

5. All of the following are associated with a poor prognosis after a head injury *except:*
   a. Age greater than 60 years
   b. The patient is a male
   c. GCS score of 3
   d. Subdural hematoma
   e. Fixed and dilated pupil

6. Symptoms of postconcussion syndrome include all of the following *except:*
   a. Dizziness
   b. Emotional lability
   c. Headaches
   d. Hemiparesis
   e. Diplopia

7. The most common cause of death in patients with severe head injuries after admission to the hospital is:
   a. Infection
   b. Uncontrolled ICP
   c. Subdural hematoma
   d. Severe skull fracture
   e. Hypotension

8. The most common sign/symptom of a head injury is:
   a. Hypotension
   b. Hypoxia
   c. Blurring of vision
   d. Diplopia
   e. Alteration in level of consciousness

9. Head-injured patients who open their eyes only to painful stimuli, utter unintelligible sounds, and pull their hands away when nailbed pressure is applied but cannot localize painful stimuli or follow commands have a GCS of:
   a. 5
   b. 6
   c. 7
   d. 8
   e. Insufficient information given to calculate GCS

10. All of the following are associated with an increased risk of an intracranial mass lesion

(e.g., a hematoma or a large contusion) *except:*
a. CSF leakage from nose
b. Age
c. Mechanism of injury
d. Fixed and dilated pupil
e. Skull fracture

Answers

1. d	6. d
2. b	7. b
3. a	8. e
4. c	9. d
5. b	10. a

39 | Musculoskeletal Injuries

JASON H. CALHOUN

KEY FEATURES

After reading this chapter you will understand:
- Fractures, including the mechanisms of injury and repair.
- Classification of fractures.
- Treatment of common fractures.
- Complications of fractures and their treatment.

Orthopedics is the treatment of musculoskeletal deformity. The word **orthopedics** derives from the Greek words **orthos** and **paidos,** originally meaning "straightening children." Today the broader sense of the words applies to the diagnosis and treatment of all bony deformities and injuries as well as to the care of associated soft tissue problems. Among these are sprains, strains, lacerations, and nerve and vessel injuries. Patient problems range from a simple ankle sprain to cervical spine fractures with quadriplegia.

In the past, bone fractures and dislocations often resulted in major disability or death. Today advances in surgical technique and antimicrobial therapy allow for better outcomes.

Fractures are often dramatic and obvious, and therefore seem to demand immediate attention. The wise physician, however, performs a thorough, rapid, systemic evaluation of the trauma victim before providing any specific care of the fracture so that associated injuries are not missed. Establishing the ABCs of trauma—airway, breathing, and circulation—precedes frac-

ture care. After necessary lifesaving measures are instituted, limb salvage is the next priority. This includes evaluation of neurovascular status, application of compression dressings to achieve hemostasis, splinting if this is required to transport the patient, and treatment of neurovascular compromise. Definitive fracture management follows, including reduction, stabilization, immobilization, and rehabilitation.

The goal of this chapter is to impart a general understanding of fracture treatment. The chapter includes an overview of the biomechanics of injury, fracture classification, soft tissue injury, and specific treatment recommendations for several common fractures. Despite many advances in the treatment of these injuries, complications and pitfalls still thwart the treatment of musculoskeletal injuries; some of these will also be reviewed.

HOW ARE BONES INJURED?

Bone fractures when it is loaded beyond its normal physiologic load. A brief explanation of the anatomy and biomechanics involved will make this clear.

Bone has a hard outer cortex that provides structural support and a soft inner medullary or cancellous bone of hemopoietic elements (Fig. 39-1). A bone's function determines its shape and strength. The long bones of the arms and legs are shaped to position the hands and move the body through joint articulations. Muscles and tendons are anchored to the bones and cross joints to move the body parts. The stress of weight-

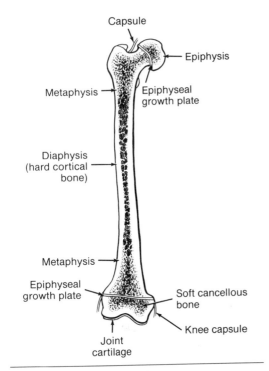

FIGURE 39-1   Anatomy of bone.

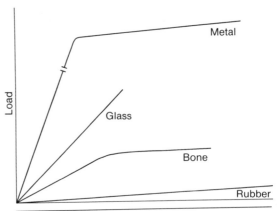

FIGURE 39-2   Load deformation curves for bone, glass, metal, and rubber.

bearing increases the strength of these bones. In contrast, the flat bones of the pelvis, skull, and the vertebra contain and protect the neural elements and viscera, and, in addition, anchor muscles. In these bones, the greater cancellous-to-cortical bone ratio allows more hemopoietic elements. This ratio reflects the blood-producing function of these bones.

A bone's response to loading is shown by a load-deformation curve (Fig. 39-2). Bone bends slightly before breaking; it is neither as brittle as glass nor as elastic as soft tissue or rubber. A bone's strength is determined by its specific ratio of mineral (hydroxyapatite) to soft tissue—collagen, elastin, osteocytes, blood vessels, and so forth—as well as by the orientation of these substances.

Wolf's law states that a bone responds to repetitive physiologic loading, such as walking, running or weight-lifting, by producing more bone to support the load. Thus bone is *anisotropic:* it is stronger in the direction that is commonly loaded than in other directions. The long bones provide axial support for the body's weight, so their greatest strength develops in response to compression loading rather than to tension or shear loading. Hence most long bone fractures occur in response to tension or shear

loading. An example of the effects of tension is when a bone is twisted or bent and a spiral, oblique, or greenstick fracture occurs (Fig. 39-3, *B, C,* and *G*); an example of the effects of loading is when a bone hits the dashboard of a car and this causes a transverse fracture (Fig. 39-3, *A*).

The combination of mineral and soft tissue and the orientation of this tissue make a bone that is *viscoelastic.* In such a structure the type of fracture produced depends on the speed with which the load is applied. A slowly applied load, for example, twisting the foot when a person steps into a hole, produces a single fracture line. However, a rapidly applied load, such as that created by a bullet, produces multiple fractures. A fracture requires a specific period of time to occur, and the energy from a rapid load spreads along multiple planes before it is possible for a single fracture line to have been completely formed. Therefore, it may be said that, in general, during a rapid or higher energy injury the bone is broken into multiple fragments (Fig. 39-3, *D* and *E*).

HOW DO FRACTURES HEAL?

Normal bone heals in an orderly histologic sequence (Fig. 39-4). Understanding this process permits the physician to provide good fracture treatment and avoid pitfalls.

When a bone breaks, the ruptured vessels in the bone (Haversian, nutrient, and endosteal vessels) and soft tissue (periosteal, muscular, and large vessels) bleed. Bleeding within the bone is tamponaded if the fracture is minimally displaced and the overlying soft tissue is intact. The

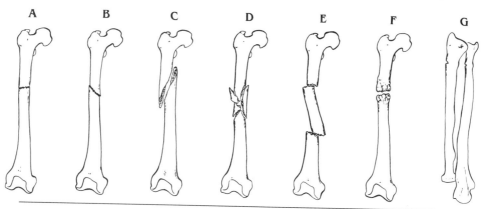

FIGURE 39-3 Types of fractures. **A,** Transverse; **B,** oblique; **C,** spiral; **D,** comminuted; **E,** segmental; **F,** pathologic; and **G,** child's greenstick.

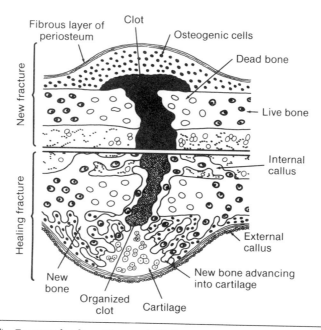

FIGURE 39-4 Fracture healing. The top half shows the histologic appearance within the first few days. The bottom half shows how the opposite half of the bone would appear within a few weeks with a healing callus of cartilage and new bone.

clot or hematoma at the fracture site extends a variable distance into the bone—usually the Haversian vessels are clotted proximally to their nearest anastomosis. This clotting and occlusion of the Haversian canal deprives some bone at the fracture site of its blood supply; this in turn results in a variable area of bone death around the fracture site.

During early fracture healing, the hematoma is transformed into the *fracture callus.* Within a few days osteogenic cells from the periosteum proliferate into the resolving hematoma and, to a lesser degree, into the marrow cavity from the endosteum. By the end of 1 week, capillaries have invaded the edges of the resolving hematoma from the periosteum, and the osteogenic cells have differentiated either into osteoblasts if they are near a rich oxygen supply (vessels) or

TABLE 39-1   Gustilo's Classification of Open Fractures

Type (Grade)	Definition	Treatment	Infection Rate (%)	Nonunion Rate (%)	Amputation Rate (%)
1	Bone puncture, clean wound, <1 cm	Irrigate and debride, culture, antibiotics, close wound immediately	0-4	2	0
2	>1 cm, minimal soft tissue damage	Irrigate and debride, culture, systemic antibiotics, wound may be left open, redebridement	2-6	8.8	0
3	Extensive soft tissue damage, contamination, wound open >8 hours	Grade 2 plus soft tissue and contamination treatment	14-23	17.5	18.7
3A	Adequate soft tissue for closure	Grade 2 plus multiple redebridements (every 48-72 hours) until wound is closed	0	12.5-27	0-2.5
3B	Extensive bone exposure or massively contaminated	Grade 2 plus multiple redebridements (every 48-72 hours) until ready for muscle flap coverage	8-59	27.7-43	5.6-17
3C	Arterial injury	Emergent arterial repair plus Grade 3A or B	57	100	59.9-78

into chondroblasts if they are in the center of the resolving hematoma and far from a good oxygen supply. After 2 weeks the osteoblasts have formed embryonic new bone trabeculae with osteocytes, and the chondroblasts have formed cartilage with chondrocytes. Over the next few weeks the cartilage is replaced by bone through *enchondral ossification:* the cartilage cells nearest the periphery mature and die as the cartilage is calcified. Blood vessels and osteoblasts then invade the calcified cartilage and replace it with new bone.

This early callus is immediately remodeled in response to the direction of loads over many weeks. During remodelling, the embryonic, cancellous, new trabecular bone is replaced with mature cortical bone. This remodelling continues for many years in response to Wolf's law. The bones of younger patients remodel more extensively than those of older patients; thus a childhood fracture may not be seen on later radiographs, whereas an adult's fracture callus is usually seen on radiographs for the rest of the patient's life.

CLASSIFICATION OF FRACTURES

Fractures are most commonly labeled by anatomic characteristics. The simplest way to discuss fractures is to describe the side of injury—right or left—and the particular bone involved (e.g., "a left tibia fracture").

Another useful classification is *open* versus *closed* fracture. A fracture with an intact overlying soft tissue envelope is closed (Fig. 39-5, *A*); a fracture in which the overlying skin and soft tissue envelope is broken is an open fracture (Fig. 39-5, *B*). In an open fracture, the break in the skin can be as small as a puncture wound, or the entire bone can be *degloved.* Of course, an open fracture carries the risk of bacterial contamination from the skin or the outside environment. Such contamination can in turn lead to a bone infection, *osteomyelitis,* that carries with it devastating functional sequelae. The size of the open wound often determines the size of the bacterial inoculum, and thus wound size plays an important role in determining the risk of infection for each particular open fracture (Table 39-1).

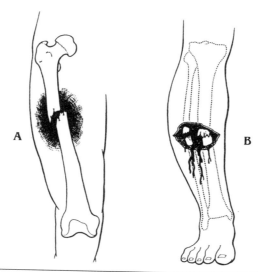

FIGURE 39-5   A, Closed right femur fracture. B, Open right tibial fracture.

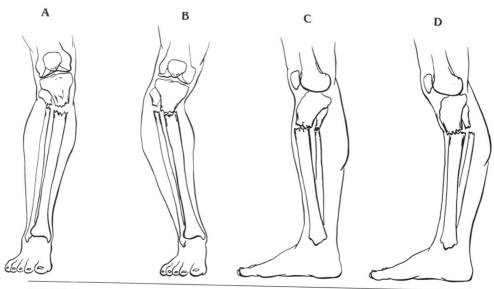

FIGURE 39-6   Fracture deformity. **A**, Valgus; **B**, varus; **C**, anterior apex or recurvatum; and **D**, posterior apex or procurvatum.

The type of deformity, the visible pattern shown by the fracture, and the anatomic location of the fracture are used to describe fractures more closely. A fracture can be angulated laterally (*valgus*), medially (*varus*), or with an anterior apex (*recurvatum*) or posterior apex (*procurvatum*) (Fig. 39-6). Specific fracture patterns include *transverse, oblique, spiral, comminuted, segmental, impacted, avulsion,* and *greenstick* fractures (Fig. 39-3). The anatomic location of a fracture in the bone, such as proximal or distal (metaphyseal), midshaft (diaphyseal), and growthplate (epiphyseal), also helps to describe fractures (Fig. 39-7).

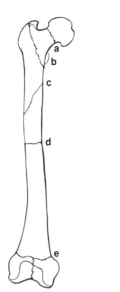

FIGURE 39-7 Nomenclature for anatomic location of femur fractures: *a,* cervical; *b,* intertrochanteric; *c,* subtrochanteric; *d,* diaphyseal; and *e,* supracondylar with intraarticular extension. Proximal (*a, b, c*), midshaft (*d*), and distal (*e*).

SOFT TISSUE INJURIES

The supranormal physiologic loads that cause bony fractures often damage adjacent soft tissue structures such as ligaments, tendons, and muscles. Ligaments are strong, fibrous structures that support tissues. Ligaments are often **sprained** (torn) as joints are stressed. These sprains most commonly occur in the ankle or knee and are classified as grade 1 for microscopic tears, grade 2 for partial tears, and grade 3 for complete tears. Complete joint dislocations, such as those of the knee or shoulder, are usually grade 3 injuries: the bones have been displaced out of the joint. Tears of muscles and their fibrous tissue anchors, tendons, are called **strains.** A strain of the Achilles tendon or hamstring muscle is also classified as grade 1, 2, or 3. It is common for a fractured extremity to be accompanied by strains or sprains.

Treatment of soft tissue injuries depends on both the joint involved and the degree of injury. Almost all ankle sprains are treated nonoperatively. Complete disruption of the ankle ligaments is rare (<5%), and only about 25% of grade 3 ankle sprains cause enough clinical problems to require surgical repair; however, a complete rupture of the Achilles tendon is usu-

ally best managed by an elective surgical repair. Knee joint injuries, especially anterior cruciate ligament disruptions, often require surgical repair. These frequently can be career-ending injuries for a professional athlete. Complete joint dislocations, such as those of the knee, may compress vessels or nerves and require emergent reduction and stabilization.

HOW ARE FRACTURES FIXED?

The basic goals of fracture management are *reduction, stabilization, immobilization,* and *rehabilitation.* If the bone fragments are displaced or angulated, they are reduced back to a more normal anatomic position to decrease future problems. What constitutes a satisfactory reduction of a fracture depends on the anatomic location of the fracture as well as on the age and functional capacity of the patient. For example, there is an obvious difference in how a professional athlete needs to function and how a sedentary octogenarian does. An intra-articular fracture (i.e., a fracture that goes into a joint) is reduced as anatomically as possible—less than 2 mm of displacement—to decrease the possibility or the degree of traumatic arthritis or joint degeneration the injury will cause. The goals of long bone fracture reduction in adults are minimal angulation (<10 degrees), minimal shortness (<2 cm difference from the contralateral uninjured limb), minimal internal or external rotation (<10 degrees), and minimal sideways displacement (<50%). In contrast, children remodel so well that fracture reduction requirements take into consideration their remodeling capability. Childhood growth plate injuries, however, carry the risk of causing growth deformities of both angulation and shortness and thus require very precise reduction and a longer follow-up than would similar injuries in adults.

Fracture reduction can be achieved by closed or open techniques. Closed reduction consists of indirectly manipulating the fracture fragments into alignment. Of course, this should follow the administration of adequate anesthesia. The manipulation is done by reversing the mechanism of injury. The physician should be constantly aware of the patient's anatomy, particularly that of the nerves and vessels. First, gentle traction of the distal extremity is done. This initial distraction must be done without any attempt at deformity correction, since the purpose of it is to distract the fracture fragments and remove any soft tissue from the fracture gap. The bone fragments are then manipulated, or reduced, and stabilized and immobilized with a cast. The position of the bone pieces is then evaluated radiographically. When a good reduction cannot be obtained with closed manipulation or maintained with a cast, open reduction is used. This means that the fracture site is surgically exposed, and the bone fragments are restored to a good position under direct vision.

The fracture fragments are stabilized with external means (cast or external fixator) or internal fixation (pins, plates, or nails). The simplest form of stabilization is a cast of plaster of paris or Fiberglas molded over a layer of soft cotton roll. Such a cast holds the bone fragments in good reduction. External fixation can be accomplished with closed reduction if small stainless steel pins (1.5 to 6 mm in diameter) are placed through the skin and into the bone fragments. Once a good reduction is obtained, the pins are clamped to a stable frame that fits over the arm or leg. External fixation is often very helpful for the stabilization of a contaminated, open fracture, a situation in which the use of a cast or internal fixation might predispose the patient to infection. With open fractures the external fixator pins are placed away from the "open" wound, thus permitting easy access to the wound for dressing changes and muscle flap coverage. Both unstable fractures—those in which bone fragments do not stay in place after reduction—and intra-articular fractures are often openly reduced and internally fixed with hardware such as screws, pins, plates, or intramedullary nails.

Fracture immobilization is needed for 1 or 2 months until the fracture callus is strong enough to allow unprotected weight-bearing. Casts and fixators are left in place until stability and healing have been demonstrated by clinical signs such as the absence of pain and gross motion at the fracture site and by radiographs demonstrating stability and healing.

Rehabilitation is important for the return of maximal functioning. Immobilization causes atrophy of muscle, tendon, ligament, and bone. To help prevent contractures and to speed recovery, the patient should follow a program of progressive weight-bearing while the cast or fixator is still in place, combined with active and passive joint motion as well as with muscle-strengthening exercises.

COMMON FRACTURES
Lower Extremity

Fractures in the foot include stress or fatigue fractures of the metatarsals and fractures of the phalanges. Both of these are often caused by kicking a night stand or stool. If undisplaced, phalanx

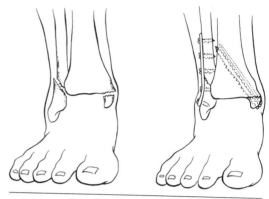

FIGURE 39-8 A bimalleolar ankle fracture treated with open reduction and internal fixation with screws and plate on the fibula and a screw and Steinmann pin on the medial malleolus. This is also called a Lauge-Hansen pronation-eversion or a Weber B.

fractures are "buddy-taped," whereas metatarsal fractures are immobilized in a short cast or hard-soled shoe. Hindfoot fractures of the talus and calcaneus are usually caused by falls from ladders or by the compressing of the foot into the floorboard in an auto accident. The surface of the talus is about 70% cartilage; therefore it has very little soft tissue attachment to provide blood supply. Displaced talus fractures disrupt the blood supply and can result in avascular necrosis of the talus. This in turn may lead to traumatic arthritis, pain, and deformity. Therefore most displaced talus fractures are treated with *open reduction* and *internal fixation (ORIF)* with screws, and the result is a lower incidence of arthritis. Fractures of the calcaneus may involve the subtalar joint and can cause long-term disability that is related to hindfoot pain. Although anatomic reduction and fixation of the calcaneus fracture is difficult, the procedure does decrease the incidence of traumatic arthritis and hindfoot deformities later.

Ankle fractures are usually caused by twisting the ankle or foot by stepping into a hole or by motor vehicle accidents (MVAs) (Fig. 39-8). This fracture is often labeled according to which of the **malleoli,** the outer edges of distal tibia, that are fractured. The lateral, medial, or posterior malleolus, or the bimalleolar or trimalleolar aspects may be involved. More elaborate classification systems are based on the biomechanics of the fracture (Lauge-Hansen) or, because the fibula is important for ankle stability, the location of the fibula fracture (Weber class). If an ankle fracture is not displaced or unstable, it can usually be treated by casting for 6 to 8 weeks. If it is displaced or unstable, usually the fibula is openly reduced and plated and the other significantly displaced malleoli are reduced and held with pins or screws.

Treatment for ankle sprains is summarized by the following acronym:

RICE-R:
Rest
Ice
Compression
Elevation
Rehabilitation

Most sprains and strains are treated this way. The exception is the high-demand patient—a professional athlete or laborer who requires a very stable joint and therefore may require immediate surgical repair.

Tibial fractures are frequently open because there is so little soft tissue over the tibia's anteromedial aspect. Car bumper and dashboard accidents as well as motorcycle accidents injure the tibia with a direct blow. Twisting injuries (e.g., those that occur when a person is skiing and the ski binding does not release) cause spiral fractures of the tibia. The resulting sharp bone ends can easily penetrate the overlying skin (Figs. 39-5, *B* and 39-6). As with all open fractures, an open tibial fracture is an orthopedic emergency. The patient requires systemic antibiotics and rapid surgical debridement and stabilization. Stabilization of a severe open tibia fracture usually requires an external fixator. The open wound is again debrided every 48 to 72 hours until only viable tissue remains. Then the wound is covered with a muscle flap. Closed tibial fractures are managed by casting unless they are irreducible or unstable. In this case either an intramedullary nail, or plates and screws, are used.

Because knee dislocations can damage the popliteal artery and nerve, they require immediate reduction, with attention to distal vascular and neurologic status. Sprains around the knee can injure the collateral ligaments, the menisci, and the anterior and posterior cruciate ligaments. Partial tears respond to RICE-R therapy; complete tears may require surgical repair.

Pelvis and Femur

Fractures about the femur and pelvis are often caused by MVAs and can be a major cause of blood loss (between 1 and 2 L) in victims with multiple traumatic injuries (Figs. 39-5, *A*, 39-7, and 39-9). Proximal femur or hip fractures are

also frequent in older patients after falls on osteoporotic bone (Fig. 39-10). Hip dislocations and pelvis fractures can damage the sciatic nerve and cause footdrop or they can injure the hip joint and cause traumatic arthritis. Stabilization of femur fractures within the first 24 hours significantly reduces the incidence of adult respiratory distress syndrome (ARDS). Stabilization is usually achieved with intramedullary nails (Fig. 39-11). Hip fractures are treated with plates and screws or, if the fracture is inside the hip capsule

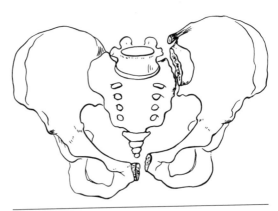

FIGURE 39-9 Pelvic fracture. Often seen with abdominal injuries; can have severe bleeding and sciatic nerve injury. Treated with external fixation and ORIF.

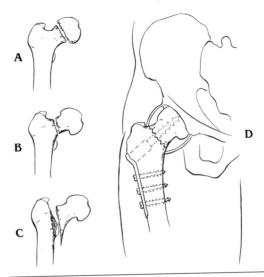

FIGURE 39-10 Hip fractures. **A**, High cervical; **B**, transcervical; **C**, intratrochanteric. **D**, Treatment of a transcervical hip fracture with a sliding hip screw with sideplate.

of an older patient, with total joint arthroplasty, the use of an artificial prosthetic joint. Pelvis fractures can be stabilized rapidly with an external fixator to tamponade bleeding and then stabilized later with ORIF. Traction was once used quite commonly for femur, hip, and pelvis frac-

tures but because of problems associated with long bed rest, such as pulmonary emboli, bed sores, poor reduction, discomfort, and muscle atrophy, internal fixation techniques are now used.

Spine

Spinal fracture-dislocations from MVAs or falls can cause paraplegia (Fig. 39-12). Yet another spinal injury, osteoporosis compression fractures in elderly patients, can be very painful (Fig. 39-12). Prevention is the best treatment for osteoporosis fractures. This includes exercise, good nutrition (adequate calcium, protein, and nutrients), and supplements (calcium, fluoride, and estrogen). When osteoporosis in compression fractures occurs, the fractures are stable and usually can be treated symptomatically with analgesics and bracing. Contemporary treatment of traumatic spinal fracture-dislocations includes early stabilization and mobilization to prevent pressure ulcers, a deformity such as kyphosis (bent back) or gibbous (acute kyphosis), and progressive neurologic compromise, such as increased pain or loss of function in partial lesions. Lumbar and thoracic spine fractures are treated with casting, or if the injury is unstable, with ORIF with rods, segmental wires, or pedicular screws and plates. Depending on the degree of stability of the injury, cervical spine fractures can be treated with a soft collar, a "halo" external fixator, or internal fixation.

Upper Extremity

Hand injuries include fractures, dislocations, and tendon and nerve lacerations. Finger dislocations are common in sports, while hand fractures and lacerations are common as a result of altercations or work injuries. Dislocations are usually re-

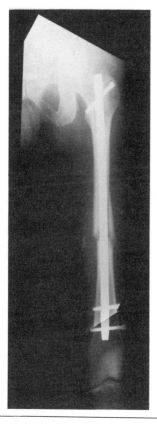

FIGURE 39-11 Radiographic view of a 34-year-old man who was injured in an automobile. Left midshaft fracture of the femur was stabilized with an intramedullary rod and interlocking screws.

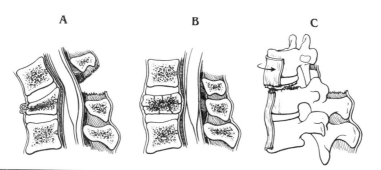

A   B   C

FIGURE 39-12 Spinal fractures. **A,** Chance, seat belt, or forward flexion fracture; **B,** axial compression fracture; and **C,** rotation/dislocation fracture.

duced after a digital lidocaine-block is instituted. (Local anesthetic epinephrine is used for digital blocks because epinephrine can cause digital artery spasm and, later, finger gangrene.) Fractures in the hand may be splinted using an aluminum finger splint or a plaster ulnar gutter splint, or, if displaced, such fractures may be reduced and pinned. Significant advances in nerve and tendon repair techniques have been made over the last two decades and, as a result, most of these injuries are now treated with early repair and protected motion.

Falls on the outstretched hand may cause wrist fractures, and forearm and elbow fractures (Fig. 39-13). If they are unstable, fractures in the wrist—such as scaphoid, lunate, and intra-articular distal radius fractures—require reduction to less than 1 mm of displacement and internal fixation. Other distal radius fractures such as the *Colle's fracture* can be managed with reduction and casting, with pins-in-plaster or external fixation. Forearm fractures in an adult and displaced elbow fractures in a child usually require ORIF (Fig. 39-14). Children's forearm fractures (see Fig. 39-3, *G*) are often treated closed.

Elbow and shoulder dislocations and humerus fractures in adults and children are usually treated closed. With these injuries, it is im-portant to avoid nerve palsy, both radial and axillary. This problem is addressed in the Pitfalls section, p. 682.

WHAT ARE SOME PITFALLS?

Any injury severe enough to fracture bone can also cause numerous other injuries. These include nerve injuries such as nerve palsy, compartment syndrome, and reflex sympathetic dystrophy; vessel injuries such as occlusion or laceration, avascular necrosis, and pulmonary embolus; and bone healing problems such as osteomyelitis, malunion, delayed union, nonunion, contractures, and conditions associated with hardware failure.

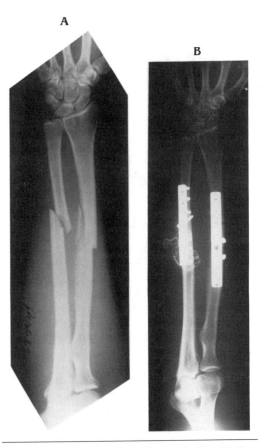

FIGURE 39-14 **A,** Same patient as in Fig. 39-11. Preoperative radiography of a both-bone forearm fracture. **B,** Intraoperative radiograph of forearm fracture stabilized with plates and screws. Note the radiopaque marker on the 4 × 4 sponge that was removed when the wound was closed (after this radiograph was taken) that demonstrates an anatomic reduction.

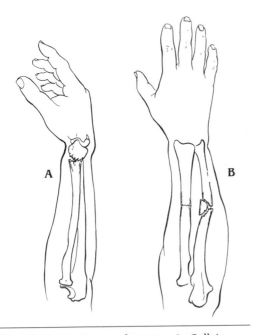

FIGURE 39-13 Forearm fractures. **A,** Colle's distal radius fracture; **B,** both-bone, midshaft forearm fracture with a butterfly fragment ulnar comminution.

Nerve Palsy

A nerve can be lacerated by bone fragments or by the object that caused the fracture. *Nerve palsy* is diagnosed during the complete and thorough neurologic examination of the extremity that should be part of the initial evaluation of any injury. The most devastating laceration of a neural structure is the division of the spinal cord with a spinal fracture: the result is paraplegia. Even with recent advances and better understanding, little can be done to reverse complete paraplegia lesions (complete division of the spinal cord). Partial and progressive paraplegia may respond to decompression (i.e., release of pressure of bone fragments on the spinal cord) and stabilization.

Upper extremity nerve palsies include brachial plexus injury that originates either at birth or from shoulder trauma; radial nerve injury related to humerus fractures; or medial or ulnar nerve palsy connected with fractures and dislocations of the elbow and wrist. All of these are generally managed with emergent reduction, followed by observation and physical therapy until functioning of the nerve returns. In the small percentage of patients (between 5% and 10%) who exhibit no improvement, tendon transfers are performed to improve function. Nerve lacerations in the hand have recently been treated with fairly good results by acute repair or nerve grafting.

In the lower extremity, there may be a posterior-tibial nerve palsy in tibia fractures or knee dislocation that can cause an insensate foot that may eventually require amputation. Both sciatic nerve injury associated with hip dislocation and superficial peroneal nerve injury in fibular or tibia fracture causes footdrop and requires emergent reduction to remove the pressure on the nerve. Treatment of footdrop may require either the use of a brace such as an ankle foot orthotic (AFO) or the surgical release of equinus (plantar-flexed foot) contracture and tendon transfer.

Compartment syndrome is caused by an increased pressure of blood, fluid and swelling into an injured muscle that is contained in a fascial compartment with a limited volume—that is, the muscle is surrounded by dense structures such as bone and fascia that limit its expansion with swelling. When the muscle can no longer swell outward, and yet blood and fluid continue to collect, the result is increased pressure within the muscle compartment. When the pressure in the muscle tissue is greater than either 30 to 40 mm Hg (of, if the patient is in shock, greater than the diastolic pressure) the small arterioles actively close and the soft-walled capillaries passively close, stopping tissue perfusion and causing ischemia. This is often seen in childhood elbow fractures (Volkmann ischemic contracture) and adult tibia fractures. However, compartment syndrome can be seen after any severe soft tissue injury, whether open or closed, or after any bone fracture of the extremities. Compartment syndrome is diagnosed by clinical signs—look for the 5 *P*'s: pain, pallor, pulselessness, paresthesia, and paralysis. The most important of these signs is increased pain that manifests both when the injured body part is at rest and during passive motion. Increased compartment pressure is confirmed by measuring the pressure with a slit catheter connected to a pressure manometer. Treatment is emergent fasciotomy to open the muscle's fascia so the muscle can swell out into the wound, relieving the increased pressure. Usually the wound is left open for a few days and then closed or skin grafted. If compartment syndrome is not treated, irreversible muscle damage starts after 4 hours, and irreversible nerve loss begins 12 hours after the beginning of the ischemia. Eventually it results in muscle loss, contractures, and nerve palsies.

Reflex sympathetic dystrophy, which used to be called causalgia, is a syndrome that is poorly understood. This diagnosis is made if a patient has persistent pain and if the swelling is greater than might reasonably be expected from the original injury. A more chronic phase of the condition results if there is an acute presentation of hyperesthesia (increased sensitivity to touch), swelling, warmth, redness, and a decreasing ability to use the limb (disuse), although this phase may be avoided if these are resolved. In this more chronic phase, there is continued pain, disuse, stiffness, coolness, and pallor. Severe disuse osteoporosis can then be seen in radiographs. The success of both prevention and treatment centers around early physical therapy and pain control. In the more chronic cases, pain control clinics are useful for management with antidepressants, sympathetic blocks, vigorous rehabilitation, and psychiatric and emotional help.

Vessel Injury

Blood flow into an extremity can be stopped by laceration or occlusion of the artery. An artery can be lacerated by bone fragments or objects causing the injury, or can be ruptured in joint dislocation, fracture displacement, or angulation. Such an injury to an artery is most commonly seen after knee dislocation, tibia and ankle fractures, and lacerations and amputations. Palpation or Doppler reading of the distal pulses and repeated checks of capillary refill—look for the clinical sign of blanch caused by finger pressure that resolves itself within 2 seconds—are essential in every physical examination of the injured patient. Tears of the inner wall of an artery (intimal wall tears), however, may not cause vessel blockage for many hours, so the pulse of these patients must be monitored for 24 to 48 hours. Certain injuries, such as severe knee dislocations, require arteriograms even if the distal pulse returns. Reduction of joint dislocations, or displaced or angulated fractures may open vessels occluded by pressure from the bone ends. If this does not occur, an emergent arteriogram, surgical exploration, and repair of the vessel are necessary.

Avascular necrosis occurs when the primary nutrient vessel to a bone is injured, causing part of the bone to die. The condition is most common in the ankle, hip, and wrist. The proximal portion of the femur, talus, and scaphoid are almost entirely intra-articular and covered with cartilage; therefore they each have few soft tissue connections to supplement their blood supply. They are each almost entirely dependent on their nutrient vessels, and thus are particularly vulnerable to the disruption of these vessels. The nutrient vessels cross the femoral neck, talar neck, and scaphoid waist (middle), so fractures through these areas cause disruption of the vessels, and the proximal portion of the bone will die. For this reason hip dislocations require emergent reduction.

Pulmonary embolism from thrombophlebitis (venous blood clots) may occur after fractures of the lower extremity and pelvis. The embolism can cause sudden respiratory arrest and death. Thrombophlebitis occurs more commonly in elderly patients. It is also common in patients whose fractures are being treated with prolonged bed rest (traction) and immobility, both of which promote venous stasis and clot formation. At the present time, the recommended techniques of fracture management include measures for preventing pulmonary embolus. Among these measures are early fracture stabilization and physical therapy to decrease venous stasis. Patients on prolonged bed rest usually receive anticoagulation therapy with heparin or warfarin (Coumadin) to prevent clot formation.

Within the first few days after a fracture occurs (usually of the femur, hip, or pelvis), fat embolism (FE) can cause adult respiratory distress syndrome (ARDS). Through some unknown mechanism, fat collects in the lung after a fracture, causing problems similar to a large pulmonary embolus. This syndrome is characterized by sudden respiratory problems that present as disorientation, fever, tachypnea, and tachycardia, and if untreated may rapidly progress to respiratory arrest. Arterial blood gas levels document hypoxia. Patients with pulmonary congestion, atelectasis, edema, and decreased lung compliance require oxygen supplementation and may also require intubation and mechanical ventilation with positive end-expiratory pressure (PEEP). Prevention of FE involves rapid mobilization after the injury. This is best accomplished by prompt fixation (<24 hours) of femur fractures. Such fixation is now possible if intramedullary nailing techniques are used.

Infection in open fractures is more common than in closed fractures. Severe soft tissue damage (see Table 39-1) and contamination increase the infection rates of fractures. The infection rate for open reduction and internal fixation on a closed fracture is about 1%. Staphylococcal and streptococcal infections are most common, but tetanus and gas gangrene from *Clostridia* bacteria from barnyards and brackish water, *Pseudomonas* infections from foot puncture wounds, and mixed infections from bite injuries are also seen. Active tetanus vaccination or prophylaxis is needed early during the treatment of an open injury. Infection rates for open fractures are reduced by gram-positive and -negative systemic antibiotics, if these are started preoperatively. Emergent debridement and jet lavage to remove contamination and necrotic tissue also reduce the likelihood of infection. Aerobic and anaerobic culture tests of the remaining tissue are performed after debridement to guide the use of postdebridement antibiotics. Large wounds (grade II or >1 cm) are usually left open for wound care. Sterile saline dressings are changed three times daily. Irrigation, debridement, and culturing are repeated every 48 to 72 hours until the wound is clean, viable, and ready for closure or muscle flap coverage. Culture test results are used to direct antibiotic choice and to determine the length of treatment.

Osteomyelitis, or bone infection, is difficult to cure because bacteria become sequestered in dead bone. Because of its mineral structure, bone has a poorer blood supply than soft tissue; therefore it is difficult to get antibiotics to reach bacteriocidal levels. Consequently, osteomyelitis is best treated by the debridement of sequestered, necrotic, or ischemic infected bone and scarred soft tissue. The debrided limb is then reconstructed with bone grafts, muscle flaps, and external and internal fixation techniques. Amputation of severely injured or infected extremities may be necessary.

Nonunion of a bone occurs when the bone ends do not heal together. Usually this happens in certain cortical long bones, such as the tibia or ulna, when there is severe soft tissue injury of the bone's diaphysis. Fracture healing normally occurs over 6 to 12 weeks. If a fracture has not healed within 3 to 5 months, it is classified as a *delayed union.* If the fracture is still not united after 5 to 6 months, it is classified as a *nonunion.* Adequate stabilization with the appropriate internal or external fixation techniques, extended casting (for up to 2 years), and use of a patient's iliac crest's cancellous bone for bone grafting are all techniques for managing delayed unions and nonunions.

When there is a malunion of a fracture, the fracture has healed in the wrong position. Angulation, rotation, shortness, and sideways displacement can all occur if the fracture has not been reduced and stabilized correctly. Patient noncompliance can also cause a malunion, whether because the patient refuses treatment or because the patient doesn't follow postreduction recommendations.

Childhood fractures that involve the growth plates can cause *growth deformities.* An angular growth deformity occurs if there is partial arrest of the growth plate. Partial or full arrest of the growth plate can cause limb shortness. A fracture of a child's growth plate needs to be very carefully reduced, and the child's progress should be closely followed with radiographic evaluation every 6 to 9 months. A growth plate arrest with a bone bar can be surgically removed and filled with a fat graft. Alternatively, angulation can be treated with corrective *osteotomies* (bone cuts); shortness can be treated by shortening the opposite limb to match the shortened one or by limb-lengthening techniques.

Contractures and *muscle atrophy* occur to some extent after any significant musculoskeletal injury. As soon as they are not used or are immobilized, muscles start to atrophy and joint capsules, ligaments, and tendons start to contract. Therefore, as soon as pain and stability

permit, physical therapy and rehabilitation are started with both active and passive range of motion activities and strengthening exercises.

Traumatic arthritis occurs after fractures occur near or in joints. Angular deformities from a malunion can cause abnormal joint stresses that also result in arthritis. Fractures involving the joint surface, even if perfectly reduced, can cause arthritis because the cartilage heals with fibrous cartilage rather than hyaline cartilage, so there will be some rough spots in the previously smooth cartilage. Comminuted intra-articular fractures usually heal with incongruities that result in arthritis. We do know that reduction of ankle fracture fragments to less than 2 mm significantly reduces the incidence of late traumatic arthritis. Symptomatic arthritis is treated with shoe and activity modifications, nonsteroidal anti-inflammatory drugs (NSAIDs), braces, canes, walkers, and crutches. If nonsurgical therapy fails to provide relief of symptoms, traumatic arthritis can be treated with total joint replacement (*arthroplasty*) or joint fusion (*arthrodesis*). Total joint replacement with plastic and metal prostheses is appropriate for older patients. Similar treatment is less appropriate for younger patients because the prosthetic components may wear out and require replacement. Fusion relieves joint pain but decreases motion and increases the demand on other joints.

Hardware failure of plates, rods, or pins can occur if the fracture does not heal fast enough. According to Wolf's law, bone has the ability to reinforce itself as it is repeatedly loaded. Unlike bone, an inert implant eventually breaks if subjected to repeated loading—much like a coat hanger that has been bent repeatedly. This is seen less often now than it once was because devices and fracture fixation techniques have improved. It is still sometimes encountered, however, in fractures of the hip, knee, and tibia.

■   ■   ■

Every medical student, regardless of the specialty the student selects, will inevitably deal with some musculoskeletal injuries in his or her practice. This chapter provides a basic approach to the evaluation of such injuries. After reading this chapter the medical student should have a general understanding of bone and soft tissue anatomy, of normal injury and healing process, of the care of common fractures, and of the possible pitfalls of treatment.

PITFALLS AND COMMON MYTHS

- The basic goals of fracture management are reduction, stabilization, immobilization, and rehabilitation.
- A thorough neurologic examination is essential because of the potential for nerve palsy and related sequelae.
- In assessing for compartment syndrome, look for these clinical signs—the 5 *P's*: pain, pallor, pulselessness, paresthesia, and paralysis.
- Frequent evaluation of capillary refill is mandatory, since an artery may be occluded or lacerated by the injury.
- Fat embolism leading to ARDS is associated with fractures of the femur, hip, or pelvis.

BIBLIOGRAPHY

Nahum AM, Melvin J. The Biomechanics of Trauma. Norwalk, Conn, Appleton-Century-Crofts, 1985.

Rockwood CA Jr, Green DP, Bucholz RW (eds). Rockwood and Green's Fractures in Adults, 3rd ed. Philadelphia, JB Lippincott, 1991.

Tsukayama DT, Gustilo RB. Antibiotic Management of Open Fractures. American Academy of Orthopaedic Surgeons, Instructional Course Lectures 39: 487, 1990.

Turek SL. Orthopaedics: Principles and Their Applications, 4th ed. Philadelphia, JB Lippincott, 1984.

CHAPTER REVIEW
Questions

1. The load-deformation curve for bone shows that it is not as _____ as glass or as _____ as metal.
2. Bone strength is determined mainly by the mineral _____.
3. Wolf's law states that bone will _____ in response to repetitive physiologic loading.
4. *Anisotropic* means that bone is _____ in the direction that it is commonly loaded.
5. The viscoelastic nature of bone means that the type of fracture depends on how _____ the bone is loaded.
6. The early fracture callus is formed by the resolving fracture _____.
7. The process of normal fracture healing is called _____.
8. After many weeks the fracture callus is _____ along stress lines.
9. Fractures in children will remodel *more/less* than fractures in adults?
10. An open fracture or compound fracture means that the _____.
11. What classification is an open fracture that has a greater than 1 cm wound with vessel injury?

12. *Valgus* means the extremity distal of the fracture is angulated _____.
13. A comminuted fracture means that it has _____ fragments.
14. A complete ankle sprain is classified as a grade _____.
15. What percent of grade 3 ankle sprains require surgical repair?
16. Treatment of displaced fractures is with _____, _____, _____, and _____.
17. ORIF stands for _____.
18. How are ankle sprains treated?
19. How are osteoporosis spine fractures treated?
20. What is the pressure that causes compartment syndrome?
21. Describe the acute presentation of reflex sympathetic dystrophy.
22. What is traumatic arthritis?
23. What is osteomyelitis?
24. What is a malunion?
25. What is a nonunion?

Answers

1. Brittle
   Strong
2. Hydroxyapatite
3. Produce more bone
4. Stronger
5. Fast
6. Hematoma
7. Enchondral ossification
8. Remodeled
9. More
10. Soft tissue envelope is broken
11. Gustilo grade 3C
12. Laterally
13. Multiple

14. 3
15. 25%
16. Reduction, stabilization, immobilization, and rehabilitation
17. Open reduction and internal fixation
18. RICE-R: rest, ice, compression, elevation, rehabilitation
19. Prevention with exercise, nutrition, analgesics, bracing
20. 30 to 40 mm Hg
21. Hyperesthesia, swelling, warmth, redness, disuse
22. Joint degeneration resulting from injury
23. Bone infection
24. A fracture that has healed incorrectly
25. A fracture that has not healed within a normal amount of time

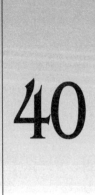

Hematuria

PAUL C. PETERS

KEY FEATURES

After reading this chapter you will understand:
- Causes of hematuria.
- Managing the patient with hematuria.
- Diagnosis and history-taking.
- The role of infection in hematuria in children.
- Hematuria in trauma victims.

WHAT IS HEMATURIA AND WHAT IS ITS SIGNIFICANCE?

Hematuria is the *appearance of erythrocytes or red blood cells (RBCs) in the urine.* The urine may appear coffee colored to bright red, depending on the age and number of RBCs in the urine (see the box on p. 685). Five-hundred RBCs per high-powered field are necessary for the human eye to perceive gross hematuria. Hemoglobinuria, myoglobinuria, and other causes of red urine must be separated from hematuria. Myoglobinuria often is associated with muscle breakdown and is one of the few conditions in which the creatinine level in the blood may be higher than the blood urea nitrogen (BUN) level.

HOW IS HEMATURIA DIAGNOSED?

Both children and adults are alarmed by the escape of their blood into the urine. Five milliliters of blood will make a quart of urine grossly red, and the patient with this sign usually comes to the doctor promptly. It is the physician's responsibility to investigate hematuria promptly and completely once its presence is confirmed by *microscopic examination of the urinary sediment.* Centrifugation of the urine in a 10-cc tapered centrifuge tube at 3000 revolutions per minute for 3 minutes, decanting the supernatant and tapping the remaining 1 or 2 ml at the bottom of the tapered test tube onto a glass slide, covering the slide with a cover slip, and examining it promptly at both low and high powers is the proper way to detect RBCs in the urine. Dipsticks (e.g., Chemstrip) dipped in the urine before centrifugation will detect the presence of the equivalent of 2 or 3 RBCs per high-powered field, but the presence of erythrocytes must be confirmed by microscopic examination.

ARE THE PHYSICAL CHARACTERISTICS OF THE RED CELLS IN THE URINE OF VALUE IN DIAGNOSIS?

Efforts continue to separate the red cells in the urine according to preglomerular origin and postglomerular or collecting system origin. The RBCs of preglomerular origin are often deformed (dysmorphic) and are microcytic with a mean corpuscular volume (MCV) of less than 92 μm^3, whereas the red cells originating in the urinary tract in Bowman's space or distal to this area are intact (isomorphic, not deformed or misshapen) and have a normal MCV of 97 + μm^3. This observation about the red cells excludes the deformation of the RBC envelope by its continued presence in hyperosmolar urine and denotes the

CAUSES OF RED URINE

Hemoglobinuria

Arsine
Aspidium
Betanaphthol
Carbolic acid (phenol)
Carbon monoxide
Chloroform
Fava beans
Hydroquinone derivatives
Mushrooms
Naphthalene
Oxalic acid
Pamaquine
Phosphorus
Phenylhydrazine
Potassium chlorate
Quinine
Snake venom
Sulfonamides
Tin compounds
Blood transfusions
Crush and burn injuries

Dark or Red Urine

Aniline dye (sweets)
Anthocyanin (beets, berries)
Antipyrine
Bile pigments
Blackberries
Congo red
Homogentisic acid
Methylene blue
Phenolphthalein
Pyridium
Rhodamine B
Urates

appearance in fresh urine. Estimation of MCV is by the Coulter counter.

Dysmorphic (preglomerular) RBCs may be thought of as having been involved in antigen-antibody reactions, glomerulonephritis, abnormal hemoglobin forms SS, SA, and SC, and Wegener's, Goodpasture's, and other immunologic syndromes, whereas *isomorphic RBCs are associated with coagulopathies, infections, and neoplasia not involving immune disorders.*

Cystoscopic examination may be indicated in patients with hematuria and isomorphic RBCs, whereas it would contribute little to ascertaining cause in patients with dysmorphic RBCs with or without proteinuria.

The *gravity of the lesion underlying the hematuria may not correlate with the magnitude of the hematuria.* An adult patient who persistently shows only one or two RBCs per high-powered, microscopic field may harbor a renal cell carcinoma, and a 20-year-old female with gross hematuria and clots may have hemorrhagic cystitis after sexual intercourse. A workup of patients with gross hematuria usually will lead to a prompt diagnosis, particularly if the patient is studied while bleeding. In investigating patients with asymptomatic microhematuria, the investigator must be thorough and persistent to pinpoint the source of the lesion in the urinary tract. Greene and associates, of the Mayo Clinic, found that an exact diagnosis of the cause of microhematuria in 500 asymptomatic patients (a mix of children and adults) could be made in 56% of them. Only 2% (11) of this group had a urinary tract neoplasm (isomorphic RBCs) as the cause of the microhematuria.

WHAT QUESTIONS SHOULD BE ASKED OF THE PATIENT ABOUT HEMATURIA?

Is the hematuria initial (meatal and urethral lesions) or total (bladder and renal origin), or is it only terminal (bladder neck and in the male prostate lesions)? Is the blood coming from the meatus not related to voiding (i.e., in cases of urethral trauma distal to the sphincter or rupture of a urethral varicosity)? Such cases are considered urethral bleeding, not hematuria. Are clots being passed? Clots are a manifestation of the *rate* of bleeding. Bright red clots indicate recent and active bleeding; dark red clots represent

TABLE 40-1   Associated Physical Findings That May Be Present With Hematuria and Their Common Causes

	Physical Findings	Causes
Eyes	Edema; conjunctival or retinal hemorrhage	(GN), drugs, (SBE), pancytopenia, platelet abnormality, leukemia
Ears	Malformations; deafness	Congenital renal anomaly, Alport's syndrome or variant
Nose	Rash	Lupus, tuberous sclerosis, Henoch-Schönlein purpura
Throat	Pharyngitis, mild or severe	Wegener's disease, (AGN)
Chest	Heart murmur; dysrhythmia	Emboli, SBE
Lungs	Rales (nodule seen on x-ray film); hemoptysis	Streptococcal infection, Wegener's disease
Abdomen	Spasm or guarding of flank	Stone
	Renal mass	Renal neoplasm, renal vein thrombosis, UPJ obstruction
	Enlarged spleen	Leukemia, idiopathic thrombocytopenic purpura, TTP
	Bruit	SBE, aneurysm, stenosis
Genitalia	Hypospadias; cryptorchidism; other anomalies	Upper tract anomalies
Extremities	Clubbing	Renal disease, congestive heart failure (CHF)
	Subinguinal petechiae	SBE
	Rash	Henoch-Schönlein purpura, glomerulo-nephritis, infectious mononucleosis
	Edema	AGN, CHF, drug ingestion

bleeding that is several or more hours old. Such clots may already be disintegrating from the action of urokinase in the urine. Long, slender clots indicate an upper tract (kidney or ureteral) origin.

Are the clots or bleeding associated with costovertebral angle pain or cramping pain in the flank or groin? *Painless hematuria with passage of clots in a patient older than 50 years indicates bladder cancer until proved otherwise.* Prostate enlargement (BPH) can cause bleeding (so does carcinoma). To determine the presence of a neoplasm or stone, ask the following: are there associated systemic symptoms of fever, chills, urgency, and dysuria; is there infection or obstruction of the urinary tract caused by a stone? It is not unusual to find a patient on the medical service who has been in the hospital 2 or 3 days with fever, chills, flank pain, hematuria, and failure of the fever to respond to antibiotic therapy who, as demonstrated by kidney, ureter, and bladder (KUB) studies, intravenous pyelogram (IVP), or CT scan, has a stone obstructing the urinary tract. Patients may know of an underlying hereditary disease that is the cause of their

hematuria and should be asked about sickle cell disease, hemoglobin C disease, glomerulo-nephritis, Berger's disease, Alport's syndrome, Wegener's syndrome, and Goodpasture's syndrome (dysmorphic RBCs may be seen in the urine) (Table 40-1).

Evidence of simultaneous bleeding in other systems besides the urinary tract may be seen. Petechiae, ecchymoses, purpuric spots associated with Rendu-Osler-Weber disease, meningococcemia, typhoid fever, leukemia, hemophilia, and blood dyscrasias may be obvious. Medications such as aspirin and nonsteroidal anti-inflammatory agents (e.g., Naprosyn, Feldene, Motrin) may be associated with renal damage and hematuria (see the box on p. 689).

WHAT IS THE ACCEPTABLE COMPLETE WORK-UP FOR HEMATURIA IN CHILDHOOD? (Fig. 40-1)

In childhood a neoplasm is seldom the cause of hematuria. Infection resulting from underlying congenital anomalies, hematuria secondary to

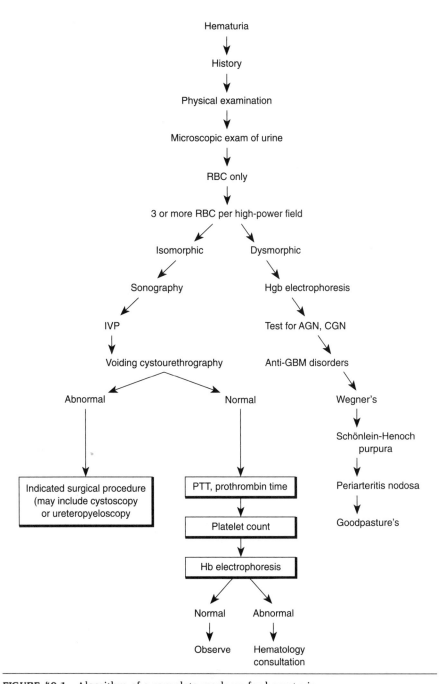

FIGURE 40-1 Algorithm of a complete work-up for hematuria.

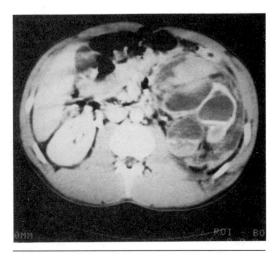

FIGURE 40-2   CT scan through the kidneys of 12-year-old child with gross hematuria following slight blow to the flank. Large hydronephrotic left kidney is seen secondary to congenital UPJ. *When bleeding is out of proportion to the magnitude of the trauma, think "preexisting disease."*

vigorous muscular exercise, and the various forms of glomerulonephritis are more common causes. *Cystoscopy is rarely needed in childhood,* especially if proteinuria accompanies the hematuria or if dysmorphic red cells are present. Ultrasonography and CT scanning more likely will assist in diagnosing the rare renal neoplasm of childhood when a mass lesion is associated with gross hematuria. Trauma as a cause of hematuria can occur at any age, but hematuria that is disproportionate to the magnitude of the trauma should cause the physician to think of preexisting disease. A commonly occurring example is gross hematuria that follows the rupture of a hydronephrotic kidney secondary to a preexisting UPJ obstruction (Fig. 40-2).

CAUSES OF HEMATURIA IN CHILDREN, YOUNG ADULTS, AND ADULTS

In childhood, infection, exercise, and glomerulonephritis predominate as the causes of hematuria (see the box on p. 689). The infection is much more common in the young girl than in the young boy, and congenital anomalies often underlie the infection. Lesions such as ureterocele, ectopic ureter, and a duplication of the collecting system, with or without reflux, comprise the ma-

jority of the causes of hematuria in younger children. In the early school-age children glomerulonephritis and trauma are the main causes of hematuria; in addition, drug ingestion, particularly of analgesic agents, may be a cause.

Stones do occur in childhood and are associated with hematuria and cramplike pain. Rarely is gross hematuria with passage of clots associated with the presence of a stone. Neoplasms do occur but are down the list as a cause of hematuria; usually they are associated with mass lesions of the kidney. Bladder transitional cell carcinomas are almost unheard of in this age group.

Parasitic infections do occur, and when sexual activity begins, urinary tract infection, particularly in teenage females, may become a cause of hematuria.

When glomerulonephritis is present, associated proteinuria usually is found. With massive proteinuria (i.e., 3 to 12 g/day), oval fat bodies, which are macrophages that have ingested lipid droplets and casts are found in the urine. Localized or generalized edema may be present, and there is often a history of antecedent respiratory infection. The signs and symptoms of anemia, fatigability, and persistent edema may portend the progression to a chronic stage of nephritis from the acute stage. The prognosis for healing in a patient with glomerulonephritis is good 95% to 99% of the time.

The child with pyuria and hematuria must be suspected of having a congenital anomaly until proved otherwise. Urine cultures are obtained and appropriate antibiotics given. Excretory urography with postvoiding films and cystourethrography performed during voiding should be considered for diagnostic purposes after infection is controlled. Seldom is cystoscopy indicated in uncomplicated cases with mild infection. It may be indicated in patients with some of the obstructive uropathies of early childhood such as ureterocele, in which case incision of the ureterocele may be all that is necessary to control the infection and hematuria. Renal biopsy is seldom indicated even in patients with glomerulonephritis except for those children who are progressing rapidly or when the nature of the vasculitis is not well defined (e.g., with periarteritis nodosa following Schönlein-Henoch purpura or in Goodpasture's or Wegener's disease). Many children with microscopic hematuria have defects in platelet function or have coagulation disorders secondary to ingestion of drugs, analgesics, or cytotoxic agents. Observation is usually all that is necessary if the offending drug cannot be discontinued.

CAUSES OF HEMATURIA IN VARIOUS AGE GROUPS

Child (<15 Years)	Young Adult	Older (>50 years) Adult
Infection	Infection	Infection
Exercise	Trauma	Neoplasm
Glomerulonephritis	Drug ingestion	Medication
Trauma	Stone	Stone
Congenital anomaly	Exercise	Enlarged prostate (in males)
Drug ingestion	Neoplasm	Renal vascular disorder
Stone	Abnormal hemoglobin level	
Neoplasm	Renal vascular disorder	
Parasite	Parasite	

Performing cystoscopy is seldom necessary in patients with mass lesions, including Wilms' tumor and neuroblastoma. Hematuria frequently occurs with Wilms' tumor, but seldom is cystoscopy or retrograde pyelography necessary in completing the necessary preoperative work-up, for ultrasonography and CT usually provide sufficient information for treatment. Metastatic bone survey is helpful in the diagnosis of neuroblastoma, which may be confused at times with Wilms' tumor, even histologically.

Renal cell carcinoma has been reported 150 to 160 times in children and is rare as a cause of hematuria in them. The work-up of a mass renal lesion usually includes the use of ultrasonography and CT rather than cystoscopy and retrograde pyelography. Transitional cell carcinoma has been reported 54 times in prepubertal children and is usually not a consideration in a child with hematuria. Recurrent gross hematuria, however, may be an indication for cystoscopic examination even in children. Stones are often associated with colicky or cramplike pain in the abdomen and hematuria, although the hematuria is usually not massive, and bleeding with bright red clots is unusual in the patient with a stone.

Parasitic infections of the urinary tract are rare before sexual intercourse begins. *Trichomonas vaginalis*, one of the most common causes of infection, is diagnosed best by cytologic study (Papanicolaou smear) of freshly voided, millipore-filtered urine. The *yeast infections that occur in childhood usually follow the use of broad-spectrum antibiotics and/or chemotherapeutic agents* for a period of time and *may be a manifestation of the diminished resistance of the child to opportunistic invaders.*

In the young adult infections predominate, and trauma first appears as a frequent cause, in contrast with the experience of older individuals in whom neoplasm, stones, prostate enlargement, and renovascular disorders predominate. In the young adult vigorous muscular exercise is often associated with "jogger's hematuria." Cystoscopic examination of these individuals often shows blood coming from both ureteral orifices after a 3- to 5-mile run. The presence of isomorphic RBCs in the urine is a further clue that the individual does not have glomerulonephritis but has hematuria secondary to running or jogging. Neoplasms begin to appear in the older young adult (i.e., in the thirties) and must be differentiated in individuals with gross hematuria. Excretory urography and a CT scan may provide the needed information. Cystoscopic examination is performed to localize the site of the hematuria, and retrograde pyelography may be of more value in diagnosing this age group than in the young adult (teens and twenties) and child. The physician must be particularly alert for the dysmorphic red cell in this age group, for it indicates an antigen-antibody mechanism's deforming the red cell membrane. Deformation of the RBC can be detected easily when RBCs in the urine that have been subjected to a Sternheimer-Malbin stain are examined. The deformation of RBCs commonly seen in patients with IgA nephropathy or Berger's disease is one of the more common causes of microhematuria in patients in this age group.

The sexually active person often is a victim of infection, and *sexually transmitted infections are major causes of hematuria in young adults.* It is at this time that a young woman begins to suffer from acute hemorrhagic cystitis. The bleeding is severe enough to cause clots, but usually only gross hematuria associated with urgency and frequency is present. Offending organisms of the coliform group are cultured from the urine 90% of the time.

Trauma is a major cause of bleeding in the 20 to 40 age group. Victims of penetrating trauma usually require exploratory surgery because of the high incidence of associated injuries. Patients with blunt trauma secondary to falls, motor vehicle accidents, or contact sports often are treated expectantly, and individuals with no history of shock and microhematuria who suffer blunt trauma nearly always are treated expectantly. Individuals with a history of hypotension (i.e., a systolic pressure of 80 or less after the injury) and with gross hematuria provide the highest yield on urologic work-up. CT is of great value in diagnosing both the blunt and penetrating trauma

patient; however, many of the penetrating trauma patients are so severely injured they must be taken immediately to surgery without time for such radiographic studies as the CT. CT is, however, of great aid in planning the management of the blunt trauma patient (Fig. 40-3).

Trauma patients with gross hematuria and/or hypotension demand immediate and complete work-up. Those patients with microscopic hematuria and no history of hypotension may be worked up promptly but often are treated expectantly with good results. The young adult and older adult with persistent microscopic hematuria and with negative sonography, CT, excretory urography, and cystoscopy results are particularly troublesome. In this circumstance the urologist is described by Lawrence Greene as being placed between the Scylla of advising a repeat, complete investigation and finding nothing

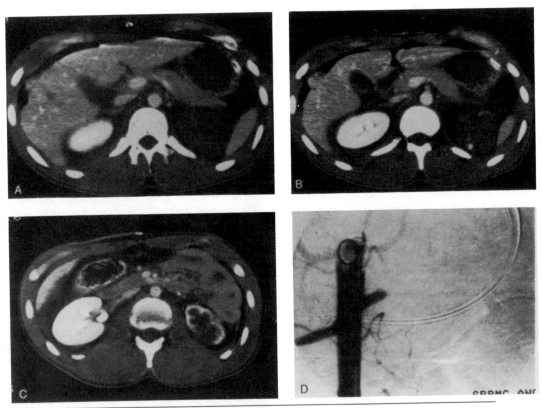

FIGURE 40-3   CT scan of a 26-year-old blunt trauma patient. Note delay in appearance of contrast material on the left, **A**, and that contrast does appear in the kidney with CT, although the main renal artery is completely disrupted, **B** and **C**. On the IVP, this left kidney would not have shown at all. Performing selective renal arteriography is indicated for trauma patients who have only fragmentary visualization, **B**, or a cortical rim sign, **C**, on CT scanning. Note complete disruption of left renal artery, **D**.

and the Charbydis of choosing to ignore the recurrent microscopic hematuria and thereby overlooking malignancy or another significant lesion. The most cost-effective work-up at the present time for children and young adults consists of excretory urography and voiding cystourethrography with postvoiding films. As mass lesions begin to appear, obtaining a battery of tests, including ultrasonography, CT scan, and occasionally MRI when vascular involvement is sought, must be considered. Collecting system lesions in the urinary tract as a cause of hematuria are best detected from cytologic techniques, brushing of the epithelium with cytologic analysis, and direct observation with cystoscopy and ureteropyeloscopy.

The presence of urinary stones in patients in the adult age group is suggested by pain and colicky, cramplike pain associated with restlessness, an inability to find a comfortable position, and the presence of microscopic hematuria. Associated pyuria is uncommon and suggests complicating factors such as infection. Calcium oxalate is the most common type of stone. Uric acid stones can be diagnosed by CT of the kidney, in which they are much more clearly delineated than they are in the excretory urogram. *Patients in the adult age group with hematuria secondary to the use of anticoagulants should be considered to have a preexisting disease until proved otherwise, and the hematuria must not be ignored.*

Hemoglobinopathies have usually been diagnosed by adulthood, but occasionally hemoglobin variance such as hemoglobin C disease or even hemoglobin SS is not discovered until hemoglobin electrophoresis is done because of recurrent hematuria. Gross hematuria often is observed by cystoscopic examination as coming from the left ureteral orifice. Hemophilia, thrombocytopenic purpura, and various blood factor deficiencies can result from medications taken by patients in this age group or from a previously undiagnosed primary abnormality. Factitious hematuria is encountered most commonly in this age group, and patients may have deep-seated emotional disturbances resulting in hematuria.

WHAT ARE THE CAUSES OF HEMATURIA IN THE ELDERLY?

Painless, gross hematuria after age 50 years is caused by cancer until proved otherwise. More than 20% of such patients have neoplasia, and primary attention must be paid to ruling it out as the cause of hematuria in patients over 50. Anticoagulant use is common in this group because of previous myocardial infarction or vascular disorders, and a high incidence of underlying urologic disease is found when these patients are examined because of recurrent hematuria initially blamed on the anticoagulant therapy.

Hematuria secondary to prostatic enlargement (BPH) is common in the male patients in the elderly group, as is cystitis in the female (often associated with atrophic changes in the vaginal and urethral mucous membranes) at this age. Cytologic studies should be done to rule out associated urothelial neoplasms, and obtaining biopsy specimens from areas of induration in the prostate is indicated, particularly when induration is associated with an elevation of the prostate specific antigen (PSA) in the blood. A biopsy to rule out carcinoma may be indicated in patients with obstructive urinary symptoms of short duration, particularly in male patients with moderate enlargement of the prostate and those with urgency, frequency, and a *clear,* microscopically normal urine. *Hematuria in the elderly patient with painless passage of clots more commonly is caused by bladder neoplasm.* Cystoscopic examination can result in localization of the site of bleeding if it is performed while the patient is actively bleeding. This procedure has been encouraged as a diagnostic maneuver by urologists for decades.

Angiography after cystoscopic localization of the bleeding to one kidney is urgently indicated in patients who show massive bleeding from the upper urinary tract. The differential diagnosis of neoplasm, aneurysm, or arteriovenous malformation and treatment by the radiologist to occlude the vessel causing the bleeding by percutaneous embolization techniques may be of great value in this patient group. The presence of hematuria with severe flank pain, obstruction, hypercalciuria, and infection should be sought in the stone patient, and a complete metabolic work-up is indicated. Any patient who develops a second stone in a 7-year period should have a complete metabolic work-up consisting of studies of the urine and blood and should follow a controlled diet to ascertain the presence of hypercalciuria, which is found in 93% of stone-forming patients. Currently the patient with a stone can be classified into one of approximately a dozen categories of diagnosis, and *a specific treatment can be recommended for each category of stone patient, resulting in a much lower rate of recurrence than when such specific therapy is not applied.*

PITFALLS AND COMMON MYTHS

- When a patient presents with a gross, painless hematuria, much information is obtained by cystoscopy at the time of bleeding. Sometimes the cystoscopy is forgotten when a complex work-up follows. This is to the detriment of the patient.
- If a patient has gross hematuria with clots and a stone, one must question whether the stone is the cause of the hematuria.
- "BPH bleeds" is an old urologic axiom, but carcinoma of the prostate can cause microhematuria. PSA testing is indicated in patients over 40 years of age along with digital rectal examination.

- A herald bleed (i.e., massive bleeding into the urinary tract, followed by a silent interval, followed by another bleeding episode) should alert the physician to an arteriovenous malformation in the kidney or a renal cell neoplasm.
- Even though the greatest yield in blunt trauma patients comes from a work-up of the patient with gross hematuria and hypotension, the nature of the injury must be remembered as a just and sufficient cause for the work-up even in a patient with microhematuria and no shock.

BIBLIOGRAPHY

Addis T. The number of formed elements in the urinary sediment of normal individuals. J Clin Invest 2: 409, 1926.

Berman LB. When the urine is red. JAMA 237:2753, 1977.

Carson CC, Segura JW, Greene LF. Clinical importance of microhematuria. JAMA 241:149, 1979.

Greene LF, O'Shaughnessy EJ Jr, Hendricks ED. Study of five hundred patients with asymptomatic microhematuria. JAMA 161:610, 1956.

McAninch JW, Carroll PR, Klosterman PW, et al. Renal reconstruction after injury. J Urol 145:932, 1991.

McInnes BK III. The management of hematuria associated with sickle hemoglobinopathies. J Urol 124: 171, 1980.

Northway JD. Hematuria in children. J Pediatr 78:381, 1971.

Pak CYC, Peters P, Hurt G, et al. Selective therapy of recurrent nephrolithiasis. Am J Med 71:615, 1981.

Sayer J, McCarthy MP, Schmidt JD. Identification and significance of dysmorphic versus isomorphic hematuria. J Urol 143:545, 1990.

CHAPTER REVIEW
Questions

1. A stone recovered from the urinary tract of a patient should be subjected to chemical analysis because:
   a. It may give a clue to a metabolic disorder.
   b. The patient is curious to know the chemical composition.
   c. It is covered by the patient's health insurance.
   d. Specific therapy is tailored for each kind of stone.

2. The highest positive yield in the work-up for hematuria in the trauma patient comes from work-up of patients with:
   a. Microhematuria and shock.
   b. Shock.
   c. Gross hematuria.
   d. Gross hematuria and shock.

3. A plain abdominal film of a patient suspected of a stone because of flank pain and microhematuria is of value because:
   a. Splenic and liver injuries may be ruled out.
   b. Ninety-three percent of stones contain calcium and will be seen on a plain abdominal film.
   c. This is the best way to see a uric acid stone.
   d. The bowel gas pattern is diagnostic of stone.

4. Painless bleeding after 50 years of age into the urinary collecting system most likely is caused by:
   a. A stone in the urinary tract.
   b. Carcinoma of the urinary bladder.
   c. Renal cell carcinoma.
   d. Carcinoma of the prostate.

5. Isomorphic red cells have normal contour and volume because:
   a. They have come into the urinary tract below Henle's loop.
   b. They are not affected by the osmolality of the urine.
   c. They have not been involved in an antigen-antibody reaction (immune reaction).
   d. They are not seen unless the patient also has Berger's disease.

6. A young black female presents with gross hematuria. Cystoscopy reveals blood coming from the left ureteral orifice. A specimen of blood is sent for observation for sickling. Which of the following should also be ordered?
   a. BUN determination
   b. Hemoglobin electrophoresis
   c. Sodium metabisulfite test
   d. Urinary osmolality determination

Answers

1. d
2. d
3. b
4. b
5. c
6. b

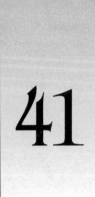

41

Obstructive Uropathy and Urinary Tract Infection

MITCHELL H. BAMBERGER
ROBERT J. IRWIN, Jr.

KEY FEATURES

After reading this chapter you will understand:
- Upper and lower urinary tract obstruction.
- The diagnosis and treatment of prostatic cancer.
- Infections of the urinary tract.

Obstruction in the urinary tract can be sudden in onset such as in the patient with a renal colic caused by an obstructing calculus or slow and insidious in nature so the patient may be asymptomatic such as in ureteral obstruction from a ureteral tumor. The physician must evaluate the entire urinary tract when signs or symptoms suggest urinary tract pathology. Urologists generally divide obstruction into two broad categories: upper or lower tract obstruction.

WHAT IS UPPER TRACT OBSTRUCTION?

Upper tract obstruction, or proximal obstruction, causes an acute pressure rise within the renal collecting system, with subsequent rise in the intratubular pressure as well. Cellular events occur that involve the release of cellular mediators, mainly prostaglandins, which in turn cause an acute rise in renal blood flow. This subsequently causes a rise in glomerular filtration rate (GFR). With a high-grade obstruction, a vicious cycle develops until one of two events occurs. The renal collecting system (e.g., the fornix) may rupture, with subsequent decompression of the col-

lecting system and the development of a collection of urine, a urinoma. If decompression does not occur within a short period after the onset of obstruction, renal blood flow decreases in a protective fashion to decrease GFR. Eventually, renal collecting system and intratubular pressures will decrease, with a decline in both renal function and GFR. This results in a progressive decrease in renal blood flow over approximately 6 weeks, after which relief of the obstruction provides little hope for the return to previously normal renal function.

What Are the Causes of Upper Tract Obstruction?

The causes of upper tract obstruction are systematically evaluated by location: either kidney or ureter. Ureteral obstruction is subdivided into intrinsic or extrinsic causes.

Renal obstruction is caused by blockage of the ureteropelvic junction (UPJ). In the adult the most common cause is a renal calculus. This obstruction is usually accompanied by a sudden onset of flank pain, which may radiate toward the groin and in men to the scrotum and testicle. Irritation of the posterior peritoneum may also cause nausea and vomiting. Infection associated with obstruction can produce fever and leukocytosis. Hematuria, either gross or microscopic, is usually present; however, it may be totally absent.

The vast majority of renal calculi are less than 1 cm; however, any size stone can obstruct the UPJ. Staghorn calculi, which conform to the shape and size of the renal collecting system, rarely obstruct the UPJ because their large size prevents progression down the ureter. Most stones between 1 and 2 cm can pass through the UPJ but probably will not pass through the ureterovesical junction (UVJ) and will produce ureteral obstruction. Calculi less than 1 cm have a 70% to 80% chance of passing spontaneously without surgical intervention.

In addition to a kidney stone, the possibility of tumor must be considered. It may be ureteral or renal in nature. A ureteral transitional cell carcinoma usually is associated with a slow onset of symptoms. In fact, many ureteral tumors are asymptomatic until the tumor is large and has extended outside the ureter. A renal tumor, most commonly a renal cell carcinoma, when originating in the lower pole, may achieve such massive size if unrecognized and likewise obstruct the renal collecting system. Other tumors originating in the renal pelvis, especially in the region of the UPJ, may grow large enough to obstruct the outflow of urine before producing other symptoms such as hematuria.

Another intrinsic form of renal obstruction is produced by an adynamic segment of ureter at the level of the UPJ. Neuronal impulses are not transmitted down the ureter in a coordinated fashion; hence ureteral peristalsis is interrupted. This usually results in significant hydronephrosis, with significant dilation of the renal collecting system. This most frequently occurs in children but occasionally can be seen in adults in the fourth to sixth decade.

There also is potential for a papilla to slough from the medullary pyramids and obstruct the outflow of urine through the UPJ. Because of *chronic infection* and *inflammation,* the papilla becomes fibrotic and inflamed. Eventually, with long-term disease the papilla becomes necrotic and falls free within the renal collecting system. If the papilla is still large enough, it may not only obstruct the UPJ but may become infected, since necrotic tissue is an excellent nidus for bacterial growth. Although this infection is not as commonly seen today as in the past, it still affects certain high-risk groups, that is, those with:

- Diabetes
- Sickle cell disease
- Tuberculosis
- Phenacetin abuse
- Chronic pyelonephritis

Very rarely UPJ obstruction is caused by a large amount of blood that has clotted within the renal pelvis. However, naturally occurring urokinase usually will slowly lyse the clots and relieve the obstruction.

An extrinsic cause of renal obstruction is associated with an aberrant blood vessel. This is frequently due to an accessory renal artery; however, anomalous renal veins or any retroperitoneal vessel may be the cause. Surgical exploration is usually required to alleviate the obstruction. If a renal artery is involved, it should not be sacrificed because the renal parenchyma supplied by this vessel would become ischemic and necrose. Accessory arteries require meticulous dissection, with division and subsequent reanastomosis of the ureter and collecting system in a fashion so that obstruction cannot recur.

Other less common causes of renal obstruction include enlarged lymph nodes with metastatic disease from retroperitoneal tumors or enlarged psoas muscles associated with athletic individuals. The differential diagnosis for upper tract obstruction is presented in Fig. 41-1.

Causes of Intrinsic Ureteral Obstruction. Intrinsic obstruction is most commonly caused by *renal calculi.* These stones pass through the UPJ but are too large to pass through the UVJ. Ureteral stones cause symptoms similar to those caused by stones obstructing the kidney itself, since it is the renal pelvic and tubular obstructions, with the development of hydronephrosis, that produce symptoms. Ureteral stones are usually differentiated by radiographic means from their renal counterparts.

Tumors, commonly transitional cell carcinomas, can cause obstruction because of their slow growth within the lumen of the ureter. Like renal pelvic tumors, these lesions usually produce few symptoms until they have nearly totally occluded the ureter and caused obstruction and have grown through the ureteral wall, which worsens the prognosis.

Other causes of intrinsic ureteral obstruction include *strictures.* These lesions are due to inflammation, with subsequent fibrosis and scarring that obstructs urinary flow and ureteral peristalsis. They can be caused by prior instrumentation for retrieving ureteral calculi, radiation treatment of the abdomen or pelvis for malignancy, or tuberculosis.

Extrinsic Lesions That Cause Ureteral Obstruction. Since the ureter is a retroperitoneal structure, the mechanism of extrinsic obstruction lies in the pathophysiology of a retroperitoneal process that impinges and/or constricts the peristaltic flow of urine down the ureter toward the bladder. The most common cause of extrinsic obstruction is *tumor*—rarely, a primary retro-

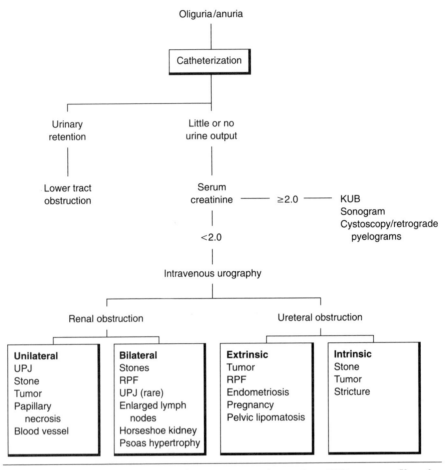

FIGURE 41-1   Differential diagnosis for upper tract obstruction. **KUB** = x-ray film of kidney, ureter, bladder; **RPF** = renal plasma flow; **UPJ** = ureteropelvic junction.

peritoneal lesion such as liposarcoma or leio-myosarcoma or, more commonly, one caused by metastasis from cervix, prostate, lung, or breast. Pelvic organ tumors such as in the cervix or prostate usually obstruct the lower third of the ureter by contiguous growth; however, **lymphatic metastases** from pelvic organ malignancies commonly obstruct the upper ureter as well.

Any **inflammatory process** involving the retroperitoneum can cause obstruction. It may be unilateral from the fibrosis of a slowly leaking abdominal aortic aneurysm. The inflammatory process from blood in the retroperitoneum slowly surrounds the ureter. The left side is more commonly affected, although both ureters may become involved. Women of childbearing years must always be asked about a history of **endometriosis.** The endometrioma can progressively obstruct the ureter, and the patient may have a history of cyclic pain associated with menses.

When bilateral obstruction occurs without aneurysmal formation or malignancy, **idiopathic retroperitoneal fibrosis,** a chronic inflammatory condition that may be associated with occult pelvic malignancy or methylsergide usage, is suspected. An intravenous urogram with bilateral ureteral medial deviation is seen. Other causes of retroperitoneal fibrosis include inflammatory bowel disease, tuberculosis, or radiation injury. There apparently is a male predominance in the fifth to seventh decade.

A common cause of obstruction on the right side that is often overlooked is **pregnancy.** It commonly occurs during the third trimester as the fetus enlarges and descends into the true pelvis. It is theorized the right side is affected more often because the sigmoid colon acts as a cushion for the left ureter. Another common cause of extrinsic obstruction is **prior pelvic surgery** such as hysterectomy or distal colon resections. The ureter is inadvertently incorporated into tissue by suture ligatures or clips. The patient may present with flank pain, acutely or even months later. Frequently, many patients develop urinary leakage through fistulous formation after the ureter has ruptured and formed a urinoma. The urine seeks the path of least resistance, and in the early postoperative period it is usually through the dissected tissue planes to the incision.

Another rare cause of extrinsic obstruction is *pelvic lipomatosis.* This is a dense deposition of fat within the pelvis, causing medial deviation of the bladder into the shape of a Christmas tree, along with lateral deviation of the ureters. It occurs primarily in overweight black males.

WHAT IS LOWER TRACT OBSTRUCTION?

Lower urinary tract obstruction generally refers to *bladder outlet obstruction.* In males this usually translates into *enlargement of the prostate by both benign and malignant processes;* however, a thorough evaluation of the entire urinary tract is necessary. Any process that obstructs the outflow of urine from the bladder, including *urethral stricture, bladder calculi, and foreign bodies,* must be considered. Urethral strictures are inflammatory processes that result from urethral infection, usually sexually transmitted disease such as gonorrhea or syphilis. In recent years iatrogenic causes from prior urethral instrumentation must be considered. This includes prior surgical resection of the prostate, cystoscopic examination of the lower urinary tract, or even the passage of a urethral catheter that may have traumatized the delicate urethral mucosa, inciting inflammation.

Women rarely present with lower urinary tract obstruction. The partial obstruction of the bladder neck by a tumor usually produces symptoms of hesitancy, intermittent voiding, postvoid dribbling, and even hematuria. In women with lower tract obstruction a pelvic bimanual examination is mandatory to rule out any mass effect, especially from the other pelvic organs. A vaginal mass may have malignant causes such as carcinoma but also may have benign causes such as a cystocoele or rectocoele.

Are There Nonanatomic Forms of Lower Tract Obstruction?

Although the vast majority of causes of urinary tract obstruction are due to an anatomic form of obstruction, occasionally obstruction without evidence of anatomic pathology is encountered. In these situations an apparent functional (or lack of function) obstruction must be considered. This occurs in patients in whom the bladder does not adequately empty; hence residual urine collects to the point at which there is essentially no effective urinary output, which may be due to a *neurologic deficit* in which the bladder cannot empty, either because of pharmacologic means or neurologic diseases.

Many *drugs* have side effects that alter bladder action. The more common ones are narcotics given for relief of postoperative pain, antihistamines for upper respiratory infections, and antipsychotics. The astute clinician must always consider a pharmacologic cause when anatomic ones are not apparent.

In addition, many patients with debilitating *neurologic diseases* have some form of bladder dysfunction, which may be due to an inability of the bladder to contract effectively, commonly seen with *diabetes.* Diabetic patients may develop a sensory deficit to the point that they do not feel a full bladder and may not even complain of any bladder symptoms. Another form of neurologic dysfunction is a lack of coordination between the detrusor muscle, which must contract to expel urine, and the sphincter, which relaxes to allow the urine to pass through the urethra. This is a rare condition called detrusor-sphincter dyssynergia. It is seen in spinal cord injury patients and those with demyelinating neurologic diseases such as multiple sclerosis. Fig. 41-2 outlines the differential diagnosis for lower urinary tract obstruction.

HOW IS THE DIAGNOSIS OF URINARY TRACT OBSTRUCTION MADE?

The first sign of urinary tract obstruction is generally a decrease in urinary output. *Oliguria is defined as production of less than 450 ml of urine within a 24-hour period. Anuria occurs when no urine is produced* within 24 hours. If the obstruction is at the level of the bladder neck or distal to it, the passage of a urethral catheter is not only diagnostic but therapeutic. After passage of a catheter, if no urine is obtained, the cause is an upper tract obstruction. However, the patient must have been adequately hydrated.

Subsequent to passage of a urethral catheter, it is essential to evaluate the patient's renal function. This is most effectively and efficiently done by obtaining serum *blood urea nitrogen (BUN)* and *creatinine levels.* Patients with a BUN/creatinine ratio of $\geq 10 : 1$ generally have a prerenal

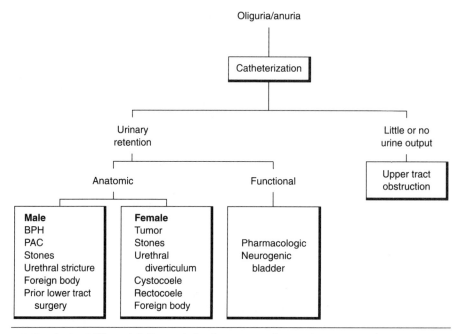

FIGURE 41-2   Differential diagnosis for lower tract obstruction. **BPH** = benign prostatic hyperplasia; **PAC** = prostatic adenocarcinoma.

or renal cause for decreased urinary output. Ratios of 10:1 or less usually are due to an obstruction.

If the creatinine level is ≤2.0 and the patient has no allergy to contrast media, it is safe to proceed with an ***intravenous urogram (IVU)***. This is the method of choice to define the upper tract anatomy and the location and cause of the obstruction. Obstruction is manifested by dilation of the calyceal collecting system (hydronephrosis). If no contrast is seen on the IVU, a high-grade obstruction exists that prevents contrast media from entering the collecting tubules, and the kidney is essentially nonfunctional. Delayed films must be obtained several hours after injection, even up to 24 hours later, to assess renal function and the anatomic cause.

When the serum creatinine level is ≥2.0 or the patient has a contrast allergy, the IVU is contraindicated. Instead a ***renal ultrasound examination*** is performed. Although the ultrasound does not provide any functional information, it is a very quick, efficient, and inexpensive method to rule out upper urinary tract obstruction and impairment. By viewing both kidneys, the collecting system can be visualized in search of hydronephrosis. If a distended renal pelvis is seen, obstruction probably exists. If further examination reveals a dilated upper ureter (hydroureter), the obstruction probably is distal to the kidney, whereas only hydronephrosis suggests obstruction at the UPJ. At this point ***a retrograde pyelogram or a renal scan*** is called for.

If the IVU fails to point to the cause of obstruction, ***cystoscopy and retrograde pyelography*** are performed, entailing passage of a catheter into the UVJ and injection of contrast material up the ureter in a retrograde fashion to delineate the anatomy and course of the ureter. Retrograde pyelography is also indicated when patients are allergic to contrast media. The dye injected is not absorbed to any significant amount to elicit an allergic response.

Nuclear renal scans are helpful in calculating differential split renal function. In addition, a radiographic obstruction seen on the IVU may not be of functional significance, but a nuclear scan with diethyltriaminepertechnetate acid (DTPA) is reliable. Not only can the function be calculated for each kidney, but the time required for half of the radioactive tracer to drain from the renal collecting system can be quantitated. This time is called the $T_{1/2}$. The normal $T_{1/2}$ is between 10 and 20 minutes. If there is any question as to whether an obstruction exists, the additional administration of furosemide (Lasix) to flush out the tracer by diuresis is helpful. If the $T_{1/2}$ after furosemide administration is less than 20 minutes, it is considered a functional obstruction of minimal significance.

If all prior diagnostic examinations fail to reveal an obstruction, a **percutaneous nephrostomy** can be inserted into the kidney to allow the anterograde injection of contrast and definition of the renal collecting system and the ureter. In addition, if a question arises as to whether the obstruction is anatomic versus functional, pressure-flow studies (Whitaker test) may be performed. The baseline renal pressure can be measured through the nephrostomy tube and should be ≤15 cm H_2O. If during a constant flow of 10 ml/min the pressure rises to ≥22 cm H_2O, obstruction exists.

HOW IS URINARY TRACT OBSTRUCTION MANAGED?

Treatment of urinary tract obstruction is based primarily on the site and cause of the obstruction. Relief should be prompt, since recovery is based on the degree and duration of the obstruction. Complete renal obstruction for greater than 6 weeks provides little hope for return to normal renal function, although the kidney has remarkable capacity to recover.

Lower tract obstruction is generally managed first by passage of a urethral catheter. If a catheter cannot be negotiated into the bladder through the urethra, suprapubic diversion is performed. Catheter placement is considered successful when urine is returned. Should urine not be obtained, injection of a small amount of contrast media through the catheter will ascertain its position. Once the correct position of the catheter is obtained and no or little urine is obtained, upper tract obstruction must be considered.

The prompt relief of lower tract obstruction (or bilateral ureteral obstruction) may elicit a **brisk diuresis of urine and electrolytes.** This is based on the accumulation of an osmotic load of electrolytes and waste products (mainly BUN) that has not been efficiently eliminated. This is usually a self-limiting process, lasting until normal serum levels are obtained. However, **if not recognized promptly, severe intravascular collapse can occur.** The patient is observed carefully for several hours once the obstruction is released, and the volume of fluid to replace is generally 0.5 ml for each milliliter of urine drained on an hourly basis. Electrolytes are replaced by measuring the urinary concentration of sodium and potassium. However, overzealous replacement

may perpetuate a diuresis. Once normal renal function has returned, the diagnostic work-up may proceed as described, with treatment based on the anatomic or functional pathophysiology.

Upper tract obstruction management is similarly based on the cause. Renal function must be maximized, especially if the kidney is to be salvaged. Ureteral obstruction can usually be treated by passage of a ureteral catheter into the renal collecting system at the same time a retrograde pyelogram is performed. If a catheter cannot be negotiated past the site of obstruction, a percutaneous nephrostomy tube can be placed, which will allow anterograde studies to diagnose the problem. In addition, relief of the obstruction hopefully will allow return of renal function, which is imperative to any renal-preserving surgery or intervention. If necessary, once a ureteral catheter or nephrostomy tube has restored renal function, differential creatinine clearances may be obtained to quantitate function. A creatinine clearance of ≤15 ml/min suggests little hope for salvageable kidney function, and nephrectomy may be the most judicious form of management.

How Does Unilateral Ureteral Obstruction Differ From Bilateral Obstruction?

In a patient with unilateral obstruction and a normally functioning contralateral kidney, there should be no sign of renal insufficiency, retention of urea, or electrolyte imbalance. Since the contralateral renal unit is unobstructed, it can maintain water and acid-base balance and excrete urea without presenting a problem to the patient. However, in a patient with bilateral ureteral obstruction and lower urinary tract obstruction, the kidneys develop hydronephrosis and are prevented from performing normal physiologic functions. The first kidney function that is impaired is urine-concentrating ability. The countercurrent mechanism of water conservation is disturbed, and initially a dilute urine is excreted. If obstruction is not relieved, it progresses to more serious renal impairment by decreasing the GFR, retaining urea, and resulting in an electrolyte and acid-base imbalance. The longer renal obstruction continues, the more urea and sodium are retained by the body, both in the intravascular space and the interstitium. Subsequently, when the obstruction is released, especially in the lower tract by placement of a urethral catheter, the solute overload promotes a brisk postobstructive diuresis and results in massive fluid and electrolyte losses in urine. If not recognized, severe hypotension can occur with serious results.

PROSTATE CANCER

In the United States prostatic adenocarcinoma (PAC) is the most common type of cancer in men. It is the second most common cause of cancer deaths in men each year. Black men have a higher incidence of PAC than white men, whereas Asian men have the lowest incidence. In autopsy studies the incidence of PAC in men over 80 years of age approaches 40% to 50%, whereas in men less than 50 it is less than 5%. Although other forms of prostate cancer such as transitional cell, squamous cell, and sarcoma exist, the following discussion focuses on PAC because of its overwhelming presence in adult men and its increasingly frequent diagnosis.

What Are the Symptoms of Prostate Cancer?

Generally, most patients who present with prostate cancer have some symptoms of lower urinary tract obstruction. Nocturia, hesitancy, increasing daytime frequency, stranguria, dysuria, gross hematuria, and urgency all suggest lower tract obstruction. Any male who has a sudden change in his voiding pattern must be considered to have prostate cancer until proven otherwise. Rectal examination is mandatory to palpate the posterior lobes of the prostate gland. Biopsy of suspicious regions should be done before any form of intervention. Approximately 25% of men will present with bony metastases, so questioning the patient for new onset of back or joint pain is imperative. Interestingly, approximately 22% of men will be diagnosed with prostate cancer only after surgical resection is performed, with diagnosis based on histologic examination by the pathologist.

What Are the Stages of Prostatic Adenocarcinoma?

The system for staging PAC most accepted and used by clinicians is based on the physical findings at presentation. This is probably the most important aspect, because treatment options are based on the clinical stage. Therefore digital rectal examination is the mainstay of diagnosis and staging of prostate cancer. However, it has been well documented that rectal examination understages the extent of the tumor approximately 50% of the time. Therefore efforts today are centered on improving staging accuracy.

When PAC is diagnosed in a patient with a normal rectal examination and clinically unsuspected gland, it is termed *stage A* disease. Tissue has been removed by either transurethral resection (TURP) or by open prostatectomy. If the tumor volume is ≤5% of the tissue and is well differentiated, it is *stage A1*. Any poorly differentiated tissue, regardless of the extent of disease, is termed *stage A2*.

When cancer is suspected by rectal examination, it is *stage B* disease. Classically, a nodule felt on examination that is ≤1.5 cm in diameter is *stage B1*. Any nodule >1.5 cm contained within one lobe of the gland is *stage B2*. When both lobes of the prostate gland are involved with cancer the *stage is B3*.

Once the cancer has spread outside the capsule of the prostate, it is *stage C* disease. When the lateral sulcus of the prostate gland is obliterated by the cancer, it is *stage C1*. Disease involving the seminal vesicles is termed *C2*. If the prostate gland is fixed and immobile, the probability of pelvic wall involvement is high, and it is now *stage C3*.

Stage D disease occurs when metastasis is apparent. Generally speaking, when the pelvic lymph nodes are involved, it is *stage D1*. Gross metastases to bones and other organs are termed *stage D2*. There is a special subsection of stage D disease, which is somewhat controversial, *stage D0*, when tumor markers are elevated. Although there may be no apparent evidence of spread, when tumor markers—acid phosphatase and/or prostatic specific antigen—are elevated, more than 50% of these patients will develop gross metastatic disease within 2 years of presentation. Hence radical curative therapy is of limited value for these patients.

Tumor Markers of Prostate Cancer. As mentioned previously, serum acid phosphatase has been the classic tumor marker for prostate cancer. Acid phosphatase is made by other tissues, including bone, liver, and pancreas. Prostatic tissue produces a specific form of acid phosphatase termed *prostatic acid phosphatase*. Prostatic acid phosphatase is produced by normal prostatic cells. It is secreted into the lumen of the prostatic glands and eliminated with the prostatic secretions. When the tubules are blocked, especially by PAC, it diffuses out of the glands into the intravascular space and is seen as an elevated serum level, which generally portends a poor prognosis, because these patients usually have micrometastases when they are initially seen by the surgeon.

Most recently, a new marker, *prostatic specific antigen (PSA)*, has had much popularity, although its role in the diagnosis and treatment of PAC is unsure and controversial. PSA is believed produced solely by prostatic cells and is more sensitive and specific than acid phosphatase or prostatic acid phosphatase. It is generally believed that high levels of PSA are associated with micrometastases; however, it is not a totally reliable diagnostic test at present. More probably, PSA is useful after treatment of PAC. Serial PSA levels are very useful and accurate in diagnosing recurrent disease after curative therapy.

Grades of Prostate Cancer. The histologic grading of prostate cancer is very useful. It is based on the grading system of Gleason and is called the *Gleason score.* It is based on the degree of differentiation of the cancer. Normal glands are lined by two or more layers of cells and have normal nuclei and shape. As cells become more anaplastic, the cells lose their normal shape, the nuclei exhibit varying degrees of shape, and mitotic figures are prominent. Eventually all semblance of glandular structure is lost. Normal glands have a score of 1, whereas the most poorly differentiated tumors are given a value of 5. Prostate cancer tends to be a heterogenous cancer, with different areas of the tumor exhibiting different degrees of differentiation. Hence two values are given for each cancer. The majority component of the cancer is given the major score, and the minority component is given the minor score. The maximal score is 9 (major = 5, minor = 4). Well-differentiated tumors have a value of 2, 3, or 4, and poorly differentiated tumors are scored 7, 8, or 9. Moderately differentiated cancers are 5, 6, or 7.

How Prostate Cancer Is Staged. After performing a careful *rectal examination,* the physician generally assigns a clinical stage to the tumor as outlined previously. *Percutaneous biopsy* is performed, either transrectally or through the perineum. Perineal biopsy is generally preferred because of the 5% to 10% incidence of fever and infection after the transrectal approach. *Tumor markers are obtained;* if the prostatic acid phosphatase level is elevated, the tumor is designated stage D0. An elevated PSA makes the clinician suspect metastases, although its usefulness in staging is uncertain at present.

Some form of upper tract evaluation is warranted. This can be accomplished by either *IVU or renal ultrasound* (provided the patient does not have microhematuria). Upper tract obstruction as evidenced by hydroureter or hydronephrosis suggests obstruction at the level of the UVJ because of extraprostatic spread.

Currently *transrectal ultrasound* is used to evaluate for extracapsular spread and spread to the seminal vesicles. In addition, it may be helpful in patients when the percutaneously guided biopsy result is either negative or inadequate. Since rectal examination can only palpate the posterior lobes, the clinician is limited in his or her evaluation of the gland. Ultrasound can visualize the anterior portion of the gland and the periurethral region where as many as 20% of cancers may originate.

A *radionuclide bone scan* is imperative. As mentioned, approximately 25% of men with prostate cancer will have bony spread. If the bone scan is positive, patients can be offered noncurative therapy to control the extent of the disease.

Provided the serum tumor markers are normal and the bone scan is negative, the next step is to evaluate the lymph nodes in the pelvis. Generally speaking, when PAC spreads, it first appears in the pelvic lymph glands, although PAC is also well known to skip the lymph glands and spread directly to the bones or other viscera. Some clinicians suggest obtaining a computed tomographic *(CT) scan of the pelvis* to evaluate the lymph glands in the obturator and external iliac regions. However, it is well documented that 20% to 25% of patients with negative CT scans will have positive lymph nodes on surgical exploration. Before the advent of CT scans, pelvic lymphangiography was popular but very difficult to perform and interpret. Reports of up to 50% inaccuracy were seen, and with development of the CT scan, the lymphangiogram fell by the wayside. Therefore a CT scan is generally obtained, but in patients in whom surgical therapy is an option, this may be omitted because the surgeon will perform a pelvic lymphadenectomy before radical curative extirpation. Should the nodes be positive for metastatic spread, the procedure is terminated. The work-up for a patient with prostate cancer is shown in Fig. 41-3. The incidence of positive lymph nodes for each stage is listed below:

Stage	Percent
A1	6
A2	22
B1	15
B2	35
C	50

How Is Prostate Cancer Treated?

For the student attempting to learn and understand the therapy for PAC, it is imperative that he or she be aware this is an area of controversy and continual debate. Therapy is based on the stage of disease and the age and physical condition of the patient. Stage A disease is believed curable.

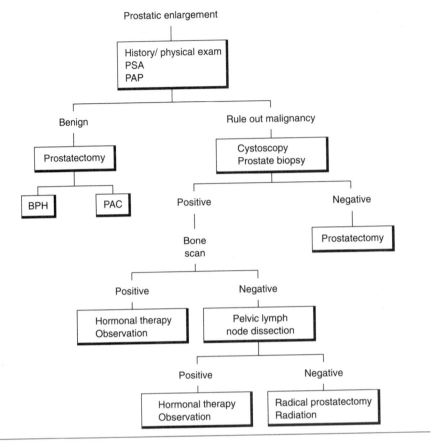

FIGURE 41-3   Work-up for prostatic cancer.

Since autopsy studies have shown such a high prevalence of unsuspected and asymptomatic disease in the elderly population, it is believed that aggressive therapy is not indicated for older patients because most of these patients will succumb to other medical problems before PAC will develop into a morbid situation. This is certainly true for stage A1 disease. However, stage A2, which has a higher incidence of pelvic lymph node spread, usually requires further therapy, especially for younger and medically sound patients. Since PAC is a radiosensitive tumor, controversy exists as to whether surgical extirpation is more beneficial than conservative radiotherapy. Well-documented studies have shown the 5- and 10-year survival rates are relatively equal for either treatment modality. Early evidence shows patients treated by radical prostatectomy may have a survival advantage after 15 years; however, this has not been well supported. Therefore for patients with an expected survival time of more than 10 years, there is no clear advantage of one form of therapy over the other. For younger

patients, especially ones less than 60 years old, surgical intervention seems a better option.

Clinical stage B disease is also a potentially curable stage as long as there is no evidence of extension outside the capsule of the prostate. Again the same arguments for treatment of stage A2 disease are valid. Younger patients are generally offered surgical therapy, since their life expectancy is longer, although many patients prefer radiotherapy.

Clinical stage C PAC may be the most difficult form of PAC to treat. By definition, clinical stage C disease means extension outside the capsule or into the seminal vesicles or even pelvic side wall fixation. These patients generally have limited 5- and 10-year survival rates. Most clinicians do not offer curative surgery for these patients. Many patients do opt for radiotherapy, because it is a means to control the local extent of their disease. Present clinical research centers mainly around stage C disease and its various treatment options.

When PAC has spread to regional lymph nodes or beyond to bones, liver, or other viscera,

TABLE 41-1 Survival Rates After Treatment for Prostate Cancer

Stage	5 Years (%)	10 Years (%)	15 Years (%)
A	60-85	40-60	15-35
B	60-85	40-60	15-35
C	35-50	10-35	0-15
D	5-30	5-10	

it is no longer a curable disease. Fortunately, PAC is also a hormonally sensitive tumor, and these patients can be treated by a variety of modalities to reduce the serum testosterone level and control the extent of disease. Although the time-honored forms of hormonal manipulation have been either bilateral orchiectomy or oral estrogen therapy, recent advances in androgen-receptor blockade and inhibition of luteinizing hormone releasing factors have made medical management quite popular and acceptable. The survival rates for all forms of treatment for PAC are shown in Table 41-1.

A comment concerning stage D0 disease is warranted. As discussed previously, an elevated serum prostatic acid phosphatase level without evidence of metastatic or lymphatic spread places the patient in this stage. Since studies have shown such high rates for recurrent disease within 2 years after curative therapy, such therapy is not currently offered for these patients. However, since there is no sign of metastatic spread, the patient may be offered observation alone. When metastatic disease occurs, the patient is treated accordingly. Clinical research has shown the 5- and 10-year survival rates for stage D0 disease are no different whether the patient is offered early endocrine therapy or observation alone. The above discussion is only meant to give the student an overview of the management of PAC and is not meant to be complete. The therapy for PAC is an ever-evolving concept and excites a controversy whenever it is mentioned.

URINARY TRACT INFECTIONS

In general, urinary tract infections (UTI) are a major cause of medical intervention in the community. In hospitals more than 40% of nosocomial infections are related to the urinary tract. A thorough knowledge of UTI management is essential to all clinicians, since many of these infections can easily be diagnosed and treated by the primary physician. More complex and complicated cases should be referred to the specialist.

What Causes UTIs?

Ascending Infection. The vast majority of UTIs are caused by ascending infection. Bacteria from the intestinal tract enter the lower urinary tract by way of colonization of the urethral openings, especially in women in whom the vagina is often colonized with enteric bacteria. Additionally, catheterization of the bladder allows bacteria to enter the urethra along the catheter, with subsequent infection. Breakdown of the natural defense mechanisms of the urinary mucosa is considered a primary event in allowing bacterial colonization and subsequent infection. Once the bladder is either colonized and/or infected, ureteral peristalsis may become dysfunctional and allow bacteria to ascend the ureter to the upper tracts.

Hematogenous Spread. Blood-borne dissemination is an infrequent cause of infection except in a few specific cases. Examples of it are bacterial endocarditis and intravenous drug use, which allows seeding of the kidney with the development of pyelonephritis. When untreated, this condition can lead to the formation of a renal abscess or carbuncle. In addition, pulmonary tuberculosis, when untreated, is the primary site for hematogenous spread to the kidneys, with subsequent development of renal tuberculosis.

Lymphatic Spread. Lymphatic spread is the least common cause of UTI in North America. Most of its infectious agents are found in the tropics or warm climates. Filarial worms such as **Wuchereria bancrofti** enter the skin through puncture wounds and travel in the lymphatics. Fibrosis and chronic inflammation produce lymphatic obstruction. The lymphatics eventually rupture and form fistulas within the kidney. In addition, because of the lymphatic obstruction, severe lower body and extremity edema (elephantiasis) occurs, affecting the legs and scrotum.

What Are the Risk Factors for UTIs?

The most common risk factor for UTI is some form of urinary tract obstruction. Patients with indwelling catheters have bladders that are colonized with bacteria. Occasionally the defense mechanisms break down and infection occurs. Patients with diabetes and other immunologic impairment are at significant risk. There is significant risk in patients with vesicoureteral reflux

**PREDISPOSING FACTORS
FOR UTIs**

Urinary tract obstruction
Indwelling catheter
Diabetes mellitus
Renal papillary necrosis
Neurogenic bladders
Pregnancy
Congenital urinary tract lesions
Vesicoureteral reflux
End-stage renal disease
Immunocompromised host

in whom urine flows in a retrograde fashion up toward the kidney during bladder emptying. Any chronic condition such as end-stage renal disease or papillary necrosis places the individual at risk. The associated risk factors are listed in the box.

How Are UTIs Classified?

Like urinary tract obstruction, a UTI is classified according to involvement of the upper or lower tracts. Most lower tract infections are readily recognizable and treatable. Upper tract infections are more complex and usually require more aggressive management, for the morbidity with upper tract infections is much greater.

What Are the Different Kinds of Upper Tract Infections?

The most common form of upper tract infection is pyelonephritis. It involves both the renal parenchyma and the collecting system. It commonly occurs from a lower tract infection with ascending infection. When the upper tract becomes obstructed and is infected as well, the infection is termed *pyonephrosis.* Many of these kidneys are not functioning at presentation. Renal calculi commonly cause the obstruction at the UPJ; however, a tumor should also be considered as a possible cause of the obstruction.

Should the infection go untreated, it may progress to form a renal abscess or carbuncle, which usually stems from a focal site of pyelonephritis or by hematogenous spread of *Staphylococcus aureus,* especially in intravenous drug abusers. If the abscess extends into the perinephric space but is contained within Gerota's fascia, it is termed a *perinephric abscess.* This is commonly

seen in infections caused by *Escherichia coli* or *Proteus.* Patients that are either diabetic or have polycystic kidneys are prone to perinephric abscess formation. The mortality rate can be as high as 50% in patients when treatment is delayed.

An unusual form of infection, xanthgranulomatous pyelonephritis, requires separate discussion. Although this is a rare infection, it most commonly occurs in diabetics and is caused by either *Proteus* or *E. coli.* Xanthgranulomatous pyelonephritis is almost universally associated with obstruction and stone formation. It commonly involves a nonfunctioning kidney, with a mass seen on radiologic evaluation. It may be confused with a renal cancer and diagnosed at surgical exploration.

Chronic pyelonephritis stems from recurrent infections in the renal parenchyma and results in cortical scarring and a contracted and shrunken kidney. It is associated with vesicoureteral reflux. The various causes of upper tract infections are seen in Fig. 41-4.

Signs and Symptoms of an Upper UTI. The most common symptoms of upper UTIs are fever, chills, and flank pain. Lower tract symptoms of dysuria, frequency, and urgency may or may not be present. Physical examination may reveal costovertebral angle tenderness. In patients with a perinephric abscess a flank mass may be palpable. In some patients the abscess will seek to drain itself to the outside through fistulous formation.

Work-Up for an Upper UTI. Initial studies for an upper UTI include obtaining a clean-catch urine specimen for analysis and culture. It must be obtained before antibiotic therapy is administered, for such therapy may lead to negative cultures. Blood studies include complete blood count (CBC), cultures, serum electrolytes, and BUN with creatinine to assess overall renal function.

A renal ultrasound, which evaluates the overall renal and pararenal anatomy, should be obtained. It is noninvasive and has minimal risks. Should the ultrasound demonstrate intrarenal pathology, an IVU should be obtained if the serum creatinine level is ≤2.0. The IVU will give some functional information about each kidney and will delineate the collecting system and ureter. The thickness of the parenchyma may be seen, which may help the clinician in diagnosing the duration of the infection. If obstruction exists, it should also be seen on the IVU. In patients with severe infections the renal function may be impaired, or the kidney may not function at all; hence the degree of visualization may be poor.

Pending the radiologic findings, further eval-

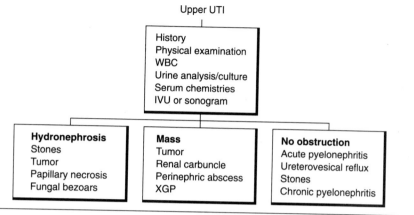

Upper UTI

| History |
| Physical examination |
| WBC |
| Urine analysis/culture |
| Serum chemistries |
| IVU or sonogram |

Hydronephrosis
Stones
Tumor
Papillary necrosis
Fungal bezoars

Mass
Tumor
Renal carbuncle
Perinephric abscess
XGP

No obstruction
Acute pyelonephritis
Ureterovesical reflux
Stones
Chronic pyelonephritis

FIGURE 41-4 Differential diagnosis for upper UTI. *WBC* = white blood cell count; *IVU* = intravenous urogram; *XGP* = xanthogranulomatous pyelonephritis.

uation may be required. Should the ultrasound or IVU demonstrate mass effect or perinephric involvement, a CT scan with contrast should be obtained to rule out perinephric abscess formation. Findings suggestive of abscess formation include a mass with fluid levels or tissue stranding within the perinephric space.

Treatment of Upper UTIs. Initial management consists of obtaining urine and blood cultures before the institution of any antibiotics. Obtaining serum electrolyte and BUN and creatinine levels is imperative to assess renal function and acid-base balance. Subsequently, antibiotics should be instituted, with the choice depending on the organisms suspected, hospital infection rates, and the patient's allergy history. Most infections can initially be treated with ampicillin (1 g every 6 hours) and gentamicin or tobramycin (1.5 mg/kg every 8 hours). Recently, ciprofloxacin has become popular, but its usefulness in complicated upper UTIs is unknown.

Should signs of obstruction or abscess be present, they must be relieved once the patient has stabilized. Occasionally, the patient may not improve with intravenous antibiotics; then only drainage will improve the patient's condition. For obstruction due to a stone, retrograde pyelography and catheterization provide an option if the patient is not septic. If the patient has an abscess or is unstable, percutaneous drainage is best. Cultures and anterograde studies, if necessary, can be obtained.

In patients with signs of poor renal function or abscess it is worthwhile to obtain a renal scan to assess both the overall function and the contralateral side. Should the function be less than 10%, nephrectomy may be necessary once the acute infection has subsided.

What Are the Different Kinds of Lower UTIs?

The most common lower UTI is cystitis. Much has been written concerning its cause. It appears that the normal mucosal defense mechanisms are impaired, allowing bacterial adherence and propagation. Cystitis occurs more commonly in women and is believed due to vaginal colonization. Older men with obstructive uropathy are also susceptible to cystitis. Children may develop lower UTIs, which mandate a thorough work-up for any congenital anomaly.

Cystitis associated with obstruction is termed *pyocystitis.* It is commonly seen in patients with poor urinary outflow such as dialysis patients in whom there is little need to empty the bladder.

The remaining types of lower UTIs are based on gender. Women may develop infections of the urethra, which may progress to form a urethral abscess. Occasionally, these abscesses spontaneously drain into the urethra, and the abscess cavity along with the fistulous tract becomes a urethral diverticulum. It may become chronically infected, obstructed, and drain in a cycle if its existence is unknown. Women can also develop infections of the genital structures such as an infected Bartholin's cyst, which may have symptoms similar to those of a UTI.

Men who develop lower UTIs but who do not have cystitis have infections of the male genital organs. Most commonly, prostatitis, which can mimic cystitis, can be diagnosed after a rectal examination. The patient may complain of perineal pain and associated bladder outlet symptoms. Should acute bacterial prostatitis go untreated, an abscess may evolve, which is palpable as a fluctuant mass during rectal examination. Care should be taken to avoid an overvigorous examination because rupture may occur, possibly causing bacteremia.

Infections within the scrotum involve the epididymis and testis. These organs are usually infected by retrograde spread down the vas deferens toward the testis. Two groups of men have this type of infection: the sexually active men over 35 years of age and the men older than 60 years who usually have obstructed symptoms as well. Men in the former group are generally infected with *Chlamydia trachomatis* or *Neisseria gonorrhoeae*. The latter group is usually infected with *E. coli*. Occasionally untreated infections can progress to abscess formation, which generally results in loss of the involved testis. Epididymitis can occur without infection of the ipsilateral testis, but it is rare for infection of the testis to occur without involvement of the epididymis. Repeated infections of the epididymis result in chronic epididymitis. Occult genitourinary tuberculosis is possible in patients with chronic epididymitis.

The mumps virus is an RNA virus that usually infects the parotid glands. On occasion, it can spread to the testis, occurring 4 to 6 days after the onset of the viral infection. It usually resolves in 7 to 10 days, but in cases of bilateral infections it may result in permanent sterility.

Urethritis is a form of lower urinary tract infection very common in the sexually active male. The same organisms as in epididymitis cause it; however, scrotal involvement will be absent. Untreated urethritis may progress to significant epididymal orchitis. The fibrosis and scarring of urethritis results in the formation of a urethral stricture.

Signs and Symptoms of Lower UTIs. When the lower urinary tract is involved, the patient may present with a wide variety of symptoms. Most commonly, frequency, dysuria, and urgency are signs of cystitis. In severely ill patients signs of sepsis with fever, leukocytosis, hematuria, and inability to urinate are common. Physical examination may reveal suprapubic tenderness or even a distended bladder in men with outlet obstruction. Pelvic examination of the female should be performed to evaluate the genitalia and exclude vaginal infections. In addition, palpation of the urethra may reveal a mass in cases of urethral diverticuli. In men scrotal pain generally refers to epididymal or testicular infection, whereas perineal pain suggests prostatic infection. Scrotal examination may reveal a tender epididymis posterior to the testis and spermatic cord tenderness near the external inguinal ring. A patient with orchitis usually presents with a globally enlarged and tender testis. Chronic or-

chitis and epididymitis must not be mistaken for a testicular tumor. A recurrent epididymal infection with negative urine cultures and no relief with antibiotic treatment is a testicular tumor until proven otherwise.

A discussion about testicular torsion is warranted. It is quite often confused with epididymal orchitis. Both are associated with testicular pain. Torsion is usually acute, and epididymitis is generally insidious in onset. The results of urinalysis are normal with torsion, whereas leukocytes are commonly seen with infection. The physical examination of a patient with torsion reveals a globally hard and tender testis. The spermatic cord may also be tender because of venous obstruction. There is usually loss of the normal cremasteric reflex with torsion. In a patient with epididymal orchitis the testis may be hard as well, but the epididymis can generally be palpated discretely from the testis. The cremasteric reflex is intact, but the spermatic cord is not typically tender. In cases in which diagnosis is unsure, a testicular scan is helpful. There will be increased blood flow with infection, whereas in torsion a photopenic area will be surrounded by hyperemia (bull's eye appearance).

In men with urethritis a urethral discharge is common, as is dysuria without other signs or symptoms. A watery discharge suggests infection by *C. trachomatis*, whereas a yellow-green discharge means *N. gonorrhoeae*. The causes of lower UTIs are seen in Fig. 41-5.

Work-Up for a Lower Tract Infection. Urinalysis and culture of a clean-catch specimen are mandatory. If a clean-catch sample is not reliable, a catheterized sample is acceptable provided the patient does not have acute prostatitis or prostatic abscess because either could cause

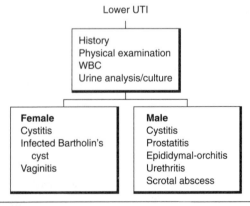

FIGURE 41-5   Differential diagnosis for lower UTI.

bacteremia. In men with symptoms referred to the scrotum, an ultrasound may be helpful in diagnosing an abscess from a testicular tumor. Transrectal prostatic ultrasound should never be performed in men with acute prostatitis or abscess. In men with obstructive outlet symptoms the work-up should proceed as described previously. In patients with fever and signs of sepsis, a CBC, serum electrolyte values, and BUN with creatinine values should be obtained, as should a radiologic upper tract study to rule out an occult upper tract infection that has been asymptomatic.

Treatment of Lower UTI. Treatment is based on the diagnosis and the physical condition of the patient. Most people can be treated as outpatients with oral antibiotics. For uncomplicated cystitis, a 5- to 7-day course of either ampicillin or trimethoprim/sulfamethoxazole is usually sufficient. In men with epididymitis or orchitis the causative organism should be known. Older men may be treated with sulfa-based drugs but usually for a longer period of time. In the sexually active age group tetracycline and its derivatives are the treatment of choice for *Chlamydia* and most of the sexually transmitted diseases.

Men with a complicated lower UTI who present with high-grade fever, extensive testicular involvement, or abscess formation must receive intravenous antibiotics and must have bed rest and scrotal elevation. For the patient with an abscess that fails to respond to treatment, incision and drainage of the abscess are required. The patient should be informed of the strong possibility that the testis probably will need resection.

UNUSUAL URINARY TRACT INFECTIONS
Genitourinary Tuberculosis

As mentioned previously, genitourinary tuberculosis (TB) is always secondary to pulmonary infection with hematogenous spread. Upper tract involvement with the kidney usually requires significant time before the kidney will be completely destroyed and may produce few symptoms if any until the end stage is reached. An abscess is formed that ruptures into the collecting system, and subsequent lower tract involvement occurs. Patients may present with a variety of complaints, typically with voiding irritability. Usually treated with oral antibiotics, the patients return with the same symptoms without relief. Constitutional symptoms such as malaise and generalized weakness are common, and night sweats certainly should alert the clinician. Occa-

sionally, the male patient presents with drainage out the scrotum. Physical examination may reveal an abscess of the epididymis that has spontaneously drained and a beaded vas deferens.

Routine urine cultures will return negative results, although the analysis will show white blood cells. This is the hallmark of genitourinary TB and is called *sterile pyuria.* Work-up should include CBC, chemistry panel with renal function tests, chest x-ray examination, IVU, and skin purified protein derivative (PPD) test. In addition, the first-voided urine should be obtained for 3 days and sent for TB culture. TB cultures require a full 6 weeks before a negative report is accepted.

Treatment consists of multidrug therapy with isoniazid (300 mg every day) and rifampin (450 to 600 mg every day) for 6 to 9 months. Longer therapy may be necessary. Pyridoxine (25 mg/day) should be administered to prevent the peripheral neuropathy associated with isoniazid treatment. In patients with upper tract obstruction therapy is dictated by the site of obstruction.

Candiduria

This yeastlike fungus is a normal inhabitant of the intestinal tract and the vagina. It infects the urinary tract either by hematogenous or retrograde spread. The organism contains pseudomycelia, which are long, threadlike structures that tend to clump together and form fungus balls. In the upper tract these balls can cause urinary obstruction. Like many other fungal infections, candiduria occurs in patients who are immunosuppressed or who have been treated with multiple antibiotics. Many of these patients also have indwelling catheters.

Candiduria is usually seen when routine urine cultures are taken for diagnosis of other lesions. Work-up should include some form of upper tract study, usually a renal ultrasound to rule out fungus balls in the renal pelves. The bladder should also be evaluated to rule out a fungal bezoar. Treatment is based on eliminating the causative factors; that is, removal of catheters when possible, termination of multiple antibiotic therapy, or tight control of diabetes. Fungal balls may require surgical extraction, although if the kidney is obstructed, percutaneous nephrostomy placement and irrigation with amphotericin B (50 mg/L) may be successful. Lower tract infection in patients that still require catheter drainage may similarly be treated with amphoteric irrigation for 5 to 7 days. Currently, fluconazole, an oral imadazole, has been successfully used in limited studies in place of amphotericin.

Schistosomiasis (Bilharziasis)

Schistosomiasis is a condition caused by a blood fluke endemic throughout Africa, the Middle East, and Asia. Three species of *Schistosoma* are *haematobium, japonicum,* and *mansoni.* The life cycle of the worm requires the adult form to reside in the pelvic and urogenital tissues of humans, in which over years it sheds eggs, which are excreted in the urine and feces. The infection occurs by penetration of the larvae into the human tissue from infected water or soil. The eggs deposited in the tissue cause a granulomatous inflammatory response with resultant fibrosis. The bladder and lower ureters are commonly involved. The incidence of squamous cell carcinoma of the bladder increases in areas endemic with schistosomiasis.

Patients may present with stones anywhere in the urinary tract but most commonly in the bladder. In addition, dysuria and hematuria occur. Diagnosis is made by detection of the eggs in the urine. An IVU to evaluate the entire collecting system is mandatory as is cystoscopy to visualize the bladder mucosa. Treatment is based on eradication of the infection, if possible, by administering metrifonate (7.5 to 10 mg/kg) three times daily for 2 weeks or longer. Obstruction of the urinary tract may require surgical intervention. Patients should be monitored for the development of squamous cell cancer of the bladder.

Filariasis

W. bancrofti are worms (i.e., nematodes) that live in human lymphatics, causing filariasis. They are endemic to the tropical climates. The life cycle of the worms requires the female to release larvae into the circulation where they are ingested by mosquito with a blood meal. They are transmitted to the next individual with the mosquito's next bite. The larvae then reside and mature in that person's lymphatics. As the worm lives in the lymphatics, it causes inflammation and fibrosis. The most common site for worms to reside in men is the lower spermatic cord and the tail of the epididymis. Subsequently, fibrosis of the scrotal lymphatics produces elephantiasis of the testicles with hydrocoele formation. In the upper tract the lymphatics of the renal hilum may become obstructed, with lymphatic rupture into a renal calyx, producing chyluria. Extensive involvement of the lower trunk may also produce obstruction and edema of the legs.

Hydrocoeles caused by filariasis will contain milky fluid and result in chyluria. Elephantiasis of the penis, scrotum, and legs is an obvious finding. Eosinophilia commonly occurs, but the diagnosis is made when the adult worms are found during histologic lymphatic biopsy. The infection is treated with diethylcarbamazine, which kills only the immature forms. There is no effective therapy for the adult worms. Surgical treatment is based on the clinical situation.

PITFALLS AND COMMON MYTHS

- Inadequate history and physical examination (especially rectal examination).
- Assuming low urinary output is due to volume depletion and not obstruction.
- Not following renal function daily with serum creatinine values in patients with obstruction.
- Waiting for culture results to return before implementing antibiotic therapy in patients with infections.
- Assuming negative cultures are due to previous antibiotic treatment in genitourinary tuberculosis and sterile pyuria.
- Assuming a catheter's not draining is due to decreased urinary output; in men the catheter balloon must be checked to ensure it is not in the prostatic urethra or blocked by clot or tissue.
- Assuming recurrent pyelonephritis is due to patient noncompliance; an abscess or infectious stone must be ruled out.
- Waiting too long before draining an abscess or relieving an obstruction.
- Not maintaining antibiotic therapy long enough for adequate treatment.
- Not following up on cultures to make sure appropriate antibiotic treatment is being administered.
- Leaving a catheter in place too long; associated with multiple antibiotic therapy, which may allow opportunistic infections to develop.

SURGICAL PHARMACOPEIA

Drug	Indications/Complications	Dosage
Pharmacologic Agents for Prostatism		
Prazosin hydrochloride (Minipress)	γ_1-blocker—orthostatic hypotension	1 mg PO bid
Terazosin hydrochloride (Hytrin)	More useful, with longer half-life	1-2 mg PO qd
Doxazosin mesylate (Cardura)	Long half-life with fewest side effects; expensive	1-2 mg PO qd
Pharmacologic Agents for Hormonal Ablative Therapy in Prostate Cancer		
Estrogens		
Diethylstilbestrol	Low cost; suppresses gonadotropin release from pituitary; increases risk of stroke, heart attack, deep venous thrombosis; can also cause painful gynecomastia	2 mg PO bid
Leutinizing Hormone-Releasing Hormone (LHRH) Agonists		
Leuprolide acetate (Lupron Depot)	Very expensive; down-regulates pituitary LHRH receptors; due to "flare" response with initial increase of testosterone, must treat with flutamide for first month	7-5 mg IM monthly
Antiandrogens		
Flutamide	Very expensive; used with LHRH agonist to prevent "flare" response; may be used in refractory cases of hormonal manipulation to combat adrenal androgens	250 mg PO tid
Pharmacologic Agents for Urinary Tract Infections (UTI)		
For Uncomplicated or Mildly Complicated UTI		
Trimethoprim/dosage 160 mg Sulfamethoxazole 800 mg (Bactrim DS, Septra DS)	Drug of choice for community-acquired UTI; although rare, can cause rash and Stevens-Johnson syndrome	One tablet PO bid
Nitrofurantoin (Macrodantin)	Less tolerated; can cause nausea, hypersensitive neuropathy, and (rarely) can cause pulmonary infiltrates, jaundice, and hemolytic anemia	50-100 mg PO qd
Norfloxacin (Noroxin)	Used strictly for UTIs; well tolerated; not as broad spectrum as the newer fluoroquinolones (e.g., ciprofloxacin)	400 mg PO bid
Ciprofloxacin (Cipro)	Broad spectrum; expensive; interferes with hepatic metabolism of theophylline and warfarin	500 mg PO bid
Methenamine mandelate (Mandelamine)	Antiseptic; converted to formaldehyde in urine; pH < 5.5; ideal as suppressive agent; should be given with vitamin C 500 mg qd to keep pH < 5.5; well tolerated; cannot use with sulfa-based medication	1 gm PO qd

Continued.

Drug	Indications/Complications	Dosage
For Complicated Urinary Tract Infections (Parenteral Antibiotics)		
Cephalosporins		
Cefazolin sodium (Kefzol)	Ideal for mild community-acquired UTI; well tolerated	1 gm IV q8h
Ceftazidime (Fortaz)	Broad spectrum; expensive; does not cover enterococcus; especially powerful against *Pseudomonas*	1-2 gm IV q8h
Aminoglycosides		
Gentamicin sulfate (Garamycin)	Good against gram-negative organisms; need to check serum levels to avoid nephrotoxicity, ototoxicity, and rare neuromuscular blockade; synergistic against gram-positive organisms	80 mg IV q8h
Monobactams		
Aztreonam (Azactam)	Strictly gram-negative coverage; well tolerated with few side effects; covers *Pseudomonas*	1 gm IV q8h
Penicillins		
Ampicillin	Inexpensive; useful for mild community-acquired UTI	2 gm IV q6h
Piperacillin (Pipracil)	Broad spectrum; covers *Pseudomonas*, anaerobes, and enterococcus; cannot use in patients with penicillin allergy	2 gm IV q6h
Fluoroquinolones		
Ciprofloxacin (Cipro)	Broad spectrum; does not cover enterococcus; caution patient about use with theophylline and warfarin	400 mg IV q12h
Antifungals		
Fluconazole (Diflucan)	Well tolerated; has almost replaced amphotericin B	100 mg IV or PO q24h
Agents Against Urethritis		
Ceftriaxone sodium (Rocephin)	Drug of choice for gonorrhea, urethritis	250 mg IM single dose
Ofloxacin (Floxin)	Single-dose oral therapy for gonorrhea only	400 mg PO single dose
Tetracycline	Drug of choice against nongonococcal urethritis (*Chlamydia*)	500 mg PO qid × 7 days
Doxycycline (Vibramycin)	Drug of choice against nongonococcal urethritis (*Chlamydia*)	100 mg PO q12h × 7 days

BIBLIOGRAPHY

Elyaderani MK, Kandzari SJ, Casteneda WR, et al. Invasive Uroradiology. Lexington, Ky, Callamore Press, 1984.

Gillenwater J. The pathophysiology of urinary obstruction. In Walsh PC, Gittes RF, Perlmutter AD, et al (eds). Campbell's Urology, 4th ed. Philadelphia, WB Saunders, 1986.

Gow JG. Genitourinary tuberculosis. In Walsh PC, Gittes RF, Perlmutter AD, et al (eds). Campbell's Urology, 4th ed. Philadelphia, WB Saunders, 1986.

Hanno PM, Wein AJ (eds). A Clinical Manual of Urology. Norwalk, Conn, Appleton-Century-Crofts, 1987.

Kunin Calvin M. Detection, Prevention and Management of Urinary Tract Infections, 4th ed. Philadelphia, Lea & Febiger, 1987.

Persky L, Kursh ED, Feldman S, et al. Extrinsic obstruction of the ureter. In Walsh PC, Gittes RF, Perlmutter AD, et al (eds). Campbell's Urology, 4th ed. Philadelphia, WB Saunders, 1986.

Resnick MI, Caldamone AA, Spirnak JP. Decision Making in Urology. St. Louis, CV Mosby, 1985.

Schoenebeck J. Fungal infections of the urinary tract. In Walsh PC, Gittes RF, Perlmutter AD, et al (eds). Campbell's Urology, 4th ed. Philadelphia, WB Saunders, 1986.

Stamey TA, Pathogenesis and Treatment of Urinary Tract Infections. Baltimore, Williams & Wilkins, 1980.

Tanagho EA, McAninch JW. Smith's General Urology, 12th ed. Norwalk, Conn, Appleton & Lange, 1988.

Von Lichtenberg F, Lehman JS. Parasitic diseases of the genitourinary system. In Walsh PC, Gittes RF, Perlmutter AD, et al (eds). Campbell's Urology, 4th ed. Philadelphia, WB Saunders, 1986.

CHAPTER REVIEW
Questions

1. Carcinoma of the prostate is most effectively diagnosed by:
   a. Determination of the serum prostatic acid phosphatase
   b. Transurethral resection of the prostate
   c. Rectal examination
   d. CEA levels

2. Oliguria is defined as:
   a. No urine for 24 hours
   b. <450 ml of urine over 24 hours
   c. <250 ml of urine over 24 hours
   d. <800 ml of urine over 24 hours

3. A patient arrives in the emergency room with a distended bladder. He is passing small amounts of bloody urine and is in intense pain. The next step in management is:
   a. Placement of a suprapubic catheter
   b. Drawing blood for serum chemistry panel and CBC
   c. Passage of a urethral catheter and obtaining a urine culture
   d. Obtaining a complete history and performing a physical examination

4. A 25-year-old male complains of left flank pain after excessive beer intake but denies pain otherwise. An IVU reveals minimal left hydronephrosis with a normal right kidney. The next step in the work-up should be:
   a. Whitaker test
   b. Renal scan with DTPA and furosemide washout
   c. Renal ultrasound
   d. Abdominal CT scan

5. A 28-year-old woman, G3P3, complains of right lower abdominal pain that occurs every 3 to 4 weeks, lasting approximately 4 days. Pelvic examination reveals a right adnexal mass. IVU shows a high-grade lower ureteral obstruction with significant hydronephrosis. The next step in management would be:
   a. Renal scan with DTPA
   b. Cystoscopy and retrograde pyelogram
   c. CT scan
   d. Percutaneous nephrostomy

6. The most likely diagnosis in the patient above is:
   a. Ureteral carcinoma
   b. Ureteral calculus
   c. Endometriosis
   d. Invasive bladder carcinoma

7. A 19-year-old male comes to the emergency room with a watery discharge for 5 days. He denies scrotal pain. The treatment of choice is:
   a. Ampicillin, 250 mg qid for 7 days
   b. Penicillin, 250 mg qid for 10 days
   c. Tetracycline, 250 mg qid for 7 days
   d. Aqueous penicillin, 4.8 million units IM

8. A 50-year-old male who recently immigrated from Egypt presents with gross painless hematuria. The most likely diagnosis is:
   a. Prostatitis
   b. Cystitis
   c. Squamous cell carcinoma of the bladder
   d. Renal cell carcinoma

9. A 22-year-old intravenous drug abuser comes to the emergency room with fever of 38.8° C (102° F) and left flank pain. Physical examination reveals a tender 15-cm mass in the left flank. The most likely diagnosis is:
   a. Left staghorn calculus
   b. Left ureteropelvic junction obstruction
   c. Left epididymitis
   d. Left perinephric abscess

10. After blood for studies and cultures has been drawn, the above patient is started on intravenous antibiotic therapy. The next step in management is:
    a. Left nephrectomy
    b. Left percutaneous nephrostomy
    c. Renal scan with DTPA
    d. Left retrograde pyelogram and ureteral catheterization

11. A 35-year-old patient with AIDS is admitted with bilateral flank pain and fever to 39.4° C (103° F). After administration of intravenous antibiotics for 3 days, the patient has not improved. An IVU shows bilateral poorly functioning kidneys with moderate hydronephrosis. The next step in management is:

a. Bilateral percutaneous nephrostomies
b. Renal ultrasound
c. Retrograde pyelograms
d. Abdominal CT scan

12. The most likely diagnosis in the above patient is:
   a. Bilateral renal calculi
   b. Bilateral ureteropelvic junction obstructions
   c. Bilateral candidial fungus balls
   d. Bilateral renal cell carcinomas

Answers

1. c. Although rectal examination understages prostate cancer, it is still the most efficient and effective method of diagnosis.

2. b

3. c. This patient is in pain and distress. Any attempt at obtaining his history and a physical examination would be useless. Blood studies can be drawn later. Suprapubic catheterization should be attempted only after urethral attempts have been made.

4. b. This young man probably has a functional ureteropelvic junction obstruction. A renal scan with furosemide washout to evaluate the $T_{1/2}$ is the next best test. A retrograde pyelogram is also possible but is an invasive study.

5. b. Retrograde pyelography not only could localize the lesion, but a ureteral catheter also could be passed to optimize renal function. A renal scan would be helpful once the obstruction has been bypassed to evaluate renal salvageability.

6. c. In this age category malignancy is unlikely, especially with the cyclic history related to her menstrual periods.

7. c. Tetracycline or its derivatives are the drugs of choice for urethritis secondary to *Chlamydia*.

8. c. Squamous cell carcinoma is endemic from Schistosomiasis in the Middle East.

9. d. Intravenous drug abusers have perinephric abscesses secondary to staphylococcal infections until proven otherwise.

10. b. Although retrograde pyelography would be helpful, in a septic patient the least amount of manipulation possible is best. This is best accomplished by drainage of the abscess by percutaneous techniques. Nephrectomy would carry a high mortality rate without prior drainage. A renal scan would be necessary to evaluate whether or not the kidney is worth saving.

11. b. This patient is not responding to traditional therapy, and an alternate diagnosis must be considered. Before aggressive intervention is attempted, a renal sonogram to assess the upper tract anatomy better would be prudent to make the diagnosis. Bilateral nephrostomies would be therapeutic and diagnostic but highly invasive in this toxic patient and would carry significant risk.

12. c. This patient is immunosuppressed, and opportunistic infections are quite common.

42

The Scrotum

H. HARLAN STONE

KEY FEATURES

After reading this chapter you will understand:
- Common skin or venereal diseases of the scrotal area.
- The best approach to a scrotal mass.
- The significance of an empty scrotum.

Abnormalities of the scrotum, in almost all instances, can be assigned to one of four categories: skin lesions, painless masses, painful masses, or an empty scrotum.

SKIN LESIONS
Sexually Transmitted Diseases

Cutaneous manifestations of sexually transmitted diseases (STDs) are primarily noted about the male external genitalia, although the penis and its glans are more frequently affected than is the scrotum. The primary lesion of *syphilis (chancre)* is a firm, nontender ulcer, a smear of which will reveal the spirochete *Treponema pallidum* on darkfield examination. Serologic tests for syphilis rarely become positive until after the ulcer has regressed or completely healed. The primary lesion of *chancroid*, on the other hand, is a tender and much softer ulcer. Microscopic examination of a smear of its exudate reveals chains of gram-negative rods, which on culture are identified as *Haemophilus ducreyi*. Both types of chancre may be associated with groin lymphadenopathy.

Treatment is based on parenteral administration of antibiotics—penicillin for syphilis, tetracycline for chancroid. However, as with all other forms of STDs, an equally important facet is the patient's sexual contacts. Any partner who could have been the source of his infection, as well as those whom he later may have infected, must also receive appropriate examination and therapy.

Lymphogranuloma venereum is caused by a virus and begins as a vesicle on the external genitalia. Shortly thereafter the primary lesion disappears, and clinical findings are then dominated by an inguinal adenopathy that usually progresses to suppuration, often discharges through the skin, and finally forms a chronic sinus. In advanced cases, multiple cutaneous fistulas may communicate with the bladder or even the rectum. Traditionally, a positive result to a Frei skin test has been the criterion for diagnosis, but at present the more specific serologic complement-fixation test is preferred. For treatment of the early stages, tetracycline is the antimicrobial agent of choice. Once extensive scarring and multiple sinus tracts have developed, radical groin dissection with correction of any resultant large soft tissue defect by a myocutaneous flap (usually based on the tensor fascia lata) offers some hope for permanent cure.

Granuloma inguinale, caused by the Donovan bacillus, progresses from an innocuous-appearing vesicle to a chronic inflammatory ulcer, usually situated in the groin or near the base of the scrotum. Regional lymphadenopathy is rare. Microscopic examination of a smear or biopsy of the resultant lesion demonstrates typical Donovan bodies of *Donovania granulomatis*. A good response can be expected from oral tetracycline or erythromycin.

Gonorrhea (*Neisseria gonorrhoeae*) produces no scrotal cutaneous lesion, although staining of the external genitalia and undergarments with the purulent urethral discharge is quite obvious. The acute urethritis is treated with parenteral penicillin or, if bacterial resistance or a history of an accelerated penicillin allergy is noted, a second- or third-generation cephalosporin is prescribed.

Early complications of gonorrhea such as prostatitis, seminal vesiculitis, and epididymo-orchitis initially respond to antibiotic therapy but may become foci for frequent exacerbations. Urethral stricture is a common complication, tends to be refractory, and is generally managed long-term by repeated dilations.

Scrotal Edema

Edema of the scrotum can be relatively minor and confined to a small area, as with some superficial infections, may be moderate and involve the entire scrotum as a consequence of pelvic vein thrombosis, or can be so massive that it is referred to as *elephantiasis*. The latter is seen following bilateral groin lymph node dissections, metastatic cancer to the same area, or parasitic infestation (filariasis) of the lymphatics.

Infection

The more severe scrotal infections are often secondary to a urethral or bladder disruption. Following extravasation of urine, the scrotum may become a huge, boggy mass with varying degrees of cellulitis or abscess. Therapy is appropriate to the type of infection and must also include a suprapubic cystostomy.

The most destructive of all forms of scrotal infection, *Fournier's gangrene,* is sudden in onset, rapidly progressing, and superficial. It is commonly associated with diabetic ketoacidosis. Treatment should include a combination of parenteral antibiotics directed against all components of the responsible mixed bacterial flora (aerobic and anaerobic). More important, however, is the absolute necessity for wide excision of all necrotic tissue. A striking feature is the sparing of testes and cords from the infection, since these scrotal contents are located in an entirely separate tissue plane. The wound is left open for later closure by a split-thickness skin graft.

Epidermoid Cancer

The first cancer ever identified as being caused by a specific carcinogen was that on the scrotum of chimney sweeps. Prolonged contact with coal tar and other organic substances account for almost half of the epidermoid carcinomas developing on and around the scrotum. Although a confirming biopsy followed by radical excision of the primary lesion in continuity with regional groin lymph nodes is the best known treatment, the 5-year survival rate is still relatively poor, at only 20%.

Miscellaneous Lesions

As with skin elsewhere, other cutaneous lesions can also be noted. Common among these are the sebaceous cyst and mite infestation (chiggers).

PAINLESS SCROTAL MASSES
Inguinal Hernia

Indirect inguinal hernias occur in patients of all ages and both sexes (Chapter 29). If there is an extension from the groin down only to the superior aspect of the scrotum, such hernias are called *funicular.* If the depth of the scrotum is reached, however, then the hernia is called complete or *scrotal.* As long as the hernia is reducible (i.e., can be pushed back into the abdomen) or as long as there is no obstruction to bowel lumen or impairment in intestinal blood supply despite the chronic incarceration, the indirect inguinal hernia presents as a painless scrotal mass that extends well up into the groin.

Scrotal Cysts

Differentiation of incarcerated bowel from one of the cystic scrotal masses is always important and can best be done by transillumination. With a strong penlight as the source of illumination, the scrotum is viewed through a special tube or paper towel cylinder, preferably in a darkened room (Fig. 42-1). Since intestine rarely contains clear fluid, only gas, and/or digestive contents, it either fails to transmit light or produces such a hazy glow that almost all details of normal scrotal contents (e.g., testis and epididymis) are obscured. Cysts, by contrast, usually contain clear or amber fluid, and thus their origin from specific scrotal structures can easily be defined.

A cyst arising from the tunica vaginalis (*hydrocele*) usually fills the entire scrotum except for its posterior attachment to the epididymis (Fig.

42-2). Occasionally the hydrocele is solely funicular; that is, it involves a residual segment of tunica vaginalis in the cord above. Hydroceles are selectively managed by excision of all portions of the sac except for posterior attachments, by excision of a portion of the sac wall so as to form a window for the insertion of a drain, or by repeated aspirations with a hypodermic needle and syringe. In infants and children, the hydrocele usually communicates with the peritoneal cavity proper via a patent processus vaginalis traversing the inguinal canal. Accordingly, treatment is based on correction of the associated indirect inguinal hernia (Chapter 29).

The *spermatocele* is derived from the epididymis itself, is much smaller than the usual hydrocele, and is perched on the epididymis in the posterior recesses of the scrotum (see Fig. 42-2). Complete excision is the preferred method of treatment. Finally, cysts can develop in the *appendix testis* or *hydatid of Morgagni.* These are on the superior aspect of the testis, just anterior to the epididymal cap. Excision is recommended only if they become symptomatic because of torsion or size.

Tumors

As a general rule, masses of the scrotum not involving the testis are seldom neoplastic and, if so, are benign. However, almost all masses of the testis proper are neoplastic, primary, and malignant. They generally appear between the ages of 20 and 35 years. The undescended testis, probably because it is already abnormal, has a twenty-fold greater predilection for developing such tumors. All spread by both direct extension into adjacent tissues and up the cord as well as by the lymphatic system. In addition, the choriocarcinoma tends to metastasize relatively early by direct vascular invasion.

Initial presentation is a scrotal mass in three fourths of patients. The remainder will have noted scrotal pain, often preceded by trauma. Work-up is based on a thorough physical examination, scrotal ultrasound, and then radical orchiectomy. Biopsy should be avoided because of its high association with both local recurrence as well as distant metastases.

Stage I tumors are confined to the scrotum; stage II lesions have extended into the retroperitoneal lymphatics (as noted on CT abdominal scan or diagnostic laparoscopy), yet have not spread above the diaphragm; stage III indicates distant metastases, especially to the lungs.

Treatment is tailored to cell type and stage

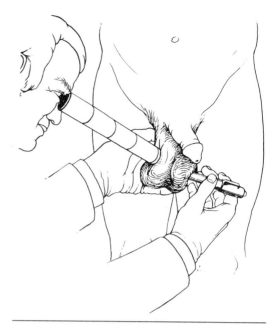

FIGURE 42-1 Technique of transilluminating the scrotum with a penlight and paper cylinder.

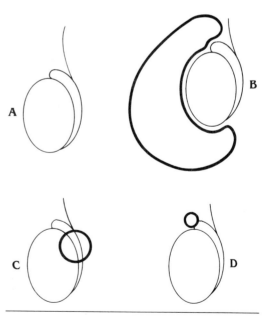

FIGURE 42-2 **A,** Normal scrotal contents in diagrammatic form. **B,** Hydrocele filling the entire scrotal sac. **C,** Spermatocele diagrammatically represented in posterior aspect of scrotum. **D,** Cyst of the appendix testis, usually found on superior aspect of testis.

TABLE 42-1   Treatment of Testicular Malignancies

Stage	Seminoma (Germinoma)	Embryonal Carcinoma and Teratocarcinoma
I	Radical orchiectomy	Radical orchiectomy *plus* retroperitoneal lymphadenectomy and systemic chemotherapy
II	As with stage I *plus* retroperitoneal radiation	As with stage I
III	As with stage I *plus* chemotherapy	Radical orchiectomy plus only chemotherapy

(Table 42-1). Recurrences and spread already above the scrotum after initial orchiectomy are diagnosed by several reliable tumor markers:

B-HCG	Beta human chorionic gonadotrophin
AFP	Alpha fetoprotein
LDH	Lactic acid dehydrogenase

Recently developed chemotherapy regimens have proved highly effective for primary therapy as well as in treatment of recurrent disease. Preferred drug combinations have included cisplatin, vinblastin (or etoposide), and bleomycin-D. At present, cure rates are reported to be above 90% and are probably the best for all solid malignancies in males.

PAINFUL SCROTAL MASSES
Mild Pain

Mildly tender masses in the scrotum include the varicocele and traumatic hematoma. Both produce a heavy, dragging sensation; both respond equally to a scrotal support. Nevertheless, there are basic differences between the two.

The *varicocele* is a collection of dilated and tortuous veins in the pampiniform plexus of the spermatic cord. Not only does the patient complain of mild discomfort, but also he is concerned about these serpentlike masses being dangerous or reducing his fertility. Although excision is usually recommended, seldom is total relief of symptoms obtained. Accordingly, it is generally best merely to explain the relatively innocuous nature of the varicocele and then to urge that the patient use a scrotal support whenever symptoms become troublesome.

The *scrotal hematoma* usually results from some type of trauma and will resolve spontaneously in time. However, if there is rapid expansion of the clot or the scrotum becomes tense, evacuation of extravasated blood and ligation of the responsible bleeding vessel is warranted.

Moderate Pain

Moderate to severe tenderness is noted when there is some component of acute inflammation to the scrotal mass. An *incarcerated inguinal hernia* becomes extremely tender if there has been vascular embracement to the entrapped bowel or mechanical intestinal obstruction has been created. The latter accounts for approximately one third of acute intestinal obstruction and generally produces the additional symptom complex of vomiting, abdominal distension, obstipation, and, at least initially, intestinal colic. X-ray films of the abdomen usually confirm the diagnosis of obstruction; the presence of distended loops of bowel with air-fluid levels can be visualized on plain films or a block to the retrograde flow of barium will be revealed on contrast enema study. Similar gas patterns and barium-filled bowel may also be seen in the scrotum.

Epididymitis and *orchitis* usually occur together if bacterial infection is the cause. An acute onset with intense swelling and pain is often seen following prostatectomy, although acute epididymo-orchitis is most commonly a complication of gonorrhea. Tuberculosis and syphilis may instead cause a more chronic inflammatory process within the testis and/or epididymis. A good response can generally be obtained by the parenteral administration of relatively specific antibiotics (e.g., penicillin for gonorrhea) and use of a scrotal support. However, once suppuration has developed or a chronic inflammation has become established (e.g., tuberculosis), epididymectomy or epididymo-orchiectomy is usually required.

The more fulminant and life-threatening bacterial infections, with primary involvement of the scrotal skin and fascial planes, were discussed under Fournier's gangrene, p. 714.

Isolated orchitis, on the other hand, is seldom caused by bacterial sepsis. Viral infection, such as mumps and pleurodynia (Coxsackie virus), are the classic examples. Bed rest, local cool compresses, and scrotal support should be maintained until all signs of active orchitis have subsided.

Severe Pain

The most exquisite and incapacitating pain of all is that associated with ***torsion of the testis*** or, to a lesser degree, torsion of its apical appendix, the hydatid of Morgagni. Usually the patient is a youth between 10 and 15 years of age and can give no logical explanation for the sudden onset of symptoms. Local tenderness is extreme, while systemic signs such as nausea, vomiting, tachycardia, pallor, abdominal or flank pain, and leukocytosis suggest a more generalized or intra-abdominal process. If the testis has incompletely descended and previously was situated high in the scrotum or even in the inguinal canal, it is virtually impossible to differentiate the torted testis from a strangulated hernia—except for the unexplained vacant scrotum below. If instead the testis is known to have fully descended, the indurated testicular mass will be seen to ride considerably higher in the scrotum than its contralateral mate. Epididymitis and orchitis can also be ruled out by the fact that sustained elevation of the scrotal mass offers absolutely no respite from the intense pain. Torsion of the appendix testis gives similar, yet less extreme, symptoms.

Surgical Correction of Torsion. Delay in surgical correction of the torsion for more than 4 hours almost guarantees infarction of the entire testis. Thus great urgency for operation must always be a prime consideration. Once infarcted, orchiectomy might as well be performed. A Silastic prosthesis can later be inserted for cosmetic purposes. If, however, a viable testis is found, it must be anchored in place with several sutures fixing the tunica albuginea to the scrotal wall. Because of the propensity for the other side to behave similarly, a bilateral orchipexy is favored by many surgeons. Torsion of the appendix testis alone is usually managed by simple excision of the lesion, regardless of tissue viability. Torsion of the appendix testis alone is usually managed by simple excision of the lesion, regardless of tissue viability.

THE EMPTY SCROTUM

Maldescent of the testis, or ***cryptorchidism,*** is defined as the inability of the testis to reach the scrotal depths without benefit of an operation. In such cases the testis will be found in the groin, within the false pelvis of the abdomen, or, rarely, in some more distant site along its normal path of descent from the urogenital ridge above. It is important that the undescended testis be differentiated from the highly retractile testis, a relatively common situation in children with an active cremaster muscle. At puberty when the gland enlarges, pure weight of the testis overcomes the cremasteric pull and allows the testis to assume its adult intrascrotal position.

Incidence of a cryptorchid testicle varies from 30% in prematurely born infants to 4% in term infants and 0.3% in young adults. The retractile testis probably accounts for the difference in percentages between infancy and adulthood.

A testicle remaining in the groin is constantly subject to trauma, while one residing within the much warmer environment of the abdomen will begin to undergo degeneration of the seminiferous tubules by the age of 5 or 6 years. By the age of 9 or 10, these microscopic changes appear to be permanent, so that impaired spermatogenesis, hypospermia, and relative infertility are the irreversible result. Leydig cell function, and thus the production of androgenic hormone, is unaffected by the elevated temperature. Accordingly, it is imperative that the truly cryptorchid testis be distinguished from the retractile one so that surgical correction can be done before the onset of tubular damage (i.e., 5 or 6 years of age).

Another consideration is the significantly greater incidence of cancer in a cryptorchid testis. The changes are 20 times those for a normally descended gland. This is not because an intra-abdominal location favors malignant degeneration (because once orchiopexy has been accomplished the incidence of cancer remains the same) but results from the fact that at least one third of undescended testes are already congenitally abnormal, which may well be the reason for their failure to have properly descended. Having the testis in a location that allows relatively easy examination should, at least theoretically, permit earlier detection of tumor growth. However, an obviously abnormal testis at the time of surgery should be removed and later replaced with a prosthesis if the contralateral side is grossly normal.

Examination. Identification of the retractile testis is quite simple. With the child supine, the index and middle fingers of the examiner's warm hand are used to sweep the groin-located testis out of the external ring and down into the scrotum, where it can be grasped by the thumb and forefinger of the other hand. Gentle traction will then prove the ability of the testis to reach the depths of the scrotum. An alternative method is to have the patient sit with his thigh and knee acutely flexed by placing his heel on the seat of the chair. A retractile testis will descend into the scrotum spontaneously. Otherwise, the testes located in the groin must be presumed to be cryptorchid, whereas absence of any suspicious mass automatically suggests an intra-abdominal location.

Treatment. Surgical correction is through a groin approach: the associated hernia sac (present in 95% of patients) is isolated, the testis is separated from it posteriorly to make the gland a retroperitoneal structure, and both the vas and spermatic vessels are then mobilized. Extra length can usually be gained by transposing the internal inguinal ring medial to the inferior epigastric vessels and thus into Hesselbach's triangle. After a pouch has been created in the scrotum, the testicle is brought down and sutured to the scrotal skin with a pullout stitch.

The often-suggested alternative of treatment—a course of chorionic gonadotropin—results in descent of the testicle by hormone-induced enlargement of the gland and thereby fatigue of its suspending cremaster muscle. Only the retractile testicle will so respond, a clear indication that such therapy is seldom, if ever, warranted. Complications from the use of chorionic gonadotropin include alterations in epiphyseal bone growth, fever, and various allergic reactions.

BIBLIOGRAPHY

Clain A (ed). Hamilton Bailey's Demonstration of Physical Signs in Clinical Surgery, 16th ed. London, Wright, 1980.

Walsh PC, Perlmutter AD, et al. (eds). Campbell's Urology, 5th ed. Philadelphia, WB Saunders, 1985.

Woolley MM. Cryptorchidism. In Ravitch MM, et al. (eds). Pediatric Surgery, 3rd ed. Chicago, Year Book Medical Publishers, 1979, pp 1399-1410.

CHAPTER REVIEW
Questions

1. Of the two primary lesions of syphilis and chancroid, which one is firm and nontender?
2. What technique of physical examination is most useful in differentiating an incarcerated hernia from a hydrocele?
3. Which tumor of the testicle has radiosensitive metastases?
4. What is the most common cause of acute epididymo-orchitis?
5. The most severe of all testicular pain is caused by what entity?
6. True cryptorchidism must always be differentiated from what normal variant before considering corrective surgery?

Answers

1. That of syphilis
2. Transillumination
3. Seminoma
4. Gonorrhea
5. Torsion of the testis
6. Retractile testis

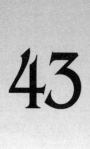

Low Back Pain

CHRISTOPHER B. SHIELDS
GEORGE RAQUE
JOHN R. JOHNSON

KEY FEATURES

After reading this chapter you will understand:
- Common causes of low back pain.
- The anatomy of the spine.
- The causes, diagnosis, and treatment of lumbar disk syndrome.
- Spinal tumors and other vertebral abnormalities.
- Infections involving the lumbar spine.

From 50% to 70% of Americans experience low back pain (LBP) at some time during their lives. Back pain constitutes the single most common cause of time lost from work, with a total estimated cost to society of $50 billion per year. Despite the magnitude of the problem, LBP remains one of the most misunderstood complaints a physician is called on to treat. Ill-planned, unsuccessful operations may result in patients with permanent physical disabilities who are unable to support themselves financially. Pain clinics are replete with patients complaining of constant back pain, searching for relief from discomfort.

The cause of LBP is multifactorial and includes diseases of the spinal column, nerves, blood vessels, and soft tissue such as ligaments, muscle, and disks. In addition, intra-abdominal or retroperitoneal diseases may also cause pain to be referred to the low back. An anatomic-pathologic classification that includes well over 95% of all causes of low back pain is outlined in the box on p. 720. The following discussion ex-

amines the most commonly encountered causes of LBP, describing symptoms, evaluation, and treatment for each disease process.

LUMBAR DISK SYNDROME

Lumbar disk disease has been recognized as a significant clinical entity for approximately 60 years. Today it is the most frequently diagnosed cause of LBP and in some sectors of industry is reaching epidemic proportions.

History

While some patients can recall a specific incident that precipitated the pain, the cause of a ruptured disk is rarely a single major injury but rather repeated episodes of mild trauma that often have been forgotten. The risk of disk herniation is increased by poor back hygiene, such as lifting weights with maximal stress on the back with the lumbar spine in the flexed or twisted position.

A ruptured disk syndrome is characterized by *pain* localized to the lumbar region, with radiation into one or both legs following a specific dermatomal distribution. Pain distribution and numbness in the most distal aspect of the leg is of great diagnostic value in identifying the level of the disk rupture (Fig. 43-1). Radicular (leg) pain may be aggravated by coughing, sneezing, and straining, activities that displace an irritated lumbar nerve root over a ruptured disk. *Paresthesias* (i.e., the sensation of pins and needles or numbness) are frequently noted in the same distribu-

COMMON CAUSES OF LOW BACK PAIN

Trauma
  Disk disease
  Vertebral fracture
  Sprains, strains
Congenital malformation
  Spondylolisthesis
Infection
  Osteomyelitis
  Epidural abscess
  Subdural abscess
Degenerative process
  Spondylosis
Neoplastic disease
  Intradural
    Intramedullary
    Extramedullary
  Extradural
Nonspinal disease
  Intra-abdominal
  Retroperitoneal
Psychogenic disease

IDENTIFYING A MALINGERING PATIENT

There is probably a greater incidence of malingering regarding low back pain than with disorders of any other body system. The clinician assessing a patient for lumbar disk syndrome must also weigh the significance of hysteria and other psychologic factors in patients for whom no organic cause can be found for their back pain. If the patient reveals increased agility when not being observed, as when getting out of bed or dressing, psychologic factors may be in play, or the patient may be malingering with a hope of some secondary financial gain, such as ongoing litigation regarding the incident that caused the back discomfort. The following tests may help the examiner to identify such a patient:

- **Straight-leg raising,** which is severely restricted when the patient is supine, and 90 degrees when sitting
- **Hemianesthesia** of the entire side of the body (leg, arm, trunk, and face) or a "glove and stocking" pattern of sensory loss in the extremities
- Diffuse weakness manifested by short bursts similar to a **clasped knife release phenomenon**

It is an unfortunate reality that litigation has played an increasingly important role in the intractable nature of some patients' symptoms, with a high percentage being miraculously cured after their legal problems have been settled. In such cases it becomes a factor of clinical judgment to distinguish those patients who will truly benefit from medical intervention.

tion as the pain, particularly in its most distal distribution. *Weakness* may result from pressure of the ruptured disk against a motor nerve root. *Impairment of bowel and bladder function* occurs rarely, and only if a large disk fragment has sequestered into the midline with compression of all nerves of the cauda equina.

Physical Examination

Abnormal physical signs are found on examination of the back and legs. Objective evidence of LBP may consist of loss of normal lumbar lordosis, paravertebral muscle spasm, scoliosis, and/or point tenderness of the spinous processes, which occurs during an acute exacerbation of back pain. Nerve root entrapment by a disk rupture causes *decreased straight-leg raising* (ability to elevate the straight leg while the patient is in the supine position) on the affected side. Forceful dorsiflexion of the foot with the leg maximally elevated greatly intensifies the leg pain (*positive bowstring sign*). *Deep tendon reflexes* may be depressed and *weakness* is often noted (see Fig. 43-1). *Numbness* may be noted in the involved dermatomes, with (1) an L5 radiculopathy causing numbness on the lateral calf, dorsum of the

foot, and medial three toes, and (2) an S1 radiculopathy affecting the posterior calf, heel, sole of foot, and lateral two toes. If present, the numbness is superimposed over the pain distribution.

Malingering or hysteria may closely mimick the lumbar disk syndrome (see the box above).

Radiographic Studies

Radiographic changes of the lumbosacral spine suggestive of disk rupture are disk space narrow-

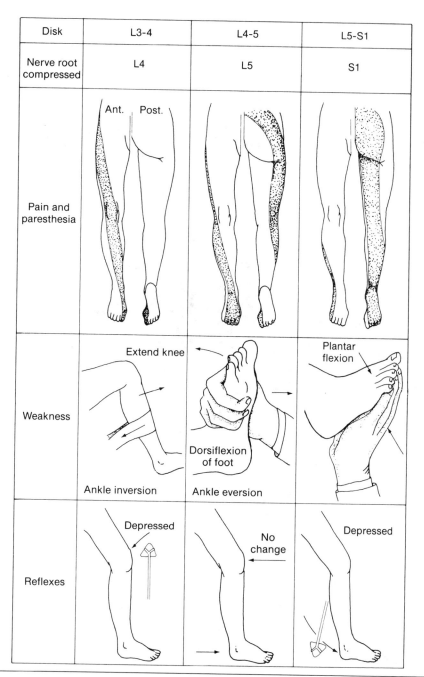

FIGURE 43-1 Areas of pain and paresthesia, weakness, and reflex changes diagnostic of lumbar nerve root compression.

ing, straightening of the normal lumbar lordosis, and lumbar scoliosis. Lumbar myelography excludes the presence of a spinal neoplasm and confirms the site of disk rupture. Myelography with iopamidol (Isovue) should be performed in the following manner:

1. The patient should be fully upright in the weight-bearing position.

2. Adequate contrast material should be placed in the subarachnoid space to fill the lumbar cistern to the bottom of L3.

3. Anteroposterior (AP), lateral, and oblique views should be obtained, and the conus medullaris should be visualized (Fig. 43-2).

Postmyelographic CT scans should always be obtained, because these provide an important addi-

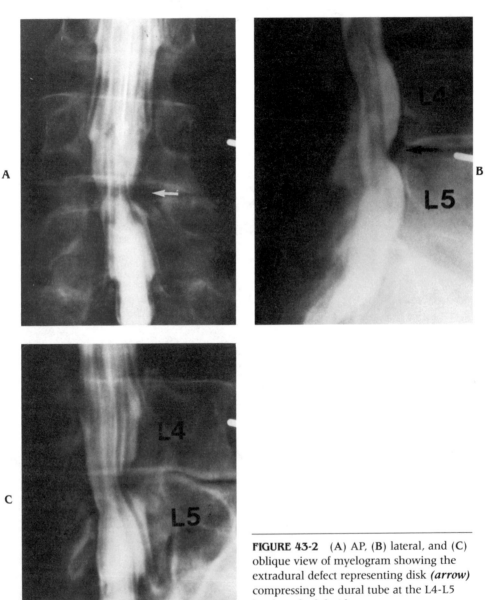

FIGURE 43-2   (A) AP, (B) lateral, and (C) oblique view of myelogram showing the extradural defect representing disk *(arrow)* compressing the dural tube at the L4-L5 level on the left side.

tion to the investigation of spinal disease. Occasionally the CT scan demonstrates a symptomatic disk fragment that has migrated through the intervertebral foramen that could not be visualized with myelography (Fig. 43-3). The coupling of the myelogram and CT is the gold standard for the diagnosis of lumbar disk disease.

A magnetic resonance imaging (MRI) scan is often used as a screening procedure. However, physicians consider this the test of choice for a simple disk rupture (Fig. 43-4). MRI is noninvasive and provides a clear delineation of the ruptured disk; however, it is of limited value in clarifying the presence of bony osteophytes and a mild disk protrusion. A degenerated disk is identified as a low signal image on a T2-weighted MRI scan as a result of its loss of water content. The finding of dehydration on MRI is frequently noted but of questionable clinical significance, and by itself is not an indication for surgery.

Treatment

Nonoperative treatment consists of analgesics, muscle relaxants, 7 to 10 days of complete bed rest, and physiotherapy (heat, massage, and ultrasound), and is performed as the first line of therapy. Pelvic traction is of limited value, because the force required to distract the lumbar intervertebral space is 150 to 170 pounds, which the patient would find intolerable. Mild analgesics such as aspirin, propoxyphene, or codeine

may be used in conjunction with diazepam (5 mg three or four times daily) for muscle relaxation. If nonoperative treatment is unsuccessful in relieving the symptoms, surgical diskectomy is performed at the appropriate level. The success of lumbar diskectomy is 90% to 95% in a simple disk rupture, without associated risk factors such as associated segmental spinal instability (SSI) or obesity. A poor result following surgery may be caused by a retained disk fragment, wrong initial diagnosis, operation at a wrong disk level, or segmental spinal instability.

If a disk fragment has been retained, or surgery was performed at the incorrect level, repeat diskectomy is necessary. If spinal instability exists, particularly if associated with severe LBP, or multiple operations have been performed at the involved level, then a spinal fusion should be performed using autogenous bone with or without metal instrumentation.

SPINAL TUMORS

Spinal tumors may be primary (arising from bone, dura, neural and glial elements, or blood vessels) or may represent extension of extra-axial tumors that metastasize to or directly invade the spinal column. Spinal tumors are either extra-

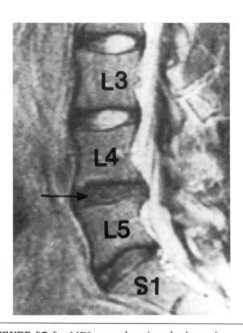

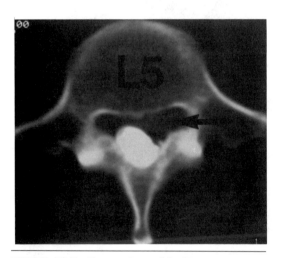

FIGURE 43-3   Postmyelographic CT scan demonstrating distortion caused by the ruptured L4-L5 *(arrow)* disk on the left side of the dural tube.

FIGURE 43-4   MRI scan showing the loss of water content at the L4-L5 disk space *(arrow)*, with compression of the anterior portion of the dural tube from the disk rupture.

dural or intradural. Extradural tumors (Fig. 43-5) tend to be malignant and include metastatic lesions from lung, breast, or prostate, as well as lymphoma and multiple myeloma. Intradural extramedullary tumors (arising within the dural sac but outside the spinal cord) are usually benign and curable (Fig. 43-6). They are best represented by (1) neurofibromas that arise from the posterior nerve roots and usually occur in men, and (2) meningiomas that arise anterolateral to the spinal cord, usually in the thoracic spine from arachnoidal elements, and most frequently occur in middle-aged women. The cell of origin of meningiomas is the arachnoidal cell, which lines the inner surface of the dura. Intramedullary intradural tumors (arising within the spinal cord) (Fig. 43-7) are usually astocytomas and ependymomas, which are slowly progressive and rarely curable lesions.

History

The clinical presentation of a tumor involving the thoracic and lumbar spine or spinal cord may mimic that of a protruded lumbar disk. However, certain characteristic features of the history may assist the physician in arriving at the correct diagnosis:

1. A history of gradually progressive pain and weakness is suggestive of a spinal cord tumor, whereas disk disease usually presents as severe exacerbations interspersed with remissions following conservative therapy.
2. The pain caused by spinal cord tumors may be aggravated by bed rest; the patient awakens at night with intense back and leg pain. Such pain is ameliorated by walking. In patients with a protruded disk, symptoms are usually aggravated by mobility and relieved by bed rest.
3. Sphincter involvement suggests a spinal cord tumor or, rarely, may be caused by a large midline disk rupture.

Special Studies

Anemia and an elevated sedimentation rate suggest metastatic epidural tumors, and the presence of urinary Bence Jones proteins and electrophoretic monophasic protein elevations indicate multiple myeloma. Serum acid phosphatase levels will be increased in metastatic prostatic cancer. Abnormal calcium and phosphorus metabolism and an increase in serum alkaline phosphatase point to metastatic tumor of the bone.

Plain spinal radiographs frequently demon-

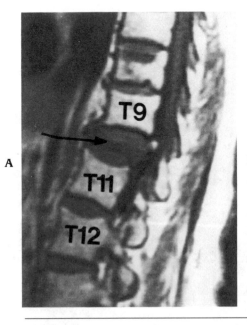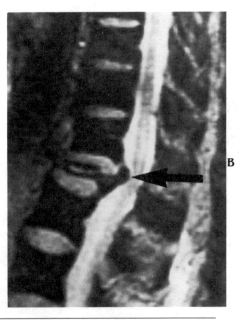

FIGURE 43-5 Metastatic lung tumor causing extradural pressure. Lateral view of an **A,** T1-weighted MRI scan showing loss of structural integrity of the T10 vertebral body *(arrow)*, and **B,** a T2-weighted MRI scan showing extradural compression of the dural tube anteriorly *(arrow)* by the collapsed T10 vertebral body and extradural tumor.

strate abnormalities in metastatic spine disease suggesting infiltration of bone, such as vertebral body compression fractures, vertebral body osteoporosis, a paraspinal soft tissue mass, and pedicle erosion. Metastatic carcinoma from the prostate and occasionally from the breast create osteoblastic deposits of bone. Neurofibromas (intradural-extramedullary) reveal subtle changes on plain x-ray evaluation, namely, scalloping of the posterior vertebral body on lateral views and enlargement of an intervertebral foramen on oblique views. MRI is of great diagnostic value in spinal tumors, accurately outlining the tumor and usually differentiating it from other types of intraspinal disease (Fig. 43-8, *A* and *B*).

MRI has virtually replaced myelography in the investigation of spinal tumors. If doubt exists as to the correct diagnosis following an MRI scan, Isovue myelography may be valuable.

If a complete spinal block by tumor is suspected either clinically or on the basis of MRI, a C1-C2 tap should be performed for instillation of metrizamide. If a block is present and contrast medium is injected via lumbar puncture, removal of the contrast may cause deterioration of neurologic function. This may result from direct pressure exerted on the spinal cord by the tumor along with caudal movement of the cord and tumor induced by cerebrospinal fluid (CSF) removal.

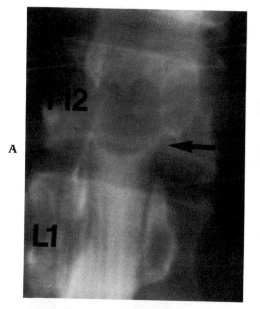

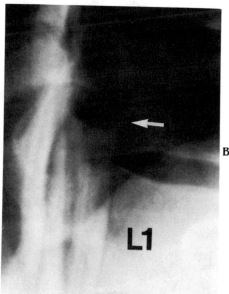

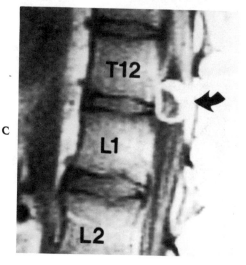

FIGURE 43-6 Intradural neurofibroma at T12. **A,** AP and **B,** lateral thoracic myelogram showing evidence of an intradural, extramedullary mass creating a meniscus-like defect of the subarachnoid space *(arrow)*. **C,** An MRI scan revealed an enhancing mass *(arrow)*.

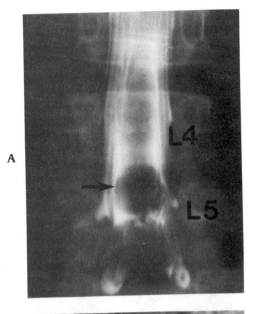

A

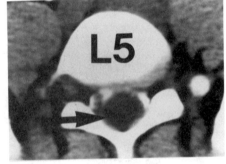

B

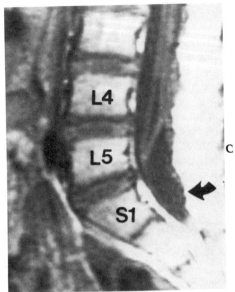

C

FIGURE 43-7   Intradural lipoma at L4-S1. **A,** AP myelogram, and **B,** postmyelographic CT scan showing the filling defect at the L4-S1 level *(arrow).* **C,** An MRI scan with a low signal indicating the presence of an intradural lipoma at the L4-S1 level.

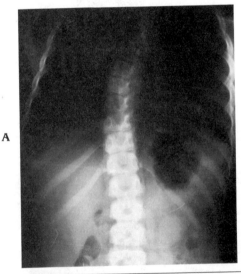

A

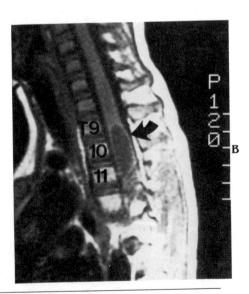

B

FIGURE 43-8   Astrocytoma of spinal cord. **A,** Plain x-ray demonstrating thoracic scoliosis (a common manifestation of spinal tumors), and **B,** an MRI scan revealing the upper end of an intramedullary lesion at T9-T10 causing expansion of the spinal cord by a mass of low density *(arrow).*

Characteristic myelographic patterns are highly suggestive of certain spinal tumors:

- An hourglass waist or smooth lateral compression of the contrast column on an AP view of the spine suggests an extradural tumor.
- A meniscus deformity of the contrast column on AP and lateral views suggests an intradural-extramedullary tumor (neurofibroma, meningioma).
- A fusiform expansion of the spinal cord suggests an intramedullary tumor (e.g., astrocytoma, ependymoma) (see the box at right).

If a tumor is identified by myelography, a post-myelographic CT scan at the level of the tumor is helpful in demarcating its extraspinal extent as well as its relationship to the spinal cord and bone (Fig. 43-9).

SPINAL TUMORS

Extradural
  Metastases (from breast, lung, prostate)
  Lymphoma
  Multiple myeloma
Intradural
  Extramedullary
    Meningioma
    Neurofibroma
    Seeding from intracranial tumor
  Intramedullary
    Ependymoma
    Astrocytoma
    Glioblastoma multiforme

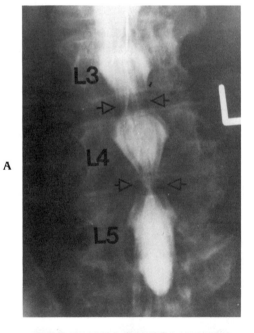

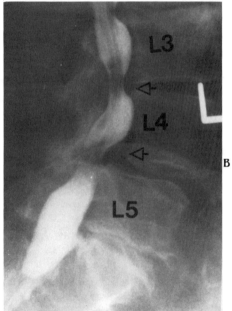

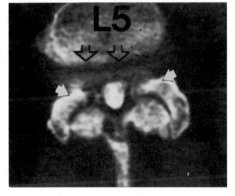

FIGURE 43-9 **A,** AP and **B,** lateral myelogram revealing marked irregularity of the contour of the dural tube *(arrows)* in the lower lumbar area, suggesting extensive lumbar spondylosis. **C,** Postmyelographic CT scan indicating that the irregularities are due to hypertrophic facet disease *(arrows),* a diffuse disk bulge.

Treatment

Operation. Spinal cord tumors are usually treated operatively. A patient with rapidly deteriorating neurologic function from an intraspinal tumor requires an emergency operation to decompress the spinal cord and remove all readily accessible tumor. If the patient is neurologically stable, operation on an elective basis is justified.

A wide decompressive laminectomy is performed with preservation of articular facets in most types of spinal tumors. If an extradural metastatic tumor exists, the laminectomy is extended to the cephalic and caudal limits of the tumor. Considering the high incidence of bony involvement and likelihood of subsequent spinal instability, patients undergoing a wide decompression operation often require concomitant spinal fusion. Either bone plus metal instrumentation or acrylic may be used to stabilize the spine affected by metastatic disease.

Resection of intradural tumors requires extensive exposure. Use of magnification with a surgical dissecting microscope allows optimal visualization, facilitating removal of these neoplasms with minimal retraction on adjacent neural structures. Complete removal of a meningioma and neurofibroma is usually possible. However, astrocytomas of the spinal cord rarely can be totally removed because of their infiltrative nature. Ependymomas often have a distinct line of cleavage from normal spinal cord and so can frequently be totally removed with little postoperative neurologic deficit.

If the vertebral bodies collapse from infiltration with tumor and cause spinal cord compression, the most direct treatment may be an anterior spinal approach. A vertebrectomy of the affected levels with removal of neoplasm is performed, along with placement of a strut graft using autogenous bone obtained from the iliac crest. This is followed by posterior stabilization using autogenous bone and instrumentation.

Irradiation. Ancillary treatment of spinal tumors by radiotherapy to the tumor bed is indicated after removal of a radiosensitive lesion. Such tumors usually are extradural and metastatic. The only radiosensitive primary intramedullary tumor is an ependymoma.

If a patient with previously diagnosed multiple myeloma, lymphoma, or a radiosensitive carcinoma develops epidural metastases with minimal or no signs of spinal cord compression, symptomatic relief may be achieved with local portals of radiation directed to the lesion. Should clinical deterioration occur during the course of radiotherapy, emergency decompressive laminectomy and steroid administration are indicated. Occasionally an intradural spinal tumor may develop in conjunction with a brain tumor, such as a cerebellar medulloblastoma or ependymoma. These tumors are friable and located adjacent to CSF pathways and seed tumor cells caudally into the spinal canal. Treatment for such a radiosensitive tumor consists of irradiation of the entire craniospinal axis. At times the intracranial tumor has not been previously recognized, and exploration of the spinal lesion calls initial attention to the primary lesion. Prophylactic irradiation to the entire cerebrospinal axis following treatment of the primary lesion is indicated.

Results

If total loss of motor, sensory, and sphincter function has developed from tumor compression on the spinal cord when the patient is initially seen, there is virtually no hope for return of function. Thus an operation is seldom indicated in this situation. The major purpose of an operation is to prevent progressive worsening of the patient's neurologic function, with little hope of regaining lost function. The prognosis for return of strength and sensation is improved if the tumor compresses the peripheral nerves constituting the cauda equina but is decreased if the spinal cord or conus medullaris is compressed by a tumor.

The prognosis for return of neurologic function also depends on the rapidity of development of spinal cord signs. Slowly progressive paraplegia over several months' time is compatible with complete recovery over a similarly prolonged period. Rapid neurologic deterioration over several hours signals a poor prognosis. Little hope of significant return can be expected after the vascular supply is compromised, with resultant cord ischemia and infarction.

LUMBAR SPONDYLOSIS

In older patients, lumbar spondylosis assumes an increasing role in the differential diagnosis of spinal disease. Even severe degrees of degenerative disease may be asymptomatic and brought into disabling reality following a seemingly trivial back injury. Osteophytes develop on the margins of vertebral bodies, as well as facets (facet hypertrophy). This combination may decrease the diameter of the spinal canal, which, if already narrowed by congenital spinal stenosis, disk rupture, or hypertrophy of the ligamentum flavum, will produce symptoms of single or multisegmental spinal stenosis. These changes also may narrow the caliber of an intervertebral foramen through which passes a spinal nerve root. Foramenal encroachment causes nerve root irritation with a clinical picture of sciatica, indistinguishable from that of a ruptured disk. Nerves at single or multiple levels may be involved by this process causing pain and paresthesias aggravated by physical activity, coughing, or sneezing. The patient with lumbar spinal stenosis often complains of a crampy, aching pain in his low back, buttocks, along with leg pain and paresthesias noted after walking for a short distance (neurogenic intermittent claudication). These symptoms are relieved by resting for a few minutes. Thus the clinical picture is similar in many ways to intermittent claudication caused by vascular insufficiency in the lower extremities.

On physical examination there is a paucity of signs elicited when the patient is at rest. After physical activity, diffuse lower limb weakness, numbness, and reflex changes may be elicited. It is assumed that such abnormal signs arise from ischemia of the cauda equina secondary to vascular compression of the blood vessels supplying these nerves. Physical exercise of the legs increases the metabolic demand of the nerves of the cauda equina. Their blood supply at rest is capable of maintaining normal function; however, blood flow to the nerves of the cauda equina during physical activity is inadequate to maintain normal metabolism of the involved neural structures, causing nerve root ischemia and the characteristic signs and symptoms. In neurogenic intermittent claudication, there are full peripheral pulses, no aortofemoral bruits, and normal blood pressure in the lower extremities.

Radiographic Studies

Plain x-ray films show narrowing of the sagittal and interpedicular diameter of the spinal canal. In the normal lumbar spine, the midsagittal diameter is 22 to 25 mm and the interpedicular diameter is 33 to 39 mm. A sagittal diameter less than 16 mm and interpedicular diameter less than 25 mm are abnormal. Encroachment of intervertebral foramina by arthritic spurs or facet hypertrophy may also be evident. Myelography may be technically difficult to perform because of a narrow canal, and insertion of the needle may cause lancinating leg pain as the needle brushes against compressed nerve roots. Myelography (see Fig. 43-8) shows (1) narrowing of the canal

diameter on AP and lateral views, (2) puddling of contrast medium adjacent to vertebral bodies, (3) decreased filling of the subarachnoid space at the disk space level, and (4) amputation of radicular axillary pouches.

Fig. 43-9 shows the value of the postmyelographic CT scan in confirming a diagnosis of lumbar spinal stenosis. This scan provides a clear image of spinal canal anatomy, demonstrating the stenotic nature of the canal and intervertebral foramina. In our experience, MRI scans are not as reliable as the CT scan in this condition, because MRI does not provide the high-quality resolution of bone provided by the CT scan.

Treatment

Treatment for spinal stenosis is both conservative and operative. The same conservative treatment is performed for this condition as for a ruptured disk: bed rest, analgesics, a bedboard, and muscle relaxants. Clinical improvement often occurs by the mechanism of decreased irritation of the involved nerve roots if radiculopathy exists. The syndrome of neurogenic intermittent claudication is infrequently relieved by conservative measures. If symptoms continue to incapacitate the patient in spite of an adequate trial of conservative treatment, an operation is performed to remodel the spinal canal. In this procedure the medial half to one third of the hypertrophied facets are removed, and diskectomy is performed if necessary. If intervertebral foramina are narrow, single- or multiple-level foraminotomies are performed. The major causes of surgical failure are continued symptoms resulting from inadequate bony decompression and segmental spinal instability arising from excessive bony decompression. If the structural integrity of the spine is maintained, spinal instability will not develop. If the degree of decompression is such that structural integrity is lost, a spinal fusion is performed to maintain adequate spinal stability. Results of this procedure in an elderly patient are highly successful. A successful outcome is achieved in 80% to 85% of patients following spinal remodelling with spinal fusion performed in selected patients.

INFECTION
Clinical Presentation

Infections of the lumbar spine region are infrequent but important causes of low back pain. Infection in this area may consist of an epidural abscess, disk space infection, or vertebral osteomyelitis. The most common causes of such infections are hematogenous seeding from a septic focus (carbuncle, furuncle, urinary tract infection, retroperitoneal infection, or septicemia), intravenous drug abuse, or following an invasive procedure (lumbar puncture or an operation). The characteristic clinical picture, regardless of which process is present, is severe low back pain. An epidural abscess may cause limitation in straight-leg raising, local tenderness of the spine, paravertebral muscle spasm, an elevated sedimentation rate, and a low-grade fever. Once the spinal cord or cauda equina is compressed, paraplegia, sensory loss, and sphincter dysfunction develop rapidly. Disk space infection and osteomyelitis may be indistinguishable from an epidural abscess; however, weakness rarely develops in the former conditions.

Diagnosis

Plain x-ray films of the lumbar spine in a patient harboring an epidural abscess are usually normal because of the relatively short progression of this disease. Disk space infection will reveal sclerosis of the margins of the vertebral bodies within 2 months after its onset. As the disk space infection enters the chronic stage, the disk space may collapse, with autofusion occurring between adjacent vertebral bodies. Plain spine x-ray films exhibit no abnormalities during the early stage of vertebral osteomyelitis, but within several weeks of its onset osteosclerosis is visualized. Bone scans often reveal evidence of increased uptake of isotope before changes are seen on plain x-ray evaluation. However, if an operation has been performed in the recent past, the significance of increased uptake of isotope is uncertain.

Lumbar myelography should be performed with extreme caution in suspected infectious processes. If the needle enters an epidural abscess, purulent material should be aspirated and studied by Gram stain and should undergo culture and sensitivity testing. Under no circumstances should the needle tract progress through the abscess into the subarachnoid space, because bacterial seeding of the CSF may result, with ensuing meningitis. If a lumbar epidural abscess is suspected, Isovue (3 ml) should be introduced via a cervical puncture to outline the upper level of a complete obstruction of the subarachnoid space. If cerebrospinal fluid is obtained from below a complete block, it is characterized by an elevated protein level, normal glucose, and variable pleocytosis (Froin syndrome).

Disk space infection or vertebral osteomyelitis may be suspected but may remain unproven on clinical and radiographic grounds. A percutaneous Craig needle biopsy of the vertebral body or the disk space under suspicion should be obtained to confirm the diagnosis. The presence of frank pus consisting of inflammatory cells confirms the infectious nature of the disease; however, bacterial cultures frequently yield negative results.

Treatment

If signs of neural compression develop as a result of an expanding epidural abscess, emergency decompressive laminectomy is imperative to drain the purulent material. Often the diagnosis of an epidural abscess is not considered preoperatively, but rather an epidural metastatic tumor or sequestered disk is suspected. If an infectious process is confirmed, high doses of a specific antibiotic should be administered intravenously for at least 4 to 6 weeks. The prognosis for return to normal neurologic function is good if paraplegia has not developed before decompression is performed. However, the outcome is poor if the patient's neurologic status has progressed to a major degree of motor and sphincter weakness. Disk space infection is treated with immobilization (bed rest, lumbar corset), analgesics, and 6 to 12 weeks of an appropriate antibiotic. Controversy exists as to the role of antibiotics in the treatment of disk space infection; however, if bacteria are cultured following an open or percutaneous biopsy of the disk space, it seems prudent to administer a prolonged course of antibiotics. The treatment of vertebral osteomyelitis is similar to that of disk space infection, with long-term administration of antibiotics and analgesic agents.

INTRACTABLE LOW BACK PAIN

Despite our best efforts to correctly diagnose the cause of low back pain, our attempts are often futile. A definitive diagnosis may not be possible, or the patient may have had an ill-advised operation performed. No evidence of organic disease may be noted either by clinical assessment or radiographic investigation, yet the patient asserts that he or she is unable to return to gainful employment. Psychologic factors often contribute to persisting complaints. Even if we exclude patients with indisputable psychopathology or those in whom secondary financial gain is an apparent factor in causing a prolongation of back pain, a sizable patient population exists with no known cause of low back pain.

Additionally, the patient may be emotionally stable at the onset of symptoms; however, after months of excruciating pain, even the most stoic patient may become depressed. Psychiatric evaluation and special neurosurgical procedures such as neural ablation or stimulation may be helpful, since medical treatment has little to offer.

Various modes of therapy such as epidural steroid injections, percutaneous rhizotomies, transcutaneous nerve stimulators, and facet rhizotomies have their advocates. An intraventricular or subarachnoid injection of morphine to relieve pain caused by metastatic cancer has proved to be of great value particularly if the patient's anticipated survival is less than 6 months. Ablative procedures or administration of narcotics is discouraged for patients with chronic low back pain of benign origin. Dysesthesias and possible motor and sphincter disturbances are potential complications of extensive rhizotomies and cordotomies. If used, these measures should be limited to desperate situations such as malignant disease and should be performed by neurosurgeons trained in the problems of chronic pain.

SURGICAL PHARMACOPEIA

Drug	Indications	Complications	Dosage
Aspirin	Mild pain, inflammation	Stomach upset, gastritis, peptic ulcer, bleeding	325-1000 mg q4h
Acetaminophen (Tylenol)	Mild pain	Less gastritis than with aspirin Hepatoxicity in very high doses	325-500 mg q4h
Ibuprofen (Motrin)	Mild to moderate pain and inflammation	Peptic ulceration, bleeding; *very rarely,* fluid retention, hepatoxicity, renal papillary necrosis	200-800 mg q4h
Naproxen (Naprosyn)	Moderate pain and inflammation	Same as with ibuprofen	250, 375, or 500 mg bid PO
Ketorlac (Toradol)	Moderate to severe pain in-hospital	Same as with ibuprofen Compatible with pain relief provided by morphine but without addictive properties	30 or 60 mg IM loading dose, then 15 or 30 mg IM or PO q6h
Codeine (with Tylenol or aspirin)	Moderate pain	Nausea, constipation, rare allergic reactions Habit forming; tolerance develops to analgesic effects; may cause drowsiness, dizziness	15-60 mg q4h PO; usually combined with 625 mg Tylenol or aspirin
Propoxyphene with Tylenol (Darvocet) Propoxyphene with aspirin (Darvon)	Moderate pain	Nausea, constipation, rare allergic reactions, physical addiction, tolerance to analgesic effects; may cause drowsiness, dizziness; more potent narcotics rarely used because of abuse potential	50 or 100 mg q4h PO combined with aspirin or Tylenol
Diazepam (Valium)	Skeletal muscle spasm	Physical and psychologic dependence may develop; may cause drowsiness, ataxia, fatigue	2-10 mg PO bid to qid (usual dose 5 mg PO qid); IM

Continued.

Drug	Indications	Complications	Dosage
Cyclobenzaprine (Flexeril)	Skeletal muscle spasm	Dizziness, dry mouth, drowsiness, rarely cardiac dysrhythmias; contra-indicated in patients with urinary retention and in patients taking mono-amine oxidase inhibitors	10 mg tid PO
Methocarbamol (Robaxin)	Musculoskeletal discomfort	Dizziness, drowsiness, lightheadedness, nausea; not a skeletal muscle relaxant; mechanism of action unknown	1500 mg qid PO for first day, then 1000 mg qid PO; IM
Chlorzoxazone (Parafon Forte)	Musculoskeletal discomfort	Drowsiness, dizziness, lightheadedness, malaise; not a skeletal muscle relaxant; mechanism of action unknown	500 mg qid PO

BIBLIOGRAPHY

DePalma AF, Rothman RH. The Intervertebral Disc. Philadelphia, 1970, WB Saunders.

Frymoyer JW. Epidemiology: Magnitude of the problem in the lumbar spine. In Weinstein JN, Wiesel SW (eds). The Lumbar Spine. Philadelphia, 1990, WB Saunders.

Horal J. The clinical appearance of low back disorders in the city of Gothenburg, Sweden. Acta Orthop Scand (suppl) 118:1-109, 1969.

Mixter WJ, Barr JS. Rupture of the intervertebral disc with involvement of the spinal canal. N Engl J Med 211:210, 1934.

Rothman RH, Simeone FA. The Spine, vols 1 and 2. Philadelphia, 1975, WB Saunders.

Shapiro R. Myelography. Chicago, 1975, Year Book Medical Publishers.

Weinstein JN, Wiesel SW. The Lumbar Spine. Philadelphia, 1990, WB Saunders.

CHAPTER REVIEW
Questions

1. Lumbosacral pain associated with herniated nucleus pulposis often:
   a. Is accentuated on motion of the segment
   b. Radiates along a specific nerve root
   c. Is accentuated by coughing or sneezing
   d. All of the above
2. Initial management of low back pain not associated with neurologic abnormalities should include:
   a. Myelogram
   b. Bed rest
   c. Muscle relaxants and analgesics
   d. Skeletal traction
3. The most common cause of low back pain in women is:
   a. Herniated nucleus pulposis
   b. Degenerative arthritis
   c. Metastatic breast cancer
   d. Acute back sprain

Answers

1. d
2. c
3. d

POSTOPERATIVE CONSIDERATIONS

PART

III

44

The Approach to the Postoperative Patient

HIRAM C. POLK, Jr.

KEY FEATURES

After reading this chapter you will understand:
- That using a checklist permits focused attention on likely problems.
- That you should develop a pattern for writing postoperative orders.
- That recognizing and admitting that a complication exists is the first step toward its correction.
- The common causes of frequent or severe complications.
- The likely temporal appearance of typical complications.

Despite significant advances in surgical practice, surgical procedures are not yet innocuous undertakings. One patient among every five undergoing a major operation also sustains a significant complication—that is, a specific disease related to the operation. The patient benefits from early detection, accurate diagnosis, and proper treatment of such an untoward and unwanted event.

The most essential psychologic factor for the physician providing good postoperative care is the realization that there is no shame in promptly admitting that a complication exists, whether it occurred as a seemingly unrelated act of God or a surgical misadventure. Surgeons who claim to perform operations without complications have either done very few surgeries or have selective forgetfulness. Immediate recognition or correction of a complication leads to good long-term surgical results in which the tempo-

rary inconvenience and aggravation are forgotten by both the grateful patient and the surgeon. It is unfortunate and inexcusable that there are a few surgeons who allow patients with correctable complications to deteriorate and die, blaming their systemic signs on a myocardial infarction or pulmonary embolism instead of admitting that a surgical complication exists. Developing the proper frame of mind and employing the appropriate scientific and clinical background information should minimize such conduct in the future generation of physicians.

Normal convalescence must be understood to judge what is and is not satisfactory progress. This is complicated, however, by the nature of the operative procedure. Operations may be evaluated or graded by length, number of blood transfusions, weight of tissue removed, or by other parameters. None of these alone is sufficient. Moyer (1972) pointed out that "the magnitude of the operation is not as important a determinant of operative risk among the aged as is the duration of the period of physiological upset attending it." For example, the extensive and relatively traumatic mastectomy seldom is associated with major systemic complications because it is a superficial procedure, dealing primarily with the body's exterior. At the other extreme is the removal of a tiny tumor near the brainstem, a precise, carefully controlled extirpation of but a few grams of tissue but associated with a very high incidence of fatal or near-fatal problems.

Resumption of normal alimentation after operation is an example of return to physiologic normalcy. Ordinarily this occurs the day after open-heart correction of a ventricular septal defect with cardiopulmonary bypass support, on the second or third day after elective resection of a major segment of the large bowel, but perhaps not until the fifth day after laparotomy for intestinal obstruction caused by adhesions. Such delay is related more closely to the organ requiring treatment and the indication for operation than to the overall trauma associated with the procedure.

A useful rule of thumb regarding satisfactory recovery from operation is that some objective evidence of progress toward normal body function should be exhibited every day. The search for such objective evidence gives rise to a variety of routines of postoperative care—not routine for its own sake but for the early evidence that these checks provide of incipient problems, when indications for a specific examination may not yet be apparent. Every visit to a postoperative patient should include:

- A review of vital signs, fluid intake and output, and other parameters (e.g., urinary sugar and acetone levels in diabetics). Precise measurement of types of fluids administered and *sources* of output should be assessed.
- Ascertaining that devices employed to assist recovery truly function properly (e.g., nasogastric tube, drains, urinary catheter, dressings, respirator, or oxygen delivery system).
- Auscultation of heart, lungs, and abdomen, as well as examination of the extremities for signs of phlebitis.
- Inspection of the wound itself.
- Consideration as to what observations and/or examinations are likely to be helpful in the next time period—specifically the judicious use of laboratory and imaging resources.
- A brief summary of these observations on the chart.

Furthermore, *every complaint* by the patient must be taken seriously and investigated to a satisfactory conclusion. *At all costs, symptomatic treatment is to be avoided because it will often mask the disease, delaying detection and diagnosis and effective treatment.* Specific examples are the use of aspirin for fever and phenothiazines for nausea and vomiting. The recommended practices have obvious common goals: the discovery, diagnosis, and treatment of complications before they progress to severe and systemically disabling conditions.

GENERAL PRINCIPLES

Postoperative orders lend themselves to the formation of a pattern of organized habitual routine procedures by both physician and nurse, reducing the potential for errors of omission (see the box below). How vigorously one should pursue diagnostic maneuvers in the ill postoperative patient has long been contended among surgeons. One hears, "She is too sick to go to x-ray." A properly attended patient can tolerate expeditious study but does not tolerate further delay in finding the precise cause of deterioration as well. Therefore definitive diagnostic procedures seldom should be withheld. A barium enema thoughtlessly performed 6 days after left colonic anastomosis may disrupt a healing anastomosis, but one need not be careless. The patient is much better served by having his or her surgeon (working side by side with the fully informed radiologist) acquire unequivocal evidence of an anastomotic leak warranting fecal diversion than by having the surgeon temporize (the so-called conservative treatment of pelvic sepsis), allowing the condition to progress because of uninterrupted fecal contamination.

As with all clinical medicine, the diagnostic approach to the ill postoperative patient is a matter of probabilities. Further, the correct diagnosis is the answer to a multifactorial equation that involves the operation itself, the disease for which the operation was conducted, any coexisting illness, surgical or anesthetic technical problems, time elapsed following operation, age of the patient, and other less frequently significant

---

A PATTERN FOR POSTOPERATIVE ORDERS

Diagnosis
Precautions (patient condition)
Activity and privileges
Vital signs
Diet
Medications
   Intravenous fluids
   Pain
   Sleep
   Bowel function
   Other, specific
Tube and drain care
Urination (initiation and volume)
Studies
   Transfusion preparation
   Procedures
   Blood chemistries, etc.

factors. Another useful rule of thumb is to consider first those reasonable possibilities most readily amenable to effective treatment. It serves the patient poorly to contemplate exotic illnesses for which no tolerable treatment is available, while a readily correctable, commonplace process becomes progressively severe. *Common things happen commonly and rare ones rarely!* The boxes immediately below reflect probable causes of two frequent postoperative problems. The box at the bottom of the column concerns a much less common problem, which is nonethe-

---

COMMON CAUSES OF POSTOPERATIVE TACHYCARDIA

Fever from any cause
Lack of a regular medication (e.g., failure to reorder digitalis postoperatively)
Relative hypotension (i.e., patient ordinarily hypertensive)
Pain or fear and apprehension

COMMON CAUSES OF POSTOPERATIVE TACHYPNEA

Pulmonary atelectasis
Pneumonia
Pulmonary embolism
Diminished lung capacity attributable to:
   Abdominal distension
   Pleural effusion

CAUSES OF PERSISTENT INTESTINAL FISTULAS

Distal obstruction
Foreign body
Noncollapsible cavity interposed
Well-epithelialized tract
Presence of cancer in the fistula
Irradiated tissue
Chronic granulomatous process

---

less remarkably disabling and may lead to the patient's death if no orderly consideration is given to the possibilities.

Agitation is another common phenomenon, particularly among elderly patients and those sustaining major trauma. Two common causes of such agitation are hypoxia and delirium tremens, which may even coexist. Objective verification of the latter is most difficult, whereas the former involves only interpretation of an arterial Po_2 value with respect to the patient's projected or known preoperative status. Certainly, correction of hypoxemia is not harmful in delirium tremens, but the combination of sedation, fluids, and vitamins commonly recommended for patients with delirium tremens is very harmful per se to a hypoxemic patient, just as surely as will be the delay involved in identifying and correcting the hypoxemia. Because hypoxemia is such a common and important postoperative problem, an algorithm for approaching this problem is provided (Fig. 44-1). Frequently one can diagnose the cause of complications with precision. When this is not possible, commonsense considerations such as the foregoing often prove extremely helpful.

POSTOPERATIVE COMPLICATIONS
How Should One Approach Postoperative Fever?

Temperature elevation may occur at any time in the postoperative period. The pattern is important, because a constant elevation may occur when inflamed tissue is removed (e.g., in acute cholecystitis), and the temperature gradually returns to normal over a period of 3 to 4 days with or without the use of antibiotics. A temperature elevation that intermittently drops to a normal level (spiking temperature) is usually more serious and implies intermittent bacteremia. In the latter instance, a thorough search for the source is crucial to normal recovery and, in many cases, may indicate the presence of an abscess or collection of pus in the wound (Chapter 45).

Spiking temperatures occurring in the early postoperative period (first 2 days) are usually pulmonary in origin. From the fourth to the seventh day, such temperatures may result from wound complications. From the sixth to the ninth day, they are commonly caused by intra-abdominal collections (pelvic or subphrenic abscess) or anastomotic leaks. Thrombophlebitis may cause fever from the sixth to the tenth day. Because fever is both common and serious in postoperative patients, Fig. 44-2 presents an algorithm for approaching this problem.

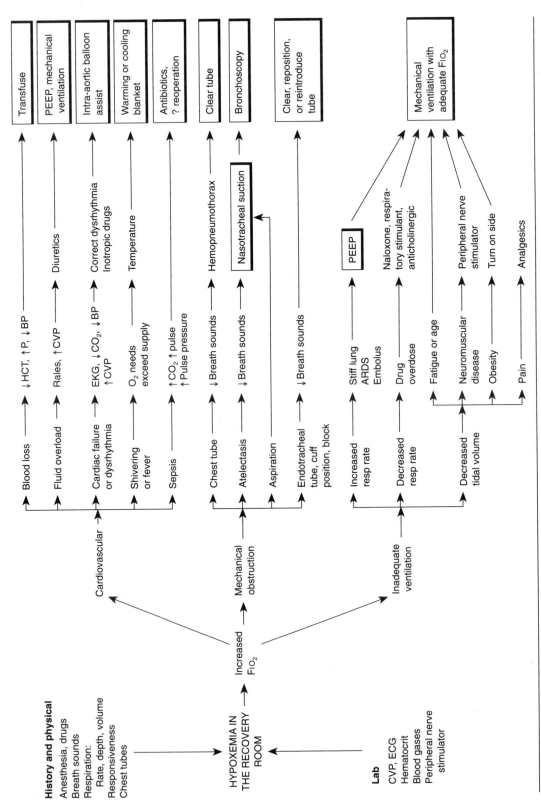

FIGURE 44-1   Treatment of postoperative hypoxemia. (From Eiseman B, Wotkyns RS. Surgical Decision Making. Philadelphia, WB Saunders, 1982.)

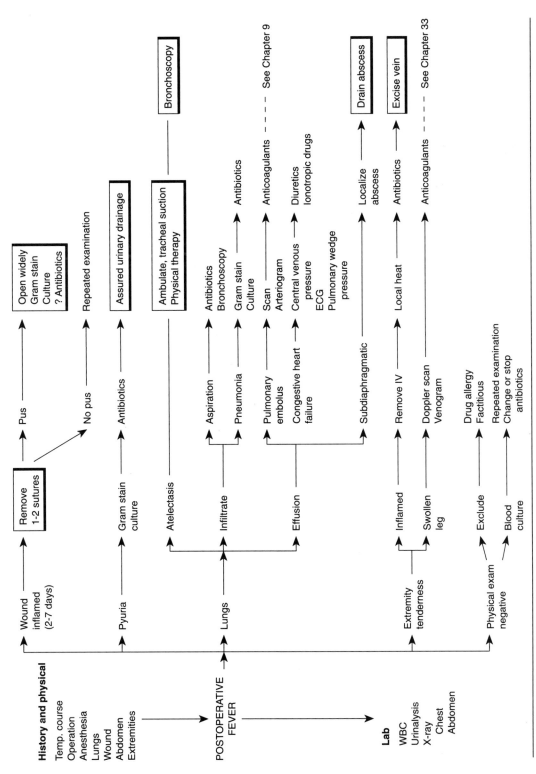

FIGURE 44-2   Treatment of postoperative fever. (From Eiseman B, Wotkyns RS. Surgical Decision Making. Philadelphia, WB Saunders, 1982.)

Renal Failure

Renal failure may occur in any critically ill patient and is the most common ultimate cause of death in patients with sepsis or those undergoing emergency aortic operations. The diagnosis is made by closely monitoring the urine and serum osmolality as well as the volume of urine excreted. The quality of the urine is as important a parameter as the volume, and high-output renal failure can be diagnosed early by measuring these osmolar ratios. By the time a rising blood urea nitrogen (BUN) is evident, complications of hyperkalemia may already have occurred. One first must ascertain that hypovolemia or dehydration is not responsible for the oliguria. Pharmacologic diuresis, if not successful, should be followed by restriction of potassium and early dialysis.

Pulmonary Complications

Pulmonary complications are frequent in all postoperative patients and may be treated simply when diagnosed. Predisposing factors in the development of atelectasis include:

Hypoventilation during anesthesia
Excessive use of narcotics
   Tracheal edema resulting from intubation or external compression (e.g., after thyroid operations)
   Thickened secretions from inadequate humidification of inspired air or dehydration
Hypoventilation postoperatively as a result of failure to produce deep inspiration
Inability to cough
   Abdominal distension from any cause
   Handling of pulmonary tissue at operation, leading to edema and alveolar damage
Aspiration, which may be either massive or subtle, caused by a malfunctioning nasogastric tube

Judicious use of coughing and tracheal toilet are indicated regularly and in all such cases vigorously. In the case of persistent or massive atelectasis, bedside bronchoscopy should be performed. This subject is discussed in detail in Chapter 48.

Overhydration and Congestive Heart Failure

Overhydration leading to early or late congestive changes in the lungs must be guarded against by careful patient monitoring. Every patient having intake and output measured should be weighed daily and this should be recorded. Usually a postoperative patient with good fluid balance will lose 1 pound every day. If this is not occurring, overhydration or a severe third space loss (see Chapter 7) may be present. The use of central venous pressure monitoring is inadequate to prevent this complication, since this technique measures, at best, right heart compensation only when fluids are administered over long periods. The patient who is judged to be at high risk merits continuing measurement of pulmonary wedge pressures with a Swan-Ganz catheter.

Embolism

Pulmonary embolism is an infrequent cause of death in some postoperative patients. Prevention by mobility in bed, early ambulation, elastic support for the legs of those predisposed to this complication (i.e., patients with a history of phlebitis), and use of anticoagulant therapy in identified high-risk groups or suspected cases are all useful in reducing the incidence of this uncommon but deadly complication.

Wound or Incisional Problems

Every surgical operation involves an incision that is in turn vulnerable to infection and dehiscence. These problems are discussed elsewhere (Chapters 45 and 49), but because of their seriousness, *they require the attention of the most senior and experienced surgeon on the team. Remember to culture all such drainage—it may be helpful tomorrow.*

Representative Problems Specific to Particular Operations

If the foregoing is a poorly disguised series of aphorisms, none bears more importance than *"Look where the hand of man has been!"* The psychologic barriers that make the surgeon's admission of a complication difficult further complicate its direct and correct relation to the technical features of the operation itself. In fact, major surgical misadventures contribute in large part to all serious postoperative complications (Table 44-1).

For example, suppose a 47-year-old man on the fifth day after operation develops upper abdominal tenderness where none existed previously. If he has undergone vagotomy and distal partial gastric resection with gastrojejunal anastomosis (Billroth II), the prime possibilities include disruption of the duodenal stump suture

TABLE 44-1   Some Common Postoperative Complications

Complication	Postoperative Days	Predisposing Causes	Diagnosis	Treatment
Fever				
Pulmonary				
Atelectasis	0-2	Inadequate respiratory effort	Response to tracheal toilet	Nasotracheal aspiration
Pneumonitis	4-10	Oversedation Chronic respiratory disease	PE, chest x-ray evaluation, examination of cultures	Bronchoscopy Antibiotics
Urinary	3-5, 8-14	Catheterization	Urinalysis, culture	Eliminate residual urine, antibiotics
Wound				
Infection	5-8	Contaminated operations	Open wound, culture	Local dressings
Dehiscence	0-2, 7-10	Early technique, late infection	Salmon pink drainage	Immediate repair
Anastomotic and deep infections	6-14	Surgical technique, blood supply	Complex, x-ray evaluation	Adequate drainage, reoperation
Oliguria	0-3	Inadequate intake		
Thromboembolism	5-14	Immobilization Abnormal veins	Leg swelling, acute cardiorespiratory failure	Local dressings, anticoagulation therapy, pulmonary therapy, angiography

line, pancreatitis related to dissection of the duodenum from the pancreas, or dehiscence of a portion of the gastrojejunostomy. Immediate study, definition, and intervention are required for the first and last possibilities. However, if his operation was a cholecystectomy, the leading possibilities for such complaints would be the collection of infected bile or blood beneath the liver (a subphrenic or, more specifically, subhepatic abscess) or pancreatitis, both of which allow for a somewhat less aggressive diagnostic and therapeutic approach.

Consider a second hypothetical situation: a 58-year-old woman develops lower abdominal pain and distention and fever on the sixth day after operation. If her operation was a total abdominal hysterectomy for leiomyomata uteri with bilateral salpingo-oophorectomy and appendectomy, pelvic abscess is the working diagnosis, allowing conservative definition and treatment. If her operation was a segmental colectomy and end-to-end colon anastomosis for adenocarcinoma of the sigmoid colon, the most worrisome cause of her symptoms would be anastomotic disruption with pelvic peritonitis. The latter requires immediate definition by careful contrast x-ray study of the colon and the performance of a diverting proximal colostomy, if the working diagnosis is confirmed.

Remote or Atypical Manifestations. The care of the complicated postoperative patient is difficult for all and often bewildering for the student. To add to that complexity, the dominant theme of postoperative patient care in the last decade has been the realization that organ dysfunction may be caused by local, systemic, or even remote infection. Among illnesses so characterized are:

- Pulmonary failure or so-called adult respiratory distress syndrome (ARDS) or posttraumatic pulmonary insufficiency
- Oliguric renal failure
- Progressive hepatic dysfunction
- Gastric mucosal failure or stress ulceration

The mechanism is now clearer; it seems likely that microemboli of platelets and/or leukocytes or other cytokines released by the infective or inflammatory process impair the function of remote organs in various ways. Support of the failing organ only temporizes the situation until the source of infection is identified and treated. Surgical drainage of that focus is often required, but one must be alert to the fact that the infective focus may be occult and very difficult to find. *Remember: a negative CT scan does not exclude the presence of an intra-abdominal abscess.*

PATTERN OF EVOLUTION

Although virtually any illness can appear at any given time, there are characteristic times at which certain postoperative complications usually appear (Table 44-2). As is true of any such guide, one must interpret these patterns thoughtfully, keeping in mind that the time periods indicated are typical, but do not exclude other possibilities. For example, in the case of infection of an abdominal incision: the typical infection evident on the fourth to seventh day after operation is usually caused by pyogenic bacteria, such as *Staphylococcus aureus* and *Escherichia coli.* However, sepsis attributable to the clostridial species appears within hours of wound closure, and streptococcal erysipelas seldom is manifested later than the 48 hours after operation. Conversely, some gram-negative bacteria may not produce typical signs of wound infection until the tenth day. A more frequent cause of late wound sepsis is the inappropriate timing and/or dosage of antimicrobial agents. Thus wound sepsis as a typical postoperative complication can occur throughout the hospital stay, or even after discharge, although more than two thirds of all abdominal wound infections become evident between the fourth and seventh days.

The respiratory system also manifests a varied pattern of evolving complications. When pre-

sented with tachypnea and fever, the respiratory tract usually is plagued by atelectasis in the first 2 days, ordinary bronchopneumonia in the intermediate period, and pulmonary embolism and infarct in the later days after operation.

CORRECTIVE THERAPY

The principles of therapy have already been discussed briefly. If ever the word *radical* was justified in describing any treatment, it is when applied to the correction of surgical complications. The uncomplicated operation is a guaranteed ticket to recovery. Even a major complication is compatible with recovery, if it is diagnosed promptly and treated effectively. An inadequately treated complication will give rise to secondary, often systemic, complications that strikingly diminish the chance for overall recovery.

Specific treatment obviously must be directed at the physiologic consequences of the illness, with appropriate consideration of the probabilities previously defined. This may be illustrated by the following example. A 53-year-old woman develops fever, leukocytosis, right upper quadrant tenderness, and a right pleural effusion 6 days after cholecystectomy for subacute cholecystitis and cholelithiasis. Her presumptive diagnosis is subhepatic or subphrenic abscess. If she appears otherwise well and continues to eat and ambulate, it would be safe to continue to observe her for a bit, which may allow for identification and resolution of more precise and specific damage. If, by contrast, she appears very ill, has an ileus and is unable to eat, becomes tachypneic, and develops an extremely rapid pulse, immediate drainage is warranted.

The first task is to recognize and admit the complication. The second is adequate and timely therapy!

TABLE 44-2   Usual Time of Appearance of Common Postoperative Complications Following Major Abdominal Surgery

Complication	Postoperative Day									
	1	2	3	4	5	6	7	8	9	10
Pulmonary	X	X								
Ear, nose, throat	X	X	X							
Urinary tract			X	X	X					
Thromboembolism						X	X	X	X	X	X
Wound infection, deep abscesses				X	X	X	X	X	X	X
Anastomotic leaks and abscesses						X	X	X		

PITFALLS AND COMMON MYTHS

- Remember where the hand of man has been: "I could not have cut the ureter, because I never even saw it."
- Don't worry about a Gram stain or a culture; it is only a *little* infection.

- He is too sick to *re*operate on.
- Everyone has fever on the third day after a major operation.

SURGICAL PHARMACOPEIA

Drug	Indications/Complications	Dosage
Parenteral		
Codeine	Constipation	60-90 mg IM q4h prn
Demerol		75-100 mg IM q4h prn
Morphine	Respiratory depression possible	10 mg IM q4h prn
		2-4 mg IV q2h prn
Oral		
Darvon		200 mg tid or qid
Ibuprofen	NSAID	400 mg tid or qid
Codeine	Constipation	90-120 mg q4h prn
Demerol		50-100 mg q4h prn
Percodan	Shorter acting	5 mg tid or qid
Dilaudid		2.5-5 mg tid or qid

NSAID = nonsteroidal anti-inflammatory drug.

BIBLIOGRAPHY

Fry DE (ed). Multiple System Organ Failure. St. Louis, Mosby-Year Book, 1992.

Martin LF, Max MH, Polk HC Jr. Failure of gastric pH control by antacids or cimetidine in the critically ill: A valid sign of sepsis. Surgery 88:59, 1980.

Moyer CA. Nonoperative surgical care. In Rhoads JE, Allen JG, et al. (eds). Surgery, Principles and Practice, 4th ed. Philadelphia, JB Lippincott, 1972, pp 293-328.

Norton LW, Eiseman B (eds). Surgical Decision Making, 3rd ed. Philadelphia, WB Saunders, 1986.

Polk HC Jr, Fry DE. Infection and fever in the surgical patient. In Hardy JD (ed). Complications in Surgery and Their Management, 4th ed. Philadelphia, WB Saunders, 1981, pp 1-19.

Sutherland FR, Temple WJ, Snodgrass T, Huchcroft SA. Predicting the outcome of exploratory laparotomy in ICU patients with sepsis or organ failure. J Trauma 29:152, 1989.

CHAPTER REVIEW
Questions

1. List in order the sequence of events to be followed in every postoperative patient visit.
2. The first diagnostic consideration in an anxious, agitated patient is:
   a. Neurogenic shock
   b. Delirium tremens
   c. Anxiety reaction
   d. Hypoxemia
   e. None of the above
3. List five factors predisposing to pulmonary complications.
4. List four common causes of postoperative tachycardia with normal blood pressure.
5. List the common causes of postoperative tachypnea.
6. List three organs that may develop clinical "failure" as a manifestation of uncontrolled infection.

Answers

1. a. Review of vital signs
   b. Evaluation of devices assisting recovery
   c. Auscultation of heart, lungs, abdomen
   d. Inspection of the wound
   e. Determination of what observations are needed next
   f. Summary of visit in the chart
2. d.
3. Any five of the following: hypoventilation in anesthesia, excessive narcotics, local tracheal edema, thickened secretions, direct lung trauma, postoperative hypoventilation, inability to cough, abdominal distension, pulmonary aspiration
4. Fever; regular medication omitted; relative hypotension (patient usually hypertensive); pain, fear, apprehension
5. Atelectasis, embolism, pneumonia, pulmonary compression resulting from abdominal distension, pleural effusion
6. Any three of the following: lung, kidney, liver, gastric mucosa

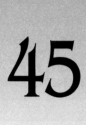

45 Postoperative Fever

DONALD E. FRY

KEY FEATURES

After reading this chapter you will understand:
- The pathophysiology of fever.
- The relationship of fever to bacterial infection.
- Whether the presence of bacteria always indicates infection.
- Translocation of bacteria.
- When fever is not associated with microorganisms.

No problem can be more vexing to the student of surgery than the diagnosis and management of a postoperative patient who has developed fever. Does the fever arise from the area of the operative procedure itself, or are remote causes responsible? Should the fever itself be treated with antipyretics? Is it important to initiate antibiotic therapy before the source of the patient's fever is identified? Answers to these questions are important to providing optimal care so the patient ultimately recovers.

Like a pilot who systematically reviews a checklist before accelerating the aircraft into flight, the student of surgery should have a checklist of the predominant causes of fever in the postoperative patient. Thus evaluation of postoperative fever can be systematized so that all realistic sources can be examined. *Since managing postoperative fever requires more than antipyretics and antibiotics, correctly diagnosing the primary provocateur of the febrile process is essential.*

WHAT IS FEVER?

Regulation of normal body temperature is under precise control by the thermoregulatory center in the hypothalamic area of the brain. Body temperature normally fluctuates within a very narrow range of $\pm 0.5°$ C and usually follows a very predictable biorhythm of maximal temperature at 6 P.M. and minimal temperature at 2 A.M. *Thus fever represents elevations of the core body temperature above these normal daily fluctuations.*

The pathogenesis of fever can be categorized as having both an *afferent* and an *efferent* limb. The afferent limb of the fever response is activated when the host is exposed to an exogenous pyrogen, such as bacteria or an endotoxin. The exogenous pyrogen stimulates the release of endogenous pyrogen principally from monocytes and macrophages. The endogenous pyrogen then travels via the circulation to stimulate receptors of the preoptic-anterior hypothalamic area of the brain. With prostaglandin metabolites (PgE) as an intermediary in the process, the thermoregulatory neurons are stimulated to an elevated thermostat level for body temperature. *The afferent limb of fever is the line of communication between phagocytic cells of the inflammatory response in the periphery and the central nervous system.*

The endogenous pyrogens from monocytes and macrophages are of several varieties. *Interleukin-1* has been the most extensively studied endogenous pyrogen, which has many effects other than stimulation of the fever response (see the box on p. 746). Tumor necrosis factor, inter-

KNOWN ACTIONS OF INTERLEUKIN-1

All are thought to have important host defense roles in the acute adaptive stress response:

Fever
Neutrophilia
Hypoferremia
Hypozincemia
Hypercupremia
Unregulates hepatic synthesis of acute phase reactants (e.g., C-reactive protein)
Muscle proteolysis
Increases amino acid oxidation
Thymocyte proliferation
Immunoglobulin synthesis
Modulates T-helper/T-suppressor cells
Enhances natural killer cell activity
Stimulates fibroblasts

leukin-6, and many other cytokines are soluble signals from macrophages to the central nervous system to cause fever. Even endotoxin as an exogenous pyrogen appears to have direct stimulatory activity on the hypothalamic receptors to provoke a febrile response.

The efferent limb of the febrile response is primarily mediated by the central nervous system. The sympathetic nervous system mediates peripheral vasoconstriction, which serves to minimize heat convection and produces the sensation of chills as interpreted by the patient. Peripheral efferent motor neurons provoke muscle contraction and shivering to promote heat production. The net consequence of the efferent response is the elevation of the core body temperature.

Fever is a nonspecific response of the host to inflammatory events within the body and is not a specific response that indicates that the patient necessarily has an infection. Infection is the activation of tissue inflammation secondary to microorganisms. Sterile inflammatory events such as crush injury and pancreatitis can activate a fever response. Since antigen-antibody complex in the presence of complement proteins can stimulate macrophage cells to produce endogenous pyrogen, autoimmune diseases and drug reactions can cause fever. Certain neoplasias may cause an inflammatory response and provoke fever (e.g., lymphoma). *Thus postoperative fever*

to the student of surgery means a focus of inflammation, which is commonly infection, that must be identified and treated.

WHEN IS POSTOPERATIVE FEVER SECONDARY TO BACTERIA FROM INFECTION?

Fever secondary to infection in a postoperative surgical patient will arise from five anatomic sites in more than 95% of patients; these sites are (1) the lung, (2) the surgical wound, (3) visceral compartments, (4) the urinary tract, and (5) intravascular devices. In patients with postoperative fever, these specific sites should be evaluated in every patient. *It is particularly important that the clinical evaluation for postoperative fever include those anatomic areas where the "hands of man" have been.* The surgical site, endotracheal tubes, Foley catheters, and intravascular devices all deserve special attention as potential locations for infectious morbidity that will explain postoperative fever.

Pulmonary Causes of Fever

Pulmonary infection in a postoperative patient can be categorized as (1) non-ventilator-associated, (2) ventilator-associated, and (3) aspiration-associated. Each has a different pathophysiology and different methods for prevention but similar treatment objectives (Fig. 45-1).

Non-ventilator-associated pneumonitis is the consequence of pulmonary atelectasis. Pulmonary atelectasis represents the most common cause of fever in the initial 24 hours after operation. The immediate postoperative influences of anesthesia, systemic analgesic effects, and painful upper abdominal incisions all result in an inadequate tidal volume, with atelectasis being a potential consequence. This complication is a particularly prevalent problem among patients with chronic obstructive pulmonary disease or long-term cigarette usage and in elderly patients.

Atelectasis represents the collapse of small bronchiolar airways and alveoli. These focal areas of collapse invariably entrap bacteria. The proliferation of entrapped bacteria results in activation of alveolar macrophages, which provokes the fever response. *If atelectasis is not effectively treated, a frankly invasive postoperative pneumonia will develop.*

Atelectasis is a clinical diagnosis. Radiographic changes of atelectasis can be identified only in the most severe cases. On physical exam-

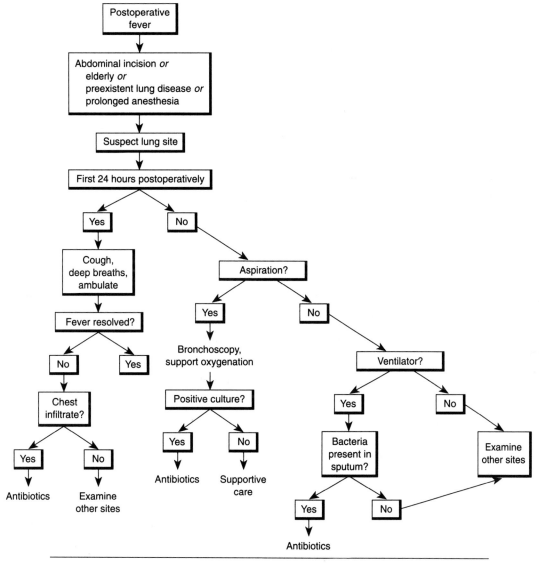

FIGURE 45-1 An algorithm for the evaluation of patients suspected of having the lung as the source of postoperative fever.

ination, the patient with atelectasis commonly is recognized as having moderate tachypnea with inadequate depth of inspiration. Rales and rhonchi are commonly found.

Atelectasis is treated not by antibiotic therapy but by reexpanding the collapsed alveoli. Coughing, deep breathing, and ambulation of the patient are imperative in the management of atelectasis. Chest physiotherapy may be helpful, and in selected refractory cases, nasotracheal suctioning may induce paroxysms of coughing. While incentive spirometry has become very popular for preventing postoperative atelecta-

sis, it is of unproven value and cannot replace coughing, deep breathing, and early postoperative ambulation.

If untreated, atelectasis progresses to invasive non-ventilator-associated pneumonitis. The diagnosis is established by chest x-ray evaluation and identification of purulent sputum. Antibiotic therapy for culture-proven or suspected organisms is necessary at this point.

Ventilator-associated pneumonia in a postoperative patient occurs when the patient has required endotracheal entubation and ventilator-assisted breathing. Such a patient usually has an edematous or impaired lung, since ventilator support has become necessary. Nosocomial pathogens gain access to the airway through the ventilator equipment or from intensive care unit personnel. Prevention requires aseptic technique in managing the endotracheal device and early weaning from the ventilator.

Diagnosis of ventilator-associated pneumonia is difficult. The pattern of fever is different than that of the non-ventilator-associated group and characteristically occurs 3 or more days after initiation of ventilator support. Management of these patients in the intensive care unit is complex, and they have multiple potential sites for fever and infection. All of these patients will have culturable bacteria from the airway after several days on the ventilator, but this may represent colonization and not necessarily invasive infection. Chest x-ray evaluation may commonly reveal infiltrates in ventilator-assisted patients yet may not be conclusive for infection. *The strongest case for the diagnosis of ventilator-associated pneumonia is the identification of bacteria within inflammatory cells by Gram stain of a tracheal aspirate.*

The treatment of postoperative fever from ventilator-associated pneumonia is aggressive tracheal suctioning and antibiotic therapy. Antibiotic therapy is quite problematic, because pathogens in these patients are characteristically resistant gram-negative rods.

Aspiration-associated pneumonitis may be from a gross aspiration event or may be subtle, such as from antacids that have been instilled into the nasogastric tube of patients in an attempt to prevent stress-associated gastritis. Aspiration results in a chemical injury to the lung, and then the patient requires ventilatory support. The pattern of events then becomes similar to that for a patient with ventilator-associated pneumonitis. *It is important to emphasize that preventive systemic antibiotics after a clinically recognized aspiration event will not prevent fever and infection but certainly may affect the ultimate pathogen that infects the patient.* For this reason, administration of preventive antibiotics after an aspiration event *is not recommended.*

Wound Infection

Wound infection is another common cause for postoperative fever. Because the bacterial contamination responsible for the wound infection occurred at the time of the operative procedure, a low-grade fever may be recognized within the first 2 days after the procedure. Fever significant enough to cause clinical concern about wound infection is usually seen on approximately the fifth postoperative day.

The diagnosis of wound infection is made by physical examination. Induration, erythema, and unusual tenderness of the surgical wound about the fourth to fifth postoperative day in the febrile patient is strong evidence to support this diagnosis. A discharge of pus from the wound establishes the diagnosis.

The treatment of postoperative fever secondary to wound infection is to remove the sutures, open the wound, and drain the pus. Fibrinous debris and deeper suture material within the subcutaneous areas may also need to be removed. Simple drainage is adequate for most infections, and administration of systemic antibiotics is not necessary. Antibiotic therapy is reserved for infections in which there is considerable necrosis of tissue or extensive cellulitis is present. Severe wound infections requiring antibiotic therapy should be cultured. Since simple wound infections usually do not require antibiotic therapy, routine culture tests in this setting are more controversial and are probably not cost effective.

What if the fever persists after opening and draining the surgical wound? This may mean that the wound was not completely drained and a residual pocket of pus remains. This commonly happens when the clinician is reluctant to open the entire wound. Fever may persist if necrotic tissue remains in the wound after it is opened, in which case additional debridement may be necessary. Obviously, if the patient has another source of fever besides the wound infection, the fever may persist. *Wound infections associated with major abdominal operations mean that the peritoneal cavity was contaminated with the same bacteria that infected the wound; ergo, beware of a coexistent intra-abdominal abscess.*

Visceral Compartment Infections

Postoperative fever secondary to infections of either of the two major visceral compartments represents a life-threatening complication. Intra-abdominal abscess or empyema of the pleural space can be difficult to diagnose and always requires more than antibiotic therapy for successful patient management.

Intra-abdominal infection as a cause of postoperative fever is most commonly identified in patients who have had major complications following elective gastrointestinal procedures or emergency abdominal operations for spontaneous gastrointestinal perforations, and in patients following penetrating trauma of the gut (Fig. 45-2). Since active infection or massive contamination is a component of the disease process in many of these patients, postoperative fever can be identified from the first postoperative day. Many of these patients will have received systemic antibiotic therapy as part of the management of acute peritonitis, and this may mask early development of the fever response. How-

ever, the development of fever on the fifth to seventh postoperative day, particularly when an intermittent spiking or "sawtooth" pattern can be identified, certainly suggests that intra-abdominal abscess may be the correct diagnosis.

The diagnosis of abdominal abscess can be quite difficult, because the abdominal examination is somewhat compromised by a painful recent surgical wound, and the abscess itself is

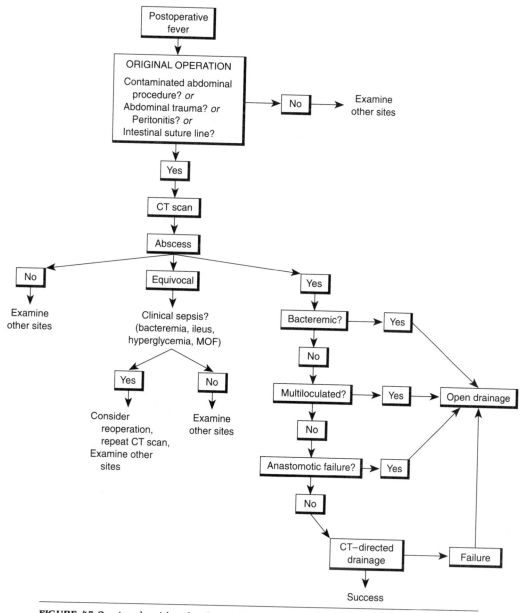

FIGURE 45-2   An algorithm for the evaluation of patients suspected of having an intra-abdominal abscess as the source of postoperative fever. *CT* = computed tomography; *MOF* = multiple organ failure.

rarely palpable. The major exception to this rule is the pelvic abscess, which can frequently be recognized on rectal examination, especially in patients after operation for a perforated appendix. Upright, supine, and lateral decubitus x-ray views are of minimal value. Computed tomography has proved to be the most effective diagnostic tool for abdominal abscess, although accuracy in the acute postoperative period can be problematic because of anatomic distortion and edema of the soft tissues. *Since diagnosis cannot always be objectively determined, surgical empiric reexploration of the abdomen must be considered in patients at reasonable risk (e.g., perforation of the colon 7 days previously) with persistent fever and a clinical septic response.*

The treatment of choice for abdominal abscess is drainage. Drainage can be achieved in selected patients with percutaneous methods using computed tomographic guidance. When abscesses are too complex, are inaccessible by percutaneous methods, or are the consequence of a failed suture line, then a conventional surgical approach is necessary. Broad-spectrum antibiotic therapy for the anticipated pathogens is always employed—but is really adjunctive therapy to effective drainage of the suppurative focus.

Empyema of the pleural space will be a source of postoperative fever in multiple-trauma patients with blunt chest trauma, patients following tube thoracostomy, and in patients with sympathetic effusions from subdiaphragmatic infections (e.g., abdominal abscess). The fever pattern is similar to that seen among patients with an intra-abdominal abscess.

Diagnosis of empyema is easier than abdominal abscess, since pleural collections of fluid are easily identified by conventional chest x-ray examination. Pleural collections of fluid must be taken seriously as sources of postoperative fever and may require diagnostic thoracentesis to document the presence of pus versus other innocent pleural fluid collections.

Like collections of pus anywhere, empyema requires mechanical drainage and cannot be managed by antibiotic therapy alone. Tube drainage of simple empyema, rib resection for more complex suppurative sites, and even pleural decortication of very large collections that threaten to restrict lung expansion may be required. Gram stains of pleural pus may identify gram-positive cocci, suggesting *Staphylococcus aureus* as the putative pathogen. Antibiotic therapy for staphylococcal infections is particularly important to facilitate resolution of these suppurative infections.

Urinary Tract Infections

Urinary tract infections commonly occur in the postoperative surgical patient, particularly in association with an indwelling Foley catheter. Urinary tract infections in the absence of bladder catheterization are usually seen only in patients who had a preoperative infection, urinary stasis secondary to prostatic hypertrophy, an anorectal procedure with urinary retention, and patients with urinary stasis after spinal anesthesia. *Fever is commonly the sole objective finding on physical examination of a patient with urinary tract infection and a Foley catheter in place.* If the Foley catheter has been removed, dysuria is the rule rather than the exception and cannot be relied on as a meaningful sign. Suprapubic tenderness may occasionally be identified, and flank tenderness can be seen with severe ascending infections within the urinary tract. Thus the urinary tract must be considered as the potential cause for fever in a postoperative patient who has no objective findings to direct suspicion elsewhere.

The diagnosis is suspected by urinalysis and is confirmed by the quantitative urine culture. The traditional threshold of 10^5 organisms per milliliter of specimen is used for the culture diagnosis, even though the validity of this may be questionable when a patient has been catheterized for a sustained period. *Beware of a severely ill patient with a septic response and a positive result on urine culture. Severe life-threatening infection rarely arises from a well-drained urinary tract.*

Antibiotic therapy is recommended for fever in patients with postoperative urinary tract infections. Hospital-acquired urinary tract pathogens are quite different from community-acquired infections. Resistant bacteria are more frequently identified in a postoperative patient and require culture and sensitivity data to direct antibiotic therapy.

Urinary stasis and active infection in the urinary bladder form a morbid combination that can result in bacteremia and septic shock. *A fever that is temporally associated with the removal of a Foley catheter may indicate the need to recatheterize the patient and effectively drain the offending source of fever.*

Infections From Intravascular Devices

The use of intravascular devices has proliferated in the care of surgical patients during the last 20 years. Peripheral intravenous lines, central venous lines, arterial lines, and Swan-Ganz catheters have now become additional portals for bacterial access to the intravascular compartment. Bacteremia from these devices is now a major consideration in the evaluation of postoperative fever.

Casual technique in the placement and management of indwelling devices and lengthy periods of peripheral intravenous catheterization result in bacterial migration down the barrel of the catheter, with resultant bacteremia. Fever from such events was classically described as "third-day fever," since peripheral intravenous lines that are present for more than 3 days have a high probability of becoming a source of bacteremia and fever.

Diagnosis of intravascular device bacteremia requires a high index of suspicion, since local findings at the catheter site may be subtle or totally absent. The abrupt onset of high, spiking fever is strong evidence of device-related infection. *A positive result to a blood culture for* **Staphylococcus aureus** *means that the postoperative surgical patient has an intravascular device bacteremia until proven otherwise.* Presence of the infection is documented by removing the device and culturing the catheter tip by the semiquantitative technique.

Treatment of intravascular device bacteremia is removal of the catheter. If *Staphylococcus aureus* is the putative organism, 7 or more days of antistaphylococcal antibiotic therapy are warranted because of potential risks of metastatic infection (e.g., endocarditis). For gram-negative infections, fever and clinical evidence of bacteremia should abruptly subside with removal of the offending device, and only limited antibiotic therapy is necessary for the 24 to 48 hours following catheter removal.

If the fever fails to respond when the catheter is removed, several considerations must be undertaken. First, the catheter may not have been the cause of the fever, or multiple variables may have been responsible for the patient's febrile course. Metastatic infection to a heart valve may have already occurred, although this eventuality is quite infrequent. *The patient may have suppurative thrombophlebitis at the site of catheter placement and may require excision of the infected vein to eliminate the pus-filled vascular structure.* Excision of the vein will be needed in about 20% to 25% of cases of device-related bacteremia.

Other Causes of Fever From Infection

The five major sites of infection just described account for the overwhelming majority of febrile events in postsurgical patients. Much less frequent causes can occur; these are summarized in Table 45-1. These causes must be considered when patients have special circumstances that predispose them to an infection and when investigation of the usual sites has yielded negative diagnostic information.

POSTOPERATIVE FEVER CAUSED BY MICROORGANISMS

Infection is the provocation of a local tissue inflammatory response secondary to the presence of microorganisms. In recent years attention has focused on a phenomenon wherein bacteria that represent normal colonization of the human body might actually gain access to the systemic circulation without causing inflammation at the site of entry and hence represent fever and a

TABLE 45-1 Unusual Infectious Sources of Postoperative Fever

Cause	Diagnosis	Treatment
Pyarthrosis	Recent trauma, tenderness, joint effusion, arthrocentesis	Drainage, antibiotics
Meningitis	Index of suspicion: recent cranial trauma, lumbar puncture	Antibiotics
Sinusitis	Index of suspicion: facial midface CT scan, aspiration	Drainage, antibiotics
Parotitis	Index of suspicion: physical examination, sialogram	Drainage, antibiotics
Hepatitis	Prior transfusion, jaundice, increased AST, ALT; positive antibody	Supportive care
Cytomegalovirus	Prior transfusion; transplant patient; jaundice; increased AST, ALT; positive CMV antibody	Acyclovir

septic response without actually causing infection in the process. The reservoir for microorganisms in this phenomenon is the human gastrointestinal tract. The phenomenon is called *translocation.*

Under normal circumstances the large number of bacteria within the gut are contained by the barrier function of the gastrointestinal tract. This barrier function is multifaceted and includes normal gut motility, mucins and IgA antibodies that prevent bacterial binding to the intestinal epithelial cells, normal anaerobic microflora, and the physical partition created by the epithelial cells and the intercellular matrix. Pathophysiologic variables that will disturb one or more of the components of barrier function can set the stage for bacteria or bacterial cell products to migrate out of the intestinal lumen and into the circulation. Fever and other expressions of the septic response will be the result.

Multiple clinical and experimental variables have been associated with microbial translocation; these include trauma, burns, shock, protein-calorie malnutrition, intestinal obstruction, prolonged antibiotic therapy, and other clinical events. Translocation appears to be primarily an event of aerobic organisms and endotoxin.

Translocation is diagnosed by a process of exclusion. A patient is deemed to have translocation if exhaustive clinical evaluation of the febrile patient has failed to identify a source of infection. Markers for translocation include positive blood cultures for *Candida* spp., *Enterococcus* spp., and *Staphylococcus epidermidis*. Obviously, if patients are receiving broad-spectrum antibiotics, recovery of organisms from blood may be severely compromised and the clinician is left with a "septic syndrome" but no definable infection.

The treatment of translocation is supportive care for the gastrointestinal barrier and antimicrobial chemotherapy for blood-borne organisms. Nutritional support appears to be an important component of therapy for these patients. Current evidence favors enteral nutritional support as opposed to the parenteral route. Enteral nutrition has the advantage of stimulating gut motility and mucin production, providing intraluminal nutrients for the gut epithelial cells, and fostering proliferation of a more normal microflora within the intestinal lumen.

Instituting antibiotic therapy for the patient in whom translocation is suspected is a precarious issue. Antibiotic therapy for anaerobic bacteria may be part of the disease by virtue of the irradication of distal gut anaerobes that are part of the functional gut barrier. Blood-borne pathogens

(e.g., *Candida* spp.) should be covered by specific antimicrobial chemotherapy. Since patients with a potential for translocation are usually at a postoperative period at which nosocomial infection is the greatest risk, and given the relative absence of anaerobes as nosocomial pathogens, empirical antibiotic therapy for these patients should not include anaerobic coverage unless specific culture data dictate otherwise.

WHEN IS POSTOPERATIVE FEVER NOT CAUSED BY MICROORGANISMS OR INFECTION?

As discussed earlier, fever is the consequence of the release of endogenous pyrogens from activated macrophage cells. The primacy of microorganisms in stimulating the febrile response is foremost in all clinicians' minds. However, any disease process that can provoke the inflammatory process and stimulate the release of endogenous pyrogen can cause fever.

Examples of nonbacterial, noninfectious causes of fever are numerous. Acute fulminant pancreatitis creates an inflammatory focus of sufficient magnitude that fever and other evidence of the systemic septic response can be identified. Major aspiration events create a chemical pneumonitis that will elicit an endogenous pyrogen release from pulmonary macrophages. Severe fractures of an extremity (e.g., femur fracture) are associated with crushed soft tissues, hematoma, and devitalized bone fragments that can provoke an inflammatory response and fever. Immediately after cardiopulmonary bypass or after hemodialysis, patients may have a febrile episode or even a "septic" event that is likely to have been secondary to the activation of the complement cascade in the wake of the patient's blood having been circulated through extracorporeal synthetic membrane units. *Macrophage stimulation and endogenous pyrogen release is a nonspecific host response as part of the inflammatory response, and it does not require bacteria or bacterial cell products.*

Still other subtle causes of postoperative fever are identified in Table 45-2. Certain malignancies, such as lymphoma, are clearly associated with fever, so that operation on these patients can be expected to have a postoperative fever response that may not reflect bacteria or infection. Similarly, patients undergoing operative procedures and who have collagen vascular diseases will have fever in the postoperative period arising from their fundamental illness and not because

TABLE 45-2 Noninfectious Causes of Fever

Cause	Diagnosis	Treatment
Drug fever	Eosinophilia	Cessation of drug
Malignant hyperthermia	Index of suspicion: intraoperative/ immediate postoperative fever to 40°-42° C	Fluid support, antipyretics, ice packs, alcohol baths, dantrolene
Thyroid storm	Clinical signs of hyperthyroidism	Propylthiouracil propranolol
Collagen vascular disease	Antinuclear antibody rheumatoid factor, muscle biopsy, nerve biopsy, etc.	Management of fundamental illness
Malignancy	Tissue diagnosis (usually lymphoma)	Antineoplastic therapy
Hypothalamic contusion	Labile body temperature, basilar skull fracture	Antipyretics, ice packs, supportive care

they are infected. In these latter two cases, the mechanism of fever may be the actual release of pyrogenic substances by the tumor (in the case of lymphoma) or may be antigen-antibody complex that is formed in the presence of complement.

Hyperthyroidism and malignant hyperthermia are two other sources of fever that share excess heat production as a basis for fever. Postoperative *thyroid storm* can occur when a patient with previously undiagnosed hyperthyroidism undergoes a major procedure and has an immediate postoperative fever and hyperthyroid crisis. Diagnosis requires a keen sense of awareness of this possibility; the suspicion is confirmed by thyroid function tests. Symptomatic temperature control through alcohol baths and antipyretics is employed, while acute management of the hyperthyroidism is undertaken on an emergent basis.

Malignant hyperthermia will be seen intraoperatively and in the immediate postoperative period secondary to anesthesia. This fulminant and life-threatening complication almost certainly is the consequence of acute heat production and is not mediated through the conventional fever mechanism of endogenous pyrogen stimulation of the thermoregulatory neurons. Cessation of anesthesia, administration of alcohol baths and ice packs, and systemic dantrolene therapy are the treatments of choice. Prompt clinical recognition so that therapy can be implemented is the critical issue to consider in this catastrophic complication of elevated body temperature.

Probably the most frequent noninfectious, non-microorganism-associated form of postoperative fever is *drug fever.* Drug fever tends to be relatively low grade in magnitude and is continuous in chart configuration. A patient with drug fever will have a fever in the range of 38° to 38.5° C but does not appear ill. The patient will commonly have an appetite and will have recovered from most sequelae of even the most extensive of operative procedures, yet the persistent, annoying fever results in the need for extensive blood cultures, x-ray evaluations, and other diagnostic studies. The diagnosis may be suggested by a mildly elevated eosinophil count. *The treatment of drug fever, which is usually secondary to antibiotic administration, is to stop the administration of the drug.*

PITFALLS AND COMMON MYTHS

- **Assumption:** Fever and a septic response are secondary to the catheterized urinary bladder because >10⁵ organisms/ml were identified on urine culture.

  Pitfall: The well-drained urinary bladder may account for mild fever problems, but not a true "septic" patient and generally not a bacteremic event. Look elsewhere for the source of fever in the septic patient.

  Exception: Elderly and immunosuppressed patients can be "septic" from any source.

- **Assumption:** Reduction of postoperative fever by antipyretics will facilitate postoperative comfort for surgical patients.

  Pitfall: Antipyretics alter the pattern of fever, which is the major clinical monitor for the assessment of treatment effectiveness.

  Exception: Severe fever greater than 40° C can have serious central nervous system sequelae and should be treated by antipyretic therapy.

- **Assumption:** A positive result shown on a computed tomogram should be obtained before a reoperation for fever secondary to intra-abdominal infection is undertaken.

  Pitfall: Computed tomography in the interval of the fifth to eighth postoperative day is commonly equivocal for diagnosis because of postoperative changes in the abdomen. Clinical judgment is critical. Reoperation can be lifesaving.

  Exception: Fever and a septic response more than 14 days after an abdominal operation are rarely secondary to undrained pus from the original procedure without convincing computed tomographic evidence.

- **Assumption:** Antibiotic coverage for aerobes and anaerobes is essential for fever from nosocomial infections following clean operative procedures.

  Pitfall: Anaerobes are uncommon nosocomial pathogens, and anaerobic antibiotic coverage (e.g., clindamycin or metronidazole) may adversely affect gut microflora with little clinical benefit and result in the potential for altered gastrointestinal barrier function.

  Exception: Aspiration pneumonia will commonly have anaerobic participation.

BIBLIOGRAPHY

Asher EF, Oliver BG, Fry DE. Urinary tract infections in the surgical patient. Am Surg 54:466-469, 1988.

Border JR, Hassett J, LaDuca J, et al. Gut origin septic states in blunt multiple trauma (ISS = 40) in the ICU. Ann Surg 206:427-446, 1987.

Caplan ES, Hoyt NJ. Nosocomial sinusitis. JAMA 247: 639, 1982.

Dinarello CA, Cannon JG, Wolff SM. New concepts on the pathogenesis of fever. Rev Infect Dis 10:168-189, 1988.

Dyess DL, Garrison RN, Fry DE. Candida sepsis: Implications of polymicrobial blood-borne infection. Arch Surg 120:345-348, 1985.

Fry DE, Clevenger FW. Reoperation for intra-abdominal abscess. Surg Clin North Am 71:159-174, 1991.

Mackowiak PA, LeMaistre CF. Drug fever: A critical appraisal of conventional concepts. Ann Intern Med 106:728-733, 1987.

Martin LF, Asher EF, Casey JM, Fry DE. Postoperative pneumonia: Determinants of mortality. Arch Surg 119:379-383, 1984.

Moore FA, Moore EE, Jones TN, et al. TEN versus TPN following major abdominal trauma-reduced septic morbidity. J Trauma 29:916-923, 1989.

Rush BF Jr, Sori AJ, Murphy TF, et al. Endotoxemia and bacteremia during hemorrhagic shock: The link between trauma and sepsis. Ann Surg 207: 549-554, 1988.

CHAPTER REVIEW
Questions

1. Which of the following bacterial species would be cultured from a patient with a ventilator-associated pneumonia?
   a. *Streptococcus pneumoniae*
   b. *Haemophilus influenzae*
   c. *Pseudomonas aeruginosa*
   d. *Bacteroides fragilis*
   e. *Candida albicans*

2. A postoperative surgical patient has had an uneventful recovery until the fourth day after the operation, at which time the patient has a fever that spikes to 39.5° C. Blood cultures and other diagnostic studies are performed. The next day the microbiology laboratory reports that all blood cultures are growing *Staphylococcus aureus*. The most likely source of this bacteremia is:
   a. Pneumonia
   b. Urinary tract
   c. Intra-abdominal abscess
   d. Wound infection
   e. Intravenous catheter

3. The most valuable objective clinical tool for diagnosis of an intra-abdominal abscess is:
   a. Rectal examination
   b. Computed tomography
   c. Upright abdominal x-ray film
   d. Spiking pattern of the fever
   e. A positive blood culture result

4. A patient has undergone an abdomino-perineal resection for a rectal cancer and has had the Foley catheter in place for 5 days. He is afebrile and the catheter is removed. Six hours later, he has rapidly developed a fever of 39° C, and the nurse reports that he has not voided since the Foley catheter was removed. Treatment for his fever is most appropriately which of the following?
   a. Start gentamicin therapy
   b. Get an infectious disease consultation
   c. Remove all intravascular devices
   d. Replace the Foley catheter
   e. Start enteral nutrition

5. A patient undergoes an inguinal hernia repair as an outpatient and returns to see you on the seventh postoperative day. He has a fever of 38.5° C. He is bitterly complaining about the pain in the wound. Examination demonstrates the wound to be very tender. The wound has a 2 cm perimeter of erythema around it. Treatment of this patient should be:

   a. Hot compresses to the wound
   b. Initiation of oral antibiotics
   c. Removal of sutures and opening the wound
   d. Obtaining a computed tomogram of the pelvis
   e. Aspirin and bed rest

6. When a patient has several positive blood cultures for *Candida albicans,* you should do all of the following except:
   a. Remove and culture the central venous catheter.
   b. Start amphotericin therapy.
   c. Consider enteral nutrition if feasible.
   d. Be certain that *Bacteroides fragilis* is covered.
   e. Perform a fundoscopic examination.

7. The use of antipyretics for fever would only be acceptable in which of the following situations?
   a. A 72-year-old man with a temperature of 38.5° C 12 hours after a transurethral prostatectomy.
   b. A 2-month-old child with a temperature of 40.5° C 3 days after placement of a ventriculoperitoneal shunt.
   c. A 45-year-old woman with a temperature of 39° C on the fourth postoperative day after a vaginal hysterectomy.
   d. A 23-year-old patient with a low-grade fever 7 days after inguinal hernia repair.
   e. A 58-year-old patient with a temperature of 39° C and an elevated cardiac output on the second postoperative day after coronary artery bypass.

8. A 37-year-old patient sustained a gunshot wound of the abdomen with a major colon injury and the presence of fecal material throughout the peritoneal cavity. The injured colon was resected, a colostomy was made, and the patient was started on ampicillin, clindamycin, and gentamicin antibiotic therapy. He remains on antibiotics for 10 days, has resumed eating, has excellent colostomy function, has a white blood cell count of 6300/mm³ but has a temperature over the last 24 hours that has averaged 38.2° C. Treatment at this time should be:
   a. Add amphotericin to the treatment regimen.
   b. Abdominal reexploration for abscess.
   c. Do nothing; colostomy patients always have fever.
   d. Examine all IV sites.
   e. Stop antibiotic therapy.

9. If fever and bacteremia were suspected as being the consequence of translocation in a critically ill patient who had been in the intensive care unit and on broad-spectrum antibiotics for 12 days, all of the following organisms would be reasonable isolates from blood culture except:
   a. *Bacteroides fragilis*
   b. *Enterococcus faecalis*
   c. *Candida albicans*
   d. *Staphylococcus epidermidis*
   e. *Enterobacter cloacae*

10. Fever is
    a. A good response
    b. Bad news
    c. A specific response to bacteria
    d. A nonspecific inflammatory response
    e. Always mediated by macrophage cells

Answers

1. c	6. d
2. e	7. b
3. b	8. e
4. d	9. a
5. c	10. d

46

Shock

GEORGE W. MACHIEDO

KEY FEATURES

After reading this chapter you will understand:
- The best clinical approach to a patient in shock.
- How to recognize when a patient is in shock.
- The pathophysiology of shock.
- The importance of monitoring, and what can be learned about the extent of the derangements in a patient in shock.
- The types of cardiovascular monitoring and their interpretations.
- Treatment of shock, including fluid therapy to improve oxygen delivery and the use of cardiotonic drugs.

Shock has been defined as a "rude unhinging of the machinery of life." Shock is one of the most quickly lethal of all of the clinical conditions that a surgeon will encounter. As we will discuss in the section on pathophysiology, since there are significant "vicious circles" set up by the body's response to shock, if the clinician does not quickly recognize that the patient is in shock and take appropriate actions to prevent further deterioration, the patient will rapidly go on to organ failure and death. In terms of the clinical management of circulatory shock, there are really six areas that need to be addressed (see the box at right). The first of these is the *recognition that the patient is in shock.* Following recognition, appropriate *monitoring techniques* must be employed. This does not always mean invasive monitoring but is frequently simple clinical observa-

tion. The basic *treatment of most types of shock* involves administration of appropriate amounts of intravenous fluid. In certain cases of cardiogenic shock, or in cases in which adequate fluid resuscitation does not return peripheral perfusion to normal, *cardiotonic agents are indicated.* There are also certain situations in which cardiac assist devices such as a left ventricular assist device (intra-aortic balloon pump) might be indicated. Additional aspects of treatment of the patient with shock include *adjunctive therapy,* such as recognition of septic foci, use of agents

---

CLINICAL MANAGEMENT OF THE PATIENT IN SHOCK

To treat the patient in shock rapidly and effectively, the clinician must:

1. *Recognize* that the patient is in shock.
2. *Monitor* the patient's condition, using noninvasive and invasive techniques as well as simple clinical observation.
3. *Treat* the patient appropriately, including the correct amount and type of fluid to be given.
4. Administer *cardiotonic agents* as appropriate.
5. Implement *adjunctive therapies* as needed.
6. *Manage* any of the postshock syndromes that may develop.

---

such as monoclonal antibodies to various mediators of shock, and appropriate management of metabolic derangements caused by shock.

As important as the management of the acute episode of shock are the recognition and *management of the various postshock syndromes.* These include (1) adult respiratory distress syndrome (ARDS), (2) acute tubular necrosis (ATN), (3) stress bleeding from gastrointestinal tract, (4) gut-mucosal function abnormalities that result in the translocation of bacteria from the GI tract into the bloodstream and mesenteric lymph nodes, and (5) hepatic dysfunction secondary to shock. When these individual organ dysfunctions are seen in the same patient, they are classed as *multiple organ failure syndrome (MOFS).* This syndrome is known to have a mortality rate approaching 75%, so it is vital that the clinician recognize and appropriately treat the patient in shock before MOFS develops.

RECOGNITION

One of the most difficult aspects in the management of the patient with shock is *recognizing* that the patient is in shock. One of the primary reasons for this difficulty is that many clinicians, those in training as well as those who have been in practice for many years, confuse the concepts of shock with hypotension or low systemic blood pressure. It is clear that many patients who are in shock will present with a lowered arterial blood pressure, but it is crucially important to understand that *shock and blood pressure are not directly related.* The reason for the dissociation between shock and blood pressure as a diagnostic tool lies in two phenomena. First, the patient may have been previously hypertensive. When a previously hypertensive patient develops a condition that will decrease the blood volume, that patient's blood pressure will fall. However, it may fall into what is classically thought of as the "normal" range. An example of this would be a previously hypertensive man who is involved in a motor vehicle accident and suffers a ruptured spleen. As that patient bleeds from the ruptured spleen, his blood pressure will gradually drift down commensurate with the blood loss. However, when the patient arrives at the emergency department, the recorded blood pressure may be 120/80. Although this is "normal" for the population as a whole, it is markedly abnormal for a patient whose previous blood pressure was 170/100, and thus would reflect inadequate perfusion.

A second and more common reason that patients in shock might not be hypotensive is the fact that the *normal defense mechanisms are designed to maintain blood pressure—at least central blood pressure—at the expense of peripheral perfusion.* As we will see when we discuss the pathophysiologic basis of shock, one of the earliest responses to a decrease in blood volume is peripheral vasoconstriction. This constricts the vasculature of the extremities and other "nonessential" circulatory beds to maintain perfusion of the brain, heart, and lungs.

Teleologically, this makes sense in that inadequate perfusion of the heart or brain will result in sudden death, whereas inadequate perfusion of the extremities can be tolerated for reasonably long periods. However, the maintenance of adequate central flow does not negate the fact that there is inadequate perfusion of large amounts of tissue in the body and that if left unchecked, this inadequate perfusion will lead to further deterioration. Therefore this phenomenon of *compensated* or *normotensive shock* must be recognized by clinical parameters other than hypotension if the patient is to be treated early on in the course of the disease process.

It is equally important to recognize that *although shock is defined as inadequate perfusion of tissues, it is not only a problem of low cardiac output.* Many of the patients seen in surgical intensive care units, particularly those in septic shock, will have markedly elevated cardiac outputs but still will have inadequate perfusion of tissues as a result of microcirculatory abnormalities. A similar phenomenon can be seen in the cirrhotic patient, in whom cardiac output will be markedly elevated as a result of intrahepatic shunting of blood. This will persist, even if the patient has a decreased blood volume, such as that seen with bleeding esophageal varices. In such a situation the patient will be hypovolemic and yet still hyperdynamic.

It is important to recognize that blood pressure and cardiac output are not only unreliable diagnostic parameters in shock, but also are not very helpful as prognostic indicators. *Neither blood pressure nor cardiac output will differ significantly between survivors and nonsurvivors of an episode of shock* until the very terminal events, when obviously in a patient who will not survive, blood pressure and cardiac output drop toward zero. However, early in the course of the shock episode, when therapy should be undertaken, there is no discriminant value in these parameters between survivors and nonsurvivors.

It is therefore important for the clinician to clearly understand the pathophysiology of shock if the goal of early recognition and treatment is to be attained.

Pathophysiology

Since we have defined shock as inadequate perfusion of tissues for the delivery of oxygen and other nutrients to individual cells in the body, it is important to look at what this definition entails. There are four major functions that need to be maintained if we are to get the ambient environmental oxygen to the cells to continue normal cellular function. These four functions include (1) free access of air to the alveolar space, (2) normal alveolar capillary gas exchange, (3) adequate delivery of oxygen to tissues, and (4) normal cellular utilization of oxygen. If any of these functions is disrupted for a significant period, *tissue hypoxia, which is the basic pathophysiologic fact of shock, will occur.* Most of our efforts, in terms of understanding the pathophysiology of shock, involve the adequate delivery of oxygen to tissues.

There are three basic types of shock. These include *hypovolemic shock,* or inadequate blood volume; *septic shock,* or shock related to the presence of infection, usually caused by gram-negative bacteria; and *cardiogenic shock,* caused by inadequacy of the pump function of the myocardium, particularly the left ventricle. Examples of clinical situations in which each of these types of shock occur can be found in the box below. It is very important to realize that these types of shock are somewhat artificial in their definition, and that in a given patient two or actually all three of the various types can be present at the same time. For example, a patient who has primarily hypovolemic shock following a motor vehicle accident with blunt trauma can rapidly develop a septic component to the shock picture if there is perforation of a hollow viscus, leading to spillage of gastrointestinal contents into the peritoneum. Similarly, a patient whose primary problem is septic shock can also be markedly hypovolemic as a result of third spacing of fluid into the interstitial and intracellular space. Similarly, a patient with sepsis might also develop myocardial dysfunction and have a combination of septic shock and cardiogenic shock. It is for this reason that the clinician needs to address basic pathophysiologic concepts, rather than labeling the patient as being in one particular type of shock and treating that to the exclusion of other causes.

A rather simplified flow diagram of the pathophysiology of shock outlining some of the "vicious circles" can be seen in Fig. 46-1. For point of discussion, it is easiest to start with the idea of a decreased blood volume, since this is the basic cause of hypovolemic shock and is frequently seen in many patients suffering from septic shock as well. It can be seen that a decreased blood volume has two primary effects on the body. First, it *decreases venous return,* which by definition *leads to a decrease in cardiac output,* since the heart can only pump the blood returned to it from the systemic circulation. At the same time, there is a *sympathoadrenal response mediated primarily through the carotid body,* which stimulates the release of catecholamines, particularly epinephrine and norepinephrine. These agents cause the vasoconstriction discussed above, which, while protecting the heart and brain for a short period, combines with a decrease in cardiac output to further *limit regional blood flow.* It is this decrease in regional blood flow that leads to the central focus of the pathophysiology of shock, the *local and cellular hypoxia.* This local hypoxia, particularly in the splanchnic circulation, leads to the release of a number of factors thought to have an adverse effect on myocardial function. These so-called myocardial depressant

---

TYPES OF SHOCK

Hypovolemic	Septic	Cardiogenic
Hemorrhage (internal or external)	Gram-negative (endotoxin)	Acute myocardial infarction
Crush injury	Gram-positive (toxic shock syndrome)	Following cardiac surgery
Burns	Fungal	Cardiomyopathy
Peritonitis		

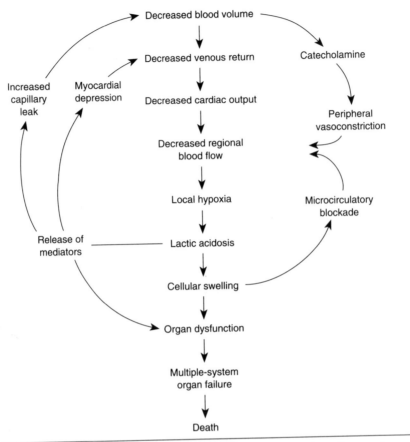

FIGURE 46-1   Pathophysiology of shock. It is apparent from the flow diagram that there are several positive feedback loops ("vicious circles") in the schema that potentiate the lethal potential of shock.

factors combine with the decrease in venous return to further decrease cardiac output, setting up the first vicious circle in shock.

The decreased regional blood flow leads to stagnation of blood within the microcirculation, causing further impediment to microcirculatory function and potentiating the local hypoxia. The tissue damage caused by the local hypoxia stimulates a cascade of mediators, many coming from the macrophage (Fig. 46-2), that are released into the circulation and have local or paracrine effects as well as systemic or endocrine effects. Among these mediators are activated complement, the interleukins, and particularly tumor necrosis factor.

All of these various factors lead to loss of fluid from the intravascular space into the interstitial space, which further decreases the effective blood volume and sets up another vicious circle.

Finally, the individual cells begin to disrupt from hypoxia and swelling. This leads to organ dysfunction, organ failure, and eventually death.

Signs and Symptoms

As can be seen from the description of the general signs and symptoms in the box on p. 761, the patient suffering from hypovolemic shock has a constellation of symptoms that result primarily from the release of catecholamines, as discussed earlier. It must be noted that nowhere in this list is the arterial blood pressure, for the reasons discussed in the introduction to this chapter. It must also be emphasized that the signs and symptoms listed here are "classic presentation" symptoms and that any and all of them may be absent in the individual patient. It is therefore important that the more subtle signs be sought.

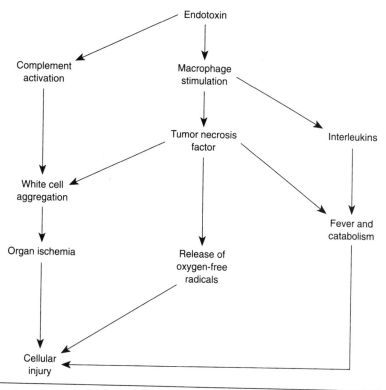

FIGURE 46-2 Cascade of mediators, the majority released from macrophages and/or activated popymorphonuclear leukocytes or lymphocytes. These mediators have a primary role in the cellular dysfunction following shock that leads to multiple organ failure syndrome (MOFS).

SIGNS AND SYMPTOMS OF SHOCK

Hypovolemic	Septic	Cardiogenic
Cool, pale skin	Warm, dry skin	Gallop rhythm
Peripheral cyanosis	Tachycardia	Pulmonary rales
Tachycardia	Fever	Distended neck veins
Tachypnea	Shaking chill	Tachycardia
Restlessness	Mental confusion	

These signs and symptoms are also seen in patients with cardiogenic shock. However, distended neck veins, the presence of a gallop rhythm on auscultation of the heart, and the presence of rales in the lung, indicative of pulmonary edema, are also frequent findings in the patient in cardiogenic shock.

The patient with septic shock presents somewhat differently. Instead of being cold and clammy, the skin is often warm and dry in septic shock. There tends to be less peripheral cyanosis, since the microperfusion of the skin is better in septic shock than in hypovolemic shock, because there is less peripheral vasoconstriction.

The other signs of shock commonly seen with hypovolemia (i.e., hyperventilation and restlessness) are also frequently seen with septic shock. The *hyperventilation results from the excessive production of lactic acid* caused by local hypoxia and the need for the body to excrete this acid load as carbon dioxide. The restlessness results from inadequate perfusion of the brain. A much more common presentation in septic shock is the sudden appearance of mental confusion and/or disorientation in a patient who has previously had a normal mental status. This is frequently seen in older individuals who are developing sepsis and can be easily confused with the changes in mental status in the elderly that are simply the result of a change in environment. It is crucial when a person has a change in mental status that cannot be explained by other reasons that a full work-up for sepsis be undertaken immediately, since if the septic process is allowed to progress to true septic shock, the mortality rate is increased by a factor of five.

MONITORING

Monitoring can be defined as the use of invasive and noninvasive technology to acquire and interpret physiologic data. It is crucial to point out that monitoring should not be synonymous with the insertion of multiple intravascular catheters, such as arterial lines and Swan-Ganz catheters. It may be as simple as careful clinical observation of a patient, but it must be done repeatedly by the same individual with careful attention to detail. The clinical observation of a patient indicating adequacy of perfusion can be followed by the parameters listed below.

Criteria of Adequate Perfusion
Normal mental status
Normal pulse rate (no beta-blockade)
Adequate urine output
Warm, pink skin
No core/extremity temperature gradient
Normal systemic vascular resistance
No lactic acidosis
Normal oxygen extraction ratio

As discussed earlier, the patient's *cerebral status* is a very sensitive indicator of adequacy of perfusion, particularly in patients with early septic shock.

The *urine output* is probably the most important single measurement in a patient with shock, particularly hypovolemic or cardiogenic shock. If a patient is making 0.5 ml/per kg of body weight of urine each hour (e.g., 35 ml/hr in a 70 kg adult), then in most cases peripheral perfusion is at least minimally adequate. An important caveat is that this does not apply in early sepsis.

Septic patients may have adequate or even supernormal urinary output while still having significantly underperfused peripheral circulation.

The relationship between *core temperature*, as measured by rectal probe or temperature-sensing urinary catheter, and the skin temperature is a good indirect measure of systemic vascular resistance. If the patient's core temperature is normal and the distal extremities are cool to the touch, there is a strong possibility that the patient is vasoconstricted and that inadequate perfusion is already present.

Arterial blood pH and serum lactate levels are excellent biochemical markers of the adequacy of perfusion. Metabolic acidosis with an elevated lactate level is almost always caused by inadequate oxygen delivery to tissues or inadequate use of oxygen by those tissues, with resultant tissue hypoxia. The difficulty with both arterial blood pH and serum lactate measurements is that they are intermittent measurements and do not give a continuous readout. Attempts have been made to use muscle surface pH as a continuous analog of arterial blood pH, but local circulatory conditions in the muscle change independent of total body perfusion and therefore the muscle surface pH is often an inadequate indicator of perfusion.

Another noninvasive technique that has been used to indirectly measure perfusion is *transcutaneous oxygen measurement.* A warmed electrode is placed on the skin and the area under the electrode becomes vasodilated. The oxygen in the skin is transmitted through to the Clark electrode in the monitor, and the actual partial pressure of oxygen is measured. This has been more successful than muscle surface pH measurements, but again depends greatly on local blood flow and often does not reflect total body circulation.

In certain patients, indirect or clinical measurements of perfusion are not adequate to diagnose and treat shock or impending shock, and it is necessary to use more invasive monitoring devices. Indications for invasive monitoring are listed in the box on p. 763. It is important to realize that high-risk surgery is not synonymous with high-tech surgery. The risk of an above-the-knee amputation in a patient with peripheral vascular disease is many times higher than the risk to a patient undergoing a coronary artery bypass graft. The risk should be estimated by careful history-taking and physical examination. If a patient has *preexisting organ dysfunction*, particularly cardiac, pulmonary, renal, or hepatic

INDICATIONS FOR
INVASIVE MONITORING*

Unresponsive hemodynamic instability
  Elderly patient
  Multiple-trauma patient
  Suspicion of sepsis
Previous organ dysfunction
  Cardiac
  Pulmonary
  Renal
  Hypertensive
High-risk surgery
Use of high levels (10 cm H_2O) of PEEP

*Established indications for the use of arterial lines and Swan-Ganz pulmonary artery catheters. These criteria are met in approximately 15% of patients in a surgical ICU, indicating that most patients can be monitored with less-invasive technology.

TABLE 46-1 Determinants of Cardiac Output

Parameter	Measurement
Preload	Pulmonary capillary wedge pressure
Afterload	Systemic vascular resistance
Contractility	Ventricular function curve
Heart rate	ECG monitor

dysfunction, then invasive monitoring is frequently indicated as a prophylactic measure in patients undergoing major surgery. For a trauma patient with preexisting organ dysfunction an intravascular monitor should be inserted soon after admission, even if he or she is hemodynamically stable when first seen, since hemodynamic instability is more likely to occur in these patients and may result from causes other than hypovolemia (e.g., cardiac failure). This could be best detected by a pulmonary artery catheter. Patients on a high level of positive end-expiratory pressure (PEEP) for ARDS frequently require invasive monitoring, since the applications of PEEP can significantly and adversely affect cardiac output to the point where inadequate perfusion of peripheral tissues can occur. Finally, patients with hemodynamic instability require invasive monitoring only if they do not respond to the initial management of that hemodynamic instability or are in one of the other high-risk groups just discussed.

Some of the uses of hemodynamic monitoring are to measure cardiac output and the determinants of cardiac output (listed in Table 46-1), to assess the magnitude of pulmonary congestion, to assess left ventricular pump performance, and to allow calculation of oxygen consumption and oxygen delivery. Table 46-1 lists the physiologic determinants of cardiac output and the clinically available technique for provid-

ing a direct measurement or an approximation of that parameter.

The first intravascular catheter normally used in a patient requiring invasive monitoring is the ***intra-arterial catheter*** or ***arterial line.*** This is most frequently placed in the radial artery and is easily inserted percutaneously. It is crucially important that an Allen test be performed before the placement of a radial artery catheter. The ***Allen test ensures the functional integrity of the palmar arch.*** Briefly, it is performed by having the patient make a fist, or if the patient is unable to do so, having an assistant passively close the hand to expel as much blood from the skin and subcutaneous tissue as possible, thereby blanching the skin. The radial and ulnar arteries are then forcibly compressed by digital pressure and the hand relaxed. While maintaining pressure on the radial artery, the pressure is removed from the ulnar artery, allowing blood to reenter the hand. If the tissue over the thenar eminence regains its normal pink color within 1 or 2 seconds, this is evidence of patency of the palmar arch, and the line can be safely placed in the radial artery with minimal fear of distal ischemia.

The benefits of arterial line insertion are that the blood pressure measurements obtained with an adequately calibrated system are more accurate in a low-flow state than those obtained by standard blood pressure cuffs. It also gives continuous measurement of blood pressure, rather than the intermittent measurements obtained with either standard cuffs of noninvasive blood pressure monitors. Another benefit of the presence of an arterial line is that it gives easy access for repeated measurements of arterial blood gases for biochemical monitoring of the circulation.

The second intravascular catheter that is normally used in monitoring patients with shock or impending shock is the ***Swan-Ganz pulmonary artery catheter.*** This catheter has the ability to measure right-sided heart pressures, including

TABLE 46-2 Interpretation of Low Cardiac Output

Cause	Parameter
Hypovolemia	Low PCWP
	High SVR
Primary cardiac failures	High PCWP
	Normal SVR
Cardiac failure secondary to vasoconstriction	High PCWP
	High SVR

TABLE 46-3 Interpretation of High Cardiac Output

Cause	Parameter
Sepsis	Low SVR
	Low oxygen extraction
Anemia	Low hematocrit
	High oxygen extraction
Posttrauma hypermetabolism	Low SVR
	Normal oxygen extraction

central venous pressure and pulmonary systolic and diastolic and wedge pressures. It also allows the measurement of cardiac output by means of the thermal dilution technique. Interpretation of the measurement of cardiac output is outlined in Table 46-2. A decreased cardiac output (less than 4 L/min or 2.2 L/min/m²) is indicative of hypovolemia if the pulmonary capillary wedge pressure (PCWP) is also low, less than 5 to 8 mm Hg. If the cardiac output is low and the PCWP is elevated, this is frequently indicative of cardiac failure. The cardiac failure may be the result of intrinsic myocardial dysfunction or may be secondary to intense peripheral vasoconstriction. It is therefore necessary to calculate systemic vascular resistance. We will discuss the appropriate calculations for this parameter in the discussion of the determinants of cardiac output.

Interpretation of an elevated cardiac output is significantly more difficult than that of a low cardiac output. The most common interpretation of a high cardiac output in a surgical patient is frequently that of sepsis. It must be remembered, however, that there are many other clinical conditions, such as cirrhosis and anemia, which can also lead to an elevated cardiac output. The most commonly seen cause of a high cardiac output in a patient following surgery or a traumatic injury is the normal hypermetabolic state that these conditions engender. It is important to recognize that any patient who has had a biologically stressful occurrence will respond to that by increasing oxygen consumption. To meet those increased metabolic demands, the cardiac output must go up proportionately. To differentiate between this normal hypermetabolic response and inappropriate elevations of cardiac output, such as those seen with sepsis, *the oxygen extraction ratio is a helpful tool.*

The body normally extracts approximately 25% of the oxygen delivered to the tissues to provide energy. *In situations of inadequate delivery this oxygen extraction ratio,* which is calculated by dividing the measured oxygen consumption by the oxygen delivery, *increases above 25%,* sometimes as high as 35% to 40%. This indicates that the body is using its reserve of circulating oxygen to meet the metabolic demands. If the *oxygen extraction ratio falls below 20%,* this usually indicates that although oxygen delivery is adequate, *oxygen consumption is being suppressed.* This is what frequently happens in a patient with sepsis. This then enables us to distinguish the various causes of an elevated cardiac output, as shown in Table 46-3.

Much more helpful than cardiac output in the management of the patient with shock are the determinants of cardiac output. As discussed briefly, these allow us to dissect out the causes for the inadequacy of perfusion, rather than just looking at perfusion itself. We will attempt to take each of the determinants and move from their physiologic underpinnings to the clinical utility of each parameter.

Preload is defined by physiologists as the length to which a contractile cell is stretched before its next contraction. Up to a given point, the strength of the contraction will be directly proportional to the amount of stretch applied to the cell. This is quite helpful to a physiologist studying a rat papillary muscle but provides little help for the clinician, since it is impossible to measure the length of each myocardial fiber. Therefore a number of assumptions must be made to convert the physiologist's definition of preload to a clinically usable measure of preload, such as pulmonary capillary wedge pressure (Fig. 46-3).

In clinical practice, the true preload of the left ventricle, the ventricle of greatest interest in a

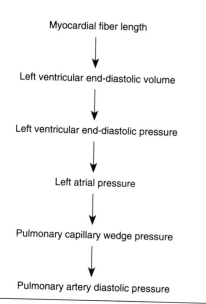

Myocardial fiber length

↓

Left ventricular end-diastolic volume

↓

Left ventricular end-diastolic pressure

↓

Left atrial pressure

↓

Pulmonary capillary wedge pressure

↓

Pulmonary artery diastolic pressure

FIGURE 46-3 Assumptions associated with the clinical measurement of preload.

consideration of the patient in shock, is the left ventricular end-diastolic volume. The greater this volume, the more stretch that is applied to the myocardial fibers and the greater the strength of the subsequent contraction. This is commonly known as *Starling's law* of the heart. However, it can be seen that while the true measure of preload is a volume measurement, what we measure clinically is a pressure measurement (PCWP). The conversion of left ventricular end-diastolic volume to left ventricular end-diastolic pressure is the major assumption made in the clinical approximation of preload.

In the normally compliant left ventricle there is a direct relationship between left ventricular end-diastolic volume and left ventricular end-diastolic pressure. However, in patients with shock, particularly septic shock or following acute myocardial infarction, the left ventricle can become less compliant. This means that for a very small increase in volume there is a disproportionately large increase in pressure. This will obviously affect the linear relationship of the two and can mislead the clinician into thinking that preload is actually rising faster than it truly is. Therefore the state of ventricular compliance must be kept in mind when preload is being used to judge the adequacy of cardiac filling. The other assumptions made in Fig. 46-3 are usually true, with the exception that in patients with mitral

valve disease, left atrial pressure does not always reflect left ventricular end-diastolic pressure. This clinical condition, however, should be recognized by history and physical examination and should not create much difficulty in managing the average patient.

The final assumption, the equivalency of pulmonary capillary wedge pressure and pulmonary diastolic pressure, is one fraught with danger in the critically ill patient. Although in the normal individual this relationship does hold, it is important to note that in any patient with pulmonary hypertension *there will be a discordance between wedge pressure and pulmonary diastolic pressure.* Pulmonary hypertension is frequently seen in critically ill patients, particularly those with hypoxemia or metabolic acidosis. Therefore the continuous measurement of PA diastolic pressure should not substitute for the intermittent measurement of wedge pressure in these patients.

One other caveat in the interpretation of wedge pressure is *position of the pulmonary artery catheter in the lung.* The lung was divided by West into three zones. In zone 1, normally seen at the apex of the lung, alveolar pressure is higher than pulmonary capillary pressure and the pulmonary capillaries are closed. If the pulmonary catheter was placed into a vessel in zone 1, the measured wedge pressure would actually be tracking alveolar pressure and not left atrial pressure. This could be highly misleading in a patient on high ventilator pressures. Fortunately, since the catheter is flow directed, it normally goes to either zone 2 or zone 3 in the lung, where intravascular pressure is higher than alveolar pressure and the capillaries are maintained in an open position. It is important, however, to check the position of the Swan-Ganz catheter after insertion to be sure that it has not been inadvertently placed in an upper or anterior position.

The next determinant of cardiac output to be discussed is *afterload.* Afterload is defined by physiologists as the impedance to ejection of blood from the left ventricle. *It is determined by the volume and mass of the blood ejected from the ventricle, as well as the compliance and total cross-sectional area of the vascular space into which the blood is ejected.* As opposed to preload in which we can actually measure a rough approximation (PCWP) of the physiologic determinant, we obviously cannot measure the total cross-sectional area of the vascular bed directly. Therefore we need to calculate an approximation

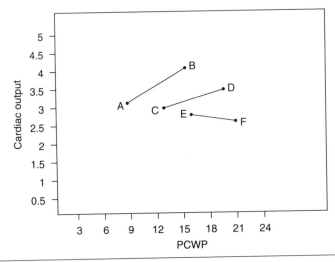

FIGURE 46-4   Graphic depiction of ventricular function curves.

of that parameter. This is done by calculating the *systemic vascular resistance (SVR)*. Normal systemic vascular resistance is between 900 and 1200 dynes/sec/cm⁵. Similar to cardiac output, this can be indexed to the body surface area. When the SVR is higher than 1200, the patient is said to be vasoconstricted, while an SVR below 900 indicates vasodilation.

The final determinant of cardiac output which is frequently used in clinical monitoring is *contractility*. Contractility is an inherent property of the myocardium that indicates the rate of contraction of the muscle, independent of both preload and afterload. We can neither measure nor calculate contractility in the clinical situation. It is for this reason that we construct ventricular function curves (Fig. 46-4) to help evaluate the contractile state of the heart. Briefly, what is done is to increase the preload and measure cardiac output or left ventricular stroke work at both the low and higher preload. *If contractility is normal, there should be a significant increase in left ventricular function with the increasing preload.* If this does not occur, it indicates a decreased contractility. More precise techniques for measuring contractility, such as the measurement of dp/dt or the rate of rise of the pressure in the left ventricle, is commonly done in cardiac catheterization laboratories but is not clinically available in most intensive care units today.

The importance of measuring contractility, or at least estimating it, is that *cardiotonic drugs that increase contractility should only be used*

when it has been proven by a ventricular function curve that the contractility is decreased. As we will discuss below one of the most common errors in the management of a shock patient is to use inotropic or vasopressor support in the presence of a low blood volume.

TREATMENT

As we discussed under pathophysiology, the most common cause of shock in clinical practice is hypovolemia. Therefore fluid administration is the cornerstone of treatment for this condition. There are several questions that must be answered when considering fluid administration for a patient in shock. These include (1) the amount of fluid to be given and (2) the type of fluid to be used.

The amount of fluid to be given (Fig. 46-5) is determined by repeated analysis of the indices of perfusion, as discussed earlier. It is very important not to use a fixed formula to estimate fluid requirements in a patient in shock, but rather to give large amounts of fluid quickly until the patient exhibits a return of normal perfusion. The parameters to be followed depend on the clinical situation. In a young individual with a healthy heart, central venous pressure and urine output may be adequate. In an older individual or one with known cardiac dysfunction, all of the invasive monitoring techniques that we discussed would be employed.

It is also important not to overresuscitate pa-

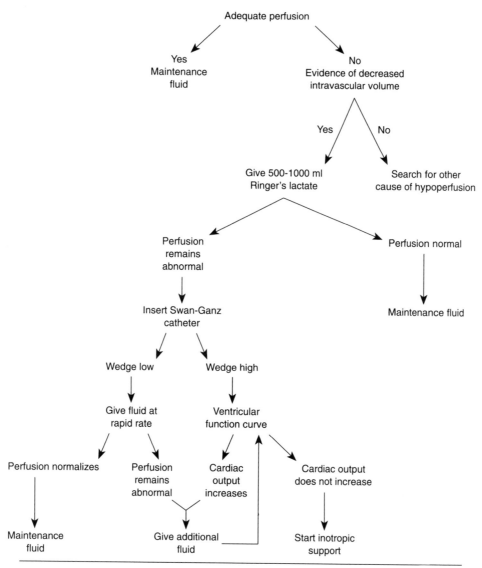

FIGURE 46-5 Algorithm outlining the use of the clinical and physiologic parameters in determining how much fluid resuscitation is required for a patient in shock.

tients. There is frequently a tendency to try to maximize the wedge pressure at levels of 12 to 15 mm Hg. This is appropriate if perfusion has not yet been returned to normal. However, *active fluid resuscitation should cease at the lowest wedge pressure that gives adequate perfusion.* Just as we cannot use blood pressure to diagnose shock, it is most important to emphasize the fact that blood pressure should not be used as an end-point of resuscitation. There is ample clinical evidence to document the fact that patients can

have an absolutely normal blood pressure and still be woefully underresuscitated. It is for this reason that cardiac output, lactic acid production, urine output, and arterial pH are all much more valuable indicators of adequacy of resuscitation than is blood pressure.

Another caveat regarding the amount of fluid to be given is to be aware of the *stiff heart syndrome.* If the myocardium has become stiffened either as a result of myocardial ischemia or interstitial fluid, a small increase in true preload will give a large increase in the measured pulmonary capillary wedge pressure. This should not be taken as evidence that volume resuscitation has been complete. If there is still evidence of inadequate perfusion, wedge pressure should be raised even higher; if the cardiac index increases, this is indicative of a positive response to fluid administration and it should be continued even at higher than "normal" preload measurements.

The type of fluid to be administered depends on the specific needs of the individual patient. Fluids can be broken down into two categories: those that replenish volume and those that replenish oxygen-carrying capacity (see the box at right). Volume resuscitative agents are usually divided into balanced salt solutions, such as Ringer's lactate, or colloid solutions, such as albumin, dextran, or hydroxethyl starch. Although this is still controversial, most clinicians feel that crystalloid resuscitation with a balanced salt solution is preferable. There are few data to suggest overall benefit of colloid resuscitation, and it is considerably more expensive than the use of a balanced salt solution, such as Ringer's lactate. When using Ringer's lactate, one must recognize that the lactate anion does not potentiate lactic acidosis. It must be recognized that the lactate in Ringer's lactate solution is sodium lactate, which is metabolized in the liver to bicarbonate and actually buffers the metabolic acidosis. This is in distinction to lactate acid or hydrogen lactate, which is being produced by the ischemic tissue.

Another major benefit of crystalloid resuscitation is that it decreases blood viscosity and replenishes the fluid lost from the extracellular space in patients suffering from shock. Both of these are helpful in improving microvascular circulatory function.

If a patient requires large volumes of resuscitative fluid (greater than 3 L in the first 8 hours), *normal saline should not be used.* The reason for this is that a liter of normal saline contains a 154 mEq of chloride. This high concentration of chloride will actually potentiate rather than correct the metabolic acidosis present in hypoperfusion by adding a nonanion gap acidosis resulting from hyperchloremia to the already existing anion gap acidosis caused by lactic acid production.

When resuscitation of oxygen-carrying capacity is necessary, the only clinically available agent is human blood. Although there has been

---

FLUID ADMINISTRATION FOR PATIENTS IN SHOCK

Fluids to Replace Volume

Crystalloid solutions
  Balanced salt solutions
    Ringer's Lactate
  Normal saline
  Hypertonic saline
Colloid solutions
  Albumin
  Dextran
  Hydroxethyl starch

Fluids to Replace Oxygen-Carrying Capacity

Whole blood
  Fresh
  Banked
Component therapy
  Packed red cells
  Fresh frozen plasma
  Platelet concentrates
Type-specific blood
O-negative blood

---

significant research on such products as stroma-free hemoglobin and fluorinated hydrocarbons, these are not clinically available at this time. The options for giving blood include the use of whole blood, either banked or fresh, packed red blood cells, O-blood, or type-specific blood. In most cases, packed red blood cells are the agent of choice to replenish oxygen-carrying capacity. In recent years, the threshold for transfusion has been lowered in many cases from a hematocrit reading of 30% (hemoglobin level of 10) to somewhat lower levels. It must be emphasized, however, that particularly in a posttrauma situation, resuscitation with packed red blood cells should be undertaken before hematocrit levels drop below 30%, since there will be a delay in the drop in hematocrit level when blood is being lost rapidly.

The next mode of therapy in a patient with shock is the use of cardiotonic agents. If volume resuscitation is unsuccessful in returning perfusion to normal and there is clear evidence that

TABLE 46-4 Cardiotonic Agents

Drug*	Dose†	Action
Dobutamine	5-25	Increase contractility
		Lower SVR
		Lower wedge pressure
Dopamine	<5	Renal vasodilator
	5-10	Increase contractility
	>10	Lower SVR
		Peripheral vasodilator
Isoproterenol	0.007-0.07	Increase heart rate
		Peripheral vasodilator
Amrinone	5-25	Increase contractility
		Lower SVR
		Lower wedge pressure

*Commonly used pharmacologic agents to provide inotropic support in patients in whom contractility has been determined to be decreased or to provide afterload reduction by inducing vasodilatation.
†All doses are μ/kg/min.

the heart is starting to fail, then the use of cardiotonic agents should be considered. The most commonly used agents are listed in Table 46-4. It is important to understand that most cardiotonic agents increase the myocardial oxygen demand and if an individual has borderline coronary artery flow, can actually induce myocardial ischemia and worsen rather than improve clinical perfusion.

CONCLUSION

Shock is clearly a clinical condition that is self-perpetuating and that, if not recognized early, monitored aggressively, and treated appropriately will lead to the death of the patient within hours. A thorough understanding of the physiologic principles underlying the monitoring and treatment of shock is crucial if the clinician is to deal appropriately with this lethal condition.

PITFALLS AND COMMON MYTHS

- Confusing hypotension with shock.
- Misinterpreting a high wedge pressure that does not reflect end-diastolic ventricular pressure because of the patient having a "stiff heart."
- Underresuscitation, particularly in patients with sepsis.
- Using invasive monitoring too late.
- Using cardiotonic agents when the patient is hypovolemic.

SURGICAL PHARMACOPEIA

Drug	Indications/Complications	Dosages*
Cardiotonics Increase cardiac output, occasionally used in cardiogenic shock		
Dopamine (Intropin)	Actions vary, depending on dose:	
	Low dose—vasodilation of renal, mesenteric, cerebral, and coronary vessels	200-500 μg/min
	Medium dose—increased force of cardiac contraction; increases myocarial oxygen requirement	500-2000 μg/min
	High dose—progressive alpha-adrenergic vasoconstriction; may increase tissue ischemia	>2000 μg/min
Dobutamine (Dobutrex)	Increases cardiac output by increasing stroke volume; also decreases afterload (SVR); increases myocardial oxygen demand, risk of tachyarrythmias in patients with atrial fibrillation	500-1500 μg/min
Isoproterenol (Isuprel)	Increases cardiac output by increased heart rate (chronotrope); also decreases afterload (SVR) and may increase venous return by decreasing venous compliance; increases myocardial oxygen demand, which may worsen myocardial infarction, tachyarrythmias	0.5 μg/min to 5 μg/min
Amrinone (Inocor)	Increases cardiac output (contractility) and decreases afterload (SVR) and preload (venous return); no measurable increase in myocardial oxygen demand; possible hepatotoxicity	10.5 mg loading, 0.35 to 0.7 mg/min
Vasoconstrictors Indicated *only* in extreme situations to maintain adequate blood pressure for perfusion of vital organs; principally used in severe septic or cardiogenic shock		
Phenylephrine (Neosynephrine)	Alpha-receptor stimulant and powerful vasoconstrictor; may result in worsening of tissue perfusion and lactic acidosis	40-60 μg/min
Norepinephrine (Levophed)	Alpha-adrenergic vasoconstrictor; also increases cardiac contractility; may result in severe tissue ischemia and worsen lactic acidosis	2-4 μg/min
Vasodilators Decrease afterload, may improve cardiac output and decrease myocardial oxygen demand; occasionally used in cardiogenic shock		
Nitroglycerin (Nitrostat)	Arterial and venous vasodilator; decreases afterload (SVR) and preload (venous return); venous effects may predominate and result in decreased cardiac output and severe hypotension	5-20 μg/min
Nitroprusside (Nipride)	Similar actions to nitroglycerin except less venous effect; major metabolite is cyanide; may result in cyanide toxicity with high doses or prolonged infusions	0.02 to 0.7 mg/min

*Dosages shown are for a normal 70 kg adult.

BIBLIOGRAPHY

Bland RD, Shoemaker WC, Abraham E, et al. Hemodynamic and oxygen transport patterns in surviving and non-surviving post operative patients. Crit Care Med 13:853, 1985.

Calvin JE, Driedger AA, Sibbald WJ. Does the pulmonary capillary wedge pressure predict left ventricular preload in the critically ill? Crit Care Med 9:437, 1981.

Dantzker D. Oxygen delivery and utilization in sepsis. Crit Care Clin 5:81, 1989.

Fiddian-Green RG. Hypotension, splanchnic hypoxia and arterial acidosis in ICU patients. Circ Shock 21:326, 1987.

Frank MM. Complement in the pathophysiology of human disease. N Engl J Med 316:1525, 1987.

Glantz SA, Parmley WW. Factors which affect the diastolic pressure-volume curve. Circ Res 42:171, 1978.

Gould SA, Rosen AL, Seigal LR, et al. Fluosol-DA as a red cell substitute in acute anemia. N Engl J Med 314:1653, 1986.

Holcroft JW, Vassar MJ, Blaisdell FW. Resuscitation of severely injured patients with 3% NaCl solution. Ann Surg 206:279, 1987.

Kaufman BS, Rackow EC, Falk JL. The relationship between oxygen delivery and consumption during fluid resuscitation of hypovolemic and septic shock. Chest 85:336, 1984.

Lewis BS, Gotsman MS. Current concepts of left ventricular relaxation and compliance. Am Heart J 99:101, 1980.

Reilly JM, Burch-Whitman C, Parker MM, et al. Characteristics of a myocardial depressant substance in patients with septic shock. Circ 76:165, 1987.

Sarnoff SJ. Myocardial contractility as described by ventricular function curves. Observations on Starling's Law of the Heart. Physiol Rev 35:107, 1955.

Schirmer WJ, Schirmer JM, Naff GB, Fry DE. Contributions of toxic oxygen intermediates to complement-induced reductions in effective hepatic blood flow. J Trauma 28:1295, 1988.

Shoemaker WC, Appel PL, Kram HB, et al. Comparison of hemodynamic and oxygen transport effects of dopamine and dobutamine in critically-ill surgical patients. Chest 96:120, 1989.

Solomkin JS, Simmons RL. Cellular and sub-cellular mediators of acute inflammation. Surg Clin North Am 63:225, 1983.

Velanovich V. Crystalloid versus colloid fluid resuscitation: A meta-analysis of mortality. Surgery 105:65, 1989.

CHAPTER REVIEW
Questions

1. Which of the following statements is true concerning the relationship of arterial blood and pressure and shock?
   a. Blood pressure is the earliest parameter to change when a patient develops shock.
   b. Although not diagnostic of shock, blood pressure is an accurate prognostic indicator of shock.
   c. Shock is defined by a low arterial blood pressure.
   d. When blood pressure returns to normal a patient is adequately fluid resuscitated.
   e. None of the above.

2. Which of the following statements concerning multiple system organ failure (MSOF) after shock is true?
   a. The presence of MSOF does not change the underlying mortality rate for an episode of shock.
   b. The mortality rate with established MSOF is 10%.
   c. The mortality rate with established MSOF is 75%.
   d. Hemorrhagic shock is more likely to cause MSOF than is septic shock.
   e. None of the above.

3. The first biochemical response to a decrease in blood volume is:
   a. Increased proteolysis
   b. Decreased antidiuretic hormone release
   c. Increased catecholamine release
   d. Decreased insulin release
   e. None of the above

4. Shock is best defined as:
   a. Inadequate blood pressure
   b. Inadequate tissue perfusion
   c. Inadequate cardiac output
   d. Inadequate blood volume
   e. None of the above

5. Which of the following causes of shock is *not* usually associated with hypovolemia?
   a. Hemorrhage
   b. Peritonitis
   c. Crush injury
   d. Cardiomyopathy
   e. Burns

6. Which of the following is *not* an early sign of shock?
   a. Tachycardia
   b. Peripheral cyanosis
   c. Hypotension
   d. Restlessness
   e. Cool pale skin

7. The single most important number to be followed in hypovolemic shock is:
   a. Serum sodium
   b. Cardiac output
   c. Urine output
   d. Plasma epinephrine level
   e. None of the above

8. Which of the following is typical of early septic shock?

	Cardiac Output	SVR	O$_2$ Extraction Ratio
a.	Normal	High	Normal
b.	Low	High	High
c.	High	High	Normal
d.	High	Low	Low
e.	Low	Low	Low

9. Conditions associated with a high cardiac output include all, *except:*

   a. Hypovolemic shock
   b. Septic shock
   c. Cirrhosis
   d. Normal response to surgery
   e. Anemia

10. Which of the following is *not* a determinant of cardiac output?
    a. Heart rate
    b. Pulmonary capillary wedge pressure
    c. Systemic vascular resistance
    d. Age
    e. Contractility

Answers

1. e	6. c
2. c	7. c
3. c	8. d
4. b	9. a
5. d	10. d

47

Surgical Bleeding and Hemostasis

JOHN A. COLLINS

KEY FEATURES

After reading this chapter you will understand:
- The key elements in the intrinsic and extrinsic coagulation cascade.
- What protects the organism from unwanted coagulation.
- How to evaluate the preoperative patient for bleeding disorders and know which studies are indicated.
- Both congenital and acquired bleeding disorders.
- Appropriate heparin therapy.
- Disseminated intravascular coagulation.
- The approach to the bleeding patient.

Hemostasis is an essential component of any surgical procedure. The incised wound with its countless severed blood vessels requires both meticulous surgical technique and an intact hemostatic mechanism for control of bleeding. A breakdown in either element can result in failure of the operation and morbidity for the patient.

NORMAL HEMOSTASIS

Understanding the normal hemostatic process is an essential first step in detecting and managing congenital or acquired bleeding disorders. Four interconnected elements comprise the hemostatic mechanism: blood vessels, platelets, coagulation, and fibrinolysis.

Blood Vessels

Vascular endothelium is normally not thrombogenic, but when injured, it promotes deposition of platelets and of thrombin by several related mechanisms. When a blood vessel is severed, smooth muscle within its wall contracts, resulting in vasoconstriction. Capillary endothelium is also contractile. Exposure of subendothelial elements such as collagen permits adherence and aggregation of platelets, which form a primary hemostatic plug. Production of fibrin is also initiated and promoted by several locally active processes. It in turn reinforces the tenuous platelet plug (Fig. 47-1).

Platelets

Platelets become activated by contact with subendothelial elements, especially collagen, in the presence of the key plasma proteins, von Willebrand's factor, and fibrinogen. Adhesion of platelets to connective tissue results in a multitude of internal changes mediated by calcium, which enters the cell and is also released from intracellular storage sites. Contraction of the platelet produces a change in shape from discoid to spherical, with multiple filamentous projections. If the stimulus is of sufficient magnitude, intracellular granules release their contents (i.e., epinephrine, serotonin, adenine nucleotides, calcium, and platelet factor 4, a heparin antagonist), which are secreted externally. Activation of membrane phospholipases by calcium initiates

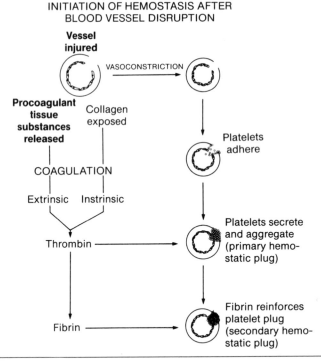

FIGURE 47-1 Formation of a primary and secondary hemostatic plug after blood vessel injury.

prostaglandin synthesis, which has profound effects on platelet activation and secretion. The substances released by adherent platelets recruit other platelets to aggregate and seal the endothelial defect, but this primary hemostatic plug is friable and must be reinforced by fibrin.

Blood Coagulation

Activation of the coagulation cascade enhances aggregation of platelets by thrombin-platelet interactions and by formation of a fibrin network to reinforce the weak platelet hemostatic plug. Coagulation is usually initiated by two distinct mechanisms that work concomitantly (Fig. 47-2).

The intrinsic pathway is activated by exposure of plasma to subendothelial material or by contact with a foreign surface. The extrinsic pathway is activated by tissue damage, with release of a procoagulant lipoprotein called *tissue factor*. The pathways converge with activation of factor X and are identical thereafter. There is crossover with activation of factor IX by the VIIa–tissue factor complex. Calcium and platelet factor 3 (a

name given to the procoagulant properties of the platelet surface, which favor the local concentration of activated clotting factors) are essential to these processes. Once fibrin is formed, it must be cross-linked for stability (a process accelerated by factor XIII).

Control Mechanisms and Fibrinolysis

The fluidity of blood is maintained by several mechanisms that prevent unwanted coagulation and dissolve thrombi once they are formed. The liver and other components of the reticulo-endothelial system remove activated coagulation factors and intermediate forms of fibrin polymers from the circulation. Plasma protease inhibitors neutralize activated coagulation factors. Thrombomodulin resides on vascular endothelium; in the presence of thrombin and calcium it accelerates the activation of protein C, which in turn acts with protein S to inactivate factors Va and VIIIa.

The fibrinolytic mechanism lyses thrombi once they are formed. Plasminogen, a protein

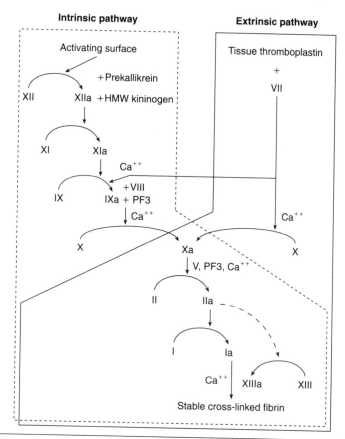

FIGURE 47-2 Intrinsic and extrinsic coagulation pathways demonstrating their convergence at Xa. *a* = activated; ***PF3*** = platelet factor 3; ***Ca*** $^{++}$ = calcium; ***HMW kininogen*** = high-molecular-weight kininogen; ***II*** = prothrombin; ***IIa*** = thrombin; *I* = fibrinogen; *Ia* = fibrin. (Modified from Brozovic M, Mibashan RS. Disorders of hemostasis in surgery. In Taylor SF [ed]. Recent Advances in Surgery, 9th ed. London, Churchill Livingstone, 1977.)

produced in the liver, is converted to its activated form, plasmin, under the influence of activators found in blood, other body fluids and tissues, and vascular endothelium. Once formed, plasmin cleaves fibrin(ogen) into multiple fragments called fibrinogen-fibrin degradation products (Fig. 47-3). Many of these products are themselves anticoagulants or lead to formation of a weak and ineffectual fibrin clot. Plasmin is inactivated by several plasma protease inhibitors and exerts most of its effect within the thrombus, where it is protected from circulating antiplasmins. Plasminogen is absorbed to the surface of newly formed clots, so most plasmin is released in proximity to fibrin. Plasmin is somewhat nonspecific, however, and can digest fibrinogen, factors II, V, and VIII, complement, and several hormones. It can also amplify coagulation by its effect on factor XII and can activate the kinin and complement systems. There are defenses against excessive production of plasmin, the most important of which may be alpha-2 plasmin inhibitor, a powerful circulating inhibitor. There are inhibitors of plasminogen activators, some of them also found on vascular endothelium. They are induced by interleukin-1, which may explain the prothrombotic effects of inflammation.

WHO SHOULD BE EVALUATED?

All patients undergoing a surgical operation or any significantly invasive procedure should be

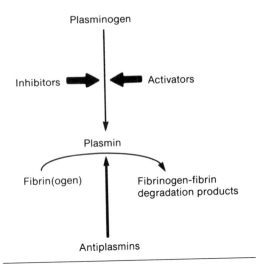

FIGURE 47-3 Fibrinolytic pathway with production of fibrinogen-fibrin degradation products.

evaluated for hemostatic function. Disagreement exists over the extent of such evaluation. Rapaport proposed a scheme that has gained wide acceptance but may not be truly practical. He proposed four patient groups. *Group 1* includes patients who have a reassuring history and physical examination who are to undergo relatively simple procedures without much bleeding expected. No laboratory screening is needed in these patients. *Group 2* patients also have a reassuring history and physical examination but are to undergo extensive surgical procedures, with the potential for significant loss of blood. A battery of hemostatic tests is proposed for such patients. Most retrospective studies have shown little or no useful information gained by such pre-operative screening in the presence of a reassuring history and physical examination. Although occasionally patients with significant hemostatic disorders not apparent on history and physical examination are detected by these tests, the incidence is very low and the expense very high. Screening in this group is commonly done but is almost always a waste of blood and money. *Groups 3 and 4* include patients who have either a history or physical examination suggesting disordered hemostasis or are to undergo procedures that mandate a completely intact hemostatic mechanism, that is, intervention in areas in which even small unexpected shedding of blood could be detrimental (eye, central nervous system); procedures that themselves impair hemo-

stasis (hypothermia, cardiopulmonary bypass, anticoagulation); or procedures that require or risk opening and closing large blood vessels or create large bleeding surfaces. Use of laboratory tests for screening such patients preoperatively seems rational. The disagreements thus exist concerning group 2, which is a large group of patients undergoing operative procedures.

METHODS OF EVALUATION
History and Physical Examination

Evaluation of the patient's hemostatic integrity should begin at the time illness is initially assessed. A thorough history should be obtained, including information about:

- Abnormal bleeding after injury, operation, childbirth, dental extractions
- Sustained bleeding after little or no trauma (e.g., nosebleeds, bleeding when brushing teeth, menorrhagia)
- Abnormal joint or muscle swelling after minor trauma
- Easy bruisability
- Drug ingestion, especially anticoagulants, drugs that alter platelet function, drugs that inhibit prostaglandin synthesis, and antibiotics
- Familial bleeding disorders

The physical examination may yield signs of a bleeding disorder. Petechiae, purpura, ecchymoses, telangiectases, splenomegaly, or swollen joints are noteworthy. Rarely, a previously undiagnosed patient with signs of cirrhosis or a collagen-vascular disease is discovered. When a bleeding problem is suspected, a thorough investigation must be undertaken before surgery can proceed.

Laboratory Tests of Hemostasis

Laboratory tests of hemostasis play an important part in screening preoperative patients, evaluating bleeding diatheses, and measuring the effects of various treatments.

Platelet Studies. Thrombocytopenia, whether congenital or acquired, may not be apparent if the patient has not been previously challenged by a significant injury. Therefore in the occasional preoperative patient who has not undergone such a challenge (which includes childbirth and dental extractions), the number of circulating platelets should be assessed. A blood smear showing six to 10 platelets per high-power field indicates adequate platelet numbers and obviates

TABLE 47-1 Factors Measured by PTT, PT, and TT and Conditions That Prolong These Tests

PTT	PTT Prolonged By	PT	PT Prolonged By	TT	TT Prolonged By
XII	Factor level	VII	Factor level		Fibrinogen
HMW-K*	decrease		decrease		decrease
Prekallikrein	Heparin		Oral anti-		Heparin
XI	Lupus anti-		coagulants		Dysfibrinogenemia
IX	coagulant		Specific factor		Fibrinogen-fibrin
VIII	Specific factor		antibodies		degradation
V	antibodies	V	Heparin		products
X	Oral anti-	X			
Prothrombin	coagulants	Prothrombin			
Fibrinogen		Fibrinogen		Fibrinogen	

*High-molecular-weight kininogen.

the need for a formal platelet count. *If the quantity of platelets is adequate but qualitative impairment is suspect (e.g., aspirin ingestion), a bleeding time evaluation should be performed.* The bleeding time is standardized by use of a template through which a superficial wound is made on the forearm while venous pressure is held constant at 40 mm Hg by a blood pressure cuff. The time until cessation of bleeding is measured and compared to that in normal individuals. Small details in technique are important in producing useful and reproducible results. The bleeding time assesses both vascular and platelet function but does not discriminate between the two. If the bleeding time is abnormal, further tests of platelet function can be done if circumstances warrant. Recently the accuracy and clinical utility of the bleeding time have been seriously questioned. Small abnormalities may be insignificant, but marked prolongation cannot be ignored. Platelet-aggregating agents such as adenosine diphosphate (ADP) can be added to platelet-rich plasma in vitro to test for characteristic patterns seen in patients with acquired and congenital platelet functional abnormalities.

Coagulation Studies. The *prothrombin time (PT),* in which a tissue extract (thromboplastin) is added to recalcified plasma, tests the extrinsic clotting mechanism (Table 47-1). The *activated partial thromboplastin time (PTT)* uses platelet-poor plasma to which calcium, phospholipid, and a surface-activating agent such as kaolin is added. The PTT measures activity of the intrinsic clotting mechanism. The *thrombin time (TT),* in which dilute thrombin is added to plasma, determines abnormalities in conversion of fibrinogen

to fibrin. The *whole-blood clotting time,* although simple and inexpensive, cannot be recommended because of its relative insensitivity. If abnormalities in PT, PTT, or TT are demonstrated, specific factor assays must be performed to identify the site of the hemostatic defect because specific replacement therapy is available.

Fibrinolytic Studies. Several tests are available to determine fibrinolytic activity, but most are indirect.

The *euglobulin lysis time* uses a fraction of plasma free of fibrinolytic inhibitors, thereby facilitating fibrinolysis. The results reflect the level of plasminogen in the original sample. *Fibrin plate lysis assays* can be modified to reflect the levels of plasminogen, plasmin, or plasmin inhibitors. The tests require 24 hours for completion unless more expensive radiolabeled substrates are used.

Other tests measure the presence of fibrin-fibrinogen degradation products by various indirect methods. More direct and precise assays for various products of fibrinolysis are being developed. They will be more quantitative and analytical and should provide better information on which to make decisions. Circulating anticoagulants are usually detected by mixing the patient's plasma with normal pooled plasma in various combinations.

CONGENITAL BLEEDING DISORDERS
Coagulation Defects

Inborn abnormalities of coagulation create lifelong bleeding problems. Functional defects of virtually all of the clotting factors have been described (but deficiency of factor XII does not lead to a bleeding tendency). Patients with inherited deficiencies often experience easy bruisability and delayed bleeding after minor trauma and may have life-threatening hemorrhage after larger injuries. Most common are the hemophilias (A and B) and von Willebrand's disease. Hemophilia A (classic hemophilia) and hemophilia B (Christmas disease) are sex-linked recessive disorders. The former has an incidence of 1 in 10,000 male births in the United States. Hemophilia A is seven to 10 times more common than hemophilia B.

In classic *hemophilia (A)* an abnormal factor VIII molecule is produced. The *PTT is elevated, but the bleeding time is normal.* Severity of the illness is directly proportional to factor VIII activity and may range from mild to severe. Hemophiliacs can pose diagnostic difficulties, for intra-abdominal hemorrhage may be clinically indistinguishable from other causes of abdominal pain, fever, and leukocytosis that require immediate operation such as appendicitis and intestinal necrosis. Often bleeding is controlled and symptoms relieved by infusion of factor VIII, and an ill-advised abdominal exploration can thus be avoided. *Factor VIII may be given as fresh frozen plasma (FFP), cryoprecipitate, or lyophilized concentrates.* The short plasma half-life of factor VIII (12 hours) and lability on storage make replacement therapy difficult. Levels of factor VIII adequate for hemostasis vary, depending on the severity of hemorrhage or the magnitude of the operation, but ones as high as 40% of normal for several days may be necessary with major operations. Replacement therapy is seriously complicated in roughly 6% of hemophiliacs by development of antibodies to factor VIII. The titer of this IgG antibody rises in response to infusion of factor VIII, thus frustrating efforts to raise factor VIII levels. In life-threatening emergencies large neutralizing doses of factor VIII may be used at the expense of a rise in antibody titer. Animal-derived factor VIII also may be used. Plasmapheresis to remove factor VIII antibody has been tried with some success. Administration of vitamin K–dependent factors (with presumed traces of activated factors) or, more recently, use of prothrombin complex concentrates screened for high thrombogenic activity has been successful.

Hemophilia B, or Christmas disease, is clinically indistinguishable from hemophilia A. It is characterized by a deficiency in factor IX activity. The *PTT is prolonged,* but again the *bleeding time is normal.* Providing replacement therapy is easier, since factor IX has a longer half-life (24 hours) and is stable on storage. Safe factor IX levels are similar to those required for factor VIII and may be obtained with FFP or lyophilized concentrates.

Von Willebrand's disease is due to a deficiency of the factor of the same name and results in impaired factor VIII activity and impaired platelet function. It is transmitted as an autosomal dominant and is the most common inherited coagulation disorder after hemophilia. Mild cases may manifest as easy bruisability, epistaxis, or menorrhagia, whereas severely affected individuals can present as do those with other hemophilia states—with joint and muscle bleeding or life-threatening retroperitoneal or gastrointestinal bleeding. Unlike the situation in hemophiliacs, the *PTT and the bleeding time are prolonged.* Transfusion of factor VIII transiently corrects the platelet defect, but, in contrast to hemophilia A, transfusion leads to a prolonged rise in factor VIII levels (72 hours) because of synthesis of new factor VIII from precursors found in the transfused plasma. FFP, cryoprecipitate, and many commercial factor VIII preparations contain both factor VIII and von Willebrand factor.

Use of plasma for treatment of factor deficiencies carries the usual risk of hepatitis. Newer methods of controlled heating may have eliminated the transmission of HIV in pooled coagulation concentrates, but not of hepatitis C. Sometimes other methods can reduce the exposure to donors. For example, administration of 1-desamino-8-D-arginine vasopressin (DDAVP) causes release of factor VIII from endothelial cells and boosts the circulatory level of the factor sufficiently to provide hemostasis in the presence of moderate challenges in patients with mild hemophilia A or von Willebrand's disease.

Platelet Defects

Congenital defects of platelet function present a clinical picture different from that of congenital coagulopathies (Table 47-2). In general, *purpuric states are not preceded by trauma,* and they occur in skin and mucosal areas. Patients are often only mildly affected and may experience a bleeding problem only after inadvertent ingestion of an antiplatelet drug or when coincident thrombocytopenia develops. *The bleeding time may or may not be prolonged,* depending on the severity of the disorder. A multitude of autosomal platelet defects has been described,

TABLE 47-2   Clinical Differences Between Congenital Platelet and Coagulation Defects

Clinical Characteristic	Coagulation Defect	Platelet Defect
Family history	Usually positive	Usually negative
Inheritance	Often sex linked	Not sex linked
Sex	Male predominance	Female predominance
Type of bleeding	Deep: muscles, joints, viscera	Superficial: skin, mucosa
Preceding trauma	Common	Uncommon
Coagulation tests	Abnormal	Normal
Bleeding time	Normal	Abnormal

and those of clinical importance fortunately are quite rare. Specific diagnosis rests on morphologic studies and characteristic responses to aggregating agents. Patients with such defects undergoing operations may require platelet transfusions perioperatively to maintain normal hemostasis.

Vascular Defects

Congenital abnormalities of the blood vessels themselves may be responsible for purpuric states, even if platelet function and coagulation are normal. Disorders such as hereditary hemorrhagic telangiectasia (Rendu-Osler-Weber disease), Ehlers-Danlos syndrome, pseudoxanthoma elasticum, and Marfan's syndrome can lead to spontaneous hemorrhage but are otherwise of little importance surgically.

ACQUIRED BLEEDING DISORDERS
Coagulation Defects

Acquired defects of hemostasis usually involve multiple rather than single components of the hemostatic mechanism. For example, *in severe liver disease (e.g., cirrhosis, hepatitis) all of the clotting factors may be reduced except for factor VIII, which is synthesized in endothelial cells.* Vitamin K–dependent factors, including prothrombin, VII, IX, and X, are most affected, whereas fibrinogen is reduced only in advanced cases. Failure of the liver to remove activators of plasminogen and hepatic production of pathologic plasminogen activators lead to increased fibrinolysis. The situation may be aggravated by failure of the liver to remove activated clotting factors from the circulation.

Correction of these hemostatic problems is difficult when bleeding occurs from varices, gas-

tritis, or peptic ulcer disease or when elective surgery is required. Replacement therapy with FFP, concentrated vitamin K–dependent factors, or exchange transfusion may be attempted, but the results are often poor.

Depletion of vitamin K–dependent clotting factors can occur with normal hepatic function. Vitamin K is formed by normal gut flora and is ingested in various foods. *With malnutrition, antibiotic sterilization of the gastrointestinal tract, or malabsorption (i.e., biliary obstruction or fistula, steatorrhea), vitamin K is depleted.* The PT and PTT are prolonged; however, they are quickly corrected in 8 to 12 hours by parenteral administration of vitamin K.

Antibodies are known to develop to specific clotting factors, particularly when there is a preexisting factor deficiency. These inhibitors prolong the PT or PTT and lead to bleeding complications. In addition to the antibody to factor VIII already described and seen also in nonhemophiliacs, inhibitors of factors V and VII and von Willebrand's factor have been detected. Antibodies usually develop after attempts at replacement therapy. Antibodies that are nonspecific are far more common and usually are not associated with significant surgical bleeding. The so-called lupus anticoagulant is an example of a nonspecific antibody. Paradoxically, this relatively common acquired "anticoagulant" is more often associated with thrombotic events.

Bleeding tendencies can be induced by anticoagulant drugs, which are used to treat thrombotic states. *Coumarin compounds inhibit the synthesis of vitamin K–dependent factors VII, IX, X, and prothrombin and also proteins C and S.* Clinical response is variable. Factor VII is first to decline (half-life, 5 hours), followed by factor IX (24 hours), factor X (40 hours), and prothrombin (72 hours). Thus development of the full anticoagulant effect may take 5 to 10 days despite prolongation of the PT before that time. Cessation of the drug results in restoration of factor levels in roughly the same order. Inadvertent coumarin excess can be treated by omitting the drug for several days until the PT once again falls to safe therapeutic levels (1½ times the control level). If the PT is greater than twice the control level or the patient is bleeding, FFP should be administered to restore coagulation to the safe range. Vitamin K used parenterally takes up to 12 hours to restore the PT to safe levels, yet its use may be desirable in patients with congestive heart failure who cannot tolerate the required volume of FFP infusions. Surgery usually can be safely performed if the PT is less than 1½ times the control level.

Heparin is a widely used anticoagulant that must be given parenterally. Heparin is a strongly anionic sulfated polysaccharide that binds to and activates a plasma cofactor, antithrombin III. Antithrombin III blocks several activated clotting factors: thrombin, XIIa, XIa, IXa, and Xa. Heparin is used when immediate anticoagulation is required in thrombotic states such as deep venous thrombosis, in pulmonary embolism, or during vascular surgery or cardiopulmonary bypass. Heparin can be rapidly reversed by protamine sulfate (1 mg protamine/100 U heparin), but because of its short plasma half-life, cessation of the drug alone usually is sufficient. *The PTT is most commonly used to monitor heparin therapy;* activated clotting time and protamine titration have also been used in cardiac surgery. The PTT may be more useful as a marker for achieving an anticoagulant effect than for indicating a danger of hemorrhage. Patients with deep venous thrombosis often seem resistant to initial doses of heparin. In such circumstances large initial doses (5000 to 10,000 U) may be needed to budge the PTT to 1½ to 2 times normal, a range for which many strive in adjusting the dose. A maintenance dose of 1000 to 3000 U/hr may be needed to maintain the PTT in this range for the first few days. Typically, the dose required then lessens. This temporal sequence may reflect low levels of antithrombin III soon after a major thrombotic event, with slow return to normal when the thrombosis is controlled.

Abnormal bleeding during the first 24 hours of administration of even large doses of heparin is unusual. *Bleeding after administration of heparin is incompletely related to dose and correlates poorly with laboratory tests* such as PTT used to "monitor" therapy. Continuous infusion of heparin is associated with a lower incidence of bleeding problems than is intermittent injection. Concurrent use of an anticoagulant or an antiplatelet drug is contraindicated because of the severe bleeding diatheses that can result. Use of heparin in patients with recent head injuries is particularly dangerous. There is increasing interest in the therapeutic use of low-molecular-weight fragments of heparin. Whether or not they have a lower incidence of bleeding complications remains unclear. Extensive evaluation is currently under way, especially in Europe.

Platelet Defects (Quantitative)

Thrombocytopenia can be caused by decreased production, increased destruction, sequestration, or dilution. Thrombocytopenia is one of the most common causes of acquired bleeding disorders, but the relationship between platelet count and clinical bleeding depends on several factors such as associated disorders and extent of injury. One of the most important factors is the functional status of the platelets. Moderate thrombocytopenia with impaired function may be much more dangerous than severe thrombocytopenia with good function. Young, large platelets tend to have excellent functional properties. Thrombocytopenia caused by accelerated destruction usually results in such a population and may have much less associated bleeding than lesser degrees of thrombocytopenia caused by impaired production, in which the circulating population tends to be senescent and hypofunctional. In most circumstances bleeding is rare if the platelet count exceeds 60,000/mm^3, but at levels of 10,000/mm^3 or less, major spontaneous central nervous system (CNS) or gastrointestinal hemorrhage can occur.

The surgeon may be called on to perform splenectomy in cases of hypersplenism or when the spleen is a site of platelet destruction in a patient with autoantibodies against platelets, (e.g., in idiopathic thrombocytopenic purpura [ITP]). Platelet transfusions (platelet-rich plasma [PRP] or platelet concentrates) are usually ineffective in raising the platelet count before splenectomy and need not be used routinely. Platelets should be available for transfusion if necessitated by profound thrombocytopenia or excessive bleeding intraoperatively, but they often are not needed if the rate of accelerated destruction is lessened by the procedure.

Platelet Defects (Qualitative)

Platelet function can be impaired in a myriad of ways. The most common cause is ingestion of a drug with antiplatelet effects. The preoperative history can often be misleading because of the danger of over-the-counter drugs containing aspirin of which the patient is unaware. *A single aspirin tablet, by irreversibly blocking prostaglandin synthesis, can prolong the bleeding time for up to 3 to 5 days.* The effect of other antiplatelet drugs such as dipyridamole, sulfinpyrazone, nonsteroidal anti-inflammatory agents, and antihistamines is less prolonged.

Solutions of dextran impair platelet aggregation by coating the platelet surface, forming complexes with plasma proteins necessary for coagulation and interfering with polymerization of fibrin. With doses above 1.5 g/kg, increased bleeding can occur.

Patients with renal failure have qualitative platelet abnormalities proportional to the degree of uremia. Although the precise defect is not known, platelet adhesiveness is clearly diminished, and levels of prostacyclin, a potent platelet inhibitor produced by vascular endothelium, are increased. Decreased platelet procoagulant activity impedes the coagulation cascade. Platelet transfusions are ineffective because they are quickly "poisoned" by the uremic milieu. Vigorous dialysis or renal transplantation can improve the platelet defect. Cryoprecipitate infusions have shown promise in shortening the bleeding time and transiently improving the bleeding tendency in patients with uremia. Cryoprecipitate may therefore be useful before invasive procedures or major surgery in uremic patients with severe bleeding tendencies. DDAVP also improves hemostasis in patients with renal failure.

Myeloproliferative diseases can result in functionally impaired platelets despite normal or even elevated platelet counts. Paraproteinemias also impair platelet function, most probably by physically coating the platelets.

Vascular Defects

Acquired vascular defects can cause purpuric states even when platelet function is normal. Immunoproliferative disorders producing abnormal proteins, drug toxicity, and allergic phenomena disrupt vascular integrity but rarely play a significant role in surgical hemostasis.

Mixed Coagulation and Platelet Defects

Disseminated intravascular coagulation (DIC) is an often catastrophic event *characterized by ongoing consumption of coagulation factors and platelets and concomitant fibrinolysis,* often widespread and uncontrolled. It occurs in several forms and settings. A subacute or chronic type is less dramatic and intense, is often associated with malignancies that produce thromboplastic material, and often responds to careful administration of heparin. The more acute forms are often much less easily characterized and controlled. Acute DIC can develop after the intravascular appearance of any of a host of thromboplastic materials. Conditions that can result in DIC include crush injury or burns; gram-negative and, less commonly, gram-positive bacterial or other (i.e., viral, malarial) infections; rapid intravascular hemolysis and vascular lesions such as vasculitides or hemangiomas; certain snake bites; and amniotic fluid embolism.

The patient often presents with purpuric lesions and bleeding from surgical wounds and intravenous sites and may develop gastrointestinal or genitourinary bleeding. Skin necrosis, peripheral gangrene, and renal necrosis can occur secondary to fibrin deposition in the microcirculation. *Diagnosis is confirmed by a characteristic blood smear with deformed red cells (schistocytes), low platelet count, prolonged PT, PTT, and TT, low fibrinogen levels, and high levels of fibrinogen-fibrin degradation products. Antithrombin III levels are usually reduced.*

When DIC apparently has a specific cause, treatment is aimed at removing the inciting cause, if possible. When DIC persists despite removal of the triggering event, heparin can be used to arrest the clotting process in the simpler forms of the disease. Often as little as 1000 U/hr is corrective. Laboratory abnormalities begin to abate after 2 to 3 hours of therapy, and bleeding usually slows or ceases shortly thereafter. Mini-heparin administration (2500 to 5000 U subcutaneously every 8 to 12 hours) may be as effective as full-dose heparin administration and has the advantage of fewer bleeding complications. When both heparin therapy and removal of the precipitating event fail to arrest DIC, replacement therapy with platelets and FFP or cryoprecipitate should be carried out. Continued failure of therapy may be due to residual fibrinogenolysis.

A particularly distressing form is the acute

DIC that occurs after serious injury or during extensive operations. It often seems multifactorial and involves hypoperfusion and damaged tissue. A prolonged period of restored perfusion and good hepatic function seems necessary to correct the process.

Fibrinolysis is a normal response to intravascular fibrin formation. In patients with DIC in whom coagulation may be massive, fibrinolysis usually is brisk and may deplete stores of fibrinogen and other clotting factors. Fibrinogen-fibrin degradation products act as anticoagulants themselves and help protect against further thrombosis. Attempts to impede fibrinolysis with such agents as epsilon-aminocaproic acid in the presence of ongoing intravascular coagulation can lead to catastrophic thrombotic complications, including unlysable clots in the genitourinary system and pulmonary embolism. *Inhibitors of fibrinolysis should be used with extreme caution, and heparin should always be used concomitantly.* Fibrinolysis rarely occurs as an isolated hemostatic derangement; for the most part it is an appropriate and protective response to the formation of fibrin.

Massive transfusion can lead to mixed platelet and coagulation factor deficiencies. Platelets lose function quickly after storage with red cells, and dilutional thrombocytopenia can occur after transfusion of several blood volumes of such blood. Fresh whole blood, PRP, or platelet concentrates can be used for replacement if needed. Prophylactic administration of platelets during massive transfusion has been proved unnecessary. Banked blood also lacks factors V and VIII, which are highly labile on storage (40% at 1 week). If mobilization of body stores or synthesis is impaired (e.g., with liver disease), these factors can be replaced with fresh whole blood or FFP. If both platelets and coagulation factors are needed, administering fresh whole blood or PRP is ideal. Again, prophylactic use is almost certainly unnecessary.

Another complex abnormality of both platelets and clotting factors is that associated with *cardiopulmonary bypass.* Roughly 4% of all patients undergoing *cardiopulmonary bypass* for open heart surgery have undue blood loss, and half of them have a definable hemostatic disorder. Coagulopathies occur secondary to *inadequate anticoagulation with heparin,* which leads to fibrin production and fibrinogen depletion. Fibrinolysis with generation of fibrinogen-fibrin degradation products may worsen bleeding, but a full-blown picture of DIC is uncommon. Excessive heparin administration or inadequate neutralization with protamine can also create a bleeding diathesis. A defect in platelet function is also common.

WHAT IS THE APPROACH TO THE BLEEDING PATIENT?

The first approach to massive bleeding should be to stop the bleeding. A rapid rate of bleeding usually requires a mechanical approach to hemostasis—immediate and rapid surgical, endoscopic, or radiologic control is chosen, depending on the circumstances. Evaluation and concern for possibly abnormal hemostatic mechanisms should be a distant second. The most common cause of intraoperative, postoperative, and post-traumatic significant hemorrhage is defective mechanical hemostasis, that is, "surgical" bleeding. No amount of coagulation components and platelets will alter such bleeding. If the injuries are great enough, a surgeon must stop them. One of the clues that this is the case is a rapid rate of bleeding. Another is relatively normal test results of coagulation and platelet count or function. (Small abnormalities commonly result from extensive transfusion or extensive tissue damage and cannot account for the bleeding described.) Even with significant abnormalities on laboratory evaluation, poor mechanical hemostasis is still possible and must always be considered, but specific correction of the defect(s), guided by appropriate laboratory studies and assisted by expert help, becomes necessary. Table 47-3 lists the pattern of abnormalities seen in various bleeding states. Once a definitive diagnosis is made, prompt therapy can be instituted.

Replacement of lost volume must be carried out at the same time, often requiring use of several sites of venous access, which must be of sufficient size. With exsanguinating hemor-

---

TREATMENT OF MASSIVE BLEEDING

1. Stop the hemorrhage.
2. Replace lost volume and red cells.
3. Replace hemostatic and coagulation components indicated by significantly abnormal laboratory tests (see Table 47-4) and/ or by clinically evident impaired hemostasis and coagulation.

rhage, infusion of red cells is mandatory; this may require use of uncrossmatched type O red cells. Too often administration of red cells is delayed until the dilutional anemia is so severe that resuscitation becomes difficult on those grounds alone. Hematocrit values less than 20% should be avoided if possible. Precious intravenous sites should not be used for prophylactic administra-

tion of platelets or coagulation factors. There is little evidence that these factors are beneficial, and exsanguinating patients need volume and red cells much more urgently. Replacement of components should be guided by appropriate laboratory tests and clinical evidence of impaired coagulation on hemostasis (see box and Table 47-4).

TABLE 47-3   Use of Screening Tests to Diagnose Acute Surgical Bleeding Disorders

Diagnosis	Platelet Count	Bleeding Time	PT	PTT	TT	Fibrin-ogen	Fibrino-lysis	Factor Assays
Massive transfusion	↓	↑	↑	↑	N	N	Absent	↓ V, VIII
DIC	↓	↑	↑	↑	↑	↓	Usually present	↓ Multiple factors
Fibrinolysis	N	N	↑	↑	↑	↓	Present	Fibrinogen
Heparin	N	N	↑	↑	↑	N	N	Normal
Congenital coagulation disorder	N	N	N or ↑	N or ↑	N or ↑	N or ↓	N	↓ Specific factor
Congenital platelet defect	N	↑	N	N	N	N	N	Normal (except in von Willebrand's disease)

↑ = prolonged; ↓ = decreased; N = normal.

TABLE 47-4   Laboratory Screening

Test	Replacement	Goal
Periodic hematocrit determination	RBC	Keep above 20%
Platelet counts	Platelet concentration	Keep above 50,000/μL
PT, PTT	FFP	Keep below 1½ times normal
Fibrinogen determination	FFP, cryoprecipitate	Keep above 200 mg/dl
Fibrin-fibrinogen split products	—	Markedly increased levels suggest DIC

RBC = red blood cells; FFP = fresh frozen plasma.

SURGICAL PHARMACOPEIA

Drug	Indications	Complications	Dosage
Heparin sodium	Rapid anticoagulation in thromboembolic disease, vascular and cardiac surgery, DVT prophylaxis	Hemorrhage and thrombocytopenia	5000 U IV bolus, then 1000-3000 U/hr to achieve PTT at 1.5 to 2 × control value; 5000 U subcutaneously q12h
Warfarin sodium (Coumadin)	Chronic anticoagulation following thrombo-embolic event	Hemorrhage	5-10 mg/day PO to achieve PT at 1.5 to 2 × control value
Protamine sulfate	Heparin antidote	Anticoagulant effect if dose is excessive	1 mg/100 U IV heparin
Vitamin K	Vitamin K deficiency and/or liver disease with elevated PT	Hypotension/anaphylaxis with IV administration	10 mg/day PO/IM × 3 days
DDAVUP	Uremia, von Willebrand's disease, following cardiac bypass surgery	Mild vasodilation, tachyphylaxis	$0.3\ \mu g/kg$ over 30 min
Dextran	Possible benefit as antiplatelet agent in vascular surgery	Bleeding, CHF, renal failure	20 ml/hr up to 3 days
Aspirin	Cerebrovascular and coronary artery disease	Gastritis, peptic ulcer disease, hemorrhage	100-300 mg/day

BIBLIOGRAPHY

Bloom AL. Physiology of blood coagulation. Hemostasis 20 (suppl 1):14, 1990.

Collins JA. Recent developments in the area of massive transfusion. World J Surg 11:75, 1987.

Esmon CT. Regulation of blood coagulation. J Biol Chem 264:4743, 1989.

Furie B, Furie BC. The molecular basis of blood coagulation. Cell 53:505, 1988.

Muller-Berghaus G. Pathophysiologic and biochemical events in disseminated intravascular coagulation: Dysregulation of procoagulant and anticoagulant pathways. Semin Thromb Hemost 15:58, 1989.

Nemerson Y. Tissue factor and hemostasis. Blood 71:1, 1988.

Rapaport SI. Preoperative hemostatic evaluations: Which tests, if any? Blood 61:229, 1983.

Reed RL, Heimbach DM, Counts RB, et al. Prophylactic platelet administration during massive transfusion. Ann Surg 203:40, 1986.

Rodgers RPC, Levin J. A critical reappraisal of the bleeding time. Semin Thromb Hemost 16:1, 1990.

CHAPTER REVIEW
Questions

1. All of the following statements are true regarding platelets *except:*
   a. Anucleate, discoid cells 2 to 3 μm in diameter
   b. Release ADP, epinephrine, serotonin from intracellular granules
   c. Life span in circulation 20 days
   d. Labile on storage
2. Which of the following tests are too insensitive for meaningful clinical use?
   a. Thrombin time
   b. Euglobulin lysis time
   c. Fibrin(ogen) degradation products
   d. Whole-blood clotting time
3. All of the following drugs have a reversible effect on platelets *except:*
   a. Aspirin
   b. Dipyridamole
   c. Sulfinpyrazone
   d. Indomethacin
   e. Dextran
4. List three mechanisms that prevent unwanted coagulation.
5. What is an indication for a preoperative bleeding time?
6. Describe the bleeding time and PTT in patients with hemophilia A, hemophilia B, and von Willebrand's disease.
7. List three abnormalities in coagulation associated with cardiopulmonary bypass.

True or false:
8. The platelet defect in patients with uremia cannot be improved with hemodialysis.
9. Massive transfusion may prolong the PT and PTT, but fibrinogen levels and TT are usually normal.
10. Warfarin effect is considered therapeutic as soon as the PT begins to rise above control levels.

Answers

1. c
2. d
3. a
4. a. Reticuloendothelial system removes activated coagulation factors.
   b. Plasma protease inhibitors neutralize activated coagulation factors.
   c. Fibrinolysis.
5. Suspected qualitative impairment of platelets
6. Hemophilia A and B: PTT is increased, and bleeding time is normal; von Willebrand's disease: PTT is increased and bleeding time is prolonged.
7. a. Inadequate heparin use
   b. Excessive heparin use or inadequate neutralization with protamine
   c. Platelet function defect
8. False
9. True
10. False

48

Critical Care

MICHAEL D. PASQUALE
FRANK B. CERRA

KEY FEATURES

After reading this chapter you will understand:

- The principles that govern the management of the critically ill surgical patient.
- How oxygen transport can be restored.
- All types of respiratory support.
- How oxygen delivery can be improved with the use of cardiac monitoring.
- The important factors in determining survival.
- The key factors that affect multiple organ failure.

Critical care has evolved in parallel with advances in surgery and medicine. This evolution can be traced back to the 1920s when the first recovery rooms were developed to care for postoperative patients. They were followed in the early 1950s by respiratory care units, originally designed for the care of poliomyelitis patients. In the late 1950s the first shock unit was developed, and in 1962 the first coronary care unit came into existence. Since that time a variety of special care units have been developed to support the postoperative patient.

Modern critical care depends on the 24-hour, on-site commitment of physicians, nurses, and health care personnel who are qualified to provide life support management. *Data suggest that postoperative deaths may be caused by physiologic problems that can be identified, described, predicted, and prevented.* Therapy for the critically ill should be defined by physiologic criteria,

and administration of therapy should be monitored to attain, prophylactically or therapeutically, optimal physiologic goals. With a combination of *source control, restoration of oxygen transport,* and *metabolic support,* there has been significant improvement in the survival rate of the critically ill patient.

Once an airway is established and ventilation assured, source control becomes the highest priority; that is, hemorrhage must be controlled, abscesses must be drained, and infection must be treated. Once source control is achieved, oxygen transport must be restored. In general, *oxygen transport depends on the integration and regulation of the lungs, circulation, and blood components.* After restoration of oxygen transport, the physician must deal with supporting the critically ill patient's metabolism.

The topics of source control and metabolic support are dealt with at length in other chapters of this text and are mentioned here only in the context of how to approach the critically ill patient. This chapter focuses on the restoration of oxygen transport through regulation of the lungs, the circulation, and the blood.

VENTILATORY SUPPORT

Before invasive hemodynamic monitoring of a critically ill patient is begun, the airway should be stabilized and adequate respiratory support provided. Respiratory injury in surgical patients is usually acute in onset and is associated with a number of primary disease processes. The initial cause of respiratory injury varies according to the disease involved; however, the final physiologic and clinical manifestations are remarkably constant. Whether respiratory failure results from an inadequate airway patency, inadequate airway protection, poor pulmonary toilet, or parenchymal injury, the final pathway is either hypoxemic, hypercarbic, or hypoxemic-hypercarbic respiratory failure. Acute respiratory failure, by definition, requires that mechanical ventilatory support be initiated.

The decision as to whether a patient is in respiratory failure and requires ventilatory support *should be based on clinical judgment combined with assessment of the patient's pulmonary status.* Indications for such support vary according to the acuity of onset of respiratory failure, the underlying disease pathology, and the patient's prognosis. Clinically, parameters have been established to evaluate tissue oxygenation, gas exchange, and the mechanics of ventilation (Table 48-1). Using these evaluations, several criteria for the diagnosis of acute respiratory failure and the need for mechanical ventilatory support have been established (Table 48-2). Others have shown that the work of breathing is more predictive in assessing the need for ventilatory support (total work is normally less than 1 kg/m/min; if greater than 1.7 kg/m/min, support is indicated).

Once the decision to intubate the patient has

TABLE 48-1 Assessing Pulmonary Function

Parameter	Derivation	Normal Value
Oxygenation Parameters		
Arterial O_2 content	$1.34 \times Hb \times Sao_2 + (0.003 \times Pao_2)$	$Cao_2 = 20$ ml/dl
Mixed venous O_2 content	$1.34 \times Hb \times Svo_2 + (0.003 \times Pvo_2)$	$Cvo_2 = 15$ ml/dl
Arteriovenous O_2 difference	$Cao_2 - Cvo_2$	$C(a\text{-}v)o_2 = 5$ ml/dl
Fractional O_2 extraction	$C(a\text{-}v)o_2/Cao_2$	0.25
Cardiac index (CI)	CO/BSA	$CI = 3$ L/min/m^2
Oxygen delivery	$Cao_2 \times CI$	$Do_2 = 600$ cc/min/m^2
Oxygen consumption	$C(a\text{-}v)o_2 \times CI$	$Vo_2 = 150$ cc/min/m^2
Carbon dioxide consumption	Direct measurement	$Vco_2 = 120$ cc/min/m^2
Respiratory quotient (RQ)	Vco_2/Vo_2	$RQ = 0.8$
Gas Exchange Parameters		
Arterial O_2 pressure	Direct measurement	$Pao_2 = 90$ mm Hg (room air)
Arterial CO_2 pressure	Direct measurement	$Paco_2 = 40$ mm Hg
Mixed venous O_2 pressure	Direct measurement	$Pvo_2 = 40$ mm Hg
		(varies at Vo_2)
Alveolar CO_2 pressure	Direct measurement	$Paco_2 = 40$ mm Hg
Alveolar O_2 pressure	$(PB - PH_2O)(Fio_2) - Paco_2/0.8$	$Pao_2 = 100$ mm Hg (room air)
		$= 650$ mm Hg ($Fio_2 = 1$)
Alveolar-arterial O_2 difference	$Pao_2 - Pao_2$	$(A\text{-}a)Do_2 = 50$ mm Hg
		($Fio_2 = 1$)
Arterial O_2 saturation	Direct measurement	$Sao_2 = 95\%$ (room air)
Mixed venous O_2 saturation	Direct measurement	$Svo_2 = 75\%$ (room air)
		(varies at Vo_2)
Shunt	$(Cco_2 - Cao_2)/(Cco_2 - Cvo_2)$	$Qs/Qt = 6\%$
Ventilation Parameters		
Tidal volume	Direct measurement	$VT = 5$ cc/kg
Vital capacity	Direct measurement	$VC = 70$ cc/kg
Functional residual capacity	Direct measurement	$FRC = 35$ cc/kg
Inspiratory force	Direct measurement	$NIF = -100$ cm H_2O
Dynamic compliance	$VT/(PIP - PEEP)$	$C_{dyn} = 70$ cc/cm H_2O
Static compliance	$VT/(\text{Pause pressure} - PEEP)$	$C_{st} = 100$ cc/cm H_2O

CO = cardiac output; BSA = body surface area; NIF = negative inspiratory force; PIP = peak inspiratory pressure.

TABLE 48-2 Criteria of Need for Ventilatory Support*

Parameter	Normal Range	Respiratory Failure
Respiratory rate	12-20/min	>35/min
Vital capacity (cc/kg)	65-75	<15
FEV_1 (ml/kg)	50-60	<10
Inspiratory force (cm H_2O)	−75 to −100	>−25
Compliance (cc/cm H_2O)	100	<20
Pao_2 (mm Hg)	80-95 (room air)	<60
$(A-a)Do_2$ (mm Hg at $Fio_2 = 1$)	25-65	>450
Shunt (%)	5-8	>20
$Paco_2$ (mm Hg)	35-45	>55 (no history of chronic obstructive pulmonary disease [COPD])
Vd/Vt	0.2-0.3	>0.6

*Mechanical ventilatory support may be used to achieve deliberate hyperventilation in patients with increased intracranial pressure and with tricyclic antidepressant overdose. Also, patients at increased risk of respiratory failure (i.e., with obesity, COPD, neuromuscular disorders, and shock) may be prophylactically mechanically ventilated postoperatively.

been made, the question of which route of intubation to use arises. The tube selected should be of sufficient size (i.e., ≥7 mm internal diameter) to allow for adequate suctioning while minimizing the airflow resistance. Orotracheal intubation is usually easier to perform than nasotracheal intubation and does not require that the patient be breathing spontaneously. Disadvantages of orotracheal intubation are that the neck usually must be hyperextended and the tube is less comfortable and less easily secured than is a nasotracheal tube. Nasotracheal intubation, on the other hand, can be done blindly with the neck in the neutral position. Longer, more narrow tubes are required. This route tends to provide better comfort for the patient, and the tube is more easily secured. Pulmonary toilet is decreased because of the narrower tube, and the possibility for nasal hemorrhage and sinusitis exists. Tracheotomy or cricothyroidotomy may also be used to establish an airway. This involves an operative procedure; however, the tracheostomy tube is comfortable and provides a means for good pulmonary toilet.

Conventional positive pressure ventilation increases the intra-alveolar pressure relative to pleural pressure, leading to lung expansion and expansion of the chest wall. The conventional management of acute respiratory failure entails endotracheal intubation and intermittent positive pressure ventilation using a mechanical ventilator that delivers tidal volumes greater than anatomic dead space. *The goals of positive pressure ventilation are:*

1. To correct hypoxemia
2. To prevent and reverse significant respiratory acidosis
3. To allow time for recovery of respiratory muscles and diaphragmatic function in a patient with obstructive lung disease
4. To allow time for institution of therapies and for treatment of the underlying disease processes.

This ventilatory technique, used most commonly in the intensive care unit (ICU), has evolved from surgical and anesthetic practice and has not changed substantially in the past 20 years. In the perioperative period the use of flow-controlled, volume-preset ventilation and large tidal volumes (10 to 15 cc/kg) has been advocated to help patients with normal lung mechanics and to prevent the microatelectasis that accompanies shallow breathing. Sufficient positive end-expiratory pressure is used to prevent desaturation of arterial blood, and the respiratory rate is adjusted to normalize pH and the partial pressure of carbon dioxide (Pco_2). These "older" standard modes of conventional positive pressure ventilation are shown in the box on p. 789 and are described below.

Control Mode Ventilation. In the control mode the ventilator delivers a preset tidal volume at a preset frequency. It is suitable only for patients who are apneic as a result of conditions such as respiratory muscle paralysis, sedation, drug overdose, or brain damage. The patient must work excessively to generate a spontaneous

OPTIONS FOR ACHIEVING ADEQUATE GAS EXCHANGE

Conventional Positive Pressure Ventilation (CPPV): Standard

Control mode ventilation
Assist-control mode ventilation
Synchronous intermittent mandatory ventilation
Continuous positive airway pressure
Positive end-expiratory pressure
Independent lung ventilation

CPPV: Alternate Modes

Inverse ratio ventilation
Airway pressure release ventilation
Pressure support ventilation
Proportional assist ventilation
Mandatory minute volume

Nonconventional Techniques

High-frequency ventilation
Constant flow ventilation
Extracorporeal membrane oxygenation
Extracorporeal carbon dioxide removal

breath, and if this mode is used in patients with airflow obstruction, dynamic hyperinflation and hemodynamic compromise can result.

Assist-Control Mode Ventilation. With the assist-control mode the ventilator provides preset tidal volumes in response to a patient's initiated effort to take a breath, and there is a preset back-up rate if no patient effort occurs. This is used as an initial mode of mechanical ventilation. The patient still is required to initiate the breath, and the patient must work to trigger the ventilator.

Synchronous Intermittent Mandatory Ventilation (SIMV). In this mode of ventilation the patient can breathe spontaneously; in addition, he or she receives a number of mechanical breaths with preset tidal volumes and at a preset rate. This mode may be used as a primary means of ventilator support or as a weaning method. During SIMV the interspersion of spontaneous breaths between machine breaths can result in more uniform intrapulmonary gas distribution. Lower mean airway pressures have also been demonstrated, when compared with those with control mode ventilation and assist-control mode ventilation. Weaning with SIMV does not necessitate changing the breathing circuit. SIMV

incorporates a demand valve that must be patient activated with each spontaneous breath and that allows delivery of the mechanical breath in concert with the patient's effort. Note that the patient still must work to initiate the breath and that minute ventilation is a combination of the effort of both the machine and the patient.

Continuous Positive Airway Pressure (CPAP). Positive pressure is maintained throughout the breathing cycle and thus functions to decrease the work of breathing. CPAP may be used as a primary ventilator mode in patients and also may be used in transition from mechanical to spontaneous breathing. There is no set delivered tidal volume or frequency.

Positive End-Expiratory Pressure (PEEP). PEEP refers to maintenance of positive pressure throughout the expiratory cycle to prevent the return of airway pressures to atmospheric pressure at end expiration. This serves to keep terminal bronchioles open and thus maintain or increase functional residual capacity (FRC). The criterion for instituting PEEP is generally hypoxia, and as a general rule, *the lowest PEEP to achieve an arterial oxygen pressure (Pao_2) of greater than 60 mm Hg at a fraction of inspired oxygen (Fio_2) of less than 0.5 without compromising oxygen delivery* is used. The main drawbacks of PEEP are associated barotrauma and a decrease in venous return.

Independent Lung Ventilation. Independent lung ventilation is a mode of support that physically separates the ventilation to each lung. It is used in patients with unilateral parenchymal lung disease in whom adequate oxygenation cannot be achieved with more conventional ventilation methods. Double-lumen tubes are used and are narrower; thus increased airway resistance and difficulty in clearing secretions may pose a problem. Two ventilators are required and must be synchronized.

■ ■ ■

Heightened awareness of the hazards of mechanical ventilation has caused many to question the use of high pressures to optimize arterial blood gas amounts. Alternative modes of conventional positive pressure ventilation have been developed in an attempt to limit pressure applied to the lung while optimizing gas exchange. These alternate modes have been used to correct gas exchange abnormalities when conventional positive pressure ventilation fails, reduce the risk of barotrauma, reduce hemodynamic compromise, enhance patient comfort, and facilitate weaning. These alternate modes of conventional positive pressure ventilation are shown in the box on p. 789 and are discussed in the following sections.

Inverse Ratio Ventilation. This is a pressure-controlled mode in which inspiratory time exceeds expiratory time, and it is used to recruit collapsed alveoli progressively and to prevent recollapse. In general, low tidal volumes and high respiratory rates are used to achieve the pressure goals, or the preset pressure maximal rate limits the tidal volume, with the minute ventilation met by an increasing rate. An inspiration:expiration (I/E) ratio greater than 1:1 during inverse ratio ventilation will impose an unnatural breathing pattern and cause discomfort. Thus these patients require sedation and/or induction of paralysis. Data showing this mode's benefit over that of conventional positive pressure ventilation are currently insufficient. With a high I/E ratio and high-frequency ventilation, there may be inducement of intrinsic PEEP, which will serve to keep alveoli open at the expense of higher mean airway pressures.

Airway Pressure Release Ventilation. In this mode continuous positive airway pressure ventilation is delivered, and the pressure intermittently decreases or releases from the preset level to either a lower level or ambient pressure. With this reduction in airway pressure, gas is allowed to leave the lungs, and carbon dioxide is eliminated. The goal of this mode of ventilation is to recruit alveoli and thereby improve oxygenation. Because of short pressure release times, inversion of the I/E ratio may result, causing patient discomfort. The release must be timed so that it occurs during expiration. To date, this mode appears more effective in improving alveolar ventilation and decreasing peak airway pressure when compared to results with conventional positive pressure ventilation.

Pressure Support Ventilation. With this mode of ventilation the ventilator delivers a preset pressure and allows the patient to determine the ultimate flow, tidal volume, inspiratory time, and frequency. The patient triggers a preset pressure sensor that allows flow of gas so that the system rapidly approaches the preset pressure level. This pressure support level is maintained until the patient's inspiratory flow decreases to a specified level (25% of peak flow or approximately 5 L/min) at which time exhalation occurs. Pressure support ventilation requires an intact respiratory drive and stable respiratory system impedance when used as the sole ventilator support. However, in patients with highly unstable respiratory drives or changeable respiratory system impedance, use of pressure support ventilation is not advisable unless backed by volume-cycled breaths because in these situations pressure support ventilation delivers variable flows. Note that with in-line nebulization treatments, patients may fail to trigger the pressure-limited breath.

Proportional Assist Ventilation. This is a closed loop positive pressure ventilation in which the ventilator changes pressure at the airway in proportion to the inspired volume (elastic assist), inspired flow (resistive assist), or both. Gain controls on the flow and volume signals determine the proportionality and therefore the degree of elastic or resistive unloading. Proportional assist ventilation unloads the patient's inspiratory work without altering the patient's breathing pattern. Although in the preliminary stage of development, proportional assist ventilation appears to have great potential because the ventilator responds automatically to varying metabolic needs, peak airway pressures are reduced, synchrony between the ventilator output and the patient's effort is achieved, and there is decreased potential for muscle atrophy. This mode cannot be used if the patient is apneic because the ventilator requires feedback from the patient.

Mandatory Minute Volume. This is a closed loop ventilation method that allows the patient to breathe spontaneously. It provides a guaranteed minute ventilation that is preset by the physician. The ventilator does not provide any assistance until the patient's minute ventilation falls below this preset level. The quality of the spontaneous minute volume is not evaluated; hence minute volume achieved by rapid shallow breathing is indistinguishable from the minute volume induced by slow deep breathing.

■　■　■

Although many modes of positive pressure ventilation have been described, the goals remain the same in all cases. Depending on patient size, clinical condition, and mode of ventilatory support, the ventilatory settings will change. The physician must set the inspired oxygen concentration, delivered tidal volume, specified respiratory rate, I/E ratio, amount of PEEP, amount of humidification, and the alarms. *The ultimate goals are an inspired oxygen concentration of less than or equal to 0.5, saturation of hemoglobin greater than 90%, peak airway pressures less than or equal to 40 cm H$_2$O, mean airway pressures less than or equal to 30 cm H$_2$O, and a pH between 7.35 and 7.50.*

The use of airway pressure therapy serves to optimize pulmonary gas exchange and minimize physiologic stress. Its use, however, may also be associated with side effects and/or complications (see the box below). Positive airway pressure potentially can decrease venous return, lower cardiac output and blood pressure, and actually worsen the ventilation-perfusion inequalities. The pulmonary and cardiovascular systems do not function as clinically separate entities. The hemodynamic effects of positive pressure ventilation can be interpreted with regard to the balance of effects on the right and left ventricular preloads and afterloads. Accordingly, determining baseline intravascular volume, cardiac function, and pulmonary mechanics before the positive pressure ventilation is important in evaluating the hemodynamic response. During positive pressure ventilation, the preload decreases because of a decrease in systemic venous return associated with the increase in intrathoracic pressure. Also, the heart is compressed within the cardiac fossa, decreasing its compliance. In addition, increases in lung volume and increases in alveolar pressure impede right ventricular outflow by increasing pulmonary vascular resistance. This may lead to dilation of the right ventricle and shift the interventricular septum toward the left, thus decreasing the compliance of the left ventricle. The combined effects lead to a decrease in left ventricular stroke volume for a given pulmonary artery pressure.

The barotrauma that is associated with airway pressure therapy allows alveolar gas to leak out of the lung parenchyma with resultant interstitial emphysema, pneumomediastinum, subcutaneous emphysema, pneumoperitoneum, and pneumothorax. The positive pressure can also injure the alveolar lining and worsen the lung injury. The physician should be aware of possible pulmonary infection, gastrointestinal bleeding, renal dysfunction, and psychologic stress.

The sedation or paralysis or both that may be required in patients treated with conventional positive pressure ventilation help decrease airway pressures by preventing agitation and keeping the patient from working against the ventilator, but they also decrease and/or eliminate respiratory drive, obscure physical examination, and prevent adequate mobilization of the patient.

■ ■ ■

Conventional positive pressure ventilation has been very effective in the treatment of many forms of respiratory failure and in improving gas exchange; however, it is associated with a num-

---

COMPLICATIONS OF VENTILATOR SUPPORT

Related to Endotracheal or Tracheostomy Tube

Intubation of mainstem bronchus (usually on right side)
Kinking of tube
Laryngeal hematoma and/or stenosis
Nasal bleeding and/or necrosis
Pharyngeal trauma and/or tooth avulsion
Airway colonization with subsequent pneumonia
Tracheal ulceration and/or subglottic stenosis
Sinusitis and/or otitis (usually with nasal intubation)
Tracheoesophageal fistula
Vocal cord injury

Related to Pulmonary Barotrauma

Arterial and/or venous air embolus
Pneumomediastinum, pneumothorax, pneumopericardium, pneumoperitoneum
Subcutaneous emphysema

Related to Cardiovascular Hemodynamics

Regional hypoperfusion with increased pulmonary vascular resistance
Impairment of preload as a result of decreased venous return with subsequent decrease in cardiac output
Decrease in renal blood flow with redistribution of flow from cortical to medullary areas (decreased glomerular filtration rate)

Other

Oxygen toxicity
Mechanical failure of ventilator

ber of hemodynamic and pulmonary complications. Also, experimental evidence suggests that large tidal volumes may produce or even worsen preexisting lung injury. In addition to the modalities mentioned and to provide support when conventional positive pressure ventilation fails, several nonconventional techniques of pulmonary support have been developed (see the box on p. 789). These techniques tend to use lower tidal volumes and lower airway pressures.

High-Frequency Ventilation. High-frequency positive pressure ventilation uses a pneumatic valve system to deliver compressed gas during inspiration while allowing passive expiration. The usual ventilator frequency is set at 60 to 120 breaths per minute with tidal volumes of 3 to 5 ml/kg and an I/E ratio of less than 0.3. High-frequency jet ventilation is a high-frequency mode in which gas is delivered under high pressures (15 to 50 psi) through a small-bore cannula (14 to 18 g) at a tidal volume of 2 to 5 ml/kg, with a frequency of 100 to 600 times per minute and an I/E ratio of 1:2 to 1:8. The jet of gas produced enters the airway at high velocity and entrains gas from the surrounding airways. Expiration is passive, and PEEP may be added. In general, increasing the airway pressure produces an increase in the tidal volume, resulting in increases in alveolar ventilation; however, use of this method may result in increased mean airway pressures and FRC because of flow limitations. At a constant driving pressure, increasing the frequency or decreasing the I/E ratio will decrease the alveolar ventilation because of a decrease in tidal volume. Increasing the frequency also leads to an increase in gas trapping. High-frequency oscillation is a mode of high-frequency ventilation in which gas is forced into the lungs during inspiration and drawn out of the lungs during expiration. The gas is delivered at a frequency of 60 to 3600 cycles per minute, with a tidal volume of 1 to 3 cc/kg.

Theoretically, gas exchange in the setting of these small tidal volumes occurs by convection and molecular diffusion. The PaO_2 is determined by the FRC. High-frequency ventilation has been used successfully in patients undergoing pneumonectomy and in patients with bronchopleural fistulas. In patients with adult respiratory distress syndrome (ARDS), however, comparisons with conventional positive pressure ventilation have shown no particular advantage for high-frequency ventilation. Also, high-frequency ventilation requires higher flow rates to achieve normocapnia and can lead rapidly to increases in lung volumes and intrathoracic pressures.

Constant Flow Ventilation. In this mode a constant flow of gas at a relatively high flow rate of approximately 1.5 to 3 L/min/kg is insufflated through the catheters, and this flow exits from the lungs via the tracheostomy tube. Gas transport is explained using a two-zone serial model of the lung. Zone 1 is just distal to the catheters. The turbulence generated by the jet's leaving the catheters is the major gas transport mechanism. Zone 2 is distal to zone 1 and is where molecular diffusion and cardiogenic oscillations are the primary gas transport mechanisms. There also may be collateral ventilation through alveolar collateral channels. Constant flow ventilation has been fairly ineffective in humans, probably secondary to the degree of collateral resistance. Also there have been problems maintaining normal arterial carbon dioxide tension ($PaCO_2$) levels.

Extracorporeal Membrane Oxygenation (ECMO). There are two components of extracorporeal gas exchange: the transfer of (1) oxygen into and (2) carbon dioxide out of the extracorporeal blood. The main objective is to provide an immediate improvement in the oxygenation of the arterial blood. Because the oxygen content of blood leaving an artificial membrane lung cannot exceed the physiologic content of arterial blood, adequate tissue oxygenation theoretically requires an extracorporeal blood flow almost equal to a relatively normal cardiac output. Thus to oxygenate without using the gas exchange surface of the lungs, virtually all of the cardiac output must go through the ECMO circuit. Venoarterial and venovenous bypass may be used. A drainage line brings blood from the patient, and it passes through an oximeter. A roller pump propels blood through the membrane oxygenator. Blood then passes through a bubble trap and outflow oximeter to the inflow catheter. Usually this method is supplemented with continuous positive pressure ventilation, with rates of 8 to 12 breaths per minute, an inspired oxygen concentration of 0.5, and a tidal volume to maintain airway pressures at less than 40 cm H_2O. ECMO has not been shown effective in adults, and the complications associated with it, bleeding and sepsis, have led to discontinuation of its use in this setting. Results in the neonate, on the other hand, have been more promising. The factors that most limit the usefulness of ECMO are not technical but relate to the ability of the lung to recover structurally and functionally after a severe insult.

Extracorporeal Carbon Dioxide Removal. This technique consists of the elimination of carbon dioxide through the extracorporeal circuit using a membrane oxygenator, concomitant with insufflation of 100% oxygen into the trachea. Significant oxygenation can be achieved through the lungs, and total elimination of metabolic carbon dioxide can be accomplished with an extracorporeal blood flow of approximately 20% to 30% of the cardiac output. There is less exposure of blood to the extracorporeal circuit (fewer bleeding complications) and more blood flow to the lungs when compared with ECMO. Extracorporeal carbon dioxide removal allows perfusion of lungs with blood that is more fully oxygenated and can be used via a venovenous circuit that uses either a roller pump or a centrifugal pump. Extracorporeal carbon dioxide removal is used in conjunction with low-frequency positive pressure ventilation (i.e., PEEP of 15 to 25 cm H_2O), 3 to 5 breaths per minute, peak airway pressure of 35 to 45 cm H_2O, and continuous flow of 1 to 2 L/min of 100% oxygen directed into the trachea through a small catheter. The main complication is bleeding secondary to the required administration of heparin. The initial results, with a survival rate of approximately 50%, have been encouraging.

When the respiratory failure has improved or resolved to a point at which the indications for mechanical ventilator support are no longer present, the patient can be weaned from the ventilator. When attempting to wean a patient from the ventilator, the physician must evaluate the overall status of the patient, state the underlying causes of respiratory failure, and determine the level of respiratory work. Weaning patients with heart failure or non-cardiogenic pulmonary edema from positive pressure ventilation may result in hemodynamic deterioration. As the mean airway pressure and the intrathoracic pressure are decreased, venous return, left ventricular afterload, and myocardial work increase. These increases may precipitate left ventricular dysfunction or worsen pulmonary edema. Thus *weaning should not be considered in the hemodynamically unstable patient or in the patient in whom both pulmonary capillary leak is present and large negative swings in intrathoracic pressure during spontaneous ventilation would be expected.* Thus it is important to correct underlying abnormalities (i.e., anemia, low cardiac output, fluid and electrolyte abnormalities, acid-base disturbances, infection, and malnutrition) before attempting weaning so that the patient's condition is optimized. Failure to do this will result in frustration, not only for the patient, but also for the ICU staff and the physician. Regardless of the ventilator mode used in weaning a

TABLE 48-3 Weaning Parameters

Parameter	Value
Minute ventilation	<10-12 L/min
Respiratory rate	<35 per minute
Tidal volume	>5 cc/kg
Vital capacity	>10 cc/kg
Inspiratory force	< − 20 cm H_2O
Frequency/tidal volume	<105 breaths/min/L
Pa_{O_2}/Pa_{O_2}	>0.35
Static compliance	>33 cc/cm H_2O

patient (e.g., intermittent mandatory ventilation, pressure support, continuous positive airway pressure), the responsibility of the ICU physician is to determine the earliest time that a patient can resume spontaneous breathing and to identify those patients in whom a trial of weaning is likely to fail. A variety of standard weaning parameters that can be measured at the bedside has been described (Table 48-3). An arterial blood gas evaluation should also be included when making the decision to wean the patient from the ventilator. Ventilator support is then slowly withdrawn while following the patient's clinical status.

The effectiveness of these parameters in predicting which patients can be weaned from the ventilator has been determined prospectively. Recently it has been shown that the frequency–tidal volume ratio is the most accurate predictor of outcome when weaning from the ventilator. In contrast, however, it has been shown that conventional parameters have not been effective in predicting outcome of weaning after a period of ventilator dependence. One study compared standard weaning parameters with the mechanical work of breathing in patients being weaned from the ventilator. (*Mechanical work of breathing* refers to the energy required to breathe spontaneously; it is a function of minute ventilation, tidal volume, lung compliance, and lung resistance.) The researchers concluded that in patients requiring prolonged (more than 24 hours) ventilatory support, the work of breathing correlated better with success of weaning than did standard parameters. These parameters do not take into account the need for airway protection and pulmonary toilet. Ultimately a clinical judgment must be made as to whether the patient can be extubated, based on the patient's ability to protect his or her airway, overall clinical status, and ability to clear secretions.

Fortunately, ventilatory support is frequently only short term (i.e., postoperative). Catastrophic medical and surgical problems requiring prolonged ventilatory support do occur, however, and in this group of patients mortality is directly related to multisystem failure. It becomes imperative then to restore oxygen transport after an adequate airway has been established and ventilation is assured. *The primary function of the cardiovascular-respiratory system in a critically ill patient is to deliver adequate amounts of oxygen to meet the metabolic demands of the body.*

MONITORING

When patients require ventilatory support, invasive hemodynamic monitoring is frequently necessary. Invasive hemodynamic monitoring serves several purposes: to help restore total body oxygen transport and analyze unexpected clinical courses; to optimize individual organ function; and as a preventive measure, to improve cardiac function before a physiologic stress such as surgery.

Invasive monitoring generally requires the use of systemic arterial catheters, central venous catheters, and pulmonary artery catheters. Central venous catheters are useful only when there is certainty that the cardiovascular abnormality present is confined to the right side of the heart. Systemic arterial catheters are used when there is need for frequent or continuous monitoring of systemic arterial blood pressure or blood gas values (for possibility of hemorrhage or septic shock and for titration of inotropic or vasoactive drugs). Pulmonary arterial catheters are used to monitor central venous pressure, pulmonary arterial pressure, pulmonary capillary wedge pressure (PCWP), cardiac output, and mixed venous blood gas values in certain situations (i.e., presence of severe, cardiopulmonary derangement, high risk of perioperative development of cardiopulmonary problems, possibility of large volume requirements or fluid shifts).

Although arterial lines can be placed in radial, brachial, femoral, or dorsalis pedis vessels, the radial line has become the site of choice secondary to the presence of collateral flow, ability to test for this collateral flow (Allen test), and the relative ease of maintaining the site.

Central venous catheters can be placed through the internal jugular, subclavian, external jugular, or cephalic veins. In general, the

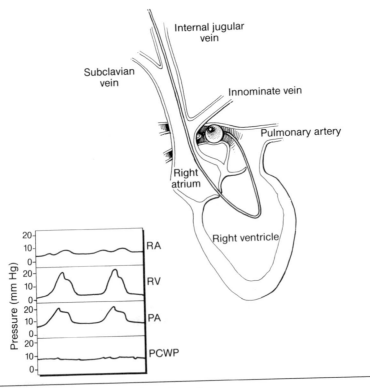

FIGURE 48-1   Pulmonary artery catheter insertion.

internal or subclavian approaches are recommended because the catheters are more easily placed and there is less incidence of subclavian vein injury and less thrombophlebitis when the catheter is in for a long period of time. The subclavian approach is associated with a higher incidence of pneumothorax but is more comfortable for the patient. The internal jugular approach is associated with a higher incidence of carotid artery injury and on the left side may damage the thoracic duct; however, the right internal jugular approach has the lowest overall complication rate and provides a straight course to the right atrium.

Pulmonary artery catheters are placed via the internal jugular or subclavian vein approach. These lines are placed via a modified Seldinger technique using either fluoroscopy and/or continuous pressure monitoring and interpretation (Fig. 48-1).

The data obtained from and complications associated with pulmonary artery catheters are shown in Table 48-4. Note that the measurement of pressure using the pulmonary artery catheter assumes that the catheter is in a West zone III region of lung and that there is a continuous, uninterrupted flow of blood from the catheter tip to the left atrium.

Regardless of the type of catheter used, invasive monitoring requires giving meticulous attention to infectious precautions. All catheters should be placed using sterile technique and standard skin preparation. These guidelines should be followed when changing catheters and catheter sites:

- Catheters should be changed over a guidewire within 24 hours of an emergent placement, if there is catheter malfunction, when doing a central venous–pulmonary artery catheter interconversion, if positive blood cultures are obtained, or if a septic clinical pattern occurs when there is no other likely source of sepsis.
- Catheters should be removed and reinserted at a new location when skin infection is determined by purulent drainage at the skin puncture site, cellulitis is present, erythema develops at the puncture site and there is a positive qualitative culture result, and if, after changing the catheter over a guidewire, bacteremia persists.

With this method of long-term management of invasive catheters, the incidence of a patient's developing sepsis is 0.3% to 0.5% per catheter per day.

TABLE 48-4 Pulmonary Artery Catheter

Indications

To assess cardiac preload, cardiac function, and oxygen delivery and consumption as a guide to treatment of the critically ill patient, that is, with adult respiratory distress syndrome, myocardial infarction, shock states, cardiac tamponade, pericarditis (constrictive), or severe mitral reflux.

Data Obtained	Normal Value
Central venous pressure	5 mm Hg
Pulmonary capillary wedge pressure	10 to 15 mm Hg
Cardiac output	5 L/min
Systemic vascular resistance	1000 dyne-sec/cm^5
Mixed venous oxygen saturation (Svo_2)	65% to 75%

Complications

Pneumothorax
Arterial injury
Venous thrombosis
Air embolism
Premature ventricular contractions
  or ventricular tachycardia
Atrial fibrillation or flutter
Right bundle branch block

Pulmonary infarct
Pulmonary artery rupture
Right ventricular perforation
Endocardial damage
Line sepsis
Balloon rupture
Catheter knotting

RESTORATION OF OXYGEN TRANSPORT

Multiple organ failure secondary to sepsis or shock is a major problem in the ICU. A mortality rate of as high as 100% is seen in patients with three failing organ systems secondary to intra-abdominal sepsis. The primary physiologic mechanism in patients with shock, whether it be from hemorrhage, trauma, sepsis, or postoperative stress states, is uneven flow that leads to inadequate tissue oxygenation. This maldistributed flow results in tissue oxygen debt that produces organ failure and subsequent death. The goal of treatment in the critically ill patient is to prevent multiple organ failure from occurring. This requires correction of maldistributed flow and restoration of adequate oxygen transport so that no oxygen debt accrues.

The need for restoration of oxygen transport is a consequence of the response to injury. Oxygen consumption falls in the initial phase of the stress response. However, with resuscitation, a phase of flow-dependent oxygen consumption ensues as the metabolic response to injury increases. This hypermetabolic phase generally peaks in 48 to 72 hours and abates within 7 to 10 days. If a complication develops (i.e., infection, ischemia, or persistent inflammatory focus), the hypermetabolic phase will recur (Fig. 48-2). The patient's response to this recurrence is one of increasing ventilation and cardiac output to increase oxygen delivery, hopefully to a level that corresponds to the magnitude of injury.

In the assessment of oxygen need, ideally tissue oxygen demand is measured and oxygen delivery ensured to meet that demand. Unfortunately, there currently is no direct method of doing this, so indirect methods are used. *The two measurements that are used are the oxygen consumption and the serum lactate levels.* In the surgical intensive care unit (SICU) the indirect Fick method is used to calculate oxygen consumption. It requires measurement of cardiac output and the arteriovenous oxygen content difference. These values can be obtained via a pulmonary artery (Swan-Ganz) catheter. With this catheter in place data can be obtained about filling pressures in the right and left sides of the heart, cardiac output, systemic vascular resistance, and mixed venous oxygen saturation (see Table 48-4). Knowing the hemoglobin value and the hemoglobin saturation in arterial blood allows calculation of the oxygen content of arterial blood (CaO_2). Mixed venous content (CvO_2) can be calculated in a like manner, and the arteriovenous oxygen difference, $C(a-v)O_2$, is obtained by subtracting mixed venous content from the arterial content:

$$CaO_2 = (1.36)(Hb)(SaO_2) + 0.0034(PaO_2)$$
$$CvO_2 = (1.36)(Hb)(SvO_2) + 0.0034(PvO_2)$$

Using the cardiac index (CI; cardiac output/body surface area) allows calculation of oxygen delivery (DO_2) and oxygen consumption (VO_2):

$$DO_2 = (CaO_2)(CI)(10)$$
$$VO_2 = (C[a-v]O_2)(CI)(10)$$

In normal, stable conditions, oxygen consumption is equal to oxygen demand, and no oxygen debt exists. In the absence of tissue hypoxia, blood lactate levels are normal (<2 mmol/L). If oxygen delivery decreases for any reason, oxygen consumption remains relatively stable over a wide range of values because the oxygen extraction ($C[a-v]O_2/CaO_2$) and the ratio of consumption to delivery increase. If, however, oxygen delivery falls below a critical level, the oxygen extraction becomes less efficient, and the oxygen consumption begins to fall. In the basal state this level is approximately 330 cc/min/m² or 8 to 10 ml/min/kg. Below this level tissue hypoxia occurs, and blood lactate levels will increase. Thus oxygen consumption is either flow independent or flow dependent, based on whether or not increasing the oxygen delivery increases the oxygen consumption (Fig. 48-3).

As mentioned, lactate levels correlate with the degree of oxygen debt and with outcome. Serial lactate measurements have also been used to assess the response to therapy in shock states. Even

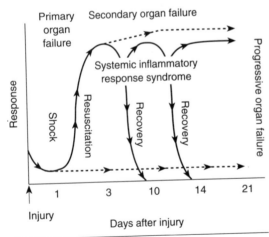

FIGURE 48-2 Inflammatory and organ failure responses to injury.

in patients with hepatic disease, perfusion failure should be the initial consideration when hyperlactemia is detected.

Thus it is assumed that oxygen delivery is meeting oxygen demand and metabolic need when there is absence of flow dependency in the lactate level of plasma. This second criterion is necessary because in certain conditions (e.g., septic shock, adult respiratory distress syndrome [ARDS], liver failure) flow-dependent oxygen consumption apparently is absent. However, the redox potential of the cells remains abnormal. This occurs secondary to a limited global oxygen extraction by the body and is characterized by a narrow $C(a-v)O_2$. The lactate-to-pyruvate ratio is also helpful because it helps identify the situation in which the concentration of lactate may be abnormally high, but the redox potential of the cell is normal (i.e., aerobic glycolysis). In hypermetabolic states pyruvate dehydrogenase is down-regulated, and levels of lactate and pyruvate increase. However, the ratio remains normal.

The body has several physiologic mechanisms by which it attempts to maintain flow-independent oxygen consumption and lactate production. The end point of these compensatory systemic and regional mechanisms is to supply oxygen to the cells so that mitochondrial oxidative phosphorylation can continue to supply the high-energy phosphates necessary for metabolic work. Systemic compensatory mechanisms refer to oxygen delivery; hence heart rate and cardiac output are increased in an attempt to increase the delivery to the tissues. Once oxygen delivery is unable to meet the metabolic demands of the body, regional (microcirculatory) mechanisms come into play. At the microcirculatory level, as local oxygen demand increases, local adenosine triphosphate (ATP) stores are depleted, and tissue adenosine levels rise. Adenosine is a potent vasodilator that reduces local precapillary sphincter tone and increases regional blood flow. This process increases tissue oxygenation and makes oxygen more available to the mitochondria. Also, there is redistribution of blood flow to organs with a higher resting oxygen extraction (heart, muscle, brain) and away from organs with a low resting oxygen extraction (skin, kidneys, viscera). Second, the capillary hematocrit level remains relatively stable over a wide range of central hematocrit values, thus protecting against anemia, whereas alterations in hemoglobin-oxygen affinity serve to enhance peripheral oxygen extraction. Finally, the amount of ambient oxygen within the cytosol that is necessary to drive oxidative phosphorylation is low, and the cells are capable of extracting more oxygen during times of increased metabolic demand.

Once these compensatory mechanisms have been used fully, further increases in metabolic activity will result in oxygen debt (i.e., supply will not meet demand). At this point anaerobic production of lactate occurs. Lactate is used as fuel by the liver and kidneys. Whenever the ability of the liver and kidneys to metabolize lactate is impaired or exceeded, systemic acidosis will occur, and lactate levels will increase. The end result of this process is further organ impairment.

In hypermetabolic models there is a higher critical oxygen delivery and thus a greater sensitivity to dysoxic injury. It has been observed in

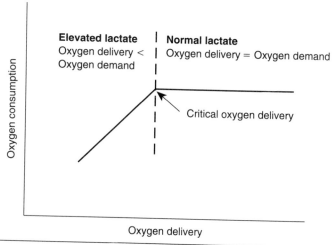

FIGURE 48-3 Normal relationship between oxygen delivery and consumption.

hypermetabolic patients that supply-dependent oxygen consumption occurred below a critical delivery of 15 cc/min/kg. This implies a pathologic supply dependency and is contrasted to physiologic supply dependency in Fig. 48-4. States of pathologic oxygen supply dependency have been noted in patients with ARDS, sepsis, and liver failure. *These patients require higher oxygen deliveries to maintain adequate tissue perfusion because at the microcirculatory level there is a failure to extract oxygen normally.* The patients then have narrowed arteriovenous oxygen differences, with normal to high mixed venous hemoglobin saturation.

It has been demonstrated that a normal oxygen consumption may actually be inadequate in critically ill patients in the postoperative period. In patients with normal preoperative baseline cardiorespiratory values, surgical trauma produces intraoperative physiologic deficits that in the immediate postoperative period lead to increased cardiac index, temperature, mean pulmonary artery pressure, and oxygen delivery. Survivors tend to have better myocardial performance with lower central venous pressure (CVP)

and PCWP and greater increases in oxygen transport. The major determinant of outcome is inadequate oxygen consumption, which leads to an oxygen debt and inability to meet metabolic needs, suggesting that in survivors the increased flow and oxygen delivery are systemic compensatory responses with survival value. In prospective trials stressed patients' outcomes were compared with respect to whether therapeutic or supranormal values were maintained in the postoperative period. These trials showed that the supranormal group had reduced morbidity, duration of hospitalization, and mortality. Further, it was shown that when calculating oxygen debt (oxygen debt = measured oxygen consumption − the preoperative oxygen consumption), a greater oxygen debt correlated with both development of multisystem organ failure and death. Of note is that forcing patients into a survivor or supranormal pattern by early aggressive therapy decreases mortality by approximately 30%. The therapeutic goals are shown in Table 48-5.

These goals have also been tested in the preoperative patient. It has been shown that by optimizing hemodynamics using a pulmonary artery

TABLE 48-5   Therapeutic Goals in the Critically Ill

Parameter	Therapeutic Goal
Cardiac index	50% greater than normal (4.5 L/min/m^2)
Oxygen delivery	Greater than normal (>600 cc/min/m^2)
Oxygen consumption	30% greater than normal (10 cc/min/m^2)
Blood volume	500 ml above normal (3.2 L/m^2 in males)
	(2.8 L/m^2 in females)

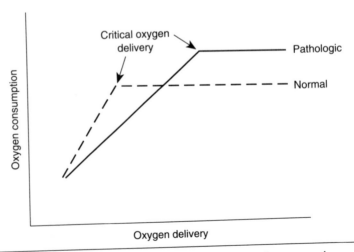

FIGURE 48-4   Normal versus pathologic oxygen delivery and consumption.

catheter "preoperative tune-up," outcome was improved in patients undergoing limb-salvage arterial surgery. The ultimate goals of the tune-up were a pulmonary capillary artery wedge pressure of 8 to 15 mm Hg, a cardiac index of greater than or equal to 2.8 L/min/m², and a systemic vascular resistance of less than 1100 dyne-sec/cm⁵. These goals were obtained using a combination of fluid loading, afterload reduction, and inotropic support. With this protocol there were significantly less adverse intraoperative events, less postoperative cardiac morbidity, and less early graft thrombosis than with the control group. The perioperative mortality rate was decreased from 9.5% in the control group to 1.5% in the study group.

If hypermetabolism develops in the postoperative critically ill patient, the ICU physician must decide who needs restoration of oxygen transport and what will be used to achieve these means. The physician must develop a systematic approach to the restoration of oxygen transport (Fig. 48-5).

In the presence of flow-dependent oxygen consumption and flow-dependent lactate production, preload should be evaluated first. Almost all critically ill patients with decreased tissue perfusion, including many in cardiogenic shock, have intravascular volume depletion. Crystalloids, colloids, or a combination of the two may be used. Packed red blood cells are used as needed, attempting to keep the hemoglobin level greater than 10 g/dl and the hematocrit level greater than or equal to 32%. It appears that colloids expand plasma volume better than crystalloids, which tend to expand the interstitial volume. In turn, hemodynamic and oxygen transport response is proportional to plasma volume. Thus prospective data indicate that optimal goals are more easily attained using colloids rather than crystalloids.

If after adequate preload is established, flow-dependent oxygen consumption and/or lactate production persists, afterload should be assessed. If the systemic vascular resistance is greater than 1100 dyne-sec and the patient is not hypotensive, afterload reduction should be undertaken. Regardless of the agent used (see the box on p. 800), therapy should be directed at improving tissue perfusion and oxygenation by dilating metarteriolar-capillary networks to provide more evenly distributed blood flow. Doses of vasodilators are titrated to effect (i.e., decrease the systemic vascular resistance to <1100 dyne-sec while keeping

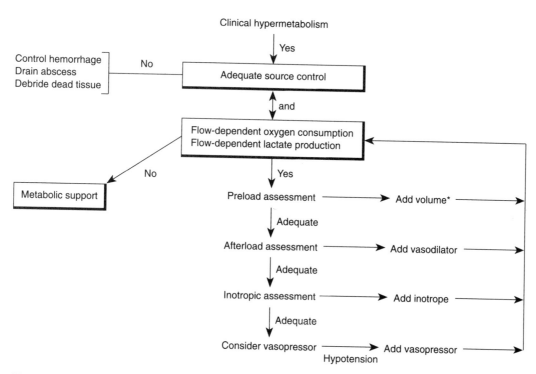

*Use PRBCs if hemoglobin is less than 10.0 g/dl.

FIGURE 48-5 Algorithm for restoration of oxygen transport.

┌─────────────────────────────────────┐

PHARMACOTHERAPY

Vasodilators

Nitroglycerin
Nitroprusside
Hydralazine
Calcium channel blockers (e.g., nifedipine)
Angiotension converting enzyme inhibitors
   (e.g., captopril)

Inotropes

Dobutamine
Dopamine (5-10 μg/kg/min)
Epinephrine
Amrinone
Dopexamine (not available in United States)

Vasopressors

Norepinephrine
Phenylephrine
Dopamine ($>$5 μg/kg/min)
Methoxamine
Metaraminol

└─────────────────────────────────────┘

the mean arterial pressure above 70 to 80 mm Hg).

If after correction of preload and afterload, flow dependence still exists, inotropic support should be considered (see box). The two most extensively studied inotropic agents are dobutamine and dopamine. Dopamine is a naturally occurring catecholamine that acts on dopaminergic and alpha- and beta-adrenergic receptors; as such, its use is associated with an increase in mean arterial pressure, heart rate, mean pulmonary artery pressure, and cardiac index. Dopamine also will increase oxygen delivery but less so than dobutamine. On the other hand, oxygen consumption has not been shown to increase significantly with the use of dopamine. Consumption is not changed significantly despite increasing delivery because the alpha effect of the drug may worsen the maldistribution of flow. However, this alpha effect makes it an excellent agent for hypotensive patients.

Dobutamine is a synthetic catecholamine with primarily beta-adrenergic properties. Dobutamine increases heart rate, cardiac index, oxygen delivery, and oxygen consumption. Also, mixed venous saturation and stroke work of the heart are increased. In contrast to dopamine, the mean pulmonary arterial pressures and the PCWPs are decreased. There apparently is no effect on mean arterial pressure. The decreased pulmonary pressures are consistent with the beta-2 effect (peripherally) and the beta-1 effect (cardiac). Thus oxygen consumption is increased secondary to improved tissue perfusion and a more evenly distributed flow. Although there has been concern about increasing myocardial oxygen consumption, it has been shown that in animal models, the increase in coronary artery blood flow and oxygen delivery to the myocardium is in excess of the increased demand for inotropy. Hypovolemia *must* be corrected before administering inotropes or vasodilators because stimulating the empty heart frequently has adverse effects on systemic perfusion and coronary artery perfusion.

Whatever volume, vasodilator, or inotrope improves oxygen consumption, that combination should be used vigorously as long as it continues to work and the clinical status improves. If therapy fails, using vasopressors in a patient with hypotension may be considered (see the box at left). They are given last because they promote lactic acidosis, increase pulmonary shunt, and increase pulmonary arterial and capillary pressures. They are useful, however, for increasing mean arterial pressure, which should be kept greater than 70 to 80 mm Hg in the previously normotensive patient. If hypertension existed preoperatively, the goal should be 80% to 90% of that pressure. By increasing the mean arterial pressure, these agents maintain coronary and cerebral blood flow, although they may compromise flow to the viscera and periphery.

Several points should be repeated with regard to data collection:

- The cardiac output should be related to the body surface area.
- The presence of anemia and/or hypoxia should be determined (maintain a hemoglobin level of 10 to 11.5 g/dl and an arterial saturation ≥90%).
- The interpretation of the mixed venous saturation is limited by the possible alteration of extraction capabilities by tissues.
- Blood lactate levels are influenced not only by production but also by elimination. Lactate levels are also increased in other conditions (i.e., seizures, diabetes mellitus, and intoxication).
- All patients should undergo a dynamic evaluation of oxygen consumption before and after a transient increase in cardiac output. This is referred to as an *oxygen consumption challenge*.

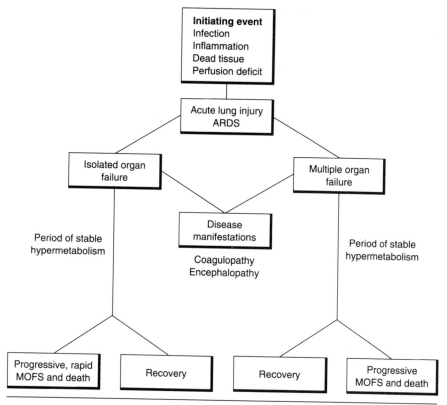

FIGURE 48-6 Multiple organ failure syndrome *(MOFS)*.

It should be done in a reasonable time period to assure that the patient's demand does not change dramatically.

Recently the following recommendations regarding oxygen transport have been made. The diagnosis of inadequate oxygen delivery states caused by absolute delivery reduction, relative reduction, or maldistribution of flow can be made in the following circumstances: (1) the patient has clinical evidence of shock with hypotension and hypoperfusion so that delivery is inadequate to meet demand; (2) elevated lactate levels in the absence of acute or chronic liver disease suggest that delivery is probably inadequate; and (3) if the mixed venous saturation is low, inadequate delivery should be suspected. If the therapeutic measures undertaken lower oxygen delivery, delivery should be returned to the pre-intervention level by whatever maneuver is appropriate (i.e., volume or inotrope). When pathologic flow dependency is suspected, performing an oxygen consumption challenge should be considered. Some measures to decrease oxygen demand are beneficial, including the use of mechanical ventilation, opiates to re-

duce pain and agitation, and cooling to treat severe hyperpyrexia. In manipulating oxygen delivery, the following steps have been recommended:

- Correction of hypoxemia and anemia
- Volume loading and afterload reduction
- Inotropic support (dobutamine)
- Vasopressor therapy if necessary
- Adjunctive inotropic therapy

MULTIPLE ORGAN DYSFUNCTION SYNDROME

The response to tissue injury has already been shown (see Fig. 48-2). With a single, uncomplicated injury, the hypermetabolic response tends to peak in 48 to 72 hours and then abate within 7 to 10 days. However, if a complication such as infection, ischemia, persistent inflammation, or persistent perfusion deficit develops, hypermetabolism will recur. After correction of the complication, the hypermetabolic response will either abate and the patient will recover, or the response will continue, multiple organs will fail, and the patient will die (Fig. 48-6).

The pathway of progressive multiple organ dysfunction syndrome (MODS) generally occurs in two forms: (1) as a primary pulmonary initiating event such as aspiration, with the multiple organ dysfunction syndrome being terminal, manifesting only within a few days of death, and (2) in patients with ARDS who are in septic shock and in whom multiple organ dysfunction syndrome is present from the time of injury. In both instances there is a period of several days to weeks of relatively stable hypermetabolism and then progression of liver and renal failure (associated with a progressive rise in serum bilirubin and creatinine levels). A third pathway recently has been identified in which liver and renal failure occurs in the absence of lung injury. In the transition to progressive multiple organ dysfunction syndrome the mortality rate increases from 40% to 60% to 90% to 100%.

Thus the clinical characterization of multiple organ dysfunction syndrome is that it occurs in a setting of a defined injury that is associated with circulatory compromise followed by a resuscitation intervention. The postresuscitation response depends on (1) the severity of injury; (2) the organ reserve of the patient at the time of injury; (3) the time lapse until the institution of effective treatment; (4) the adequacy of treatment; and (5) the number and severity of subsequent injuries and complications. This postresuscitation response manifests as hypermetabolism, with a patient with primary organ dysfunction such as ARDS requiring mechanical ventilation. Secondary organ injuries and failure such as liver and kidney dysfunction can then manifest. The hypermetabolism may abate without progressive organ dysfunction or may continue as progressive organ failure and result in death.

■ ■ ■

In conclusion, it has been shown that when the principles of source control, restoration of oxygen transport, and metabolic support are adhered to, morbidity and mortality rates can be significantly reduced in critically ill patients. This chapter has outlined a rational approach to the restoration of oxygen transport as it fits in the overall care of the ICU patient. Also, the multiple organ dysfunction syndrome has been discussed as it applies to the critically ill patient.

SURGICAL PHARMACOPEIA

Drug	Indications and Action	Complications	Dosage
Nitroglycerin	Reduce myocardial oxygen demand for ischemic heart disease a. Reduction in venous tone; increasing preload b. Decrease in systemic vascular resistance (SVR) c. Decreased afterload Treatment of congestive heart failure (CHF)	Hypotension, tachycardia, headaches, and, rarely, bradycardia	IV initial dose 5 μg/min, then +5 μg/min q2-3 min (1.0-2.0 μg/kg/min) until response is noted; occasionally 200 μg/min may be needed to relieve chest pain Sublingual: 0.4 mg q5min × 3; if no response call physician
Nitroprusside	Treatment of severe pump failure in hypertensive and normotensive patients who experience a marked reduction in cardiac output associated with increased systemic vascular resistance Action: Direct acting vasodilator acts on both venous and arterial vessels	Hypotension, hypoxemia, increased blood level of thiocyanate and cyanide	Adults: 15-200 μg/min IV Children: 0.1-8 μg/kg/min IV

Drug	Indications and Action	Complications	Dosage
Hydralazine	Management of chronic hypertension May be used to treat hypertension emergency; useful for acute glomerulonephritis or eclampsia *Action:* Direct acting vasodilator, reduces SVR; little effect on capacitance vessels (venous system)	Tachycardia, hypotension, flushing, headache, myocardial ischemia, fluid retention, SLE syndrome	Adult: 20 mg IV over 2 min Additional doses of 40-80 mg at 10 min intervals until desired blood pressure is attained or a total dose of 300 mg is reached PO: 200-400 mg in bid or qid doses
Calcium channel blocker	Angina, arrhythmias, hypertension *Action:* Reduce intracellular calcium concentrations in cardiac and smooth muscle cells of coronary and systemic vasculature a. Nifedipine: hypertension b. Diltiazem: angina or hypertension c. Verapamil: arrhythmias	See PDR for numerous possible complications	Nifedipine: 10-20 mg PO tid; initial dose 10 mg PO tid Diltiazem: 60 mg PO q6h Verapamil: 240-480 mg daily tid or qid
Angiotensin-converting enzyme inhibitors	Essential and renal hypertension *Action:* Inhibitor of angiotensin-I-converting enzyme	Captopril: rashes, pruritus, loss of taste, proteinuria, increased serum K^+ levels	Captopril: 25-50 mg PO tid; may increase to 150 mg PO tid See PDR for additional angiotensin-converting enzyme inhibitors
Ionotropes			
Dobutamine	Short-term therapy to increase CO in patients with severe congestive heart failure *Action:* Active on β_1; is less active on β_2 and α	Nausea, headaches, palpitation, chest pain, and shortness of breath	2-20 μg/kg/min IV
Dopamine	Shock associated with acute heart failure; congestive heart failure Promotes diuresis in early stages of acute oliguric renal failure *Action:* dose dependent <5 μg/kg/min activates dopaminergic response in renal and mesenteric vascular beds to cause vasodilation	Nausea, vomiting, headaches, anginal pain, tachyarrhythmia	1-20 μg/kg/min IV

Continued.

Drug	Indications and Action	Complications	Dosage
Dopamine—cont'd	5-10 μg/kg/min Dopaminergic and β; increases CO, heart rate, and myocardial contractility 10-20 μg/kg/min: increased β_1, but decreasing alpha activity		
Amrinone	Severe congestive heart failure Mechanism of action unknown	Headaches, hypotension, anorexia, GI disturbances, reduced taste and smell, thrombocytopenia	IV bolus 0.75 mg/kg followed by infusion of 5-10 μg/kg/min
Vasopressors			
Norepinephrine	Treatment of shock when potent vasoconstrictor is needed to maintain adequate tissue perfusion *Action:* Positive ionotrope, chronotrope and potent constrictor of resistant and capacitance vessels	Extravasation may produced local skin necrosis; risk is reduced if phentolamine (Regitine) is used in conjunction with Levophed bitartrate Headaches, anxiety, weakness, palpitations, respiratory distress	0.02-0.20 μg/kg/min IV
Phenylephrine bitartrate	Potent vasoconstrictor		1.0-5.0 μg/kg/min IV

BIBLIOGRAPHY

Abrams JH, Cerra FB, Holcroft JW. Cardiopulmonary monitoring. In Critical Care—Care in the ICU. New York, Scientific American, 1989.

Berlauk JF, Abrams JH, Gilmour IJ, et al. Preoperative optimization of cardiovascular hemodynamics improves outcome in peripheral vascular surgery: A prospective randomized clinical trial. Ann Surg 214:289, 1991.

Cain SM. Assessment of tissue oxygenation. Crit Care Clin 2:537, 1986.

Cerra FB. Multiple organ failure syndrome. In Disease of the Month. 1992. (in press)

Dhainaut JF, Edwards JD, Grootendorst AF, et al. Practical aspects of oxygen transport: Conclusions and recommendations of the roundtable conference. Intensive Care Med 16S2:S179, 1990.

Eyer S, Brummitt C, Crossley K, et al. Catheter-related sepsis: Prospective, randomized study of three methods of long-term catheter maintenance. Crit Care Med 18:1073, 1990.

Fenwick JC, Dodeck PM, Ronco JJ, et al. Increased concentrations of plasma lactate predicts pathologic dependence of oxygen consumption on oxygen delivery in patients with adult respiratory distress syndrome. J Crit Care 5:81, 1990.

Gilbert J, Erian R, Soloman D. Use of survivors cardiorespiratory values as therapeutic goals in septic shock. Crit Care Med 18:1304, 1990.

Kruse JA, Zaidi SJ, Carlson RW. Significance of blood lactate levels in critically ill patients with liver disease. Am J Med 83:77, 1987.

Sassoon CSH. Positive pressure ventilation: Alternate modes. Chest 100:1421, 1991.

Shoemaker WC, Appel PL, Bland R. Use of physiologic monitoring to predict outcome and to assist in clinical decisions in critically ill postoperative patients. Am J Surg 146:43, 1983.

Shoemaker WC, Appel PL, Kram HB. Oxygen transport measurements to evaluate tissue perfusion and titrate therapy: Dobutamine and dopamine effects. Crit Care Med 19:672, 1991.

Shoemaker WC, Appel PL, Kram HB, et al. Prospective trial of supranormal values of survivors as therapeutic goals in high risk surgical patients. Chest 94:1176, 1988.

Villar J, Winston B, Slutsky AS. Non-conventional techniques of ventilatory support. Crit Care Clin 6:579, 1990.

Vincent JL. The relationship between oxygen demand, oxygen uptake, and oxygen supply. Intensive Care Med 16S2:S145, 1990.

Yang KL, Tobin MJ. A prospective study of indexes predicting the outcome of trials of weaning from mechanical ventilation. N Engl J Med 324:1445, 1991.

CHAPTER REVIEW
Questions

1. The patient is a 70-year-old female who 5 days earlier underwent a right hemicolectomy for a cecal carcinoma. She is reportedly having difficulty breathing, and the nursing staff believe she may have aspirated. On arriving at the patient's room, you find she is apneic. How would you establish an airway and ensure adequate gas exchange? Be sure to consider your approach to this patient while she is on the surgical floor and during transport to the ICU. Comment on the ventilator settings you would select.

2. The above patient is diagnosed as having aspiration pneumonia. Over the next 48 hours her pulmonary status deteriorates. Despite increases in PEEP and FIO_2, she is unable to maintain 90% arterial saturation, and her peak airway pressure has increased to 60 cm H_2O. You decide to attempt inverse ratio ventilation. Describe this mode of ventilation, commenting on its advantages and disadvantages.

3. The patient improves over the next week, and she is slowly weaned from the ventilator using an intermittent mandatory ventilation mode. What parameters would you use to determine whether or not the patient could be extubated?

4. A 65-year-old male is brought to the ICU after sigmoid colon resection with an end-colostomy and mucous fistula for a perforated diverticulum. On arrival in the ICU the patient has a systolic blood pressure of 110 mm Hg, pulse rate of 110, respiratory rate of 24 breaths/min, and temperature of 37.2° C (99° F). He has produced only 10 ml of urine in the past 3 hours. You decide to place a pulmonary artery catheter. Discuss the data that can be obtained with this catheter.

5. The patient mentioned in question 4 has a body surface area of 2 m², a cardiac output of 8 L, a hemoglobin level of 10 g/dl, an arterial saturation of 96%, and a mixed venous oxygen saturation of 60%. Calculate the oxygen delivery index, oxygen consumption index, and the arterio-venous oxygen difference.

6. In the critically ill patient adequacy of resuscitation is best gauged by:
   a. Systolic blood pressure
   b. Pulse rate
   c. Absence of flow-dependent oxygen consumption
   d. Urinary output
   e. Mixed venous oxygen consumption

7. True or false: the risks of preoperatively "tuning" a patient outweigh the potential benefit and therefore should not be done in high-risk patients.

8. Discuss the rationale behind the recommended approach to restoring oxygen delivery.

9. The initial agent of choice for inotropy is:
   a. Dopamine
   b. Dobutamine
   c. Amrinone
   d. Norepinephrine
   e. Epinephrine

10. With progressive multiple organ dysfunction syndrome, the mortality rate is approximately:
   a. 25%
   b. 50%
   c. 75%
   d. 90%

Answers

1. Initially, an airway (oropharyngeal or nasopharyngeal) should be established, and the patient should be ventilated with a bag-mask device and 100% oxygen. Adequate suction equipment should be made available, and plans for intubation should be made. Nasal intubation should not be attempted because the patient described is apneic. After oral intubation is completed, the patient is ventilated by the bag-tube method while being transported to the ICU. Again 100% oxygen is used. When the patient arrives in the ICU, she is connected to the ventilator, and settings are determined. Appropriate ventilator settings in this patient would be an FIO_2 of 100%, a tidal volume of 12 cc/kg, intermittent mandatory ventilation of 16 (because the patient is apneic, there is

probably no advantage in using the assist-control mode), I/E ratio of 1:4, and PEEP of 5 cm H_2O. Further changes should be made based on the patient's arterial blood gas values, airway pressures, hemodynamic status, and significant chest x-ray film changes.

2. Inverse ratio ventilation is a pressure-controlled mode in which inspiratory time exceeds expiratory time. This mode is used to recruit alveoli and in doing so, to increase the arterial oxygen saturation. Characteristically, lower tidal volumes and higher frequencies are used with this mode. In this way peak airway pressures are limited, and adequate ventilation is achieved. A disadvantage of this mode is that inverse ratio ventilation may cause discomfort to the patient, requiring sedation and at times even paralysis. Also, auto-PEEP may be induced at a higher frequency ventilation, which will serve to increase the mean airway pressures.

3. When preparing to wean the patient, the first thing to consider is whether or not the underlying abnormality that led to intubation has been corrected. If it has, you must ensure that the patient's condition has been optimized. When this has been done, several bedside parameters have been found useful for determining whether or not the patient will successfully wean from the ventilator (see Table 48-3). Finally, a clinical judgment must be made as to whether or not the patient will be able to protect his or her airway and control secretions. If all these conditions are met, the patient most likely will tolerate extubation.

4. The pulmonary artery catheter allows determination of whether or not the patient has adequate preload (as determined by estimating the PCWP), inotropy (as reflected by the cardiac index), and afterload (as determined by calculating the systemic vascular resis-tance). Also, the function of the right side of the heart is reflected by the CVP. Finally, the oxygen delivery and consumption data can be calculated and interventions made to ensure the absence of flow-dependent consumption.

5. Refer to the following calculations:

$$Do_2 = (1.36)(10 \text{ g/dl})(0.96) \times 4 \text{ L/min/m}^2 \times 10 = 522 \text{ cc/min}$$

$$Vo_2 = (1.36)(10 \text{ g/dl})(0.96 - 0.6) \times 4 \text{ L/min/m}^2 \times 10 = 163 \text{ cc/min}$$

$$C(a\text{-}v)o_2 = (1.36)(10 \text{ g/dl})(0.96 - 0.6) = 4$$

6. The best way to assess adequacy of resuscitation is to ensure absence of flow-dependent oxygen consumption and flow-dependent lactate production.

7. False. In a prospective study at the University of Minnesota, a significant reduction in perioperative mortality and morbidity rates was shown in patients undergoing a preoperative tune-up before peripheral vascular surgery. On the other hand, complications associated with the tune-up itself were not frequent. The benefits were found to outweigh the risks of the tune-up.

8. The approach outlined in this chapter is one of correcting hypoxemia and anemia first, followed by appropriate volume loading or unloading and afterload manipulation. Then consideration for inotropic support is given. Finally, vasopressor therapy is considered. With this approach, myocardial oxygen consumption is minimized; thus the potential myocardium at risk also is minimized. The hope is to improve flow to the body without imposing too vigorous a demand on the heart.

9. Dobutamine

10. d

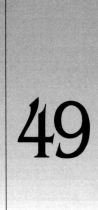

49

Infection

H. HARLAN STONE

KEY FEATURES

After reading this chapter you will understand:
- The pathophysiology of infection.
- How infection is spread.
- The general principles of treatment of infection.
- Specific types of infections, including peritonitis and gangrene.
- Some causes of postoperative fever.
- Viral infections of significance to surgeons, including hepatitis.

Surgeons have treated wound infections since earliest recorded history. Subsequently, minor operations and eventually even major procedures, such as limb amputation, were carried out. However, infection was expected as an almost universal outcome of any break in the body's protective skin mantle until the past century.

Because of infection, some intricate surgical procedure would culminate in wound sepsis, disruption of a critical suture line, and eventual patient death as a consequence. With the introduction of the germ theory and antisepsis and refinements in anesthesia, operations of greater magnitude were undertaken, with even greater prospects for success. It was only then that infection was perceived in its true role—the constant enemy.

Despite these strides, until mankind establishes an entirely germ-free environment, surgeons will have to continue to battle the possibility of bacterial sepsis and attempt to control such an infection once it has evolved.

In addition, in the last decade the scourge of HIV infection and acquired immunodeficiency syndrome (AIDS) have put both the population at large and the surgical team at risk.

PATHOPHYSIOLOGY OF INFECTION

For an infection to develop, three factors must exist: (1) an inoculum of pathogens of sufficient number and virulence, (2) a nutrient medium on which microbes can thrive, and (3) some alteration in host resistance must occur, thereby limiting the body's capacity to combat invasive infection. The relative importance of any one factor changes from time to time with respect to species of pathogen, type of culture medium provided, and the variety as well as magnitude of impairment in host defenses. Rarely does a single factor become overpowering, except under extreme and unusual circumstances.

Inoculum

The smallest number of bacteria required to cause infection varies from species to species. The greater the virulence of the individual pathogen, the fewer the number of microbes needed to initiate an infection. For example, there is a striking difference between highly infective type A *beta-hemolytic streptococci* and the relatively innocuous *Bacillus subtilis* or even some nonpathogenic diphtheroid. However, what an inoculum lacks in quality (i.e., specific factors of virulence or infectivity) can often be made up by quantity (i.e., absolute numbers in the inoculum). Likewise, a single species may have many strains that differ significantly in virulence, and even a single strain can pass through certain phases when infectivity has been almost entirely lost. For example, *Clostridium* spores may not demonstrate any ability to infect for relatively long periods, yet once aroused, the same strain can rapidly activate or adapt critical enzyme systems or other biologic mechanisms so as to establish a lethal gas gangrene.

Not only do pathogens vary in invasiveness with respect to a specific host, but also differences in susceptibility to infection occur among different tissues or organs of a single host. For example, pneumococci can cause a serious pneumonia but essentially never produce a wound infection.

Single species in a mixed bacterial inoculum can either enhance or reduce the virulence of other individual components. Some microbe pairs, such as the anaerobic *Peptostreptococcus* and the aerobic *Staphylococcus aureus*, greatly augment the infectiveness of one another (as in *Meleney's cellulitis or gangrene*) despite marked differences in their environmental requisites for cell multiplication and tissue invasiveness when the two are separate. In such cases, each species appears to be immune to the toxic factors elaborated by the other. The phenomenon is generally referred to as *bacterial symbiosis.* The resultant *synergistic infection* has more than a mere additive increase in pathogenicity and lethality.

On the other hand, since no single species is resistant to all other species, certain bacteria in a mixed flora can be destroyed by elaborated toxins or actual overgrowth by some other pathogen. Therefore, in a wound infected by a multiplicity of microbes, the population may change to a single bacterial species or to a mixture of only a relatively few compatible species.

There is a basic difference between bacterial *colonization* and *invasive infection.* It is a change in status that cannot easily be measured, yet the distinction is crucial, because it determines whether there is (1) local bacterial invasion of adjacent tissues, (2) absorption of bacterial products leading to local or systemic impairment in host defenses, and (3) the likelihood of primary wound healing. Generally, if the bacterial population of an open wound exceeds 1000 organisms per gram of tissue, per milliliter of exudate, or per square millimeter of surface area, mere colonization no longer exists. When the population exceeds 100,000 organisms per simi-

lar base of measurement, infection has assuredly been established and may even have become life threatening.

Nutrient Medium

In addition to any inoculum, there must also be some form of pablum from which the pathogens gain nourishment. Accumulations of blood or blood products, areas of necrosis, or even exposed healthy tissues with limited local resistance offer ideal sources of nutrition for infecting bacteria. Only one other component in the environment is necessary for active bacterial existence, and that is water. Although bacteria are unicellular forms, they have no greater requirements for life than do humans—that is, food and water. Thus, if infection is to be avoided, the surgeon must endeavor to remove all nonviable tissue and to obliterate any space with the potential for accumulation of blood or serum.

Infection seldom arises in closed areas of ecchymosis, contusion, or fracture unless the deeper wound and its clot have been exposed to bacterial invasion through a break in the skin, as occurs with operation, attempts at aspiration, or fistulization via a drain. In addition, there is a significant difference between infection rates for a blood clot developing in an open wound or in a wound that has been drained and the same hematoma in a nonviolated closed space. A traumatic or surgically incised wound has a higher incidence of infection whenever any sizable clot is allowed to accumulate, irrespective of whether wound closure was performed under the relatively sterile conditions of an operating room or with little attention to antiseptic details—despite the use of antibiotics or other antiseptic measures.

Host Resistance

Host resistance is of utmost importance in reducing the likelihood of subsequent infection following a given bacterial inoculation. Even highly virulent microorganisms will have little effect if host resistance against them is great and if local nutrients for bacterial growth are lacking. On the other hand, in the presence of an adverse change in host defenses or a failure to possess resistance against a certain bacterial species, infection can arise only after minimal inoculation of a surface offering little nutritional support.

Local Resistance. Resistance can be categorized as local or general. Local resistance depends on the exclusion of such nutrient factors as blood or serum that might collect in the so-called dead space of a wound or cavity and that functionally will obstruct free access of various anti-infectious moieties of the host (i.e., histiocytes). Such phagocytes then fail to reach the local area of bacterial inoculation in sufficient time or numbers to prevent infection. Accordingly, this dead space provides both the potential for nutrition and a restriction in the host defense mechanism. Other considerations in local resistance are primarily based on tissue immunity. For example, the upper respiratory tract is colonized primarily by gram-positive organisms, while the anus and rectum contain almost exclusively anaerobes and gram-negative rods. Despite these great concentrations of potentially infectious bacteria, seldom are infections caused by the usual local flora. Only the most virulent gram-positive cocci create infections in the upper air passages. Likewise, except for instances in which there has been a break in the mucosal lining of the anorectum, gram-negative rods alone rarely cause an infection in that area. Furuncles, or the so-called boils that develop over the buttocks, are almost never caused by some gram-negative rod but by a gram-positive coccus (*Staphylococcus aureus*).

Systemic Resistance. A multitude of systemic factors are active in host resistance. Indeed, research into methods for enhancing host defense is most promising. These factors include various components of the phagocytic system, production of antibodies and other related humoral factors, and the ability of the host to neutralize toxic enzymes elaborated by the invading pathogens.

Phagocytes are of several different types. *Tissue histiocytes* are not fixed but wander about those intercellular spaces that contain interstitial fluid. Local infection increases both their number and activity. The same is true of *neutrophilic granulocytes,* yet these phagocytes are blood borne and arrive by passage through the walls of congested capillaries. More *fixed phagocytes,* such as the Kupffer's cells lining hepatic sinusoids, cull out pathogens as well as other foreign products that have reached the bloodstream. Phagocytes accomplish their mission by ameboid ingestion of particulate matter, whether infectious or autogenous waste products, followed by enzymatic digestion of such substances within vacuoles, and finally total eradication of residual infectious particles by absorption into their own cytoplasm. Often, however, ingested bacteria or bacterial products are sufficiently potent to destroy the challenging phagocyte before ingestion or afterward by breakdown of the vacuole wall

with release of contained destructive lysozymes (i.e., phagocyte-lysing enzymes).

Lymphocytes also play a major role in host resistance. Of the two component systems, non-thymic-dependent (*B-cell*) lymphocytes function primarily through their production of circulating antibody (*humoral immunity*) and are responsible for control of extracellular bacterial challenges. Both nonspecific and highly antigen-specific moieties are involved. Common mechanisms of action are neutralization of toxins, co-adaptation of infecting cells, disruption of pathogen cell membranes, and tagging and thereby identification of pathogens as being foreign substances now subject to phagocytic ingestion. Such functions are mediated by B-cell lymphocyte production of various *immunoglobulins,* particularly gamma globulin.

The other component, *cellular immunity,* is based on thymic-dependent lymphocytes. There are multiple subsets of these so-called *T-cell* lymphocytes. Convenient groups for reference include:

Killer cells: able to destroy cellular pathogens as well as other foreign cells
Helper cells: activate phagocytes and augment both phagocyte and killer cell function
Suppressor cells: limit and effectively terminate the inflammatory response

Elaborated factors that control as well as become the effector mechanisms for T-cell activity include:

Interleukin 1 and 2
Fibronectin
Tumor necrosis and growth factors
Interferon
Prostaglandin E
Complement
Calcium
Various cytokines

Their presently presumed interactions are given in Fig. 49-1. Host resistance against viruses, fungi, and intracellular bacteria resides in this latter system.

HOW IS INFECTION SPREAD?

The patient would almost certainly die if infection were not checked by a set of normally responsive local as well as systemic host defense mechanisms. Medical and surgical therapy designed to increase host resistance may be implemented, but unless such treatment is appropriate

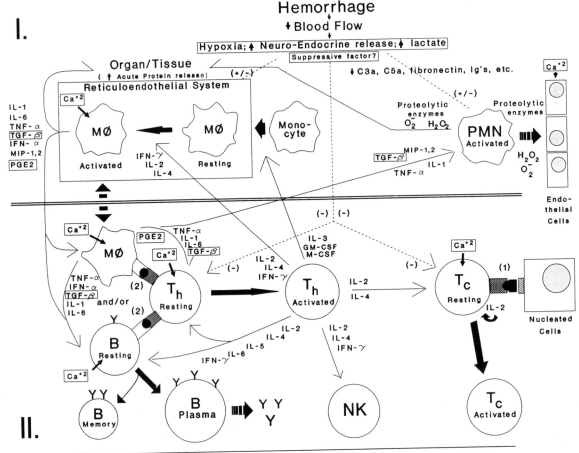

FIGURE 49-1   Flow chart of interactions of cytokines and other factors involving B- and T-cell lymphocytes.

and timely, it may prove detrimental rather than beneficial. For example, incision for drainage of an intra-abdominal abscess at too early a stage—before the process has been confined or walled off—can potentially spread the infection to uninvolved areas and thereby worsen the patient's condition.

Despite various antiinfectious measures, the natural course for any infection is to expand. There are many ways in which this may take place:

- By continuity, there is direct invasion into adjacent tissues and organs in immediate proximity.
- Extension may also occur along tissue planes that offer no obstacle to actual dissection by purulent exudate. Examples are the tendon sheath, areolar spaces between finite fascial planes, and the free flow permitted throughout

a body coelom, such as the abdomen or hemithorax.

- External drainage may occur spontaneously. Since this expels infectious material from the body, the desired end has been achieved. Resolution of the process can now take place.
- Drainage from within an organ or specific anatomic area into its confining or adjacent body cavity may also occur; yet this event considerably worsens the infection by extension without the advantages of external drainage. Examples are the spontaneous leak or operative spill of an intra-abdominal abscess, perforation in acute appendicitis, and rupture of a lung abscess into the free pleural space.

Under normal circumstances, products of infection are absorbed into lymphatic as well as venous channels. Hyperemia surrounding an infected lymph channel, even though the peripheral site of its origin appears innocuous, is called *acute lymphangitis* (or, colloquially, blood poisoning). The enlarged, tender, and inflamed nodes to which it drains signify *acute lymphadenitis*. These involved lymph nodes may later abscess and accordingly progress to *suppurative lymphadenitis*. Finally, invasion of vascular channels leads to *bacteremia* and subsequently the more feared *septicemia*, with spread throughout the body and eventually death if unabated.

HOW IS INFECTION DIAGNOSED?

It is of utmost importance that a culture be taken of any significant or potentially significant infection. If there is great urgency for initiating therapy, a smear and Gram stain of any available infected material can be used as a guide until the culture report is available. Only by knowing the species of pathogen and, in many cases, its individual antibiotic sensitivities can appropriate and rational antimicrobial treatment be given. For this reason, cultures should always be processed for both anaerobic and aerobic growth. Identification of the responsible species will then indicate the most likely source of the infection. Treatment can thereby be directed toward ultimate cure, prevention of a recurrence in the present location, and eradication of the same infection from some more distant area. It will also demonstrate the carrier state, so that spread of infection to other individuals can be prevented.

ANTIBIOTIC TREATMENT OF INFECTION

Different antimicrobial agents have different sites of action. Some destroy bacteria by punching holes in the cell wall (e.g., penicillins, cephalosporins); others act as detergents and disrupt the cell membrane (e.g., polymyxin); and still others interfere with amino acid replication during protein synthesis (e.g., aminoglycosides, macrolides). Finally, several antimicrobials (primarily the sulfonamides) block one or more metabolic steps in the production of some critical substrate (e.g., folic acid). To counter such antagonism, pathogens develop resistance to the antimicrobial or its adverse effects along one of several lines: elaboration of an enzyme to block or destroy the antibiotic (e.g., penicillinase and cephalosporinase representing the so-called beta-lactamases), passive transfer of chromosome-like resistance factors (R factors), actual mutation to a resistant strain, activation of latent biochemical

mechanisms, or acquisition of a critical substrate from its immediate environment rather than depending upon self-production.

The various bacteria pathogenic to humans have certain distinguishing characteristics with respect to source and site of infection, presentation of the infection, and specific types of antibiotics to which they are generally susceptible. Detailed sensitivities are listed in the box on p. 812.

For parenteral therapy, appropriate antibiotics are administered at doses that will provide blood levels exceeding by at least twofold the usual bacteriocidal concentrations for known or suspected pathogens. The antimicrobial agent is then readministered every fourth to sixth pharmacologic half-life of the agent (e.g., at 4- to 24-hour intervals). Therapy continues for a minimum of 3 days and is discontinued when signs of active infection are no longer evident. Beyond the tenth day of treatment, questions arise about the antibiotic selected—the appropriateness of its spectrum, the evolution of pathogen resistance, the drug's failure to penetrate the site of infection, and the need for surgical debridement or drainage instead. Signs that are useful in confirming eradication of infection, in order of increasing reliability, are fever, leukocyte count, and percent of immature granulocytes on differential white blood cell smear.

Topical and oral antimicrobial agents are useful in certain cases but must be understood to have variable absorption according to agent and status of the barrier surface (e.g., gut mucosa, granulating wall, and so on).

For prophylaxis against wound infection in surgery, perioperative antibiotics are indicated as follows:

- Although complicating infection is uncommon, when it occurs, the mortality or lifetime morbidity rate is exceedingly high (cardiac, peripheral vascular, major joint procedures)—generally, the "clean case."
- When infection is a common complication of potentially contaminated surgery (alimentary tract, biliary, and gynecologic procedures)—the "clean contaminated" and "contaminated" cases.
- Whenever there is significant impairment in host defenses (e.g., an immunosuppressed patient).

Appropriate antibiotics should be in the blood and tissues at risk in continuous bacteriocidal concentrations throughout the period from wound opening to its closure. A useful guide is to

SELECTION OF ANTIBIOTICS FOR MOST SURGICAL INFECTIONS*

Aerobic Gram-Positive Cocci and Bacilli

Penicillin and its analogs
Cephalosporins (first, second, and third
  generations)
Macrolides (erythromycin, lincomycin, and
  clindamycin)
Tetracyclines
NOTE: Penicillin-resistant *Staphylococcus*—
  Penicillin analogs, second and third
  generation cephalosporins
Methicillin-resistant *Staphylococcus*—
  Vancomycin
Enterococcus—Penicillin G plus tobramycin or
  gentamicin

Aerobic Gram-Negative Cocci

Penicillin
Cephalosporins (first and second generation)
Tetracycline
NOTE: Meningitis—Chloramphenicol

Aerobic Gram-Negative Bacilli

Aminoglycosides
Cephalosporins (second and third generation)
Certain penicillin analogs—Ampicillin,
  amoxacillin, carbenicillin, and ticarcillin
Chloramphenicol
Quinolones (Ciprofloxacin)
Monobactams (Aztreonam)
NOTE: *Pseudomonas* and certain resistant gram-
  negative rods—Tobramycin, gentamicin, and
  amikacin—or Quinolone or Monobactam
Salmonella—Chloramphenicol and ampicillin
Shigella—Ampicillin, tetracycline, and
  chloramphenicol

Anaerobes

Metronidazole
Macrolides (erythromycin, clindamycin, and
  lincomycin)
Cephalosporins (selective second and third
  generation only)
Chloramphenicol
Certain penicillin analogs (carbenicillin and
  ticarcillin)
Tetracycline
NOTE:*Clostridium difficile*—Vancomycin,
  metronidazole

Fungi

Topical—Nystatin, chlortrimazole, and
  amphoteracin B
Parenteral—Amphoteracin B and fluconazole

**Other Specific Pathogens (not all
inclusive)**

Actinomycetes—Penicillin, erythromycin, and
  tetracycline
Chancroid—Tetracycline
Mycobacteria tuberculosis and atypical
  mycobacteria—Isoniazid plus rifampin,
  streptomycin
Mycoplasma—Macrolides (erythromycin) and
  tetracyclines
Rickettsia—Tetracyclines and chloramphenicol
Spirochetes—Penicillin, tetracycline, and
  erythromycin
Vibrio—Tetracycline, chloramphenicol, and
  erythromycin

*According to pathogen, in decreasing order of preference.

repeat the dose of agent every second pharmacologic half-life. Once the skin has been closed,
there is no further need for antibiotic prophylaxis.

It cannot be overemphasized that under certain conditions, any area of the body can become
infected by any one or a multiplicity of bacterial
species. Although initial treatment of infection is
always directed against anticipated pathogens
based on the present clinical findings, only culture will allow identification of less commonly
occurring bacteria in any given septic state.

CLASSIFICATION OF SURGICAL INFECTION

Infection presents clinically in several different
ways, depending on individual species of bacteria, the area of the body affected, preexisting local factors (e.g., trauma, blood supply), patient
response to injury, and host resistance to infection. Nevertheless, signs of inflammation are almost always present, either at the site of infection
itself or along its immediate periphery. These
findings include pain and tenderness as caused
by irritation of local nerve endings, increased

temperature and redness secondary to hyperemia of the vascular response, and local swelling as a result of the edema of inflammatory exudation.

Cellulitis

Definition and Pathology. When the inflammatory response is diffuse and without extensive tissue necrosis or loculation of purulent exudate, the process is called *cellulitis.* In these circumstances, the vascular component of inflammation is extreme. Complications merely reflect the natural course of the disease and include conversion of areas within the initial inflammation to gangrene, formation of small isolated abscesses, and eventual bacteremia progressing to frank septicemia.

Cause. The usual case of isolated cellulitis is caused by infection by the hemolytic *Streptococcus* or *Staphylococcus aureus.* Occasionally both species are present, thereby creating a symbiosis. In other types of infection, there is almost always a margin of cellulitis at the interface between area of infection and surrounding normal host tissue. However, pure cellulitis is itself a common form of infection. The more virulent form of such a streptococcal infection is generally called *erysipelas.*

Treatment. Treatment consists of administration of a parenteral antibiotic known to be specifically effective against gram-positive cocci. Penicillin, some penicillin analog, a cephalosporin or a macrolide (e.g., erythromycin) should be chosen initially and then continued, unless the patient's clinical course fails to show improvement or primary cultures demonstrate an antibiotic-resistant species. Observation of the area of inflammation is always warranted so as to allow detection at an early stage of any major complication, such as gangrene or abscess formation. Support measures include rest and elevation of the infected part to facilitate both lymphatic and venous drainage. The application of local heat to further increase vasodilation and thereby augment the vascular response of inflammation is seldom necessary, although it is almost routinely prescribed. With appropriate antibiotic therapy, elevation, rest, and time, cellulitis almost always responds and promptly resolves.

Phlegmon

Definition and Pathology. When inflammation is relatively diffuse, yet there are small foci of necrotic tissue as well as multiple tiny pockets of accumulated pus, the infection is generally called a *phlegmon.* The process initially appears identical to cellulitis, but there is subsequent progression to innumerable microscopic abscesses, which in turn are often followed by extensive tissue destruction. Such compartmentalization of infection is the result of tissue plane division by interposing fibrous strands not degradable by pathogen enzymes.

Cause. The usual causative organism is *Staphylococcus aureus,* possibly in combination with a virulent strain of *Streptococcus.* Aerobic gram-negative rods plus various anaerobes can produce a similar clinical picture.

Treatment. Initial treatment of a phlegmon is identical to that for cellulitis—elevation, rest, and appropriate parenteral antibiotics. If significant necrosis develops, extensive debridement will then be required. Usually the minute abscesses are resorbed, although several may conglomerate into one or two pockets of suppuration that must be drained. In general, the phlegmon is a more destructive, fulminant, and refractory process than is cellulitis. A good example is the *carbuncle,* a subcutaneous infection of the posterior scalp, nape of the neck, or upper trunk. In some such cases, surgical excision of all overlying skin is the only method by which adequate debridement and effective drainage can be achieved.

Abscess

Definition and Pathology. When infection is confined to a single anatomic space by a wall of granulations, necrotic bits of tissue and purulent exudate then collect into one or more macroscopic cavities. The inflammatory process is thus said to have suppurated and thereby to have formed an *abscess. Pus,* or the purulent fluid contained within the abscess, is composed of destroyed host tissue, living and dead bacteria, various components of the phagocytic system (primarily neutrophilic granulocytes), and extracellular fluid. The process initially begins with a wound or in an area of established inflammation. There is almost immediate progression into one or more larger pockets. Surrounding this process is an area of relatively intense inflammation, the confining wall being a cellulitis. Debris of both host and invading bacteria collect as purulent exudate in the central cavity of the abscess, whereas interaction between viable bacteria and host defenses primarily occurs in the peripheral area of intense inflammation.

Cause. Although abscesses can be caused by almost any bacterial species, the usual culprits are hemolytic *Staphylococcus aureus* and various aerobic gram-negative rods, the latter commonly in synergy with various anaerobic species.

Treatment. Basic to the treatment for all abscesses is drainage. However, any channel thus provided for escape of purulent exudate must establish direct fistulization of the abscess to the outside through a relatively wide opening and with an absolutely dependent position so that gravity will be effective in guaranteeing pus discharge. Incomplete drainage results in persistence of the infection, continued absorption of bacterial toxins, and even greater local destruction of tissues. Nothing is ever gained by a small puncture wound or by aspiration of the abscess cavity. If dependent drainage cannot be obtained, then some form of suction should be instituted to overcome the adverse influence on free flow now created by gravity. Not only should the incision for drainage be made in accordance with cosmetic lines in an attempt to minimize unsightly scarring, but it also should be so placed as to reduce the likelihood or magnitude of contamination to other areas by its purulent discharge.

Antibiotics play only a secondary role in the treatment of abscesses. However, if sepsis resulting from an undrained abscess has reached major proportions, parenteral antibiotics serve a useful function by destroying such bacteria as have already invaded or as continue to seed the bloodstream until appropriate drainage can be accomplished. Antibiotic coverage similarly protects the host against the same bacteria that are massaged into vascular channels during the procedure of abscess drainage. Any mechanical scrubbing or forceful irrigation of an abscess cavity further increases the severity of the associated bacteremia, while a pack snugly inserted into the abscess not only causes transient bacteremia but also obstructs the free drainage of pus. Thus the importance of a wide, direct, and dependent tract for abscess drainage cannot be overemphasized.

The fistulous communication between abscess and body surface should be kept open by insertion of a relatively pliable, nonirritating foreign body. For this purpose, a piece of rubber dam or soft tubing is generally used. The tract is maintained until the abscess cavity has completely collapsed. At that point, the drain is advanced daily in a stepwise fashion so that healing progresses from the base. Should the tract close

first at the skin surface, pus once again will accumulate and thus the abscess recurs.

Gangrene

Definition and Pathology. Infectious gangrene is caused by the action of microbial enzymes directly on otherwise healthy tissues or indirectly by thrombosis of nutrient blood vessels serving the area. Often both processes occur simultaneously. The destruction of tissue is sufficiently extensive to produce visible necrosis. According to the species of bacteria, tissue infected, and general resistance of the host, *infectious gangrene* varies considerably with respect to rapidity and depth of necrosis as well as to systemic manifestations of the septic process.

The several types of infectious gangrene are best categorized on the basis of oxygen requirements of the individual bacteria and multiplicity of different invading species.

Aerobic Gangrene

Cause. Aerobic gangrene is usually caused by a highly virulent strain of hemolytic streptococci. Such infections have been epidemic during wartime, have accounted for the majority of cases of classic hospital gangrene, and were undoubtedly the cause of puerperal sepsis as noted by Semmelweiss. With proper isolation of wounds, use of aseptic technique, and appropriate antibiotic therapy, epidemics of aerobic streptococcal gangrene have almost become a thing of the past. Nevertheless, cases do still occasionally develop and demand the immediate intravenous administration of penicillin (or cephalosporin or tetracycline, if the patient is allergic to penicillin) in relatively massive doses. Certain highly virulent strains of *Staphylococcus aureus* can produce a similar infection (e.g., *scalded skin syndrome*).

Other forms of monobacterial aerobic gangrene occur with infections resulting from several other species (e.g., *Pseudomonas* burn wound necrosis of pyoderma gangrenosa, anthrax, *Yersinia pestis*, and tularemia). However, with the exception of those caused by *Pseudomonas aeruginosa*, other forms of aerobic infectious gangrene now occur relatively infrequently.

Treatment. Regardless of the infecting organism, treatment requires wide debridement of all necrotic tissues, parenteral administration of antibiotics appropriate to the pathogen, and delayed wound closure.

Anaerobic Gangrene

Cause and Pathology. Anaerobic gangrene is well represented by the gas bacillus *Clostridium* perfringens and its related species. Although not as common in civilian practice or even during wartime as it once was, *gas gangrene* occasionally develops in wounds that have been neglected and/or heavily contaminated by soil or feces. The onset is usually sudden, and there is rapid progression of the necrotizing process. Tissues become dark, cool, and brawny; areas of hemorrhage develop at the margin of the infection; local pain is intense; drainage from the wound is brackish and watery; tissues are crepitant from gaseous emphysema of the fascial planes; the patient has an exceedingly high fever, is usually irrational, and is frequently jaundiced; and the wound has a distinct, nauseatingly putrid odor that, once noted, can never be forgotten.

Treatment. For treatment to be adequate, there must be so thorough a debridement that absolutely all necrotic and infected tissues are included in the surgical specimen. The wound is then left open to increase local oxygen tension and thereby retard growth of any remaining gas bacilli. Massive doses of penicillin are given intravenously, with the object of combatting progression of the infection through bactericidal concentrations of antibiotic in adjacent tissues as well as in the open wound itself. In recent years, the hyperbaric oxygen tank has been advocated for drenching the tissues in oxygen through immersion of the patient in pure oxygen at a pressure of 3 atmospheres. However, critical evaluation of the method has failed to confirm as great a benefit as was initially claimed.

Synergistic Gangrene

Cause and Pathology. Synergistic gangrene is produced by the symbiosis of two or more bacterial species, with the resultant infection being more fulminant than either individual pathogen could cause alone. Many combinations have been documented since the first recognized synergistic infection was reported by Meleney—a progressive recalcitrant ulcer (Meleney's cellulitis) caused by the combination of the aerobic *Staphylococcus aureus* and anaerobic *Peptostreptococcus.* Other symbiotic partners producing characteristic infections include a fusiform bacillus and spirochete, the duo causing a persistent ulcerative infection of the gingiva (generally referred to as *trench mouth*), several sets of gram-positive cocci, producing destructive lesions about the nose and mouth (cited as *cancrum oris, noma,* and others), and various combinations of anaerobes and aerobic gram-negative rods causing infections of subcutaneous tissues (*necrotizing fasciitis*) or muscle and supporting structures beneath the deep enveloping fascia (*necrotizing cellulitis*).

Overall, most bacterial synergisms consist of two components—one aerobic, the other anaerobic. The anaerobes are generally the primary pathogen and contribute those destructive enzymes that establish and then make the infection so fulminant as well as refractory to routine measures of therapy. The major, if not sole, purpose of the aerobe is to create and maintain a local microenvironment conducive to continued life and propagation of the anaerobes through near-total oxygen extraction from local tissues. Thus both components are absolute necessities to the infection—the anaerobe for virulence, the aerobe to sustain the anaerobe. Elimination of either partner will disrupt the symbiotic relationship and accordingly revert the process to a relatively benign infection. Nevertheless, it is the aerobe that, on invading the bloodstream, causes the attendant bacteremia and thus lethal septic shock.

Treatment. Synergistic gangrene demands the same basic treatment as do other forms of necrotizing infection: immediate debridement of all nonviable tissue, delayed wound closure (usually by skin grafting), and massive intravenous doses of appropriate antibiotics. Depending on the amount of tissue necrosis and therefore the extent of debridement required, major deformity and loss of function can result unless energetic measures are instituted at an early stage. Incomplete debridement always leads to local recurrence of infection and is routinely followed by progression into previously uninvolved tissues.

Toxemia

Definition and Pathology. Although essentially all infection is based on tissue penetration and subsequent host absorption of various bacterial toxins, certain forms of sepsis have a small and relatively innocuous-appearing primary focus, and yet their virulence factors (*exotoxins*) exert a significantly destructive and generally disruptive influence on metabolic and/or physiologic functions of the host. Accordingly, such infections are appropriately referred to as *toxemias.*

Cause. The classic example is *tetanus,* in which the site of toxin production is usually an otherwise inconsequential minor wound. Nevertheless, systemic manifestations of toxin absorption are profound and frequently lethal. In tetanus toxemia, the central nervous system is primarily affected; the stages in clinical progression are irritability, muscle spasm, convulsions, coma, and death from respiratory arrest.

The other two relatively common and equally life-threatening exotoxemias are **diphtheria,** arising from infection of the pharynx by *Corynebacterium diphtheriae* (a cardiac toxin producer), and *Pseudomonas* wound sepsis, with toxin being absorbed usually from an extensively colonized burn wound. The latter directly inhibits various antiinfectious functions of the reticuloendothelial system.

Treatment. Initial treatment of any toxemia should include massive doses of intravenously administered antibiotic appropriate to the infecting species, correction of fluid and electrolyte deficits to make general anesthesia safer, and administration of specific antitoxins, preferably of human origin, if such are available. As soon as the patient's condition permits, wide excision of the site of infection, when feasible, with delayed wound closure is the only reliable method of eradicating the process. As with abscesses and infectious gangrene, all nonsurgical measures are merely supportive and serve only to prepare the patient for operation—the definitive step in therapy for patients with tetanus and *Pseudomonas* toxemia.

Septicemia

Definition and Pathology. When bacteria have invaded the bloodstream either through infection or by contamination of intravascular monitoring or treatment devices, **bacteremia** is said to have occurred. If this progresses to propagation of bacteria within the bloodstream, actual **septicemia** has been established and becomes the greatest threat of that originating infection. Prior disease changes in the endothelial lining of cardiovascular structures then provide ideal sites for metastatic infection to complicate the bacteremia.

Bacteria may also form the nidus of a clot, which can propagate and then embolize to some more distant locus in the vascular system. Such an origin of metastatic abscesses is called a **mycotic embolism.**

In addition to the septic state caused by growth of bacteria within the bloodstream, bacterial enzymes and tissue breakdown products (particularly components of erythrocytes and leukocytes), if circulating, exert profound humoral influences on various organ systems. Examples are peripheral pooling of blood, heart failure, intravascular coagulopathy, and a multiplicity of other poorly understood phenomena. Characteristic vasomotor responses, and then

TABLE 49-1   Clinical Differentiation of Septicemias

	Gram-Positive	Gram-Negative
Clinical Sign/Parameter		
Sensorium	Irrational	Rational
Temperature	Spiking 39°-40° C	Sustained, 38°-39° C
Blood pressure	Gradual fall	Gradual fall until sudden shock
Urine flow	Gradual fall	Low until sudden anuria
Jaundice	Often	Rare
WBC	>16,000	10,000-16,000
Urine microscopic	—	—
Wound	Dissolution of granulations	Focal necrosis of granulations
Wound odor	Sour/sweetish	—
Usual source	Soft tissues	Peritoneum
	IV site	Urinary tract
	Respiratory	Wound
		Pulmonary
Antimicrobials for Therapy		
	Penicillin	Aminoglycoside
	Penicillin analog	Cephalosporin
	Cephalosporin	Monobactam
	Tetracycline	Quinolone

circulatory collapse secondary to gram-negative bacteremia and septicemia, are referred to as *endotoxemia*. In fact, individual reactions to different bacterial toxins as well as host catabolic products create somewhat specific clinical syndromes that can be used to differentiate among gram-positive, gram-negative, anaerobic, and fungal septicemia (Table 49-1).

Cause. Any invasive bacterial infection may culminate in septicemia.

Treatment. Unless the focus seeding the bloodstream is eradicated, bacteremia will persist and may progress to septicemia. Thus, as soon as is practical, abscesses must be drained, necrotic tissue excised, and responsible venous cannulas eliminated. Equally important is the parenteral administration of antibiotics with known activity against the specific pathogens presumed to be present in the blood (see Surgical Pharmacopeia, p. 825). Blood infections can generally be separated into broad pathogen types by the patient's clinical course, although culture of both site of origin and the blood itself are required to substantiate an initial clinical assumption. Choice of antibiotic may then need to be altered when more specific information regarding species and antimicrobial sensitivities is available.

Other treatment measures are directed toward correction of dehydration, electrolyte derangements, acidosis, septic shock if present, and any obvious failure in a critical organ system. Monoclonal antibody specific for endotoxin has shown promise in reducing the likelihood and severity of lethal physiologic derangements in patients with gram-negative sepsis.

COMMON FORMS OF INFECTION

Certain infections, such as those of the skin and hand, warrant relatively detailed description as to differential diagnosis and management. These problems are relatively common, and their respective treatment methods are well established. In addition, identification of the infection responsible for postoperative fever, particularly that following laparotomy, is an important and frequently encountered problem.

Skin Infections

Cellulitis. Cellulitis of the skin and subcutaneous tissues is identical to cellulitis occurring elsewhere. However, the original site of infection is usually marked by a wound or some break in the protective skin through which invading bacteria have gained access to deeper structures. Treatment consists of elevation, rest, and administration of pathogen-specific antibiotics.

Endotoxemia	Anaerobic	Fungal
Irrational	Irrational	Rational
Falling, hypothermia	Spiking to 39°-40° C	Sustained, 38°-39° C
Sudden shock	Gradual fall	Gradual fall
Sudden anuria	Gradual fall	Gradual fall
—	Common	Rare
<6000	>14,000	>14,000
—	—	Yeast
Enlarging focal necrosis	Extensive necrosis, gangrene	Occasional focal necrosis
—	Putrid	—
Peritoneum	Peritoneum	Alimentary
Urinary tract	Perineal area	IV cannula
Wound	Pulmonary	
Aminoglycoside	Clindamycin	Nystatin (oral)
Cephalosporin	Erythromycin	Amphotericin B
Quinolone	Chloramphenicol	Fluconazole
	Metronidazole	

Furuncle. The furuncle begins with infection of a skin appendage (sebaceous gland, hair follicle, or sweat gland) and progresses to an intradermal abscess with subcutaneous extension. The process is generally confined to a relatively small area and eventually will drain spontaneously after necrosing the overlying skin. *Staphylococcus aureus* alone or in combination with hemolytic streptococci is the usual pathogen. Recurrences suggest an altered host resistance (e.g., from diabetes or reticuloendothelial diseases) or that the individual is a carrier of staphylococci and repeatedly reinoculates himself. The usual endemic foci are the nasopharynx and tonsillar fossa, seldom with either area showing any sign of obvious infection. Eradication of the carrier state requires appropriate systemic antibiotics and, more importantly, the nasal insufflation of a pathogen specific topical antimicrobial agent.

Hidradenitis. As a result of differences in gland structure and function or changes in local skin conditions, infections of the various skin appendages present with equally diverse clinical pictures. For example, *hidradenitis* is an infection of sudoriferous glands of the axilla. It is frequently precipitated by irritating underarm deodorants, tends to localize into one or more abscesses, and usually recurs unless the underarm is kept clean and deodorant use is restricted.

Pilonidal Abscess. The pilonidal cyst or abscess is caused by obstruction to a hair follicle in the intergluteal crease of a relatively hirsute patient. With accumulation of skin secretions and debris, a cyst develops, and infection almost uniformly follows. Drainage is then required for control of the acute inflammatory process, while excision of both the cyst and its arborizing communications is reserved for a later time as an elective procedure when all evidence of acute infection has disappeared.

Cysts. *Sebaceous cysts* arise from obstructions to the neck of sebaceous glands, develop over the face, scalp, neck, and upper aspect of the trunk, and frequently become infected. Drainage, with release of both purulent exudate and infected sebum, is then required. Once the acute inflammatory process has resolved, residual cyst and scar are excised in continuity with an ellipse of overlying skin.

Carbuncle. The carbuncle, as mentioned previously, is a more extensive infection of dermis and subcutaneous tissue. As with other phlegmonous inflammations, division of all partitioning fibrous septa with conversion of the process thereby into a single abscess pocket is required. Occasionally, overlying necrotic skin must also be excised.

Folliculitis. Folliculitis is a staphylococcal infection of hair follicles. It is prone to develop in patients with heavy growth of hair generally or in areas where hair is coarse, such as the beard, axilla, and suprapubic region. The infection tends to persist and even spread until both topical and systemic antibiotics are administered to control the immediate local infection as well as to eradicate the carrier state.

Hand Infections

Similar to other areas of the body, infections of the hand can present as any one of several types of inflammation, although cellulitis and abscess are the most common. Abscesses are drained as detailed below, while cellulitis is treated with antibiotics alone unless complicated by abscess formation. Additional therapeutic measures, irrespective of the type of infection, should always include antibiotics, elevation, and splinting the hand in the position of function. Whenever the hand is not in a splint, only active motion is allowed.

Hand infections usually develop in specific anatomic spaces, spread along predetermined fascial planes, and in general pose a greater threat to loss of function rather than loss of life. Characteristically, swelling of the palmar aspect is caused by infection on that same side of the hand, whereas dorsal swelling may instead be mere edema consequent to volar infection. Delay in drainage can be most costly to future hand use; yet inappropriate and poorly placed incisions can do even greater and inexcusable harm to important nerves and tendons. As a general rule, most drainage procedures on the hand proper and for tendon sheaths at any level should be done in the operating room under general anesthesia with the benefit of a dry field as provided by tourniquet.

Paronychia. *Paronychia* is an infection of the soft tissues of the nail margin. Other more colloquial terms used to describe the process are *runaround* and *whitlow* for the fingers and *ingrown nail* for the toes. There is burrowing beneath the eponychium as well as under the nail itself, particularly at its edges. If infection is restricted to a small area amounting to less than half of the nail margin, a limited incision may be tried under local anesthesia. More extensive infection, however, requires separation of nail from nail bed and then avulsion of the nail from beneath the eponychium.

Felon. Infection of the pulp space of the fingertip is called a *felon*. The resultant abscess is confined to a small area bounded by fibrous septa passing between skin and bony phalangeal tuft. Rather than spreading into adjacent subcutaneous pockets, the infection often erodes into the phalanx below and causes a resorptive osteomyelitis generally called a **bone felon.** Treatment is by midlateral drainage (Fig. 49-2), care being taken to sever all obstructing fibrous bands without destroying fingertip alignment or placing a tender scar on the finger's working surface.

Web Space Infections. Infection in the web space between fingers generally develops in the areolar tissue just between adjacent palmar calluses. As a small abscess forms, the inflammation then dissects dorsally between metacarpal heads and creates a satellite abscess on the back of the hand. This is called a **collarbutton infection.** Drainage of one pocket is never sufficient; both

must be opened (Fig. 49-3). Dorsally, a longitudinal incision is placed between metacarpal prominences, while on the volar aspect, the web space is opened horizontally to avoid putting a scar in palmar skin.

Thenar Space Infections. The palmar aspect of the hand can be divided into two major compartments where deep infections tend to localize. The **thenar space** lies between thumb and second metacarpal. Abscesses here cause a volar swelling that abducts and externally rotates the thumb. Since direct drainage through palmar skin can cause injury to the median nerve, the appropriate incision is one placed dorsally in the first web space (Fig. 49-3). Then by blunt dissection, the abscess cavity can be reached, and yet both nerve and radial artery are avoided.

Midpalmar Space Infections. The **midpalmar**

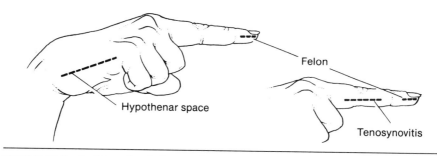

FIGURE 49-2 Incisions for drainage of tenosynovitis and other finger infections.

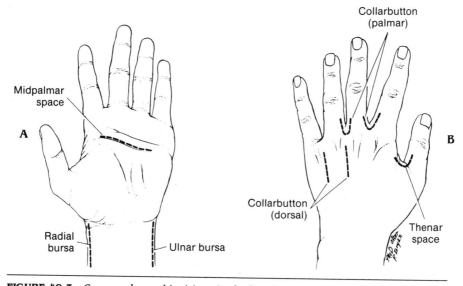

FIGURE 49-3 Commonly used incisions in the hand. **A,** Palmar view. **B,** Dorsal view.

space lies medial to the second metacarpal on the volar aspect of the hand. Although infection of the area will obliterate the normal palmar hollow, dorsal edema can be so massive as to almost overshadow its true ventral location. An indirect route to abscess drainage is impractical. Accordingly, the incision is made straight through volar skin with care being taken to cut along the normally occurring midpalmar or distal palmar crease so as to obviate any later disabling contracture (Fig. 49-3).

Tenosynovitis. Tenosynovitis, or infection of an individual tendon sheath, is characterized by fusiform swelling of the involved finger, which in turn is held in slight flexion, resists all motion because of pain, and exhibits exquisite percussion tenderness along the anatomic course of the tendon. Initially cellulitis is present and may resolve with parenteral antibiotics. However, if inflammation persists or if the question arises as to purulent fluctuance, drainage should be carried out as soon as possible. For the fingers, midlateral incisions are placed down to and including the tendon sheath (see Fig. 49-2); in the hand, an approach similar to that used to expose the midpalmar space is used.

Other Infections. Tendon sheaths of the fifth finger and thumb frequently communicate with similarly lined sacs at the wrist. These are, respectively, the ulnar and radial bursae. Infection can extend from the thumb, along its flexor tendon sheath to the radial bursa, then across at the wrist to the ulnar bursa, and down the fifth finger tendon sheath to the little finger. These are called *horseshoe abscesses* and require individual drainage, as with infections of the separate tendon sheaths (Fig. 49-3).

Postoperative Fever

At some time during their postoperative course, patients often become febrile; yet such an event cannot be attributed indiscriminately to infection warranting administration of an antibiotic. Although infections of the incision and coelom proper are common complications, there are many other and relatively frequent causes of postoperative fever.

Infections nevertheless do develop during the postoperative period, especially in the patient whose abdomen has been contaminated by bacteria as a result of disease or trauma. Four areas are primarily suspect and for simplicity can be referred to as the "four W's". They are the wind, the water, the veins (a somewhat corrupted "W"), and the wound. More specifically, these represent pneumonia or pulmonary problems, uri-nary tract infections, thrombophlebitis, and infection of the surgical incision and/or cavity subjected to operation. Only by investigating each of these areas can the true cause of postoperative sepsis be identified.

Pulmonary. Postoperative respiratory tract infections are usually based upon retained and thereby obstructing bronchial secretions, pulmonary insufflation with hospital pathogens during assisted ventilation, or both. An effective cough is most important in prevention as well as in therapy, because it is the single best method for clearing secretions. Otherwise, atelectasis develops and then progresses gradually into pneumonia. Antibiotics alone consistently fail on both counts, because only after the bronchopulmonary tree has been relieved of obstruction will infectious processes resolve. On the other hand, antibiotics can be lifesaving. At the very least, bacteremia is temporarily controlled until pulmonary sepsis has responded to the combination of improved bronchial drainage and antibiotic therapy.

Although physical examination is useful for general evaluation, a chest x-ray evaluation is a more accurate means of gauging the extent and severity of pneumonia. A Gram stain of the sputum serves as reliable a guide as is available for directing initial antimicrobial therapy, yet the antibiotic regimen may need to be changed when culture and sensitivities on the sputum have been reported. On many occasions, ventilatory support becomes an equally important consideration. Patients with borderline pulmonary function may have been so compromised by operation, respiratory muscle splinting because of the incision, or pneumonia itself that energetic ventilatory therapy may well be the prime determinant in their eventual survival.

Urinary. Hematogenous seeding of the urinary tract by otherwise insignificant circulating bacteria occurs almost routinely during the act of glomerular filtration. Indwelling catheters, however, for either urinary tract decompression or urine collection allow retrograde inoculation with even more dangerous pathogens, i.e., those from the hospital environment. With stasis of urine flow, whether from dehydration or mechanical obstruction, acute infection usually develops. Should the patient have previously maintained a heavily colonized urinary tract or have symptomless chronic urinary tract infection, an acute exacerbation routinely ensues.

Diagnosis is made by urinalysis, particularly the microscopic examination demonstrating presence of bacterial or white cell casts, and urine culture for both colony count and antibiotic sensitivities. Bacterial counts equal to or greater than 100,000 organisms per milliliter are absolutely diagnostic, although colony counts even as low as 2000 per milliliter can be noted in acute infection. Dysuria, urgency, frequency, and flank tenderness may not be discernible despite active infection. In any event, either dehydration and/or urinary tract obstruction are almost always present.

Treatment requires that an antibiotic be administered appropriate initially to a Gram stain of the urine and subsequently to results of culture sensitivities, that the patient be sufficiently well hydrated to produce a suitable urine output, and that any obstruction to urine flow must be relieved by diversion or anatomic correction.

Venous. In the past postoperative thrombophlebitis seldom had a bacterial cause, since pathologically it was more of a bland phlebothrombosis than an inflammatory thrombophlebitis and accordingly was associated with a high incidence of pulmonary embolism. Following the introduction of synthetic and relatively inert intravenous cannulas, parenteral fluid therapy is now continued for much longer periods than in all probability is actually necessary. There also has been a greater tendency for irritating medications to be given intravenously. The result has led to the almost routine development of postoperative phlebitis, as manifested either by intense local inflammation without true sepsis or by a cannula-seeded bacteremia in the absence of significant reactive phlebitis.

Treatment of chemically induced phlebitis is merely supportive. The intravenous catheter is removed, and the limb is elevated as well as put at rest. Similar measures are used in patients with bacteremia. If bacteremia persists or initially there is septicemia—usually caused by *Staphylococcus aureus*—the cannula wound is opened widely and a parenteral antistaphylococcal agent is given. The preferred antibiotics are either one of the penicillinase-resistant penicillins or a cephalosporin. However, cultures taken before initiating antimicrobial therapy may dictate a change in parenteral agent if instead some resistant microbe is identified, e.g., *Candida albicans* or methicillin-resistant *Staphylococcus aureus*.

Wound. The wound, represented by both the surgical incision and the body coelom explored (e.g., peritoneal cavity), is the most common site of postoperative infection. The incidence is greater when significant contamination has occurred, either because of a break in sterile technique during operation or because of autoinoculation by the disease process itself.

The postoperative day on which a given wound infection produces identifiable and thus diagnostic local signs varies according to the incubation period of bacteria responsible for the infection and use of specific antiseptic measures,

TABLE 49-2   Postoperative Wound Infections

Onset (postoperative days)	Usual Pathogen	Wound Appearance	Other Signs
1-3	*Clostridium perfringens* and related species	Brawny, hemorrhagic, cool, gaseous crepitation, putrid exudate, intense local pain	High sustained fever (39°-40° C); irrational; leukocytosis >15,000/mm³; jaundice.
2-3	*Streptococcus*	Erythematous, warm, tender, occasionally hemorrhagic with blebs, serous exudate	High spiking fever (to 39°-40° C); irrational at times; leukocytosis >15,000/mm³; rarely, jaundice
3-4	*Staphylococcus*	Erythematous, warm, tender, purulent exudate	High spiking fever (to 38°-39° C); irrational at times; leukocytosis 12,000-20,000/mm³
>4	Symbiotic (usually anaerobes plus gram-negative rods)	Erythematous, warm, tender, focal necrosis, putrid exudate	Moderate to high fever (38°-40° C); mentation variable; leukocytosis >15,000/mm³; occasionally, jaundice
>6	Gram-negative rod	Erythematous, warm, tender, purulent exudate	Sustained moderate fever (38°-39° C); rational; leukocytosis 10,000-16,000/mm³

such as parenteral antibiotics (Table 49-2). As a general rule, the earlier the onset of clinical sepsis, the more destructive and life-threatening the infection becomes. Pure anaerobic or streptococcal cellulitis appears 2 or 3 days postoperatively, staphylococcal wound infection usually within 3 to 4 days, and symbiotic and gram-negative rod sepsis after 4 or 5 days (see Table 49-2).

Treatment of the infected surgical incision is straightforward. The wound must be opened for adequate drainage, the patient positioned so as to provide reliable dependent drainage, and, if tissue necrosis is extensive, careful debridement performed. The wound is then allowed to close spontaneously by contracture, with split skin grafts, or through rotation of a pedicled flap—the individual technique being selected for appropriateness to the size, type, and location of surface defect.

The chances of postoperative infection developing in a heavily contaminated wound can be diminished by use of various technical maneuvers during operation as well as timely and appropriate drug chemotherapy. Delayed primary wound closure on the third postoperative day and instillation of topical antimicrobial agents directly into the primarily closed wound are relatively effective and generally reduce the incidence of infection in the surgical incision to less than a third of what would have been expected otherwise. In cases where wound contamination is predictable, however, appropriate parenteral antibiotics provide a moderate degree of prophylaxis against subsequent wound infection if such agents are given in sufficient time before operation to establish bactericidal levels in local tissues and extracellular fluid from the moment of incision to final wound closure. In addition, if the area from which anticipated autoinoculation occurs is known, procedures and medications to minimize such contamination are always indicated. The most common application of this final principle is mechanical bowel cleansing and oral administration of nonabsorbable antimicrobial agents during preoperative preparation of the patient for elective colon surgery. Nevertheless, antibiotic use must always be selective, never indiscriminate, as even greater problems are caused by the evolution of antibiotic-resistant strains of bacteria.

Peritonitis. Postoperative peritonitis is initially either generalized or confined primarily to a specific region of the abdomen. As time elapses and as both the host defenses and administered antimicrobial agents come into play, the inflammatory process tends to become localized into one or more individual abscesses. Failure of protective adhesions to develop and thereby to restrict the inflammation to a given area of the abdomen is usually associated with a persistence of peritonitis and often death. As a general rule, operation under these circumstances is indicated only to correct any cause for continuing peritoneal contamination, to close a complicating evisceration, or to drain specific abscesses.

Pathogens isolated from peritonitis are generally those harbored normally in the colon or biliary tract, i.e., gram-negative rods with or without various anaerobic species. (Gastric perforations usually contaminate with gram-positive cocci and rods.) Accordingly, aminoglycosides, cephalosporins, and certain synthetic penicillins with or without agents active against anaerobic species are the more reliable antibiotics to be used until specific culture and sensitivity tests have dictated otherwise. In symbiotic infections, aerobic bacteria are generally those responsible for patient death, whereas anaerobic participation correlates with a predilection for persistent or recurrent sepsis. Multiple antibiotics may be required to give the desired, more complete spectrum for patient protection. Because of paralytic ileus, antibiotics are given parenterally with intravenous fluid and electrolyte therapy.

Postoperative peritonitis is basically related to the size and virulence of the bacterial inoculum. Thus infection often follows operations for already established intra-abdominal sepsis and whenever major contamination occurs during surgery. Intraoperative blood levels of appropriate bacteriocidal antibiotics significantly reduce the incidence of subsequent peritoneal infection in such cases by killing off potential pathogens. Meticulous cleansing of the abdominal cavity likewise tends to reduce the magnitude of inoculum below the infectious minimum. The value of abdominal drains is moot, for although purulent material may be discharged during the postoperative phase, the drain serves only to evacuate from a small portion of peritoneum and is itself a foreign body, which itself favors the evolution of infection by inward migration of hospital pathogens.

There are three general areas to which most intra-abdominal infections localize: (1) the *true pelvis,* (2) the *midabdomen,* i.e., the region situated between pelvis and transverse mesocolon and including the lateral gutters, and (3) the *subphrenic space,* i.e., that portion of abdomen immediately above the transverse mesocolon but below the diaphragm.

Intra-abdominal Abscess. The most common site for such localization is the pelvis. A gloved finger inserted into the rectum readily identifies any pelvic abscess. If there is uncertainty, however, rectal examinations should be repeated at frequent intervals. Any suspicious mass can be aspirated transrectally. The mid-abdominal abscess usually develops in one of the lateral gutters situated on either side of the vertebral prominence, often with communication to a similar purulent collection via the false pelvis. Mass and/or tenderness on careful abdominal palpation and spontaneous drainage through the incision (*subfascial abscess*) are characteristic, although an earlier diagnosis can often be made by scrutiny of plain x-ray films of the abdomen. Doubtful cases can further be resolved by noting any telltale extraluminal air-fluid level on lateral decubitus views or by better definition on CT scan. Infection within the subphrenic space is more difficult to document. Abscesses, however, contain material similar to that found within the cecum—water, bacteria, organic debris, and gas—and thus the x-ray film appearance can be almost identical. In doubtful cases, a CT scan should be ordered.

Pelvic abscesses may be drained rectally if a firm synthesis exists between the abscess wall and rectum. Otherwise, extraperitoneal lateral drainage is safer. With respect to other areas, that is, the midabdominal and subphrenic spaces, drainage should be gained through an extraperitoneal approach with an attempt at assured dependency to guarantee the beneficial effects of gravity. Most abscesses can be drained in this way by CT guided percutaneous catheter insertion—that is, provided another surgical procedure is not required, debridement of necrotic tissue is unnecessary, and a phlegmonous mass of pancreas or colon is not part of the process. However, when the locus of life-threatening sepsis is uncertain or if there has been failure to gain a complete response to extraperitoneal drainage alone, then a laparotomy with a search of all intra-abdominal spaces must be performed to avoid overlooking a correctable process. When true dependent drainage cannot be obtained, sump suction should be used.

Fungal Sepsis. Although relatively uncommon, generalized fungal infection carries an inordinately high mortality rate in the surgical patient, probably because of a failure either to suspect its presence or to institute appropriate therapy. Use of topical and/or parenteral antibacterial agents not only predisposes toward the development of fungal sepsis, but also generally guarantees a persistence of such infection if antibiotics are continued.

Sporotrichosis and aspergillosis usually arise by systemic invasion from a colonized wound. Treatment requires radical wound excision, topical antifungal agents (nystatin), and often parenteral therapy (amphotericin B or fluconazole). *Candida* sepsis, on the other hand, originates by seeding via a contaminated intravenous set or through yeast translocation from a heavily colonized small intestine. The primary focus must likewise be eradicated, usually by discontinuation of the intravenous set or with oral antifungal agents, respectively. Parenteral therapy may also be given but is probably of little value in comparison with the almost curative effect of eliminating the source of invasion and discontinuing systemic antibacterial drugs.

VIRAL INFECTIONS OF SURGICAL SIGNIFICANCE

Two separate viral infections have taken on major surgical importance during the past decade. Not only does each pose a set of surgical problems, but also both put the surgeon and the entire patient care team at considerable risk.

Viral Hepatitis

At present, no less than five different viruses are known to cause human hepatitis; these are identified as A through E.

Hepatitis A (HAV). A small RNA virus (enterovirus) is responsible for the condition once referred to as *infectious hepatitis.* Spread is usually through ingestion, with a relatively brief incubation period of 2 to 4 weeks. It has a unique predilection for preschool nurseries and kindergartens, appears to be transmitted by food handlers, and is primarily carried in uncooked food. Poor sanitation, as is prevalent in the third world, has a close correlation with its incidence. Theoretically hepatitis A can be spread through blood transfusion or even an incidental needlestick.

Most cases run an anicteric course, although if jaundice does occur, the patient is most infectious before the onset of icterus. Presently there is no proven vaccine, but transient passive protection can be gained by the administration of gamma globulin.

Hepatitis B (HBV). The old term *serum hepatitis* was used to denote infection by a relatively large DNA virus that would cause a more severe form of hepatitis after a period of several months' incubation following inoculation through transfusion, needlestick, or intimate sexual contact. The responsible virus is made up of a core (HB_cAg, which can be identified only by the presence of the antibodies it has induced), an identifiable central core antigen (HB_eAg, which can be isolated and thereby reflects presence of active circulating virus), and a surface coat, referred to as *surface antigen* (HB_sAg, antibodies against which document an immune response gained either by active virus or vaccine). Approximately two thirds of patients never develop jaundice; one tenth become chronic carriers, with potential for infecting others; a fourth progress to cirrhosis, with its disability and potential for death from chronic liver disease or hepatic malignancy.

There are two hepatitis B vaccines available for active immunization, both having been produced by recombinant technology. After three doses, approximately 97% of recipients will develop antibodies against surface antigen, and this uniformly conveys immunity. The necessity for a booster dose has yet to be determined.

Hepatitis C (HCV). In the past patients with negative test results for hepatitis A and B were classified as having *non-A, non-B hepatitis.* However, at present there is a specific serologic test, which unfortunately may not yield a positive result for anti-HCV antibodies until 6 to 18 months after exposure. The infection is primarily spread by blood transfusion, although needlesticks and intimate sexual contacts also provide a means for transmission. Half of the patients so infected become chronic carriers. There is no vaccine available that would convey either active or passive immunity.

Hepatitis D (HDV). *Delta hepatitis* appears to be unable to cause hepatitis alone, but is a co-infective virus with many cases of hepatitis B. It also can create a carrier state.

Hepatitis E (HEV). In the third world, especially during monsoon season, epidemics of non-A, non-B hepatitis occur and appear to be caused primarily by hepatitis E. As yet is has not been diagnosed in patients in the continental United States.

AIDS

Human immunodeficiency virus (HIV) is an RNA agent (retrovirus) that acts on nuclear DNA through reverse transcriptase. Once infected years may pass before symptoms develop. Such clinical manifestations are caused, as the name implies, by an immune-depressed state. Specifically the virus kills T-lymphocytes, with the result that relatively uncommon infections, from such pathogens as *Pneumocystis carinii* and cytomegalic virus, as well as certain tumors (i.e., lymphoma and Kaposi's sarcoma), arise. Because of a lack of appropriate host resistance, the infections persist and eventuate in death.

HIV can be transmitted by transfusions (those given between 1979 and 1984 before routine donor screening and blood bank testing), multipartner unprotected sex, and even needlesticks. Unfortunately, at least 6 months elapses from the time of inoculation until circulating antibody can be detected in the blood. Risk to the health care worker is quite high, but not as great as with hepatitis B. To date, only three patients have been documented to have become infected by a single health care worker.

For both hepatitis and AIDS, several basic facts must be kept in mind. First, the blood and body fluids of all patients should be assumed to be infectious. Accordingly, *universal precautions* must be practiced for protection against both AIDS and hepatitis. Even if all patients could be tested for these viral infections, many cleared individuals may still be infectious, because several months must elapse before diagnostic serology becomes positive. Fortunately, for hepatitis B there is a reliable means of immunization.

SURGICAL PHARMACOPEIA

Drug	Indications/Complications	Dosage
Penicillins		
Methicillin (Staphicillin, Celbenin)	*Indication:* Penicillin-resistant gram-positive cocci and bacilli *Adverse effects:* Hypersensitivity, leukopenia, nephropathy, hemolytic anemia, hemorrhagic cystitis	2 g q4h IV
Nafcillin (Unipen, Nafcil)	*Indication:* Penicillin-resistant gram-positive cocci and bacilli *Adverse effects:* Bone marrow depression, granulocytopenia	2 g q4h IV
Oxacillin (Prostaphlin, Bactocil)	*Indications:* Penicillin-resistant gram-positive cocci and bacilli *Adverse effects:* Anemia, nephropathy, neutropenia	2 g q4h PO
Mezlocillin (Mezlin)	*Indications:* Gram positive: including enterococcus; gram negative: including *Pseudomonas* sp, *Enterobacter* sp, *Klebsiella, Serratia;* anaerobes: including *Bacteroides fragilis* *Adverse effects:* Bone marrow depression, hypersensitivity	3 g q4h IV
Piperacillin (Pipril, Pipracil, Pentcillyn, Avocin)	*Indications:* Gram positive: including enterococcus; gram negative: including *Pseudomonas* sp, *Enterobacter* sp, *Klebsiella, Serratia;* anaerobes: including *Bacteroides fragilis* *Adverse effects:* Bone marrow depression, hypersensitivity	3 g q4h IV
Dicloxacillin (Dynapen, Pathocil)	*Indications:* Gram positive, especially resistant staphylococci	125-500 mg q6h
Penicillin G	*Indications:* Aerobic: Gram-positive cocci, bacilli; anaerobic: gram-negative cocci, *Actinomycites;* spirochetes *Adverse effects:* Hypersensitivity, bone marrow depression	600,000-1.2 million units/day IV, IM
Ampicillin	*Indications:* Aerobic: Gram-positive cocci, bacilli; aerobic: gram-negative bacilli, *Shigella, Salmonella* *Adverse effects:* Hypersensitivity, bone marrow depression	500 mg q6h IM, IV, PO
First-Generation Cephalosporins		
Cephalothin (Seffin, Keflin)	*Indications:* Aerobic: Gram-positive cocci, bacilli; aerobic: Gram-negative cocci *Adverse effects:* Hypersensitivity, neutropenia, nephrotoxicity	1-2 g q4h IV
Cefazolin (Ancef, Zolicef, Kefzol)	*Indications:* Aerobic: Gram-positive cocci, bacilli; aerobic: Gram-negative cocci *Adverse effects:* Hypersensitivity, neutropenia, nephrotoxicity	1-2 g q6h IV
Cephradine (Velocef, Anspor)	*Indications:* Aerobic: Gram-positive cocci, bacilli; aerobic: Gram-negative cocci *Adverse effects:* Rash, leukopenia	1 g q12h PO
Cephalexin (Keflet, Keflex)	*Indications:* Aerobic: Gram-positive cocci, bacilli; aerobic: Gram-negative cocci *Adverse effects:* Rash, leukopenia	0.5 g q6h PO

Continued.

Drug	Indications/Complications	Dosage
Second-Generation Cephalosporins		
Cefoxitin (Mefoxin)	*Indications:* Aerobic: Gram-positive cocci, bacilli; aerobic: Gram-negative cocci, bacilli; anaerobes *Adverse effects:* Hypersensitivity reaction, neutropenia, hypoprothrombinemia, thrombocytopenia	2 g q6h IV
Cefaclor (Ceclor)	*Indications:* Aerobic: Gram-positive cocci, bacilli; aerobic: Gram-negative cocci *Adverse effects:* Rash, neutropenia	1 g q8h PO
Cefonicid (Monocid)	*Indications:* Aerobic: Gram-positive cocci, bacilli; aerobic: Gram-negative cocci, bacilli; anaerobes *Adverse effects:* Hypersensitivity reaction, neutropenia, hypoprothrombinemia, thrombocytopenia	2 g q24h IV
Cefotetan (Cefotan)	*Indications:* Aerobic: Gram-positive cocci, bacilli; aerobic: Gram-negative cocci, bacilli; anaerobes *Adverse effects:* Hypersensitivity reaction, neutropenia, hypoprothrombinemia, thrombocytopenia	2-3 g q12h IV
Third-Generation Cephalosporins		
Ceftazidime (Fortaz)	*Indications:* Aerobic: Gram-positive cocci, bacilli; aerobic: Gram-negative cocci, bacilli; anaerobes variable *Adverse effects:* Hypersensitivity reaction, neutropenia, hypoprothrombinemia, thrombocytopenia	2 g q8h IV
Cephoperazone (Cefobid)	*Indications:* Aerobic: Gram-positive cocci, bacilli; aerobic: Gram-negative bacilli; anaerobes variable *Adverse effects:* Hypersensitivity reaction, neutropenia, hypoprothrombinemia, thrombocytopenia	2 g q8h IV
Ceftriaxone (Rocephin, Nitrocephin)	*Indications:* Aerobic: Gram-positive cocci, bacilli; aerobic: Gram-negative bacilli; anaerobes variable *Adverse effects:* Hypersensitivity reaction, neutropenia, thrombocytopenia	1 g q12-24h IV
Ceftizoxime sodium (Cefizox)	*Indications:* Aerobic: Gram-positive cocci, bacilli; aerobic: Gram-negative bacilli; anaerobes variable *Adverse effects:* Hypersensitivity reaction, neutropenia, thrombocytopenia	3 g q4h IV
Cefotaxime (Claforan)	*Indications:* Aerobic: Gram-positive cocci, bacilli; aerobic: Gram-negative bacilli; anaerobes variable *Adverse effects:* Hypersensitivity reaction, neutropenia, thrombocytopenia	2 g q4h IV
Other Antibiotics		
Erythromycin	*Indications:* Aerobic: Gram-positive cocci, bacilli; aerobic: Gram-negative *Vibrio, Mycoplasma, Legionella*; anaerobes: Gram-positive *Actinomycetes*; spirochetes (aerobic or anaerobic) *Adverse effects:* Allergic reactions, cholestatic hepatitis, abdominal cramps, nausea and vomiting	1 g q6h IV 0.5 g q6h PO

Drug	Indications/Complications	Dosage
Clindamicin (Cleocin)	*Indications:* Aerobic: Gram-positive cocci, bacilli; anaerobes *Adverse effects:* Neutropenia, pseudomembranes, colitis	900 mg q8h IV
Chloramphenicol (Chloromycetin)	*Indications:* Aerobic: Gram-negative cocci meningitis; aerobic: Gram-negative bacilli, *Salmonella, Shigella, Vibrio;* anaerobes: *Rickettsia* *Adverse effects:* Aplastic anemia, neuropathy	600 mg q6h IV 500 mg q6h PO
Tetracycline	*Indications:* Aerobic: Gram-positive cocci, bacilli; aerobic: Gram-negative cocci, *Chancroid, Mycoplasma, Shigella, Vibrio;* anaerobes: Gram-positive *Actinomycetes;* spirochetes (aerobic or anaerobic); *Rickettsia* *Adverse effects:* Abdominal discomfort, phototoxicity, hepatic toxicity, deposition in calcified tissues	500 mg q12h IV 500 mg q6h PO
Vancomycin (Vancocin, Vancoled)	*Indications:* Methicillin-resistant staphylococci; *Clostridium difficile* *Adverse effects:* Fever, red-man syndrome, ototoxicity, nephrotoxicity	1 g q12h IV 125 mg q6h PO
Minocycline (Minocin)	*Indications:* Aerobic: Gram-positive cocci, bacilli; aerobic: Gram-negative bacilli, cocci, *Mycoplasma; Rickettsia* (aerobic); anaerobes *Adverse effects:* Abdominal discomfort, phototoxicity, hepatic toxicity, deposition in calcified tissues	100 mg q12h PO
Isoniazid (Nydarzin, Laniazid, Teebaconin)	*Indications: Mycobacterium tuberculosis* and atypical mycobacteria *Adverse effects:* Rash, fever, jaundice, neuritis	300 mg q day PO
Rifampin (Rifadin, Rimactane, Rifocin)	*Indications: Mycobacterium tuberculosis* and atypical mycobacteria *Adverse effects:* Jaundice	600 mg q day PO
Ciprofloxicin (Cipro)	*Indications:* Aerobic: Gram-negative bacilli *Adverse effects:* Abdominal discomfort, rash	750 mg q12h PO, IV
Axtreonam (Azactam)	*Indications:* Aerobic: Gram-negative bacilli (used in place of aminoglycosides) *Adverse effects:* Hypersensitivity, neutropenia, oligemia, seizures	2 g q6h IV
Streptomycin	*Indications: Mycobacterium tuberculosis* and atypical mycobacteria (when used with other agents) *Adverse effects:* Ototoxicity, nephrotoxicity	0.5-2.0 g/day IM
Amphotericin B (Fungizone)	*Indications:* Fungi *Adverse effects:* Fever, azotemia; if given rapidly, seizures, ventricular dysrhythmias, hypotension, anaphylaxis, cardiac arrest can result	Topical: 35 mg IV: every 24-48h
Fluconozol (Diflucan)	*Indications:* Fungi *Adverse effects:* Headache, nausea, exfoliative dermatitis, hepatotoxicity	100-200 mg q24h PO
Nystatin (Mycostatin)	*Indications:* Candidiasis (cutaneous, vaginal, oral) *Adverse effects:* Well tolerated	Topical
Metronidazole (Flagyl, Metryl, Protostal, Satric, Metro)	*Indications:* Anaerobes; parasites: *Giardia, Trichomonas, Entamoeba histolytica;* aerobes: Gram-negative *Helicobacter jejuni (C. jejuni)* *Adverse effects:* Metallic taste, pancreatitis, seizures, ataxia, neutropenia	Loading dose 1 g IV; then 500 mg q6h IV or 500 mg q6h PO

Continued.

Drug	Indications/Complications	Dosage
Imepinim and cilastatin (Primaxin)	*Indications:* Aerobes: Gram-positive (including *Nocardia*) and gram-negative cocci, bacilli; anaerobes: Gram-positive and gram-negative cocci, bacilli *Adverse effects:* Neutropenia, oliguria, hepatic toxicity, seizures, abdominal discomfort	1 g q6h IV
Aminoglycosides		
Gentamicin (Garamicin)	*Indications:* Aerobic: Gram-negative bacilli; *Enterococcus* (when given with penicillin G) *Adverse effects:* Ototoxicity, nephrotoxicity, neuromuscular blockade	3-5 mg/kg/day given q8h IV
Tobramicin (Nebcin)	*Indications:* Aerobic: Gram-negative bacilli; *Enterococcus* (when given with penicillin G) *Adverse effects:* Ototoxicity, nephrotoxicity, neuromuscular blockade	3-5 mg q8h IV
Amikacin (Amiken)	*Indications:* Aerobic: Gram-negative bacilli; *Enterococcus* (when given with penicillin G) *Adverse effects:* Ototoxicity, nephrotoxicity, neuromuscular blockade	350 mg q8h IV

BIBLIOGRAPHY

Clowes GHA Jr (ed). Symposium on Response to Infection and Injury. Parts I and II. Surg Clin North Am 56:801, 1976.

Cohen PT, Sande MA, Volberding PA. The AIDS knowledge base. Waltham, Mass, Medical Publishing Group of the Massachusetts Medical Society, 1990.

Conte JE Jr, Jacob LS, Polk HC Jr. Antibiotic Prophylaxis in Surgery. A Comprehensive Review. Philadelphia, JB Lippincott, 1984.

Howard RJ. Host defense against infection. Parts I and II. Curr Probl Surg 17:267, 1980.

Polk HC Jr. Further clarification of the pathogenesis of human pulmonary failure. Surg Gynecol Obstet 150:727, 1980.

Polk HC Jr (ed). Infection and the Surgical Patient. Edinburgh, Churchill Livingstone, 1982.

Polk HC Jr, Fry DE. Infection and fever in the surgical patient. In Hardy JD (ed). Complications in Surgery and Their Management. Philadelphia, WB Saunders, 1981.

Polk HC Jr, Malagoni MA. Chemoprophylaxis of wound infections. In Simmons RL, Howard RJ (eds). Surgical Infectious Disease, 2nd ed. Norwalk, Conn, Appleton-Century-Crofts, 1983.

Pollock AV. Surgical wound sepsis. Lancet 1:1283, 1979.

Stone HH, Bourneuf AA, Stinson LD. Reliability of criteria for predicting persistent or recurrent sepsis. Arch Surg 120:17, 1985.

Stone HH, Kolb LD, Currie CA. *Candida* sepsis: Pathogenesis and principles of treatment. Ann Surg 179:697, 1974.

Stone HH, Martin JD Jr. Synergistic necrotizing cellulitis. Ann Surg 175:702, 1972.

Ziegler EJ, Fischer CJ Jr, Sprung CL, et al. Treatment of gram negative bacteremia and septic shock with HA-1A human monoclonal antibody against endotoxin. N Engl J Med 324:429, 1991.

CHAPTER REVIEW
Questions

1. List three requirements for development of an infection.
2. The most common cause of surgical wound infection is:
   a. Failure to use enough soap to wash skin
   b. Dressings that were not put on properly
   c. Contamination during operation
   d. Retractor trauma to wound
   e. Patient anergy
3. The most important step in treating an established infection is to:
   a. Start antibiotics at once
   b. Identify the pathogenic organism
   c. Stimulate the patient's immune system
   d. Lower the patient's temperature
4. The most important step in treating an abscess is:
   a. Hot soaks
   b. Drainage
   c. Broad-spectrum antibiotics
   d. Elevation
   e. Immobilization
5. Anaerobic gangrene should be treated primarily by:
   a. High-pressure oxygen therapy
   b. Specific antitoxins
   c. Penicillin
   d. Radical debridement
   e. Improvement in arterial flow
6. A felon is:
   a. A closed-space infection of the pulp space of the fingertip
   b. Pus under a fingernail
   c. Infection of a skin appendage
   d. Involves the flexor tendon
   e. An infection in the palm of the hand
7. Postoperative fever beginning 12 hours after operation is usually caused by:
   a. Contamination of the intravenous cannula
   b. Urinary tract infection
   c. Atelectasis
   d. Wound dehiscence
   e. Overhydration
8. The most reliable protection for the surgeon against hepatitis B is:
   a. Universal precautions
   b. Gamma globulin
   c. Active immunization
   d. Acyclovir
   e. Double-gloving

Answers

1. a. Inoculum of pathogenic organisms
   b. Nutrient medium
   c. Local or systemic alteration in host resistance
2. c
3. b
4. b
5. d
6. a
7. a
8. c

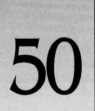

50

Basic Principles of Hand Surgery

MICHAEL L. BENTZ
J. WILLIAM FUTRELL

KEY FEATURES

After reading this chapter you will understand:
- The basic approach in evaluating a hand injury begins with an accurate history and examination.
- The physical examination includes evaluation of the vascular and nerve supply.
- The importance of reviewing the anatomy of the hand.
- Nerve and tendon injuries.
- How to diagnose common tendon lacerations.
- Common fractures, burns, amputations, and infections.

The hand is a complex and versatile structure. Acute and chronic hand problems can safely be addressed by using basic principles. Particularly for acute hand injuries, the application of these principles as the initial intervention is the most important determinant of long-term outcome. This chapter defines the basic principles of hand surgery and relates them to the practical management of hand pathology.

WHAT IS THE INITIAL APPROACH TO A HAND INJURY?

Evaluation of the injured hand begins with a thorough history and physical examination. The history should include relevant medical problems, medications, allergies, occupation, and hand dominance. Documentation of previous

hand injuries and baseline function is important. The mechanism of injury for blunt and penetrating trauma should be well described. The examination of the hand should take place in a clean, well-lighted site. Saline solution irrigation, sterile dressings, and a method of elevating the extremity should be readily available. If a patient is uncooperative or too anxious to permit a thorough hand examination, it is often better (in the absence of ischemia) to re-examine the patient at another time. The pediatric patient occasionally requires examination with him or her under anesthesia in the operating room.

The hand is examined in an orderly fashion starting with observation. The hand should be inspected for color, posture, and the digital cascade. Open wounds should be measured and described in detail (i.e., linear or stellate, transverse or longitudinal, clean or dirty). Areas of contusion, ecchymosis, or edema should be noted. Open wounds in the hand are classified as "tidy" or "untidy." Tidy wounds represent clean lacerations with minimal associated tissue injury. They have little bacterial contamination and frequently can be repaired primarily. Untidy wounds are caused by crush or avulsion injuries and demonstrate significant tissue injury, necessitating delayed definitive wound care. If there is obvious ongoing bleeding at the start of the examination, the extremity should be elevated and digital pressure used to control the bleeding site. A tourniquet is rarely indicated for control of bleeding in the extremity. Blind clamping of bleeding sites with a hemostat is ***never*** acceptable because of the risk of associated nerve injury. Local cleansing is helpful in visualizing specific injuries; however, thorough cleansing usually requires the use of local anesthesia; therefore it is critical to complete a thorough sensorimotor examination before administering any anesthetic in the hand. The wound should be irrigated with normal saline solution, using a 30-ml syringe and a 20-gauge angiocatheter. Debridement should be limited only to obviously nonviable tissues. Tetanus prophylaxis and antibiotic therapy should be initiated. Antibiotic treatment is indicated for most open wounds or for any wound in a diabetic patient.

After examination, wounds should be dressed with sterile gauze dressings moistened with normal saline solution. Tidy wounds should undergo one layer of primary repair using 4-0 or 5-0 simple nylon sutures. (Subcutaneous absorbable sutures are never required in the hand.) All hand injuries should be splinted in the position of safety with 20 degrees of extension at the wrist, 70 degrees of metacarpophalangeal joint flexion, and 0 to 10 degrees of interphalangeal joint flexion. The thumb should be positioned in palmar abduction.

How Is the Hand Anesthetized?

The hand can be anesthetized by local anesthetic infiltration into the wound, by digital block, or by a combination of individual nerve blocks. Plain lidocaine is the usual choice of local anesthetic because of its rapid onset of action. Lidocaine with epinephrine should never be used in the distal extremity because of the risk of tissue loss caused by vasospasm and vasoconstriction. Using a 25- or 27-gauge needle, local anesthetic can be infiltrated into the wound margin for wounds located on the palm or dorsum of the hand. Lacerations of the digits are best managed by digital blocks, which are performed by injecting 1 ml of lidocaine into the volar surface of the web space on either side of the affected digit to a level approximately 1 cm into the web space. This will isolate the site where the common digital nerve bifurcates into the proper digital nerves of the adjacent digits. Lidocaine (1 ml) should also be injected over the dorsum of the finger at the level of the proximal phalanx to anesthetize the dorsal sensory branches.

A median nerve block is performed by injecting 3 ml of 1% lidocaine between the palmaris longus tendon and the flexor carpi radialis tendon at the level of the proximal wrist crease. An ulnar nerve block is similarly performed at the level of the proximal wrist crease just radial to the flexor carpi ulnaris tendon. A radial nerve block is performed by injecting 1% lidocaine on the radial aspect of the radial artery at the level of the proximal wrist crease. Care must be taken in the latter two nerve blocks to avoid the respective adjacent arteries to prevent intense vasospasm. If the needle induces paresthesias, it should be withdrawn so that no local anesthetic is injected directly into the nerve. Any combination of the above digital and/or isolated nerve blocks can be performed to anesthetize the hand for thorough cleansing and wound repair.

HOW IS HAND VASCULARITY ASSESSED?

The only urgent emergency in hand surgery is a devascularized hand or digit. Generally, vascularity can be assessed by noting the presence of pink digits and nail beds. Capillary refill should be tested, turning a blanched nail bed pink within 2 to 3 seconds. The digits should also be evaluated for warmth. Arterial inflow to the hand should be assessed by the Allen's test. It is performed by occluding both the radial and ulnar arteries at the wrist, following which the patient flexes and extends the digits several times to partially exsanguinate the hand. While maintaining ulnar artery occlusion, the radial artery is released, allowing perfusion of the digits. This maneuver is repeated while maintaining radial artery occlusion and allowing ulnar artery perfusion to occur. The relative time to refill should be noted, since the ulnar artery is the dominant arterial inflow of the hand. For a more objective measurement of hand perfusion, Doppler assessment of individual vessels can be performed. Evidence of devascularization or lack of perfusion is a surgical emergency and should be treated by immediate consultation with a hand surgeon.

HOW ARE SPECIFIC NERVES EXAMINED?

Injuries to the nerves of the hand or the digits can be classified into three general categories: neurapraxia, axonotmesis, and neurotmesis. **Neurapraxia,** the temporary cessation of nerve conduction, is generally caused by a contusion of the nerve. Nerve conduction is temporarily blocked, but the integrity of the axons is not disturbed. Sensory loss and motor paralysis are temporary, generally lasting only a few weeks, and there is usually complete return of nerve function. More severe trauma to the nerve results in the injury of **axonotmesis.** Axonal fibers are interrupted, resulting in complete loss of motor and sensory function of the nerve. Surrounding connective tissue tubules, however, are not disrupted. In this injury distal wallerian degeneration occurs, and axonal regeneration through the existing tubular structures results in complete return of nerve function over an appropriate period of time. Total disruption of the nerve, either by laceration or severe crush injury, is called **neurotmesis.** Complete motor and sensory paralysis is observed, and the nerves do not recover spontaneously unless formal nerve repair is carried out (Table 50-1).

At the time of injury the examiner can determine only that there is loss of nerve function. In the operating room a detailed examination of the nerve under magnification will provide information about the severity of the nerve injury. An understanding of the mechanism of trauma, however, may lead the physician to the correct diagnosis. The diagnosis of specific nerve injuries requires a meticulous examination of the nerve's motor and sensory distribution. Fig. 50-1 dem-

onstrates the most common sensory distribution of the ulnar, radial, and median nerves in the hand.

The median nerve supplies sensation to the radial half of the palm and to the thumb, index, and long fingers. The proper digital nerves send dorsal branches to supply sensation to the dorsum of the digits distal to the proximal interphalangeal joint. The only motor function of the median nerve in the hand distal to the wrist is provided by the recurrent motor branch to the thumb and branches to the radial two lumbricales. The location of this branch can be found by drawing a line parallel to the wrist crease from the metacarpal phalangeal joint of the thumb across the palm to where the line intersects with the oblique palmar crease. Examination for loss of motor function of the median nerve involves laying the hand on a table dorsal side down and elevating the thumb out of the plane of the hand. Palpation of the thenar eminence will indicate function in the abductor pollicis brevis and flexor pollicis brevis muscles. In 20% of patients oppo-

TABLE 50-1   Classification of Nerve Injuries

	Morphology	Symptoms	Prognosis
Neurapraxia (first degree)	Axons intact	Complete loss of motor and sensory function	Complete recovery in several days to a few weeks
Axonotmesis (second degree)	Axons divided but connective tissue tubules intact	Complete motor and sensory paralysis	Complete recovery after nerve regeneration occurs
Neurotmesis	Axons and tubules divided	Complete motor and sensory paralysis	No recovery

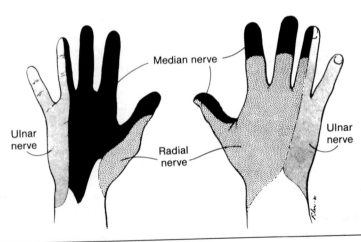

FIGURE 50-1   Common distribution of radial, ulnar, and median nerves.

sition of the thumb is provided by a branch from the ulnar nerve. Longstanding median nerve paralysis produces flattening of the thenar eminence and an adduction contracture of the thumb because of the unopposed adductor pollicis muscle, which is innervated by the ulnar nerve.

The sensory distribution of the ulnar nerve includes a small ulnar palmar cutaneous branch and digital nerves to the little finger and the ulnar half of the ring finger. The dorsal sensory branch supplies the entire ulnar side of the dorsum of the hand, including the little and ring fingers. The motor branch divides from the sensory branches at the pisiform bone and transverses the palm, innervating the muscles of the hypothenar eminence, the interossei, the ulnar lumbricales, and, finally, the adductor of the thumb. Motor function of the ulnar nerve in the hand can be tested by placing the hand palm down and asking the patient to adduct and abduct the fingers. Abduction of the fifth finger is tested while palpating the hypothenar eminence. The first dorsal interosseous muscle can be examined by having the patient radially abduct the index finger and palpating the muscle in the web space. A careful examination of the motor function of the ulnar nerve is essential to diagnose an isolated injury. Late paralysis results in the claw-hand deformity, with hyperextension of the fourth and fifth metacarpal phalangeal joints and flexion contractures of the proximal interphalangeal joints caused by paralysis of the ulnar intrinsic muscles. The index and long fingers do not form a claw deformity because the radial lumbricale muscles are innervated by the median nerve.

The radial nerve is purely sensory in the distal portion of the wrist and hand. It courses dorsally and proximally to the distal radius and supplies sensation to the thumb-index web space and to the dorsum of the thumb, index, and long finger as far as the proximal interphalangeal (PIP) joint. The nerve may be injured during resection of a dorsal wrist ganglion. Neuromas of this nerve can lead to disabling, intractable causalgia.

Most nerve lacerations should be repaired using an operating microscope. In general, clean lacerations can be repaired at the time of injury or within a week of injury. Minimal, if any debridement of the nerve ends is required when the laceration is caused by a knife or glass. In crush injuries the nerve should be surgically debrided (proximally) until healthy fascicles are observed. In untidy wounds, especially those caused by severe trauma, the nerve may be injured more proximally and distally than is initially appreci-

ated. Delayed primary repair (within 2 weeks) or secondary repair is the more prudent choice in these cases. During the initial treatment, however, the nerve ends may be grossly approximated to prevent nerve retraction.

Secondary repair involves debridement until healthy nerve tissue with an identifiable fascicular pattern is observed. Adequate mobilization of the nerve ends is required to allow tensionfree repair. Radical mobilization of the nerve, however, deprives it of its segmental blood supply. A gap of 2 cm or greater is an indication for a nerve graft. If the nerve ends can be approximated with 8-0 nylon sutures, the tension is usually acceptable. Attempts to overcome tension by flexing the wrist and elbow will only lead to increased scar formation at the repair site once mobilization is begun.

Digital nerves can be repaired as distal as the distal interphalangeal (DIP) joint, at which point the nerve arborizes. Only one or two sutures of 10-0 nylon are required to give accurate approximation if fascicular groups are present. This is accomplished by inspection of the fascicular bundle pattern under magnification, followed by accurate alignment by epineural and/or fascicular sutures (Fig. 50-2). If the nerve is grossly intact but contused, the patient should be observed for at least 6 months before secondary procedures are contemplated. Injuries to motor nerves in the proximal forearm and above the elbow require a prolonged period of time before nerve regeneration progresses to the muscle in the hand. Early tendon transfer should be considered to prevent the claw deformity caused by injury to the ulnar nerve and to provide opposition by the thumb in median nerve injuries.

What Is a Nerve Compression Syndrome?

Nerve compression syndromes result in characteristic clusters of signs and symptoms caused by compression of a specific nerve at a specific location. The sensory and motor deficits are predictable, based on the point of compression, and are suggestive of the site of nerve injury. A thorough understanding of the sensory and motor contributions of the ulnar, radial, and median nerves is essential to understanding and detecting nerve compression syndromes. Compression of the median nerve at the wrist, *carpal tunnel syndrome,* is a frequent occurrence characterized by numbness and paresthesia over volar aspect of the thumb, index, and middle fingers, and radial half of the ring finger. The patient may complain

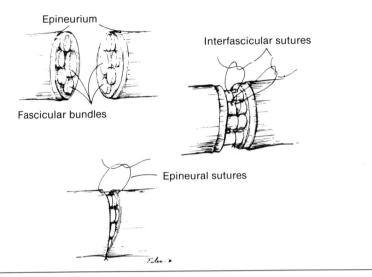

Epineurium

Interfascicular sutures

Fascicular bundles

Epineural sutures

FIGURE 50-2 Grouped fascicular nerve repair.

of pain in the hand and weakness that is often worse in the morning or night. Phalen's test, placing the wrist in acute flexion, is useful in reproducing the symptoms. Tinel's sign manifests as "electrical shocks" and is generated by tapping along the course of the nerve to identify the point of dysfunction. Nerve conduction testing may help in diagnosing questionable cases. If untreated, loss of sensation, paralysis, and thenar-muscle wasting can occur. The syndrome is caused by compression of the median nerve within the rigid confines of the carpal canal. Causes include an anomalous sublimis or palmaris muscle, rheumatoid synovitis, trauma, mass lesions, and metabolic disturbances such as myxedema or pregnancy. The definitive treatment is surgical release of the flexor retinaculum.

Compression of the anterior interosseous nerve can also occur. The anterior interosseous nerve is a motor branch of the median nerve arising 4 to 6 cm distal to the elbow. The nerve innervates the flexor pollicis longus muscle, the flexor profundus to the index and long fingers, and the pronator quadrants. Compression of this nerve can be caused by tendinous bands, the deep head of the pronator teres muscle, or from the archlike origin of the flexor digitorum sublimis muscle. Symptoms of anterior interosseous nerve compression are pain (often referred to the forearm) and weakness or loss of thumb and index finger flexion. The pronator quadratus muscle is tested with the elbow flexed to eliminate the action of the pronator teres muscle. It is necessary to release compression of this nerve as

it passes between the two heads of the pronator teres or beneath the flexor sublimis muscle.

The ulnar nerve can be compressed at the wrist, the **ulnar tunnel syndrome,** by such anomalies as duplicated hypothenar muscles or an accessory palmaris longus muscle. The usual cause, however, is a posttraumatic ganglion in Guyon's canal. A patient with it can present with purely motor symptoms such as weakness and a weak key pinch. Less frequently, the sensory branch is involved, presenting with paresthesias over the fourth and fifth fingers. Surgical release of the volar carpal ligament is indicated if symptoms persist.

Ulnar nerve compression at the elbow, **cubital tunnel syndrome,** often causes pain in the forearm that radiates to the little and ring fingers. It can include weakness of grip or frank paralysis of the ulnar intrinsic muscles. The nerve can be irritated by spurs of bone within the cubital groove. Trauma can be the source of chronic neuritis. Symptoms of cubital tunnel syndrome differ from those of ulnar nerve compression at the wrist, principally by their progressive nature. If the symptoms include paresthesia over the dorsum of the hand, the elbow is the most likely cause. Treatment consists of transposing the nerve out of the cubital tunnel to a subcutaneous or submuscular position.

The radial nerve can be compressed along its course, **radial tunnel syndrome,** by the fibrous edge of the supinator muscle, by the radial recurrent vessels, or by fibers of the flexor digitorum superficialis muscle. In a patient with radial tunnel syndrome pain is the chief complaint, and it is referred to the elbow. The "middle-finger test" is positive when the elbow, wrist, and fingers are held in full extension and pressure is placed on the dorsum of the middle finger, producing pain in the forearm. The posterior interosseous nerve innervates the wrist and digital extensor muscle and the extensor and abductor muscles of the thumb. Symptoms include pain and weakness. The sensory branch is not involved, thereby distinguishing this entity from higher radial nerve lesions.

HOW DO EXTENSION TENDON INJURIES PRESENT?

Isolated extensor tendon lacerations can generally be treated in the emergency room. Because extensor tendons have a short excursion, the cut ends are easily retrieved from the wound edges and can be sutured with mattress nylon sutures. Unrepaired lacerations of the extensor tendons will cause characteristic deformities, depending on the level of the injury (Fig. 50-3). Open or closed injury at the DIP joint may cause a severed extensor tendon. A "mallet finger" results, manifesting as a flexion deformity of the DIP joint with inability to extend the distal phalanx. This deformity can occasionally be repaired by suturing the extensor tendon with mattress nylon sutures. A closed injury resulting in avulsion of the extensor tendon is treated by splinting the distal joint in hyperextension with or without Kirschner wire fixation. Ideally, the extensor tendon will be avulsed from the distal phalanx, including a portion of the condyle of the bone. This injury is well treated by open reduction and fixation of the bony fragment.

Extensor tendon lacerations over the PIP joint may result in a "boutonniere deformity," consisting of DIP joint hyperextension and PIP joint flexion. A boutonniere deformity is caused by a disruption of the central extensor tendon slip and volar displacement of the lateral bands between the axis of the PIP joint. This injury usually involves the oblique retinacular ligaments and the central slip of the extensor tendon. These tendons flex the PIP joint and pull the DIP joint into hyperextension. The treatment of this laceration involves suture repair of the central slip and reapproximation of the lateral bands on the dorsum of the digit. Although this procedure is often possible in the patient with an acute injury, older injuries generally require more complex surgical reconstruction.

Extensor lacerations proximal to the PIP joint

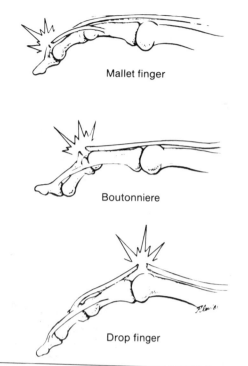

FIGURE 50-3 Deformities caused by extensor tendon lacerations.

generally involve the central slip of the extensor tendon. Intertendinous bands between the adjacent digits often allow the patient to extend the injured digit partially. In favorable circumstances these injuries can be repaired primarily in the emergency room. Extensor tendon injuries should be splinted for 4 to 6 weeks to prevent rupture of tendon repairs.

HOW DO FLEXOR TENDON INJURIES PRESENT?

The diagnosis of flexor tendon injury is made by careful examination. In repose the fingertips form a gentle curve, with increasing flexion of the PIP and DIP joints. If a flexor tendon is lacerated, the finger will fall out of this curve and straighten, becoming apparent on inspection. Individual testing of the superficialis and profundus tendons will subsequently confirm this initial impression. Each digit should be tested separately. The profundus tendons flex the distal joints of the fingers. In addition, they flex all joints proximal to their insertion, including the wrist. Each digit should be tested separately. The superficialis tendon flexes the PIP joint. To test this tendon, the profundus tendon must be blocked by holding the other fingers in extension while the patient is asked to flex the involved finger (Fig. 50-4). Only the PIP joint will flex if the tendon is intact. To test the profundus tendon, block the PIP joint and look for flexion at the DIP joint (Fig. 50-5). Flexion of the metacarpophalangeal joints is due to the intrinsic muscles of the hand and will be present when both sublimis and profundus tendons are lacerated. Flexor tendon lacerations should be repaired under ideal conditions with tourniquet control. Depending on the relative position of the digits at the time that the laceration is incurred, the proximal and distal tendon ends may retract a considerable distance from the wound edge.

Frequently, the proximal tendon will have retracted into the palm or the wrist. To minimize the chances of this occurrence, the hand should be splinted in extreme wrist flexion until definitive repair is completed.

In tidy wounds flexor tendons may be repaired primarily. Delayed primary repair (up to 14 days) is indicated if the wound is contaminated or if appropriate facilities are not available. After that time, shortening of the proximal muscle belly may prevent primary repair. Secondary tendon grafting is an acceptable repair technique in these delayed cases.

The repair of flexor tendon lacerations is classified according to the level of injury (Fig. 50-6). Zone 1 lacerations (within 1 cm of the insertion of

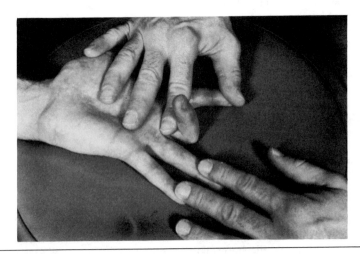

FIGURE 50-4   Assessment of flexor digitorum profundus integrity.

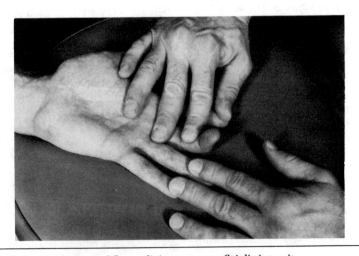

FIGURE 50-5   Assessment of flexor digitorum superficialis integrity.

the profundus tendon) can be treated by primary repair or by advancing the tendon to the distal phalange and reinserting it with a pullout wire. Additional methods of treatment for this injury include tenodesis or arthrodesis of the DIP joint if the tendon cannot be repaired. It is essential that sublimis tendon function not be compromised in treating a distal profundus injury.

Flexor tendon lacerations in zone 2 require special expertise to achieve maximal function. This "no-man's land" injury is treated by primary repair of both the sublimis and profundus tendons. More proximal injuries in zones 3, 4, and 5 are generally treated by primary tendon repair.

Attention must be given intraoperatively to preserving the flexor pulleys, especially in the proximal phalanx (A_2) and the middle phalanx (A_4) (Fig. 50-7) to prevent bow stringing of the tendon. Early mobilization of the tendon after repair is a useful method of preventing adhesions between the tendon and surrounding structures. The preferred method of suture technique in flexor tendon repairs is the one that does not cause ischemic necrosis of the tendon ends (Fig. 50-8). This is accomplished with a 4-0 nylon suture oversewn with a running 6-0 nylon suture.

After primary repair, the hand is immobilized for 3 weeks before active flexion is initiated. Kleinert's early mobilization technique uses active extension and passive flexion with rubber band traction to prevent adhesions between the healing flexor tendon and the surrounding sheath. In both instances careful active flexion is begun after 3 weeks. The tendon repair must be protected from severe strain for a total of 12 weeks.

HOW ARE BONE AND JOINT INJURIES ASSESSED?

Careful physical examination can diagnose many common bone and joint injuries, although these injuries are difficult to evaluate adequately in the presence of swelling. Obvious deformity should be noted, and an area of ecchymosis may suggest an underlying fracture. Point tenderness is suggestive, but not diagnostic, of a fracture. Radiography should be used to assess all injuries. Radiographs are particularly sensitive for bony injuries but may not show fractures on the initial

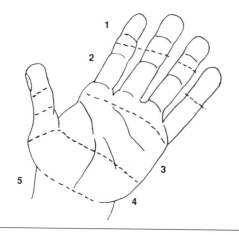

FIGURE 50-6 Zones of flexor tendon injury.

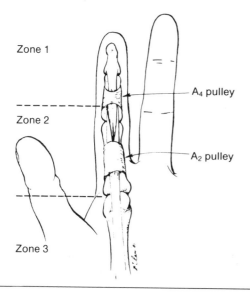

FIGURE 50-7 Flexor pulleys must be preserved in the repair of flexor tendon lacerations.

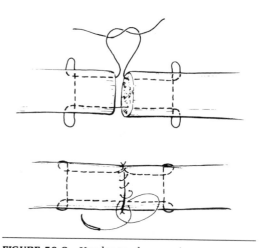

FIGURE 50-8 Kessler tendon repair.

films. Therefore when a fracture is suspected but not evident radiographically, the patient should be immobilized as if there were a fracture. Repeat radiographic evaluation several weeks later frequently shows the suspected fracture. The radiographic appearance of dislocations is also helpful in diagnosing joint injuries when used as a compliment to the evaluation for motion, laxity, and joint stability.

How Are Hand Fractures Treated?

Treatment of fractures of the hand varies according to the location of the fracture and the amount of displacement, rotation, angulation, and shortening. Fractures of the distal phalanx can frequently undergo closed reduction and splinting for 3 weeks. Articular fractures of the DIP joint may include avulsion of the extensor or flexor tendon insertions. These fractures should be treated with open reduction and fixation of the tendon with a pullout wire, although some advocate splinting in hyperextension. Frequently the volar plate is involved in articular joint surface injuries, and it should be suspected in dorsal dislocations. Open reduction of articular fractures allows for anatomic reduction of the fracture with fixation by either a fine Kirschner wire or circumferential wire technique. When more than 25% of an articular surface is involved in an intra-articular fracture, significant joint stiffness or osteoarthritis may result if the fracture is not anatomically reduced. Fractures of the proximal or middle phalanx not involving articular surfaces generally can be managed by closed reduction and percutaneous Kirschner wire fixation. Two crossed Kirschner wires are generally used to control fragment rotation. If closed reduction is not satisfactory, open reduction and Kirschner wire fixation is necessary.

The most common metacarpal fracture is the "boxer's fracture," which involves volar angulation of the metacarpal head. Closed reduction and immobilization in an ulnar gutter splint is usually adequate, although Kirschner wire fixation may be necessary. Rotational deformity should be identified by physical examination. (A rotation deformity is noted with the digits in flexion so that the involved digit is not parallel to the adjacent digits.) Fractures of the carpal bones can be difficult to diagnose by physical examination or initial radiographs. These fractures can be quite debilitating if inadequately treated. Common fractures include those of the scaphoid and the lunate. Both have a high rate of nonunion if not anatomically reduced because of tenuous vascularity.

WHY ARE FINGERTIP INJURIES SO SIGNIFICANT?

Fingertip injuries are the most common hand problem presenting in the emergency room. Management of fingertip injuries should be geared to provide the patient with a painfree, well-padded distal digit that has adequate sensation for fine motor activity. Fingertip injuries are classified according to the amount of absent soft tissue and the relationship of the volar pad to digital length. Lacerations or crush injuries without loss of soft tissue require only minimal debridement and simple closure. Pulp loss may be transverse or oblique, with either a greater volar or dorsal defect (Fig. 50-9). When the injury involves a soft tissue loss less than 1 cm², most wounds will contract and heal by secondary intention with an excellent functional and aesthetic result. When the distal phalanx is exposed, a rongeur should be used to debride exposed bone, preserving as much length as possible. If a larger amount of soft tissue is missing, a combination of bony debridement and flap coverage is indicated. Local flaps available in this area include volar and lateral V-Y advancement flaps and rotation flaps. Adjacent flaps include the cross-finger flap and the thenar flap in which the digit is placed into flexion and sutured to a pedicled skin flap on the thenar eminence.

Isolated nail bed injuries should be treated by

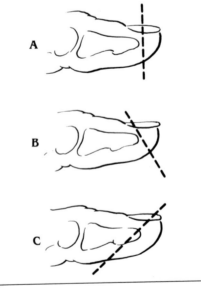

FIGURE 50-9 **A,** Transverse guillotine amputation. **B,** Oblique amputation with greater preservation of volar skin. **C,** Oblique amputation with volar loss extending proximally.

removal of the nail plate and primary repair of the nail bed with fine absorbable 6-0 chromic suture. The nail itself or a small piece of non-adherent dressing or suture wrapper should be placed back into the nail fold as a stent. The nail should also be removed for any subungual hematoma that encompasses more than 30% of the surface area of the nail bed.

HOW ARE EXTREMITY AMPUTATIONS MANAGED?

The definitive management plan for amputated digits that are not replantable should allow maximal residual function. Length should be preserved whenever possible, but only when adequate sensate soft tissue is available. Amputations between the eponychial fold and the middle of the proximal phalanx of the thumb should be shortened and stable skin coverage provided. Amputations proximal to the midportion of the proximal phalanx result in a thumb too short for useful function and require delayed definitive reconstruction.

Index finger amputations distal to the middle of the middle phalanx should be treated by preserving length and soft tissue coverage. More proximal amputations commonly result in the exclusion of the index finger by the patient. Shortening and closure provide the ultimate procedure of choice because many patients will return for secondary amputation. For middle, ring, and little fingers, preservation of length is not as significant because these digits are more involved with power grip. In closing these wounds, the volar pad should be advanced toward the dorsal surface after bone shortening. If amputation is required, tendons should be cleanly cut and allowed to retract, condyles should be trimmed, and digital nerves should be cleanly divided and buried.

What Amputated Digits Should Be Reattached?

All patients with amputated digits should be evaluated by a hand surgeon for individual consideration for replantation. Indications for replantation include patient age less than 55 years, thumb amputation, multiple digit amputation, hand amputation, forearm amputation, and any amputation in a pediatric patient. Absolute contraindications to replantation include associated life-threatening injuries, severe crush or avulsion injuries, segmental amputations, debilitating systemic illness, significant prior injury to the same extremity, and severe contamination of the tissues. Relative contraindications to replantation include psychiatric illness that prohibits full patient cooperation in postoperative and rehabilitation phases and single-digit amputations with a warm ischemic interval greater than 12 hours.

How Should Amputated Digits Be Stored and Transported?

Improper transportation of digits can prevent successful replantation. The amputated part should be debrided of any gross contaminating foreign body, after which it should be rinsed with saline solution. The part should be wrapped in sterile gauze moistened with saline solution and placed in a clear plastic bag. This plastic bag should be placed on ice, preventing direct contact of ice and tissue. (Dry ice should not be used, since the digit should not be allowed to freeze.) As soon as convenient, definitive radiographs should be obtained, not only of the patient's proximal extremity but also of the amputated part. Although the overall success of replantation procedures is in excess of 75%, even the most motivated patients exhibit postoperative joint stiffness, tendon adhesions, impaired sensibility, and cold intolerance. Many of these patients will require several procedures to optimize postoperative function.

WHAT KIND OF INFECTIONS OCCUR IN THE HAND?

Hand infections are caused by a large variety of agents and can lead to serious sequelae. An accurate history and a bacteriologic diagnosis are essential in treating these infections. The most common finger infection is *paronychia,* which occurs in the space between the nail plate and the eponychium. The majority of these infections are caused by *Staphylococcus aureus* and should be treated with surgical drainage. After achieving digital block anesthesia, a vertical incision is made along the lateral margin of the nail plate, and the eponychium is elevated from the base of the nail. The nail base may then be excised, leaving the remainder of the plate intact.

A *felon* is an infection of the pulp space that occurs either at the volar pad or laterally in the fingertip. Incision and drainage of this space must be carried out with attention to the course of the digital nerves. A midlateral incision is performed, dividing the septum between the pulp skin and the distal phalanx to drain the infection properly. Making longitudinal incisions in the center of the volar digital pulp will avoid the digital nerves but leaves a scar in a sensitive, sensate area.

Purulent tenosynovitis of the flexor tendon sheaths has a significant morbidity rate if not treated properly. The diagnostic hallmark of tenosynovitis is swelling of the digit, tenderness to palpation over the flexor tendon sheath, and pain in the hand with passive extension of the digit. When a tendon sheath infection is diagnosed, surgical drainage should be carried out immediately. By the time an abscess localizes in these aggressive infections, loss of the flexor tendon may have occurred. A small transverse incision is made at the distal palmar crease and the flexor sheath opened. A second midlateral incision is made distally, and a catheter is introduced into the sheath. Through-and-through irrigation with an antibiotic solution is carried out for 48 hours, after which the catheter is removed. Additional therapeutic measures include immobilization and elevation. Tendon sheath infections may rupture into thenar or hypothenar spaces. These infections should be drained and treated aggressively with antibiotics, elevation, and splinting.

Why Are Human Bites of the Limb Threatening?

Human bites pose particularly high-risk infections in the hand. These injuries are usually the result of a violent assault. This history is frequently not offered and must be suspected by the physician. An incisor wound sustained with the hand flexed into a fist will penetrate the digit through a different tract than the wound observed with the digits extended. Late sequelae of such an undiagnosed injury may include septic arthritis and joint destruction. The most frequent organisms found in human bites of the hand are *S. aureus* and streptococci. *Eikenella corrodens*, a common oral pathogen, is responsible for particular virulent infections in the hand. Human bites presenting as fresh, superficial abrasions (without deep tissue penetration) can be treated on an outpatient basis with oral antibiotics, warm soaks, and frequent examination. If there is any concern about compliance, the patient should be admitted to the hospital for careful surveillance. Patients with wounds with cellulitis on presentation should be admitted for intravenous antibiotic therapy. Debridement may be required if no improvement is noted within 24 hours. All hand infections should be splinted in the position of safety and elevated. Antibiotic coverage should be broad initially, then tailored to the specific culture and sensitivity.

HOW IS THE BURNED HAND TREATED?

Treatment of hand burns can be divided into acute and chronic phases. Acute management is geared toward preventing burn sequelae, including tissue loss, scar contracture, and joint stiffness. Cool saline solution compresses should be applied early to minimize edema and pain. Burns should be dressed with moist saline solution gauze in preparation for definitive care. Topical agents such as silver sulfadiazine (Silvadene) should not be applied until the patient is examined by a hand or burn surgeon. Patients with first-degree burns are initially seen with red skin and intact epidermis, second-degree burns with blistering and dermal exposure, third-degree burns with leathery full-thickness wounds that usually lack sensation, and fourth-degree burns with exposed bone. Blisters should be left intact if small because they provide the optimal biologic dressing. Infected collections under blisters should be drained and the blisters debrided. Superficial second-degree burns can be treated by washing the hand with soap and water and then dressing the wound with a nonadherent gauze. A light dressing will allow the patient to fully flex and extend all of the joints. Complete healing of these wounds is expected by 7 to 10 days.

Deep second- and third-degree burns require good clinical judgment in their management. Areas of deep second-degree injury may be intermixed with full-thickness skin loss. Burns of deeper structures, including veins and tendons, require extensive measures to ultimately restore function. Of utmost importance is the continual assessment of circulation to the hand and the digits. This may be done with the Doppler ultrasound flowmeter if pulses cannot be palpated. Midlateral digital escharotomies and release of the flexor retinaculum in the palm and wrist are indicated if circulation is compromised. The wound can be treated with topical antimicrobial agents such as silver sulfadiazine.

Proper splinting in the position of safety is essential in postburn patients to prevent contractures of the joints, leading to residual stiffness. Vigorous physical therapy is necessary to maintain mobility and reduce edema.

In patients with deep second-degree burns the surgeon must choose between early excision and grafting of the burn wound or spontaneous eschar separation and epithelialization. The latter technique has the potential for leaving the hand with unstable scars, which may result in scar contractures or delayed healing. Throughout the time of wound healing, vigorous physical therapy is necessary.

Early tangential excision of the burn wound, followed by split-thickness skin grafting, is performed within the first 10 days after a burn injury. A dermatome knife is used to excise the burn serially until dermal bleeding is encountered. Hemostasis is achieved with topical thrombin and epinephrine-soaked gauze, after which a split-thickness skin graft is applied. After 5 days, physical therapy is instituted. This technique has the advantage of promoting early healing and joint mobility, with decreased pain. In addition, stable skin coverage is provided. Full-thickness burns should be excised and a graft of flap coverage provided.

CHRONIC CONDITIONS OF THE HAND

De Quervain's disease, or stenosing tenovaginitis of the first dorsal compartment, is characterized by pain during motion of the thumb. The pain may be referred to the forearm and accompanied by weakness in functions requiring wrist or thumb motion. The pain is caused by synovial inflammation of the abductor pollicis longus and extensor pollicis brevis tendons at the radial styloid. Finkelstein's test is performed by asking the patient to grasp the thumb in the palm and then to deviate the wrist ulnarly. Pain occurring over the first compartment is usually diagnostic. Treatment is by steroid injections and immobilization. Occasionally release of the first compartment and synovectomy are required.

Trigger fingers are caused by a nodule on the flexor tendon, usually caused by tenosynovitis. The nodule restricts gliding of the tendon through the tendon sheath at the level of the metacarpophalangeal (MCP) joint. The usual symptoms are locking of the finger in the flexed position. There is usually tenderness in the area of the sheath, and a nodule may be palpable when the finger is flexed. The condition is relieved by steroid injections. Surgical treatment requires incision of the A_1 pulley.

Dupuytren's disease is a proliferation of the palmar fascia characterized by nodules and cords along the longitudinal fibers. Often they extend across the MCP and PIP joints, causing joint contractures. The cause of Dupuytren's disease is unknown. The disease is hereditary, occurs most frequently in Caucasian men, and is more severe in epileptic and alcoholic patients. Surgery is indicated only when the nodules are tender or for a flexion contracture. The longitudinal fascial bands may be incised (fasciotomy) or excised. Limited fasciectomy with excision of involved skin may be indicated in recurrent disease.

Rheumatoid arthritis is a disease of synovial tissue that affects joints and tendons in the proliferative stage. The synovium becomes inflamed, causing pain and tenderness of the joints. The wrist and the MCP and PIP joints are usually involved. Progression of the disease leads to joint destruction, bone erosion, and tendon rupture. In the late stages of the disease synovial activity has burned itself out, resulting in joint fibrosis, stiffness, and deformity. In the early stages surgery is directed at resecting the destructive synovium in joints and surrounding tendons. Tightening loose joint capsules, centralizing subluxed extensor tendons, and splinting are useful in correcting ulnar drift at the MCP joint. Boutonniere and swan-neck deformities of the fingers are corrected by repositioning subluxed tendons. In more severe cases, however, joint replacement and fusions are required to restore balance and proper hand function.

Psoriasis also causes severe joint destruction and is distinguished from rheumatoid arthritis by distal joint involvement and characteristic skin and nail changes. *Osteoarthritis* also affects the DIP joints, often presenting with exostoses called *Heberden's nodes.* Other systemic diseases with manifestations in the hand include *gout* and *scleroderma.* Each of these systemic diseases has characteristic clinical presentations that can be confirmed by appropriate laboratory studies. Many patients have severe deformities, yet they are often able to function well. Treatment should be directed to the most disabling of these deformities and to the systemic disease.

Ganglions, the most common hand tumors, are outpouchings or cysts of synovial tissue. They commonly arise from joint spaces, tendon sheaths, or the tendon itself. Common sites for ganglions to arise are the dorsum of the DIP joint (mucous cyst), the flexor tendon of the digits at the MCP joint level, and the volar and dorsal aspect of the wrist. Dorsal wrist ganglions often originate from a fenestration in the scapholunate ligament. Excision of ganglions in a formal operative setting is recommended when they cause symptoms or interfere with normal function. Awareness of the anatomy of adjacent tissues is essential to avoid injury to these structures and allow complete excision of the lesion.

PITFALLS AND COMMON MYTHS

- There is no substitute for a complete and thorough physical examination. In the absence of frank ischemia of the hand or digits, wounds can be closed and the patient re-examined remotely when he or she is more cooperative. Examinations should be performed in clean, well-lighted areas with appropriate instrumentation immediately available. Physical examination of the hand requires meticulous attention to detail.
- Vascular inflow should always be defined by an Allen's test. Delayed capillary refill or presumed vascular insufficiency should never be ascribed to vasospasm.
- Tendon injuries require splinting of the hand to minimize proximal segment retraction into the palm. The thickness of the cast should be indirectly related to the patient's therapeutic compliance.
- A complete sensorimotor examination should be completed before the administration of any local anesthetic agent that would only mask any deficits.
- When the physical examination suggests a bone or joint injury, in the absence of significant radiographic findings, the hand should be treated as though a fracture or joint injury is present. Most hand injuries require simple radiographic evaluation, including anteroposterior and lateral films to look for fracture, dislocation, or foreign body.
- Always follow the principles of aggressive wound care, gentle tissue handling, adequate immobilization, and elevation when treating hand injuries.

BIBLIOGRAPHY

Bentz M (ed). Care of the acutely injured hand. Trauma Q 6:1-86, 1990.

Conn HF. Current Therapy. Philadelphia, WB Saunders, 1983.

Converse JM (ed). Reconstructive Plastic Surgery. Philadelphia, WB Saunders, 1977.

Flatt AE. The Care of the Rheumatoid Hand. St. Louis, CV Mosby, 1974.

Grabb WC, Smith JW (eds). Plastic Surgery, 3rd ed. Boston, Little, Brown & Co, 1980.

Green D (ed). Operative Hand Surgery. New York, Churchill Livingstone, 1988.

Lister GD. The Hand: Diagnosis and Indications. Edinburgh, Churchill Livingstone, 1977.

Lister GD, Kleinert HE, et al. Primary flexor tendon repair followed by immediate controlled mobilization. J Hand Surg 2:441, 1977.

Mann RJ, Hoffeld T, Farmey C. Human bites of the hand: Twenty years experience. J Hand Surg 2:97, 1977.

May J, Littler J (eds). Plastic Surgery—The Hand. Philadelphia, WB Saunders, 1990.

O'Brien B McC. Microvascular Reconstructive Surgery. Edinburgh, Churchill Livingstone, 1977.

Salisbury RE, Pruitt BA. Burns of the Upper Extremity. Philadelphia, WB Saunders, 1976.

Seddon H. Surgical Disorders of the Peripheral Nerves, 2nd ed. Edinburgh, Churchill Livingstone, 1975.

Sood R, Bentz M, Shestak K, et al. Extremity replantation. Surg Clin North Am 71:317-329, 1991.

Spinner M. Injuries to the Major Branches of Peripheral Nerves in the Forearm, 2nd ed. Philadelphia, WB Saunders, 1978.

Sunderland S. Nerves and Nerve Injuries, 2nd ed. Edinburgh, Churchill Livingstone, 1979.

Terzis J. Neural microsurgery. In Daniel RK, Terzis J (eds). Reconstructive Microsurgery. Boston, Little, Brown & Co, 1977.

CHAPTER REVIEW
Questions

1. The optimal dressing for a burn on the hand before transfer to a burn center is:
   a. Silver sulfadiazine (Silvadene)
   b. Silver nitrate
   c. Mafenide acetate (Sulfamylon)
   d. Normal saline solution
2. Which of the following injuries represents a surgical emergency?
   a. Tendon laceration
   b. Nerve laceration
   c. Ischemic digit
   d. Exposed bone
3. A laceration across the volar surface of the ring finger's proximal phalanx should be anesthetized by:
   a. Local wound infiltration with lidocaine
   b. Digital block of adjacent web spaces
   c. Median and ulnar nerve blocks
   d. Topical lidocaine
4. An Allen's test should be performed before which of the following procedures?
   a. Hand examination
   b. Arterial blood gas evaluation
   c. Insertion of arterial monitoring line
   d. All of the above
5. A laceration of the median nerve at the wrist would be expected to produce each of the following except:
   a. Numbness of the thumb, index, and long fingers
   b. Inability to oppose the thumb
   c. Thenar atrophy
   d. Claw deformity
   e. Numbness on the radial one half of the palm
6. All of the following statements about ganglions are true except:
   a. They arise from joint or tendon sheath synovium.
   b. They frequently recur after excision.
   c. They are the most common tumor of the hand.
   d. The sensory branch of the radial nerve can be injured during their removal.
   e. Excision of ganglions is safely performed in the office.
7. Each of the following statements concerning pyogenic flexor tenosynovitis of the finger is true except:
   a. The primary symptoms are diffuse swelling and tenderness of the digit, with pain on extending the digit.
   b. Systemic symptoms of fever are often absent.
   c. Warm soaks and antibiotics are effective treatment.
   d. The infection carries the potential for necrosis of the flexor tendon.
   e. The cause is often a puncture wound.
8. Which of the following statements concerning fingertip injuries are true?
   a. Loss of the fingertip where bone is exposed is best treated with local advancement flaps.
   b. Split-thickness skin grafts regain sensibility after approximately 6 months.
   c. Fingertip loss in children may be left to granulate and epithelialize with excellent cosmetic results.
   d. Preservation of digit length with a cross-finger flap is indicated when the thumbnail is intact.
9. All of the following statements concerning digital replantation are true except:
   a. All multiple digit amputations and amputated thumbs should be replanted.
   b. The index finger is the most important digit to replant in single digit amputations.
   c. Warm ischemia time for amputated extremities should not exceed 6 hours.
   d. In replantation surgery all structures possible should be repaired primarily.
   e. An amputated part should be wrapped in a sterile gauze, sealed in a waterproof bag, and packed in regular ice before replantation.

Answers

1. d. Saline solution dressings are most appropriate for acute burns in preparation for transfer to a burn center for definitive management. These dressings allow thorough reexamination and evaluation by the primary burn team. Silver sulfadiazine is commonly used for topical burn antisepsis after the initial evaluation. Silver nitrate and mafenide acetate (Sulfamylon) have been used historically for the treatment of burns but are particularly painful and cause metabolic acidosis, respectively.
2. c. An ischemic digit is the only true hand surgery emergency, although exposed bone or open fractures require aggressive irrigation and debridement. Both nerve and tendon lacerations can be repaired in a delayed primary fashion.

3. b. Digital block anesthesia is ideal for digital lacerations and is performed at adjacent web spaces on either side of the lacerated digit. Local wound infiltration in the digits is risky because of the threat of vascular compromise. Combined median and ulnar nerve blocks would provide adequate anesthesia for this laceration but are more risky. Topical lidocaine is ineffective in adequately anesthetizing nonmucosal wounds that require suturing.

4. d. An Allen's test should be performed before any invasive arterial procedure is contemplated. Similarly, an Allen's test should be performed as part of the routine hand examination. If pulses are not palpable at the wrist, Doppler ultrasound can be used to perform the Allen's test.

5. d. The median nerve supplies sensation to the thumb, index and long fingers, and radial half of the ring finger. The palmar cutaneous branch supplies the radial half of the palm. Motor loss includes inability to oppose the thumb with concomitant thenar atrophy. The claw deformity is caused by paralysis of ulnar-nerve innervated intrinsic muscle and consists of hyperextension of the MCP joints.

6. e. Ganglions are synovial sacs that arise from joints or tendon sheaths. They are the most common hand tumor and frequently recur because of inadequate excision. Dorsal wrist ganglions arise from the scapholunate ligament. The dorsal sensory branch of the radial nerve is often injured in excising these ganglions. Surgery should be performed under operating room conditions with a tourniquet available.

7. c. Pyogenic flexor tenosynovitis of the finger is an infection of the tendon sheath that can ultimately result in necrosis of the tendon. The symptoms are pain on passive extension of the finger with diffuse tenderness and swelling. Systemic symptoms are usually absent. Appropriate treatment consists of incision and drainage of the tendon sheath with antibiotic irrigation. Once the infection has become established, systemic antibiotic therapy alone is not sufficient.

8. All are true.

9. b. All multiple digits and thumb amputations should be replanted if possible. Single-digit amputations except the thumb rarely regain adequate function to justify their replantation. The index finger is readily excluded by a patient in favor of the long finger. All structures, including tendons and nerves, should be repaired primarily when possible.

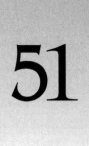

51

Basic Plastic Surgery

STEPHEN J. MATHES

KEY FEATURES

After reading this chapter you will understand:
- How a wound heals.
- The techniques of wound closure.
- Common skin grafts and flaps and their construction.
- Injury to the face.

Restoration of form and function in all body regions that have congenital and acquired deformities requires surgical manipulation of tissue. The specialty of plastic surgery is dedicated to the skillful use of principles of surgery to achieve this goal. The fundamentals of wound closure are the basis for management of traumatic, infectious, neoplastic, genetic, and aesthetic defects.

HOW DOES A WOUND HEAL?

When skin continuity is lost as a result of trauma, disease, or surgery, the open wound is subject to contamination by bacteria and fluid loss from the exposed wound surface. The initial inflammatory response to skin injury results in migration of leukocytes, fibroblasts, and undifferentiated mesenchymal cells into the wound. If the wound edges are approximated, epidermal cells migrating from the basal epithelial layer at the wound edge will bridge the gap in 24 to 48 hours. During the subsequent proliferative stage, fibroblasts produce scar tissue. Scar tissue is essential to provide structural integrity to the regenerated

epithelium. This period of fibroplasia is characterized by collagen synthesis. This phase of wound healing starts at 4 to 5 days after injury and continues approximately 6 weeks with the majority of collagen deposition accruing in the initial weeks following injury. Finally, collagen fibers realign from a random to an organized pattern and intramolecular cross-linking between collagen fibers occurs during the process of scar maturation. During this maturation phase, collagen production and lysis occur simultaneously during an extended period of wound remodeling.

When the inflammatory and proliferative phases of wound healing are prolonged because of failure to achieve wound closure or as a result of infection, scar formation will be increased. Although all wounds undergo contraction, a biologic process in which open wounds shrink, delay in skin closure accentuates the process. *Wound contraction* appears to be related to the presence of fibroblasts with properties similar to smooth muscle. These *myofibroblasts* are present during the fibroblastic phase of wound healing and will reduce the size of the wound left open. The process of wound contraction may be helpful in wounds in the abdomen, chest, and back, but in the face and extremities such contraction results in excessive pull on adjacent normal structures. Scar formation that limits the motion of tissue or loss of excursion of a joint is known as *contracture.*

Abnormalities of scar maturation may also result in increased scar formation. If the rate of collagen production exceeds the rate of collagen lysis, hypertrophic scar will result. When the resultant scar extends into adjacent normal tissue, this scar is known as a *keloid.*

WOUND CLOSURE
General Principles

Techniques of wound closure vary from simple or direct closure to more complex techniques, ranging from use of skin grafts to flaps. Failure to close a wound, whether it is a result of surgical procedure or trauma, allows progressive bacterial contamination and wound desiccation and sets the stage for increased scar formation. Factors that determine timing of wound closure include:

- Etiology
- Bacterial contamination
- Circulation

A clean surgical wound of the face is immediately closed with sutures. A wound from blunt trauma may require debridement of devitalized tissue before closure. The extent of bacterial contamination is a function of both the cause of the wound and the timing of closure. A human bite of the hand, a farm injury, or an appendectomy incision for removal of a ruptured appendix have excessive bacterial contamination, and immediate closure will often result in wound infection. If a wound has been open for 6 to 8 hours, bacterial contamination may exceed 10^5 bacteria. When wound closure is delayed or bacterial contamination is extensive, the technique of delayed secondary wound closure is used. After wound debridement and 3 to 5 days of antibiotic therapy, the wound is closed.

When skin circulation is impaired because of excessive trauma or underlying vascular disease, immediate closure is not advisable. Restoration of normal wound circulation or removal of tissue with poor circulation must precede wound closure. When the wound duration is less than 6 hours, bacterial contamination minimal (less than 10^5) and wound circulation intact, immediate wound closure is indicated.

Technique

Suture closure of wounds should provide both accurate skin approximation and an environment that minimizes scar formation during the subsequent process of wound healing (Fig. 51-1, *A*). Careful skin approximation will allow epithelialization across the wound gap within 24 to 48 hours. Buried sutures are used to approximate fascia and dermis. These layers provide temporary wound strength until the proliferation and maturation phases of wound healing are completed. Selection of a nonreactive suture material for approximation of the fascia, dermis, and skin will reduce the body's inflammatory response to the buried suture, which represents a foreign body. Permanent sutures (i.e., Prolene) or slow-absorbing sutures (i.e., monofilament polyglyconate or polydioxanone) are used to restore fascial continuity. Polyglycolytic absorbable sutures placed in the dermis will provide strength to the skin closure with minimal tissue reactivity. Sutures placed directly through the skin are re-

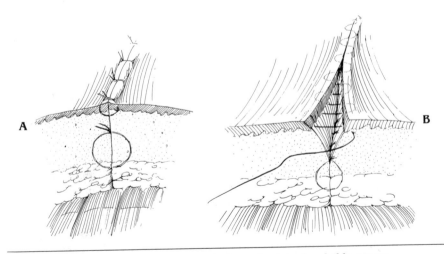

FIGURE 51-1 Simple suture technique. **A,** Deep, buried, absorbable suture approximates dermis; interrupted skin suture provides epidermal approximation. **B,** Running subcuticular suture technique.

quired only for delicate skin approximation. As skin sutures pass through the epidermis, a wound is established. Early removal of these sutures prevents epidermal growth into the suture tract and avoids stitch marks. The use of a subcuticular suture approximates the skin edges without injuring the skin adjacent to the wound (Fig. 51-1, *B*). Nonreactive, nonabsorbable sutures such as nylon (4-0 to 6-0) are preferred for skin closure. In most areas, suture removal is possible within 5 to 7 days after skin closure.

When direct wound closure is not possible because of the absence of skin, closure must await the process of wound contraction and epithelialization from wound edges or skin must be added to the defect from another source. Skin is supplied either as a graft or a flap. Unlike a flap, a skin graft does not contain its own nutrient circulation and depends on revascularization from the wound base. Selection of the method of wound coverage is based on multiple factors: (1) size of the wound, (2) circulation at the base of the wound, (3) specific reconstructive requirements to provide form and function, (4) donor site morbidity, and (5) complexity of the technique.

SKIN GRAFTS

A portion of skin may be removed from one part of the body and transplanted to an area of skin deficiency or absence in another distant site. This graft either includes only a superficial layer of skin (split-thickness skin graft) or the entire skin layer (full-thickness skin graft). Since the graft is separated from its circulation, it requires revascularization from the wound base. Skin grafting represents the least complex technique available for wound coverage and is frequently used for wound closure.

Use of a specialized knife or dermatome allows excision of the epidermis and part of the dermis from skin (Fig. 51-2). The donor site, which retains the deep dermis, heals spontaneously in 10 to 14 days by epithelialization from the epidermal lining of sweat glands and hair follicles that reside in the deep dermis and subcutaneous tissue. A split-thickness skin graft placed in the wound initially survives by plasmic circulation and heals by capillary in-growth from the wound base. If the wound base has inadequate circulation because of scar, chronic infection, or vascular insufficiency, a skin graft will not survive on the recipient site.

Since the donor site of a split-thickness skin graft heals spontaneously, skin grafting is used when large skin defects are present. This method of skin wound closure is particularly important in skin replacement in the burn wound. Factors that prevent the "take," or revascularization, of the skin grafts include:

- Presence of necrotic tissue
- Infection
- Vascular insufficiency

Specific examples of vascular insufficiency include the chronic radiation wound, exposed bone devoid of periosteum, and peripheral vascular disease. When the wound has a deep cavity or has exposure of vital structures (heart, viscera, nerves), the thin coverage of a split-thickness skin graft often is not durable and frequently fails to restore form and function.

The donor site for the split-thickness skin graft has minimal morbidity. If the graft is removed from the buttock, abdomen, or posterior thigh, the donor site is concealed by clothing. Wound closure by skin grafts is the simplest and most versatile method of wound management when direct skin approximation is not possible.

A full-thickness skin graft contains both epidermis and dermis. Since the donor site requires suture closure, the size of this graft is limited. A full-thickness graft is frequently used in the face for several reasons: (1) skin from the neck and preauricular or postauricular regions are of a color and thickness similar to those of most facial defects, (2) the donor site, when closed directly, is not readily apparent, and (3) a full-thickness skin graft with the entire dermis undergoes less

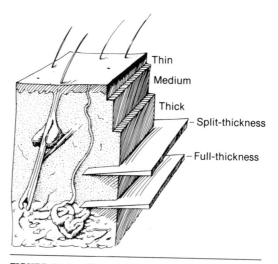

FIGURE 51-2 Skin grafts. Cross section of skin demonstrates varying thickness of split- and full-thickness skin grafts.

contraction than a split-thickness skin graft. Failure of revascularization is more common in the full-thickness skin graft. This potential for skin graft loss and the small graft size generally limit use of the full-thickness skin graft to the face and hands.

FLAPS

A flap is a composite of tissue that may include skin, subcutaneous tissue, and deep fascia or muscle that is elevated from its normal site based on a source of circulation located at its base. The flap base is either left intact or is isolated only on its vascular source as an island flap. A flap is either designed adjacent to the wound (rotation or transposition flap) or from another site adjacent to the wound but within reach of the wound (interpolation flap). The flap donor site requires either direct closure or use of skin grafts. Indications for flap use include (1) inadequate skin for direct wound closure, (2) inadequate local wound circulation for use of skin grafts (e.g., radiation-induced wound, exposed bone), (3) exposed vital structures (e.g., cranial bone defects), (4) contracture sites (e.g., neck or axillary burn contracture, (5) contour deformity, and (6) special requirements (e.g., scalp defects). If a wound has inadequate circulation, a flap may be the only method to provide skin that will survive in the defect. When located adjacent to the wound, a flap's skin has characteristics similar to those of the defect and often provides an excellent reconstruction. Wound contraction is much less than occurs after use of a skin graft.

Since a flap must initially maintain its own circulation, a flap is classified based on its source of circulation (Fig. 51-3). Direct skin perfusion is based on a subdermal vascular plexus. *Random-pattern flaps* are based on perfusion through this subdermal plexus of vessels originating from underlying muscle and fascia. Because such a flap is not based on a specific vascular pedicle, its size is limited to a length-width ratio of 2:1. This flap is most often used for small defects when adjacent skin circulation is normal. Two small flaps designed at 60% angle from the wound are frequently used as Z-plasty flaps to allow scar release. The *rhomboid flap* is another example of a local random flap that allows closure of a small defect with direct closure of the donor site.

The requirements for a larger flap and the unavailability of local tissue adjacent to the wound requires design of a flap with its special vascular pedicle distant to the wound site. The subdermal plexus receives its circulation from two sources: musculocutaneous perforating vessels and intermuscular vessels that enter the deep fascia. Thus a flap may be designed based on a muscle or deep fascia, which has unique advantages when compared with the random-pattern flaps: (1) its circulation is more reliable, (2) it is not limited to a specific length-width ratio, (3) a vascular pedicle can be used that is located distant to the wound site, and (4) the potential for design as an island flap.

The fasciocutaneous flap is based on intermuscular pedicles that course beneath the fascia and provides fasciocutaneous perforating vessels to skin. Specific vascular pedicles course along the deep fascia permitting design of overlying skin as either a standard flap or an axially oriented island flap. Axially oriented fasciocutaneous flaps have been identified in the scalp, face, groin, and extremities. Specific examples include the lateral-based forehead flap (superficial temporal artery), medial-based forehead flap (supraorbital and supratrochlear arteries), the deltopectoral flap (second, third, and fourth anterior perforating branches of the internal mammary artery) and the groin flap (superficial circumflex iliac artery). Both the lateral forehead flap and the deltopectoral flap have been used for reconstruction of oral and facial defects. The medial forehead flap, the classic flap originally described in 750 B.C. in India for total nasal reconstruction, is still used today for this purpose. In the upper extremity, the lateral arm flap and radial forearm flap are used both as local transposition flaps and for microvascular composite tissue transplantation. In the lower extremity, fasciocutaneous flaps based on the anterior tibial, posterior tibial, and peroneal arteries are available for coverage of lower extremity defects.

Muscle and musculocutaneous flaps are now commonly used for coverage of complex wounds (Fig. 51-3). The majority of the muscles receive a major or dominant vascular pedicle adjacent to either the muscle's origin or insertion. Release of the muscle from its bone or fascial attachments distant to the site of entrance of the vascular pedicle into the muscle allows transposition of the muscle to another site without disruption of its circulation. The point of rotation occurs at the site of entrance of the vascular pedicle into the muscle. The arc of rotation of muscle depends on the length of the muscle (Fig. 51-4). In all body regions muscles have been identified that have a pattern of circulation suitable for transposition as a flap.

Since superficial muscle provides circulation directly to overlying skin through musculocutaneous vessels, a segment or island of skin may be transposed with the muscle as a musculocutaneous flap. If the muscle is transposed without skin, the exposed portion of muscle at the wound site is covered with a skin graft. Muscle and musculocutaneous flaps are useful for reconstruction of wounds where local circulation is absent or vital structures are exposed. The donor site of the muscle or musculocutaneous flap is generally closed directly. Although the transposed muscle cannot always perform its intended locomotor function, synergistic muscles are almost always available to maintain normal function.

Muscle and musculocutaneous flaps have

been identified to reconstruct specific problem wounds and defects. The pectoralis major and trapezius musculocutaneous flaps are now routinely used to provide coverage after major head and neck tumor extirpation. Likewise, the pectoralis major muscle is transposed into the anterior mediastinum after debridement of the infected sternum. The latissimus dorsi and rectus abdominis musculocutaneous flaps are used to provide both skin and muscle in breast reconstruction after mastectomy, whether modified or radical.

The rectus abdominis has a dual circulation from the superior epigastric artery and vein via

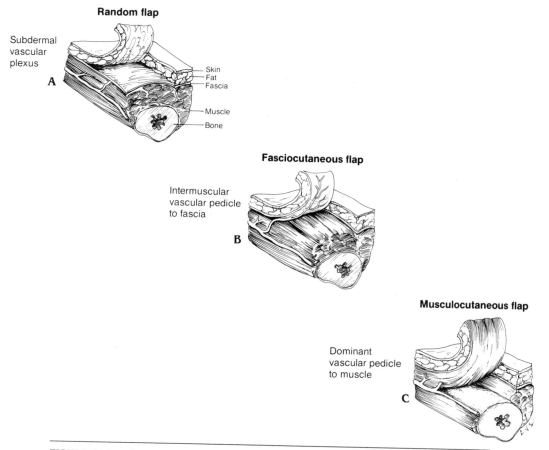

FIGURE 51-3 Flaps. **A,** Random flap. Flap consists of skin and subcutaneous tissue nourished by skin fascial and musculocutaneous perforating vessels entering the flap base. **B,** Fasciocutaneous flap. Flap is nourished by specific vascular pedicles that enter deep fascia as intermuscular vessels. Skin included with deep fascia is nourished by vascular connections (fasciocutaneous perforating vessels) between the fascia and skin. **C,** Musculocutaneous flap. Flap is nourished by major or dominant vascular pedicles entering muscle at the flap base. The skin island included with the muscle flap is nourished by vascular connections (musculocutaneous perforating vessels) between muscle and skin.

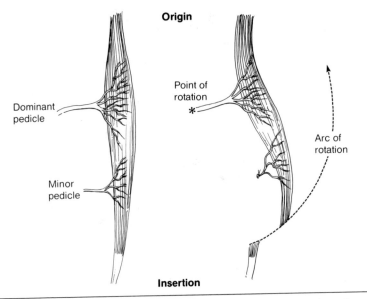

FIGURE 51-4 Muscle or musculocutaneous flap arc of rotation. Note that after release of muscle insertion and division of minor pedicles, if present, the flap is elevated to the dominant pedicle, which determines the point of rotation. Muscle length and location of the pedicle determine the extent of the arc of rotation.

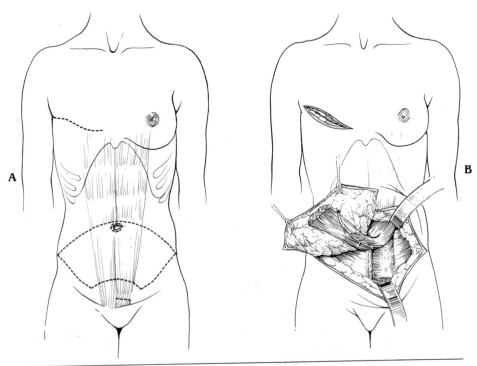

FIGURE 51-5 Autogenous breast reconstruction with transverse rectus abdominis musculocutaneous flap (TRAM flap). A, The skin island between umbilicus and pubis will provide skin and subcutaneous tissue for breast reconstruction. B, TRAM flap is elevated with flap based on superior pedicle to rectus muscle (superior epigastric artery and vein).

the internal mammary vessels and the inferior epigastric artery and venae comitantes via the external iliac vessels. In breast reconstruction, a skin island is designed between the umbilicus and pubic hair line and is elevated with the underlying rectus abdominis muscle. When transposed beneath the remaining superior abdominal skin, the flap provides both the skin to restore the missing breast skin envelope and the required fatty tissue to replace the breast mound (Fig. 51-5). This technique provides a breast reconstruction without the necessity of an implant and allows direct closure of the donor site in the abdomen, thereby improving the abdominal contour. An inferior-based rectus abdominis musculocutaneous flap based on the inferior epigastric vessel is used to reconstruct defects in the groin and pubis after radical groin dissection and pelvic tumor extirpative procedures.

Posterior thigh muscles and the gluteus maximus muscle are now routinely used for coverage of pelvic defects after abdominoperineal resections and for coverage of chronic pressure sore wounds occurring on pelvic skin. The gastroc-nemius and soleus muscles will provide coverage of complex open tibial fractures. Muscle flaps are now used in combination with sequestrectomy for management of chronic osteomyelitis. With the availability of muscle flaps for single-staged reconstruction in all body regions, aggressive tumor extirpation or debridement of chronic infected wounds is accomplished with confidence that reliable, immediate wound coverage is available.

TRANSPLANTATION OF COMPOSITE TISSUE

Flap transposition is now possible with the use of microsurgical techniques. Muscle, musculocutaneous, and fascial flaps have a specific arc of rotation based on the site of entrance of the major vascular pedicle into the flap. The artery and vein in these vascular pedicles have external lumen diameters in the range of 0.8 to 3.0 mm. With the use of the operating microscope, it is now possible to completely remove the flap from its site of origin and restore circulation to the flap

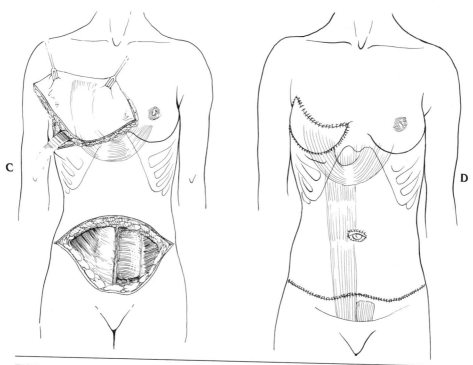

FIGURE 51-5, cont'd C, TRAM flap inset. Flap passes beneath the superior abdominal skin and enters the skin and breast defect at the mastectomy site. **D,** The final result includes an autogenous breast mound and closure of the abdomen, which is now devoid of redundant abdominal skin and fatty tissue.

by anastomosis of the flap vessels to receptor vessels identified at the site of the defect. When local fasciocutaneous or muscle flaps are not available, a suitable flap from a distant site is transplanted directly into the complex wound.

Large defects of the scalp and distal lower extremity are frequently difficult to close using local flaps. The skull or the tibia often does not have adequate local circulation to support a skin graft. Transplantation by microvascular techniques of a distant flap, such as muscle or omentum, will provide required tissue for wound coverage. Microvascular transplantation of specialized tissue is now possible for defect reconstruction. In facial palsy, distant muscles are transplanted to the face with both microvascular revascularization and repair of the muscle's motor nerve to suitable receptor nerves in the face. A segment of jejunum transplanted to the neck may be used to replace scarred or absent cervical esophagus. The radial forearm flap, with its minimal subcutaneous tissue and long vascular pedicle, is ideally suited for reconstruction of intraoral defects. A segment of fibula or the iliac crest based on its vascular pedicle may be transplanted to the mandible or long bones to replace a missing segment of bone with a vascularized graft, thus restoring bone continuity. Microvascular techniques are now widely used for both wound closure and reconstruction.

HOW IS TISSUE EXPANDED?

Tissue expansion has recently been appreciated as a method to cover wounds. Ideally, wound closure is accomplished with skin adjacent to the wound. This skin has similar thickness and color. Placement of a silicone balloon connected to a reservoir beneath the skin and subcutaneous tissue at the wound edge allows for increase in skin dimensions. Saline is injected transcutaneously into the reservoir at frequent intervals. With gradual filling of the silicone implant, the skin is stretched without interruption of the dermal fascial circulation. After 6 to 8 weeks the implant is removed, and the stretched skin will advance to close the defect or allow use of the tissue as a flap for reconstruction of a defect (Fig. 51-6). This method is particularly useful where the skin has unique characteristics that cannot always be provided by a distant flap source, such as the chest wall skin for breast reconstruction after mastectomy or for closure of a defect in hair-bearing tissue such as the scalp.

The basic principles of wound closure apply to all congenital and acquired surgical defects. Specific reconstructive requirements are identified for each wound. If direct wound approximation is not feasible, wound closure is accomplished with the simplest method that restores form and function without donor site morbidity.

MAXILLOFACIAL TRAUMA

To achieve an optimal outcome, a systematic approach to maxillofacial trauma is necessary. Potential injuries of the cervical vertebrae and other life-threatening injuries must be sought in the initial evaluation of the patient. Management of associated soft tissue, nerve, and skin injuries

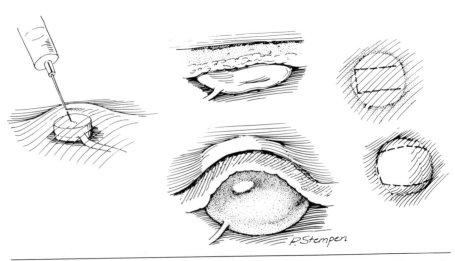

FIGURE 51-6 Skin expansion. Saline injected into silicone bag via connected reservoir gradually stretches skin with resultant increase in flap size.

usually requires immediate attention. A multidisciplinary approach, with neurosurgery for management of associated intracranial injury and ophthalmology for ocular injuries, is required for management of complex facial injuries.

The facial bones are evaluated through physical examination and radiologic studies. Asymmetry in the nose, malar eminence, or forehead may indicate fractures of the nasal, zygoma, or frontal bones, respectively. On examination of the eye and orbit, either intrinsic eye injury or fractures of the orbital wall or floor may be found. Blowout fractures of the orbital walls may result in enophthalmos or dystopia (uneven vertical placement of the globes), and an orbital floor fracture may result in a loss of upward vertical gaze because of entrapment of the inferior rectus muscle. Dental occlusion must be evaluated; any change in the patient's normal bite can indicate maxillary and/or mandibular fractures.

Severe midface trauma results in fractures that may separate the midface from the cranium at different levels; these are classified according to LeFort levels (Fig. 51-7). A LeFort I fracture separates the lower maxilla from the midface and occurs through the piriform aperture, including the hard palate and pterygoid process. LeFort II fractures separate the maxilla with the attached nasal bones from the frontal and zygomatic bones, with the fracture occurring along the nasofrontal suture, floor of the orbit, zygomaticoaxillary sutures, and pterygoid processes. A LeFort III fracture or craniofacial dysjunction separates the maxilla and inferior orbital bones from the skull, with the fracture occurring through the zygomaticofrontal and nasofrontal suture lines and through the orbital floor. Physical examination of the patient with a LeFort fracture will demonstrate movement of the maxilla with associated crepitus.

Radiologic examination of suspected injuries includes cervical spine films in addition to posterior-anterior and Waters' views of the face. A panoramic view of the mandible is helpful in demonstrating mandibular fractures as well as the status of the teeth. Computed tomography is now routinely used for evaluation of the craniofacial skeleton, especially for fractures of the skull, orbits, midface, and mandibular condyles.

Facial lacerations are generally repaired at the time of initial evaluation. Nasal septal hematomas should be drained to avoid destruction of septal cartilage, with subsequent perforation or saddle deformity of the nose. Extensive fractures may require urgent management, particularly if

the patient's airway is obstructed or if bleeding is uncontrollable; reduction of fracture sites in the midface will frequently stop the bleeding. Initial airway management may require intubation or tracheotomy.

After the patient is stabilized, specific fracture management is performed immediately or within 3 to 5 days after facial edema has resolved. If necessary, fractures may be reduced as late as 10 to 14 days after injury before early healing and remodeling begin to interfere with the ability to achieve anatomic reduction. The basic principles of fracture management include wide exposure of the facial skeleton through incisions hidden in the hair, natural creases, or within the mouth, followed by anatomic reduction whenever possible. Miniplating and lag screw techniques have made rigid fixation of facial fractures possible, and there is increasing use of open reduction followed by plate fixation of

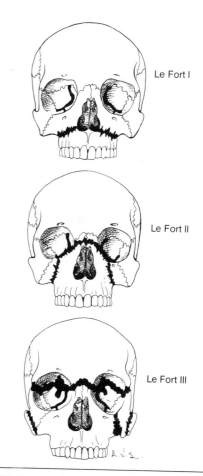

FIGURE 51-7 LeFort classification of midface fractures.

facial fractures. Missing bone is replaced by bone grafts when necessary.

Fractures of the orbital floor (blowout fractures) require the release of any entrapped extraocular musculature and placement of a synthetic or autogenous graft to support the orbital contents. Displaced fractures of the zygoma generally require open reduction and fixation. Failure to achieve proper bony alignment will result in depression of the malar eminence and enophthalmos. Most nasal fractures can be treated with closed reduction and splinting to avoid posttraumatic nasal deformity.

LeFort III complex naso-orbital and frontal sinus fractures require use of a transcoronal incision in which the anterior scalp and forehead skin are elevated and retracted over the midface to allow direct vision of the frontal bone, orbits, and nasoethmoid regions. More extensive fractures of this type frequently require both plating of fractured segments (or wiring) and immediate bone graft techniques to provide additional support and replace missing segments of bone.

Fractures of the tooth-bearing bones (i.e., maxilla or mandible) demand restoration of normal occlusion for proper treatment. Occlusion is restored through the use of arch bars that attach to the maxillary and mandibular teeth and that are subsequently wired together in intermaxillary fixation (IMF), to reestablish the pretraumatic relationship of the teeth. Because of the pull of the powerful muscles of mastication on the fracture segments, open reduction and fixation of mandibular fractures or alveolar splinting within the oral cavity is generally required in conjunction with IMF. Isolated mandibular fractures are managed by a combination of intermaxillary fixation (IMF) and direct reduction and fixation of the fracture site with either wires or screws and plates. Condylar fractures can usually be treated with a brief period of IMF, followed by controlled early motion, but cases in which the condylar head is displaced from the temporal fossa may require open reduction and fixation.

With recognition and precise reduction and fixation of facial fractures, facial function and normal appearance are preserved.

BIBLIOGRAPHY

Anthony JP, Mathes SJ, Alpert BS. The muscle flap in the treatment of chronic lower extremity osteomyelitis: Results in patients over 5 years posttreatment. Plast Reconstr Surg 88:311, 1991.

Ariyan S. The pectoralis major myocutaneous flap: A versatile flap for reconstruction in head and neck. Plast Reconstr Surg 63:73, 1979.

Edgarton MT Jr. Replacement of lining to oral cavity following surgery. Cancer 4:110, 1951.

Gruss JS, MacKinnon SE. Complex maxillary fracture: Role of buttress reconstruction and immediate bone grafts. Plast Reconstr Surg 78:9, 1986.

Hartrampf CR, Scheflan M, Black PW. Breast reconstruction with a transverse abdominal island flap. Plast Reconstr Surg 69:216, 1982.

Jurkiewicz MJ, Krizek T, Mathes S, Ariyan S. Plastic Surgery: Principles and Practice. St Louis, CV Mosby, 1990.

LeFort R. Experimental study of fractures of the upper jaw. Parts I and II. Plast Reconstr Surg 50:497, 1972.

LeFort R. Experimental study of fractures of the upper jaw. Parts I and II. Plast Reconstr Surg 50:600, 1972.

Manson PN, Hoopes JE, Su CT. Structural pillars of the facial skeleton: An approach to the management of LeFort fractures. Plast Reconstr Surg 66:54, 1980.

Mathes SJ, Abouljoud M. Wound healing. In Davis JH, Foster RS Jr, Gamelli RL (eds). Clinical Surgery. St Louis, CV Mosby, 1987.

Mathes SJ, Bostwick J III. A rectus abdominis myocutaneous flap to reconstruct abdominal wall defects. Br J Plast Surg 30:282, 1977.

Mathes SJ, Nahai F. Classification of the vascular anatomy of muscles: Experimental and clinical correlation. Plast Reconstr Surg 67:177, 1981.

Mathes SJ, Nahai F. Clinical Applications of Muscle and Musculocutaneous Flaps. St Louis, CV Mosby, 1981.

McCraw JB, Dibbell DG, Carraway JH. Clinical definition of independent myocutaneous vascular territories. Plast Reconstr Surg 60:341, 1977.

Radovan C. Tissue expansion in soft-tissue reconstruction. Plast Reconstr Surg 74:482, 1984.

CHAPTER REVIEW
Questions

1. In which of the following patients is a delay in skin closure justified?
   a. Human bite of the hand
   b. Two-hour-old facial laceration
   c. Shotgun wound to medial thigh
   d. Site of excision of sebaceous cyst
2. List in order the sequence of events in healing of sutured skin laceration.
   a. Wound maturation
   b. Inflammatory phase
   c. Migratory phase
   d. Fibroplasia
3. Which of the following represents an advantage of the split-thickness skin graft over the full-thickness skin graft?
   a. Covers large surface area
   b. Less wound contraction
   c. Normal skin color and thickness
   d. Normal hair growth at graft sites
4. Select one of the following techniques: (1) split-thickness skin or (2) full-thickness skin graft for closure of the following wounds:
   a. Twenty-percent full-thickness burn to anterior trunk
   b. Excision of 2 × 2 cm basal cell carcinoma from lower eyelid
   c. Excision of a 4 × 5 cm giant hairy nevus from back
   d. Avulsion of part of upper eyelid
5. Select one of the following techniques: (1) random-pattern flap or (2) musculocutaneous flap, for each of the following wounds:
   a. 2 × 3 cm cheek defect after excision of congenital nevus
   b. Composite resection of floor of mouth and mandible for squamous cell carcinoma
   c. Coverage of open proximal tibial fracture site
   d. Osteoradionecrosis of sternum after radiation therapy for lymphoma

Answers

1. a, c
2. b, c, d, a
3. a
4. a. (1)
   b. (2)
   c. (1)
   d. (2)
5. a. (1)
   b. (2)
   c. (2)
   d. (2)

52 Basic Otolaryngologic Surgery

STANLEY E. THAWLEY

KEY FEATURES

After reading this chapter you will understand:
- Physical examination of the ear, nose, and throat.
- How do you differentiate acute from chronic ear infections?
- Hearing loss.
- Common nose and throat problems.
- Diseases of the salivary glands.
- What are the diagnostic clues to the presence of laryngeal cancer?

Otolaryngology is the surgical subspecialty dealing with diseases and surgery of the head and neck. Otolaryngologists deal with problems of the ear, nose, and throat, facial plastic, facial trauma, and tumors of the head and neck area and perform reconstructive surgery of the head and neck.

HOW IS THE EAR, NOSE, AND THROAT AREA EXAMINED?

The *required instruments* for the examination are an otoscope, tuning fork, headlight, tongue blade, laryngeal mirror, and nasal speculum. The *external ear* is examined for deformities, trauma, skin lesions, injection, and swelling. The otoscope is used to examine the ear canal and tympanic membrane. The ear pinna may be gently retracted posteriorly and superiorly to straighten the canal. The *ear canal* may be cleaned of cerumen with a small curette, but care must be used

to avoid trauma to the skin and eardrum. Injection, swelling, and tenderness may be noted in the canal with infections such as external otitis (swimmer's ear). The *tympanic membrane* should be identified as a grey-white semitransparent membrane. The malleus is the most easily identifiable structure. It extends from the top to the center of the drum, the umbo. The light reflex is in the anteroinferior quadrant. It is only for identification. Its presence does not indicate a normal drum, nor does its absence indicate an abnormality. The color of the drum should be noted. There may be injection typical of infection or an amber opaque quality seen with fluid within the middle ear space (serous otitis). The eardrum has a normal variety of appearances (e.g., very thin, almost transparent to very thick with white scars [tympanosclerosis]). Eardrum mobility can be evaluated by sealing the canal with the ear speculum and applying a small amount of air pressure with the pneumatic attachment. This evaluation is important, especially in children when eardrum mobility is limited by fluid within the middle ear space.

The *tuning fork test* helps differentiate types of hearing loss. A 500- to 1000-cycle vibrating tuning fork is held approximately 6 to 8 inches away from the external ear and then is placed on the skull directly behind the ear (mastoid bone). In patients with normal hearing and neurosensory hearing loss the fork should be heard better through the ear canal than behind the ear on the mastoid bone (*air conduction is greater than bone conduction*). If the tuning fork is heard better behind the ear on the mastoid bone, the ear has a conductive hearing loss (**bone conduction is greater than air conduction**). The indication of " + " or " − " is confusing and best is not used. In the **Weber test** the vibrating fork is placed on the forehead. The sound will be heard louder in the ear that hears better in patients with neurosensory hearing loss and in the ear with poorer hearing in patients with conductive hearing loss.

The **nose** is examined with a light source and a nasal speculum. An otoscope and large ear speculum may also be used. Care should be taken to avoid contact with the sensitive nasal mucosa. The inferior turbinate is visualized as a rounded area in the inferior aspect of the nasal cavity. It is a normal structure and should not be confused with a nasal polyp. The quality of the nasal mucus should be noted as clear like saliva, thick, purulent, bloody, excessive, or dry. The nasal membrane is noted as normal pink, injected, or swollen.

The **oral examination** should start with the lips anteriorly and progress posteriorly to the soft palate–tonsil area. After the lips are examined, using a tongue blade and light source, the sulci lateral and medial to the teeth, the area beneath the tongue, the floor of the mouth, the tongue, the lateral buccal mucosa, the hard and soft palates, and the tonsils are examined. The floor of the mouth, the tongue, and the base of the tongue posterior to the circumvallate papillae should be palpated. The point of entry of the ducts of the parotid and submaxillary glands should be noted in the lateral buccal mucosa and the anterior floor of the mouth. A normal finding often mistaken for a tumor is the bony bulge in the center of the hard palate (torus palatinus).

The **pharynx** is visualized by pushing the tongue inferiorly with a tongue blade. The gag reflex is usually avoided if the posterior tongue is not touched. The remainder of the pharynx and larynx is visualized with a laryngeal mirror and headlight. Indirect **nasopharyngoscopy** is performed by placing a small laryngeal mirror in the posterior pharynx and aiming it superiorly as a light is directed on it. This allows visualization of the nasopharynx, the adenoid area, and the eustachian tube openings. Indirect **laryngoscopy** is performed by grasping the tongue and pulling it forward. A warmed laryngeal mirror is placed on the soft palate, and light, which reflects inferiorly, is focused on it, and the laryngeal and pharyngeal structures are visualized (Fig. 52-1). The epiglottis is apparent as a thin, curved white structure extending up from the larynx. Inferiorly is the airway with the vocal cords appearing as two thin white bands. Posteriorly the aryte-

noid area and posterior pharyngeal wall are visualized. The pyriform fossae are crevices of mucosa just lateral to the larynx within the lateral wall of the pharynx. The laryngeal examination is difficult, takes practice, and may not be feasible in some patients because of a strong gag reflex. This area can be examined with a small flexible fiberoptic scope that is passed through the nose.

- The posterior wall of the ear canal is seen first because of the anterior angulation of the ear canal. Avoid mistaking the posterior wall for the eardrum by following the canal anteriorly.
- The bulbous structure seen in the anterior nose is the inferior turbinate. Do not confuse it for the middle turbinate, which is more superior, or a nasal polyp.
- The gag reflex frequently can be avoided by not depressing the tongue posterior to the circumvallate papillae.

EAR CONDITIONS
Why Are Swimmers Susceptible to Ear Infections?

External otitis (swimmer's ear) is a skin infection of the ear canal. It is usually secondary to excessive moisture in the external ear canal, which creates a condition conducive to infection. The most common offending organisms are *Pseudomonas*, *Proteus*, and *Staphylococcus*. Symptoms are itching and pain. The ear canal reddens and swells, and the external ear frequently becomes tender to manipulation. Treatment consists of cleaning the ear canal and using antibiotic eardrops. The ear canal should be kept dry, and if the infection is associated with cellulitis or perichondritis of the periauricular tissues, systemic antibiotics should be used along with the topical therapy. Prevention consists of drying the ear canal and not allowing moisture to remain in the canal.

What Are the Signs and Symptoms of Acute Ear Infections?

Acute otitis media most commonly occurs in infants and children, but it can occur in patients of any age. If frequently follows an upper respiratory tract infection and is associated with increasing ear pain, a sensation of fullness in the ear, hearing loss, fever, and chills. The eardrum first shows dilation of the blood vessels of the malleus, followed by dullness and hyperemia. The eardrum may bulge because of the pressure from retained secretions in the middle ear, and it

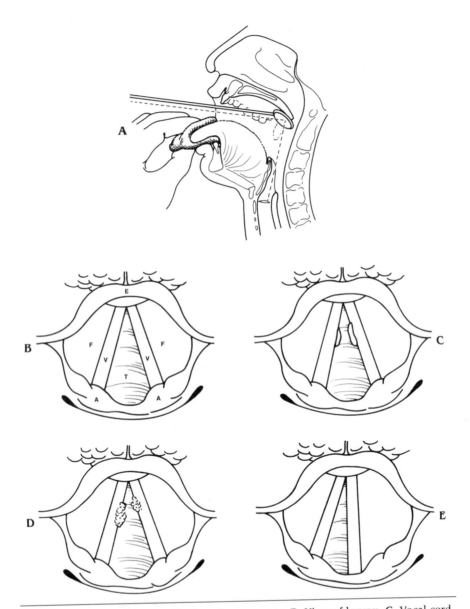

FIGURE 52-1 **A,** Technique of indirect laryngoscopy. **B,** View of larynx. **C,** Vocal cord nodules. **D,** Carcinoma of the true vocal cord. **E,** Paralysis of the left true vocal cord.

also may rupture. The disease should be differentiated from bullous myringitis, which is an infection associated with bullae on the eardrum. The usual infecting organisms in patients with acute otitis media are pneumococci, streptococci, staphylococci, and *Haemophilus influenzae*. Treatment consists of analgesics and systemic antibiotics. *Myringotomy* (incision of the eardrum) may be indicated if the infection does not resolve promptly or if there is associated bulging of the eardrum, continued pain or fever, increased hearing loss, vertigo, or facial paralysis. Myringotomy with the placement of ear ventilation tubes may be performed for patients with recurrent otitis, especially if it is associated with hearing loss.

What Distinguishes Chronic Ear Infections From Acute Ear Infections?

Chronic otitis media is characterized by persistent perforation of the tympanic membrane and is associated with recurrent or persistent purulent ear infections. The recurrent infections can be induced by poor eustachian tube function or can result from an associated mastoid disease. If the perforations are at the margin of the eardrum or in the superior attic area, ingrowth of squamous epithelium into the middle ear and mastoid bone (*cholesteatoma*) may erode bone and surrounding structures and produce repeated infections and possible complications. *Chronic otitis media frequently requires surgical therapy.* This surgery usually involves patching of the eardrum perforation (tympanoplasty) and may involve reconstruction of the middle-ear ossicles, removal of the cholesteatoma, and removal of the chronically infected bone in the mastoid air cells (mastoidectomy).

The possible *complications* of both acute and chronic otitis media are conductive and/or neurosensory hearing loss, mastoiditis, facial paralysis, meningitis, labyrinthitis, epidural and subdural abscess, brain abscess, sigmoid sinus thrombophlebitis, and petrous apicitis (Fig. 52-2).

Why Does Fluid Accumulate in the Middle Ear Space?

Serous otitis media can occur at any age but is more common in the young child up to 8 to 10 years of age. Accumulation of serous or mucoid fluid in the middle-ear space can be caused by (1) obstruction of the eustachian tube, preventing normal ventilation of the middle ear, (2) incom-plete resolution of otitis media, (3) allergic transudate of serous fluid in the middle-ear space, and (4) sudden barometric pressure changes in the middle ear (barotitis media) such as experienced in flying or diving. The accumulation of fluid in the middle ear produces symptoms of hearing loss and a full, plugged feeling in the ear. Examination reveals a meniscus fluid level or air fluid bubbles seen through the eardrum. The eardrum appears thickened, and there are characteristic amber discoloration and impaired mobility of the eardrum when viewed with a pneumatic otoscope. *Tympanometry* provides an objective measurement and a graph of the eardrum mobility. Cancer of the nasopharynx with obstruction of the eustachian tube must be ruled out in unilateral serous otitis media in an adult. Treatment consists of eustachian tube inflations, topical nasal decongestants, and oral antihistamines and decongestants. Underlying problems of nasal allergy and nasal or sinus infections should also be treated, and tonsillectomy or adenoidectomy may sometimes be necessary. If serous otitis is persistent or unresponsive to medical therapy, especially if it is associated with recurrent ear infections or conductive hearing loss, myringotomy and placement of ventilating tubes may be necessary.

- The physical appearance of the eardrum in a patient with serous otitis may have only subtle amber color changes.
- Serous otitis may produce hearing loss without infection.

What Are the Different Types and Causes of Hearing Loss?

The various types of hearing loss are classified as sensorineural, conductive, mixed, and functional. Diagnosis of the type of hearing loss is obtained by careful history and examination along with an audiologic test (Table 52-1). The tuning-fork tests are used to distinguish conductive loss and nerve-type loss. Audiometric tests (pure-tone, speech, and special site-of-lesion testing) provide quantitative measurements of hearing loss. Evoked response audiometry (ERA) is a method of quantitative testing for hearing losses in patients such as young children who are unresponsive to normal audiometric tests. It may also help locate the site of the lesion in patients with neurosensory hearing loss.

Sensorineural (nerve, perceptive) deafness is due to abnormal function of the cochlea, cranial nerve VIII, or the auditory cortex. *Presbycusis* is a common sensorineural hearing loss in elderly

TABLE 52-1   Hearing Loss

	Sensorineural	Conductive
Disease location	Cochlea, cranial nerve VIII, brain	Ear canal, eardrum, middle-ear ossicles
Eardrum appearance	Normal	May be abnormal
Tuning fork test	Air conduction better than bone conduction	Bone conduction better than air conduction
Weber test	Heard better in better ear	Heard better in worse ear
Cause	Age, noise trauma, meningitis, congenital, inner ear trauma	Serous otitis, otitis media, otosclerosis, cerumen
Treatment	Hearing aid, cochlear implant	Medicine, surgery
Prognosis	Stable or progressively worse	Correctable with treatment
Prevention	Protection from sound	Treatment of causative disease

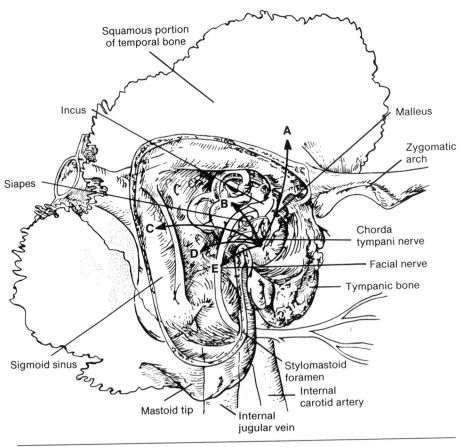

FIGURE 52-2   Complications of otitis media. *A,* Meningitis, brain abscess. *B,* Labyrinthitis. *C,* Sigmoid sinus thrombophlebitis. *D,* Mastoiditis. *E,* Facial nerve paralysis.

people that occurs as gradual progressive deterioration occurs in the organ of Corti within the cochlea. Other causes of nerve deafness in adults include exposure to loud noises, ingestion of ototoxic drugs, temporal bone trauma, labyrinthine infections, circulatory problems of the inner ear, and tumors of cranial nerve VIII or the cerebellopontine angle. The physician is usually not able to restore neurosensory hearing loss once it occurs.

Prevention of nerve deafness is therefore an important concept. Nerve hearing loss caused by ***acoustic trauma*** can be avoided by prevention of exposure to loud noise, either by avoiding the source of the noise or by wearing ear protectors. Prompt treatment of bacterial central nervous system infections and severe febrile illnesses and the avoidance or discontinuance of ototoxic drugs are important in the prevention of neurosensory hearing loss. Any adult with unexplained unilateral neurosensory hearing loss should be carefully studied for the possibility of an ***acoustic neuroma.*** This study usually involves special site-of-lesion audiologic testing, evoked response testing, and MRI scans of the internal auditory canal. Many adults with neurosensory hearing loss are helped by wearing a hearing aid after appropriate diagnosis and testing. Neurosensory hearing loss commonly is associated with decreased discrimination of sounds, even when the sound is adequately heard. It is particularly worse in noisy environments. New computer programmable hearing aids offer customized fittings based on the patient's particular frequency pattern of hearing loss.

Neurosensory deafness should be suspected and diagnosed early in children with histories of congenital anomalies, rubella, and other fetal infections, in any child with a birth weight less than 1500 g, and in children with elevated indirect bilirubin concentrations. In children the effective management of neurosensory deafness includes early diagnosis, auditory rehabilitation, and education. A hearing aid and speech reading for the child and education programs for both the child and the parents are usually essential in the child's rehabilitation. A few patients with severe neurosensory hearing loss who are not helped by a hearing aid may be candidates for an electronic inner ear implant.

Conductive deafness indicates malfunction of the conductive mechanism of the ear and includes any problems with the external ear, the eardrum, or the middle-ear ossicles. Common causes of conductive deafness include impacted cerumen in the ear canal, acute otitis media, chronic otitis media, serous otitis media, ear trauma, and fixation of the stapes (otosclerosis). Treatment for conductive hearing losses involves correction of the condition that prevents conduction of sound waves to the inner ear. This treatment may include simple removal of ear canal cerumen, myringotomies to release the fluid from the middle ear in patients with serous otitis, patching a perforation of the eardrum, or surgical correction of otosclerosis in which the fixed stapes is replaced with a mobile prosthesis. ***Mixed deafness*** refers to various combinations of neurosensory and conduction deafness. ***Functional deafness*** refers to hearing loss in which no organic lesion can be detected. Frequently, people with functional deafness are malingerers who can be detected by special audiologic evaluation.

- Poor speech development in a child may be the result of hearing loss.

What Causes Tinnitus?

Tinnitus is the sensation of an abnormal noise in the ear. ***Objective tinnitus*** is uncommon and usually is caused by transmitted vascular vibrations from blood vessels close to the ear. It can also be produced by rhythmic rapid contractions of the muscles of the soft palate or middle ear. The examiner can hear the sound through a stethoscope placed over the patient's ear or occasionally can see movement of the eardrum or palate. ***Subjective tinnitus*** commonly occurs. Its presumed cause is damage to the nerve endings in the cochlea; the sensation is usually described as a ringing, cricket, or hissing noise. Tinnitus usually accompanies high-frequency neurosensory hearing loss and is commonly considered an expected associated symptom of presbycusis. It may occur in patients with hypertension, drug toxicity, anemia, arteriosclerosis of the inner ear, and Ménière's disease. If possible, treatment is directed at the underlying cause. In severe cases a hearing aid type of tinnitus masker may be beneficial.

Does Vertigo Always Indicate Ear Disease?

Vertigo is a sensation of turning or spinning in which the patient experiences a distinct sense of motion in relation to his or her environment. It must be distinguished from dizziness, which is a feeling of faintness, unsteadiness, or wavering. True vertigo usually indicates a disorder of the inner ear or its central connections. It can be associated with various medical and neurologic disorders. *When evaluating a patient with vertigo, try to differentiate between vertigo of peripheral origin and that of central origin. Peripheral vertigo* produces a definite sensation of movement. The vertigo attacks are severe and paroxysmal and last from minutes to days; they usually are accompanied by spontaneous nystagmus and autonomic nervous system signs of nausea, vomiting, and sweating (Table 52-2). *In almost 80% of patients with vertigo the cause is peripheral.* In comparison to the peripheral type, central vertigo is mild and more like a sensation of unsteadiness. It is vague, with no specific onset or termination; lasts for weeks, often with no apparent nystagmus; and may be associated with loss of consciousness, seizures, or other neurologic signs (Table 52-3). The differential diagnosis of vertigo is usually accomplished by history and physical examination. It can be confirmed by various tests, including audiography, CT or MRI scans of the brain and internal auditory canal, and electronystagmography, which measures vestibular function based on caloric responses.

What Is Ménière's Disease, and How Is It Treated?

Ménière's disease (labyrinthine hydrops) presents a triad of symptoms that include episodic vertigo, fluctuating sensorineural hearing loss, and tinnitus. The cause is either overproduction or underabsorption of endolymph of the inner ear. The vertiginous spells last from a few minutes to several hours. Differential diagnosis is usually confirmed by special diagnostic audiometry and electronystagmography. Medical therapy consists of sodium restriction, diuretics, antihistamines, and vestibular suppressants. In cases associated with severe deafness, procedures that destroy the vestibular portions of the acoustic nerve may be recommended to prevent further attacks of vertigo. In patients with reasonably good hearing, endolymphatic shunt operations may be recommended to relieve the vertigo and preserve hearing.

- A common mistake is to label everyone who is dizzy as having Ménière's disease.

What Is the Most Common Type of Facial Paralysis?

Facial paralysis may be due to a number of causes at various locations along the facial nerve. The central nervous system portion of the facial nerve may be affected by infections, various neurologic

TABLE 52-2   Peripheral-Labyrinthine Vertigo

Disease	Characteristics
Ménière's disease	Tinnitus, episodic vertigo, sensorineural deafness
Viral labyrinthitis	Recent upper respiratory infection
Benign positional paroxysmal vertigo	Only occurs with positional changes; brief episodes
Bacterial labyrinthitis	Chronic otitis with cholesteatoma
Ototoxicity	From streptomycin ingestion
Aging changes	Vestibular counterpart of aging hearing loss

TABLE 52-3   Central-Nonlabyrinthine Vertigo

Disease	Characteristics
Acoustic neuroma	Produces vestibular symptoms and deafness from cranial nerve VIII dysfunction
Brain tumors	Associated with other neurologic signs
Multiple sclerosis	Classic triad is nystagmus, intention tremor, and scanning speech
Epilepsy	Temporal lobe seizures
Vascular insufficiency	Vertebrobasilar artery compression or subclavian steal syndrome
Medications	Alcohol, barbiturates, antihistamines

syndromes, and vascular accidents. Within the internal auditory canal the nerve may be affected by tumors or by trauma. Within its course through the ear and mastoid region, the nerve may be affected by acute and chronic ear infections, trauma, and surgical injury. As the nerve runs distally through the parotid gland to supply the facial muscles, it may be affected by parotid tumors, trauma, and surgical injury during parotidectomy. *Bell's palsy* is the most common type of peripheral facial paralysis. Its cause is unknown, and most patients spontaneously recover facial motion within 2 weeks to 6 months. The treatment of Bell's palsy is controversial, ranging from medical therapy with steroids to surgical therapy with facial-nerve decompression. Many patients with facial paralysis caused by accidental injury to the nerve can be rehabilitated by surgical anastomosis of the transected nerve or by grafting of the major segment of the nerve or other reinnervation procedures.

What Is the Possible Extent of Injury From Ear Trauma?

Hematoma of the ear pinna can be produced by blunt injury to the external ear, which may result in a hematoma beneath the perichondrium of the ear. Incision and drainage are necessary to prevent possible ear-cartilage necrosis, with resultant *cauliflower ear deformity.* Frequently foreign bodies are placed within the ear canals of young children and mentally disturbed patients. Removal of these *foreign objects* should be performed under good visualization and with excellent control of the patient. In very young children removal of a foreign body may necessitate use of a surgical microscope and administration of a general anesthesia. *Traumatic perforations of the eardrum* can result from slaps on the ear and can occur when cotton-tip applicators are used to clean the ear. Most of these perforations heal spontaneously, but the patient should be referred to an otolaryngologist for evaluation of any possible hearing loss and possible associated injuries such as dislocation of the middle-ear ossicles.

- Care should be used by the physician when removing cerumen from the ear because trauma can easily occur.

NASAL CONDITIONS
What Are the Most Common Causes of Nasal Congestion?

Acute viral rhinitis (common cold) is the most frequent cause of nasal congestion. The patient complains of malaise, headache, nasal congestion with rhinorrhea, and sneezing. The nasal mucosa is injected and edematous. Treatment options include rest, fluids, aspirin, nasal sprays, oral antihistamines or decongestants, saline solution gargles, cough suppressants, and use of a vaporizer. Most untreated colds resolve within 5 to 7 days unless a secondary infection occurs.

Allergic rhinitis (hay fever) is another common cause of nasal congestion. It is characterized by a watery nasal discharge, itching of the nasal mucosa, and sneezing and may be associated with conjunctival itching and lacrimation. The nasal mucosa is pale, blue, and edematous. A smear of the nasal secretions reveals increased

numbers of eosinophils. The specific allergic stimulus can be determined by skin tests and immunologic tests such as the radioallergosorbent test (RAST). Treatment consists of avoidance of the offending agent, antihistamines, decongestants, cortisone nasal sprays, and control of the environment at work and home. An alternative method is hyposensitization or desensitization to the specific allergenic stimulus.

A third common cause of nasal congestion is excessive use of nasal sprays for relief of nasal congestion *(rhinitis medicamentous).* Most medicated decongestant nasal sprays should not be used for more than 1 week. Prolonged use of nasal sprays results in chronic rhinitis secondary to the irritative effects of the nasal spray. Discontinuance of use of the nasal spray results in an initial aggravation of congestion symptoms, followed by a return of normal nasal function, usually within 3 to 4 weeks. Nasal congestion can also be caused by the side effects of drugs such as reserpine and some tranquilizers and may be associated with pregnancy.

- Patients who use excessive decongestant nasal sprays are considered addicted, and their symptoms will worsen initially from withdrawal of the medicine.

What Are the Common Causes of Nasal Obstruction?

In early childhood nasal obstruction can be caused by *choanal atresia,* a condition in which the posterior aperture of the nose fails to open normally secondary to embryologic failure. Patients with bilateral involvement may have severe respiratory distress at birth. The diagnosis is usually made by failure to pass a soft rubber catheter through the nose; diagnosis is confirmed by radiologic study. Surgical therapy is necessary to restore the patency of the posterior choanae.

Encephaloceles and meningoceles may present as *intranasal masses* producing nasal obstruction. These structures are usually in the roof or dorsum of the nose. All such nasal masses should be carefully studied radiographically before either removal or biopsy is attempted. Nasal obstruction associated with foul-smelling discharge may occur with a *foreign body* within the nose. This is not uncommon in young children.

Nasal obstruction occurring in a child from *hypertrophy of adenoid tissue* is not unusual. A child presents with mouth breathing, and his or her parents usually describe snoring during sleep. The patient has hyponasal speech, and the presence of large adenoids is suspected if the soft palate is depressed or has limited elevation. The diagnosis is made by digital palpation of the nasopharynx or lateral soft tissue x-ray films of the nasopharynx.

Nasal polyps frequently occur in cases of longstanding allergic rhinitis. Nasal polyps result when the polypoid hypertrophied mucosa of the nose or the adjacent sinus protrudes into the nose. If nasal polyps are found in a child, cystic fibrosis should be suspected. Turbinates should not be confused with nasal polyps. If polyps do not respond to medical therapy, they may require surgical removal.

A *deviated nasal septum* is commonly a normal finding, but it may also produce nasal obstruction. This obstruction may occur secondary to nasal trauma with acute subluxation of the nasal septum, or it may be secondary to mild nasal trauma earlier in life, producing changes in the growth of the nasal septum that result in a deviated nasal septum years after the initial injury. In addition to nasal obstruction, a deviated septum may impinge on the middle turbinate area, aggravating sinusitis. Surgical therapy allows relief of the nasal obstruction by straightening the nasal septum.

Why Do Nosebleeds Occur?

The majority of nosebleeds originate from the vascular plexus (Kiesselbach's plexus) in the *anterior* nasal septal mucosa. Nosebleeds are usually produced by dryness of the anterior septal mucosa, with cracking leading to epistaxis. They occur more frequently in the cold, dry winter air and frequently are initiated by nose picking. Treatment consists of external digital pressure and the use of a vasoconstricting nasal spray. *Anterior nasal packing* may be necessary as may cautery of the bleeding site. Prevention includes moisturizing the nasal mucosa with a saline solution nasal spray and discontinuance of nose picking.

Posterior epistaxis is much less common, usually occurs in elderly patients, and may be associated with hypertension. Posterior epistaxis is usually more severe and more difficult to control and treat than anterior epistaxis. If posterior epistaxis is severe, *posterior nasal packing* is applied. This is accomplished by inserting a standard posterior nasal pack in the nasopharynx or by inserting a balloon catheter, inflating the balloon partially, and holding the balloon in place in the nasopharyngeal area (Fig. 52-3). This procedure is usually supplemented by anterior nasal packing. These patients must be hospitalized and

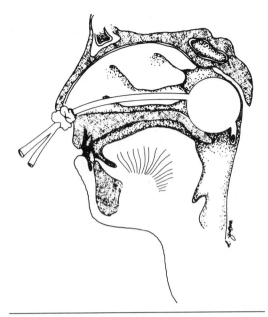

FIGURE 52-3   Control of posterior epistaxis with balloon catheter.

observed for hypoxia, and supplemental oxygen should be given. If bleeding persists despite adequate therapy, especially after the packing has been removed, *ligation of specific feeding vessels* for both anterior and posterior epistaxis may be necessary. Patients with recurrent nasal hemorrhage who have coagulopathies or friable blood vessels such as with leukemia or uremia usually are treated with absorbable gelatin sponge (Gelfoam) packs soaked in topical thrombin. If recurrent or severe epistaxis occurs in a young boy, especially if it is associated with nasal obstruction, an *angiofibroma* should be suspected.

- Most nosebleeds occur anteriorly and can be controlled by using a decongestant nasal spray and by compression of the anterior septum.

How Are Most Nasal Fractures Treated?

Most nasal fractures can be treated adequately by *closed reduction* with the patient under local anesthesia. Nasal trauma may be associated with a hematoma beneath the perichondrium of the nasal septum. This may result in a *nasal septal hematoma,* which should be incised and drained early before it becomes infected and produces a septal abscess. *Septal abscess* may be associated with necrosis of the septal cartilage, resulting in *septal perforation* and possibly collapsing deformities of the nose. *Cerebrospinal rhinorrhea*

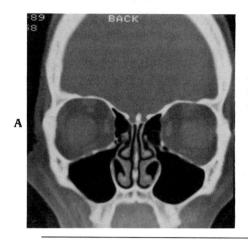 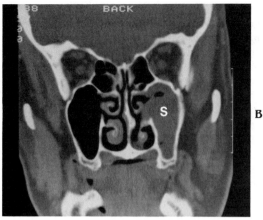

FIGURE 52-4   **A,** Normal CT scan of sinuses. **B,** CT scan demonstrating sinusitis (abnormal sinus = *S*).

should be suspected in any patient with watery discharge from the nose, especially after nasal trauma. This discharge usually will cease spontaneously; however, surgical therapy may be necessary if the cerebrospinal fluid rhinorrhea persists, especially if it is associated with complications such as meningitis.

What Area of the Nasal Vestibule Most Likely Will Be Infected?

Inflammation of the nasal vestibule may occur secondary to chronic dermatitis or from the trauma of picking or wiping the nose. Commonly folliculitis or a furuncle develops secondary to infection of the root of the hairs in the nasal vestibule. These infections can be quite painful and can be serious in patients with diabetes mellitus, even resulting in septic thrombosis of the cavernous sinus. Treatment consists of applying local antibiotic ointments and administering systemic antibiotics.

What Are Contributing Factors in Chronic Sinusitis?

Sinus infections may follow an acute upper respiratory infection, a cold, or allergic rhinitis or may result from exacerbation of a chronic recurrent sinus infection. Some cases are secondary to sudden changes in atmospheric pressure such as in flying or diving (barosinusitis). Frequently, multiple sinuses are involved in a single infection, but the infection may be limited to a single sinus. Patients usually complain of headache, facial pain, and nasal congestion and obstruction. There is usually a purulent nasal and postnasal discharge. Maxillary sinusitis may produce pain

in the teeth, and ethmoiditis frequently produces headaches in the periorbital area. X-ray films frequently reveal clouding of the involved sinuses. Treatment consists of administering oral nasal decongestants and systemic antibiotics and applying local heat and topical nasal decongestants. After the acute inflammation has subsided, maxillary sinus irrigation may be indicated for residual infected mucus that the sinus does not expel. In cases of chronic recurrent sinusitis, contributing factors may be allergic rhinitis, nasal polyps, altered immunologic status, and structural problems such as an enlarged turbinate or deviated nasal septum. The accurate anatomic diagnosis of chronic sinusitis has been greatly improved by use of the CT scan (Fig. 52-4). Surgery to promote drainage of the involved sinuses may be necessary and may involve the removal of polyps, septal surgery to relieve an obstructing nasal septum, or the creation of openings in the sinus. The precision of endoscopic sinus surgery has greatly improved the therapy of this common chronic disease.

- Excessive prolonged use of decongestant nasal spray may produce many symptoms suggestive of chronic sinusitis.

What Are the Indications for Tonsillectomy and Adenoidectomy?

In the past many children had their tonsils and adenoids removed, but today fewer tonsillectomies and adenoidectomies are performed because of more rigid criteria for surgical indications. ***Indications*** for tonsillectomy include recurrent tonsillitis, especially streptococcal infections, peritonsillar abscess, recurrent pyogenic cervical adenitis, persistent oral obstruction and dysphagia, and suspected tonsillar tumor. Indications for adenoidectomy include persistent nasal obstruction with mouth breathing and recurrent otitis that is especially unresponsive to the use of ear ventilation tubes. Combined tonsillectomy and adenoidectomy are indicated in patients with marked tonsillar and adenoidal hypertrophy with resultant cor pulmonale. Children who have *sleep apnea syndrome,* with excessive daytime sleepiness and poor school performance secondary to markedly enlarged tonsils and adenoids, frequently are helped by tonsillectomy and adenoidectomy. In adults the obstructive sleep apnea syndrome is treated by removal of enlarged tonsils and excessive tissue of the uvula and soft palate. This procedure may prevent obstruction of this area during sleep and frequently decreases snoring.

- Children have relatively larger tonsils than adults. Tonsils generally decrease in size until young adulthood. Adults who have hypertrophied tonsils and recurrent tonsillitis are more likely than a child to have recurrent infections on a long-term basis.

What Are the Factors Involved in Salivary Gland Infections?

Suppurative parotitis usually occurs in elderly, dehydrated patients. Pus can be expressed from the parotid duct as it enters the mouth. *Staphylococcus aureus* is the usual causative pathogen. Treatment consists of hydration and intravenous antibiotics. If parotitis is unresponsive to medical therapy, surgical drainage is necessary. Salivary gland infections (*sialadenitis*) may become recurrent. They may be secondary to scarring or stricture of the salivary gland ducts and may be associated with dilation of the ductal structures (*sialectasia*) and resultant stasis. Occasionally they are associated with lymphoepithelial disease (Sjögren's syndrome, Mikulicz's syndrome). The salivary ducts may become obstructed by *salivary stones (sialolithiasis).* These patients present with pain in the duct and glandular area, with distention of the involved gland and resultant infection. Stones occur in the submandibular salivary glands more frequently than in the parotids. Stones are often multiple and frequently can be removed intraorally. For chronic recurrent infections, removal of the submandibular or parotid gland may be necessary.

A *mass in the salivary gland* is suspect for neoplasm if it persists and does not disappear with appropriate therapy or if it enlarges. Most parotid gland tumors are benign. Tumors of the submaxillary gland or minor salivary glands of the oral mucosa are more likely to be malignant than are those of the parotid gland.

- A mass in the tail of the parotid gland may be confused for a superior cervical node.

What Symptoms Do Laryngeal Problems Produce?

A patient with a disorder of the larynx usually presents with changes in voice quality or breathing problems. In the newborn or small infant *laryngomalacia* may be present, which is characterized by inspiratory stridor more marked in the supine position but relieved in a prone position. The disorder is due to immature fibrocartilaginous development and inadequate support of the larynx, permitting the larynx to collapse on itself with inspiratory efforts. The disease is self-limiting and usually resolves spontaneously within 1 to 2 years. Children up to approximately 10 years of age may present with difficulty in breathing secondary either to *croup* or *epiglottiditis.* Laryngeal *papillomas* are benign, wartlike growths that can involve any part of the larynx and occur most commonly in children. They produce hoarseness and occasionally become large enough to produce airway obstruction. Usually they require multiple excisions and are characterized by their tendency to recur. They may be removed by using a microscope with a laser, which creates minimal vocal cord scarring.

What Benign Causes Produce Laryngeal Lesions in Adults?

Nodules of the vocal cords are thickened areas, which usually result from vocal abuse and frequently occur in singers. They may respond to voice rest and speech therapy if they are treated early, but persistent cases may require endoscopic removal, followed by speech rehabilitation. *Polyps* of the vocal cords are hypertrophied tissue on the cords. This hypertrophy may be secondary to chronic laryngitis, smoking, chronic vocal abuse, allergies, or chronic upper respiratory infections with postnasal drainage. The condition producing the polyps is treated, and frequently the polyps are removed by laryngoscopy. Diffuse thickening and edema of the vocal cords may produce deepening of the voice quality in patients with hypothyroidism. These patients usually respond quickly to appropriate thyroid-replacement medication and seldom require surgical intervention.

What Is the Most Common Risk Factor for Laryngeal Cancer?

Any patient with *hoarseness* lasting longer than 3 weeks should be examined by indirect laryngoscopy to rule out tumor of the larynx. *Dysplasias* of the vocal cords frequently have a plaquelike appearance and are usually secondary to overgrowth of the surface epithelium (hyperkeratosis). Often it is impossible by physical appearance to distinguish malignant degeneration of the vocal cords from simple dysplasias. In these patients direct endoscopic *biopsy* must be performed. Most cases of dysplasia and laryngeal cancer occur in patients who are excessive smokers. *Squamous cell carcinoma,* the most common malignant tumor of the larynx, may occur on the true vocal cords, the supraglottic or subglottic areas. Patients with *tumors on the true vocal cords* usually present early with hoarseness. *Lesions on the false cords,* or epiglottis, may cause only a sore throat or muffled voice quality. Patients frequently will present with both hoarseness from the primary laryngeal cancer and a mass in the neck secondary to involvement of lymph nodes with metastatic cancer. Depending on the stage of the tumor, treatment is irradiation alone or surgery alone, or both irradiation and surgery may be necessary. If surgery is necessary for these tumors, some cases are treated by partial removal of laryngeal structures, thus preserving laryngeal speech. Other cases require complete total laryngectomy, with resultant loss of normal laryngeal speech. Speech can be restored by using speech therapy to learn esophageal voice or by voice restoration surgery.

- The classic triad of a malignant tumor of the larynx is hoarseness, ipsilateral neck mass (cervical node metastasis), and referred pain in the ipsilateral ear.

What Type of Voice Quality Does Laryngeal Paralysis Produce?

Patients with vocal cord paralysis also present with hoarseness. Any lesion that involves the recurrent laryngeal nerve in its course along the vagus nerve from the brainstem through the neck and to the larynx can produce paralysis of the vocal cord. Patients usually have a *breathy, airy voice quality,* and they sometimes will *aspirate* food and saliva because of the incompetency of the glottic sphincter area of the true vocal cords. *Conditions that produce paralysis* include tumors at the base of the skull, lung tumors, thyroid tumors, esophageal lesions, tumors of the larynx, cardiac disease, mediastinal disease, and aortic aneurysms. If no cause is found, careful follow-up observation is necessary. If vocal cord function is not recovered spontaneously, the vocalization and sphincter functions of the true vocal cord can be improved by injection of Teflon paste into the paralyzed cord. It pushes the free margin of the paralyzed cord toward the midline and improves its opposition with the opposite functional vocal cord.

- In a significant number of cases the cause of vocal cord paralysis is idiopathic. Careful investigation of the route of the recurrent laryngeal nerve will provide the diagnosis of many cases.

BIBLIOGRAPHY

Baloh RW. Dizziness, Hearing Loss, and Tinnitus: The Essentials of Neurotology. Philadelphia, FA Davis, 1984.

Cummings CW, Fredrickson JM. Otolaryngology—Head and Neck Surgery, Vols 1-3. St. Louis, CV Mosby, 1986.

DeWeese DD, Saunders WH, Schuller DE, et al. Otolaryngology—Head and Neck Surgery. St. Louis, CV Mosby, 1988.

Gates GA. Current Therapy in Otolaryngology—Head and Neck Surgery, 4th ed. Toronto, Brian C Decker, 1990.

Lee KJ. Essential Otolaryngology, 4th ed. New York, Medical Examination Publishing, 1987.

Paparella MM, Shumrick DA, Gluckman JL, et al. Otolaryngology, Vols 1-3, 3rd ed. Philadelphia, WB Saunders, 1991.

Rice DH, Schaefer SD. Endoscopic Paranasal Sinus Surgery. New York, Raven Press, 1988.

Suen JY, Wetmore SJ. Emergencies in Otolaryngology. New York, Churchill Livingstone, 1986.

Thawley SE, Panje WR. Comprehensive Management of Head and Neck Tumors, Vols 1 and 2. Philadelphia, WB Saunders, 1987.

CHAPTER REVIEW
Questions

1. What are the causes of serous otitis media?
2. In what condition is determination of eardrum mobility especially important?
3. What are the results of tuning fork tests in an ear with conductive hearing loss?
4. If the nasopharynx and/or larynx cannot be examined by the indirect mirror examination, how can these areas be visualized?
5. What is the predisposing condition for external otitis?
6. What conditions can result from persistent serous otitis?
7. What is the most common surgical procedure for preventing recurrent otitis media and persistent serous otitis?
8. What is a cholesteatoma?
9. What is the most common hearing loss in elderly patients?
10. What is the most common method for preventing sensorineural hearing loss?
11. Which type of tinnitus is more common—subjective or objective?
12. What type of hearing loss is produced by serous otitis?
13. What condition should be ruled out in an adult with unilateral serous otitis?
14. What comprises the triad of symptoms in Ménière's disease?
15. What type of vertigo is more common—peripheral or central?
16. What are the characteristics of peripheral vertigo?
17. What is the most common type of peripheral facial paralysis?
18. What type of deformity can hematoma of the external ear produce?
19. What type of topical nasal medicine produces chronic rhinitis?
20. What conditions arouse suspicion of posterior choanal atresia?
21. What are nasal polyps, and if they occur in a child, what disease should be suspected?
22. What area of the nose most commonly bleeds?
23. What advances have helped in the diagnosis and treatment of chronic sinusitis?
24. What comprises the treatment for suppurative parotitis?
25. What must be ruled out in patients with persistent hoarseness?
26. What is the major risk factor for laryngeal cancer?
27. How is the gag reflex decreased in the oral exam?
28. How is mobility of the eardrum determined?
29. What are common causes of nasal stuffiness?
30. What are the predisposing factors for sinus infections?

Answers

1. Obstruction of the auditory tube, incomplete resolution of otitis media, allergic transudate in middle ear, and atmospheric pressure changes
2. Serous otitis in children
3. Bone conduction will be greater than air conduction; Weber test will lateralize to the ear with conductive hearing loss.
4. Use of a small flexible fiberoptic scope
5. Persistent moisture in the ear canal
6. Hearing loss and recurrent otitis media
7. Myringotomy with placement of ear ventilation tubes
8. Ingrowth of squamous epithelium into the middle ear and mastoid bone
9. Presbycusis, a type of neurosensory hearing loss that occurs from aging changes within the cochlea
10. Sound protection
11. Subjective
12. Conductive
13. Tumor of the nasopharynx
14. Episodic vertigo, fluctuating sensorineural hearing loss, tinnitus
15. Peripheral (in approximately 80% of cases)
16. Attacks are severe, paroxysmal, usually accompanied by nystagmus and nausea
17. Bell's palsy
18. Cauliflower ear deformity
19. Excessive use of decongestant nasal sprays produces rhinitis medicamentous.
20. Stridor in breathing and inability to pass catheter through nose
21. Nasal polyps are hypertrophy of the nasal-sinus mucosa. If they occur in a child, cystic fibrosis should be suspected.
22. Anterior septum
23. Sinus CT scans and endoscopic sinus surgery
24. Hydration, antibiotics, and drainage (if necessary)

25. Tumor of the larynx
26. Smoking
27. Avoid pushing on the tongue posterior to the circumvallate papillae.
28. By a pneumatic otoscope and tympanometry

29. Common cold, allergic rhinitis, excessive use of nasal spray
30. Upper respiratory infection, cold, allergic rhinitis, previous sinus infection

53 Basic Surgical Techniques

HOWARD S. NEARMAN
JERRY M. SHUCK

Achieving competence in basic surgical techniques requires a thorough knowledge of the related anatomy. The surgeon must gain experience under adequate supervision. What we present here, therefore, provides only a background and the rudiments necessary for the student of surgery. Not all of the techniques described here may be mastered by everyone. We have attempted, however, to describe basic techniques needed for good patient care.

INDUCING LOCAL ANESTHESIA

Local anesthetic agents may be used to ensure patient comfort while performing minor invasive procedures. The extent of the area anesthetized and the duration of the block depend on the type of agent, its concentration, and the total volume injected. Table 53-1 lists common agents used.

To produce local anesthesia, a small (no. 25 or 26) needle is used to raise an intradermal wheal, extending the intracutaneous injection linearly or circumferentially, depending on the need (Fig. 53-1). The anesthetic solution should be injected ahead of the advancing needle to minimize patient discomfort. It is important to deliver the solution intradermally to achieve satisfactory epidermal anesthesia. Further anesthetic can be injected subcutaneously if necessary.

Figures redrawn from Shuck J, Nearman H. In Davis J, et al. Clinical Surgery. St Louis, CV Mosby, 1987.

CENTRAL LINES

Central venous access may be needed to administer solutions or medications that cannot be given through a peripheral line (hyperalimentation, vasopressors, chemotherapy), deliver fluids when peripheral access is difficult or insufficient (large bore catheters for rapid fluid resuscitation), or monitor central venous pressure.

Access to the central venous system may be obtained through the basilic vein in the arm, the internal jugular vein, or the subclavian vein. The choice among these approaches may be highly subjective and based on personal experience. However, each site has certain advantages and disadvantages, and the clinician should be familiar with all three approaches.

Peripheral central access may be used when the potential complications of the internal jugular or subclavian approaches must be avoided. Trauma victims in hemorrhagic shock may have collapsed central veins, and a peripheral cutdown may be the most reliable way to obtain rapid venous access. Since bleeding is more easily controlled, it is also the preferred route for patients with a coagulopathy. Central catheters inserted via peripheral sites can cause axillary vein thrombosis and have a high rate of infection; therefore their use should be limited to 48 to 72 hours if possible.

The subclavian approach provides fast access to the central venous system and is thus the preferred route in emergency situations. In addition,

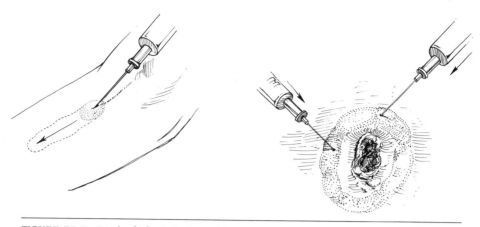

FIGURE 53-1 Methods for injection of local anesthetic solution.

TABLE 53-1 Doses of Local Anesthetics for Infiltration and Nerve Blocks

Drug	Concentration (%)	Duration	Maximum Dose
Bupivacaine (Marcaine)	0.5	5-7 hr	200 mg
Lidocaine (Xylocaine)	1-2	1-2 hr	500 mg
Mepivacaine (Carbocaine)	1-2	1-2 hr	500 mg
Procaine (Novocain)	2-4	½ hr	1000 mg
Tetracaine (Pontocaine)	0.1-0.25	2-3 hr	75 mg

subclavian lines have a low incidence of sepsis and are easy to maintain and comfortable for the patient, making them preferable for the administration of total parenteral nutrition. Although the rate of successful cannulation of the subclavian vein is high in experienced hands, the incidence of serious complications such as pneumothorax and arterial laceration is also significant.

Alternatively, the internal jugular vein is safer to access, although the success rate may not be as high. Carotid artery puncture remains the main complication.

Strict sterile technique should be maintained for elective line placement, regardless of the approach selected. The site is prepared and draped, and the operator should don cap, mask, gown, and sterile gloves. Local anesthesia should be used for initiation of the procedure, as well as for suturing the catheter in place. Lines inserted in emergency situations under suboptimal sterile conditions should be replaced within 24 hours.

Peripheral Central Venous Line

Catheter Length
Premeasured from the site of insertion to the sternum

The median or basilic veins should be used because their course toward the subclavian vein is usually direct and presents no anatomic obstruction to passage of a catheter. If the upper arm is unsuitable, then the cephalic vein in the deltopectoral groove may be chosen (Fig. 53-2).

With the arm fully extended, a tourniquet is applied to the upper arm. Percutaneous insertion may proceed if an appropriately sized vein is identified. The selected site is prepared and draped, and local anesthetic is infiltrated. A needle-clad catheter is used to cannulate the vein; blood return along the length of the catheter indicates successful placement. With the needle held fixed in place with one hand, the catheter is passed through the needle into the vein with the other (Fig. 53-3). The tourniquet is then released, the needle withdrawn, and the catheter fixed in place.

If the percutaneous technique proves unsuccessful, peripheral central venous catheterization should proceed by direct venous cutdown. Using a no. 15 scalpel, a 3 to 4 cm incision is made transverse to the axis of the vein. The underlying tissue is carefully dissected in a direction parallel to the course of the vein to minimize risk of tearing until the structure is identified. About 4 cm of the vein is exposed, and 3-0 sutures are placed distally and proximately to isolate the segment (Fig. 53-4). The distal suture is then tied to occlude venous flow. With traction on the distal tie, the vein is incised longitudinally with a no. 11 scalpel blade. The catheter is passed through a separate stab wound just below the incision and inserted directly through the venotomy site (Fig. 53-5). With the catheter in satisfactory position, the proximal suture is gently tied and the incision closed.

Subclavian Line

Catheter Lengths

Right 15-17 cm
Left   18-20 cm

The patient is placed in the Trendelenburg position to distend the central veins and lessen the risk of air embolism during catheter introduction. A rolled towel is placed between the shoulder blades to elevate the vein more anteriorly, and the patient's head is turned toward the opposite side (Fig. 53-6). A wide sterile preparation is used, including the shoulder, neck, and upper chest. After infiltrating the skin with local anesthetic, a 22-gauge needle is used to carry anesthetic through the subcutaneous tissue and into the periosteum of the inferior portion of the clav-

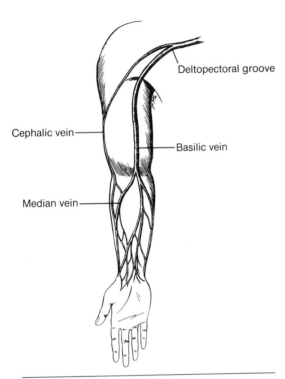

FIGURE 53-2 Anatomy of upper extremity veins used for central venous access.

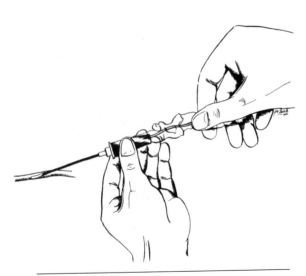

FIGURE 53-3 Percutaneous peripheral central venous catheter insertion.

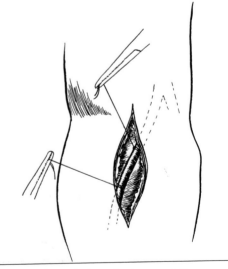

FIGURE 53-4 Isolation of vein segment.

icle. The bevel of the needle is aligned with the markings on the syringe so that the orientation of the bevel can be readily ascertained. The insertion site is approximately 2 cm inferior and lateral to the angle where the first rib angles beneath the clavicle. The needle is advanced, bevel up, parallel to the chest wall, staying as close as possible to the underside of the clavicle, aiming just above the sternal notch. Gentle negative pressure is maintained on the syringe until blood is aspirated. At that point the needle is advanced another 0.5 cm and the syringe rotated 180 degrees so the bevel is directed downward. After checking again for proper blood return, the syringe is removed and a gloved hand placed over the needle hub. Using the Seldinger technique, a flexible guidewire is inserted through the needle into a central position. The needle is removed completely, and the catheter is inserted into the vein over the guidewire. The guidewire is then withdrawn and the catheter sutured in place. Free flow of blood should be confirmed by aspiration before starting infusion of fluids.

Internal Jugular Line

Catheter Lengths
Right 15-17 cm
Left   18-20 cm

Anterior Approach. This is also referred to as "the top of the triangle" approach and is probably the safest method of central venous catheterization. After placing the patient in the Tren-

delenburg position, the neck is extended and the head turned toward the opposite side. A wide sterile preparation of the neck and upper chest should be done. The needle entrance site is located at the apex of the triangle formed by the clavicle at the base and the sternal and clavicular heads of the sternocleidomastoid muscle. Identification may be made easier if the patient is able to lift the head against resistance, outlining the musculature. Local anesthetic is infiltrated and a 22-gauge "finder" needle is initially used to identify the location of the internal jugular vein. This is done to minimize the chance of inadvertent puncture of the carotid artery with a large-bore needle. The needle is attached to a 3 or 5 ml syringe and is inserted at a 30-degree angle to the skin, aiming at the ipsilateral nipple (Fig. 53-7). Once venous blood is obtained, the location is noted by both direction and depth of penetration of the needle. The larger-bore needle is then passed along the same line as the "finder," maintaining the bevel upward. When the internal jugular vein is identified, the Seldinger technique is used as described above to insert the catheter.

Posterior Approach. In this approach, the site of introduction of the needle is just inferior to the junction of the external jugular vein and the posterior border of the clavicular head of the sternocleidomastoid muscle. Again, a 22-gauge needle should be used to identify the vein. The needle is directed toward the sternal notch, keeping the syringe parallel to the coronal plane of the patient, as shown in Fig. 53-8. The technique is

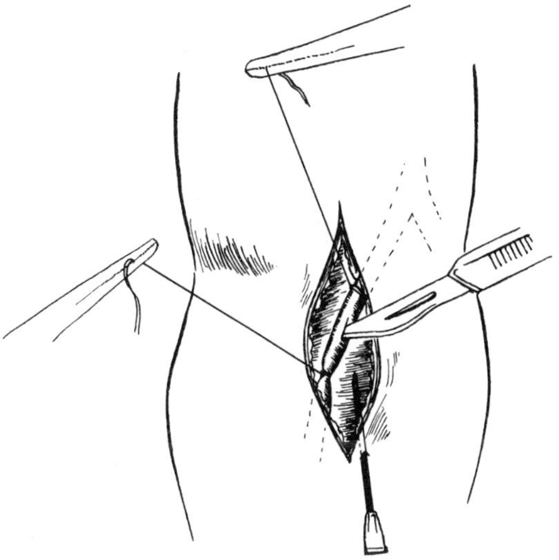

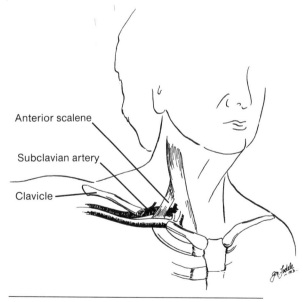

Anterior scalene

Subclavian artery

Clavicle

FIGURE 53-5   Incision of vein for catheter insertion.

FIGURE 53-6   Position for subclavian vein cannulation.

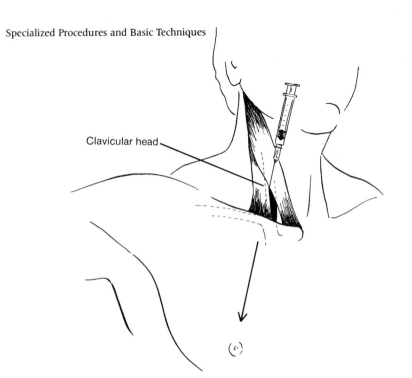

Clavicular head

(c)

FIGURE 53-7   Anterior approach to internal jugular vein.

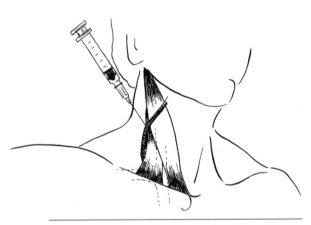

FIGURE 53-8   Posterior approach to internal jugular vein.

otherwise the same as just outlined for the anterior approach.

ARTERIAL LINES

Indwelling arterial lines allow continuous accurate blood pressure monitoring and easy sampling of arterial blood. Several different sites may be used, depending on the clinical circumstances. The radial artery is the most frequently used site and has the least potential for complications. An Allen test may be used to assess the collateral circulation, although a satisfactory result is still no guarantee against distal ischemia. Both radial and ulnar arteries are simultaneously occluded with the thumbs, and the patient is asked to open and close the hand several times until it blanches (Fig. 53-9). With the hand open, compression of the ulnar artery is released and the hand checked for return of color. If the entire hand does not regain color within 7 seconds, collateral circulation through the palmar arch may be inadequate, and proceeding with radial artery cannulation is unsafe.

The dorsalis pedis artery may also be used for arterial cannulation. Collateral circulation may be checked in a manner similar to that described for the radial artery. The dorsalis pedis and posterior tibial arteries are compressed, the posterior tibial artery is then released, and the great toe checked for return of color.

Central placement of an arterial catheter may be desirable for monitoring the patient in severe shock, or when peripheral sites are unobtainable. Either the femoral or axillary arteries are readily accessible and may be used for this purpose. The brachial artery is used as a last resort, since it carries with it the highest incidence of complications.

Arterial catheterization requires careful sterile

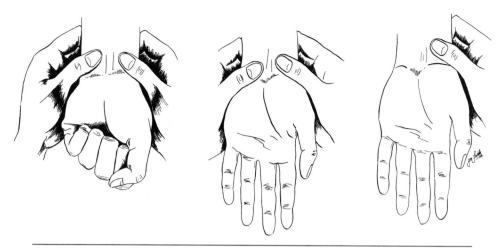

FIGURE 53-9   Allen test to evaluate collateral circulation.

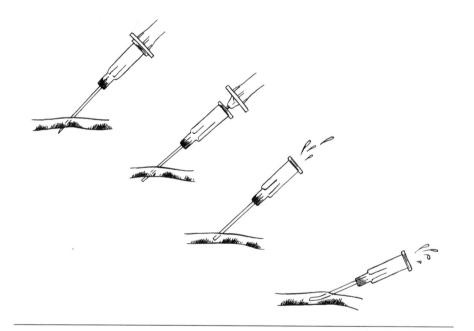

FIGURE 53-10   Through-and-back technique for arterial cannulation.

preparation and draping of the indicated site. A mask and gloves are worn, and a local anesthetic is used for both insertion and suturing of the catheter.

For peripheral arterial cannulation, the selected extremity should be relatively immobilized distally. For radial artery catheterization, the hand and lower arm are taped to an armboard and a roll placed between the board and the dorsiflexed wrist. Similarly, the foot may be plantarflexed, and taped down to a short board.

A 20-gauge catheter-clad needle is inserted at a 45-degree angle to the skin and advanced parallel to the course of the vessel until arterial blood flashes back into the hub. At this point, the artery is transfixed by advancing the needle-catheter assembly another 1 cm or so until the blood return ceases. The needle is removed, leaving the catheter in place. The catheter is then slowly pulled back until arterial flow is obtained, at which point the catheter is quickly advanced up into the artery (Fig. 53-10).

Alternatively, the catheter-clad needle may be inserted by first puncturing the proximal wall of the artery, as described above, obtaining arterial blood flashback. The catheter is then threaded over the needle and advanced up into the vessel. This technique does not puncture the back wall of the artery as does the above technique; however, it is technically more difficult to perform successfully.

Central catheter insertion requires use of the Seldinger technique. A Potts-Cournaud needle is inserted percutaneously into the artery. Following identification of the intended vessel, a guidewire is threaded centrally and the needle removed. A 3.0 or 4.0 French catheter is then inserted into the artery over the guidewire and the guidewire removed.

After the catheter is hooked up to pressure tubing and checked for aspiration of arterial blood, the system is flushed and the catheter secured to the skin.

PULMONARY ARTERY BALLOON FLOTATION CATHETER

The pulmonary artery balloon flotation, or Swan-Ganz, catheter is a more advanced form of hemodynamic monitoring than the central venous pressure determination. A pulmonary artery (PA) catheter allows measurement of left-sided as well as right-sided filling pressures, cardiac output, and continuous mixed venous oximetry. The PA catheter may be inserted through any central venous site; however, the right internal jugular vein is the preferred route, because it presents a straight course to the right side of the heart.

The patient should be attached to continuous electrocardiographic (ECG) monitoring before insertion of the PA catheter. Central venous access is obtained via one of the techniques described previously. An 8.5 or 9.0 French sheath-dilator assembly is introduced into the vein via the Seldinger technique, and the dilator is removed. A sideport/hemostasis valve is attached to the dilator and the assembly sewn in place. Attention is then turned toward sterile preparation of the PA catheter. The distal and proximal lumens are flushed with heparinized saline and the distal lumen hooked up to a pressure transducer. The balloon is inflated with 1.5 cc of air and observed for leaks. Finally, the catheter is threaded through the catheter contamination shield, which is then pulled back to a proximal position along the catheter.

While maintaining sterile technique, the catheter is inserted through the hemostatic valve into the vein, advancing it about 20 cm. At this point, a central venous pressure tracing should be noted on the monitor, and the balloon carefully inflated. The catheter may then be advanced through the right side of the heart while observing the pressure tracing and ECG (Fig. 53-11). The catheter usually reaches a wedge position at approximately 50 cm from the right internal jugular or subclavian vein, 55 cm from the left internal jugular or subclavian vein, and 70 cm from the femoral vein. On reaching the wedge position, the balloon is deflated and a pulmonary artery tracing should promptly return. The catheter contamination shield is advanced distally

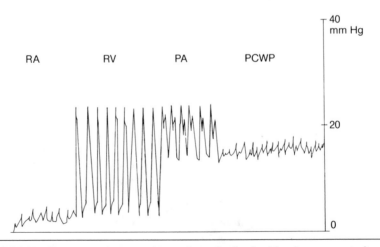

FIGURE 53-11 Representative pressure tracings obtained with advancement of pulmonary artery catheter. **RA** = right atrium; **RV** = right ventricle; **PA** = pulmonary artery; **PCWP** = pulmonary capillary wedge pressure.

and locked onto the hemostatic valve, with care not to move the catheter itself. A chest x-ray evaluation must be performed to confirm that the catheter is in the correct position and that no complications of insertion have occurred.

ENDOTRACHEAL INTUBATION

Airway control is crucial in the management of the critically ill or injured patient. Endotracheal intubation is usually the best route for establishing emergency airway access; however, hypoxic patients must have their lungs adequately ventilated with mask and bag before intubation is attempted. Orotracheal intubation is the easiest and quickest method of endotracheal intubation and is therefore preferred when rapid intubation is required. Nasotracheal intubation is indicated when direct laryngoscopy is not possible, such as in cervical spinal injury or severe temporomandibular disease. For patients with facial trauma or coagulopathy nasal intubation should not be attempted.

Orotracheal Intubation

The patient's head is placed in the sniffing position with the neck flexed, occiput elevated, and head tilted slightly backward (Fig. 53-12). If time allows, topical anesthetic may be used to anesthetize the tongue and posterior pharynx of the awake patient. Sedatives and/or narcotics may also be used to help achieve optimal intubating conditions if clinical circumstances dictate.

All equipment should be checked for proper functioning. A mask-bag unit is attached to an oxygen source, and a Yankauer tip is connected to suction. An appropriately sized endotracheal tube is selected (Table 53-2), and the balloon cuff is checked. A malleable stylet may be placed within the tube, making sure the tip of the stylet does not protrude beyond the end of the tube.

The patient is ventilated with 100% oxygen for 2 to 3 minutes, and the mouth opened. The laryngoscope is held in the left hand, and the blade inserted gradually down into the hypopharynx. The tip of a curved blade is advanced into the groove between the base of the tongue and the epiglottis, while the tip of a straight blade is placed beyond the epiglottis (Figs. 53-13 and 53-14). In either case, the vocal cords are then exposed by lifting the laryngoscope upward and

TABLE 53-2   Endotracheal Tube Sizes

Patient	Tube Diameter
Adult male	8.0-8.5 mm
Adult female	7.5-8.0 mm
Neonate	3.5 mm
Premature infant	2.5 mm
Children	Age 5 years: 5.5 mm
	Each 2 years older: 0.5 mm increase
	Each 2 years younger: 0.5 mm decrease

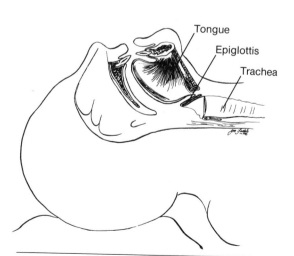

FIGURE 53-12   Sniffing position for orotracheal intubation.

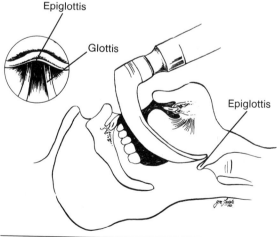

FIGURE 53-13   Exposure of the vocal cords—curved blade.

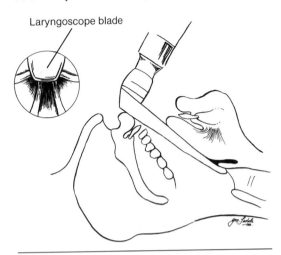

Laryngoscope blade

FIGURE 53-14   Exposure of the vocal cords—straight blade.

Intubation of the trachea may be accomplished using a blind technique, or under direct visualization. In the blind approach in a spontaneously breathing patient, the tube is advanced slowly while listening for breath sounds through its end. As the tube nears the glottic opening, the sounds increase in intensity. The tube is then pushed through the cords during inspiration. Sudden cessation of breath sounds implies that the tube has possibly entered the esophagus; the tube is withdrawn back into the pharynx, and another attempt made. If direct visualization is used, a laryngoscope is inserted in the manner described. The tip of the endotracheal tube is visualized and is grasped either above or below the balloon with a Magill forceps. The tube is then advanced and guided directly through the cords into the trachea. Once the trachea is successfully intubated, the cuff is inflated and breath sounds are checked, as described above.

forward. The endotracheal tube is then gently inserted to a depth at which the tip lies approximately 4 cm below the level of the cords. After the laryngoscope and the stylet are removed, the cuff of the tube is inflated until no air leak occurs during manual bagging, and the tube is taped or tied in place. Proper placement of the tube may be evaluated by listening for equal breath sounds on both sides of the chest as well as noting the absence of breath sounds over the gastric area. A chest x-ray film should be taken to confirm the position.

Nasotracheal Intubation

All the equipment mentioned for orotracheal intubation, except for the stylet, should be made ready. The patient should be placed in a semi-sitting position, with the head neutral; if this is not possible, the patient should be supine with the neck slightly flexed. If cervical injury is suspected, nasotracheal intubation must be undertaken without manipulation of the neck. In a nonemergent situation the selected nostril should be prepared with either cocaine or cetacaine and phenylephrine to produce anesthesia and decrease mucosal swelling. The tube is inserted with the bevel pointed toward the septum, then gently advanced posteriorly until the nasopharynx is reached. If the left nostril is used, the tube should be rotated 180 degrees at this point so that its curvature conforms to the shape of the airway.

CRICOTHYROTOMY

There may be occasions when emergency airway access is needed and endotracheal intubation cannot be accomplished or is contraindicated. In such cases, cricothyrotomy is the procedure of choice.

The patient should be supine, with the neck hyperextended and a rolled towel under the shoulders. The neck is prepared and draped, and the operator dons mask, cap, gown, and sterile gloves. The cricothyroid membrane, which lies between the thyroid and cricoid cartilages, is identified (Fig. 53-15), and, if time permits, local anesthetic is infiltrated. A 2 cm midline transverse incision is made with a no. 11 blade through skin and membrane. A clamp or dilator is then inserted into the trachea and spread. The tracheostomy tube is placed into the trachea, directing it caudally. After removing the instrument, the cuff on the tracheostomy tube is inflated, and breath sounds are checked bilaterally. The tube is then secured by suturing it to the skin, or by placing umbilical tapes through the slots in either wing of the tube and tying them around the patient's neck.

FIBEROPTIC BRONCHOSCOPY

The flexible fiberoptic bronchoscope is a valuable tool for diagnostic evaluation and therapeutic management of airway problems. In a nonintubated patient, fiberoptic bronchoscopy may be performed by either the transoral or transnasal

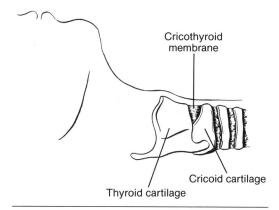

FIGURE 53-15 Landmarks for identification of cricothyroid membrane.

approach. The patient should be sitting, and aerosolized lidocaine or cetacaine should be sprayed into the posterior pharynx and upper airway. For the transnasal route, the more-patent nostril is anesthetized with cocaine or cetacaine and phenylephrine; for the transoral route the tongue is also sprayed with topical anesthetic. The bronchoscope is lubricated and passed either through the nose or a Guedel oral airway down into the tracheobronchial tree.

The supine position is usually used in an intubated patient. The endotracheal tube must be at least 8 mm in internal diameter to admit the standard adult bronchoscope and still have room enough to allow effective ventilation. A swivel adaptor with a rubber bronchoscope cap is inserted between the endotracheal tube and the ventilator tube. Lidocaine solution is injected down the endotracheal tube; the bronchoscope is lubricated and then inserted through the port of the adaptor. Additional lidocaine may be needed during the bronchoscopic procedure to keep the airway anesthetized and prevent the cough reflex.

FOLEY CATHETER

Male Patients. The patient should be supine with his legs slightly apart. Sterile gloves are worn. The penis is cleansed and a sterile drape applied around the shaft. The foreskin is retracted and the urethral meatus carefully washed. After thoroughly lubricating the tip of the Foley catheter, the penis is gently stretched at a right angle to the body. The catheter is inserted with constant gentle pressure the entire length

up to the balloon sidearm. If no urine return is obtained, the catheter is injected with 25 to 50 ml of sterile saline. Free return of fluid confirms catheter position in the bladder. The balloon is then inflated with the proper amount of sterile water, and the catheter is slowly withdrawn until the balloon is seated against the bladder neck. The catheter is then attached to a closed sterile drainage system and fixed to the patient's leg.

Female Patients. The patient should be supine with her knees and hips flexed and legs abducted. Sterile gloves are worn. The labia and urethral orifices are prepared and draped. The labia are separated, and the lubricated catheter is gently passed through the urethral meatus approximately 10 cm up into the bladder. The catheter position is confirmed as described in the preceding section, and the balloon is inflated. The catheter is connected to a closed sterile drainage system, and fixed to the leg.

PERICARDIOCENTESIS

Aspiration of fluid from the pericardial space is performed for diagnostic purposes and for relieving cardiac tamponade. A mask, cap, gown, and sterile gloves are worn, and the patient's lower chest and abdomen are prepared and draped. The patient is positioned with the upper body elevated at a 20- to 30-degree angle, allowing the heart to drop away from the chest wall.

After infiltrating with local anesthetic, a pericardiocentesis needle is attached to a 10 ml syringe and is inserted into the skin just below the xiphoid. Lead V of a 12-lead ECG is connected to the needle with a sterile alligator clip; the needle assembly is passed beneath the left costal arch and slowly advanced toward the suprasternal notch, making an angle of 30 to 45 degrees to the skin (Fig. 53-16).

The ECG should be monitored as the needle assembly is slowly advanced. A sudden "give" may be felt as the pericardium is entered, and fluid should be aspirated. If PR or ST segment elevation is noted on the ECG, epicardial contact may be present and the needle should be withdrawn slightly and repositioned. After the appropriate amount of pericardial fluid is obtained, the needle assembly is removed and a dressing applied.

NASOGASTRIC TUBE

With the patient in a sitting position, a well-lubricated nasogastric tube is placed into the

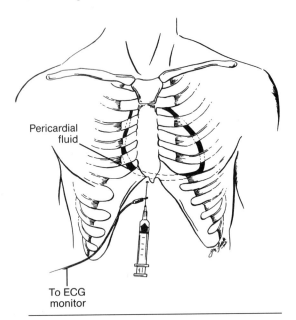

Pericardial fluid

To ECG monitor

FIGURE 53-16   Subxiphoid approach to pericardiocentesis.

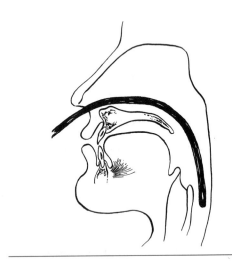

FIGURE 53-17   Nasogastric tube directed parallel to the palate.

nose, being careful to assess which is the more patent nostril. The tube should not be aimed upward, but rather kept parallel to the palate. This allows the tube to follow the nasal canal most directly to the posterior choanae (Fig. 53-17). When the tube reaches the nasopharynx, the patient should be asked to swallow continuously. Sips of water may be offered if the patient is able to cooperate and the risk of aspiration low.

The tube is slowly advanced until the second black mark on the tube is at the nose, corresponding to approximately 55 cm (the distance from the dentate line to the esophagogastric junction is about 40 cm). The tube is then taped in place.

If the patient coughs violently or experiences respiratory distress during placement attempts, it is likely that the trachea has been intubated and the tube should immediately be removed. Placement can be checked by rapidly instilling 10 to 20 cc of air into the lumen while listening for gurgling over the stomach area with a stethoscope. Aspiration of at least 50 ml of bile-stained fluid from the lumen is also good evidence of correct tube position. If any doubt exists concerning tube placement, an x-ray film using portable equipment will confirm it. In addition, an x-ray evaluation is essential if any fluids or medications are to be administered via the tube.

SENGSTAKEN-BLAKEMORE TUBE

The Sengstaken-Blakemore tube is used to control documented upper gastrointestinal bleeding from gastric or esophageal varices. The patient should be in a sitting position; if this is not possible because the patient is in shock, the supine position with slight head elevation may be used. The balloons should be checked for proper functioning and the tube generously lubricated. The tube may be inserted either through the mouth or the nose. It is advanced slowly beyond 50 cm, at which point 50 cc of air is injected into the gastric balloon to confirm placement by auscultation. Because it is imperative that the gastric balloon be well within the stomach before being fully inflated, a confirming abdominal x-ray film may be obtained.

With the tube in satisfactory position, the gastric balloon is slowly inflated by injecting an additional 200 to 250 cc of air. The balloon lumen is clamped, and the tube is withdrawn until resistance is felt, indicating that the balloon has been seated up against the esophagogastric junction. A foam cube is placed around the tube and against the nose, and the tube is taped to maintain traction.

If the bleeding is not controlled by this maneuver, it may be necessary to inflate the esophageal balloon. A Y connector is attached to the esophageal balloon lumen, with one end connected to a syringe, the other to a manometer. The esophageal balloon is then inflated to 30 to 40 mm Hg, and the lumen is clamped (Fig. 53-18). In either case, a nasogastric tube must be

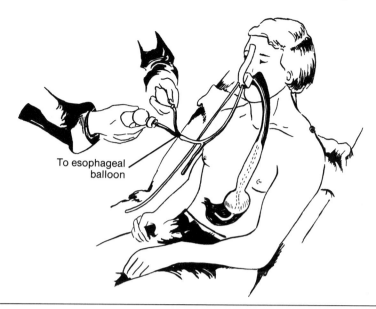

To esophageal
balloon

FIGURE 53-18   Sengstaken-Blakemore tube—inflation of esophageal balloon.

inserted into the esophagus above the inflated balloon to drain secretions and lessen the risk of aspiration. When the bleeding is controlled, the esophageal balloon may be deflated; the patient should be observed for 24 hours. The gastric balloon may then be deflated if no further bleeding occurs, and the Sengstaken-Blakemore tube left in place another 24 hours while the patient is monitored for evidence of bleeding.

ABDOMINAL TAP AND LAVAGE

Indications for peritoneal lavage continue to evolve. As with any invasive diagnostic procedure, some thought should be given to indications. If criteria are met for emergency operation in a patient with traumatic injuries, a lavage would be superfluous. However, if one determines that if the lavage yields negative results the patient will not be operated on immediately, then the diagnostic study is very valuable.

There are compelling arguments regarding penetrating abdominal trauma that suggest that the changing physical picture on examination of the patient and close observation obviate the need for a lavage. Most people agree that lavage is most useful in blunt abdominal injury.

Debate continues whether open (via cutdown in the midline with the patient under anesthesia) or percutaneous trochar is the best method to introduce the lavage catheter. In either case, a no. 11 blade is used to make a small incision 3 to 4 cm below the umbilicus after sterile preparation. In pregnant patients or in patients with expanding hematomas from pelvic fracture, this procedure can be performed above the umbilicus and should be done using the open technique. A stylet or trochar can then be inserted gently at a 45-degree angle heading toward a point below the sacral promontory. The cut-down method is performed in this same site using a small incision carried down through the midline fascia. The peritoneum is opened under direct vision through a purse string. A dialysis catheter is inserted using either a special trochar or under direct visualization (Fig. 53-19). Aspiration of free-flowing blood in excess of 10 ml precludes the need for lavage. Otherwise, a liter of Ringer's lactate is allowed to run into the peritoneal cavity by gravity.

Gentle abdominal movement and deep breathing will distribute the fluid, and siphon retrieval is recommended. As much fluid as possible is removed and examined for gross blood (which indicates a positive result) or a pink color requiring microscopic and quantitative counts of red blood cells, white blood cells, debris, enzymes, etc. There is little agreement about what is "positive," mandating exploration. Various authors state that anywhere between 1000 and 100,000 cells are used as the criterion. Generally accepted positive criteria include 50,000 red cells, 500 white cells, and any evidence of bile, amylase, cellulose fragments, or fecal material.

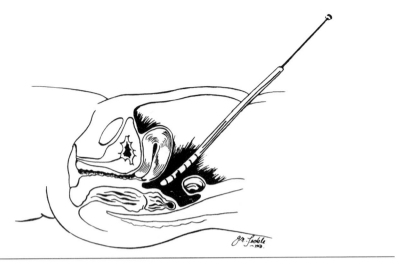

FIGURE 53-19   Insertion of dialysis catheter into peritoneum.

THORACENTESIS AND CHEST TUBES

Sampling and removing pleural collections can be diagnostic or therapeutic. Thoracentesis is primarily diagnostic. The relief of tension pneumothorax can occasionally be lifesaving. Sampling fluids may help the clinician differentiate transudates from purulent exudates, hemorrhage, malignancy, or lymphatic fluid. Removal of a large quantity of fluid may allow lung expansion and improve ventilation. In fact, in a posttraumatic situation, the early complete emptying of the pleural cavity may reduce the incidence of empyema and fibrothorax.

Chest tubes are inserted for a number of important indications. The treatment of pneumothorax after injury or diagnostic procedures generally requires a tube. For small pneumothoraces, the use of a percutaneous catheter can also be helpful. Tension pneumothoraces may require more than one chest tube. If this condition is suspected, the chest tube should be inserted before confirmation by chest x-ray evaluation. Occasionally a chest tube is necessary when prolonged ventilation is required in the treatment of pulmonary contusion, particularly when positive end-expiratory pressure (PEEP) may be required.

The safest and fastest site for tube insertion is the second intercostal space in the midclavicular line. This is sometimes necessary after injury when tension pneumothorax or hemopneumothorax is suspected. Ideally, the tube should be placed in the most dependent portion of the pleural cavity. The seventh intercostal space is recommended, in the posterior axillary line. If

the patient can tolerate it, the sitting position may be used for needle or tube insertion, allowing ready access to the posterior axillary area; otherwise, the patient is placed supine.

For inserting all needles and chest tubes, a surgical field with appropriate preparation, aseptic technique, and use of gloves and mask is mandatory. After the skin is infiltrated with local anesthetic, a longer needle is used to inject anesthetic down through all layers to the pleura itself. A thoracentesis needle is inserted after a three-way stopcock and appropriate tubing has been connected. Once fluid is aspirated, a Kelly clamp can be placed on the needle so that it will hold its position (Fig. 53-20). Using the stopcock, large volumes of fluid can be removed and allowed to run into a sterile container for diagnostic studies. The needle is removed after deep aspiration and a small bandage is placed over the hole.

For chest tube insertion, a wide area is infiltrated with local anesthetic, and an incision is made parallel to the rib. It is important to stay along the upper border of the rib below when going through the interspace, because the neurovascular bundle courses just below the rib. A 2 cm transverse incision is taken through all layers of the intercostal space. Once the knife enters the pleura, it becomes apparent with a short sucking sound being heard. A Kelly clamp can then be inserted to spread the wound.

Before placing the tube, the surgeon may insert an exploring finger, particularly when the site of insertion is low on the chest wall. This prevents injury to the diaphragm. In addition, if there was no free flow of fluid when the needle was inserted, it is important to know whether

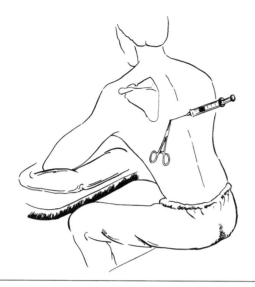

FIGURE 53-20   Thoracentesis in seated patient.

pleural adhesions are directly under the chest tube site if lung injury is to be avoided.

The tube should be clamped so that once it is in place, a sucking wound does not develop before connection to water seal or suction. The connecting tubing is then directed to either a simple water seal bottle or to one of the more elaborate suction-collection devices. At this point, the wound should be closed snugly around the chest tube. The suture should close

the wound and then be tied around the tube with several knots. A small dry, sterile dressing is placed.

Closed water-seal suction is adequate for most clinical situations. However, currently there are many modified versions of the classic three-bottle suction that are plastic, disposable, and allow easy measurement of effluent.

The chest tube should remain in place only as long as it is performing an important function. Generally if there has been no loss of air, fluid, or blood of any measurable amount for 24 hours, the tube is removed. The longer it remains, the greater the risk of infection. If pneumothorax or hemothorax persists but the tube is no longer draining, it should be removed and another tube inserted. The procedure should be explained carefully to the patient so that the patient can cooperate and not be startled by the brief discomfort from chest tube removal. Aseptic technique should be employed when removing the chest tube. The dressing is removed, and the suture attached to the tube is cut. The petrolatum gauze underneath the dressing should be held in the left hand and placed against the skin so that it will stack over the wound when the tube is withdrawn. The patient should be allowed to take several deep breaths; after a complete exhalation the tube is quickly slid out. A chest x-ray film is taken to be sure that a pneumothorax did not occur during the removal of the chest tube. This dressing should not be changed for at least 48 hours so that the wound can seal.

PITFALLS AND COMMON MYTHS

- The tip of the central venous catheter should **not** be pushing up against the lateral wall of the superior vena cava or positioned within the atrium, because the repetitive pulsation associated with myocardial contraction may cause perforation.
- Care must be taken every time the balloon on the pulmonary artery catheter is inflated to obtain a wedge pressure. The balloon should be inflated slowly, using only as much volume as is necessary to obtain a wedge tracing. *Pulmonary artery rupture is a potentially fatal complication* that is more common in patients with pulmonary artery hypertension.
- An air leak associated with an endotracheal tube is not always the result of a damaged or underinflated balloon cuff. If the tube is im-

properly positioned too high in the trachea, the balloon may lie between the vocal cords. In this case, further inflation of the cuff will not stop the leak, and may cause tube dislodgement or cord damage. The balloon should be deflated and the tube carefully pushed a few centimeters further down into the trachea, checking for breath sounds afterward.
- Patients with chest tubes are often transported to and from the operating room, radiology department, and/or the intensive care unit. It is vitally important to pay careful attention to all components of the chest tube system during transport to prevent disconnection and minimize the risk of developing tension pneumothorax.

BIBLIOGRAPHY

Davis J. Technical Skills in Patient Care. In Shuck JM, Nearman HS. Clinical Surgery. St Louis, CV Mosby, 1987.

May HL. Emergency Medical Procedures. New York, John Wiley & Sons, 1992.

Norwood S, Ruby A, et al. Catheter-related infections and associated septicemia. Chest 99:968, 1991.

Root HD, Hauser CW, McKinley CR, et al. Diagnostic peritoneal lavage. Surgery 57:633, 1965.

Suratt PM, Gibson RS. Manual of Medical Procedures. St Louis, CV Mosby, 1982.

Swan HJC, Ganz W. Use of balloon flotation catheters in critically ill patients. Surg Clin North Am 55:501, 1975.

Vander Salm TJ, Cutler BS, Wheeler HB. Atlas of Bedside Procedures. Boston, Little, Brown & Co, 1979.

CHAPTER REVIEW
Questions

1. Nasotracheal intubation is the procedure of choice in patients who:
   a. Require rapid intubation
   b. Have a severe coagulopathy
   c. Suffer cervical spinal injury
   d. Receive facial trauma
   e. Need a large tube for suctioning pulmonary secretions
2. The following statements regarding Sengstaken-Blakemore intubation are true, *except*:
   a. The esophageal balloon is inflated first for the treatment of bleeding esophageal varices.
   b. The Sengstaken-Blakemore tube is not indicated in the treatment of massive bleeding from gastritis.
   c. Proper inflation of the gastric balloon requires approximately 250 cc of air.
   d. It is mandatory to insert a separate nasogastric tube into the esophagus, above the esophageal balloon.
   e. The Sengstaken-Blakemore tube should be left in place for 24 hours after balloon deflation to monitor for recurrence of bleeding.
3. Which of the following is true concerning chest tube placement?
   a. The safest place for insertion is the sixth intercostal space, anterior axillary line.
   b. Trocars are recommended for ease of insertion.
   c. Pleural catheter placement is effective for hemothorax.
   d. Suspicion of metastatic cancer is a contraindication.
   e. Removal of chest tubes should follow a deep exhalation.
4. Peritoneal lavage is recommended for abdominal trauma in the following situations:
   a. Stab wound with evisceration
   b. Gunshot wound of the epigastrium
   c. Mild pain in a child who has fallen from a bicycle
   d. Unexplained shock and unconsciousness
   e. None of the above

Answers

1. c
2. a
3. e
4. d

Index

A

ABA; *see* American Burn Association
Abbreviated Injury Scale (AIS), 607-608
Abdominal abscess, postoperative fever and, 749-750
Abdominal distention, of newborn, 642
Abdominal epilepsy, 566
Abdominal hernias, 545
Abdominal masses
  with actual or impending rupture, 510-511
  appendicitis and, 512-513
  arteriography in evaluation of, 509-510
  associated with bacteremia, 510
  associated with gastrointestinal obstruction, 511
  auscultation in evaluation of, 507
  carcinoma of gallbladder and, 517-518
  change in size of, 506, 507
  choledochal cyst and, 518
  classification of, 504
  colon carcinoma and, 513-514, 515
  contour of, 507
  diagnostic studies of, 504-510
  discovery of, 506
  diverticulitis and, 514-516
  empyema of gallbladder and, 517
  examination of, 507
  extrahepatic biliary system and, 517-518
  fallopian tubes and, 529
  fluctuation and, 507
  gallbladder and, 517-518
  gastrointestinal system and, 506
  gynecologic system and, 506
  hydrops of gallbladder and, 517
  intraperitoneal, 511-512
  liver and, 516-517
  mesentery and, 516
  mucocele and, 512-513
  omentum and, 516
  operative intervention for, 504-510
  ovaries and, 529-530
  palpation in examination of, 507
  pancreas and, 519-522
  patient history and, 506-507
  pelvic, 528-530
  periampullary carcinoma and, 518
  pulsation of, 507
  rectal examination in evaluation of, 507
  retroperitoneal masses and, 519-522, 528
  secondary to obstructive disease, 522
  secondary to renal cystic disease, 522-524
  secondary to renal infections, 524-525
  secondary to renal neoplasms, 525-527
  small intestine, 511-512
  spleen and, 518-519
Abdominal masses—cont'd
  stomach carcinoma and, 511
  systematic approach to, 506
  urinary system and, 506-507
  uterus and, 528-529
Abdominal migraine, abdominal pain and, 566
Abdominal musculature, congenital absence of, 635
Abdominal pain
  acute, 422-459
  acute appendicitis and, 427-429
  approach to patient in, 426-427
  carcinoma of colon and rectum and, 514
  cholecystitis and, 429-437
  colonic diverticulitis and, 443-446
  diagnosis of, 423-424
  distribution of, 423
  free intraperitoneal perforations of GI tract and, 446-448
  intestinal obstruction and, 449-455
  ischemic colitis and, 449
  ischemic small bowel disease and, 448-449
  jaundice and, 465
  origin of, 422-427
  pancreatitis and, 437-443
  patient history and, 423-424, 561
  physical examination and, 424-426, 561
  physiology of, 422-427
  psychogenic, 566
  rarely requiring surgery, 561-570
  Zollinger-Ellison syndrome and, 213
Abdominal tap and lavage, 881, 882
Abdominal trauma
  blunt, 613-615
  operation and, 615-616
  preoperative preparation of patient with, 615
Abdominal Trauma Index (ATI), 608
Abdominal wall
  anterior, hernias of, 542-544
  pain arising from, 561-564
Abdominal wall test for pain, 561-564
Abnormal bowel movements, 481-503
Abscess
  abdominal, 749-750
  anorectal, 554-556
  appendiceal, appendicitis and, 429
  breast, treatment of, 389
  horseshoe, 820
  intra-abdominal, 822-823
  lung, hemoptysis and, 306-307
  nephric, 524-525
  pancreatic, 441, 520-521
  pelvic; *see* Pelvic abscess
  perinephric, 524-525, 704

Abscess—cont'd
  peripharyngeal, 261
  peritonsillar, 261
  pilonidal, 818
  retropharyngeal, 261
  septal, 864
  subfascial, 823
  subphrenic, appendicitis and, 428
Accommodation response, 484
Acetaminophen (Tylenol), 731
  with codeine, 235
Acetylcysteine (Mucomyst), 160
Achalasia, 292, 297-299
Acid secretory tests, duodenal ulcer and, 206
Acid-base balance, 127-130
  role of lung in, 154
Acidosis, coarctation of aorta and, 343
Acoustic neuroma, 861
Acoustic trauma, nerve deafness caused by, 861
Acquired bleeding disorders, 779-782
Acquired hernia, 533-534
Acquired immunodeficiency syndrome (AIDS), 824
  blood transfusion and, 17, 18
  Kaposi's sarcoma and, 269-270
Actinomycin D, 234
Activated T-cells (NF-AT$_c$), transplantation and, 243
Adalat (nifedipine), 377
Addison's disease, jaundice and, 465
Adenocarcinoma, 283-284
  of kidney, 525
Adenoid tissue, hypertrophy of, 863-864
Adenoidectomy, indications for, 865-866
Adenoma
  adrenal, 182
  bronchial, 188, 309
  pleomorphic, 262
  of thyroid gland, 166, 179
Adenomatous polyps, 494
Adenomyosis uteri, 528
Adhesion molecules, transplantation and, 243
Adhesions, intestinal, 497, 498
Adjuvant chemotherapy for breast cancer, 396-397, 399
Adrenal adenoma, 182
Adrenal carcinoma, 182
Adrenal glands
  anatomy of, 180
  evaluation of, for neoplasms, 73-74
  tumors of, 180-183
Adrenal hyperplasia, adrenal tumors and, 181-182
Adrenalectomy, operative approaches for, 188
Adult polycystic kidney disease, 524
Adult respiratory distress syndrome (ARDS), 149, 158-159
  fracture of femur and, 676, 680
Aerobic gangrene, 814
Afferent limb of fever, 745-746
Afferent nerves, 422-423
Afterload, cardiac output and, 765
AIDS; *see* Acquired immunodeficiency syndrome
Airway
  establishment of, 609
  upper, obstruction to, 612
Airway compromise, 41
Airway pressure release ventilation, 790
AIS; *see* Abbreviated Injury Scale

Alanine transferase (ALT), 467
Albumin-globulin ratio, 467
Albuterol, 160
Alcoholics, liver transplantation and, 251
Aldactone (spironolactone), 193, 376
Aldomet (methyldopa), 376
Aldosteronoma, 184-185
Alfentanil hydrochloride (Alfenta), 47, 58
Alkaline phosphatase, 467
Allen test, 763
Allergic reactions, 618
Allergic rhinitis, 863
Allogeneic graft in transplantation, 241
Alpha-adrenergic agents, centrally acting, 376
Alpha-adrenergic-blocking agent, 376
Alprazolam (Xanax), 235
ALT; *see* Alanine transferase (ALT), jaundice and
Alternogel (Mylanta), 629
Amaurosis fujax, 381
Ameloblastoma, 269
American Burn Association (ABA), 624
American Cancer Society (ACS), 68
American College of Radiology, 67
American Joint Committee for Cancer Staging and End
    Results Reporting, 266
American Society of Anesthesiologists (ASA), physical
    status classification of, 19, 29
American Thyroid Association, 283
Amidate (etomidate), 47, 55
Amides, anesthesia and, 43, 57
Amikacin (Amiken), 828
Aminoglycosides, 828
  urinary tract infections and, 710
Aminophylline, 160
Amnesia, retrograde, 660
Amphotericin B (Fungizone), 827
Ampicillin, 710, 825
Amputation, fingertip, 838-839
Amrinone lactate (Inocor), 56, 769, 770, 804
Anaerobic gangrene, 814-815
Anal atresia in infants, 644-645, 646-647
Anal canal, 549
Anal canal carcinoma, 552-553
Anal fissure, 550-551
Analgesia, patient-controlled (PCA), 51-52
Analgesics
  intramuscular, 51
  intravenous, 57-59
  oral, 51
  used in cancer management, 235
Anaplastic adenocarcinoma of thyroid, 284
Anatomic dead space, 150
Ancef (cefazolin), 456, 825
Anectine (succinylcholine chloride), 49, 58
Anemia
  carcinoma of colon and rectum and, 514
  deglutition and, 292
  preexisting, operative risk and, 16-17
Anesthesia
  ASA Physical Status Classification and, 29
  brachial plexus, 46
  liability of surgeon and, 53
  epidural, 45
  general, 46-48
  informed consent and, 52-53

Anesthesia—cont'd
  laboratory tests required for, 29
  local; *see* Local anesthesia
  monitored, 42
  neuromuscular blockade in, 48-49
  and postanesthetic care, 49-52
  preanesthetic evaluation and, 28-29
  preoperative medication and, 30-31
  preoperative preparation for, 28-32
  regional, 45-46
  subarachnoid, 45
  techniques of, 41-49
Anesthesiologist
  liability of surgeon for anesthesia delivered by, 53
  postoperative visit of, 52
Anesthetics
  for hand injuries, 831
  induction, 55
  inhalation, 48, 55-56
  intravenous, 46-48
  local; *see* Local anesthesia
Aneurysm
  aortic, 526-527
    diagnosis and treatment of, 363-365
  cirsoid, 259
  of sinus of Valsalva, 347
  ventricular, 356
Angina
  aortic stenosis and, 344
  Ludwig's, 261-262
  Vincent's, 262
Angina pectoris
  diagnosis of, 350
  reflux esophagitis and, 291
  surgical treatment of, 353-355
  treatment for, 350-355
Angiodysplasia
  colonoscopy for, 91
  gastrointestinal bleeding and, 417
Angiofibroma, epistaxis and, 864
Angiography
  in detection of GI bleeding, 78, 79
  jaundice and, 472
Angioma, 597
Angioplasty
  balloon, 353
  femoral artery, 78-80
  percutaneous transluminal, 80
  percutaneous transluminal coronary, 351, 353
  popliteal artery, 78-80
Angiosarcoma, Kaposi's, 597
Angiotensin, arterial blood pressure and, 370
Angiotensin-converting enzyme inhibitors, 803
Anglechick prosthesis, 116
Anisotropic bone, 670
Anorectal abscesses, 554-556
Anorectal anatomy, 547-549
Anorectal fistulas, 554-556
Anorectal melanoma, 553
Anspor (cephradine), 825
Antacids, burns and, 629
Antiandrogens, prostate cancer and, 709
Antibiotics
  for abdominal pain, 455-456
  abdominal trauma and, 615

Antibiotics—cont'd
  broad-spectrum, 456
  infection and, 826-828
  prophylactic systemic, 474
  treatment of infection with, 811-812
  urinary tract infections and, 710
Anticholinergics, anesthesia and, 54
Anticholinesterases, anesthesia and, 54
Antiemetics used in cancer management, 235
Antifungals, urinary tract infections and, 710
Antigen, transplantation, immune response to, 241-245
Antigen-presenting cells (APCs), transplantation and, 242
Antihypertensives, anesthesia and, 54
Anti-IL-2 strategies, transplantation and, 247-248
Antilymphocyte globulin
  Minnesota, 246
  transplantation and, 246-247, 252
Antimicrobials, topical, burns and, 628-629
Antimicrosomal (MCHA) antibodies, 166
Antiplatelet drugs, 781
Anti-tac, transplantation and, 248
Antithyroglobulin (TGHA) antibodies, 166
Antithyroid drugs for Graves' disease, 173-174
Anuria, 697
Anus
  defecation and, 483
  squamous cell carcinoma of, 552-553
Aorta, 363-367
  coarctation of; *see* Coarctation of aorta
Aortic aneurysm, 526-527
  diagnosis and treatment of, 363-365
Aortic dissection, 365-367
Aortic regurgitation, 317, 324-325
Aortic rupture, aortic dissection and, 366
Aortic stenosis (AS), 317, 322-324, 331, 344, 345
Aortic valve disease, 322-325
Aortopulmonary window, 334-335
APCs; *see* Antigen-presenting cells
Appendiceal abscess, appendicitis and, 429
Appendicitis
  acute, 427-429
    laparoscopy for, 102-104
  left-side, 514
  postoperative complications of, 428-429
Appendix, abdominal masses and, 512-513
Apple core carcinoma involving ascending colon, 495
Apresoline (hydralazine), 54, 376, 377, 803
Apudomas, 192
Arch anomalies, 347
ARDS; *see* Adult respiratory distress syndrome
Arduan (pipecuronium), 49, 58
Arsenic poisoning, 567
Arterial baroreflex, 370
Arterial catheterization, 149
Arterial line, 763, 874-876
Arteriography
  in evaluation of abdominal masses, 509-510
  for bleeding, 83
  for limb ischemia, 576-578
  pulmonary, 81-82
Arteriovenous fistula, 592
Arteriovenous malformation
  gastrointestinal bleeding and, 417
  lower extremity swelling and, 592

Arteriovenous malformation—cont'd
  arteriovenous fistulas in, 592
  treatment of, 592
Arteritis
  giant cell, 569
  temporal, 569
Arthritis
  rheumatoid, 568
  traumatic, fracture and, 681
Arthrodesis, 681
Arthroplasty, 681
AS; *see* Aortic stenosis
ASD; *see* Atrial septal defect
Aspartate transferase (AST), 467
Asphyxia, respiratory tract burns and, 260
Aspiration, patient at risk for, intubation of, 37
Aspirational pulmonary disease, 293
Aspiration-associated pneumonitis, 748
Aspirin, 731, 784
  effect of, on bleeding time, 781
Assist-control mode ventilation, 789
AST; *see* Aspartate transferase
Asthma, 21
Astrocytoma of spinal cord, 725, 726
Atelectasis, 21, 746-748
ATGAM, transplantation and, 246
Atheroma, carotid bifurcation, 382
ATI; *see* Abdominal Trauma Index
Ativan (lorazepam), 47, 55, 235
Atracurium (Tracrium), 49, 58
Atresia
  anal, in infants, 644-645, 646-647
  choanal, 637
  esophageal, 640-641, 642
  intestinal, 642-643
Atrial septal defect (ASD), 329, 330, 332
Atrioventricular canal, common, 333
Atropine, 54, 160
Auscultation in evaluation of abdominal masses, 507
Autologous blood donation, recombinant human
    erythropoietin and, 18
Avascular necrosis, fracture and, 680
Avocin (piperacillin), 825
Avulsion fracture, 673
Axid (nizatidine), 217
Axilla, palpation of, 385
Axonotmesis, 831, 832
Azactam (aztreonam), 710, 827
Azathioprine (Imuran), in transplantation, 245, 246,
    247, 248, 251, 252
Aztreonam (Azactam), 710, 827

B

Bacitracin ointment, 628
Back pain, low, 719-732
  intractable, 730-731
Bacteremia, 811, 816
  abdominal masses associated with, 510
Bacteria
  from infection, postoperative fever secondary to,
      746-751
  intestinal, metabolic effects of, 481, 482
Bacterial colonization, invasive infection and, 808
Bacterial enteritis, diarrhea and, 493
Bacterial pneumonia, hemoptysis and, 306

Bacterial symbiosis, 808
Bactocil (oxacillin), 825
Bactrim DS (sulfamethoxazole), 709
Balloon angioplasty, 353
Balloon dilation, esophagogastroduodenoscopy and, 89
BAO; *see* Basal acid output
Barbiturates, anesthesia and, 47, 54-55
Barotrauma, pulmonary, 791
Basal acid output (BAO), 206
Basal cell carcinoma, 553, 597, 598
Basilar skull fracture, 613, 654, 655
Bassini hernia repair, 539
BCAA; *see* Branched-chain amino acids
B-cell lymphocytes, infection and, 809
Bell's palsy, 862
Benadryl (diphenhydramine), 235
Benign cystosarcoma, treatment of, 390
Benign lesions of breast, treatment of, 389-390
Benign neoplasms of soft tissues, 602-603
Benign skin lesions, 596-597
Benzocaine (Hurricane), 43, 57
Benzodiazepines, anesthesia and, 47, 55
Benzothiadiazine diuretics, 376
Beta-adrenergic-blocking agents, 376
Betamethasone, 184
Bilateral breast cancer, 398
Bilateral hyperplasia, aldosteronoma and, 185
Bile, components of, 464
Bile acids, 464
Bilharziasis, 708
Biliary atresia, liver transplantation and, 251
Biliary cholesterol, 464
Biliary decompression, preoperative, 474
Biliary phospholipids, 464
Biliary system, extrahepatic, 517
Biliary tract, contrast radiology of, 470-472
Bilious vomiting, 642
Bilirubin, normal metabolism of, 461-464
Billroth I, 212
Billroth II, 212
Bimanual palpation in examination of oral cavity, 258
Biochemical tests in assessment of nutritional status,
    138-139
Biopsy
  of intraoral tumors, 265-266
  liver, 473
Bite
  human, of hand, 840
  snake, 564, 567
  spider, 564, 567
Bladder, 562-563, 566
Blakemore-Sengstaken tube, GI bleeding and, 408
Blalock-Hanlon procedure, transposition of great
    arteries and, 339
Blalock-Taussig procedure
  tetralogy of Fallot and, 339
  tricuspid atresia and, 337
Bleeding
  arteriography in evaluation of, 83
  gastrointestinal; *see* Gastrointestinal bleeding
  massive, treatment of, 782-783
  rectal; *see* Rectal bleeding
  surgical, and hemostasis, 773-785
Bleeding diathesis, trauma and, 617
Bleeding disorders, 777-782

Bleomycin (Blenoxane), 234
Blind loop syndrome, 485, 487
Bloating, dumping syndrome and, 212
Blood
    administration of, trauma and, 611
    in urine, 684-693
    vomiting of, 87
Blood clots in urine, 685-686
Blood coagulation, 774, 775
Blood deficiencies, correction of, 474
Blood flow, interruption of, 612-613
Blood pressure
    normal, isolated postoperative tachycardia associated
        with, 737
    trauma and, 613
Blood supply, inadequate, delayed healing and, 608,
        609
Blood transfusion
    autologous, 18
    risk of, 17-18
Blood vessels in normal hemostasis, 773, 774
Bloody discharge from breast, 68
Blowout fractures, 854
Bochdalek, foramen of, hernia through, 544-545,
        639
Body fluid
    anatomy of, 122-123
    classification of changes in, 125-131
    volume changes in, 125, 126
Body temperature; *see also* Fever
    burn injury and, 621
    of infants, 631
Boerhaave's syndrome, 291-292
Bombesin, 204-205, 222
Bone
    anatomy of, 670
    anisotropic, 670
    injuries to, 669-683
    viscoelastic, 670
Bone felon, 819
Boutonnière deformity, 835
Bowel
    absorptive capacity of, measurement of, 485
    hypoxic paralysis of, 498
    postirradiated, GI bleeding and, 418
    preoperative preparation of, 474
Bowel gangrene in infants, 651-652
Bowel habits, altered, 514
Bowel movements, abnormal, 481-503
Bowen's disease, 553, 598
Bowstring sign, positive, 720
Boxer's fracture, 838
Brachial plexus anesthesia, 46
Brain
    lesions of, 657-658
    referred abdominal pain and, 562-563, 565-566
Brain injury, secondary, 658
Branched-chain amino acids (BCAA), 142-144
Breast
    bloody discharge from, 68
    cancers metastatic to, 390
    cystosarcoma phylloides of, 390
    fat necrosis of, 390
    fibrous disease of, 389-390
    lump in; *see* Lump in breast

Breast—cont'd
    malignant lesions of, 390-398
    Paget's disease of, 399, 553
Breast abscess, 389
Breast cancer
    bilateral, 398
    breast reconstruction and, 395-396
    dietary factors and, 391
    geographic incidence of, 391
    hormone binding and, 399
    with inflammation, 398
    invasive lobular carcinoma, 395
    male, 397
    nipple discharge and, 398, 399
    postoperative irradiation for, 398
    pregnancy and, 398
    staging and prognosis of, 391, 393-397
    TNM classification of, 391, 392
    treatment options for, 391-399
    tumor markers and, 390-391
Breast lesion
    benign, treatment of, 389-390
    needle localization and, 68-71
Breast palpation, 68, 69
Breast self-examination (BSE), 388
Breath, shortness of, 302
Breathing, 150-152
    mechanical work of, 793
Brevital (methohexital), 47, 54
Brodie-Trendelenburg test, 590, 592
Bronchial adenoma, 188, 309
Bronchiectasis, 21
    cylindrical, 307
    cystic, 307
    hemoptysis and, 307-308
    pneumonia and, 306
    saccular, 307
Bronchiolitis, obliterative, 253
Bronchogenic carcinoma, 309-310
Bronchoscopy, fiberoptic, 878-879
BSE; *see* Breast self-examination
Budd-Chiari syndrome, 411
Buerger's disease, 573
Bundle of His, injury to, 347
Bupivacaine (Marcaine; Sensorcaine), 43, 57, 871
Burn
    body temperature and, 621
    calculating body surface area involved in, 621, 623
    caloric requirements of patient with, 627
    cardiopulmonary resuscitation of patient with, 624
    care of, 624, 625-627
    chemical, 260
    electrical injury and, 260, 622
    fluid requirements for patient with, 624-625
    full-thickness, 621, 622, 626-627
    of hand, 840-841
    infected, 627
    intravenous access and, 624
    major, 624, 626
    minor, 624
    moderate uncomplicated, 624
    of oral cavity, 260
    partial-thickness, 621, 622
    pathophysiologic changes in, 620-621
    pulmonary injury and, 621, 622-624

Burn—cont'd
  respiratory tract, 260
  rule of nines and, 621, 623
  superficial, 621
Burned nasal hair, respiratory tract burns and, 260
Burr holes, diagnostic, 663-664
Butorphanol tartrate (Stadol), 57

C

Calan (verapamil), 377
Calcification, metastatic, 176
Calcineurin, transplantation and, 243-244
Calcitonin, 135
Calcitoninoma, 497
Calcium abnormalities, 130
Calcium channel blocker, 803
  hypertension and, 377
Calcium gluconate, 135
Calcospherites, 169
Calculi, renal, 695
Callus, fracture, 671-672
Caloric requirements; *see also* Nutritional support
  burn injury and, 627
Cancer; *see also* Carcinoma; Neoplasms; Oncology;
    Tumors
  adjuvant treatment for, 231
  breast; *see* Breast cancer
  clinical management of, 227-233
  clinical staging of, 227, 228-230
  comparison of therapeutic approaches, 231, 232
  cure for, definition of, 226
  epidermoid, 714
  gastric, 216
  growth rate of, 223-224
  incidence of, by site and sex, 230
  initiator state of, 220
  laryngeal, 867
  metastatic to breast, 390
  nonsurgical treatment of, 230
  oral, 264-269
  physiology of, 229
  promoter agent of, 220
  propensity to metastasize, 224-225
  prostate; *see* Prostate cancer
  skin; *see* Skin cancer
  thyroid, nonsurgical treatment of, 73
Cancer surgery
  as adjuvant therapy, 231
  biologic basis for, 225-227
  curability of solid neoplasms and, 225-226
  debulking procedures in, 230
  and follow-up care, 232-233
  lymph nodes and, 229-230
  maintaining records of, 231-232
  palliative, 230
  patient preparation for, 228
  preoperative evaluation in, 227-228
  prophylactic, 225
Cancrum oris, 815
Candiduria, 707
Capillary hemangioma, 259
Captopril (Capoten), 377
Carafate (sucralfate), 217
Carbocaine hydrochloride (mepivacaine), 43, 57,
  871

Carbohydrates
  absorption of, in GI tract, 483
  gastroduodenal digestion and absorption and, 197-198
Carbon dioxide in laparoscopy, 96, 97
Carboxyhemoglobin levels, elevated, respiratory tract
    burns and, 260
Carbuncle, 813, 818
Carcinoembryonic antigen (CEA), 222
  medullary thyroid cancer and, 172
Carcinogens, 220, 221
Carcinoid syndrome, 188-189
Carcinoid tumors, 188-189
Carcinoma; *see also* Cancer; Neoplasms; Oncology;
    Tumors
  adrenal, 182
  anal canal, 552-553
  basal cell, 553, 597, 598
  bronchogenic, 309-310
  of colon and rectum, 494-496, 513-516
    Dukes staging system for, 495, 496
  endometrial, 528
  epidermoid, 552
    of oral cavity, 264-265
  of esophagus; *see* Esophagus, carcinoma of
  of fallopian tubes, 529
  of gallbladder, 517-518
  of head of pancreas, 477-478
  intraepidermal, 553
  of liver, 516, 517
  lung; *see* Lung cancer
  of pancreas, 519-520
  of parathyroids, 177
  periampullary, 477-478, 518
  renal cell, 525
  squamous cell; *see* Squamous cell carcinoma
  stomach, 511, 512
  of thyroid gland; *see* Thyroid cancer
Cardiac catheterization, 350
Cardiac output, shock and, 763, 764
Cardiac tamponade, 616
  acute, clinical shock and, 362
  with heart failure, trauma and, 612
Cardiac transplantation, 252
  indications for, 361
  orthotopic, 361-362
  rejection and, 362
Cardiogenic shock, 759, 770
Cardioplegia, 354
Cardiopulmonary bypass, 320
  abnormalities of platelet and clotting factors and, 782
Cardiopulmonary function, preoperative preparation,
    474
Cardiopulmonary operative risk factors, 19-22
Cardiopulmonary resuscitation, burn injury and, 624
Cardiospasm, 297-299
Cardiothoracic derangements, 610
Cardiotonics, shock and, 770
Cardiovascular hemodynamics, complications of
    ventilator support related to, 791
Cardura (doxazosin mesylate), 709
Carnett's test, 561-564
Carotid bifurcation atheroma, 382
Carpal tunnel syndrome, 833-834
Castration, breast cancer and, 398
Catabolic state, delayed healing and, 608, 609

Catapres (clonidine), 376
Cathecholamines, anesthesia and, 56
Catheter
  central venous, 33-34, 794-795
  Foley; *see* Foley catheter
  intra-arterial, in intraoperative monitoring, 33
  pulmonary artery, 34, 794-795
  pulmonary artery balloon flotation, 876-877
  Swan-Ganz, 876-877
  systemic arterial, 794-795
Cauliflower ear deformity, 863
Cavernous hemangioma, 259
CBD stones; *see* Common bile duct stones
CCK; *see* Cholecystokinin
CCK-PZ; *see* Cholecystokinin-pancreozymin
CD4+ cells, transplantation and, 242-243, 244, 245
CD8+ cells, transplantation and, 244, 245
CD3 complex, transplantation and, 243
CEA; *see* Carcinoembryonic antigen
Cefaclor (Ceclor), 826
Cefazolin (Ancef; Kefzol; Zolicef), 456, 710, 825
Cefizox (ceftizoxime sodium), 826
Cefobid (cephoperazone), 826
Cefonicid (Monocid), 826
Cefotan (cefotetan), 826
Cefotaxime (Claforan), 456, 826
Cefoxitin sodium (Mefoxin), 455, 826
Ceftazidime (Fortaz), 710, 826
Ceftizoxime sodium (Cefizox), 826
Ceftriaxone (Nitrocephin; Rocephin), 710, 826
Celbenin (methicillin), 825
Cell cycle, 221
Cellular immunity, infection and, 809
Cellular rejection, transplantation and, 244
Cellulitis, 817
  infection and, 813
  Ludwig's angina and, 261
  Meleney's, 808
  necrotizing, 815
Cellulose, GI tract and, 483
Central lines, 870-874
Central nervous system, lesions of, 562-563, 565-566
Central obesity, in Cushing's syndrome, 375
Central parenteral nutrition (CPN), 144
Central venous catheter, 33-34, 794-795
Cephalexin (Keflet; Keflex), 825
Cephalosporine, 825, 826
  urinary tract infections and, 710
Cephalothin (Keflin; Seffin), 825
Cephoperazone (Cefobid), 826
Cephradine (Anspor; Velocef), 825
Cerebral hypoxic spells, 331
Cerebral infarction, tetralogy of Fallot and, 339
Cerebral status, shock and, 762
Cerebritis, 659
Cerebrospinal rhinorrhea, 865
Cerebrovascular disease
  clinical evaluation of, 382
  spectrum of, 380-381
Certified registered nurse anesthetist (CRNA), 53
Cervical masses, congenital, 272, 274
Cervical spine, damage to, 611-612, 617
Cervical teratoma in infants, 638
Cetacaine (tetracaine hydrochloride), 43, 57
Chancre, syphilis and, 713

Chancroid, 713
Chemical burns of oral cavity, 260
Chemotherapeutic agents
  common, 234-235
  mechanism of action of, 231
Chemotherapy
  adjuvant, for breast cancer, 396-397, 399
  for intraoral tumors, 267-268
Chest
  flail, trauma and, 612
  trauma to, 616
Chest pain
  acute myocardial infarction and, 355-356
  of cardiovascular origin
    aorta and, 363-367
    ischemic heart disease and, 349-357
    left ventricular assist devices and, 359-361
    orthotopic cardiac transplantation and, 361-362
    pericardium and, 362-363
    pulmonary embolism and, 367-368
    ventricular aneurysms and, 357-359
  pericarditis and, 362
  pleuritic, pneumonia and, 302
  radiographic examination and, 308-309
Chest tubes, thoracentesis and, 882-883
Child abuse, trauma to head and, 659-660
Children; *see also* Infant
  head injuries of, 659-660
  hematuria in, 686-691
Child's classification of hepatic reserve, 412, 413
Chills, jaundice and, 465
Chlorambucil, 234
Chloramphenicol (Chloromycetin), 827
Chloroprocaine (Nesacaine hydrochloride), 43, 57
Chlorothiazide (Diuril), 376
Chlorzoxazone (Parafon Forte), 732
Choanal atresia
  in infants, 637
  nasal obstruction and, 863
Cholangiography
  intravenous, 472
  laparoscopic, 106, 108
  operative, role of, in common duct exploration, 437
  oral, 472
Cholangitis, sclerosing, jaundice and, 477
Cholecystectomy
  indications for common duct exploration at, 433
  laparoscopic, 104-111, 436-437
Cholecystitis
  acute, 429-433
    treatment of, 433, 434
  chronic, 433-437
  recurrent, 433-437
Cholecystokinin (CCK), 200, 203, 204-205
Cholecystokinin-pancreozymin (CCK-PZ), 198, 202
Choledochal cyst, 518
Choledochoduodenostomy
  jaundice and, 476
  reimplantation, 476
Choledocholithiasis, ERCP and, 106
Choledochostomy, role of, 437
Choledochotomy, jaundice and, 475
Cholestasis, 460
  intrahepatic, 469
Cholestatic jaundice, 465-466

Cholesteatoma, 859
Cholesterol, biliary, 464
Cholesterol stones, 464
Christmas disease, 778
Chyme, short bowel syndrome and, 485
Cimetidine (Tagamet), 30, 193, 217
Ciprofloxacin (Cipro), 709, 710, 827
Cirsoid aneurysm, 259
Cisplatin, 234
Citanest (prilocaine), 43
Claforan (cefotaxime), 456, 826
Claudication
    angioplasty for, 79-80
    chronic ischemia and, 572
    neurogenic, limb ischemia and, 573-574
    venous, limb ischemia and, 574
Cleft lip, 258
Cleft palate, 258
Clindamicin (Cleocin), 827
Clinical stage; *see* Staging
Clonidine (Catapres), 376
Closed fracture, 672
Closed head injuries, 658-659
Clots, blood, 685-686
Coagulation cascade, 774, 775
Coagulation defects, 777-778
    platelet defects and, 779, 781-782
Coagulation studies
    in evaluation of hemostasis, 777
    liver function and, 467-468
Coarctation of aorta, 330-331, 342-344, 365
    hypertension and, 374
Cocaine, 43, 57
Codeine, 743
Coin lesions, 309-310
Colace (docusate sodium), 559
Cold, common, 863
Cold storage solutions, for transplantation, 239, 240
Colectomy, laparoscopic-assisted, 118-120
Colic, lead, 567
Colitis
    ischemic, 449
    pseudomembranous, 487
    ulcerative; *see* Ulcerative colitis
Collagen diseases, 562-563, 568-569
Collagen vascular disease, fever and, 753
Collarbutton infection, 819
Colles' fracture, 678
Collins solution, transplantation and, 239
Colloid nodules of thyroid, 166
Colon
    abdominal masses and, 513-516
    absorptive functions of, 481, 482
    common operations of, 444-446
    diverticular disease of, gastrointestinal bleeding and, 416-417
    malrotation of, in infants, 645
    volvulus of, 454-455
Colon cancer, 494-496, 513-516
    colonoscopy in surveillance of, 91
Colon disease, laparoscopy for, 118-120
Colon resection, laparoscopic, 118-120
Colonic diverticulitis, 443-446
Colonic pseudoobstruction, 499

Colonic underperfusion, gastrointestinal bleeding and, 417-418
Colonoscopy, 90-92
    complications of, 91-92
    indications for, 90-91
    limitations of, 91
    therapeutic procedures performed with, 91
Coma, hypercalcemia and, 176
Comminuted fracture, 670, 671, 673
Common bile duct (CBD) stones
    extraction of, under laparoscopic guidance, 109-111
    removal of, ERCP and, 89-90
Common cold, 863
Common duct stones, retained, jaundice and, 476
Common duct stricture, jaundice and, 476-477
Compartment syndrome, fracture and, 679
Compazine (prochlorperazine), 235
Compensated shock, 758
Compliance, effective, of lung-thorax system, 151
Computed tomography (CT)
    in evaluation of abdominal masses, 507, 508
    guidelines for, 63-64
    jaundice and, 470
    versus magnetic resonance imaging, 61-67
Concussion, 660
    initial evaluation and treatment of, 662
Conductive deafness, 861
C'1-esterase deficiency, 568
Congenital bleeding disorders, 777-779
Congenital cervical masses, 272, 274
Congenital diaphragmatic hernia, 544-545
Congenital goiter in infants, 638
Congenital heart disease, 329-348
    aneurysms of sinus of Valsalva in, 347
    aortic stenosis in, 331, 344
    aortopulmonary window in, 334-335
    arch anomalies in, 347
    atrial septal defects in, 330, 332
    coarctation of aorta in, 330-331, 342-344
    congenital mitral valve disease in, 346-347
    coronary arteriovenous fistula in, 347
    Ebstein's malformation in, 341
    endocardial cushion defects in, 333
    heart block in, 347
    hypoplastic left heart syndrome in, 341-342
    origin of both great arteries from right ventricle in, 336
    origin of left coronary artery from pulmonary artery in, 347
    patent ductus arteriosus in, 330, 334
    physiologic considerations of, 329-330
    pulmonary atresia with intact ventricular septum in, 338
    pulmonary stenosis in, 331, 344-346
    tetralogy of Fallot in, 331, 338-339
    total anomalous pulmonary venous connection in, 335-336
    transposition of great arteries in, 330, 339-340
    tricuspid atresia in, 331, 337-338
    truncus arteriosus in, 336-337
    vascular rings in, 347
    ventricular septal defects in, 330, 333-334
Congenital hernia, 533
Congenital lesions of oral cavity, 258-260
Congenital lobar emphysema in infants, 639

Congenital mitral valve disease, 346-347
Congestive heart failure, 330-331
    aneurysm of sinus of Valsalva and, 347
    coarctation of aorta and, 343
    postoperative, 740
    transposition of great arteries and, 339
    truncus arteriosus and, 336-337
Consciousness, level of, trauma and, 613
Consent, informed; *see* Informed consent
Constant flow ventilation, 792
Constipation, 497-501
    colonoscopy for, 90-91
    definition of, 483
    hypercalcemia and, 176
Constrictive pericarditis, 363
    abdominal pain and, 562-563, 565
Continent ileal pouch procedure, 488
Continuous hypothermic perfusion, transplantation and, 241
Continuous positive airway pressure (CPAP), 789
Contractility, cardiac output and, 766
Contractions, haustral, 483
Contracture, 608, 681, 845
Contrast radiology of biliary tract, jaundice and, 470-472
Contrast studies of gastrointestinal tract, 473
Contrast x-ray evaluation of abdominal masses, 509
Control mode ventilation, 788-789
Contusions of brain, severe head trauma and, 657-658
Convalescence, normal, 735
Conventional positive pressure ventilation (CPPV), 788, 789
Converting enzyme inhibitors, hypertension and, 377
Coombs' test, jaundice and, 468
COPD, 21
Core temperature, shock and, 762
Coronary arteriovenous fistula, 347
Coronary artery bypass grafting, 354
Coronary artery revascularization, 355
Corticosteroids, transplantation and, 252
Cortisone acetate, 184, 193
Cough
    persistent, chest x-ray examination and, 308-309
    pulmonary lesions and, 302-314
Cough reflex, 302
Coumadin (warfarin sodium), 784
Courvoisier's sign, 518
CPAP; *see* Continuous positive airway pressure
CPN; *see* Central parenteral nutrition
CPPV; *see* Conventional positive pressure ventilation
Cramping, dumping syndrome and, 212
Cricothyrotomy, 878
Critical care
    invasive hemodynamic monitoring in, 794-795
    multiple organ dysfunction syndrome in, 801-802
    restoration of oxygen transport in, 796-801
    ventilatory support in, 786-794
Crohn's colitis, colonoscopy for, 91
Crohn's disease, 488-490
    indications for surgery in, 489, 490
Croup, 866
Cryptorchidism, 717-718
CT; *see* Computed tomography
Cubital tunnel syndrome, 834
Curare, 58

Cushing's syndrome
    diagnosis of, 181
    hypertension and, 375
    medullary cancer of thyroid and, 171
    pathophysiology of, 181
    postoperative management of, 183
    preoperative management of, 183
Cutaneous melanoma, 599-602
Cutaneous striae, Cushing's syndrome and, 375
Cyanosis
    Ebstein's malformation and, 341
    esophageal rupture and, 292
    pulmonary atresia with intact ventricular septum and, 338
    pulmonary stenosis and, 346
    tetralogy of Fallot and, 338
    transposition of great arteries and, 339
    tricuspid atresia and, 337
    truncus arteriosus and, 336
Cyanosis, congenital heart defects associated with, 335-342
Cyclobenzaprine (Flexeril), 732
Cyclophilline, transplantation and, 246
Cyclophosphamide (Cytoxan), 234
Cyclosporine, transplantation and, 245-246, 248, 251, 252
Cylindrical bronchiectasis, 307
Cylindroma, 309
Cyst
    breast, treatment of, 389
    choledochal, 518
    dermoid, 263
    in hydatid of Morgagni, 715
    multilocular, of kidney, 524
    odontogenic, 263
    omental, 516
    ovarian, 529-530
    pilonidal, 818
    renal, 523-524
    retention, 262
    scrotal, 714-715
    sebaceous, 597, 818
    simple, of kidney, 523
    synovial, 603
    thyroglossal duct, 259
    of thyroid, 166
Cystic bronchiectasis, 307
Cystosarcoma, benign, treatment of, 390
Cystosarcoma phylloides of breast, treatment of, 390
Cytochrome P-450 enzymes, transplantation and, 246
Cytomegalovirus, postoperative fever and, 751
Cytotec (misoprostol), 217
Cytotoxic crossmatch, transplantation and, 245
Cytoxan (cyclophosphamide), 234

D

Dactinomycin, 234
Dalton's law, 152
Darvocet, 731
Darvon, 731, 743
Data base, 9
DDAVUP, 784
de Quervain's disease, 841
Deafness, 859-861
Decerebrate posturing, head injury and, 661

Decorticate posturing, head injury and, 661
Deep thrombophlebitis, 585-588
Deep venous insufficiency, 591-592
Defecation, 483-484
  abnormal, etiology of, 496
Deglutition, difficulties in, 289-301
Dehydration in infants, correction of, 632
Delta hepatitis, 824
Demerol (meperidine hydrochloride), 59, 455, 743
Dentate line, characteristics defined by, 548
Deoxyspergualin, transplantation and, 245
Depolarizing neuromuscular blockers, 48
Depression, hypercalcemia and, 176
Dermatomyositis, abdominal pain and, 569
Dermoid cysts, 263
Desflurane, 55
Deviated nasal septum, 864
Dexamethasone, 184, 193
Dextran, 784
Dextrose, insulin with, 135
Dextrose solutions, total parenteral nutrition and, 142
DHG; *see* Diffuse hemorrhagic gastritis
Diabetes
  abdominal pain and, 562-563, 567-568
  type 1, pancreas transplantation and, 249, 250
  watery diarrhea syndrome and, 190
Diabetic acidosis, 568
Diabetic foot, 574
Diabetic ketoacidosis, 567-568
Diabetic neuropathy, limb ischemia and, 574
Diagnostic imaging modalities, 61-85
Dialysis versus kidney transplantation, 248
Diaphragm, trauma to, 616
Diaphragmatic hernia
  congenital, 544-545
  in infants, 639-640
  traumatic, 545
Diarrhea
  causes of, 496
  definition of, 483
  diagnostic approach to, 484-485
  explosive, dumping syndrome and, 212
  exudative, 485
  idiopathic, 496
  incontinence and, 496
  medullary cancer of thyroid and, 171
  non-insulin-producing islet cell tumors associated with, 497
  osmotic, 484-485
  secretory, 485
  sphincter spasm and, 496
  tenesmus and, 496
  watery diarrhea syndrome and, 190
  Zollinger-Ellison syndrome and, 213
Diazepam (Valium), 30, 47, 55, 235, 731
Dibenzyline (phenoxybenzamine hydrochloride), 193
DIC; *see* Disseminated intravascular coagulation
Dicloxacillin (Dynapen; Pathocil), 825
Diethylstilbestrol, 709
Diffuse hemorrhagic gastritis (DHG), 410
Diflucan (fluconazole), 710, 827
Digits, amputation of, 839
Diiodotyrosine (DIT), 164
Dilaudid, 743
Diphenhydramine (Benadryl), 235

Diphenoxylate/atropine (Lomotil), 235
Diphtheria, 816
Diplopia, postconcussion syndrome and, 660
Diprivan (propofol), 47
Direct inguinal hernia, 536, 538
Direct vasodilators, hypertension and, 376
Dislocation, pelvic, 616-617
Disseminated intravascular coagulation (DIC), 781-782
Distal aortic dissection, 365
Distention, gastric outlet obstruction and, 210
DIT; *see* Diiodotyrosine
Diuretics
  benzothiadiazine, 376
  for hypertension, 376
  loop, 376
  potassium-sparing, 376
Diuril (chlorothiazide), 376
Diverticula
  esophageal, 299-300
  of small and large intestine, 443, 444
Diverticular disease of colon, gastrointestinal bleeding and, 416-417
Diverticulitis, 443, 444, 514-516
  colonic, 443-446
Dizziness, postconcussion syndrome and, 660
Dobutamine (Dobutrex), 56, 769, 770, 803
Docusate sodium (Colace; Surfak), 559
Dopamine (Intropin), 56, 769, 770, 803-804
Double outlet–right ventricle, 336
Double-lung transplantation, 252-253
Doubling time, tumor growth and, 224
Down's syndrome, endocardial cushion defects in, 333
Doxacurium (Neuromax), 49
Doxazosin mesylate (Cardura), 709
Doxorubicin, 234
Doxycycline (Vibramycin), 710
Drinking, epidermoid carcinoma of oral cavity and, 264
Drop finger, 835
Droperidol, 59
Drug fever, 753
Dukes staging system for carcinoma of colon and rectum, 495, 496, 513
Dumping syndrome, 212-213, 214-215
Duodenal obstruction in infants, 642, 643
Duodenal ulcer
  choice of operation for, 210-212
  diagnosis of, 206-207
  gastrointestinal bleeding and, 408-410
  indications for operation in, 209
  management of, 207
  parietal cell vagotomy for, 212
  pathophysiology of, 203-206
  truncal vagotomy, 211-212
Duodenum, surgical anatomy of, 196-197
Dupuytren's disease, 841
Duragesic patches, 235
Duranest (etidocaine hydrochloride), 43, 57
Dynapen (dicloxacillin), 825
Dysphagia
  arch anomalies and, 347
  difficulties in swallowing and, 290
  esophageal carcinoma and, 292
Dysplasia of vocal cords, 867

E

Ear
  cauliflower deformity of, 863
  examination of, 856-867
  removal of foreign objects from, 863
  swimmer's, 857
Ear infections, 857-863
  acute, 857-859
  chronic, 859
Ear trauma, injury caused by, 863
Eardrum, traumatic perforation of, 863
Ebstein's malformation, 341
Ecchymosis, trauma and, 613
ECMO; *see* Extracorporeal membrane oxygenation
Ectopic ACTH syndrome, 181, 182
Ectopic pregnancy, 529
Ectopic salivary glands, 262
Edecrin (ethacrynic acid), 135, 376
Edema
  respiratory tract burns and, 260
  scrotal, 714
Edrophonium chloride, 54
Effective compliance of lung-thorax system, 151
Efferent limb of fever, 745-746
Efudex (5% fluorouracil cream), 559
EGF; *see* Epidermal growth factor
Elderly persons, hematuria in, 691
Electrical burns of oral cavity, 260
Electrical injury, burn injury and, 622
Electrocoagulation, esophagogastroduodenoscopy and, 88
Electrolytes
  abnormalities in, 130-131
  gastric, 200, 201
  maintenance requirements for
    for infants, 632
    intraoperative, 40
Elephantiasis, 714
Embolism
  mycotic, 816
  pulmonary; *see* Pulmonary embolism
  versus thromboembolism, 571, 572
Embolization to solid organs from clots in heart, abdominal pain and, 565
Emotional lability, postconcussion syndrome and, 660
Emphysema, 21
  congenital lobar, in infants, 639
Empyema
  of gallbladder, 517
  of pleural space, postoperative fever and, 750
  pneumonia and, 306
Emulsification, 198
Encephalocele in infants, 636
Endocardial cushion defects, 333
Endocardial fibroelastosis, congenital mitral valve disease and, 346-347
Endochondral ossification, fracture healing and, 672
Endocrine abnormality, imaging of, 71-75
Endocrinology, surgical, 162-195
Endometrial carcinoma, 528
Endometriosis, 528-529
  ureteral obstruction and, 696
Endoscopic retrograde cholangiography, jaundice and, 470-472

Endoscopic retrograde cholangiopancreatography (ERCP), 87, 89-90
  choledocholithiasis and, 106
  chronic pancreatitis and, 485, 486
  obstructive jaundice and, 478
Endoscopy
  colonoscopy in, 90-92
  endoscopic retrograde cholangiopancreatography in, 89-90
  esophagogastroduodenoscopy in, 87-89
  flexible sigmoidoscopy in, 92
  instrumentation in, 86-87
  percutaneous endoscopic gastrostomy, 92-93
  in surgical practice, 86-94
  upper gastrointestinal, 87-89
Endothelene, transplantation and, 246
Endotoxemia, 817
Endotracheal intubation
  complications of, 38
  indications for, 37
  in intraoperative monitoring, 35-38
  technique for, 877-878
Endotracheal tube, complications of ventilator support related to, 791
Endovaginal ultrasound, 75
Energy needs, calculation of, in nutritional support, 141
Enflurane, 56
Enteral nutrition, 140
  results of, in surgical patients, 24
Enteritis
  causes of, 493
  regional, 511-512
  staphylococcal, 487
Enterocolitis, necrotizing; *see* Necrotizing enterocolitis
Enteroglucagon, 204-205
Enterohepatic circulation, 463
Ephedrine sulfate, 56
Epidermal growth factor (EGF), 222
Epidermoid carcinoma, 552, 714
  of oral cavity, 264-265
Epididymitis, 716
Epidural anesthesia, 45
Epidural hematoma, 657
Epidural opioids in postoperative pain management, 52
Epigastric hernia, 543
Epigastric pain, 89
Epiglottiditis, 866
Epilepsy, abdominal, 566
Epinephrine, 56, 57
  local anesthetics and, 44-45
Epiplocele, 543
Epispadias in infants, 635-636
Epistaxis, 864
Epulis, 262-263
ERCP; *see* Endoscopic retrograde cholangiopancreatography
Erysipelas, 813
Erythrocytes in urine, 684-693
Erythromycin, 203, 826
Erythroplasia, epidermoid carcinoma of oral cavity and, 264
Escharotomies, 626-627
Esidrix (hydrochlorothiazide), 376
Esmolol hydrochloride, 54
Esophageal atresia in infants, 640-641, 642

Esophageal diverticula, 299-300
Esophageal hiatal hernia, 544
Esophageal reflux, laparoscopy for, 116-118
Esophageal rupture, 291-292
Esophageal variceal hemorrhage, gastrointestinal
    bleeding and, 411-414
Esophagitis, 544
    gastrointestinal bleeding and, 414-415
    reflux, 291, 296-297
Esophagogastroduodenoscopy
    electrocoagulation in, 88
    gastrointestinal bleeding and, 408
    heater probe in, 88
    indications for, 87
    laser therapy in, 88-89
    ligation in, 88
    role of, in UGI bleeding, 87
    sclerotherapy in, 87-88
    therapeutic endoscopic procedures in, 87-89
Esophagus
    carcinoma of, 292, 294
        treatment of, 295-296
    trauma to, 616
Esters, anesthesia and, 43, 57
Estrogens, prostate cancer and, 709
Ethacrynic acid (Edecrin), 135, 376
Etidocaine hydrochloride (Duranest), 43, 57
Etomidate (Amidate), 47, 55
Euglobulin lysis time in evaluation of hemostasis, 777
Exotoxins, 815
Expiratory reserve volume, 151
Exstrophy in infants, 635-636
Extensor tendon injuries of hand, 835
External otitis, 857
Extracellular fluid, 122-123, 125, 126
Extracorporeal carbon dioxide removal, 792-794
Extracorporeal membrane oxygenation (ECMO), 640,
    792
Extrahepatic biliary system, abdominal masses and, 517
Extramammary Paget's disease, 553
Extubation in postanesthesia care, 49-50
Exudative diarrhea, 485

F

Face
    moon, Cushing's syndrome and, 375
    trauma to, 617
Facial fractures, 852-854
Facial lacerations, 853
Facial paralysis, 862-863
Factitial enteritis, diarrhea and, 493
Fallopian tubes
    abdominal masses and, 529
    abdominal pain and, 562-563, 566-567
Familial Mediterranean fever, abdominal pain and,
    562-563, 569
Familial medullary carcinoma syndrome, medullary
    cancer of thyroid and, 171
Family history, jaundice and, 465
Famotidine (Pepcid), 30, 217
Fascial cutaneous flaps, 848, 849
Fasciitis, necrotizing, 815
Fasting
    acute state of, 139
    before surgery, 31-32

Fat necrosis of breast, treatment of, 390
Fatigue, hypercalcemia and, 176
Fats
    absorption of, in gastrointestinal tract, 483
    gastroduodenal digestion and absorption and,
        198-200
Feeding tubes, placement of, esophagogastro-
    duodenoscopy and, 89
Felon, 818-819, 839-840
Femoral artery angioplasty, 78-80
Femoral hernia, 536, 538, 542
Femoral pulses, weak or absent, coarctation of aorta
    and, 343
Femur, fracture of, 676-677
Fentanyl citrate (Sublimaze), 47, 59
Ferguson hernia repair, 540, 541
Fever
    afferent limb of, 745-746
    definition of, 745-746
    drug, 753
    efferent limb of, 745-746
    familial Mediterranean, 562-563, 569
    jaundice and, 465
    pericarditis and, 362
    postoperative, 737, 739, 741
        caused by microorganisms, 751-752
        infection and, 820-823
        noninfectious causes of, 752-753
        secondary to bacteria from infection, 746-751
    pulmonary causes of, 746-748
    surgical patient with, imaging of, 71, 83
Fever curve, type of sepsis and, 618
Fiberoptic bronchoscopy, 878-879
Fiberoptic endoscopy; see Endoscopy
Fibrin plate lysis assays in evaluation of hemostasis, 777
Fibrinolysis, 774-775, 782
Fibrinolytic studies in evaluation of hemostasis, 777
Fibroadenoma, 388
    giant, treatment of, 390
    treatment of, 389
Fibroblastic growth factor, 222
Fibrocystic breast condition, 389-390
Fibroplasia, healing and, 608
Fibrosis, idiopathic retroperitoneal, 528
Fick equation, 34
Fick method, indirect, oxygen consumption and, 796
Filariasis, 708
Finger
    amputation of, 839
    drop, 835
    mallet, 835
    trigger, 841
Fingertip injuries, 838-839
Fissure, anal, 550-551
Fistula
    anorectal, 554-556
    arteriovenous, role of, in arteriovenous malformation,
        592
    coronary arteriovenous, 347
    gastrocolic, percutaneous endoscopic gastrostomy
        and, 93
    horseshoe, 556
    intestinal, persistent, 737
    surgery for, 556
    tracheoesophageal, in infants, 640-641

Fistula-in-ano, 555
Fistulectomy, 556
Fistulotomy, 556
Fixed phagocytes, infection and, 809
FK-506, transplantation and, 245, 246, 247, 248, 252
Flagyl (metronidazole), 456, 827
Flail chest, trauma and, 612
Flaps, 848-851
    fascial cutaneous, 848, 849
    muscle, 848-851
    musculocutaneous, 848-851
    random-pattern, 848, 849
    rhomboid, 848
    transverse rectus abdominis musculocutaneous,
      850-851
Flexeril (cyclobenzaprine), 732
Flexible sigmoidoscopy, 92
Flexor tendon injuries of hand, 835-837
Flocculation tests, liver function and, 467
Floxin (ofloxacin), 710
Fluconazole (Diflucan), 710, 827
Fluid
    and electrolyte exchange, physiology of, 123-125
    extracellular, 122-123, 125, 126
    intracellular, 122, 123
    in middle ear space, 859
Fluid management
    intraoperative, 39, 133
    postoperative, 133-134
    preoperative, 132-133
Fluid resuscitation, burn injury and, 624-625
Fluid volume, regulation of, arterial blood pressure and,
    370
Fluoroquinolones, urinary tract infections and, 710
5% Fluorouracil cream (Efudex), 559
Fluorouracil (5-FU), 234
Flutamide, 709
Foley catheter, 879
    insertion of, abdominal trauma and, 615
Follicular adenocarcinoma of thyroid, 283-284
Follicular cancer of thyroid, 169-171
Folliculitis, 818
Fontan operation
    hypoplastic left heart syndrome and, 342
    tricuspid atresia and, 338
Food poisoning, abdominal pain and, 562-563, 567
Foot, diabetic, 574
Foramen
    of Bochdalek, hernia through, 544-545, 639
    of Morgagni, hernia through, 544
    of tentorium cerebelli, 656
    of Winslow, hernia through, 545
Foregut obstruction, 451, 452, 453
Fortaz (ceftazidime), 710, 826
Fournier's gangrene, 714
Fracture
    avascular necrosis and, 680
    avulsion, 673
    blood loss and, 616
    blowout, 854
    boxer's, 838
    classification of, 672-673
    closed, 672
    Colles', 678
    comminuted, 670, 671, 673

Fracture—cont'd
    compartment syndrome and, 679
    contracture and muscle atrophy and, 681
    delayed union of, 681
    facial, 852-854
    of femur, 676-677
    greenstick, 670, 671, 673
    growth deformities and, 681
    hand, treatment of, 838
    hardware failure of plates and, 681
    healing of, 670-672
    hip, 676-677
    immobilization of, 674, 675
    impacted, 673
    infection and, 680
    lower extremity, 675-676
    management of, 674-675
    of mandible, 260
    of maxilla, 260
    nasal, 864-865
    nerve palsy and, 679
    nonunion of, 681
    oblique, 670, 671, 673
    open, 616, 672
      classification of, 672
    of orbital floor, 854
    osteomyelitis and, 680-681
    pathologic, 670, 671
    pelvic, 616-617, 676-677
    pulmonary embolism and, 680
    reduction of, 674-675
    reflex sympathetic dystrophy and, 679
    rehabilitation of, 674, 675
    segmental, 670, 671, 673
    skull, 616, 654-656
      basilar, 613, 654, 655
    soft tissue injuries and, 674, 676
    spinal, 677
    spiral, 670, 671, 673
    stabilization of, 674, 675
    talus, open reduction and internal fixation of,
      675
    transverse, 670, 671, 673
    traumatic arthritis and, 681
    upper extremity, 677-678
    vessel injury and, 679-681
    wrist, 678
Fracture callus, 671-672
Full-thickness burn, 621, 622, 626-627
Full-thickness skin graft, 847-848
Functional deafness, 861
Fungal sepsis, 823
Fungizone (amphotericin B), 827
Furosemide (Lasix), 135, 376
Furuncle, 818
Fusiform aneurysm, 363, 364

G

Gadolinium (Magnevist), 83
Gallbladder
    abdominal masses and, 517
    carcinoma of, 517-518
    empyema of, 517
    hydrops of, 517
Gallbladder disease, laparoscopy for, 104-111

Gallium-67 scanning, versus indium-111 leukocyte scanning, 71
Gallstone ileus, 454
Gallstones, 464
    risk factors for prevalence of, 464
Ganglion, 603, 841
Gangrene
    aerobic, 814
    anaerobic, 814-815
    of bowel, in infants, 651-652
    degree of, operative risk and, 16
    Fournier's, 714
    gas, 815
    infection and, 808
    infectious, 814-815
    synergistic, 815
Gangrenous hernia, 532
Gangrenous intestinal obstruction in infants, 651
Garamycin (gentamicin sulfate), 710, 828
Gas exchange in lung, 152-153
Gas gangrene, 815
Gastric acid secretion, physiology of, 200-203
Gastric anacidity, watery diarrhea syndrome and, 190
Gastric cancer, 216
Gastric electrolytes, 200, 201
Gastric motor activity, physiology of, 200
Gastric ulcer
    diagnosis of, 208
    gastrointestinal bleeding and, 411
    indications for operation in, 209
    management of, 208
Gastrin, 203, 204-205
    gastrinomas and, 189
Gastrinoma, 189, 207, 213, 497
Gastritis, hemorrhagic, gastrointestinal bleeding and, 410
Gastrocolic fistula, percutaneous endoscopic gastrostomy and, 93
Gastroduodenal defensive factors, 206
Gastroduodenal digestion and absorption, physiology of, 197-200
Gastroduodenal physiology and peptic ulcer disease, 196-219
Gastroduodenostomy, 212
Gastroenterostomy and truncal vagotomy, 211-212
Gastrointestinal bleeding
    angiodysplasia and, 417
    arteriovenous malformation and, 417
    chronic, 418-419
    colonic underperfusion and, 417-418
    detection of, with angiography, 78, 79
    diagnosis of, 407-408
    diverticular disease of colon and, 416-418
    duodenal ulcer and, 408-410
    esophageal variceal hemorrhage and, 411-414
    esophagitis and, 414-415
    etiology of, 403, 404
    gastric ulcers and, 411
    hemoptysis and, 302
    hemorrhagic gastritis and, 410, 411
    hemorrhoids and, 418
    initial clinical approach to, 404-407
    from lower gastrointestinal tract, 416-418
    Mallory-Weiss' syndrome and, 415-416
    patient history in, 407

Gastrointestinal bleeding—cont'd
    physical examination in, 407-408
    physiology of, 403-404
    polyps and, 418
    postirradiated bowel and, 418
    radiology in, 408
    from small intestine, 416
    ulcerative colitis and, 417
Gastrointestinal endocrine tumors, 188
Gastrointestinal evaluation of abdominal masses, 509
Gastrointestinal hormones, 203, 204-205
Gastrointestinal obstruction
    of later infancy, 649-651
    masses associated with, 511
Gastrointestinal secretions, composition of, 125
Gastrointestinal system, abdominal masses and, 506
Gastrointestinal tract
    carbohydrate absorption and, 483
    cellulose and, 483
    contrast studies of, 473
    fat absorption and, 483
    free intraperitoneal perforations of, 446-448
    protein absorption and, 483
    transit in, affect of on bowel movements, 483-484, 485
    water absorption and, 482-483
Gastroschisis, 544
    in infants, 635-636
    surgical repair of, 635
Gastrostomy, 145
Gaviscon, 300
GCS; see Glasgow Coma Scale
General anesthesia, 46-48
Genitourinary system, lesions of, abdominal pain and, 562-563, 566-567
Genitourinary tuberculosis, 707
Gentamicin sulfate (Garamycin), 710, 828
Giant cell arteritis, abdominal pain and, 569
Giant fibroadenoma, treatment of, 390
Gingiva, upper, tumors of, 267
Gingivitis, 262
GIP, 204-205
Glasgow Coma Scale, 607, 660, 661
Glucagon, 203, 217
Glucagonoma, 497
Glucagonoma syndrome, 191-192
Glucocorticoid equivalencies, 184
Gluconeogenesis, 141
Glycopyrrolate, 30, 54
Goiter, congenital, in infants, 638
Gonorrhea, 714
Goodsall's rule, 555
Gout, manifestations of, in hand, 841
Graft, skin; see Skin graft
Granulocytes, neutrophilic, infection and, 809
Granuloma, reparative, 262-263
Granuloma inguinale, 713-714
Graves' disease, 164
Greenstick fracture, 670, 671, 673
Groin hernias, 536-538
Growth deformities, fracture and, 681
Growth factors, relationship of, to cancer, 221, 222
Growth plates, fractures and, 681

Guanethidine (Ismelin sulfate), 376
Gustilo's classification of open fractures, 672
Gynecologic system, abdominal masses and, 506

H

Halcion (triazolam), 235
Halothane, 56
Halsted hernia repair, 539
Hand
    anesthetics and, 831
    bone and joint injuries of, assessment of, 837-838
    burns of, 840-841
    chronic conditions of, 841
    extensor tendon injuries of, 835
    flexor tendon injuries of, 835-837
    fractures of, treatment of, 838
    human bites in, 840
    nerve compression syndromes of, 833-835
    nerves of, examination of, 831-835
    vascularity of, assessment of, 831
Hand infections, 818-820, 839-840
Hand injury, initial approach to, 830-831
Hand surgery, basic principles of, 830-844
Hard palate, tumors of, 267
Harris-Benedict equations, estimation of energy needs by, 141
Hashimoto's thyroiditis, 166
Haustral contractions, 483
Hay fever, 863
Head injury
    of children versus adults, 659-660
    closed versus penetrating, 658-659
    diagnostic studies and, 663-664
    factors determining outcome after, 665-666
    hyperventilation and, 665
    increased intracranial pressure and, 664-665
    infection and, 665
    initial evaluation and treatment of, 661-664
    patient history and, 662-663
    severe, management of, 664-665
    signs and symptoms of, 660-661
Head trauma, severe, common brain lesions from, 657-658
Headache, postconcussion syndrome and, 660
Healing, 608, 609
Hearing loss, 859-861
Heart, abdominal pain and, 565
Heart block, 347
Heart disease
    classification of, 319, 320
    ischemic; see Ischemic heart disease
Heart failure
    cardiac tamponade with, trauma and, 612
    origin of left coronary artery from pulmonary artery and, 346
    physiologic classification of, 317
    right-sided, Ebstein's malformation and, 341
Heart murmur
    acquired, valve disease in, 315-328
    congenital, 329-348
Heart transplantation; see Cardiac transplantation
Heartburn
    antacids for, 300
    difficulties in swallowing and, 290-291
    hiatal hernia and, 292

Heart-lung transplantation, 252-253
Heater probe, esophagogastroduodenoscopy and, 88
Heavy metal poisoning, abdominal pain and, 562-563, 567
Heberden's nodes, 841
Helper cells, infection and, 809
Helper T-lymphocytes, transplantation and, 242-243
Hemangioma, 259, 262, 597
    capillary, 259
    cavernous, 259
    sclerosing, 259
Hematemesis, esophageal rupture and, 292
Hematocrit level, 403-404
Hematologic disorders amenable to splenectomy, 518-519
Hematoma
    epidural, 657
    nasal septal, 864
    scrotal, 716
    subdural, 656-657
Hematuria
    in adults, 688-691
    causes of, 684, 685
    in children, 686-691
    diagnosis of, 684
    in elderly persons, 691
    painless, 686
    physical characteristics of red cells in, 684-685
    pyuria and, 688-689
    secondary to prostatic enlargement, 691
    sexually transmitted infections and, 689-690
    trauma and, 690-691
    urinary stones and, 686, 688, 691
Heme, bilirubin metabolism and, 461
Hemigastrectomy, truncal vagotomy with, for duodenal ulcer, 212
Hemodynamic changes
    improper patient positioning and, 41
    in postanesthesia care, 49-52
Hemodynamic management, intraoperative, 39
Hemolytic disease, abdominal pain and, 562-563, 569
Hemolytic jaundice, 460
Hemophilia A, 778
Hemophilia B, 778
Hemoptysis
    bacterial pneumonia and, 306
    bronchiectasis and, 307-308
    causes of, 302, 304
    chest x-ray examination and, 308-309
    diagnosis of, 302-304
    evaluation of, 304-305
    life-threatening, management of, 305-306
    lung abscess and, 306-307
    massive, definition of, 306
    pulmonary infarction and, 307
    pulmonary lesions and, 302-314
    pulmonary tuberculosis and, 308
    treatment of, 305-306
Hemorrhage
    esophageal variceal, gastrointestinal bleeding and, 411-414
    fracture and, 616
    as indication for operation in peptic ulcer disease, 209
    intracranial, 656-657
    lacerations of oral cavity and, 260

Hemorrhage—cont'd
  management of, trauma and, 609, 613
  rate of, gastrointestinal bleeding and, 404
  subarachnoid, 656
Hemorrhagic gastritis
  diffuse, 410
  gastrointestinal bleeding and, 410
Hemorrhagic shock, massive hemoptysis and, 306
Hemorrhoidal tag, 549
Hemorrhoids
  external, 557, 559
  gastrointestinal bleeding and, 418
  internal, 557-559
Hemostasis
  evaluation of, 775-777
  laboratory tests of, 776-777
  normal, 773-775
  surgical bleeding and, 773-785
Hemothorax, 156, 616
Henderson-Hasselbalch equation, 127
Heparin, 160, 593, 780
  inadequate anticoagulation with, coagulopathies and, 782
Heparin sodium, 784
Heparin-induced thrombocytopenia, 368
Heparin-induced thrombosis, 368
Hepatic reserve, Child's classification of, 412, 413
Hepatitis
  chronic active, liver transplantation and, 251
  delta, 824
  infectious, 823
  non-A, non-B, 824
  postoperative fever and, 751
  serum, 823-824
  viral, 823-824
    test for, 468-469
Hepatitis A (HAV), 823
Hepatitis B (HBV), 823-824
  blood transfusion and, 18
Hepatitis C (HCV), 824
  blood transfusion and, 17-18
Hepatitis D (HDV), 824
Hepatitis E (HEV), 824
Hereditary skin cancers, 599
Hernia
  abdominal, 545
  acquired, 533-534
  of anterior abdominal wall, 542-544
  classification, 532
  complications of, 534
  congenital, 533
  definition of, 532
  diaphragmatic, 544-545
  direct inguinal, 536, 538
  epigastric, 543
  femoral, 536, 538, 542
  gangrenous, 532
  groin, 536-538
  hiatal; see Hiatal hernia
  incarcerated, 532
  incisional, 544
  indirect inguinal, 536, 537-538
  in infants, 639-640
  inguinal; see Inguinal hernia
  internal, 545

Hernia—cont'd
  of Littre, 532
  pathogenesis and diagnosis of, 533-534
  repair of, 535-542
    indications for, 534
  Richter's, 532
  rupture of, 534
  scrotal, imaging of, 75
  sliding, 532
  spigelian, 544
  strangulated, 532
  treatment of, 534-536
  types of, 536-545
Hernia reduction, 532
  en masse, 532
  nonoperative, 534-535
Herniation, uncal, 656
Herniorrhaphy, 535-536
  laparoscopic, 120
Herpes simplex, 262
Hesselbach's triangle, direct inguinal hernia and, 538
Heterotopic transplantation, 237, 241
HEV; see Hepatitis E
Hiatal hernia, 292, 293, 294, 296-297, 298
  esophageal, 544
  esophageal carcinoma and, 292
Hidradenitis, 818
High midgut obstruction, 451-454
High-frequency positive pressure ventilation, 792
High-output renal failure, postoperative, 134
Hindgut obstruction, 452, 454
Hip fracture, 676-677
Hirschsprung's disease in infants, 646-648
Histiocytes, tissue, infection and, 809
HIV; see Human immunodeficiency virus
HLA complex; see Human leukocyte antigen (HLA) complex
Hoarseness
  laryngeal cancer and, 867
  persistent, chest x-ray examination and, 308-309
Hormone binding, breast cancer and, 399
Hormones, gastrointestinal, 203, 204-205
Horseshoe abscess, 820
Horseshoe fistula, 556
Host defenses, tumor aggressiveness and, 224
Host resistance, infection and, 808-809
Human immunodeficiency virus (HIV), 824
Human leukocyte antigen (HLA) complex in transplantation, 241
Humoral immunity, infection and, 809
Humoral rejection, transplantation and, 244
Hurricaine (benzocaine), 43, 57
Hydatid of Morgagni, cysts in, 715
Hydralazine (Apresoline), 54, 376, 377, 803
Hydramnios, maternal, intestinal obstruction of newborn and, 641-642
Hydration, preoperative preparation of jaundiced patient and, 474
Hydrocele, 714-715
Hydrocephalus, meningocele and, in infants, 636
Hydrochloric acid, 135
Hydrochlorothiazide (Esidrix; Hydrodiuril; Oretic), 376
Hydrocortisone, 184
Hydrocortisone acetate 1% and pramoxine hydrochloride 1% (ProctoCream-HC), 559

Hydrodiuril (hydrochlorothiazide), 376
Hydronephrosis, 522
Hydropneumothorax, esophageal rupture and, 292
Hydrops of gallbladder, 517
Hydroxyzine hydrochloride (Vistaril), 30, 59
Hyperaldosteronism
    hypertension and, 375
    primary, 184
Hyperbilirubinemia
    conjugated, 461
    unconjugated, 461
Hypercalcemia, 130
    causes of, 177
    primary hyperparathyroidism and, 175
    watery diarrhea syndrome and, 190
Hypercapnia, 21
Hypercarotinemia, jaundice and, 464-465
Hypergastrinemia, 213
Hyperkalemia, 130
Hypermagnesemia, 131
Hypernatremia, 126-127, 132-133
    postoperative, 134
Hypernephroma, 524
Hyperparathyroidism
    primary, 175-180
        diagnosis of, 172, 176, 177
        hypercalcemia and, 176-177
        localization of parathyroid adenomas in, 178-179
        location of abnormal parathyroid glands in, 177-178
        pathology of, 177
        principles of exploration in, 179
        serum calcium level and, 176
    secondary, 175
Hyperplasia
    adrenal, adrenal tumors and, 181-182
    bilateral, aldosteronoma and, 185
Hypertension, 370-378
    coarctation of aorta and, 374
    Cushing's syndrome and, 375
    diagnosis of, 370, 371-372, 373
    drugs in control of, 376-377
    essential, 372-374
    hyperaldosteronism and, 375
    pathophysiology of, 370-371
    pheochromocytoma and, 185-186, 375
    renal artery stenosis and, 374
    surgically correctable, 372, 373, 374-375
    unilateral renal parenchymal disease and, 374-375
    upper extremity, coarctation of aorta and, 343
Hyperthermia, malignant, fever and, 753
Hyperthyroidism, 73
    fever and, 753
Hypertonic citrate solution, transplantation and, 239, 240
Hypertrophy of adenoid tissue, nasal obstruction and, 863-864
Hyperventilation, head trauma and, 665
Hypocalcemia, 130
    hypoparathyroidism and, 179
Hypocapnia, 21
Hypokalemia, 130
    watery diarrhea syndrome and, 190
Hypomagnesemia, 131
Hyponatremia, 126, 132-133
    postoperative, 134

Hypopharynx, examination of, 258
Hypophosphatemia
    hyperparathyroidism and, 177
    primary hyperparathyroidism and, 175
Hypoplastic left heart syndrome, 341-342
Hypospadias in infants, 636
Hypothalamic contusion, fever and, 753
Hypothermia, organ preservation and, in transplantation, 238-239, 241
Hypothyroidism, 73
Hypovolemic shock, 759
Hypoxemia
    congenital heart defects and, 331
    postoperative, 737, 738
Hypoxia, 21
    tetralogy of Fallot and, 338, 339
Hypoxic paralysis of bowel, 498
Hytrin (terazosin hydrochloride), 709

I

^{131}I metaiodobenzylguanidine (^{131}I MIBG), 187
^{123}I metaiodobenzylguanidine (^{123}I MIBG), 74, 83
Ibuprofen (Motrin), 731, 743
Iceberg effect, bronchial adenomas and, 309
ICP; *see* Intracranial pressure
Idiopathic retroperitoneal fibrosis, 528
    ureteral obstruction and, 696
IL-2 toxins, transplantation and, 248
Ileocecal intussusception, 512
Illness
    cumulative, rating scale for, 23
    duration of, operative risk and, 14-16
    natural history of, 10
Imepinim and cilastatin (Primaxin), 456, 828
Immobilization of fracture, 674, 675
Immune response to transplantation antigens, 241-245
Immunity
    cellular, infection and, 809
    humoral, infection and, 809
Immunoglobulins, infection and, 809
Immunologic tests in assessment of nutritional status, 139
Immunosuppressive therapy, transplantation and, 245-248
Impacted fracture, 673
Implantable pumps, intra-arterial chemotherapy and, 268
Imuran (azathioprine), transplantation and, 245
Incarcerated hernia, 532
Incisional hernia, 544
Incisional problems, postoperative, 740, 741
Incontinence, abnormal defecation and, 496
Independent lung ventilation, 789
Inderal (propranolol hydrochloride), 193, 376
Indirect inguinal hernia, 536, 537-538
Indium-111 leukocyte scanning, 83
    versus gallium-67 scanning, 71
Induction anesthetic agents, 55
Infant
    abdominal distention in, 642
    absence of normal meconium stool in, 642
    anal atresia in, 644-645, 646-647
    bowel gangrene in, 651-652
    cervical teratoma in, 638
    choanal atresia in, 637

Infant—cont'd
   congenital absence of abdominal musculature in, 635
   congenital goiter in, 638
   congenital lobar emphysema in, 639
   correction of dehydration and electrolyte deficits in, 632
   daily caloric requirements for, 633
   defects in body mantle of, 633-635
   diaphragmatic hernia in, 639-640
   duodenal obstruction in, 642, 643
   duplications of intestinal tract in, 650-651
   encephalocele in, 636
   epispadias in, 635-636
   esophageal atresia in, 640-641, 642
   exstrophy in, 635-636
   gangrenous intestinal obstruction in, 651
   gastrointestinal obstructions in, 649-651
   gastroschisis in, 635-636
   Hirschsprung's disease in, 646-648
   hydrocephalus in, 636
   hypospadias in, 636
   intestinal atresia in, 642-643
   intestinal obstruction in, 641-648
   intussusception in, 649-650
   maintenance requirement for water and electrolytes in, 632
   malrotation of colon and, 645
   massive pneumoperitoneum in, 640
   Meckel's diverticulum in, 650
   meconium ileus in, 645-646
   meningocele in, 636
   metabolic rate of, 632, 633
   myelomeningocele in, 636
   necrotizing enterocolitis in, 651-652
   omphalocele in, 633-635
   Pierre-Robin syndrome in, 637-638
   pneumothorax in, 639
   pyloric stenosis in, 649
   rachischisis in, 636
   respirations of, 631
   respiratory distress syndromes in, 636-641
   strangulating midgut volvulus in, 651
   temperature control of, 631
   tracheoesophageal fistula in, 640-641
   tracheomalacia in, 638
Infantile polycystic kidney disease, 524
Infarction
   myocardial; *see* Myocardial infarction
   pulmonary, hemoptysis and, 307
Infection
   abscess and, 813-814
   acquired immunodeficiency syndrome and, 824
   antibiotic treatment of, 811-812
   bacteria from, postoperative fever secondary to, 746-751
   burn injury and, 627
   cellulitis and, 813
   collarbutton, 819
   common forms of, 817-823
   delayed healing and, 608, 609
   diagnosis of, 811
   ear; *see* Ear infections
   fracture and, 680
   gangrene and, 808, 814-815
   hand, 818-820

Infection—cont'd
   host resistance and, 808-809
   human immunodeficiency virus and, 824
   inoculum and, 807-808
   intra-abdominal, postoperative fever and, 748-749
   from intravascular devices, postoperative fever and, 750
   invasive, bacterial colonization and, 808
   of lumbar spine region, 729-730
   malnutrition and, 139
   midpalmar space, 819-820
   nutrient medium and, 808
   of oral cavity, 261-262
   pathophysiology of, 807-809
   phlegmon and, 813
   postoperative fever and, 751, 752-753, 820-823
   pulmonary, 21
      recurrent, arch anomalies and, 347
   risk factors for, in elective biliary tract operations, 433
   salivary gland, 866
   scrotal, 714
   septicemia and, 816-817
   severe head trauma and, 665
   skin, 817-818
   surgical, classification of, 812-817
   thenar space, 819
   toxemia and, 815-816
   trauma and, 617, 618
   urinary tract; *see* Urinary tract infections
   viral, 823-824
   viral hepatitis and, 823-824
   visceral compartment, postoperative fever and, 748-750
   web space, 819
   wound; *see* Wound infection
Infectious gangrene, 814
Infectious hepatitis, 823
Inferior vena cava filters, 82
Inflammation, 608
   cellular component of, 608
   of fallopian tubes, 529
   vascular portion of, 608
Inflammatory bowel disease, colonoscopy for, 91
Inflammatory breast carcinoma, 398
Inflammatory neck masses, 272-277, 278
Informed consent
   anesthesia and, 52-53
   for needle localization, 70
Ingrown nail, 818
Inguinal hernia, 714
   direct, 536, 538
   incarcerated, 716
   indirect, 536, 537-538
   in infants, 649
Inhalation anesthetics, 48, 55-56
Initiator state of cancer, 220
Injection sclerotherapy for varicose veins, 591
Injury; *see also* Trauma
   ear trauma and, 863
   electrical, burn injury and, 622
   head; *see* Head injury
   local response to, 608
   musculoskeletal, 669-683
   pulmonary, 621, 622-624

Injury—cont'd
    systemic management of, 609-610
    systemic response to, 609, 610
Injury Severity Scale (ISS), 607-608
Inocor (amrinone lactate), 56, 769, 770
Inoculum, infection and, 807-808
Inositol 1,4,5-triphosphate (IP$_3$), transplantation and,
    243
Inotropes, anesthesia and, 56
Inspiratory reserve volume, 151
Inspiratory vital capacity, 151
Insulin growth factors I and II, 222
Insulin with dextrose, 135
Insulinoma, 190
Interferons, 223
Interleukin-1, 245, 745, 746
Interleukin-2 (IL-2), transplantation and, 247-248
Intermittent positive-pressure breathing device, 155-156
Internal hernias, 545
Internal jugular line, 873-874
Interventional radiology, 75-78
Intestinal adhesions, acute constipation and, 497, 498
Intestinal atresia in infants, 642-643
Intestinal bacteria, metabolic effects of, 481, 482
Intestinal fistulas, persistent, 737
Intestinal obstruction, 449-455
    foregut, 451, 452, 453
    gangrenous, in infants, 651
    high midgut, 451-454
    hindgut, 452, 454
    low midgut, 452-454
    of newborn, 641-648
    partial small bowel, 454
    strangulation, 452, 455
Intestinal tract, duplications of, in infants, 650-651
Intestine
    large, 483
    small; see Small intestine
Intra-abdominal abscess, 822-823
Intra-abdominal infection, postoperative fever and,
    748-749
Intra-aortic balloon pump, 359
Intra-arterial catheter, 763
    in intraoperative monitoring, 33
Intra-arterial chemotherapy for intraoral tumors, 268
Intracellular fluid, 122, 123
Intracranial arteries, anatomy of, 380, 381
Intracranial hemorrhage, 656-657
Intracranial pressure (ICP), increased, severe head
    trauma and, 664-665
Intractability, duodenal ulcer and, 210
Intraepidermal carcinoma, 553
Intramuscular analgesics, in postoperative pain
    management, 51
Intranasal masses, nasal obstruction and, 863
Intraoperative fluid management, 133
Intraoperative fluid therapy, 39
Intraoperative hemodynamic management, 39
Intraoperative monitoring, anesthesia and, 32-41
    fluid therapy and, 39-40
    hemodynamic management and, 39
    ventilatory support and, 38
Intraoperative physiologic support, 32-41
Intraoperative ventilatory support, 38
Intraoral lesions, 257-271

Intraoral tumors, multimodal therapy for, 268, 269
Intraperitoneal masses, 511-512
Intraperitoneal perforations, free, of gastrointestinal
    tract, 446-448
Intrathecal opioids in postoperative pain management,
    52
Intravascular devices, infections from, postoperative
    fever and, 750
Intravenous access, burn injury and, 624
Intravenous anesthetics, 46-48
Intravenous cannula, trauma and, 611
Intravenous conscious sedation, administration of,
    42-43
Intravenous line, placement of, abdominal trauma and,
    615
Intrinsic bowel disease, malabsorption resulting from,
    488-494
Intropin (dopamine), 769, 770
Intussusception
    ileocecal, 512
    in infants, 649-650
    surgical repair of, 650
Invasive hemodynamic monitoring in critical care, 794
Invasive infection, bacterial colonization and, 808
Inverse ratio ventilation, 790
Iodine-123 versus technetium-99m sodium
    pertechnetate, 71-72
Ionotropes, 803-804
Irradiation to neck, relationship of, to thyroid cancer,
    169-170
Irritable bowel syndrome, 501
Ischemia
    acute, 571-572
    chronic, 572
    following fracture, 616
    limb; see Limb ischemia
    origin of left coronary artery from pulmonary artery
        and, 347
Ischemic colitis, 449
Ischemic heart disease
    acute myocardial infarction and, 355-357
    angina pectoris and, 350-353
    coronary artery revascularization and, 355
    natural history of, 349-350
    symptoms of, 349
Ischemic lower extremity, 571-583
Ischemic small bowel disease, 448-449
Islet transplantation, 250-251
Ismelin sulfate (guanethidine), 376
Isoflurane, 56
Isoniazid (Laniazid; Nydarzin; Teebaconin), 827
Isoproterenol (Isuprel), 769, 770
Isoptin (verapamil), 377
ISS; see Injury Severity Scale
Isuprel (isoproterenol), 769, 770

J

Jatene operation, transposition of great arteries and,
    340
Jaundice
    acute cholecystitis and, 433
    choledochoduodenostomy in, 476
    choledochotomy in, 475
    cholestatic, 465-466
    classification of, 461

Jaundice—cont'd
  common duct stricture and, 476-477
  diagnosis of, 464-466
  diagnostic imaging techniques in, 469-473
  endoscopic retrograde cholangiopancreatography in,
      470-472, 478
  hematologic tests in, 468-469
  hemolytic, 460
  indications for surgical intervention in, 473-474
  liver biopsy in, 473
  liver transplantation and, 477
  obstructive, 469
    nonoperative relief of, 478
  papillotomy and, 478
  patient history in, 465-466
  percutaneous transhepatic cholangiography in, 470
  periampullary carcinoma and, 477-478
  physical examination in, 466
  posthepatic, 460
  retained common duct stones and, 476
  sclerosing cholangitis and, 477
  stenting and, 478
  surgical, 460
  surgical approach to patient with, 474-478
  transduodenal sphincteroplasty in, 475-476
Juxtaglomerular apparatus, 184

K

Kaposi's angiosarcoma, 597
Kaposi's sarcoma, 597
  in oral cavity, 269-270
Kayexalate (sodium polystyrene sulfonate), 135
Keflet (cephalexin), 825
Keflex (cephalexin), 825
Keflin (cephalothin), 825
Kefzol (cefazolin sodium), 456, 710, 825
Keloid, 597, 846
Keratosis, 596-597
  epidermoid carcinoma of oral cavity and, 264
Kernohan's notch, 656
Kessler tendon repair, 837
Ketamine (Ketalar), 47, 55
Ketorolac (Toradol), 58, 731
Kidney
  abdominal masses and, 522
  abdominal pain and, 562-563, 566
  adenocarcinoma of, 525
  anatomy of, 522
  multicystic, 524
  multilocular cysts of, 524
  simple cysts of, 523
Kidney disease, polycystic, 524
Kidney transplantation, 248-249
Killer cells, infection and, 809

L

Labetalol (Normodyne; Trandate), 54, 376, 377
Laboratory tests
  preoperative, operative risk and, 24-25
  required for anesthesia, 29
  selection of anesthetic technique and, 42
Labyrinthine hydrops, 862
Lacerations of oral cavity, 260
Lactose intolerance, abdominal pain and, 562-563, 568
Lag, healing and, 608

Laniazid (isoniazid), 827
Laparoscopic cholangiography, 106, 108
Laparoscopic cholecystectomy, 104-111, 436-437
Laparoscopic colon resection, 118-120
Laparoscopic herniorrhaphy, 120
Laparoscopic Nissen fundoplication, 117
Laparoscopic stapling devices, 98, 115, 119
Laparoscopic vagotomy, 112-116
Laparoscopic-assisted colectomy, 118-120
Laparoscopy
  for acute appendicitis, 102-104
  for benign or malignant colon disease, 118-120
  diagnostic and therapeutic, 95-121
  for esophageal reflux, 116-118
  for gallbladder disease, 104-111
  instrumentation for, 96-98
  patient preparation for, 98-99
  for peptic ulcer disease, 111-116
  requirements of, 96-98
  use of, in general surgery, 100-102
Laparotomy, exploratory, jaundice and, 466
Large intestine, transit in, effect of, on bowel
    movements, 483
Laryngeal cancer, 867
Laryngeal lesions, 866-867
Laryngeal nerve, superior, injury to, 180
Laryngeal papilloma, 866
Laryngeal paralysis, voice quality and, 867
Laryngomalacia, 866
Laryngoscopy, 857, 858
Larynx
  examination of, 258
  squamous cell carcinoma of, 867
Laser
  intravascular use of, 80-81
  YAG, esophagogastroduodenoscopy and, 88
Laser coagulation, colonoscopy and, 91
Laser therapy, esophagogastroduodenoscopy and, 88-89
Lasix (furosemide), 135, 376
Lazaroids, head injury and, 665
Lead colic, abdominal pain and, 567
Lead poisoning, abdominal pain and, 567
Lean body mass, 139
LeFort levels of facial fractures, 853-854
Left coronary artery, origin of, from pulmonary artery,
    347
Left ventricular assist devices, 359-361
Left ventricular end-diastolic pressure (LVEDP), 34
Left ventricular end-diastolic volume (LVEDV), 34
Left ventricular failure, aortic stenosis and, 344
Left-side appendicitis, 514
Left-to-right shunts, defects associated with,
    332-335
Leg, swelling of; see Swelling, lower extremity
Leriche syndrome, 572
Lesions
  of central nervous system, abdominal pain and,
      565-566
  coin, 309-310
  of genitourinary system, abdominal pain and,
      562-563, 566-567
  intraoral, 257-271
  localized in thorax, abdominal pain and, 562-563,
      564-565
  of peritoneum, abdominal pain and, 567

Lesser sac collections, 520, 521
Leukoplakia, epidermoid carcinoma of oral cavity and, 264
Leuprolide acetate (Lupron Depot), 709
Leutinizing hormone-releasing hormone (LHRH) agonists, prostate cancer and, 709
Levophed bitartrate (norepinephrine bitartrate), 56
Levophed (norepinephrine), 770
LHRH; *see* Leutinizing hormone-releasing hormone agonists
Lidocaine hydrochloride (Xylocaine), 43, 57, 871
Life expectancy of aged patient, operative risk and, 14
Ligament, sprain of, 674, 676
Ligation, esophagogastroduodenoscopy and, 88
Limb ischemia, 571-573, 581-583
Linear fracture of skull, 654
Lingual thyroid, 258-259
Lip, cleft, 258
Lip tumors, 266, 267
Lipid emulsions, total parenteral nutrition and, 142
Lipoma, 602-603
Littre, hernia of, 532
Liver
    abdominal masses and, 516-517
    carcinoma of, 516, 517
    enzymatic functions of, jaundice and, 466-467
    excretory functions of, 468
    metabolic functions of, 467-468
Liver biopsy, 473
Liver transplantation, 251-252
    jaundice and, 477
Living related donor (LRD), 241, 250
Lobar emphysema, congenital, in infants, 639
Local anesthesia, 57, 870, 871
    complications of, 44
    difference between monitored anesthesia care and, 42
    epinephrine and, 44-45
    systemic toxicity of, 43-44
Local resistance, infection and, 808-809
Lomotil (diphenoxylate/atropine), 235
Loop diuretics, 376
Lopressor (metoprolol), 376
Lorazepam (Ativan), 30, 47, 55, 235
Low back pain, 719-732
    intractable, 730-731
Low midgut obstruction, 452-454
Lower esophageal complex, 289, 290
Lower extremity
    fracture of, 675-676
    ischemic, 571-583
LRD; *see* Living related donor
Ludwig's angina, 261-262
Lumbar disk syndrome, 719-723
    history of, 719-720
    physical examination and, 720, 721
    radiographic studies of, 720-723
    treatment of, 723
Lumbar hernia, 545
Lumbar spondylosis, 728-729
Lump in breast, 384-402
    aspiration of mass in, 388
    biopsy of, 389
    clinical approach in, 386-389
    cytologic examination of, 388-389
    diagnosis of, 384-389

Lump in breast—cont'd
    patient history in, 384
    physical examination in, 384-386
Lung
    anatomy of, 302, 303
    carcinoma of, 21
    gas exchange in, 152-153
    lesions localized to, abdominal pain and, 564-565
    role of, in acid-base balance, 154
Lung abscess, hemoptysis and, 306-307
Lung cancer, 309-310
Lung resection, 20, 22
Lung water accumulation, intraoperative change in pulmonary compliance and, 39
Lupron Depot (leuprolide acetate), 709
LVEDP; *see* Left ventricular end-diastolic pressure
LVEDV; *see* Left ventricular end-diastolic volume
Lycopenemia, jaundice and, 465
Lye, chemical burns of oral cavity and, 260
Lymph nodes
    cancer surgery and, 229-230
    in head and neck, 276
Lymphadenitis
    acute, 811
    suppurative, 811
Lymphangioma, 597
Lymphangitis, acute, 811
    lower extremity swelling and, 593
Lymphatic abnormalities, lower extremity swelling and, 592-593
Lymphatic system, diseases of, lower extremity swelling and, 592-593
Lymphocytes
    B-cell, 809
    host resistance and, 809
Lymphocytic thyroiditis, 166
Lymphogranuloma venereum, 713
Lymphoma, metastasis of to breast, 390
Lysodren (mitotane o,p'-DDD), 193

M

Macrodantin (nitrofurantoin), 709
Magnesium abnormalities, 130-131
Magnesium deficiency, 131
Magnesium excess, 131
Magnetic resonance imaging (MRI)
    versus computed tomography, 61-67
    guidelines for, 63-64
Magnevist (gadolinium), 83
Major histocompatibility complex (MHC) in transplantation, 241
Malabsorption, gastrointestinal tract and
    abnormal substances in stool and, 486-487
    bacterial enteritis and, 493
    chronic pancreatitis and, 485-486
    Crohn's disease and, 488-490
    decreased transit time due to neoplasms and, 493-494
    defective digestion and, 485-486
    enteritis and, 493
    mechanical short circuits and, 487-488
    obstruction of pancreatic duct and, 486
    resulting from intrinsic bowel disease, 488-494
    resulting from rapid transit, 486-487
    short bowel syndromes and, 487-488
    ulcerative colitis and, 490-493

Maldescent of testis, 717-718
Male breast cancer, 397
Malignancy, fever and, 753
Malignant hyperthermia, fever and, 753
Malignant lesions of breast, treatment of, 390-398
Malignant melanoma, 597
  metastasis of, to breast, 390
Malignant mixed tumors, 268-269
Malignant skin lesions, 597-602
Malignant soft tissue neoplasms, 603-604
Mallet finger, 835
Mallory-Weiss' syndrome, gastrointestinal bleeding and, 415-416
Malnutrition, 139
Malrotation of colon in infants, 645
Mammography, 67-68, 83
  American Cancer Society's recommendations for screening examinations by, 68
  equipment for, 67
  significant findings on, 68
  types of cancers detected by, 68
Mandatory minute volume, 790
Mandelamine (methenamine mandelate), 709
Mandible, fracture of, 260
MAO; *see* Maximal acid output
Marcaine hydrochloride (bupivacaine), 43, 57, 871
Marfan's syndrome, 365, 366
Marginal ulcer, 213, 214-215
Marjolin's ulcer, 598
Masses, neck; *see* Neck masses
Massive pneumoperitoneum in infants, 640
Maternal hydramnios, intestinal obstruction of newborn and, 641-642
Maxilla, fracture of, 260
Maxillofacial trauma, 852-854
Maximal acid output (MAO), duodenal ulcer and, 206
Maximal expiratory flow rate, 151
Maximal midexpiratory flow, 151
Maximal voluntary ventilation, 151
McBurney's point, acute appendicitis and, 427
MCHA antibodies; *see* Antimicrosomal antibodies
MCT; *see* Medullary adenocarcinoma
McVay hernia repair, 541
Mechanical fragility test, jaundice and, 468
Mechanical work of breathing, 793
Meckel's diverticulum in infants, 650
Meconium ileus in infants, 645-646
Meconium stool, normal, absence of, intestinal obstruction of newborn and, 642
Mediastinal tumors, 312, 313
Medical anti-shock trousers (MAST), 616
Medullary adenocarcinoma (MCT) of thyroid, 284
Medullary cancer of thyroid, 171-172
Mefamide (sulfamylon), 628
Mefoxin (cefoxitin sodium), 455, 826
Megacolon, toxic, 493
Melanin spots on lips, multiple, Peutz-Jeghers syndrome and, 258
Melanoma
  anorectal, 553
  cutaneous, 599-602
  malignant, 390, 597
Melena, 418
  upper gastrointestinal bleeding and, 87
Meleney's cellulitis, 808

Melphalan, 235
Memory loss, postconcussion syndrome and, 660
MEN; *see* Multiple endocrine neoplasia
MEN-I syndrome, 189
Ménière's disease, 862
Meningeal inflammation, radiculitis from, abdominal pain and, 565
Meningitis
  cerebrospinal rhinorrhea and, 865
  postoperative fever and, 751
Meningocele in infants, 636
Menstrual history, abdominal pain and, 566
Meperidine hydrochloride (Demerol), 30, 59, 455
Mepivacaine (Carbocaine; Polocaine), 43, 57, 871
6-Mercaptopurine, transplantation and, 245
Mercury poisoning, abdominal pain and, 567
Mesenteric tumors, primary, 516
Metabolic abdominal crises, abdominal pain and, 567-569
Metabolic acidosis, 128, 129
Metabolic alkalosis, 128-130
Metabolic rate of infants, 827, 828
Metamucil (psyllium hydrophilic mucilloid), 559
Metaproterenol, 160
Metastases, pulmonary, resection of, survival after, 232
Metastatic calcification, hypercalcemia and, 176
Methenamine mandelate (Mandelamine), 709
Methicillin (Celbenin; Staphcillin), 825
Methimazole for Graves' disease, 173-174
Methocarbamol (Robaxin), 732
Methohexital (Brevital), 47, 54, 55
Methotrexate, 234
Methyldopa (Aldomet), 376
Methylprednisolone, 184
Metoclopramide hydrochloride (Reglan), 30, 59, 217, 235
Metocurine (Metubine), 49
Metoprolol (Lopressor), 376
Metro (metronidazole), 827
Metronidazole (Flagyl; Metro; Metryl; Protostal; Satric), 456, 827
Metryl (metronidazole), 827
Metubine (metocurine), 49
Mezlin (mezlocillin), 825
Mezlocillin (Mezlin), 825
MHC; *see* Major histocompatibility complex
MHC class II molecules, transplantation and, 242
Microadenoma, pituitary, 181, 182, 183
Micronutrients, total parenteral nutrition and, 142
Microorganisms, postoperative fever and, 751-752
Midazolam (Versed), 30, 47, 55
Middle ear space, fluid in, 859
Midpalmar space infections, 819-820
Migraine, abdominal, abdominal pain and, 566
Minipress (prazosin hydrochloride), 376, 709
Minnesota antilymphocyte globulin, 246
Minocycline (Minocin), 827
Misoprostol (Cytotec), 206, 217
MIT; *see* Monoiodotyrosine
Mithramycin, 135
Mitotane o,p'-DDD (Lysodren), 193
Mitral regurgitation (MR), 316, 320-322
Mitral stenosis, 316, 318-320
Mitral valve disease, 318-322
Mitral valve reconstruction, 322

Mitral valve replacement, 322
Mixed deafness, 861
Mixed tumors
  malignant, 268-269
  of oral cavity, 262
Mixed venous oxygen saturation in intraoperative
    monitoring, 34
MODS; *see* Multiple organ dysfunction syndrome
MOFS; *see* Multiple organ failure syndrome
Moles, 596
Monitored anesthesia care (MAC), difference between
    local anesthesia and, 42
Monobactams, urinary tract infections and, 710
Monocid (cefonicid), 826
Monoiodotyrosine (MIT), 164
Moon face, Cushing's syndrome and, 375
Morbidity, operative risk and, 18-22
Morgagni, foramen of, hernia through, 544
Morphine, 30, 235, 743
Morphine SQ, 235
Morphine sulfate, 59, 455, 628
Mortality, operative risk and, 12-18
Motilin, 203, 204-205
Motrin (ibuprofen), 731
Mouth
  anatomy of, 257
  trench, 262, 815
MR; *see* Mitral regurgitation
MRI; *see* Magnetic resonance imaging
MS Contin, 235
Mucocele, abdominal masses and, 512-513
Mucomyst (acetylcysteine), 160
Mucosa, reddening of small area of, epidermoid
    carcinoma of oral cavity and, 264
Multicystic kidneys, 524
Multilocular cysts of kidney, 524
Multimodal therapy for intraoral tumors, 268, 269
Multiple endocrine neoplasia (MEN), type IIA,
    medullary cancer of thyroid and, 171
Multiple endocrine neoplasia (MEN), type IIB,
    medullary cancer of thyroid and, 171-172
Multiple organ dysfunction syndrome (MODS),
    801-802
Multiple organ failure syndrome (MOFS), 758
Muromonab-CD3 (Orthoclone OKT3), transplantation
    and, 247
Muscle
  atrophy of, fracture and, 681
  strain of, 674, 676
Muscle damage, improper patient positioning and, 41
Muscle flaps, 848-851
Muscle relaxants, 48, 49
Musculocutaneous flaps, 848-851
Musculoskeletal injuries, 669-683
Mustard procedure, transposition of great arteries and,
    340
Mycostatin (Nystatin), 827
Mycotic embolism, 816
Myelomeningocele in infants, 636
Mylanta (alternogel), 629
Mylicon-80, 300
Myocardial infarction
  abdominal pain and, 562-563, 565
  acute, symptoms of, 355-356
  natural history of, 356

Myocardial infarction—cont'd
  origin of left coronary artery from pulmonary artery
      and, 347
  treatment for, 356-357
Myofascial syndromes, abdominal pain and, 564
Myofibroblasts, wound healing and, 845
Myomata, uterine, 528
Myringotomy, 859

N

Nafcillin (Nafcil; Unipen), 825
Nail, ingrown, 818
Nalbuphine hydrochloride (Nubain), 58
Naloxone hydrochloride (Narcan), 59
Naproxen (Naprosyn), 731
Narcan (naloxone hydrochloride), 59
Nasal congestion, 863-867
Nasal fractures, 864-865
Nasal hair, burned, respiratory tract burns and, 260
Nasal obstruction, 863-864
Nasal polyps, 864
Nasal septal hematoma, 864
Nasal septum, deviated, 864
Nasogastric tube
  insertion of, abdominal trauma and, 615
  technique for inserting, 879-880
Nasogastric tube feeding, 145
Nasopharyngoscopy, 857
Nasopharynx, examination of, 258
Nasotracheal intubation, 37-38, 878
National Surgical Adjuvant Breast Project (NSABP), 393
Natural history of illness, 10
Natural killer (NK) cells, tumor lysis and, 223
Nausea, hypercalcemia and, 176
Nebcin (tobramicin), 828
Neck
  irradiation to, relationship of, to thyroid cancer,
      169-170
  trauma to, 617
Neck masses
  diagnostic approaches in evaluation of, 278-279
  treatment of, 279-281
  visual inspection of, 278-279
Necrolytic migratory erythema, diabetes mellitus and,
    191, 192
Necrotizing cellulitis, 815
Necrotizing enterocolitis
  in infants, 651-652
  surgical repair of, 651-652
Necrotizing fasciitis, 815
Needle localization, breast lesion and, 68-71
Negative nitrogen balance, delayed healing and, 608,
    609
Nelson's syndrome, 183
Nembutal (pentobarbital), 54-55
Neoadjuvant chemotherapy for breast chemotherapy,
    396-397
Neonatal cranial ultrasound, 75
Neoplasms; *see also* Cancer; Carcinoma; Oncology;
    Tumors
  benign, of soft tissues, 602-603
  decreased transit time in gastrointestinal tract due to,
      493-494
  malignant soft tissue, 603-604
  of oral cavity, benign, 262-263

Neoplasms—cont'd
  renal, abdominal mass secondary to, 525-527
  of small intestine, 494
  solid, curability of, cancer surgery and, 225-226
Neoplastic lesions in head and neck, 272-277, 278
Neosporin ointment, 628
Neostigmine, 54
Neosynephrine (phenylephrine), 770
Nephric abscess, 524-525
Nephroblastoma, 525-526
Nerve blocks, peripheral, with local anesthetics in
      postoperative pain management, 52
Nerve compression syndromes of hand, 833-835
Nerve damage, improper patient positioning and, 41
Nerve deafness, 859-861
Nerve entrapment, abdominal pain and, 562-563, 564
Nerve palsy, fracture and, 679
Nerve sheath tumors, 603
Nerves of hand, injuries to, 831-835
Nesacaine hydrochloride (chloroprocaine), 43, 57
Neurapraxia, 831, 832
Neuroblastoma, 526
Neurogenic claudication, limb ischemia and, 573-574
Neurologic deficit, 381
Neurologic examination, trauma and, 613
Neuroma, 263
  acoustic, 861
Neuromax (doxacurium), 49
Neuromuscular blockers, 48-49
Neuropathy, diabetic; see Diabetic neuropathy
Neurotensin, 204-205
Neurotmesis, 832
Neutrophilic granulocytes, infection and, 809
Nevi, 596
Newborn; see Infant
NF-AT$_c$; see Activated T-cells
Nifedipine (Adalat; Procardia), 54, 377
Nipple, retraction of, breast cancer and, 386
Nipple discharge, breast cancer and, 398, 399
Nipride (nitroprusside), 377, 770
Nissen fundoplication, laparoscopic, 117
Nitro-bid (nitroglycerine), 377
Nitrocephin (ceftriaxone), 826
Nitrofurantoin (Macrodantin), 709
Nitrogen balance
  definition of, 141
  negative, delayed healing and, 608, 609
Nitrogen needs, determining, in nutritional support
      plan, 141
Nitroglycerine (Nitro-bid; Nitrostat; Tridil), 54, 377, 770,
      802
Nitroprusside (Nipride; Nitropress), 54, 377, 770, 802
Nitrostat (nitroglycerine), 377, 770
Nitrous oxide, 56
  in laparoscopy, 96
Nizatidine (Axid), 217
NK cells; see Natural killer cells
Nodules of vocal cords, 866
Non-A, non-B hepatitis, 824
  blood transfusion and, 17-18
Nondepolarizing neuromuscular blockers, 48, 49
Non-small-cell carcinoma of lung, 313
Nonspecific immunity, tumor lysis and, 223
Nonsteroidal anti-inflammatory drugs (NSAIDs), peptic
      ulcer disease and, 208-210

Non-ventilator-associated pneumonitis, 746
Norcuron (vecuronium), 49, 58
Norepinephrine (Levophed), 770, 804
Norepinephrine bitartrate (Levophed bitartrate), 56
Norfloxacin (Noroxin), 709
Normodyne (labetalol), 376, 377
Normotensive shock, 758
Noroxin (norfloxacin), 709
Norwood operation, hypoplastic left heart syndrome
      and, 342
Nose, examination of, 857-859
Nosebleeds, 864
Novacor left ventricular assist system, 360
Novocain (procaine), 871
NSABP; see National Surgical Adjuvant Breast Project
NSAIDs; see Nonsteroidal anti-inflammatory drugs
Nubain (nalbuphine hydrochloride), 58
Nutrient medium, infection and, 808
Nutrition
  central parenteral, 144
  enteral; see Enteral nutrition
  parenteral; see Parenteral nutrition
  preoperative preparation of jaundiced patient and,
      474
Nutritional states, 139-140
Nutritional status, assessment of, 138-139
Nutritional support
  calculating energy needs in, 141
  central parenteral nutrition in, 144
  indications for, 140-141
  oral and gastric feeding in, 145
  routes to deliver nutrition by, 144-146
  setting priorities in, 141
  standard orders for, 144
Nydarzin (isoniazid), 827
Nystatin (Mycostatin), 827

O

Oat-cell carcinoma of lung, 312
Obesity, central, Cushing's syndrome and, 375
Oblique fracture, 670, 671, 673
Obliterative bronchiolitis, heart-lung transplantation
      and, 253
Obstipation, 497-501
Obstruction as indication for operation in peptic ulcer
      disease, 210
Obstructive disease, abdominal mass secondary to, 522
Obstructive jaundice, 469
  nonoperative relief of, 478
Obstructive lung diseases, 154
Obstructive uropathy, 694-712
Occupation, jaundice and, 465
Octreotide acetate (Sandostatin), 203, 212, 217
Odontogenic cysts, 263
Odor
  foul, Vincent's angina and, 262
  of necrotic tumor mass in oral cavity, 258
Ofloxacin (Floxin), 710
Ogilvie's syndrome, 499-500
OKT3 monoclonal antibody, transplantation and, 247,
      252
Oliguria, 697
Omental cysts, 516
Omental tumors, 516
Omentum, torsion of, 516

Omeprazole (Prilosec), 193, 201, 207, 217
Omphalocele, 544
    in infants, 633-635
Oncogenes, relationship of, to cancer, 222, 223
Oncogenesis, 220-221
Oncology, 220-236
    defense mechanisms in, 222-225
    molecular events in, 221-222
    oncogenesis and, 220-221
Oncovin (vincristine), 235
Open fracture, 616, 672
Open reduction and internal fixation (ORIF) of
        fractures, 675
Operability, lung cancer and, 310-312
Operative risk
    age and, 13-14
    assessment of, 22
    cardiopulmonary problems and, 19-22
    determination of, 12-22
    duration of illness and, 14-16
    evaluation of, 8-27
    influence of degree of suppuration and/or gangrene
        on, 16
    life expectancy of aged patient and, 14
    morbidity and, 18-22
    mortality and, 12-18
    nutritional status and, 22-23
    preexisting anemia and, 16-17
    preoperative laboratory testing and, 24-25
    pulmonary clinical problems and, 21
    risk for postoperative complications and, 22-23
Opiates, anesthesia and, 58-59
Opioids
    anesthesia and, 47
    epidural, in postoperative pain management, 52
    intrathecal, in postoperative pain management, 52
Oral analgesics in postoperative pain management,
        51
Oral cancer, 264-268
    treatment of, 266-267
Oral cavity
    anatomy of, 257-258
    benign neoplasms of, 262-263
    burns of, 260
    congenital lesions of, 258-260
    examination of, 258
    infections of, 261-262
    injuries of, treatment of, 260
    Kaposi's sarcoma in, 269-270
    lacerations of, 260
    malignant lesions of, 264-268
    staging of cancer in, 266-267
Orbital floor, fractures of, 854
Orchitis, 716
Oretic (hydrochlorothiazide), 376
Organ preservation in transplantation, 237-241
Organ preservation solution, transplantation and,
        239-241
ORIF; *see* Open reduction and internal fixation
Orotracheal intubation, 877-878
Orthoclone OKT3 (muromonab-CD3), transplantation
        and, 247
Orthopedics, 669-683
Orthotopic cardiac transplantation, 361-362
Orthotopic transplantation, 237, 241

Osmolar concentration, acute changes in, 126-127
Osmotic diarrhea, 484-485
Osmotic fragility test, jaundice and, 468
Osteoarthritis, manifestations of, in hand, 841
Osteomyelitis
    fracture and, 680-681
    open fracture and, 672
Ostium primum defect, 332
Otitis, external, 857
Otitis media, 859, 860
Otolaryngology, 856-869
Outcome, measurement of, 9
Ovarian cysts, 529-530
Ovarian tumors, 530
Ovaries
    abdominal masses and, 529
    abdominal pain and, 562-563, 566-567
Overhydration, postoperative, 740
Oxacillin (Bactocil; Prostaphlin), 825
Oxycodone (Percocet; Percodan), 235
Oxygen consumption
    level of, in assessment of oxygen need, 796
    relationship of, with respiration, 148-150
Oxygen delivery, relationship of, with respiration,
        148-150
Oxygen extraction ratio, 764
Oxygen transport, restoration of, 796-801

P

PAC; *see* Prostatic adenocarcinoma
Pacemaker, heart block and, 347
PAD; *see* Percutaneous abscess drainage
PADP; *see* Pulmonary artery diastolic pressure
Paget's disease, 399, 553
Pain
    abdominal; *see* Abdominal pain
    arising from abdominal wall, 561-564
    chest; *see* Chest pain
    epigastric, 89
    esophageal rupture and, 292
    gnawing, burning, midepigastric or right upper
        quadrant, duodenal ulcer and, 206
    limb ischemia and, 571-573
    parietal, 423
    rest, ischemia and, 572-573
    right upper quadrant, postcholecystectomy bile
        collection and, 76
    visceral, 423
Pain management, postoperative, 51-52
Painless hematuria, 686
PAK; *see* Pancreas transplantation after successful kidney
        transplant
Palate
    cleft, 258
    hard, tumors of, 267
Pallor, dumping syndrome and, 212
Palmaz stent, 80
Palpation
    bimanual, in examination of oral cavity, 258
    in evaluation of abdominal masses, 507
Pancreas, 196
    abdominal masses and, 519-522
    carcinoma of, 519-520
    carcinoma of head of, jaundice and, 477-478
    common operations on, 442, 443

Pancreas transplantation, 249-250
    after successful kidney transplant (PAK), 249
Pancrease MT (pancrelipase), 456
Pancreatectomy, 486
Pancreatic abscess, 441, 520-521
Pancreatic disease as indication for endoscopic
        retrograde cholangiopancreatography, 89
Pancreatic endocrine tumors, 188
Pancreatic islets, transplantation of, 250-251
Pancreatic mass, 441-442
Pancreatic pseudocyst, 441-442
Pancreaticojejunostomy, 486
Pancreatitis, 437-443, 520-521, 522
    acute, 437-441
        acute cholecystitis and, 433
        pancreatic mass and, 441-442
        Ranson's criteria, 441
    chronic, 442-443, 485-486
    pseudocysts and, 521-522
    relapsing, 442
    subacute, 442
Pancrelipase (Pancrease MT), 456
Pancuronium (Pavulon), 49, 58
PAOP; see Pulmonary artery occlusion pressure
Papillary adenocarcinoma of thyroid, 283
Papillary cancer of thyroid, 169, 170
Papilloma, laryngeal, 866
Papillotome, wire-guided, 478
Papillotomy, obstructive jaundice and, 478
Paracecal hernia, 545
Paraduodenal hernia, 545
Paraesophageal hernia, 544
Parafon Forte (chlorzoxazone), 732
Paraganglioma, 185
Paralysis
    facial, 862-863
    hypoxic, of bowel, 498
    laryngeal, voice quality and, 867
Paralytic ileus, trauma and, 618
Parasitic enteritis, diarrhea and, 493
Parathyroid hormone (PTH), 175
Parathyroid-related polypeptide (PRP), hypercalcemia
        and, 176
Paraumbilical hernia, 543
Parenchymal liver disease, jaundice and, 466
Parenteral fluids
    composition of, 131
    and electrolyte therapy, 122-137
Parenteral nutrition, 140-147
    results of, in surgical patients, 24
Paresthesias, lumbar disk syndrome and, 719-720, 721
Parietal afferent nerves, 422
Parietal cell vagotomy for duodenal ulcer, 212
Parietal pain, 423
Parkland formula, fluid resuscitation and, 625
Paronychia, 818, 839
Parotitis
    postoperative fever and, 751
    suppurative, 866
Partial small bowel obstruction, 454
Partial thromboplastin time (PTT) in evaluation of
        hemostasis, 777
Partial-thickness burn, 621, 622
Patent ductus arteriosus (PDA), 329, 330, 334, 335
Pathocil (dicloxacillin), 825

Pathologic fracture, 670, 671
Patient
    physical status of, selection of anesthetic technique
        and, 42
    positioning of
        endotracheal intubation and, 35-36
        intraoperative, improper, 40-41
        responsibility for, 41
    preference of, in selection of anesthetic technique, 42
Patient presentations, symptom-based, 255-732
Patient-controlled analgesia (PCA), 51-52
Pavulon (pancuronium), 49
PCA; see Patient-controlled analgesia
PDA; see Patent ductus arteriosus
PDGF; see Platelet-derived growth factor
PDPH; see Postdural puncture headache
Pediatric surgical emergencies, 631-652
PEEP; see Positive end-expiratory pressure
PEG; see Percutaneous endoscopic gastrostomy
Pelvic abscess, 823
    appendicitis and, 428
Pelvic fracture or dislocation, 616-617
Pelvic hernias, 545
Pelvic lipomatosis, ureteral obstruction and, 697
Pelvic masses, 528-530
Pelvis, fracture of, 676-677
Penetrating head injuries versus closed head injuries,
        658-659
Penicillin G, 825
Penicillins, 825
    urinary tract infections and, 710
Pentcillyn (piperacillin), 825
Pentobarbital (Nembutal), 30, 54-55
Pentothal (thiopental), 47, 55
Pepcid (famotidine), 217
Peptic ulcer disease
    gastroduodenal physiology and, 196-219
    indications for operation in, 209-210
    laparoscopy for, 111-116
    nonsteroidal anti-inflammatory drugs and, 208-210
Peptide YY, 204-205
Perceptive deafness, 859-861
Percocet (oxycodone), 235
Percodan (oxycodone), 235, 743
Percussion in evaluation of abdominal masses, 507
Percutaneous abscess drainage (PAD), 76-78
Percutaneous endoscopic gastrojejunostomy, 146
Percutaneous endoscopic gastrostomy (PEG), 92-93
Percutaneous needle biopsies, 77-78
Percutaneous transluminal angioplasty, 80
Percutaneous transluminal angioplasty catheter, 580,
        582
Percutaneous transluminal coronary angioplasty
        (PTCA), 351, 353, 356
Perforation as indication for operation in peptic ulcer
        disease, 209-210
Perforin, transplantation and, 244
Periampullary carcinoma, 518
    jaundice and, 477-478
Perianal and rectal complaints, 547-560
Perianal regions, malignancies of, 552-553
Periarteritis nodosa, abdominal pain and, 568-569
Pericardial effusions, chronic, 363
Pericardial tamponade, acute, 362-363
Pericardiocentesis, 879, 880

Pericarditis, constrictive, 363
   abdominal pain and, 562-563, 565
Pericardium, 362-363
Perinephric abscess, 524-525, 704
Periodic disease, abdominal pain and, 569
Perioperative cardiac risk, multifactorial assessment of, 19, 20
Peripharyngeal abscess, 261
Peripheral central venous line, 871-872
Peripheral nerve blocks with local anesthetics, 52
Peripherally acting sympatholytic agents, hypertension and, 376
Peristalsis in small intestine, 483
Peritoneum, lesions of, abdominal pain and, 567
Peritonitis, postoperative, 822
Peritonsillar abscess, 261
Person-years of life, measurement of, 9, 10, 11, 12
Peutz-Jeghers syndrome, 258
Phagocytes
   fixed, infection and, 809
   infection and, 809
Phalen's test for carpal tunnel syndrome, 834
Pharynx, 857
Phenergan (promethazine hydrochloride), 59
Phenoxybenzamine hydrochloride (Dibenzyline), 193
Phenylalanine mustard, 235
Phenylephrine bitartrate, 804
Phenylephrine hydrochloride, 56
Phenylephrine (Neosynephrine), 770
Pheochromocytoma, 172, 185-188
   hypertension and, 375
Phlebitis, trauma and, 618
Phlegmasia alba dolens, 585
Phlegmasia cerulea dolens, 585
Phlegmon, infection and, 813
Phosphate, increased, in urine, primary hyperparathyroidism and, 175
Phosphate buffered sucrose, transplantation and, 239, 240
Phospholipids, biliary, 464
Physician, preference of, in selection of anesthetic technique, 42
Pierce-Donachy pump, 360
Pierre-Robin syndrome, 259-260, 637-638
Pigment stones, 464
Pilonidal abscess, 818
Pilonidal disease, 551-552
Pilonidal sinus, 551
Piperacillin (Avocin; Pentcillyn; Pipracil; Pipril), 456, 710, 825
Pipercuronium (Arduan), 49, 58
Pipracil (piperacillin), 456, 710, 825
Pipril (piperacillin), 825
Pit viper bite, abdominal pain and, 564
Pituitary microadenoma, 181, 182, 183
Plastic surgery, 845-855
Platelet defects, 778-779, 781, 782
Platelet studies in evaluation of hemostasis, 776-777
Platelet-derived growth factor (PDGF), 222
Platelets in normal hemostasis, 773-774
Pleomorphic adenoma, 262
Plethysmography in evaluation of limb ischemia, 576
Pleural effusion, 21

Pleural space
   air or fluid in, abdominal pain and, 564
   empyema of, postoperative fever and, 750
Pleurisy, pneumonia and, 302
Pleuritic chest pain, pneumonia and, 302
Pneumatocele, pneumonia and, 306
Pneumonia, 158
   bacterial, hemoptysis and, 306
   complications of, 306
   restrictive lung defects and, 155
   ventilator-associated, 747-748
Pneumonitis
   aspiration-associated, 748
   lung abscess and, 306
   non-ventilator-associated, 746
Pneumoperitoneum
   in laparoscopy, 99
   massive, in infants, 640
   peptic ulcer disease and, 210
   percutaneous endoscopic gastrostomy and, 93
Pneumothorax, 156, 616
   in infants, 639
   tension, 39
      trauma and, 612
Poisoning, 562-563, 567
Polocaine (mepivacaine), 43
Polycystic kidney disease, 524
Polydipsia, hypercalcemia and, 176
Polypectomy, colonoscopy and, 91, 92
Polypeptideoma, vasoactive intestinal, 497
Polyps, 263
   adenomatous, 494
   gastrointestinal bleeding and, 418
   nasal, 864
   of vocal cords, 866
Polyuria, hypercalcemia and, 176
Pontocaine (tetracaine hydrochloride), 43, 57, 871
Popliteal artery angioplasty, 78-80
Porphyria, acute intermittent, 568
Portal-systemic shunts, 413-414
Portography, splenic, 472-473
Positive end-expiratory pressure (PEEP), 789
Positive pressure ventilation, 788, 789
   high-frequency, 792
Postanesthesia care, 49-52
Postanesthesia recovery room, 50-51
Postconcussion syndrome, 660
Postdural puncture headache (PDPH), 45
Posterior fossa tumors, abdominal pain and, 565-566
Postgastrectomy syndromes, 212-216
Posthepatic jaundice, 460
Postirradiated bowel, gastrointestinal bleeding and, 418
Postoperative complications, 733-884, 737-742
   common, usual time of appearance of, 742
   corrective therapy for, 742
   risk for, operative risk and, 22-23
Postoperative fever; see Fever, postoperative
Postoperative fluid management, 133-134
Postoperative hypoxemia, 737, 738
Postoperative orders, 736-737
Postoperative pain management, 51-52
Postoperative patient, approach to, 735-744
Postoperative pulmonary complications, 156-158
Postoperative tachycardia, isolated, associated with normal blood pressure, 737

Postoperative tachypnea, 737
Postoperative thrombophlebitis, 821
Posturing, 661
Potassium abnormalities, 130
Potassium-sparing diuretics, 376
PP, 204-205
Prazosin hydrochloride (Minipress), 376, 709
Preanesthetic preparation, 28-29
Prednisolone, 184
Prednisone, 135, 184
    transplantation and, 245-248, 251, 252
Pregnancy
    breast cancer and, 398
    ectopic, 529
    ureteral obstruction and, 696
Preload, cardiac output and, 764-765
Preoperative considerations, 1-254
Preoperative fluid management, 132-133
Preoperative laboratory testing, operative risk and,
    24-25
Preoperative preparation for anesthesia, 28-32
Preoperative pulmonary evaluation, 154-156
Presbycusis, 859-861
Preservation solution, transplantation and, 239-241
Pressure necrosis, trauma and, 618
Pressure support ventilation, 790
Prilocaine (Citanest), 43
Prilosec (omeprazole), 193, 217, 300
Primary hyperaldosteronism, 184
Primary hyperparathyroidism, 175-180
Primaxin (imepinim and cilastatin), 456, 828
Procaine hydrochloride (Novocain), 43, 57, 871
Procardia (nifedipine), 377
Prochlorperazine (Compazine), 235
Procidentia, 557
ProctoCream-HC, 559
Proctofoam-HC, 559
Prolonged neurologic deficit, 381
Promethazine hydrochloride (Phenergan), 59
Promoter agent of cancer, 220
Prophylactic oophorectomy, breast cancer and, 398
Propofol (Diprivan), 47-48, 55
Proportional assist ventilation, 790
Propoxyphene
    with aspirin (Darvon), 731
    with Tylenol (Darvocet), 731
Propranolol hydrochloride (Inderal), 193, 376
Propylthiouracil for Graves' disease, 173-174
Prostaphlin (oxacillin), 825
Prostate cancer, 700-703
Prostatic acid phosphatase, prostate cancer and, 700
Prostatic adenocarcinoma (PAC), 700-703
Prostatic enlargement, hematuria secondary to, 691
Prostatic specific antigen (PSA), prostate cancer and,
    700-701
Prostatic ultrasound, 75
Protamine sulfate, 784
Protein
    absorption of, in gastrointestinal tract, 483
    gastroduodenal digestion and absorption and, 198,
        199
Prothrombin time (PT) in evaluation of hemostasis, 777
Proto-oncogenes, 222
Protostal (metronidazole), 827
Proximal aortic dissection, 365

PRP; see Parathyroid-related polypeptide
Pruritus, cholestatic jaundice and, 465-466
Pruritus ani, 552
PS; see Pulmonic stenosis
PSA; see Prostatic specific antigen
Psammoma bodies, papillary cancer of thyroid and, 169
Pseudocyst
    acute pancreatitis and, 521-522
    pancreatic, 441-442
Pseudomembranous colitis, 487
Pseudoobstruction, colonic, 499
Psoriasis, manifestations of, in hand, 841
Psychogenic abdominal pain, 566
Psychosis, hypercalcemia and, 176
Psyllium hydrophilic mucilloid (Metamucil), 559
Pulmonary arteriography, 81-82
Pulmonary artery catheter, 794-795
    balloon flotation catheter, 876-877
    in intraoperative monitoring, 34
    Swan-Ganz, 763-764
Pulmonary artery diastolic pressure (PADP), 34
Pulmonary artery occlusion pressure (PAOP), 34
Pulmonary atresia with intact ventricular septum, 338
Pulmonary barotrauma, complications of ventilator
    support related to, 791
Pulmonary causes of fever, 746-748
Pulmonary compliance, intraoperative change in, 38-39
Pulmonary complications, postoperative, 156-158, 740
Pulmonary embolism
    cause of, 367, 588
    fracture and, 680
    lower extremity swelling and, 588-589
    treatment of, 367-368, 589
    postoperative, 740
    prevention of, 589
    symptoms of, 588-589
Pulmonary function
    assessment of, 787
        clinical approach to, 154
        intraoperative factors influencing, 156
        testing of, 154-156
Pulmonary hypertension, 307, 334-335, 343
Pulmonary infarction, hemoptysis and, 307
Pulmonary infection, 21
    postoperative fever and, 820
    recurrent, arch anomalies and, 347
Pulmonary injury, burn injury and, 621, 622-624
Pulmonary insufficiency, trauma and, 617
Pulmonary metastases, resection of, survival after, 232
Pulmonary nodules, solitary, 309-310
Pulmonary perfusion, 153-154
Pulmonary stenosis, 336, 344-346
Pulmonary tuberculosis, hemoptysis and, 308
Pulmonic stenosis (PS), 331
Pulse, trauma and, 613
Pulse oximetry, 32-33
Pupil, size and reactivity of, trauma and, 613
Purpura, Schönlein-Henoch, abdominal pain and, 569
Purulent tenosynovitis, 840
Pus
    abscess and, 813
    in peritonsillar space, peritonsillar abscess and, 261
Pyarthrosis, postoperative fever and, 751
Pyelonephritis, 524-525
Pylephlebitis, appendicitis and, 428-429

Pyloric stenosis in infants, 649
Pyonephrosis, 704
Pyrosis, difficulties in swallowing and, 290-291
Pyuria
    hematuria and, 688-689
    sterile, 707

Q

Quinsy throat, 261

R

Rachischisis in infants, 636
Radial tunnel syndrome, 834-835
Radiation enteritis, diarrhea and, 493
Radiculitis from meningeal inflammation, abdominal
    pain and, 565
Radioactive iodine therapy for Graves' disease,
    174-175
Radiology
    contrast, of biliary tract, jaundice and, 470-472
    interventional, 75-78
Radionuclide liver scans, jaundice and, 472
Random-pattern flaps, 848, 849
Ranitidine hydrochloride (Zantac), 30, 193, 217
Ranula, 258
Rapamycin, transplantation and, 245, 247
Rastelli procedure, transposition of great arteries and,
    340
RBCs; see Red blood cells
Rebound tenderness, abdominal pain and, 424
Recombinant human erythropoietin, autologous blood
    transfusion and, 18
Rectal and perianal complaints, 547-560
Rectal bleeding; see also Gastrointestinal bleeding
    carcinoma of colon and rectum and, 514
    colonoscopy for, 90
    upper gastrointestinal bleeding and, 87
Rectal examination, 549-550
    in evaluation of abdominal masses, 507
Rectal prolapse, 557
Rectum
    anatomy of, 547-548
    carcinoma of, 494-496, 513-516
    defecation and, 483-484
Recurrent ulcer, 213, 214-215
Red blood cells (RBCs) in urine, 684-693
Reddening of mucosa, epidermoid carcinoma of oral
    cavity and, 264
Reduction, fracture, 616, 674-675
Reflex sympathetic dystrophy, fracture and, 679
Reflux esophagitis, 291, 296-297
Regional anesthesia, 45-46
Regional enteritis, 511-512
Registry of the International Society for Heart and Lung
    Transplantation, 253
Reglan (metoclopramide hydrochloride), 30, 59, 217,
    235
Regurgitation, difficulties in swallowing and, 291
Rehabilitation of fracture, 674, 675
Reimplantation choledochoduodenostomy, 476
Rejection, types of, in transplantation, 237, 244
Relaxing incision, hernia repair and, 535
Renal artery stenosis, hypertension and, 374
Renal calculi, ureteral obstruction and, 695
Renal cell carcinoma, 525

Renal cystic disease, abdominal mass secondary to,
    522-524
Renal cysts, 523-524
Renal failure
    postoperative, 740
    trauma and, 617
Renal infections, abdominal mass secondary to, 524-525
Renal mass, systematic evaluation of, 523; see also
    Kidney
Renal neoplasms, abdominal mass secondary to,
    525-527
Renal parenchymal disease, unilateral, hypertension
    and, 374-375
Renin, arterial blood pressure and, 370
Renin-angiotensin system, 184, 185
Reparative granuloma, 262-263
Resectability, lung cancer and, 310-312
Reserpine, 376
Residual volume, 151
Resistance, 808-809
Respiration, 148
    in infants, 631
    relationship of, with oxygen delivery and oxygen
        consumption, 148-150
    trauma and, 613
Respiratory acidosis, 128, 129, 154
Respiratory alkalosis, 128, 129, 154
Respiratory distress syndromes in infants, 636-641
Respiratory function and support, 148-161
Respiratory quotient (RQ), 148
Respiratory sounds, obstructed, arch anomalies and, 347
Respiratory tract burns, 260
Rest pain, ischemia and, 572-573
Resting metabolic expenditure (RME), 141
Restoril (temazepam), 235
Restrictive lung disease, 21, 154
Retained common duct stones, jaundice and, 476
Retention cyst, 262
    in oral cavity, 258
Retraction, of nipple, breast cancer and, 386
Retrograde amnesia, concussion and, 660
Retrograde pancreaticojejunostomy, chronic pancreatitis
    and, 486
Retroperitoneal diseases, 528
Retroperitoneal fibrosis, idiopathic, 528
Retroperitoneal masses, 519-522
Retroperitoneal tumors, 528
Retropharyngeal abscess, 261
Reversible ischemic neurologic deficit (RIND), 381
Revised Trauma Score (RTS), 607
Rheumatoid arthritis
    abdominal pain and, 568
    of wrist, 841
Rhinitis, 863
Rhinitis medicamentous, 863
Rhomboid flaps, 848
Rib tip syndrome, 564
Richter's hernia, 532
Rifampin (Rifadin; Rifocin; Rimactane), 827
Right ventricle, origin of both great arteries from, 336
Right-sided heart failure, Ebstein's malformation and,
    341
Rimactane (rifampin), 827
RIND; see Reversible ischemic neurologic deficit
RME; see Resting metabolic expenditure

Robaxin (methocarbamol), 732
Rocephin (ceftriaxone), 826
Rocephin (ceftriaxone sodium), 710
Rolaids, 300
Roux-en-Y gastrojejunostomy, 216
RQ; *see* Respiratory quotient
RS-61443, transplantation and, 245, 247, 248
RTS; *see* Revised Trauma Score
Rule of nines, burn injury and, 621, 623
Runaround, 818
Rupture, abdominal masses with actual or impending,
    510-511

S

Saccular aneurysm, 363, 364
Saccular bronchiectasis, 307
SAH; *see* Subarachnoid hemorrhage
Saline solution, 134
Salivary glands
    ectopic, 262
    infections of, 866
Salmonella food poisoning, abdominal pain and, 567
Sampling response, 483-484
Sandostatin (octreotide acetate), 193, 212, 217
Sarcoma
    Kaposi's, 597
    soft tissue, cell of origin of, 603, 604
    treatment of, 390
Satric (metronidazole), 827
Scalded skin syndrome, 814
Scar formation, wound healing and, 845
Schilling test, blind loop syndrome and, 487
Schistosomiasis, 708
Schönlein-Henoch purpura, abdominal pain and, 569
Scleroderma
    abdominal pain and, 568
    manifestations of, in hand, 841
Sclerosing cholangitis, jaundice and, 477
Sclerosing hemangioma, 259
Sclerotherapy
    esophagogastroduodenoscopy and, 87-88
    injection, for varicose veins, 591
Scopolamine, 54
Scrotal edema, 714
Scrotal hematoma, 716
Scrotal hernia, imaging of, 75
Scrotal swelling, painless, evaluation of, 74-75
Scrotum, 713-718
Sebaceous cyst, 597, 818
Secobarbital (Seconal), 30, 55
Seconal (secobarbital), 30, 55
Secondary hyperaldosteronism, primary
    hyperaldosteronism and, 185
Secondary hyperparathyroidism, 175
Secretin, 204-205
Secretory diarrhea, 485
Sedation, intravenous conscious, administration of,
    42-43
Seffin (cephalothin), 825
Segmental fracture, 670, 671, 673
Sellick maneuver, 37
Sengstaken-Blakemore tube, 880-881
Senning procedure, transposition of great arteries and,
    340
Sensorcaine (bupivacaine), 43

Sensorineural deafness, 859-861
Sepsis
    fungal, 823
    type of, fever curve and, 618
Septal abscess, 864
Septic shock, 759, 770
Septicemia, 811, 816-817
Septra DS (sulfamethoxazole), 709
Serotonin, 204-205
Serum cholesterol level, liver function and, 468
Serum gastrin measurements, duodenal ulcer and,
    206-207
Serum hepatitis, 823-824
Serum lactate level in assessment of oxygen need, 796
Sexually transmitted diseases (STDs)
    cutaneous manifestations of, on male genitalia,
        713-714
    hematuria and, 689-690
Shock
    acute cardiac tamponade and, 362
    cardiac output and, 763, 764
    cardiogenic, 759, 770
    cardiotonic agents for, 769
    cerebral status and, 762
    clinical management of, 757
    compensated, 758
    core temperature and, 762
    esophageal rupture and, 292
    fluid administration in, 768
    hemorrhagic, massive hemoptysis and, 306
    hypovolemic, 759
    monitoring in, 762-766
    normotensive, 758
    pathophysiology of, 759-760
    preexisting organ dysfunction and, 762-763
    recognition of, 758-762
    septic, 759, 770
    signs and symptoms of, 760-762
    strangulated intestinal obstruction, 455
    tissue hypoxia and, 759
    transcutaneous oxygen measurement and, 762
    treatment of, 766-769
    types of, 759
    urine output and, 762
Short bowel syndrome, 485, 487-488
Shortness of breath, pulmonary neoplasm and, 302
Shouldice hernia repair, 540, 541
Shunt, left-to-right, defects associated with,
    332-335
Sialadenitis, 866
Sialectasia, 866
Sialolithiasis, 866
Side-to-side pancreaticojejunostomy, chronic
    pancreatitis and, 486
Sigmoid volvulus, colonoscopy for, 91
Sigmoidoscopy, flexible, 92
Silver sulfadiazine (Silvadene), 628
Simultaneous pancreas-kidney transplantation (SPK),
    249, 250
SIMV; *see* Synchronous intermittent mandatory
    ventilation
Single-lung transplantation, 252-253
Sinus
    pilonidal, 551
    of Valsalva, aneurysm of, 347

Sinusitis
  chronic, 865
  postoperative fever and, 751
Sipple's syndrome, 284
  medullary cancer of thyroid and, 171
  neuroma and, 263
Skeletal damage, improper patient positioning and, 41
Skin
  retraction of, over breast cancer, 385
  squamous cell carcinoma of, 597
Skin cancer, 597-602
  hereditary, 599
  incidence and mortality rates for, 597
Skin damage, improper patient positioning and, 41
Skin graft, 847-848
Skin infections, 817-818
Skin lesions
  benign, 596-597
  biopsy of, 595-596
  malignant, 597-602
Skull, trauma to, 616
Skull fracture, 654-656
SLE; *see* Systemic lupus erythematosus
Sleep apnea syndrome, 866
Sleep disturbances, postconcussion syndrome and, 660
Sliding hernia, 532
Small bowel disease, ischemic, 448-449
Small bowel obstruction, partial, 454
Small intestine
  abdominal masses in, 511-512
  blood loss from, 416
  neoplasms of, 494
  obstruction of, 497, 498
  transit in, effect of, on bowel movements, 483
Small-cell carcinoma of lung, 313
Smoking, epidermoid carcinoma of oral cavity and, 264
Snake bite, 564, 567
Sodium bicarbonate, 134, 628
Sodium citrate, 30
Sodium exchange, 123-125
Sodium polystyrene sulfonate (Kayexalate), 135
Soft tissue injuries, fractures and, 674
Soft tissue neoplasms, 602-604
Solitary pulmonary nodules, 309-310
Somatostatin, 203, 204-205
Somatostatin analogue (Sandostatin), 193
Somatostatinoma, 497
SOSSUS; *see* Study of Surgical Services in the United
    States
Spermatocele, 715
  imaging of, 75
Sphincter spasm, abnormal defecation and, 496
Sphincteroplasty, transduodenal, jaundice and,
    475-476
Spider bite, abdominal pain and, 564, 567
Spigelian hernia, 544
Spiking temperatures, 737
Spinal cord, lesions of, 562-563, 565
Spinal cord injury, 616
Spinal fracture, 677
Spinal tumors, 723-728
Spine, cervical, trauma to, 617
Spiral fracture, 670, 671, 673
Spironolactone (Aldactone), 193, 376
SPK; *see* Simultaneous pancreas-kidney transplantation

Spleen, 518-519
Splenectomy, hematologic disorders amenable to,
    518-519
Splenic portography, jaundice and, 472-473
Split-thickness skin graft, 847-848
Spondylosis, lumbar, 728-729
Sprain of ligament, 674, 676
Squamous cell carcinoma
  of anus, 552-553
  of larynx, 867
  of skin, 597, 598
Squatting, tetralogy of Fallot and, 338
Stabilization of fracture, 616, 674, 675
Stadol (butorphanol tartrate), 57
Staging, cancer, effect of on survival, 9
Staphcillin (methicillin), 825
Staphylococcal enteritis, 487
Staphylococcal food poisoning, abdominal pain and,
    567
Starling's law, 756
Stasis ulcer, 591
Steatorrhea, 484
Stein-Leventhal syndrome, 530
Stent
  obstructive jaundice and, 478
  Palmaz, 80
  placement of, ERCP and, 90
  use of, in vascular system, 80
Sterile pyuria, 707
Steroids, transplantation and, 245
Stiff heart syndrome, 767-768
Stomach
  anatomic division of, 196
  blood supply of, 197
  carcinoma of, abdominal mass and, 511, 512
  surgical anatomy of, 196-197
Stones, hematuria and, 686, 688, 691
Stool
  abnormal substances in, 486-487
  bacterial flora of, 481, 482
  composition of, 481-482
  evaluation of, 485
  formation and transit of, physiology of, 481-484
  normal meconium, absence of, intestinal obstruction
    of newborn and, 642
Strain of muscle, 674, 676
Strangling, Pierre-Robin syndrome and, 259
Strangulated hernia, 532
Strangulation obstruction, 452, 455
Streptokinase, 593
Streptomycin, 827
Striae, cutaneous, Cushing's syndrome and, 375
Strictures, ureteral obstruction and, 695
Stroke, 379-383
Study of Surgical Services in the United States
    (SOSSUS), 4
Stupor, hypercalcemia and, 176
Subarachnoid anesthesia, 45
Subarachnoid hemorrhage (SAH), 656
Subclavian line, 872-873
Subdural hematoma, 656-657
Subfascial abscess, 823
Sublimaze (fentanyl citrate), 47, 59
Submucosal mass, slow-growing, mixed tumors and,
    262

Subphrenic abscess, appendicitis and, 428
Substance P, 204-205
Subtotal pancreatectomy, chronic pancreatitis and, 486
Succinylcholine chloride (Anectine), 49, 58
Sucralfate (Carafate), 206, 217
Sufentanil (Sufenta), 47, 59
Sulfamethoxazole (Bactrim DS; Septra DS), 709
Sulfamylon (Mefamide), 628
Superficial burn, 621
Superficial thrombophlebitis, 584-585
Superior laryngeal nerve injury, 180
Suppressor cells, infection and, 809
Suppuration, degree of, operative risk and, 16
Suppurative lymphadenitis, 811
Suppurative parotitis, 866
Supraclavicular masses, 272
Surface antigen, 824
Surfak (docusate sodium), 559
Surgeon, liability of, anesthesia and, 53
Surgeons, number of, 7
Surgery
    attitude for action in, 5-6
    fasting before, 31-32
    general, laparoscopy and, 100-102
Surgical attitudes, history, and ethics, 3-7
Surgical bleeding and hemostasis, 773-785
Surgical compromise, improper patient positioning and, 40
Surgical techniques, basic, 870-884
Surital (thiamylal), 47
Suture technique, 846-847
SVR; see Systemic vascular resistance
Swallowing, difficulties in, 289-301
Swan-Ganz pulmonary artery catheter, 763-764, 876-877
Sweating, dumping syndrome and, 212
Swelling
    lower extremity, 584-594
    in posterior area of tongue, Ludwig's angina and, 261
Swimmer's ear, 857
Symbiosis, bacterial, 808
Sympatholytic agents, hypertension and, 376
Sympathomimetics, anesthesia and, 56
Synchronous intermittent mandatory ventilation (SIMV), 789
Syncope, aortic stenosis and, 344
Synergistic gangrene, 815
Synovial cysts, 603
Syphilis, 713
Systemic arterial catheter, 794-795
Systemic lupus erythematosus (SLE), abdominal pain and, 568
Systemic resistance, infection and, 809
Systemic vascular resistance (SVR), 766

T

T_4; see Thyroxine
T_3; see Tri-iodothyronine
T-lymphocytes, helper, transplantation and, 242-243
Tachycardia
    dumping syndrome and, 212
    postoperative, isolated, associated with normal blood pressure, 737
Tachypnea, postoperative, 737
Tag, hemorrhoidal, 549

Tagamet (cimetidine), 193, 217
Talus fracture, open reduction and internal fixation of, 675
Taussig-Bing syndrome, 336
Technetium-99m sodium pertechnetate versus iodine-123, 71-72
Technetium-99m sulphur colloid liver scans, 472
Technetium-99m-HIDA (Tc-HIDA) liver scans, 472, 473
Technetium-99m-labeled red blood cells, liver scans and, 472
Teebaconin (isoniazid), 827
Teeth, trauma to, 260
Temazepam (Restoril), 235
Temperature; see also Fever
    core, shock and, 762
    spiking, 737
Temporal arteritis, abdominal pain and, 569
Tenesmus, abnormal defecation and, 496
Tenosynovitis, 819, 820
    purulent, 840
Tension pneumothorax, 39
    trauma and, 612
Tentorium cerebelli, foramen of, 656
Teratoma, cervical, in infants, 638
Terazosin hydrochloride (Hytrin), 709
Tertiary waves in esophagus after barium swallow, dysfunction of propulsive action of muscles of esophagus and, 299
Testes
    imaging of, 74-75
    maldescent of, 717-718
    torsion of, 717
Tetanus, 815
Tetanus toxoid, 629
Tetracaine hydrochloride (Cetacaine; Pontocaine), 43, 57, 871
Tetracycline, 710, 827
Tetralogy of Fallot, 329-330, 331, 338-339
TGHA antibodies; see Antithyroglobulin antibodies
Thenar space infections, 819
Theophylline, 160
Thiopental (Pentothal), 47, 55
Thoracentesis and chest tubes, 882-883
Thoracic aortic aneurysms, 364-365
Thoracoabdominal aortic aneurysms, 365
Thorax, lesions localized in, abdominal pain and, 562-563, 564-565
Throat
    examination of, 857-859
    quinsy, 261
Thrombin time (TT) in evaluation of hemostasis, 777
Thrombocytopenia, heparin-induced, 368
Thromboembolism versus embolism, 571, 572
Thrombolytic therapy, indications for, 81
Thrombophlebitis
    deep, 585-588
    postoperative, 821
    superficial, 584-585
Thrombosis, heparin-induced, 368
Thymol turbidity test, liver function and, 467
Thyroglossal duct cyst, 259
Thyroid
    adenoma of, 166
    anaplastic adenocarcinoma of, 284
    anatomy of, 162-163

Thyroid—cont'd
  arterial supply to, 162
  cysts of, 166
  diagnostic tests of function of, 164-166
  follicular adenocarcinoma of, 283-284
  lingual, 258-259
  malignant lesions of, 166
  medullary adenocarcinoma of, 284
  nodules, 166-169
  normal physiology of, 163-164
  palpable abnormality of, diagnosis of, 72-73
  papillary adenocarcinoma of, 283
  radioiodine scans of, 167
  undifferentiated adenocarcinoma of, 284
Thyroid cancer, 281-286
  age and, 281-282
  anaplastic, 171
  clinical evaluation of, 284
  detection of, 281
  diagnosis of, 281-282
  follicular, 169-170
    treatment of, 170-171
  follow-up of patient with, 285-286
  isolated nodule and, 282
  laboratory evidence for, 282-283
  medullary, 171-172
  nonsurgical treatment of, 73
  papillary, 169, 283
    treatment of, 170-171
  past medical history and, 281
  pathologic types of, 283
  patient history and, 281-282
  physical examination in, 282
  relationship of irradiation of neck to, 169-170
  sex and, 281-282
  therapeutic options for, 284-285
  treatment of, 281
  types of, 169-172
  undifferentiated, 171
Thyroid storm, 175, 180
  fever and, 753
Thyroiditis, 166
  acute, 166
  granulomatous, 166
  Hashimoto's, 166
  lymphocytic, 166
Thyroid-stimulating hormone (TSH), 164
Thyrotoxicosis, 164, 172-175
  Graves' disease and, 173-175
Thyrotropin-releasing hormone (TRH), 164
Thyroxine (T_4), 163-164, 165
TIA; see Transient ischemic attack
Ticarcillin disodium and clavulanate potassium
    (Timentin), 456
Tidal volume, 150, 151
Time zero, identification of, 9
Timentin (ticarcillin disodium and clavulanate
    potassium), 456
Tinnitus, 861
Tissue expansion, wound coverage and, 852
Tissue factor, 774
Tissue histiocytes, infection and, 809
Tissue plasminogen activator, 593
TNM classification of breast cancer, 391, 392
TNM system of classification, 266

Tobramicin (Nebcin), 828
Toluidine blue, ability of lesion to take up, intraoral
    tumors and, 265
Tongue
  anatomy of, 257
  swelling in posterior area of, Ludwig's angina and, 261
  tumors of, 266-267
Tonsillectomy, indications for, 865-866
Topical antimicrobials, burns and, 628-629
Toradol (ketorolac), 58, 731
Torsion, of testis, 717
Torus palatinus, 259, 262
Total anomalous pulmonary venous connection,
    335-336
Total body surface area (TBSA), burn injury and,
    621-622, 623
Total pancreatectomy, chronic pancreatitis and, 486
Total urine nitrogen (TUN), 141
Toxemia, 815
  infection and, 815-816
Toxic megacolon, 493
TR; see Tricuspid regurgitation
Tracheoesophageal fistula in infants, 640-641
Tracheomalacia in infants, 638
Tracheostomy tube, complications of ventilator support
    related to, 791
Tracrium (atracurium), 49, 58
TRAM flaps; see Transverse rectus abdominis
    musculocutaneous flaps
Trandate (labetalol), 376, 377
Transcutaneous oxygen measurement, shock and, 762
Transduodenal sphincteroplasty, jaundice and, 475-476
Transforming growth factor 2 (TGF2), 222
Transforming growth factor B (TGFB), 222
Transfusion, blood; see Blood transfusion
Transfusion, massive, platelet and coagulation factor
    deficiencies and, 782
Transient ischemic attack (TIA), 381
Transient neurologic episodes, 380-381
Transit in gastrointestinal tract
  abnormalities in, 485
  decreased, due to neoplasms, 493-494
  effect of, on bowel movements, 483-484
  rapid, malabsorption resulting from, 486-487
Translocation, 752
Transplantation, 237-254
  cardiac; see Cardiac transplantation
  of composite tissue, wound coverage and, 851-852
  heart-lung, 252-253
  heterotopic, 237, 241
  historical aspects of, 237, 238
  immune response to transplantation antigens in,
    241-245
  immunosuppressive therapy and, 245-248
  islet, 250-251
  kidney, 248-249
  liver, 251-252
  major histocompatibility complex and, 241
  organ preservation in, 237-241
  orthotopic, 237, 241
  pancreas, 249-250
Transplantation antigens, immune response to, 241-245
Transposition of great arteries (TGA), 330, 337, 339-340
  corrected, 347-348
Transverse fracture, 670, 671, 673

Transverse guillotine amputation, 838
Transverse rectus abdominis musculocutaneous (TRAM) flaps, 850-851
Trauma
  abdominal; *see* Abdominal trauma
  acoustic, nerve deafness caused by, 861
  drawing blood and, 611
  ear, injury caused by, 863
  head, severe, common brain lesions from, 657-658
  hematuria and, 690-691
  management of, 609-610
  monitoring and recording vital signs and, 611
  multiple, 610-613
  physical examination and, 611-613
  physiology of, 608-609
  postoperative complications of, 617-618
  preparation of intravenous cannula and, 611
  preparation of patient for examination and treatment and, 611
  role of team leader in management of, 610-611
  scoring systems for, 607-608
Trauma center levels, 606-607
Traumatic diaphragmatic hernia, 545
Travel, jaundice and, 465
Trench mouth, 262, 815
Triamcinolone, 184
Triazolam (Halcion), 235
Tricuspid atresia, 331, 337-338
Tricuspid insufficiency, Ebstein's malformation and, 341
Tricuspid regurgitation (TR), 326-327
Tricuspid stenosis, 325-326
Tricuspid valve disease, 317, 325-327
Tridil (nitroglycerine), 377
Trigger fingers, 841
Tri-iodothyronine (T_3), 163-164, 165
Trimethoprim, 709
Truncal vagotomy
  and drainage (TV&D) for duodenal ulcer, 211-212
  gastroenterostomy and, 211-212
  with hemigastrectomy for duodenal ulcer, 212
Truncus arteriosus, 336-337
TSH; *see* Thyroid-stimulating hormone
TT; *see* Thrombin time
Tuberculosis
  genitourinary, 707
  hemoptysis and, 308
  indications for surgical resection in, 308
Tubocurarine, 49
Tumor aggressiveness, host defenses and, 224
Tumor biology, 220-236
Tumor markers
  breast cancer and, 390-391
  prostate cancer and, 700-701
Tumors; *see also* Carcinoma
  adrenal, adrenal hyperplasia and, 181-182
  of adrenal glands, 180-183
  gastrointestinal endocrine, 188
  of hard palate, 267
  intraoral, 268, 269
  laryngeal, 867
  lip, 266, 267
  mediastinal, 312, 313
  mesenteric, 516
  mixed; *see* Mixed tumors
  mixed, of oral cavity, 262

Tumors—cont'd
  nerve sheath, 603
  omental, 516
  ovarian, 530
  pancreatic endocrine, 188
  posterior fossa, abdominal pain and, 565-566
  retroperitoneal, 528
  scrotal, 715-716
  spinal, 723-728
  of tongue, 266-267
  of upper gingiva, 267
  ureteral obstruction and, 695-696
  on vocal cords, 867
  Wilms', 525-526
Tums, 136, 300
TUN; *see* Total urine nitrogen
Tuning fork test, 856-857
TV&D; *see* Truncal vagotomy and drainage
Tylenol (acetaminophen), 731
  with codeine, 235
Tympanic membrane, 856
Tympanometry, 859

U

UGI endoscopy; *see* Upper gastrointestinal endoscopy
Ulcer
  duodenal; *see* Duodenal ulcer
  gastric; *see* Gastric ulcer
  marginal, 213
  Marjolin's, 598
  peptic; *see* Peptic ulcer disease
  recurrent, 213
  stasis, 591
Ulcerative colitis, 490-493
  colonoscopy for, 91
  gastrointestinal bleeding and, 417
Ulnar tunnel syndrome, 834
Ultrasonography
  in evaluation of abdominal masses, 507-509
  jaundice and, 470
Ultrasound
  Doppler, in evaluation of limb ischemia, 574-576
  endovaginal, 75
  neonatal cranial, 75
  prostatic, 75
Umbilical hernia, 542, 543
Uncal herniation, 656
Unconsciousness, prolonged, evaluation and treatment of, 662
Undifferentiated adenocarcinoma of thyroid, 284
Unilateral renal parenchymal disease, hypertension and, 374-375
Unipen (nafcillin), 825
Universal precautions, 824
University of Washington (UW) solution, transplantation and, 240-241
Upper airway, obstruction to, trauma and, 612
Upper extremity, fracture of, 677-678
Upper gastrointestinal (UGI) endoscopy, 87-89
Upper gingiva, tumors of, 267
Uremia, abdominal pain and, 562-563, 568
Ureter, abdominal pain and, 562-563, 566
Ureteral obstruction, 695-700

Urethritis, 706, 710
Urinary system, abdominal masses and, 506-507
Urinary tract infections (UTI), 694-712
    ascending infection and, 703
    classification of, 704
    hematogenous spread of, 703
    lower, 705-707
    lymphatic spread of, 703
    postoperative fever and, 750, 820-821
    risk factors for, 703-704
    upper, 704-705
Urinary tract obstruction
    diagnosis of, 697-699
    lower, nonanatomic forms of, 697
    management of, 699-700
    trauma and, 618
    upper, 694-697
Urine
    red blood cells in, 684-693
    trauma and, 610
Urine output, shock and, 762
Urine urea nitrogen (UUN), 141
Urobilinogen, urinary excretion of, 463
Urokinase, 83, 593
Uropathy, obstructive, 694-712
Uterine myomata, 528
Uterus
    abdominal masses and, 528-529
    abdominal pain and, 562-563, 566-567
UTI; see Urinary tract infections
UUN; see Urine urea nitrogen
UW solution; see University of Washington solution

V

VAD; see Ventricular assist device
Vagotomy
    anterior, 116
    laparoscopic, 112-116
    parietal cell, for duodenal ulcer, 212
    posterior truncal, 116
    truncal; see Truncal vagotomy
Valium (diazepam), 30, 47, 55, 235, 731
Valsalva, sinus of, aneurysm of, 347
Vancomycin (Vancocin; Vancoled), 827
Varicocele, 716
    imaging of, 75
Varicose veins, 589-592
Vascular autoregulation, arterial blood pressure and, 370
Vascular defects, 779, 781
Vascular malformations of oral cavity, 259
Vascular rings, 347
Vascular system, use of stents in, 80
Vasoactive intestinal polypeptideoma, 497
Vasoconstrictors
    anesthesia and, 57
    shock and, 770
Vasodilators
    direct, hypertension and, 376
    shock and, 770
Vasopressin, 83
    pharmacologic effects of, 412
Vasopressors, 804
Vecuronium (Norcuron), 49, 58
Vein stripping for varicose veins, 591

Veins
    diseases of, lower extremity swelling and, 584-588
    varicose; see Varicose veins
Velocef (cephradine), 825
Venous claudication, limb ischemia and, 574
Ventilation
    airway pressure release, 790
    assist-control mode, 789
    constant flow, 792
    control mode, 788-789
    high-frequency positive pressure, 792
    independent lung, 789
    inverse ratio, 790
    maximal voluntary, 151
    positive pressure, 788
    pressure support, 790
    proportional assist, 790
    relationship of, with perfusion, 153-154
    synchronous intermittent mandatory, 789
Ventilator therapy, forms of, 157, 158
Ventilator-associated pneumonia, 747-748
Ventilatory support, 157
    complications of, 791
    criteria of need for, 787, 788
    in critical care, 786-794
    intraoperative, 38
    weaning parameters and, 793
Ventral hernia, 542, 543-544
Ventricular aneurysms, 356, 357-359
Ventricular assist device (VAD), 359-361
Ventricular septal defect (VSD), 329, 330, 333-334
Verapamil (Calan; Isoptin), 377
Verner-Morrison syndrome, 190
Verruca vulgaris, 596
Versed (midazolam), 47, 55
Vertigo
    ear disease and, 861-862
    postconcussion syndrome and, 660
Vibramycin (doxycycline), 710
Videoendoscopy, 86
Vincent's angina, 262
Vincristine (Oncovin), 235
VIP, 204-205
Vipoma, 190
Viral hepatitis, 823-824
    test for, 468-469
Viral infections, 823-824
Viral rhinitis, acute, 863
Visceral afferent nerves, 422
Visceral compartment infections, postoperative fever and, 748-750
Visceral pain, 423
Viscoelastic bone, 670
Vision, blurring of, postconcussion syndrome and, 660
Vistaril (hydroxyzine hydrochloride), 59
Vital capacity, 151
Vitamin D, 136
Vitamin K, 784
Vitamin K-dependent factors, 779
Vocal cords
    polyps of, 866
    visualization of, endotracheal intubation and, 36
Volume abnormalities, 132
Volume deficit, 125, 126
Volume excess, 125, 126, 134

Volume fluid changes in body fluid, 125, 126
Volvulus of colon, 454-455
Vomiting
    bilious, intestinal obstruction of newborn and, 642
    of blood, upper gastrointestinal bleeding and, 87
    gastric outlet obstruction and, 210
    hypercalcemia and, 176
Von Willebrand's disease, 778
VSD; *see* Ventricular septal defect

W

Warfarin sodium (Coumadin), 593, 784
Warts, 596
Water
    absorption of, in gastrointestinal tract, 482-483
    maintenance requirements for, for infants, 632
Water exchange, 123, 124
Watery diarrhea syndrome, 190
Weakness, hypercalcemia and, 176
Weaning parameters, ventilatory support and, 157, 793
Web space infections, 819
Weight loss, deglutition and, 292
Wermer's syndrome, 216
Wheezing, chest x-ray examination and, 308-309
Whitlow, 818
Whole-blood clotting time, 777
Wilms' tumor, 525-526
Winslow, foramen of, hernia through, 545
Wolf's law, 670
Wound, 608
    arrest of hemorrhage in, 609
    cleansing of, 609

Wound—cont'd
    closure of, 846-847
    debridement of, 609
    disruption of, trauma and, 618
    dressing of, 609
    healing process of, 845-846
    selective closure of, 609
Wound contraction, 845
Wound infection
    appendicitis and, 428
    postoperative, 740, 741, 821-822
    postoperative fever and, 748
Wrist
    fracture of, 678
    rheumatoid arthritis of, 841

X

Xanax (alprazolam), 235
Xanthogranulomatous pyelonephritis, 525
Xenogeneic graft in transplantation, 241
X-ray examination, abdominal trauma and, 615
Xylocaine (lidocaine hydrochloride), 43, 57, 871

Y

YAG laser, esophagogastroduodenoscopy and, 88

Z

Zantac (ranitidine hydrochloride), 193, 217
ZE syndrome; *see* Zollinger-Ellison syndrome
Zinc sulfite turbidity test, liver function and, 467
Zolicef (cefazolin), 825
Zollinger-Ellison (ZE) syndrome, 189, 213-216